Randall E. Harris, MD, PhD

Professor, Colleges of Public Health and Medicine
Director, Center of Molecular Epidemiology & Environmental Health
Division of Epidemiology & Departments of Pathology & Emergency Medicine
The Ohio State University Wexner Medical Center
Columbus, Ohio

EPIDEMIOLOGY
OF CHRONIC DISEASE

Global Perspectives

SECOND EDITION

JONES & BARTLETT
LEARNING

World Headquarters
Jones & Bartlett Learning
5 Wall Street
Burlington, MA 01803
978-443-5000
info@jblearning.com
www.jblearning.com

Jones & Bartlett Learning books and products are available through most bookstores and online booksellers. To contact Jones & Bartlett Learning directly, call 800-832-0034, fax 978-443-8000, or visit our website, www.jblearning.com.

Substantial discounts on bulk quantities of Jones & Bartlett Learning publications are available to corporations, professional associations, and other qualified organizations. For details and specific discount information, contact the special sales department at Jones & Bartlett Learning via the above contact information or send an email to specialsales@jblearning.com.

15101-5

Production Credits
VP, Product Management: Amanda Martin
Director of Product Management: Cathy Esperti
Product Manager: Sophie Fleck Teague
Product Specialist: Carter McAlister
Senior Project Specialist: Vanessa Richards
Project Specialist: Robert Furrier
Senior Marketing Manager: Susanne Walker
Manufacturing and Inventory Control Supervisor: Amy Bacus
Composition: codeMantra U.S. LLC
Project Management: codeMantra U.S. LLC
Cover Design: Kristin E. Parker
Rights & Media Specialist: Maria Maimone
Media Development Editor: Shannon Sheehan
Cover Image (Title Page, Section Opener, Chapter Opener):
 © Andrew Brookes/Getty Images
Printing and Binding: LSC Communications
Cover Printing: LSC Communications

Library of Congress Cataloging-in-Publication Data
Names: Harris, Randall E., author.
Title: Epidemiology of chronic disease: global perspectives / Randall E. Harris, MD, PhD, Director, Center of Molecular Epidemiology and Environmental Health College of Public Health, Division of Epidemiology The Ohio State University Medical Center, College of Medicine, Departments of Emergency Medicine & Pathology The Ohio State University Medical Center, Columbus, Ohio.
Description: Second edition. | Burlington, MA: Jones & Bartlett Learning, [2020] | Includes bibliographical references and index.
Identifiers: LCCN 2018059324 | ISBN 9781284151015 (paperback: alk. paper)
Subjects: LCSH: Chronic diseases—Epidemiology. | World health—Statistics.
Classification: LCC RA644.5 .H37 2020 | DDC 616/.044—dc23
LC record available at https://lccn.loc.gov/2018059324

6048

Printed in the United States of America
23 22 21 20 19   10 9 8 7 6 5 4 3 2 1

Contents

Chapter 42   Epidemiology of Obesity 609

Chapter 43   The Epidemiology of Thyroid Disease: *Hyperthyroidism* and *Hypothyroidism* 647

SECTION IV Epidemiology of Neurological Diseases 751

Chapter 48 Epidemiology of Alzheimer's Disease 753

Chapter 49 Epidemiology of Parkinson's Disease. 775

Chapter 50 Epidemiology of Multiple Sclerosis 791

Chapter 51 Epidemiology of Epilepsy. 805

Preface

This second edition of *Epidemiology of Chronic Disease: Global Perspectives* is written for all students and teachers of the health sciences, particularly those in epidemiology, public health, and medicine. Its main purpose is to present current and comprehensive information on epidemiology, etiology, pathogenesis, risk factors, and preventive factors of common chronic diseases. In writing the new edition of this book, I have made liberal use of the internet and drawn upon worldwide information to address the global landscape of chronic diseases.

This new edition has 56 chapters that are organized into five distinct sections beginning with an introductory chapter on the "*epidemiologic transition*" whereby chronic diseases have replaced acute infectious conditions concurrent with improved health care and increasing longevity in many populations of the world. Subsequent sections cover cardiovascular and cerebrovascular diseases (coronary heart disease, myocardial infarction, sudden cardiac death, stroke, congestive heart failure, peripheral artery disease and aortic aneurysms, venous thromboembolism and pulmonary embolism, and hypertension), major forms of cancer (lung cancer, laryngeal cancer, head and neck cancer, esophageal cancer, stomach cancer, colon cancer, pancreatic cancer, liver cancer, breast cancer, ovarian cancer, vulvar and vaginal cancer, cervical cancer, prostate cancer, testicular cancer and other male genital cancers, bladder cancer, kidney cancer, sarcoma, malignant melanoma, lymphoma, leukemia, and brain tumors), diseases of the respiratory tract (chronic obstructive pulmonary disease and asthma), metabolic and digestive diseases (diabetes mellitus, obesity, thyroid disease, kidney disease, and liver disease), musculoskeletal diseases (osteoporosis and arthritis), neurodegenerative diseases (Alzheimer's disease, Parkinson's disease, schizophrenia, epilepsy, multiple sclerosis, and suicide), and finally three major infectious diseases (tuberculosis, malaria, and HIV disease) that often manifest as chronic conditions.

I have added new chapters on sudden cardiac death, congestive heart failure, peripheral artery disease and aortic aneurysms, and venous thromboembolism and pulmonary embolism. Important new findings are discussed, such as the association of post-traumatic stress disorder with suicide and the emerging crisis of antibiotic resistance in tuberculosis and other chronic infections. Epidemiologic findings and references have been updated throughout this book.

Each chapter follows a similar format, with subsections describing diagnostic criteria, historical perspectives, the global burden of disease, population differences and time trends in incidence, prevalence, disability and mortality, mechanisms of pathogenesis, risk factors, preventive factors, and opportunities for disease prevention and control. Key epidemiologic studies and findings are presented in chronological order with supporting evidence and references selected to guide readers for further study. It is assumed that students and readers are building on a knowledge base of basic epidemiology and human biology. The text blends the traditional elements of epidemiology with human anatomy, physiology, and molecular biology. The text is accompanied by an online instructor's manual with recommended questions and answers drawn from each of the chapters.

It is my hope that the text will provide a forum for examining current hypotheses regarding chronic disease epidemiology. Subsections of each chapter focus on controversial topics in the epidemiology of each disease. This format facilitates active student discussion of molecular mechanisms of disease pathogenesis and the relevant epidemiologic issues pertaining to the prevention and control of chronic diseases.

In essence, the new edition of this book, like the first, is an amalgamation of a long-standing continuum of the exchange of ideas and information with many colleagues in the fields of medicine, public health, epidemiology, biostatistics, genetics, pathology, and molecular biology. This new edition will continue to reflect my own experiences in medicine, epidemiology, and public health, and I am deeply indebted to mentors, colleagues, and particularly students who have contributed to my education, research, and teaching over the past four decades.

▶ What Is New and Improved?

Epidemiology of Chronic Disease: Global Perspectives, Second Edition presents the current epidemiology and global burden of each of the 56 major diseases. This new edition contains the most recent information available on the epidemiology of major cardiovascular diseases; cancers; respiratory, metabolic, and musculoskeletal conditions; and neurodegenerative diseases complete with updated figures, tables, and global maps. The section on cardiovascular and cerebrovascular disease includes four new chapters on the epidemiology of congestive heart failure, peripheral artery disease and aortic dissection, venous thromboembolism and pulmonary embolism, and sudden cardiac death. The new epidemiology of cancer section contains widely updated materials to provide in-depth information on cancers that affect 28 regions of the body.

- **New Chapters.** The new edition includes 13 new chapters to include more information on Epidemiology of Sudden Cardiac Death (Chapter 5), Epidemiology of Heart Failure (Chapter 7), Epidemiology of Aortic Aneurysm and Dissection (Chapter 8), and Epidemiology of Venous Thromboembolism and Pulmonary Embolism (Chapter 9). There are also nine new chapters on cancer epidemiology including Epidemiology of Laryngeal Cancer (Chapter 14), Epidemiology of Cancers of the Lip, Oral Cavity, and Pharynx (Chapter 15), Epidemiology of Cancer of the Corpus Uteri (Chapter 23), Epidemiology of Vaginal, Vulvar, and Anal Cancer (Chapter 25), Epidemiology of Testicular Cancer (Chapter 27), Epidemiology of Carcinoma of the External Male Genitalia (Chapter 28), Epidemiology of Cancers of the Thyroid and Parathyroid (Chapter 31), Epidemiology of Adrenal Cancer (Chapter 32), and Epidemiology of Nonmelanoma Skin Cancer (Chapter 34).

- **Global Burden of Disease.** This new edition incorporates the most recent data from the World Health Organization, the Institute of Health Metrics and Evaluation, the International Agency for Cancer Research, and other international organizations to characterize important global patterns and trends in the epidemiology of each disease. Updated world maps and figures are used to display global patterns and trends in disease prevalence, incidence, mortality, and disability-adjusted life years.

- **U.S. Burden of Disease.** Each chapter includes a section on the burden of disease in the U.S. population based on current data from the National Institutes of Health, the American Heart Association, the American Cancer Society, and other national organizations.

- **Risk Factors.** Published studies from the recent literature are discussed regarding new findings on risk factors and preventive factors that impact the pathogenesis of disease.

- **Pathogenesis.** Current mechanisms of pathogenesis of each disease are discussed and depicted in each chapter.

- **Disease Prevention and Control.** The most recent and effective programs of disease prevention and control are presented in each chapter.

- **Instructor Resources.** Instructors using the text will have online access to updated lecture slides, outlines, and test banks with answers for each chapter.

Randall E. Harris, MD, PhD
Professor, Colleges of Public Health and Medicine
Director, Center of Molecular Epidemiology &
Environmental Health
Division of Epidemiology & Departments of
Pathology & Emergency Medicine
The Ohio State University Wexner Medical Center
Columbus, Ohio

Contributors

Susanne K. Scott, PhD, MPH
Belgium, Wisconsin

Zachary M. Harris, MD, Fellow
Pulmonary, Critical Care and Sleep Medicine
Department of Internal Medicine
Yale School of Medicine
Yale University
New Haven, Connecticut

© Andrew Brookes/Getty Images

Epidemiologic Transition and Epidemiology of Cardiovascular Diseases

© Andrew Brookes/Getty Images

CHAPTER 1

Global Epidemiology of Chronic Diseases: The Epidemiologic Transition

▶ Global Pandemic of Chronic Diseases

A silent pandemic of chronic diseases is gradually enveloping the world population, spreading to all corners of the globe. This distinct spectrum of human afflictions is systemically replacing infectious and parasitic diseases as the leading cause of morbidity and mortality worldwide, thereby producing one of the greatest public health challenges of all time. According to global cause-specific mortality data reported by the *Institute of Health Metrics and Evaluation* noncommunicable (chronic) disorders such as coronary heart disease, stroke, cancer, chronic obstructive pulmonary disease (COPD), diabetes mellitus type 2, neurodegenerative disease, and renal failure accounted for 39.5 million of the 54.7 million deaths (72%) for which a cause was identified during 2016 (Ritchie & Roser, 2018). This compares with 10.6 million deaths (19%) due to communicable (infectious) diseases, maternal, neonatal, and nutritional diseases, and 4.6 million deaths (8%) from injury including homicide, suicide, conflict, and terrorism. As shown in **FIGURE 1.1**, trends in the annual number of deaths in these three categories during 1990–2016 reflect a steady increase in annual deaths from noncommunicable diseases concurrent with a steady decline in annual deaths from

communicable, maternal, neonatal, and nutritional diseases, whereas the annual number of deaths from injury has remained stable (Ritchie & Roser, 2018; WHO, 2009a, 2017c).

The following excerpts from the 2008 WHO global report entitled *Preventing Chronic Diseases: A Vital Investment* capture the essence of the global pandemic of chronic diseases (Reprinted from WHO, 2008a).

"Chronic diseases are the leading causes of death and disability worldwide. Disease rates from these conditions are accelerating globally, advancing across every region and pervading all socioeconomic classes. The World Health Report 2002 "Reducing Risks, Promoting Healthy Life" indicates that the mortality, morbidity and disability attributed to the major chronic diseases currently account for almost 60% of all deaths and 43% of the global burden of disease. By 2020 their contribution is expected to rise to 73% of all deaths and 60% of the global burden of disease. Moreover, 79% of the deaths attributed to these diseases occur in the developing countries. Four of the most prominent chronic diseases, cardiovascular diseases (CVD), cancer, chronic obstructive pulmonary disease (COPD), and type 2 diabetes, are linked by common and preventable biological risk factors, notably high blood pressure, high blood cholesterol and overweight, and

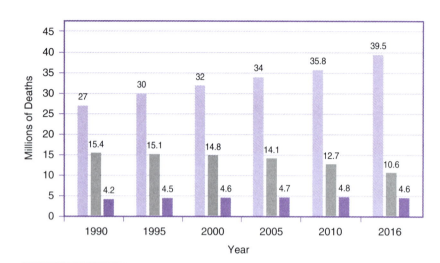

FIGURE 1.1 Global Trends in Deaths from Noncommunicable and Communicable Diseases and Injuries, 1990–2016.

Data from WHO. (2009a). *World health statistics, 2009*. Geneva, Switzerland: WHO; WHO. (2017). *World health statistics, 2017*. Geneva, Switzerland: WHO; Ritchie, H., & Roser, M. (2018). "Causes of Death". Published online at OurWorldInData.org. Retrieved from https://ourworldindata.org/causes-of-death [Online Resource]

by related major behavioral risk factors: unhealthy diet, physical inactivity, and tobacco use. Action to prevent these major chronic diseases should focus on controlling these and other key risk factors in a well-integrated manner."

The global pandemic of chronic diseases has emerged in concert with the changing demography of the world population. Overall, the world birth rate exceeds the death rate, and the number of living individuals on the planet continues to increase. At the same time, more and more people are living to older ages thereby creating the phenomenon of "global aging." Aging populations are particularly evident in the industrialized and developed nations of the world, such as Japan, Italy, and Germany, where the proportion of elderly people (over 65 years of age) has increased from approximately 10% to 20% in the past half century (Hayutin, 2007). In large developing nations such as China and India, the proportion of elderly people is also expected to increase from current levels of about 5% to nearly 10% in the next few decades. In smaller underdeveloped nations where less than 5% of the people currently live beyond 65 years of age, population aging is also progressing, but at a slower pace. As a general consequence of the aging world population, long-term mechanisms of pathogenesis are more likely to cause disease late in life, thus resulting in vastly increased rates of chronic diseases, particularly among the elderly.

▶ Increase in World Population

As of July 1, 2017, The Department of Economic and Social Affairs of the United Nations Secretariat

estimated that the world population consisted of 7.55 billion living human beings (World Population Prospects, 2017). In that year, approximately 60 million people died and 140 million new babies were born, a net gain of 80 million people. Based upon projections of death rates and birth rates, the world population is expected to increase to nearly 9 billion people by the year 2040 (**FIGURE 1.2**).

▶ Aging of the World Population

The world population is not only increasing in number, but it is also growing older. Two demographic parameters are driving these phenomena: *longevity is increasing and the fertility rate is decreasing.* Studies at the World Health Organization (WHO, 2009a) and the Stanford Center of Longevity (Hayutin, 2007) clearly show that people around the world are living longer and women are having fewer children.

▶ Increasing Longevity (Life Expectancy)

The average life expectancy (also called longevity) for members of the world population born during 2010–2015 is 71 years (68 years for men and 73 years for women) (CIA, 2017). In the past half century, life expectancy has increased dramatically throughout the world, particularly in populations of developing nations. Since 1950, life expectancy in highly populated nations such as China and India has increased from approximately 40 years to nearly 70 years (**FIGURE 1.3**).

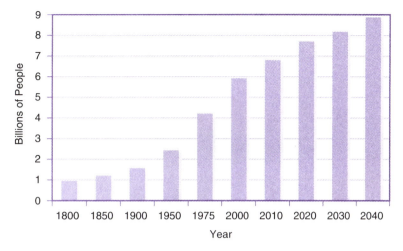

FIGURE 1.2 World Population.

Data from the United States Census Bureau. (2018). International Data Base. (estimates for 2020–2040 are based on curvilinear regression).

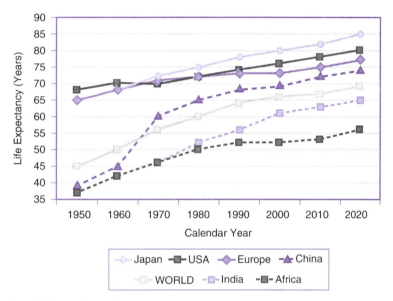

FIGURE 1.3 Longevity Trends in Selected Populations.

Data from United Nations Department of Economic and Social Affairs, Population Division. (2017). *United Nations World Population Prospects: 2017 revision.* New York, NY: United Nations. National Center for Health Statistics, 2017, USA.

In lesser developed nations, particularly those of central Africa where acute infectious and parasitic diseases prevail and greatly reduce the survival of children and young adults, life expectancy is much less, currently only about 50 years. In highly developed nations such as Japan, the United States, and European countries, longevity now approaches or surpasses 80 years and deaths are more likely due to chronic diseases of old age. The Japanese people currently enjoy the greatest longevity, about 82 years. Longevity in the United States currently stands at 79 years, only slightly higher than the average of the more developed nations (**FIGURE 1.4**).

Life expectancy is the average number of years that a newborn could expect to live if he or she were to pass through life *subject to the age-specific death rates of the population of interest for the past year.*

Derivation of life expectancy is usually presented as a "*two-step*" process. For large populations, life expectancy is calculated by *first constructing a life table and recording the number of deaths and survivors that occur in a given year for successive intervals of the life span.* The number of deaths and survivors and corresponding age-specific death rates are usually tabulated for ages 0–1 years, 1–5 years, and successive 5-year age groups for ages 5 and above. From these data, a second life table is then constructed to represent the entire mortality experience from birth to death for a hypothetical cohort of 100,000 infants born alive and subject to the age-specific death rates that prevail in the population of interest for a particular year. Using the data from this second life table for 100,000 hypothetical individuals, life expectancy is simply calculated as the average years of life for all members since birth

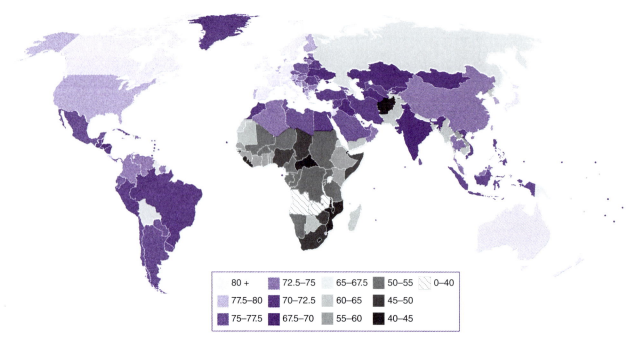

FIGURE 1.4 Global Longevity, 2011.

Data from CIA World Factbook, 2011 Estimates of Life Expectancy at Birth (Years).

(e.g., life expectancy = total years of life for all members of the life table divided by the total number of persons at birth, *Life Expectancy = Σ years of life/100,000*). Life expectancy (longevity) at birth is therefore the mean years of life for individuals based entirely on the age-specific death rates for the population and year of interest (Colton, 1974).

▶ Gender Differences in Longevity

Throughout the world, life expectancy (longevity) for women is 5–10 years greater than for men. With some exceptions in nations where high maternal death rates prevail due to lack of prenatal care, women have lower death rates and better survival at every age. In the industrialized world, improvements in prenatal care have reduced maternal mortality during the childbearing years thereby widening the gender gap in longevity during much of the 20th century. For example, the gender divergence in longevity in the U.S. population gradually increased from about 2 years in 1900 to approximately 8 years in 1970, after which the difference shrank back to about 6 years, currently 81 years for women versus 75 years for men (**FIGURE 1.5**). The slight shrinkage of the U.S. gender gap during the past 40 years is believed to reflect equalizing smoking rates among men and women (Pampel, 2002).

The survival differential favoring females actually begins at conception. Only about 90% of male fetuses survive to birth compared to nearly 100% of female

fetuses. While precise causative factors for this disparity remain unclear, the relatively high rates of spontaneous abortions, miscarriages, and stillbirths among male fetuses could be due to hormonal incompatibilities of the male genotype in a milieu of female hormones such as estrogen and progesterone throughout gestation (Austad, 2006). At the other end of the life span, approximately 70% of individuals over 90 years of age are female, and remarkably, about 90% of centenarians (individuals over 100 years of age) are female (Perls, Hutter Silver, & Lauerman, 1999).

While no single factor can satisfactorily explain the clear survival advantage of women throughout life, certain environmental and biological differences are worth pointing out. The longer life span of women compared to men is undoubtedly related to gender differences in lifestyle. Despite the fact that men are, on average, bigger, stronger, faster, and more economically self-sufficient, their lifestyle choices and risky health behaviors obviously confer a clear survival advantage to women. In general, men have greater exposure to classical risk factors of disease such as tobacco and alcohol and, as a consequence, are more likely to die earlier from associated chronic conditions such as cardiovascular disease, lung cancer, chronic obstructive pulmonary disease, and cirrhosis of the liver. Men are also more likely to die from injuries, whether unintentional (motor vehicle or occupational accidents) or intentional (suicide, homicide, or war). Reciprocally, women have traditionally been the "*sentinels of health*" for their families and communities at large. Due to their instinctive "*nurturing maternal instinct,*" women tend to take better care

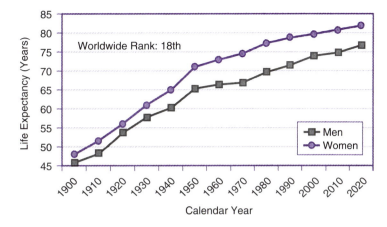

FIGURE 1.5 Life Expectancy, the United States, Women and Men.

Data from United Nations Department of Economic and Social Affairs, Population Division. (2017). *United Nations World Population Prospects: 2017 revision*. New York, NY: United Nations. National Center for Health Statistics, 2017, USA.

of themselves and make healthier lifestyle choices than men, thus contributing to their longer life span.

Hormonal differences between men and women may also influence their differences in lifestyle and longevity. Men are greater risk-takers than women, particularly during the years of young adulthood when circulating levels of testosterone are highest. The biological effects of androgens and estrogens differ dramatically. Androgens have vasoconstrictive and inflammatory effects in blood vessels consistent with higher rates of cardiovascular disease in men whereas estrogens exert opposite effects and are thus cardioprotective in women, particularly during their reproductive years (Blackman et al., 2002; Parker et al., 2009). Moreover, gender differences in the balance of estrogens and androgens appear to confer heightened immunity and more resistance to infectious and degenerative diseases in women throughout life (Austad, 2006).

▶ Aging and Disease

Aging is a complex process involving a decline in physiological processes that are essential for life. As humans age, there is heightened susceptibility to life-threatening acute and chronic diseases. A characteristic "death curve" is depicted in **FIGURE 1.6**. The data points represent approximate all-cause annual mortality rates estimated for successive 10-year age brackets for the U.S. population of 2002 (National Vital Statistics System, 2002). Note that the risk of death is elevated in the early years up to 5 years of age, after which there is a relatively long subtle increase in the risk of death until approximately 40 years of age, after which all-cause mortality exponentially rises for all successive age brackets.

Aging can thus be viewed as the general deterioration in human health over the life span generally associated with development of debilitating and

life-threatening disease processes. Indeed, aging has been defined as the spectrum of changes that render human beings progressively more likely to die (Medawar, 1952). As shown in **FIGURE 1.7**, the prevalence of major chronic diseases (arthritis, heart disease, cancer, diabetes mellitus type 2, and chronic obstructive pulmonary disease) rises exponentially with age. It is obvious that the phenotype of human aging is one in which practically any system, tissue, or organ can fail, resulting in debilitation and death (Austad, 1997; MacNee, Rabinovich, & Choudhury, 2014; Strehler, 1999). Nevertheless, it is important to stress that aging is not merely a collection of diseases. Rather, certain pathologic conditions progress in parallel with the aging process while others, such as asthma, remain constant or even decline late in life.

▶ Aging of Human Cell Populations

Aging is a complex and controversial subject. The aging phenomenon appears to be driven by deterioration in cellular health. The human body consists of tens of trillions of cells. This huge population of cells is divisible into subpopulations, each consisting of billions of cells that comprise certain anatomic structures, organs, and tissues. These component cell populations exist in a state of relative homeostasis performing the essential functions of life.

Studies of aging suggest that different cellular populations comprising the human body of a single individual do not all age at the same rate. Acceleration of the aging phenomenon in even one critical cell population may create a "weak link" for the entire system resulting in debilitation and death. However, as pointed out by Hayflick, the aging process does not share its elemental features with any particular disease

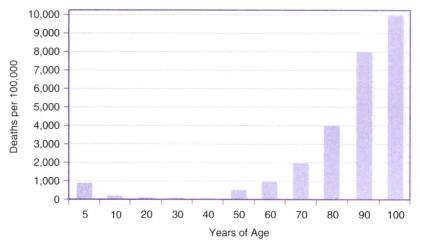

FIGURE 1.6 Characteristic Death Curve Modeled on the U.S. Population 2002.

Data from Aris, E. (2004). United States life tables, 2002. *National Vital Statistics Reports*, *53*(6), 1–40.

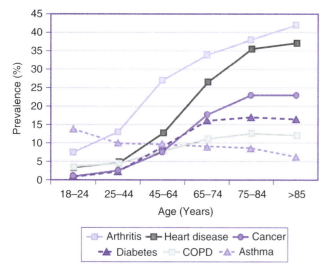

FIGURE 1.7 Prevalence of Selected Chronic Conditions Expressed as Percentages, as a Function of Age for the U.S. Population (2002–2003 Dataset).

Data from National Center for Health Statistics, Data Warehouse on Trends in Health and Aging, 2003.

(Hayflick, 2007). This observation led him to state that, "*the fundamental aging process is not a disease but it increases vulnerability to disease.*" To paraphrase, aging may be the cause but not necessarily the effect of a disease process.

The preservation of homeostasis among populations of normally functioning cells in the human body depends primarily upon the balance of cell death and cell replacement. If cells die faster than they are replaced, then the progressively greater demands placed upon those cells that remain may eventually lead to pathologic changes and rapid deterioration in cellular health. Any one of multiple intrinsic and extrinsic factors capable of upsetting the balance of cell death and cell replacement may therefore have considerable impact on the aging phenomenon, particularly for those cell populations that do not

normally undergo cell division (e.g., neurons and mature muscle cells).

Programmed cell death (called apoptosis) and cell division are tightly regulated by genetic factors; nevertheless, both processes are also subject to modulation by extracellular as well as intracellular molecular factors. Aging may thus result from extrinsic or intrinsic factors that cause an accumulation of cellular and tissue damage, or alternatively, changes in gene expression related to DNA damage and somatic mutations, epigenetic factors such as methylation or acetylation of DNA, or structural modification of DNA by the intrinsic biological clock that regulates the number of cell divisions (e.g., telomere shortening in chromosomes) (Campisi, Kim, Lim, & Rubio, 2001). The etiology of the aging phenomenon therefore appears similar to most complex human traits. Aging is influenced by genetic and environmental factors that interact to produce significant phenotypic variability. Two key theories of aging are briefly discussed in the following sections: one involves the energy rich microenvironment of the cell and the other the genetically controlled biological clock of cell division.

▶ Free Radical Theory of Aging

More than half a century ago, Denham Harman developed the free radical theory of aging (Harman, 1956). His theory states that aging is a consequence of accumulating oxidative damage to cells and cellular components over time (reviewed in Beckman & Ames, 1998). Harman later extended his theory to include mitochondrial production of free radicals during normal cellular respiration (Harman, 1972).

Free radicals and oxidants, commonly called reactive oxygen species (ROS), are highly unstable

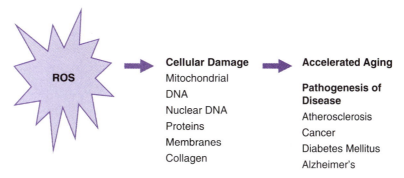

FIGURE 1.8 Free Radical Theory of Cell Damage, Aging, and Chronic Disease.

reactive molecules that can damage many vital cellular components (**FIGURE 1.8**). Rebecca Gerschman and colleagues discovered that ROS can originate from exogenous sources such as ultraviolet and ionizing radiation and were the first to suggest that free radicals are toxic agents (Gerschman, Gilbert, Nye, Dwyer, & Fenn, 1954).

ROS can be formed by exogenous processes such as irradiation and inflammation as well as normal cell metabolism. These short-lived molecules include superoxide, peroxide, hydroxyl radicals, and reactive nitrogen species such as peroxynitrite, all of which are unstable and readily react with DNA to cause a variety of structural genetic alterations including base pair mutations, rearrangements, deletions, insertions, and DNA sequence amplification. While DNA mutations, alterations, and chromosomal abnormalities increase with age in mice and other laboratory animals, damage to nuclear diploid DNA by ROS remains an unproven cause of aging (Ames, Shigenaga, & Hagen, 1993).

Oxidative phosphorylation is responsible for energy production within the mitochondria of virtually all cells. Since this process continually produces ROS such as superoxide and hydrogen peroxide, and since mitochondria possess haploid DNA unprotected by histones, many advocates of the free radical theory of aging consider that oxidative damage to mitochondria and the mitochondrial DNA has a primary role in the aging process (Barja & Herrero, 2000; de Grey, 1997; Harman, 1972; Linnane, Marzuki, Ozawa, & Tanaka, 1989).

Certain nutraceutical agents have gained favor as free radical scavengers that offer some protection against oxidation and the formation of ROS. These include ascorbic acid (vitamin C), tocopherol (vitamin E), carotenes, melatonin, and antioxidant enzymes such as superoxide dismutase (SOD), catalase, and glutathione peroxidase that are capable of degrading ROS into inert compounds (Ames, Cathcart, Schwiers, & Hochstein, 1981).

▶ Telomere Shortening and Aging

Cell division is an extraordinarily precise process that gives rise to daughter cells that have *almost* exactly the same genetic constitution as their progenitors. However, with every cell division, there is incomplete duplication of the chromosomal tips (called telomeres). Successive cell divisions therefore result in shortening of chromosomes until a point is reached where the daughter cells are no longer capable of dividing (called the "*Hayflick Limit*" after its discoverer). Since cells that reach their Hayflick Limit cannot replicate, the balance of cell replication and cell death is interrupted and cellular health may deteriorate. This is the basis of the *Telomere Theory of Aging*; namely, as an ever-increasing percentage of cells reach their Hayflick Limit and are unable to reproduce, then defense, maintenance, and repair of the body becomes increasingly impaired. Thus, telomere attrition due to the Hayflick Limit could account for most of the decline in functional efficiency of cell populations and increases in vulnerability to chronic diseases that characterize the aging phenomenon (de Magalhaes & Faragher, 2008; Hayflick, 1985, 2007).

▶ Declining Fertility Rate in Women

Over the past half century, the worldwide fertility rate (the average number of births per woman during the childbearing years) has been cut in half, from 5.0 in the 1950s to 2.5 in the 21st century (**FIGURE 1.9**). The decline in fertility rates has been sharpest in the most populous nations such as China, India, and Russia. For example, the fertility rate in China, which has the world's largest population (1.38 billion), decreased from more than 6 in 1970 to 1.6 births per woman in 2017, well below the worldwide

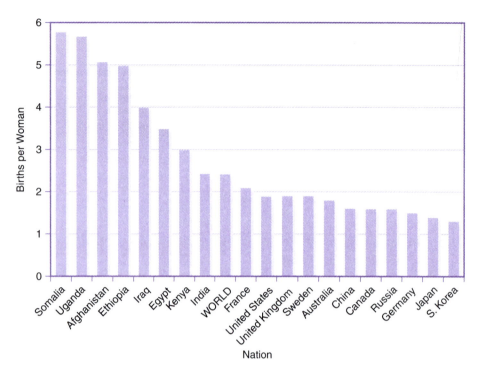

FIGURE 1.9 Selected Fertility Rates, 2017.

Data from Central Intelligence Agency (CIA). (2017). *The world factbook*. Washington, DC: U.S. Central Intelligence Agency.

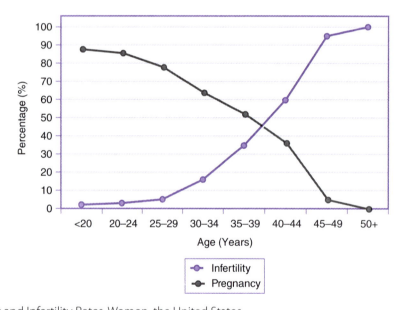

FIGURE 1.10 Pregnancy and Infertility Rates, Women, the United States.

Data from Menken, J., Trussell, J., & Larsen, U. (1986). Age and infertility. *Science, 233,* 1389–1394; Rowe, T. (2006). Fertility and a woman's age. *Journal of Reproductive Medicine, 51*(3), 157–163.

replacement rate of 2.1. There are areas of Africa and the Middle East where fertility rates have remained high with populations consisting of predominately children and young adults. In industrialized nations such as Canada, Germany, Great Britain, and Japan, fertility rates are now well below the replacement rate. In the United States, the fertility rate has decreased from 3.5 in the 1960s to 1.9 currently, only slightly below the replacement rate. Worldwide birth control has likely contributed to the general decline in the global fertility rate (Hayutin, 2007).

A woman's potential for childbearing begins to gradually decline between 20 and 30 years of age and then exponentially decreases until the end of the reproductive years at menopause (Menken, Trussell, & Larsen, 1986; Rowe, 2006; **FIGURE 1.10**). Widespread use of effective contraceptives, the accessibility of medical abortion, and the shifting paradigm for women to pursue professional careers rather than start families have combined to delay their having children. As a consequence of these factors, the reproductive window of childbearing years has been pushed back and dramatically reduced in women around the world. Furthermore, certain family planning incentives and policies such as China's "*one child policy*" in 1979 have further contributed to the steep decline in fertility in large populations of the world. These factors have all contributed to the global decline in fertility rates, particularly in the industrialized world (Hayutin, 2007).

▶ Chromosomal Aneuploidy and Ovarian Reserve

Biological factors that reduce fertility in the aging female include increased chromosomal aneuploidy and diminished ovarian reserve with each successive menstrual cycle. As a woman ages, an ever-increasing proportion of the eggs she releases during each successive menstrual cycle are aneuploid (contain an abnormal number of chromosomes) and thus highly prone to spontaneous miscarriage.

The ovarian reserve (the remaining viable eggs in the ovaries) of each woman generally begins to decline about 15 years prior to menopause. Depletion of the ovarian reserve of eggs with aging is also an exponentially expanding phenomenon resulting in the markedly decreased fertility of women in their fifth decade of life. Notably, cigarette smoking is one of the most common and important factors, which has been found to decrease ovarian reserve (Parker et al., 2009).

▶ Epidemiologic Transition

It is obvious that many developing and developed nations throughout the world are experiencing marked increases in life expectancy and decreases in fertility. This "*demographic transition*" has produced populations with a relative abundance of geriatric individuals compared to younger people, and it is occurring in concert with a closely related phenomenon called the "*epidemiologic transition.*"

In general, all nations of the world are in various stages of "*epidemiologic transition*," defined as the transition from acute infectious, parasitic, and nutritional deficiency diseases as the predominant causes of morbidity and mortality to a predominance of noninfectious chronic diseases (Omran, 1971). This worldwide epidemiologic transition is undoubtedly a consequence of the improving economic standards of many nations, which has translated into better health and greater longevity for their native populations. Important contributing factors include adequate caloric intake throughout life, improved sanitation, vaccination against common infectious microbes,

effective antibiotics to combat bacterial and parasitic diseases, effective drugs to reduce hypertension and other physiological disturbances, better health education for promotion of healthier lifestyles, advances in medical education, progress in medical technology, and overall improvements in healthcare systems.

From a historical perspective, until the beginning of the 20th century, epidemics of communicable (infectious) and parasitic diseases such as typhoid, cholera, smallpox, diphtheria, tuberculosis, bubonic plague, yellow fever, malaria, and influenza were the main causes of morbidity and mortality in all countries of the world. Although certain infectious and parasitic diseases such as tuberculosis and malaria remain epidemic in Third World countries, industrialization and progressive modernization of many nations have resulted in major improvements in housing, sanitation, water supply, nutrition, and health care. The discovery and availability of antibiotics and vaccines have radically changed the profile of diseases, initially in developed countries and later in many developing countries. Consequently, these improvements in medicine and public health have led to dramatic reductions in mortality from infectious and parasitic diseases.

Paradoxically, concurrent with decreases in morbidity and mortality from infectious and parasitic conditions, there has been a remarkable increase in the prevalence of chronic noncommunicable diseases such as cardiovascular disease, hypertension, stroke, chronic obstructive pulmonary disease, type 2 diabetes, and neurodegenerative pathologies such as Alzheimer's disease.

While good health coupled with increasing longevity is generally viewed as beneficial, it is also clear that the epidemiologic transition has produced a concomitant rise in chronic pathogenic processes typically manifested later in life. Cellular damage to vital tissues, organs, and systems of the human body by ROS, atherosclerosis, carcinogenesis, chronic inflammation, allergic reactions, insulin insensitivity, autoimmune reactions, and immunosuppression has produced a world pandemic of chronic diseases and conditions. Furthermore, the escalating burden of heart disease, cancer, hypertension, stroke, emphysema, chronic bronchitis, obesity, diabetes mellitus (type 2), cirrhosis of the liver, arthritis, autoimmune disease, kidney disease, and neurodegenerative disorders such as Alzheimer's disease is threatening to overwhelm the healthcare systems of many nations. As pointed out by Ernst L. Wynder, such chronic disease processes appear to be spurred by *metabolic overload* due to intake of high-calorie diets with excessive fats and carbohydrates coupled with insufficient exercise and addictive use of tobacco and alcohol (Wynder, 1994).

Fortunately, such metabolic insults are fundamentally preventable or correctable since they are largely controlled by personal behavior and lifestyle (please see discussion in the section on Global Prevention of Chronic Diseases).

It has become apparent that epidemiologic transitions are not necessarily unidirectional, and should best be viewed as continuous transformation processes wherein some diseases may disappear while others may reappear. A case in point is the reemergence of infectious diseases in high-income nations due to antibiotic or drug resistance of pathogenic bacteria, viruses, and other microbes. Epidemiologic transitions therefore reflect complex and dynamic patterns of health and disease due to demographic, socioeconomic, technological, cultural, environmental, and biological changes.

It is also important to realize that the populations of many less-developed nations continue to manifest relatively short average life spans due to the impact of failing healthcare systems coupled with unstable governance, war, and pestilence. For example, life expectancy in sub-Saharan Africa is only about 45 years, largely due to infectious and parasitic diseases such as HIV/AIDS, tuberculosis, and malaria that produce life-threatening acute conditions such as diarrhea, pneumonia, and anemia. The following sections discuss the diseases and conditions that cause death in the world population, and address the disparate profiles of disease among nations according to their economic status.

▶ Global Death Rates

Crude annual death rates for the nations of the world are shown in **FIGURE 1.11**. The figure for annual death rates for the world is derived from crude rates published by the World Health Organization in 2009 based upon data collected during 2002–2007 (CIA, 2009; WHO, 2009a). It is stressed that crude rates are not adjusted for differences in the age distributions of the different populations. Hence, some populations with relatively more young people may have lower death rates than populations with more old people. Nevertheless, certain conclusions can be drawn by comparing the crude death rates among nations.

What is painfully obvious is that among the relatively young populations of central and southern Africa (sub-Saharan Africa), the death rates are the highest in the world. Compared to developed nations such as the United States, Canada, Japan, Great Britain, Australia, and many European nations, whose populations have far more older people, individuals in African nations such as Swaziland, Botswana, Angola, Niger, Chad, Mozambique, and Zimbabwe have a 3–4 times higher risk of dying. Even greater disparities in the crude death rates are apparent in the populations of sub-Saharan Africa (more than 20 deaths per 1000) compared to those of the Mediterranean populations of northern Africa (less than 4 deaths per 1000).

In sub-Saharan Africa, conditions of hunger and malnutrition cause life-threatening diarrhea in infants and children, killing 5 million every year before they

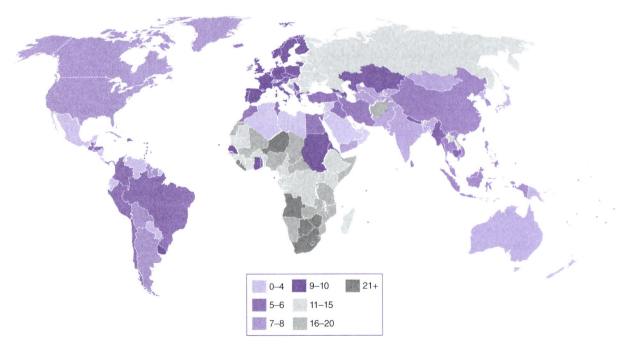

0–4	9–10	21+
5–6	11–15	
7–8	16–20	

FIGURE 1.11 Global Death Rates, 2006.

Data from: CIA World Factbook, 2006 Estimates of Crude Death Rates per 1,000. Reprinted with permission: World Health Organization, 2009a: Annual Death Rates per 1,000.

reach the age of 5 years. Parasitic diseases such as malaria are left untreated, killing 1 million more children annually before they reach the age of 15 years. Infectious diseases such as HIV, hepatitis, and tuberculosis ravage the health of young adults, killing nearly 3 million young adults each year before they reach the age of 45 years. Wars and strife due to political unrest kill 100,000 more young adults every year. And if an individual manages to live through these early afflictions, chronic conditions such as cardiovascular disease, stroke, diabetes, chronic obstructive pulmonary disease, and others manifest early and kill 3 million more adults before they reach the age of 65 years. Indeed, of the 60 million deaths that occur every year in the world population of approximately 7.5 billion, nearly 20%, about 12 million, occur in the central/southern African population of 0.8 billion people. Hence, just a single stratification of the world data divides individuals into two camps of death risk: populations residing in sub-Saharan Africa with crude average death rates exceeding 20 per 1000 per year, and the rest of the world with an average rate less than 10 per 1000 per year (Adetunji & Bos, 2006; Baingana & Bos, 2006; Bradshaw & Timaeus, 2006; Hill & Amouzou, 2006; Rao, Lopez, & Herned, 2006).

Other nations with high death rates include Afghanistan and member nations of the Russian Federation. The crude annual death rate in Afghanistan (nearly 20 per 1000) reflects a war-torn impoverished population with little access to health care. The Afghanistan population has high rates of infant and maternal mortality, childhood mortality from malnutrition, and mortality in young adults from violence and diseases caused by addiction to tobacco, alcohol, and illicit drugs such as cocaine and opium (Duckett, 2005; WHO, 2009a).

In Russia, overall mortality has increased sharply since the disbanding of the Soviet Union during 1985–1991. Crude death rates for the Russian population during the 1980s were on par with other industrialized nations (about 8 per 1000) but have since increased reaching a peak of nearly 15 per 1000 in 2010. Recent studies have found a link between excessive alcohol consumption and mortality, particularly among men of working age. For example, Leon and colleagues reviewed the drinking habits of 2835 men from the industrial city of Izhevsk who died at ages 25–54 years during 2003–2005 compared to 3078 age-matched living controls. Results revealed that 51% of the men who died consumed *nonbeverage alcohol* (e.g., aftershave) or were problem drinkers compared to 13% of controls. Alcohol-related deaths included cirrhosis of the liver, hepatitis, certain malignancies (hepatocellular cancer, pancreatic cancer, and esophageal cancer), cardiovascular disease, accidents, and violence (homicide and

suicide). The investigators estimated that 43% of deaths in men aged 25–54 years in Izhevsk were attributable to hazardous drinking (Leon et al., 2007).

In a recent study, a team of international investigators examined the drinking and smoking habits of 48,557 decedents from three Russian industrial cities (Tomsk, Barnaul, and Biysk) who died at ages 15–74 years during 1990–2001. Alcohol-related deaths included accidents, violence, heart disease, aerodigestive tract cancer, liver cancer, tuberculosis, pneumonia, hepatitis, liver cirrhosis, and pancreatic disease. Excess alcohol consumption accounted for 52% of all deaths at ages 15–54 years and 18% of deaths at later ages. The investigators concluded that alcohol and tobacco account for the large difference in adult mortality between Russia and other industrialized nations (Zaridze et al., 2009).

▶ Global Epidemiology of Disease

FIGURE 1.12 shows the number of deaths due to specific diseases based upon estimated cause-specific mortality rates published by the *Institute of Health Metrics and Evaluation* for the world population during 2016 (Ritchie & Roser, 2018). About 1 in 3 deaths (17.65 million) were caused by conditions of the cardiovascular system (ischemic heart disease, myocardial infarction, sudden cardiac death, stroke, congestive heart failure, valvular disease, cardiomyopathy). Strokes which caused 10% of deaths (5.5 million) are included as a subcategory within cardiovascular diseases. Cancers caused 16.3% of deaths (8.9 million) and infectious/parasitic diseases (pneumonia, diarrhea, HIV, tuberculosis, malaria) caused 14.2% of deaths (7.8 million).

Chronic noncommunicable diseases (heart disease, stroke, cancer, COPD; noninfectious digestive disease such as liver cirrhosis, diabetes, neurological disorders such as Alzheimer's disease, and chronic renal failure) caused approximately 72% of all deaths (39.5 million) whereas relatively acute conditions (infectious and parasitic diseases, accidents, violence, perinatal disease [low birth weight and failure to thrive], maternal conditions, congenital anomalies, and malnutrition) accounted for the remaining 28% of deaths (15.2 million) worldwide.

Diseases and conditions afflicting the human race show profound disparities arising from the prevailing environmental conditions and population susceptibilities. A crude but effective discriminant of the disease profile of a population is its economic status. Estimates of relative mortality for specific diseases in high-income

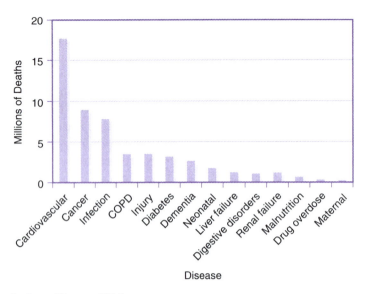

FIGURE 1.12 Worldwide Deaths from Disease, 2016.

Data from Ritchie, H., & Roser, M. (2018). "Causes of Death". Published online at OurWorldInData.org. Retrieved from https://ourworldindata.org/causes-of-death [Online Resource].

nations versus low-income nations derived from WHO data are given in **FIGURES 1.13** and **1.14**.

In high-income nations such as the United States, Japan, Canada, Australia, Great Britain, France, Germany, Italy, Finland, and Sweden, approximately 75% of deaths are due to noncommunicable chronic diseases such as heart disease (21%), cancer (19%), stroke (10%), chronic obstructive pulmonary disease (10%), diabetes mellitus (6%), and other chronic conditions (9%). The remaining 25% of deaths in these populations are attributable to relatively acute conditions such as pneumonia, influenza, or other infections (16%) and accidents (8%), suicide, or homicide (2%).

The profile of life-threatening diseases for low-income nations differs markedly from that of high-income nations (Figures 1.13 and 1.14). In nations such as Afghanistan, Bangladesh, Cambodia, Central African Republic Chad, Democratic Government of Congo, Laos, Ethiopia, Guinea, Haiti, Laos, Liberia, Madagascar, Mali, Mozambique, Nepal, Niger, Rwanda, Somalia, Sudan, Tanzania, Uganda, Tanzania, Yemen, and Zambia, approximately 60% of deaths are attributable to relatively acute conditions such as infectious and parasitic diseases (24%), perinatal disease (16%), violence (10%), malnutrition (5%), and maternal or other acute conditions (5%). Remaining deaths are attributable to conditions associated with chronic disease processes such as heart disease (15%), cancer (12%), stroke (8%), and COPD (5%).

Remarkably, more than 5 billion people (about 75% of the world population) reside in the low-income nations represented in Figure 1.14 (United Nations Department of Economic and Social Affairs, Population Division, 2017). These populations exist on less than $3 per person per day and have *little or no access* to clean water, proper sanitation and sewer systems, adequate nutrition, and health care.

In **FIGURE 1.15**, deaths from acute disease, chronic disease, and injury are further stratified according to the 2008 gross national income (GNI) per capita. The GNI groupings were calculated using the World Bank Atlas method for nations with populations exceeding 30,000 people (World Bank, 1993). Based on its 2008 GNI per capita, every economy was classified as low income, middle income (subdivided into lower-middle income and upper-middle income), or high income. The GNI groups translated into U.S. dollars are as follows: low income, $975 or less; lower-middle income, $976–$3855; upper-middle income, $3856–$11,905; and high income, $11,906 or more.

Enormous differences are evident in the profiles of death-causing diseases according to economic level (Figure 1.15). Poverty with its attendant poor hygiene, malnutrition, inferior education, heavy use of tobacco and alcohol, and lack of access to effective health care is associated with acute diseases that tend to impact younger generations. Reciprocally, greater prosperity is associated with chronic diseases more likely to impact older individuals through improved public health practices (e.g., vaccination against infectious agents, adequate nutrition, higher education, avoidance of tobacco and alcohol, and more effective health care). Unfortunately, the latter scenario has created in many populations "*metabolic overload of caloric intake*" leading to an epidemic of obesity and related chronic diseases of adults and the elderly.

It is noteworthy that in lower-middle-income nations with large populations, such as India and

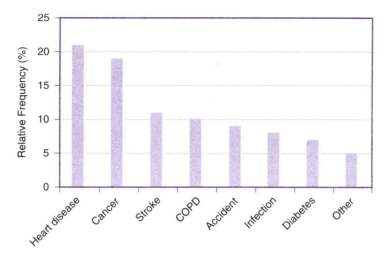

FIGURE 1.13 Relative Mortality for High-Income Nations.

Data from WHO. (2009a). *World health statistics, 2009*. Geneva, Switzerland: WHO.

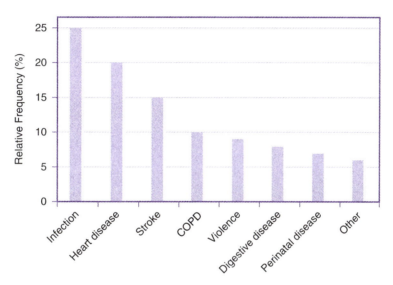

FIGURE 1.14 Relative Mortality for Low-Income Nations.

Data from WHO. (2009a). *World health statistics, 2009*. Geneva, Switzerland: WHO.

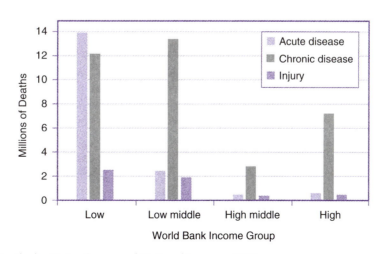

FIGURE 1.15 Worldwide Deaths by Major Cause and National Income, 2008.

Data from WHO. (2008a). *Chronic diseases: A vital investment*. Geneva, Switzerland: WHO.

China, deaths from chronic diseases now outnumber deaths from acute conditions by more than fivefold, and even in low-income nations, the number of deaths from chronic diseases is approaching that of acute conditions. In higher-middle-income nations such as Poland, Russia, Mexico, and Argentina, mortality from chronic disease far outstrips that from acute disease. Their profile is similar to the mortality pattern of high-income nations such as Sweden, the United States, the United Kingdom, Germany, and Japan. These trends reflect the tremendous worldwide impact of the *epidemiologic transition*.

A disturbing trend in more prosperous nations is the heavy and indiscriminate use of antibiotics in the treatment of bacterial infections. Selection forces in these populations therefore favor the accumulation of resistant bacterial genes and plasmids resulting in the reemergence of certain infectious agents due to their evolving antibiotic resistance (e.g., *methicillin resistant staphylococcus aureus*, or *MRSA*).

Risk Factors and Mortality

Worldwide mortality rates can also be examined according to major risk factors that are known to cause disease. Two major risk factors, tobacco and obesity, rival one another as perhaps the greatest public health menaces of all time. Another devastating menace to the status of public health is the problem of undernutrition which currently impacts millions of children, particularly in the underdeveloped nations of the world.

Global Tobacco Pandemic

Several comprehensive reports have addressed the global pandemic of disease resulting from tobacco addiction (Doll, Peto, Boreham, & Sutherland, 2004; Guindon & Boisclair, 2003; Jha, Chaloupka, Corrao, & Jacob, 2006; Peto et al., 1996; WHO, 2009b, 2015). According to estimates from these sources, 100 million people died from tobacco addiction (primarily cigarette smoking) during the 20th century, and if current smoking rates and trends prevail, 1 billion people will die from tobacco addiction in the 21st century. Estimates of smoking prevalence among individuals 15 years of age or older are 8–15 times higher in males than females in the populations of Africa, the Middle East, Asia, and the Western Pacific whereas female smoking rates are trending higher and may eventually approach male rates in the Americas and Europe (**FIGURE 1.16**). Worldwide, approximately 34% of men and 6% of women smoke, accounting for approximately 6 million deaths annually (**FIGURE 1.17**).

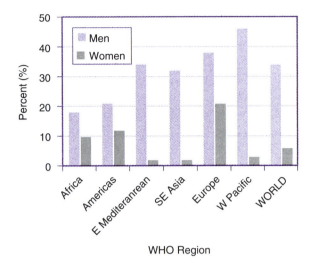

FIGURE 1.16 Worldwide Smoking Prevalence: 2016.
Data from WHO. (2017). *Global health observatory (GHO)*.

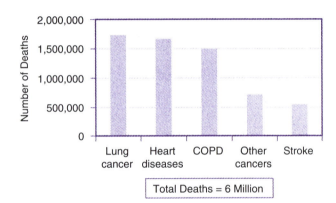

FIGURE 1.17 Worldwide Deaths Attributable to Cigarette Smoking, 2017.
Data from WHO. (2017). *Report on the global tobacco epidemic*.

Prevention and Control of Tobacco Use

Recently, an international program of tobacco control titled the *Tobacco Free Initiative (TFI)* was ratified and implemented through the auspices of the World Health Organization to curb the epidemic of tobacco-related diseases throughout the world (WHO, 2009b). In addition to careful monitoring of tobacco use and prevention policies and their effectiveness in reducing tobacco-related morbidity and mortality, the *WHO TFI* advocates specific guidelines for the prevention of tobacco use and control of tobacco products. These are: (1) primary prevention of initiating the smoking habit by early health education programs, (2) warning about the dangers of tobacco through hard-hitting antitobacco ads and graphic warnings on tobacco packaging, (3) protecting people from tobacco smoke by advocating smoke-free environments, (4) offering effective help to quit tobacco use through counseling and medications, (5) enforcing bans on tobacco advertising, promotion, and sponsorship, and, finally,

(6) raising taxes on tobacco to generate revenues to support the program.

Global Obesity Pandemic

The phenotype of an obese individual is characterized by an unnatural excess of body fat. This condition is commonly assessed by the body mass index (BMI) also known as the "*Quetelet Index*" calculated as weight in kilograms divided by the square of height in meters (kg/m²). In adults, a BMI of 30 or more is defined as obese. In children, obesity is defined as weight above the 95th percentile for age-gender-specific growth charts.

As shown in **FIGURE 1.18**, approximately 11% of men and 15% of women are obese in the world population reflecting the global pandemic of over-nutrition and metabolic overload (WHO, 2017c). The condition is particularly prominent in the developed nations

of the Americas and Europe (e.g., in the Americas, about one in four men and one in three women are in the obese category). According to surveys conducted by the WHO in 2016, there are more than 650 million clinically obese adults in the world population. Furthermore, the obesity pandemic is not restricted to adults as the world population now contains more than 41 million children under the age of 5 years that are either overweight or obese (International Obesity Task Force, 2010; WHO, 2017a, 2017b).

Obesity with its associated lipid engorgement of the fat cell (adipocyte) population often produces adverse metabolic effects on blood pressure, cholesterol, triglycerides, and insulin resistance. Based on the results of recent epidemiologic investigations of diverse populations (Calle, 2007; Interheart, NCI bulletin), it is evident that as the BMI climbs above 30, there are corresponding risk increases in several chronic diseases including cardiovascular disease (hypertension, myocardial infarction, and stroke), chronic arthritis, type 2 diabetes, gallbladder disease, gastroesophageal reflux disease, and several cancers (Caballero, 2007; Calle, 2007; de Courten, Bennett, Tuomilehto, & Zimmet, 1997; Fisichella & Patti, 2009; Leach, Baumgard, & Broom, 1973; Zimmet & Alberti, 2006) (**FIGURE 1.19**). Gravid obesity (BMI > 40) has been found to be associated with greater than a two-fold increase in the risk of all-cause mortality in both men and women (Calle, 2007).

Life-threatening conditions associated with obesity include hypertension, atherosclerosis, and hypercholesterolemia leading to catastrophic cardiovascular and cerebrovascular events such as myocardial infarction and stroke, insulin resistance resulting in type 2 diabetes, heightened carcinogenesis, and development of certain types of malignant tumors, especially the hormonally related and large-bowel cancers. Nonfatal

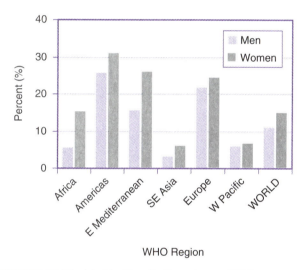

FIGURE 1.18 Worldwide Obesity Prevalence: 2016.

Data from WHO. (2016). *Global health observatory*. Geneva, Switzerland: World Health Organization.

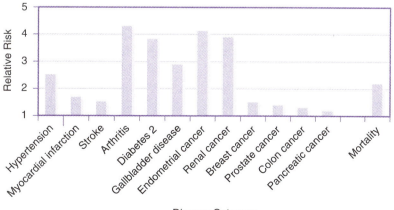

FIGURE 1.19 Obesity and Risk of Disease.

Data from WHO. (2008a). *Chronic diseases: A vital investment*. Geneva, Switzerland: WHO; Caballero, B. (2007). The global epidemic of obesity: An overview. *Epidemiologic Reviews, 29*, 1–5; Calle, E. E. (2007). Obesity and cancer. *BMJ, 335*(7630), 1107–1108.

but debilitating health conditions associated with obesity include gastroesophageal reflux disease (GERD), cholelithiasis (genesis of gallstones), urolithiasis (genesis of kidney stones), and degenerative osteoarthritis.

The fundamental cause of obesity is an imbalance of energy input versus energy output. It should be realized that the development of obesity is *usually* not an acute process, but rather one that requires years or even decades of energy imbalance involving a sustained excess of calories consumed versus calories expended. Two primary risk factors are evident: (1) increased consumption of high-calorie foods, particularly simple carbohydrates and other foods high in saturated fats and sugars, and (2) lack of sufficient physical activity. The inevitable consequence of calories taken in exceeding calories burned is obesity.

Societal changes and related behaviors are driving the obesity epidemic. With the globalization of food markets and continuing urbanization of the world population, low-calorie diets with abundant complex carbohydrates are rapidly being replaced by high-calorie diets with a high proportion of fats and sugars. At the same time, sedentary lifestyles characterized by little or no physical activity have become commonplace in the populations of modernized nations.

The International Obesity Task Force (IOTF) was established in 1996 to raise awareness and develop approaches to combat the emerging global pandemic of obesity. The IOTF membership consists of experts in the field of obesity research and represents 43 national organizations. The IOTF collaborates closely with the World Health Organization and other international health organizations concerned about the obesity problem.

The IOTF initiative on the prevention and management of obesity has four main goals: (1) to increase the awareness among governments, healthcare professionals, and the community that obesity is a serious medical condition and a major health problem with substantial economic costs; (2) to provide evidence and guidance for the development of better prevention and management strategies; (3) to secure the commitment of policy makers to action; and (4) to foster the development of national, regional, and international structures that will enable and support the implementation of action on overweight and obesity.

The IOTF recommends several long-term strategies for the prevention and treatment of obesity and obesity-related diseases. Treatment centers incorporating effective weight loss programs should be developed with well-trained staff to ensure effective support to help individuals safely lose weight and maintain their optimum weight. Existing healthcare facilities

should strive to develop and maintain an integrated team of physicians, dieticians, physical therapists, and other healthcare professionals, plus the necessary resources for the accurate diagnosis and effective treatment and management of obesity and obesity-related diseases.

A key element for success is primary prevention through promotion of healthy diets and regular physical activity beginning with health education programs initiated early in life. The following consensus statement from the British Medical Association is timely:

> "Such interventions at the family or school level will need to be matched by changes in the social and cultural context so that the benefits can be sustained and enhanced. Such prevention strategies will require a coordinated effort between the medical community, health administrators, teachers, parents, food producers and processors, retailers and caterers, advertisers and the media, recreation and sport planners, urban architects, city planners, politicians, and legislators. Environments that encourage healthy eating and active living are vitally important. The focus of such strategies should be to make it easier for the public to make healthy choices. Such strategies require funding for implementation, but should ultimately lead to a reduction in the costs from obesity related ill health."

Global Undernutrition and Malnutrition

More than 50% of deaths in children under 5 years of age are attributable to conditions related to malnutrition and starvation (Caulfield, de Onis, Blössner, & Black, 2004; Pelletier, Frongillo, Schroeder, & Habicht, 1995). Global estimates of relative cause-specific mortality rates are shown for malnourished and underweight children under the age of 5 years in **FIGURE 1.20** (WHO, 2008b). Underweight children suffer from malnutrition and near starvation, and are highly predisposed to infectious and parasitic diseases leading to diarrhea, dehydration, energy depletion, immunosuppression, and death. Such conditions currently exist in epidemic proportion in low-income nations, particularly in sub-Saharan Africa.

Overall, the proportion of children under 5 years of age with stunted growth (defined as height for age more than two standard deviations below the WHO Child Growth Standards median) declined from 39% in 1990 to 22% in 2017. However, progress has been uneven and in 2017, there were an estimated 150 million children exhibiting stunted growth, and

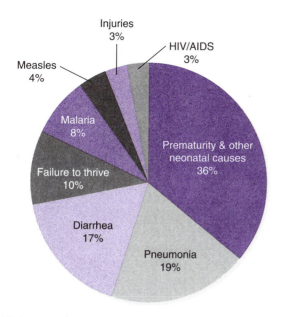

FIGURE 1.20 Relative Mortality Associated with Malnutrition and Underweight in Children Less than 5 Years of Age.

Data from WHO. (2008b). *Global tuberculosis control 2008 report*. Geneva, Switzerland: WHO; WHO, UNAIDS, UNICEF. (2008). *Towards universal access: Scaling up priority interventions in the health sector: Progress report 2008.*

50 million of these undernourished children suffered from wasting (defined as weight more than two standard deviations below normal). Furthermore, in 2017, 303,000 women died from complications of pregnancy or childbirth, 99% of them in developing countries primarily in the populations of sub-Saharan Africa (UNICEF-WHO, 2018).

Reducing child mortality increasingly depends on approaches to improve neonatal survival. Globally, an estimated 46% of deaths among children under 5 years of age occur in the first month of life, most in the first week. Countries making the least progress are generally those affected by high prevalence rates of malnutrition and low birth weight, HIV/AIDS, indigenous infectious and parasitic diseases such as tuberculosis and malaria, economic hardship, and conflict.

In recent years, there has been considerable progress in reducing mortality among children. During 1990–2016, the annual number of deaths among children under age 5 years fell from 12.8 million to 4.6 million, a reduction of 64%. Much of the progress in reducing child mortality can be attributed to improved nutrition particularly during gestation and the neonatal period, increased immunization coverage against common infectious diseases such as measles, antiretroviral therapy for HIV/AIDS, use of oral rehydration therapies during episodes of diarrhea, use of insecticide-treated mosquito nets and access to combination therapies to combat malaria, efforts to eliminate disease due to *Haemophilus influenzae* type B infection, and ready access to clean water and

sanitation facilities. However, because the availability and use of proven interventions at the community level remain low in impoverished populations, nearly 13,000 children under age 5 still die every day in the world population (UNICEF, 2017).

▶ Body Mass and All-Cause Mortality

While no single biological factor can satisfactorily explain the disparate profiles of disease-specific mortality for different nations, there is one factor that does provide a crude but effective discriminant of all-cause mortality. Perhaps surprisingly, that factor is the body mass index (or Quetelet index) defined as weight in kilograms divided by height^2 in meters; $BMI = kg \; wt/(m \; ht)^2$. Its potential value as a measure of disease versus health is that BMI is a continuous variable that is easily calculated for every individual. The expectation is that low values are associated with nutritional deficiencies and high values with nutritional excesses.

FIGURE 1.21 shows all-cause mortality rates for adult men and women by eight categories of BMI ranging from extremely underweight (<14) to morbidly obese (>35) based upon a review of epidemiologic studies of 34 different populations from around the world. These data clearly reflect a U-curve for both genders where the optimum value corresponding to the lowest all-cause mortality is a BMI range of 21–25. As with most physiological factors, BMI shows a window of homeostasis wherein the potential for good health is optimized and individuals with a BMI that is either too low or too high significantly increase their risk of dying. In particular, high BMI carries a fivefold increase of dying from obesity-linked conditions such as cardiovascular disease, stroke, diabetes, pulmonary disease, renal disease, and selected cancers such as breast cancer, colorectal cancer, and prostate cancer.

▶ Disability-Adjusted Life Years (DALY)

The *Disability-Adjusted Life Years* (*DALY*) is a measure of overall disease burden, expressed as the *number of years lost due to ill-health, disability, or early death*. The measure was originally developed by Christopher Murray and Alan López at Harvard University in order to characterize the overall burden of disease in

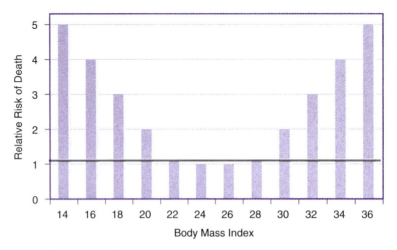

FIGURE 1.21 Body Mass Index and Mortality: Window of Homeostasis.

populations (Murray & López, 1990, 1994). The World Health Organization subsequently adopted the measure in its *Global Burden of Disease Studies*.

The DALY is now widely used in the field of public health to assess the impact of death and disability in populations. This parameter is designed to extend the concept of potential years of life lost due to premature death to include equivalent years of "healthy" life lost due to states of poor health or disability. One DALY represents *one lost year of healthy life* and the sum of DALYs for all individuals of a population therefore quantifies the "gap" between current health status and ideal health where the entire population lives to an advanced age, free of disease and disability. The DALY therefore attempts to quantify mortality and morbidity in a single, common metric.

Traditionally, health liabilities were expressed as the expected or average number of *Years of Life Lost (YLL)*. This measure does not take into account the impact of disability or the number of years an individual lives with a severe disability. The population DALY for a disease or health condition is thus calculated as the sum of the years of life lost due to premature mortality in the population and the *Years Lost Due to Disability (YLD)* for incident cases of the specific health condition:

$$DALY = YLL + YLD$$

The YLL in a population for a particular disease is the product of the average life expectancy at average age of death for all individuals who died from that disease during a certain period of time (e.g., 1 year). The basic formula for YLL for a given cause, age, and gender is thus

$$YLL = N \times L_1$$

where N is the number of individuals who died from the disease in the population during the time period (year) of interest and L_1 is their standard life expectancy in years. Standard life expectancies for different ages are currently based upon life tables for the Japanese population, which has the highest biological life expectancy (80 years for men and 82.5 years for women).

To estimate YLD in a population for a particular disease in a particular time period, the average duration of disease (L_2) in years is weighted by a factor (DW) that reflects the severity of the disease on a scale from 0 (perfect health) to 1 (dead). The basic formula for YLD is thus

$$YLD = I \times DW \times L_2$$

where I denotes the number of new cases of disease, DW is the disability weight, and L_2 is the average duration of disease.

In calculating DALYs, the years of future life lost are weighted according to the formula

$$f(y) = 0.16243\, y e^{-0.04 y}$$

where y = the age at death or diagnosis of disease. This technique gives less weight to years of future life lost during periods of lesser productivity in the life span (childhood and late in life) and greater weight to years of future life lost during periods of higher productivity (late adolescence and adulthood). Furthermore, since a year of present life is considered more important than a year of future life, years of future life lost are discounted (reduced) at a standard rate of 3% per annum. Population estimates of DALYs for specific diseases are usually presented for a particular year per either 1000 or 100,000 inhabitants (Murray & López, 1990, 1994, 1997).

Global Disability Life Years DALY: All Causes

In 1997, Murray and López reported results of the first Global Burden of Disease Study using a standardized approach to epidemiologic assessment based upon estimates of DALY for various regions of the world. Estimates were calculated by age and gender for 107 disorders based upon cause-specific mortality and incidence rates, average age at onset, duration of disease, and severity of disability. Of the total DALY, 44% were due to communicable, maternal, perinatal, and nutritional disorders, 41% were due to noncommunicable diseases, and 15% were due to injuries. Among noncommunicable diseases, neurologic disease accounted for 10.5%, cardiovascular disease 9.7%, and cancer 5.1%, of the total DALY. Communicable, maternal, perinatal, and nutritional disorders accounted for two-thirds of the disease burden in sub-Saharan Africa while noncommunicable diseases accounted for 80% of the burden in established market economies. The highest disease burdens were in sub-Saharan Africa and India (21.4% and 20.9% of the global DALY total, respectively). The authors noted that "*developing countries carried almost 90% of the global disease burden yet were recipients of only 10% of global health care funding*" (Murray & López, 1997).

FIGURE 1.22 depicts the worldwide pattern of DALY in 2004. The average DALY across all regions was 237 per 1000 persons, of which about 60% was due to years of life lost from premature death and 40% due to years of healthy life lost due to disability from nonfatal diseases (WHO, 2009c).

In the nations of sub-Saharan Africa, the DALY are more than twofold higher than the rest of the world, largely due to high mortality rates from both acute and chronic conditions as discussed earlier in this chapter. Higher than average DALY are also evident in the war-torn nations of Afghanistan and Iraq.

The DALY and contributions of years of life lost due to premature death (YLL) and years of healthy life lost due to disability (YLD) are contrasted for various regions of the world as shown in **FIGURE 1.23**. In regions with the highest DALY (Africa, East Mediterranean, and Southeast Asia), premature deaths account for more than two-thirds of the DALY whereas in Europe, America, and the Western Pacific, premature deaths and disability each account for roughly half of the disease burden. This pattern clearly reflects the impact of the *epidemiologic transition*, vis-à-vis the greater disease burden of communicable diseases and maternal, perinatal, and nutritional conditions in developing nations compared to the noncommunicable diseases that are more prominent in developed nations. For example, in the nations of sub-Saharan African, over 70% of the DALY are due to *communicable diseases* such as HIV, tuberculosis, and malaria, whereas in the nations of North America, Western Europe, and Australasia, just the opposite is true and over 70% of the DALY are due to *noncommunicable diseases* such as ischemic heart disease, cancer, chronic obstructive pulmonary disease, diabetes, and neurological conditions (Murray & López, 2013).

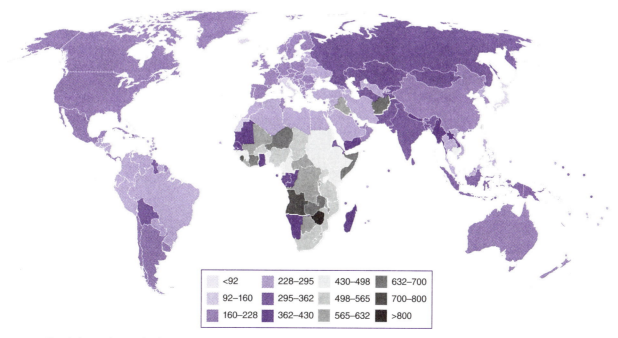

<92	228–295	430–498	632–700
92–160	295–362	498–565	700–800
160–228	362–430	565–632	>800

FIGURE 1.22 Disability-Adjusted Life Years, 2004.

Data from World Health Organization (2018). *The global burden of disease: 2004 update.* Geneva: WHO. Available at www.who.int/evidence/bod

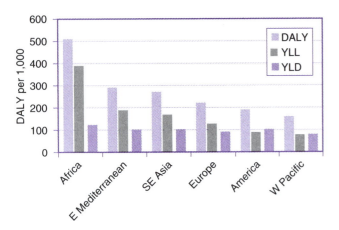

FIGURE 1.23 DALY, YLL, YLD by Region.

Data from WHO. (2009c). *Death and DALY estimates for 2004 by cause for WHO Member States: Persons, all ages*. Geneva, Switzerland: WHO.

Global Prevention of Chronic Diseases

Four major groups of chronic diseases: cardiovascular diseases, cancers, chronic respiratory diseases, and diabetes represent the greatest burden to human health. These four diseases are the world's biggest killers, causing an estimated 36 million deaths each year and approximately 60% of all deaths globally.

Fortunately, these diseases are largely preventable. Up to 80% of heart disease, stroke, and type 2 diabetes, and over 30% of cancers can be prevented by eliminating shared risk factors, mainly tobacco addiction, unhealthy diet and obesity, sedentary lifestyle, and the harmful use of alcohol.

However, unless appropriately addressed with well-designed and effective disease prevention and health promotion programs, the mortality and disease burden from these health problems will continue to increase. WHO projects that, globally, deaths from these conditions will increase by 10%–20% over the next 10 years. Due to high rates of smoking and alcohol abuse, increasing intake of diets ladened with salt, fat, and sugar, and a deficit in the access to health care, the populations of developing nations in Africa, Asia, and the Middle East are particularly susceptible.

Action for Prevention

Though proven cost-effective strategies currently exist to prevent and control the growing health burden of chronic diseases, high-level commitment, and concrete action are often missing or underfunded at the national level. On a global basis, it will be necessary to raise the priority accorded to chronic diseases, and develop and implement effective disease prevention and health promotion strategies and policies for the populations at risk. There is an immediate call for the

international public health communities to lobby and mobilize politicians, other international and regional agencies such as the United Nations Development Programme (UNDP), the United Nations Children's Fund (UNICEF), WHO, and the World Bank, and other international nongovernmental agencies to address the socioeconomic, behavioral, nutritional, and public health issues that have led to the current chronic disease epidemic. A multidisciplinary approach by governments that involves multiple ministries such as health, finance, education, sports, and agriculture can all contribute to a reversal of the underlying socioeconomic causes of the problem (Alberti et al., 2004; Simpson, Tuomilehto, Lindstrom, Shaw, & Zimmet, 1997; WHO, 1999; WHO, UNAIDS, UNICEF, 2008; Zimmet, 1999, 2000; Zimmet, Alberti, & Shaw, 2001; Zimmet, Shaw, & Alberti, 2003).

Effective interventions should obviously target tobacco use, unhealthy diets, physical inactivity, and excessive alcohol consumption. Programs must also be implemented to promote research and develop international partnerships for the prevention and control of chronic diseases. To this end, improved registration systems of vital statistics are needed in order to monitor the incidence, prevalence, and mortality of chronic diseases, as well as their determinants, and to evaluate progress at the national, regional, and global levels (WHO, 1999, 2008a).

The World Health Organization, working closely with its 193 Member States, has developed an Action Plan to prevent chronic diseases from occurring and to help the millions who are already affected to cope with these lifelong illnesses. This Action Plan, endorsed at the 61st World Health Assembly in May 2008, builds on the report of the Global Strategy for the Prevention and Control of Noncommunicable Diseases, 53rd World Health Assembly, May 2000. Key components of the plan are addressed in the following statement by Dr. Ala Alwan, Assistant Director-General, Noncommunicable Diseases and Mental Health, World Health Organization (Alwan, 2008).

"The action plan builds on the WHO Framework Convention on Tobacco Control and the WHO Global Strategy on Diet, Physical Activity, and Health. The Action Plan provides Member States, WHO, and the international community with a roadmap to establish and strengthen initiatives for the surveillance, prevention, and management of noncommunicable diseases. Furthermore, the Action Plan highlights the pressing need to invest in noncommunicable disease prevention as an integral part of sustainable socioeconomic development.

NCD prevention is an all-government responsibility. Considerably more gains can be achieved by influencing policies of nonhealth sectors than by health policies alone. All stakeholders will need to intensify and harmonize their efforts to avert these preventable conditions and to save millions from suffering needlessly and dying prematurely."

For every individual, effective prevention of chronic disease is contingent upon the total avoidance of major known risk factors. Many of these risk factors are well established and primary prevention is straightforward; avoidance of cigarette smoking (and other forms of tobacco addiction), avoidance of excessive alcohol consumption, control of blood pressure by avoidance of high-salt fat-laden diets, control of blood glucose by avoidance of high carbohydrate (sugar based) diets and foods with high glycemic indices, maintenance of body weight within normal limits, intake of calories matched to energy expenditure, daily intake of antioxidant and anti-inflammatory nutraceutical agents (fresh fruits and vegetables), daily aerobic exercising, daily stress release, and maintenance of a positive attitude in meeting life's challenges.

References

Adetunji, J., & Bos, E. R. (2006). Levels and trends in mortality in sub-Saharan Africa: An overview. In E. D. Jamison, R. G. Feachem, M. W. Makgoba, E. R. Bos, F. K. Baingana, K. J. Hofman, & K. O. Rogo (Eds.), *Disease and mortality in Sub-Saharan Africa* (2nd ed., pp. 11–14). Washington, DC: The World Bank.

Alberti, G., Zimmet, P., Shaw, J., Bloomgarden, Z., Kaufman, F., Silink, M., & Consensus Workshop Group. (2004). Consensus Workshop Group: Type 2 diabetes in the young: The evolving epidemic: The International Diabetes Federation consensus workshop. *Diabetes Care, 27*, 1798–1811.

Alwan, A. (2008). *2008–2013 Action plan for the global strategy for the prevention and control of noncommunicable diseases.* Geneva, Switzerland: World Health Organization.

Ames, B., Cathcart, R., Schwiers, E., & Hochstein, P. (1981). Uric acid provides an antioxidant defense in humans against oxidant- and radical caused aging and cancer: A hypothesis. *Proceedings of the National Academy of Sciences USA, 78*(11), 6858–6862.

Ames, B. N., Shigenaga, M. K., & Hagen, T. M. (1993). Oxidants, antioxidants, and the degenerative diseases of aging. *Proceedings of the National Academy of Sciences USA, 90*(17), 7915–7922.

Aris, E. (2004). United States life tables, 2002. *National Vital Statistics Reports, 53*(6), 1–40.

Austad, S. N. (1997). *Why we age: What science is discovering about the body's journey through life.* New York, NY: John Wiley & Sons.

Austad, S. N. (2006). Why women live longer than men: Sex differences in longevity. *Gender Medicine, 3*(2), 79–92.

Baingana, F. K., & Bos, E. R. (2006). Changing patterns of disease and mortality in Sub-Saharan Africa: An overview. In E. D. Jamison, R. G. Feachem, M. W. Makgoba, E. R. Bos, F. K. Baingana, K. J. Hofman, & K. O. Rogo (Eds.), *Disease and mortality in Sub-Saharan Africa* (2nd ed., pp. 1–10). Washington, DC: The World Bank.

Barja, G., & Herrero, A. (2000). Oxidative damage to mitochondrial DNA is inversely related to maximum life span in the heart and brain of mammals. *FASEB Journal, 14*(2), 312–318.

Beckman, K. B., & Ames, B. N. (1998). The free radical theory of aging matures. *Physiological Reviews, 78*, 547–581.

Blackman, M. R., Sorkin, J. D., Münzer, T., Bellantoni, M. F., Busby-Whitehead, J., Stevens. T. E., … Harman, S. M. (2002). Growth hormone and sex steroid administration in healthy aged women and men: A randomized controlled trial. *JAMA, 288*(18), 2282–2292.

Bradshaw, D., & Timaeus, I. M. (2006). Levels and trends of adult mortality. In E. D. Jamison, R. G. Feachem, M. W. Makgoba, E. R. Bos, F. K. Baingana, K. J. Hofman, & K. O. Rogo (Eds.), *Disease and mortality in Sub-Saharan Africa* (2nd ed., pp. 31–42). Washington, DC: The World Bank.

Caballero, B. (2007). The global epidemic of obesity: An overview. *Epidemiologic Reviews, 29*, 1–5.

Calle, E. E. (2007). Obesity and cancer. *BMJ, 335*(7630), 1107–1108.

Campisi, J., Kim, S. H., Lim, C. S., & Rubio, M. (2001). Cellular senescence, cancer and aging: The telomere connection. *Experimental Gerontology, 36*(10), 1619–1637.

Caulfield, L. E., de Onis, M., Blössner, M., & Black, R. E. (2004). Undernutrition as an underlying cause of child deaths associated with diarrhea, pneumonia, malaria, and measles. *American Journal of Clinical Nutrition, 80*, 193–198.

Central Intelligence Agency (CIA). (2009). *The world factbook.* Washington, DC: U.S. Central Intelligence Agency.

Central Intelligence Agency (CIA). (2017). *The world factbook.* Washington, DC: U.S. Central Intelligence Agency.

Colton, T. (1974). *Statistics in medicine.* Boston, MA: Little, Brown and Company.

de Courten, M., Bennett, P., Tuomilehto, J., & Zimmet, P. (1997). Epidemiology of NIDDM in non-Europids. In K. G. M. M. Alberti, R. A. DeFronzo, & P. Zimmet (Eds.), *International textbook of diabetes mellitus* (2nd ed., pp. 143–170). Chichester, United Kingdom: Wiley.

de Grey A. D. (1997). A proposed refinement of the mitochondrial theory of aging. *Bioessays, 19*(2), 161–166.

de Magalhaes, J. P., & Faragher, R. G. (2008). Cell divisions and mammalian aging: Integrative biology insights from genes that regulate longevity. *Bioessays, 30*(6), 567–578.

Doll, R., Peto, R., Boreham, J., & Sutherland, I. (2004). Mortality in relation to smoking: 50 years' observations in male British doctors. *BMJ, 328*(7455), 1519.

Duckett, P. (2005). Globalized violence, community psychology and the bombing and occupation of Afghanistan and Iraq. *Journal of Community & Applied Social Psychology, 15*, 414–423.

Fisichella, P. M., & Patti, M. G. (2009). Gastroesophageal reflux disease and morbid obesity: Is there a relation? *World Journal of Surgery, 33*, 2034–2038.

Gerschman, R., Gilbert, D. L., Nye, S. W., Dwyer, P., & Fenn, W. O. (1954). Oxygen poisoning and X-irradiation: A mechanism in common. *Science, 119*(3097), 623–626.

Guindon, G. E., & Boisclair, D. (2003). *Past, current and future trends in tobacco use* (pp. 13–16). Washington, DC: The International Bank for Reconstruction and Development, The World Bank.

Harman, D. (1956). Aging: A theory based on free radical and radiation chemistry. *Journal of Gerontology, 11*(3), 298–300.

Harman, D. (1972). A biologic clock: The mitochondria? *Journal of the American Geriatrics Society, 20*(4), 145–147.

Hayflick, L. (1985). The cell biology of aging. *Clinics in Geriatric Medicine, 1*(1), 15–27.

Hayflick, L. (2007). Entropy explains aging, genetic determinism explains longevity, and undefined terminology explains misunderstanding both. *PLoS Genetics, 3*(12), e220.

Hayutin, A. (2007). Graying of the global population. *Public Policy & Aging Report, 17*(4), 12–17.

Hill, K., & Amouzou, A. (2006). Trends in child mortality. In E. D. Jamison, R. G. Feachem, M. W. Makgoba, E. R. Bos, F. K. Baingana, K. J. Hofman, & K. O. Rogo (Eds.), *Disease and mortality in Sub-Saharan Africa* (2nd ed., pp. 15–30). Washington, DC: The World Bank.

International Obesity Task Force. (2010). *Obesity the global epidemic.* London, United Kingdom.

Leach, R. E., Baumgard, S., & Broom, J. (1973). Obesity: Its relationship to osteoarthritis of the knee. *Clinical Orthopaedics, 1973,* 93271–93273.

Leon, D. A., Saburova, L., Tomkins, S., Andreev, E., Kiryanov, N., McKee, M., & Shkolnikov, V. M. (2007). Hazardous alcohol drinking and premature mortality in Russia: A population based case-control study. *Lancet, 369*(9578), 2001–2009.

Linnane, A. W., Marzuki, S., Ozawa, T., & Tanaka, M. (1989). Mitochondrial DNA mutations as an important contributor to aging and degenerative diseases. *Lancet, 1*(8639), 642–645.

MacNee, W., Rabinovich, R. A., & Choudhury, G. (2014). Aging and the border between health and disease. *European Respiratory Journal, 44,* 1332–1352.

Medawar, P. B. (1952). *An unsolved problem of biology.* London, United Kingdom: H. K. Lewis.

Menken, J., Trussell, J., & Larsen, U. (1986). Age and infertility. *Science, 233,* 1389–1394.

Murray, C. J. L., & López, A. D. (1990). Global and regional cause-of-death patterns in 1990. *Bulletin of the World Health Organization, 72,* 447–480.

Murray, C. J. L., & López, A. D. (1994). Quantifying disability: Data, methods and results. *Bulletin of the World Health Organization, 72,* 481–494.

Murray, C. J. L., & López, A. D. (1997). Global mortality, disability, and the contribution of risk factors: Global Burden of Disease Study. *Lancet, 349*(9063), 1436–1442.

Murray, C. J. L., & López, A. D. (2013). Measuring the global burden of disease. *New England Journal of Medicine, 369,* 448–457.

National Vital Statistics System. (2002). *Centers for Disease Control and Prevention.* Washington, DC: National Center for Health Statistics.

Omran, A. R. (1971). The epidemiological transition: A theory of the epidemiology of population change. *Milbank Memorial Fund Quarterly, 49,* 509–538.

Pampel, F. (2002). Cigarette use and the narrowing sex differential in mortality. *Population and Development Review, 28,* 77–104.

Parker, W. H., Broder, M. S., Chang, E., Feskanich, D., Farquhar, C., Liu, Z., … Manson, J. E. (2009). Ovarian conservation at the time of hysterectomy and long-term health outcomes in the Nurses' Health Study. *Obstetrics & Gynecology, 113,* 1027–1037.

Pelletier, D. L., Frongillo, E. A. Jr., Schroeder, D. G., & Habicht, J.-P. (1995). The effects of malnutrition on child mortality in developing countries. *Bulletin of the World Health Organization, 73,* 443–448.

Perls, T. T., Hutter Silver, M., & Lauerman, J. F. (1999). *Living to 100: Lessons in living to your maximum potential at any age.* New York, NY: Basic Books.

Peto, R., Lopez, A. D., Boreham, J., Thun, M., Heath, C., & Doll, R. (1996). Mortality from smoking worldwide. *British Medical Bulletin, 52,* 12–21.

Jha, P., Chaloupka, F. J., Corrao, M., & Jacob, B. (2006). Reducing the burden of smoking worldwide: Effectiveness of interventions and their coverage. *Drug and Alcohol Review, 25*(6), 597–609.

Rao, C., Lopez, A. D., & Herned, Y. (2006). Causes of death. In E. D. Jamison, R. G. Feachem, M. W. Makgoba, E. R. Bos, F. K. Baingana, K. J. Hofman, & K. O. Rogo (Eds.), *Disease and mortality in Sub-Saharan Africa* (2nd ed., pp. 43–58). Washington, DC: The World Bank.

Ritchie, H., & Roser, M. (2018). "Causes of Death". Published online at OurWorldInData.org. Retrieved from https://ourworldindata.org/causes-of-death [Online Resource]

Rowe, T. (2006). Fertility and a woman's age. *Journal of Reproductive Medicine, 51*(3), 157–163.

Simpson, R. W., Tuomilehto, J., Lindstrom, J., Shaw, J. E., & Zimmet, P. (1997). Prevention of type 2 diabetes. In R. A. DeFronzo, E. Ferranini, H. Keen, & P. Zimmet (Eds.), *International textbook of diabetes mellitus* (3rd ed., pp. 1899–1913). Chichester, United Kingdom: John Wiley.

Strehler, B. L. (1999). *Time, cells, and aging* (3rd ed.). Larnaca, Cyprus: Demetriades Brothers.

UNICEF. (2017). *Levels and trends in child mortality.* Report 2017. New York, NY: UNICEF Publications.

UNICEF-WHO-The World Bank. (2018, May). *Joint child malnutrition estimates 2018 Edition—Interactive Dashboard* (UNICEF, New York; WHO, Geneva; The World Bank, Washington, DC).

UNICEF-WHO-The World Bank, United Nations. (2018). *Trends in maternal mortality: 1990 to 2015.* WHO, UNICEF, UNFPA, World Bank Group and the United Nations Population Division.

United Nations Department of Economic and Social Affairs, Population Division. (2017). *United Nations World Population Prospects: 2017 revision.* New York, NY: United Nations.

United States Census Bureau. (2018). International Data Base.

WHO. (1999). *The World health report 1999: Making a difference.* Geneva, Switzerland: WHO.

WHO. (2008a). *Chronic diseases: A vital investment.* Geneva, Switzerland: WHO.

WHO. (2008b). *Global tuberculosis control 2008 report.* Geneva, Switzerland: WHO.

WHO. (2009a). *World health statistics, 2009.* Geneva, Switzerland: WHO.

WHO. (2009b). *Report on the global tobacco epidemic, 2009.* Geneva, Switzerland: WHO.

WHO. (2009c). *Death and DALY estimates for 2004 by cause for WHO Member States: Persons, all ages.* Geneva, Switzerland: WHO.

WHO. (2015). *Report on the global tobacco epidemic, 2015.* Geneva, Switzerland: WHO.

WHO. (2017a). *Global strategy on diet, physical activity & health, childhood overweight and obesity, 2017*: WHO.

WHO. (2017b). *Obesity and overweight, 2017.* Geneva, Switzerland: WHO.

WHO. (2017c). *World health statistics, 2017.* Geneva, Switzerland: WHO.

WHO, UNAIDS, UNICEF. (2008). *Towards universal access: Scaling up priority interventions in the health sector; Progress Report 2008.*

World Bank. (1993). *World development report 1993: Investing in health: World development indicators.* Oxford, United Kingdom: University Press Oxford.

World Population Prospects: The 2017 Revision. Department of Economic and Social Affairs, United Nations, 2017.

Wynder, E. L. (1994). Principles of disease prevention from discovery to application. *International Journal of Public Health, 39*(5), 167–172.

Zaridze, D., Brennan, P., Boreham, P., Boroda, A., Karpov, R., Lazarev, A., … Peto, R. (2009). Alcohol and cause-specific mortality in Russia: A retrospective case-control study of 48,557 adult deaths. *Lancet, 373*(9682), 2201–2214.

Zimmet, P. (1999). Diabetes epidemiology as a trigger to diabetes research. *Diabetologia, 42,* 499–518.

Zimmet, P. (2000). Globalization, coca-colonization and the chronic disease epidemic: Can the doomsday scenario be averted? *Journal of Internal Medicine, 247,* 301–310.

Zimmet, P., Alberti, K. G., & Shaw, J. (2001). Global and societal implications of the diabetes epidemic. *Nature, 414,* 782–787.

Zimmet, P., Shaw, J., & Alberti, K. G. (2003). Preventing type 2 diabetes and the dysmetabolic syndrome in the real world: A realistic view. *Diabetic Medicine, 20,* 693–702.

Zimmet, P. Z., & Alberti, G. M. M. (2006). Introduction: Globalization and the non-communicable disease epidemic. *Obesity, 14,* 1–3.

CHAPTER 2

Global Epidemiology of Cardiovascular Disease

▶ Introduction

Cardiovascular disease (CVD) in its various forms is the leading cause of death worldwide, ranking first in both developing and developed nations. During 2016, 17.9 million people died from CVD (8.5 million women and 9.4 million men), approximately 31% of all reported deaths in that year. These data reflect a 42% increase from the 12.6 million CVD deaths reported in 1990. The largest increase in CVD deaths occurred in regions of Southern Asia including India where there were at least 1.8 million more CVD deaths in 2013 than 1990, an increase of 97% (Ritchie & Roser, 2018; Roth et al., 2015, 2017).

Even though the number of CVD deaths has increased dramatically in the world population, age-standardized mortality rates due to CVD have declined in all high-income nations and many middle-income nations. In fact, CVD death rates by age have remained steady or declined in all regions of the world with the exception of certain areas of Western sub-Saharan Africa. As a result of worldwide progress in the prevention and therapy of CVD, the global age-standardized mortality rate due to CVD declined by 22% during the period 1990–2010, from 393 deaths per 100,000 in 1990 to 307 deaths per 100,000 in 2010. Nevertheless, progress has slowed in the past few years and the current global CVD mortality rate has plateaued at around 286 deaths per 100,000 (Roth et al., 2017). **FIGURE 2.1** shows the distribution of age-standardized CVD mortality rates by country for 2015.

Rates are lowest (<200 per 100,000) in populations of the Americas, Western Europe, Scandinavia, Australia, New Zealand, and Japan, and highest (>500 per 100,000) in Russia, Eastern Europe, and Central and Southern Asia. Japan had the lowest rate among industrialized nations, 95 per 100,000, and among all nations, war-torn Afghanistan had the highest rate, 830 per 100,000 (Roth et al., 2017).

Concurrent with increasing longevity throughout the world population, the burden of CVD no longer has greater impact in the developed world. According to the most recent World Health Organization (WHO) data, more than 80% of all CVD deaths occurred in developing (low and middle income) countries compared to developed (high income) countries (Bowry, Lewey, Dugani, & Choudhry, 2015; WHO, 2009, 2010). **FIGURE 2.2** shows the marked excess of CVD deaths in low and middle-income countries compared to high-income countries (14.7 million versus 3.2 million).

CVD not only causes death but can also result in severe disability, particularly among those who survive a myocardial infarction or stroke. One measure of overall disease burden that is commonly used to measure the impact of *both* death and disability is *disability-adjusted life years* (DALY). The DALY extends the concept of *potential years of life lost due to premature death* (YLL) to include *years of healthy life lost due to disability* (YLD). In other words, the DALY combines mortality and morbidity into a single common measurement calculated as DALY = YLL + YLD.

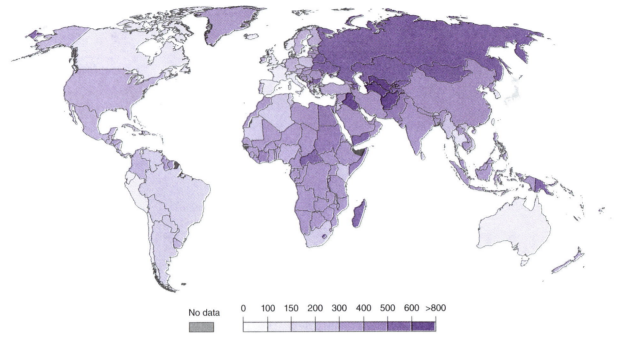

No data   0   100   150   200   300   400   500   600   >800

FIGURE 2.1 Cardiovascular Disease Mortality Rates by Country, 2016.

Reproduced from Institute for Health Metrics and Evaluation, Global Burden of Disease. Our World in Data Organization.

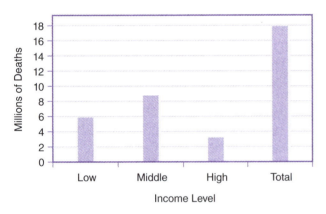

FIGURE 2.2 Global CVD Mortality.

Data from Bowry, A. D. K., Lewey, J., Dugani, S. B., & Choudhry, N. K. (2015). The burden of cardiovascular disease in low and middle income countries: Epidemiology and management. *Canadian Journal of Cardiology, 31*(9), 1151–1159; World Health Organization. (2010). *World Health Organization statistical information system (WHOSIS)*. Geneva, Switzerland: World Health Organization. Countries are grouped by national annual income per capita: Low: < $826, Middle: $826–$10,065, High: > $10,065.

FIGURE 2.3 depicts the burden of CVD measured by DALY where one DALY is equivalent to the loss of 1 year of healthy life (WHO, 2009). Clearly, the CVD burden is higher in many of the developing nations of Asia, South America, and Africa (DALY > 5100 per 100,000) than in the more advanced societies of North America, Europe, and Australia (DALY < 3000 per 100,000). The composition of DALY also varies by economic region. Developing nations with high DALY rates suffer more lost years of healthy life due to premature death from CVD (60%–70%) whereas developed nations lose more years of healthy life due to disability from CVD (50%–60%).

▶ Spectrum of Cardiovascular Disease

Categorization of the pathologies underlying CVD is complex since the primary disease processes are often interdependent. Even so, more than 95% of all CVD can be categorized according to a few major pathologic conditions (Braunwald, Zipes, Libby, & Bonow, 1997). Furthermore, more than 75% of deaths from CVD are attributable to either ischemic heart disease culminating in myocardial infarction or stroke culminating in cerebral infarction. These two conditions, ischemic heart disease and stroke, account for nearly one quarter of all deaths worldwide.

The approximate global number of deaths due to the various forms of CVD is shown in **TABLE 2.1**. Of the 17.9 million deaths attributable to CVD every year, 8.9 million are due to ischemic (coronary) heart disease resulting in sudden cardiac death (sudden unexpected death caused by loss of heart function) or acute myocardial infarction (heart attack); 6.3 million are due to cerebrovascular disease (stroke); and an additional 1 million are due to hypertensive disease (which often results in congestive heart failure). The remaining deaths are due to rheumatic heart disease and inflammatory conditions (myocarditis, endocarditis, and pericarditis), aortic aneurysms, pulmonary emboli, and other cardiovascular conditions. Major diseases and conditions in the spectrum of CVD are briefly defined

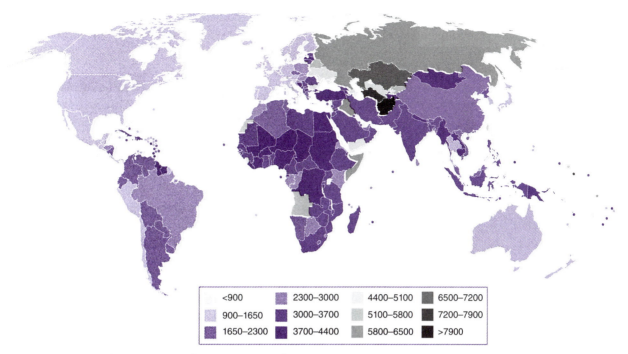

FIGURE 2.3 Cardiovascular Disease: Disability-Adjusted Life Years (DALY), 2004.

Data from World Health Organization. (2008). *The global burden of disease: 2004 update.* Geneva: WHO. Available at www.who.int/evidence/bod. Age-standardized DALY from cardiovascular disease by country (per 100,000 inhabitants). Disability-adjusted life years (DALY) are rates per 100,000 people that combine years of life lost (YLL) due to premature disease mortality in the population and the years lost due to disability (YLD) for incident nonfatal cases of the disease (DALY = YLL + YLD). One DALY represents the loss of 1 year of healthy life.

TABLE 2.1 Relative Mortality due to Cardiovascular Disease, 2016		
Ischemic (coronary) heart disease	8.92 million	50%
Cerebrovascular disease (stroke)	6.33 million	35%
Hypertensive heart disease	0.96 million	5%
Rheumatic heart disease	0.32 million	2%
Myocarditis/cardiomyopathy	0.35 million	2%
Atrial fibrillation	0.19 million	1%
Peripheral vascular/aortal disease	0.22 million	1%
Other conditions	0.63 million	4%
Total	17.92 million	

Data from CVD were estimated from worldwide data published by Roth, G. A., Johnson, C., Abajobir, A., Abd-Allah, F., Abera, S. F., Abyu, G., . . . Murray, C. (2017). Global, regional, and national burden of cardiovascular diseases for 10 causes, 1990 to 2015. *Journal of the American College of Cardiology, 70*(1), 1–25; Watkins, D. A., Johnson, C. O., Colquhoun, S. M., Karthikeyan, G., Beaton, A., Bukhman, G., . . . Roth, G. A. (2017). Global, regional and national burden of rheumatic heart disease, 1990–2015. *New England Journal of Medicine, 377,* 713–722. Other conditions include heart failure, pulmonary embolism, endocarditis, pericarditis, non-rheumatic heart valve disease, congenital heart disease.

in the following paragraphs, and separate chapters of this text are devoted to the epidemiology of these conditions.

Ischemic Heart Disease (Coronary Heart Disease) is caused by narrowing and obstruction of one or more blood vessels supplying the heart muscle itself (the myocardium). Ischemia means lack of oxygen (obviously due to the absence or lack of blood without which the heart muscle quickly dies). The catastrophic culminating event of obstructive coronary heart disease is a myocardial infarction (heart attack), which is frequently fatal. Coronary heart disease is almost always due to the presence of atherosclerotic plaque that impedes blood flow in one or more of the small caliber arteries of the heart. The development of atherosclerotic plaque (a process called atherogenesis) begins early in life and progresses over many years (usually decades) throughout the life span. Atherosclerotic plaque may develop over time in one or more coronary arteries eventually leading to stenosis and obstruction; or plaque may develop in a larger artery upstream (e.g., the aorta) that may rupture producing plaque remnants and thrombotic fragments (blood clots) that travel to smaller vessels such as the coronary arteries where they lodge and become obstructive. The process of atherogenesis is discussed in some detail in a following section of this chapter.

Sudden Cardiac Death refers to sudden, unexpected death caused by the abrupt loss of heart function. This condition classically involves malfunction of the electrical system of the heart triggered by atherosclerotic occlusion of coronary blood vessels, ischemia, and infarction of segments of the myocardium. It should be obvious that sudden cardiac death cardiac arrest can occur coincident with a myocardial infarction, or during recovery from a myocardial infarction. Nevertheless, in developed countries such as the United States that have advanced emergency services, more than 75% of acute myocardial infarctions *do not* lead to sudden cardiac arrest. Nevertheless, autopsy studies reveal the presence of ischemic heart disease and focal areas of infarcted myocardium in more than 80% of individuals who suffer sudden cardiac arrest. Other heart conditions may also disrupt the heart's rhythm and result in sudden cardiac arrest. These include a thickened or weakened heart muscle (cardiomyopathy), heart failure, arrhythmias, particularly ventricular fibrillation, and an abnormal pattern of heart rhythm such as Long Q-T syndrome. Other causes include cardiomyopathies and congenital anomalies. Most sudden cardiac deaths are caused by interruption of normal heart rhythm which disables the ability of the heart to pump blood, and without immediate treatment (cardiopulmonary resuscitation (CPR)) and defibrillation, death occurs in minutes.

Myocardial Infarction (Heart Attack) is caused by acute obstruction of a coronary artery, usually one in which blood flow is already compromised by the presence of significant atherosclerotic plaque. Most infarcts of the myocardium arise due to ischemic heart disease as a consequence of long-standing atherosclerosis. There is controversy regarding the exact sequence of events leading to a myocardial infarction, and it is likely that there is considerable variability in the process from patient to patient. One proposed

scenario involves rupture of an atherosclerotic plaque followed by platelet aggregation and possibly thrombotic occlusion in key coronary arteries (e.g., the right or left anterior descending or the left circumflex artery). Albeit, the end result of a myocardial infarction, is significant necrosis of the myocardium which can quickly progress to arrhythmia and sudden cardiac death.

Cerebrovascular Disease (Stroke) is caused by acute disruption of the blood supply to the brain due to either blockage (ischemic stroke) or rupture of a blood vessel (hemorrhagic stroke). As with ischemic heart disease, strokes are usually caused by atherosclerotic plaque either developing in place or dislodged from a larger (upstream) artery. Plaque rupture, platelet aggregation, and thrombotic occlusion may all be involved.

Hypertensive Heart Disease occurs when the heart continually pumps against high resistance in the peripheral circulatory system. Resistance to blood flow in the peripheral arteriolar system increases with the constriction of blood vessels (vasoconstriction). The effects of vasoconstriction and increased resistance to blood flow are measured by the blood pressure. Regulation of blood pressure is complex and involves the kidneys and other organs. Hypertension is defined as systolic blood pressure exceeding 140 mm Hg and/or diastolic blood pressure exceeding 90 mm Hg. As the peripheral resistance to blood flow increases, the heart (particularly the left ventricle) must work harder to maintain cardiac output. This sequence leads to left ventricle hypertrophy and dilatation and may cause the pooling of blood in the left ventricular chamber (left-sided congestive heart failure). If there is long-standing high blood pressure in the lungs (pulmonary hypertension), the right ventricle may undergo hypertrophy leading to right-sided congestive heart failure *(cor pulmonale)*. Other factors, particularly ischemic heart disease, may contribute to and exacerbate hypertensive heart disease and congestive heart failure.

Congestive Heart Failure is the sequela of antecedent pathologies of the cardiovascular system, primarily (but not limited) to ischemic heart disease and hypertension. This condition is defined as failure of the heart to pump blood at a rate commensurate with the requirements of the body. The life-threatening effects of congestive heart failure are congestion, edema, and hypoxia, not only in the heart itself but also in the lungs, kidneys, brain, liver, and other vital organs. Congestive heart failure is often divided into left-sided versus right-sided failure. Left-sided failure most often arises due to the combination of ischemic damage to the myocardium from coronary atherosclerosis plus peripheral hypertension requiring greater contractile force of the left ventricle to maintain cardiac output. Right-sided failure *(cor pulmonale)* can develop as a consequence of intrinsic lung disease (e.g., chronic obstructive pulmonary disease) and heightened blood pressure in the pulmonary circulation or may arise from progressive edematous changes in the lungs due to left-sided heart failure. In either case, the right ventricle encounters increased contractile resistance and is subject to hypertrophy, dilatation, and failure.

Rheumatic Heart Disease refers to damage to the heart valves and/or the myocardium caused by a persistent infection with beta hemolytic streptococcal A bacteria. The infectious process typically begins as an acute pharyngitis. Rheumatic fever develops as a sequela to the infection and involves inflammatory immune reactions in the heart and joints.

Inflammatory Heart Disease refers to inflammatory conditions of the heart other than rheumatic heart disease. Inflammatory heart disease encompasses viral myocarditis (viral infection of the myocardium), bacterial endocarditis (bacterial infection of the endocardium, the inner lining of the heart chambers), and pericarditis (infection of the pericardial membranes that surround the heart). Infectious agents may attack the myocardium directly or alternatively and may stimulate an autoimmune inflammatory response in the myocardium. A variety of viruses, bacteria, protozoa, and other microbes may be involved, especially in the immunocompromised patient.

Peripheral Artery Disease is caused by obstruction of the arteries (usually by atherosclerotic plaque) supplying the arms and legs. This condition is often a forerunner of ischemic heart disease due to atherosclerosis.

Aortic Aneurysms are abnormal dilatations of the aorta. These balloon-like outpouchings of the aorta arise primarily due to severe atherosclerosis and hypertension that produce thinning and necrosis of the artery wall. Long-standing aortic aneurysms are highly prone to rupture and discharge of blood into surrounding tissues and body cavities. Such dissecting aortic aneurysms are frequently fatal.

Deep Venous Thrombosis refers to obstructive blood clots in peripheral veins of the legs (veins carry blood back to the right atrium of the heart). Thrombotic material can dislodge and travel through the pulmonary arteries to the lungs, resulting in a life-threatening pulmonary embolism.

Congenital Heart Disease refers to malformation of anatomic structures (e.g., septal defects, abnormal heart valves) at birth due to genetic factors or gestational events.

▶ Declining Mortality from Cardiovascular Disease in Developed Countries

CVD is the predominant cause of death and disability throughout the industrialized world as well as in many developing nations. Nevertheless, in developed countries such as the United States, Great Britain, Australia/New Zealand, and Western European nations, deaths from CVD have declined dramatically in the past several decades. Declining CVD mortality in the United States is illustrative of this trend. In the past four decades, steep declines are evident for coronary heart disease and stroke, the two leading causes of CVD deaths (**FIGURE 2.4**). The declining trend in CVD mortality is undoubtedly due to major advances in the prevention and treatment of hypertension, ischemic heart disease, diabetes, heart failure, and related conditions that predispose to fatal heart attacks and strokes. Indeed, it is estimated that more than half of the deaths due to CVD could be prevented through health promotion and disease prevention activities including cost-effective healthcare policies and individual actions to reduce exposure to major risk factors such as high blood pressure, high cholesterol, elevated blood glucose, obesity, and smoking (Anand & Yusuf, 2011; Mensah et al., 2017; Sanderson et al., 2007; Sidney et al., 2016).

▶ United States Mortality from Cardiovascular Disease

Despite the approximate 70% decline in deaths from ischemic heart disease and stroke during the past

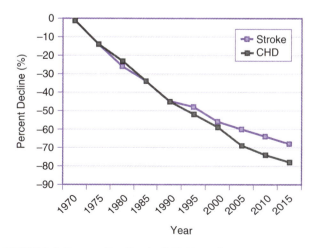

FIGURE 2.4 Percent Decline in CVD Mortality.

Data from National Heart, Lung and Blood Institute (NHLBI, 2012). *Morbidity and mortality: 2012 chart book on cardiovascular, lung and blood diseases.* Bethesda, MD: National Institutes of Health; Mensah, G. A., Wei, G. S., Sorlie, P. D., Fine, L. J., Rosenberg, Y., Kaufmann, P. G. M., … Gordon, D. (2017). Decline in cardiovascular mortality: Possible causes and implications. *Circulation Research, 120,* 366–380; Sidney, S., Quesenberry, C. P., Jr., Jaffe, M. G., Sorel, M., Nguyen-Huynh, M. N., Kushi, L. H., …, Rana, J. S. (2016). Recent trends in cardiovascular mortality in the United States and public health goals. *JAMA, 1*(5), 594–599.

40 years, CVD remains the leading cause of death in the United States (as well as most other developed nations). In 2015, CVD claimed approximately 832,024 U.S. lives (30.7% of all deaths) and more than 157,000 CVD victims (19%) died before reaching age 65 years. Ischemic/coronary heart disease caused 366,801 deaths in 2015 and is the single leading cause of death in the United States today (Heron et al., 2009; Murphy, Xu, Kochanek, Curtin, & Arias, 2017).

According to recent survey data published by the American Heart Association, approximately 37% of adults over 20 years of age (92.1 million) are living with one or more forms of CVD. Prevalent conditions among living American adults include high blood pressure (84.7 million), type 2 diabetes mellitus (23.4 million), myocardial infarction (7.4 million), stroke (6.6 million), and heart failure (6.5 million). More than one-third of these individuals have two or more forms of CVD, which synergistically increases their risk of developing a secondary catastrophic cardiovascular event (e.g., fatal myocardial infarction, stroke, or end-stage congestive heart failure) (Benjamin et al., 2017; Levy, 1993; Mozaffarian et al., 2015).

▶ Epidemic of Congestive Heart Failure in the United States

One form of CVD that has markedly increased rather than decreased in the United States and other developed nations during the past 40 years is congestive heart failure (Bleumink et al., 2004). As shown in **FIGURE 2.5**, the hospitalization rate for congestive heart failure has increased more than fourfold for adults 65 years and older and more than twofold for younger adults in the United States since 1970 (Blecker, Paul, Taksler, Ogedegbe, & Katz, 2013; National Heart, Lung and Blood Institute, 2009). According to recent survey data from the National Health and Nutrition

Examination Survey (NHANES), the number of adults living with heart failure in the United States increased from 5.7 million in 2009–2012 to 6.5 million in 2011–2014 (Benjamin et al., 2017). This condition occurs when the heart pumps insufficient blood to meet the metabolic demands of the body. It is effectively diagnosed and monitored by measuring cardiac output as the ejection fraction of the lower heart chambers (ventricles) by using electrocardiography and other imaging techniques. The normal adult range for the ejection fraction is 50%–70% and congestive heart failure is indicated when the ejection fraction falls below 50%.

Many interactive factors are undoubtedly responsible for the epidemic of congestive heart failure in the United States and other developed nations. Congestive heart failure represents the end stage of a web of pathogenic events of CVD including ischemic/coronary heart disease, atherosclerosis, hypertension, type 2 diabetes, and inflammation (He et al., 2001). Indeed, improvements in the detection and treatment of these conditions have led to a significant increase in overall survival. It is estimated that more than 81 million Americans are living with two or more forms of CVD, and as more and more patients survive CVD and live longer, their risk of developing congestive heart failure increases. Furthermore, the prevalence of certain risk factors, particularly type 2 diabetes and obesity, has increased in parallel with the rising rates of congestive heart failure.

▶ Gender and Ethnic Differences in Cardiovascular Disease in the United States

Striking gender and ethnic differences are present in the rates of CVD and its spectrum of component

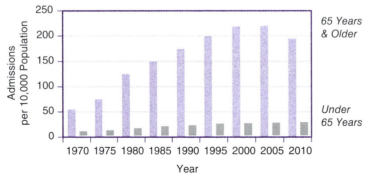

FIGURE 2.5 Hospitalization Rates for Congestive Heart Failure, 1970–2010, United States.

Data from National Heart, Lung and Blood Institute (NHLBI, 2009). *Morbidity and mortality: 2009 chart book on cardiovascular, lung and blood diseases*. Bethesda, MD: National Institutes of Health.

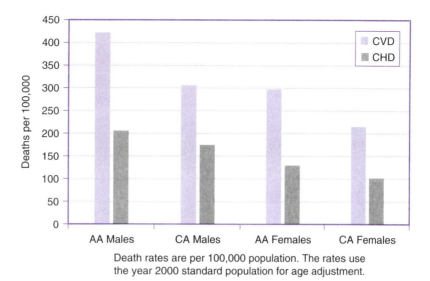

FIGURE 2.6 Cardiovascular Disease (CVD) and Coronary Heart Disease (CHD): United States, 2006.

Data from Heron, M., Oyert, D. L., Murphy, S. L., Xu, J., Kochanek, K. D., & Tejada-Vera, B. (2009). Deaths: Final data for 2006. *National Vital Statistics Reports, 57*(14), 1–134.

conditions. **FIGURE 2.6** shows the 2006 U.S. mortality rates for CVD and coronary/ischemic heart disease (CHD) for men and women of African American and Caucasian American ethnicity. For each stratum, CHD constitutes approximately half of the CVD mortality burden. The excess mortality among men compared to women is evident for each ethnic group (e.g., men are at an approximately 40% higher risk of dying from any form of CVD than women). The excess CVD mortality in the African American population is also striking (e.g., in gender-specific comparisons, African Americans have 38% higher CVD mortality than Caucasian Americans). These population disparities in cardiovascular health have persisted over several decades and reflect not only differences in exposure to the risk factors, but also inadequacies of the healthcare system for the early detection and efficacious treatment of CVD in subpopulations of Americans. The elimination of such disparities will require aggressive action focused on prevention and therapy in high-risk populations (Freeman & Payne, 2000; Graham, 2015).

▶ Epidemiologic Transition of Cardiovascular Disease

Major causes of death and disability have undergone an epidemiologic transition from predominantly nutritional deficiencies and infectious diseases in underdeveloped nations to chronic degenerative diseases such as CVD, cancer, and type 2 diabetes in more advanced societies. Yusuf and colleagues divide the international patterns of CVD into four distinct stages of the epidemiologic transition: (1) excess rheumatic heart disease and other inflammatory conditions in children and young adults in populations of sub-Saharan Africa, rural Southeast Asia, and South America, (2) excess hypertensive heart disease in young and middle-aged adults in populations of China and urban Asia, (3) rapidly increasing ischemic (coronary) heart disease and cerebrovascular disease in populations of India, Latin America, and Russia, and (4) declining CVD among adults in populations of North America, Western Europe, Australia, and New Zealand (Yusuf, Reddy, Ôunpuu, & Anand, 2001).

While CVDs afflict men and women of all socioeconomic classes in all geographic areas of the world, the prevalence of known CVD risk factors, and corresponding disease rates are highest and on the increase in the developing world. As a consequence, the most populous nations of the world have not yet progressed to stage 4 of the epidemiologic transition. As pointed out by Sanderson and colleagues in their review of the global burden of CVD:

Although the mortality rate of cardiovascular diseases and prevalence of major cardiovascular risk factors has generally decreased in economically developed countries, the corresponding mortality rate, and risk prevalence has substantially increased in China, other East Asian societies and now India, which have been under-going rapid demographic, social and, economic changes.

(Sanderson et al., 2007)

Furthermore, CVD often strikes middle-aged adults, and as a result, families spiral into a cycle of poverty as they lose their primary breadwinners to death or severe disability (Anderson & Chu, 2007). Such premature death and disability reflect a virtual pandemic of CVD, and if current trends continue, the annual death toll will approach 20 million in the developing world by the year 2020 (WHO, 2005).

▶ Risk Factors for Cardiovascular Disease

The stages in the epidemiologic transition of CVDs have occurred in response to shifts in risk factor profiles for specific cardiovascular conditions. The classical risk factors for CVD include tobacco addiction, hyperlipidemia (high low-density lipoprotein cholesterol and low high-density lipoprotein cholesterol), diabetes type 2 with hyperglycemia (increased blood glucose), hypertension, and inflammatory conditions of the heart and blood vessels. The inflammatory biomarker, C-reactive protein (CRP), has also been proven to be of value in predicting the development of CVD.

There is also convincing epidemiologic evidence that CVD risk is increased by consuming a diet high in saturated fats, being markedly overweight or obese, and maintaining a sedentary lifestyle with little physical activity. These risk factors tend to cluster in populations thereby synergistically elevating the risk to much higher levels. The time-lag effect of risk factors for CVD means that the full effect of past exposure to behavioral risk factors, especially among children, will be seen only in the future. Unless preventive and management efforts are embraced worldwide, the global burden of CVD death and disease will continue to rise (Anderson et al., 2010; MacKay & Mensah, 2004). **TABLE 2.2** provides a listing of the major and contributing CVD risk factors, each of which is discussed in subsequent chapters.

The global rise in CVD in developing nations reflects increases in the risk factors listed in Table 2.2: Heightened consumption of westernized diets, declining physical activity levels, and increased tobacco addiction as a result of industrialization, urbanization, economic development, and market globalization. People of these nations are consuming a more energy-dense, nutrient-poor diet and are less physically active. Imbalanced nutrition, reduced physical activity, and increased tobacco addiction are the key lifestyle factors. High blood pressure, high blood cholesterol, obesity, and type 2 diabetes are among the major biological risk factors. Unhealthy dietary

TABLE 2.2 Selected Risk Factors for Cardiovascular Disease

Major Risk Factors
1. Tobacco addiction
2. Elevated LDL cholesterol
3. Low HDL cholesterol
4. High blood pressure
5. Elevated blood glucose
6. Elevated C-reactive protein
7. Obesity*
8. Physical inactivity*
9. Dietary factors*

Contributing Risk Factors
1. Low socioeconomic status*
2. Elevated prothrombotic factors: Fibrinogen, PAI-1
3. Markers of infection or inflammation
4. Elevated homocysteine
5. Elevated lipoprotein(a)
6. Psychological factors (depression, anger proneness, hostility, stress, acute life-events) and breakdown in social structures (loss of social support and cohesion)*

PAI indicates plasminogen activator inhibitor.

*Predisposing risk factors: A predisposing risk factor is presumed to work, at least in part, through impact on other risk factors that act directly. For example, obesity raises blood pressure, causes dyslipidemia, and increases blood glucose. It is likely that some of the contributing risk factors also have direct effects.

practices include the high consumption of saturated fats, salt, and refined carbohydrates, and reciprocally, the low consumption of fruits and vegetables, whole grains and nuts, and certain types of unsaturated fats (e.g., omega-3 fatty acids). Furthermore, individuals in the developing world have the "double jeopardy" of increased chronic disease prevalence combined with persistently high rates of infectious diseases, leading to exceedingly high overall morbidity and mortality (Jamison et al., 2006).

Primary Prevention of Cardiovascular Disease

Primary prevention is the avoidance of known CVD risk factors. For example, individuals who never initiate the smoking habit markedly reduce their risk. Other lifestyle changes that have proven beneficial to cardiovascular health include cessation of tobacco use, aerobic exercising for at least 30 minutes daily, maintaining optimal body weight, and consuming a diet low in sodium, carbohydrates, saturated and total fats that is more weighted toward unsaturated fats, fruits, vegetables, whole grains, and omega-3 fatty acids. Compelling evidence indicates that the following strategies listed in **TABLE 2.3** are effective in preventing CVD and in helping manage the disease.

The most cost-effective methods of reducing CVD rates involve population-wide efforts to reduce modifiable risk factors through multiple economic and educational policies and programs. Food labeling for nutritional content; educational programs to promote decreased consumption of saturated fats, trans-fatty acids, and sodium; targeting and penalizing tobacco use; and campaigns advocating regular aerobic physical activity for weight reduction and control have proven effective in certain populations (Anderson et al., 2010).

Tertiary Prevention of Cardiovascular Disease

Individuals who have already experienced a cardiovascular event such as a heart attack or stroke are at high risk of suffering recurrence or death. Such individuals have numerous interventions available to them including nonpharmaceutical lifestyle modifications including regular aerobic exercising and dietary changes (e.g., restriction of salt, sugar, refined carbohydrates, and transition of the fatty acid profile to include less saturated fats and more polyunsaturated fats such as omega-3 fatty acids). Safe and effective weight reduction programs typically involve reduced caloric intake and increased fiber in the diet combined with a regular program of aerobic physical activity (Weight Control Information Network, 2010).

Pharmaceutical modalities include aspirin use, blood pressure modification, statin medication for hyperlipidemia, and specific medications to regulate blood glucose. In addition, there are several intensive techniques that are used in patients with CVD, such as coronary stenting and coronary artery bypass grafting for ischemic heart disease, and thrombolytics for cerebrovascular disease.

Global Prevention of Cardiovascular Disease

Until recently, CVD has been largely absent from the international consciousness, overshadowed by public health concerns about HIV/AIDS and other infectious diseases. As recently as 2000, CVD was conspicuously absent from the United Nation's Millennium Development Goals. CVDs are largely preventable through public health strategies and evidence-based risk factor interventions. International, national, and community programs are needed to ensure that these

---

TABLE 2.3 Strategies for the Prevention of Cardiovascular Disease

- Avoid smoking or using any form of tobacco.

- Maintain a healthy weight.

- Practice at least 30 minutes of aerobic physical activity daily.

- Limit energy intake from total fats and shift fat consumption away from saturated fats to unsaturated fats and toward the elimination of trans-fatty acids.

- Increase consumption of omega-3 fatty acids from fish oil or plant sources such as olive oil.

- Consume a diet high in fruits, vegetables, nuts and whole grains, and low in refined grains.

- Avoid excessively salty or sugary foods.

- Limit alcohol consumption to one drink daily.

interventions reach the individuals most at risk. The World Health Organization has called for a global partnership of nationwide public health campaigns and high-risk intervention strategies (WHO, 2005). In 2016, a new initiative, "Global Hearts," was launched by WHO to scale up prevention and therapeutic measures designed to reduce the global burden of CVD.

This collaborative effort joins the forces of WHO with the United States Centers for Disease Control and Prevention and several other international partners, including the World Heart Federation, the World Stroke Organization, the International Society of Hypertension, and the World Hypertension League (WHO, 2016).

References

Anand, S. S., & Yusuf, S. (2011). Stemming the global tsunami of cardiovascular disease. *Lancet, 377*(9765), 529–532.

Anderson, C. F., & Chu, E. (2007). Expanding priorities-confronting chronic disease in countries with low income. *The New England Journal of Medicine, 356*(3), 209–211.

Anderson, J., Parker, W., Steyn, N. P., Grimsrud, A., Kolbe-Alexander, T., Lambert, E. V., & Mciza, Z. (2010). *World Health Organization global strategy on diet, physical activity and health: Interventions on diet and physical activity: Executive summary*. Geneva, Switzerland: World Health Organization.

Benjamin, E. J., Blaha, M. J., Chiuve, S., Cushman, M., Das, S. R., Deo, R., … Muntner, P. (2017). Heart disease and stroke statistics–2017 update: A report from the American Heart Association. *Circulation, 135*, e146–e603.

Blecker, S., Paul, M., Taksler, G., Ogedegbe, G., & Katz, S. (2013). Heart failure associated hospitalizations in the United States. *Journal of the American College of Cardiology, 61*(12), 1259–1267.

Bleumink, G. S., Knetsch, A. M., Sturkenboom, M. C. J. M., Straus, S. M., Hofman, A., Deckers, J. W., … Stricker, B. H. (2004). Quantifying the heart failure epidemic: Prevalence, incidence rate, lifetime risk and prognosis of heart failure: The Rotterdam Study. *European Heart Journal, 25*(18), 1614–1619.

Bowry, A. D. K., Lewey, J., Dugani, S. B., & Choudhry, N. K. (2015). The burden of cardiovascular disease in low and middle income countries: Epidemiology and management. *Canadian Journal of Cardiology, 31*(9), 1151–1159.

Braunwald, E., Zipes, D. P., Libby, P., & Bonow, R. (1997*). Braunwald's heart disease: A textbook of cardiovascular medicine* (5th ed.). Philadelphia, PA: WB Saunders Company.

Freeman, H., & Payne, R. (2000). Racial injustice in health care. *NEJM, 342*(14), 1045–1047.

Graham, G. (2015). Disparities in cardiovascular disease risk in the United States. *Current Cardiology Reviews, 11*(3), 238–245.

He, J., Ogden, L. G., Bazzano, L. A., Vupputuri, S., Loria, C., & Whelton, P. K. (2001). Risk factors for congestive heart failure in US men and women: NHANES I epidemiologic follow-up study. *Archives of Internal Medicine, 161*(7), 996–1002.

Heron, M., Oyert, D. L., Murphy, S. L., Xu, J., Kochanek, K. D., & Tejada-Vera, B. (2009). Deaths: Final data for 2006. *National Vital Statistics Reports, 57*(14), 1–134.

Jamison, D. T., Breman, J. G., Measham, A. R., Alleyne, G., Claeson, M., Evans, D. B., … Musgrove, P. (2006). *Disease control priorities in developing countries* (2nd ed.). Washington, DC: World Bank.

Levy, D. (1993). A multifactorial approach to coronary disease risk assessment. *Clinical and Experimental Hypertension, 15*(6), 1077–1086.

MacKay, J., & Mensah, G. (2004). *The atlas of heart disease and stroke*. Geneva, Switzerland: World Health Organization.

Mensah, G. A., Wei, G. S., Sorlie, P. D., Fine, L. J., Rosenberg, Y., Kaufmann, P. G. M., … Gordon, D. (2017). Decline in cardiovascular mortality: Possible causes and implications. *Circulation Research, 120*, 366–380.

Mozaffarian, D., Benjamin, E. J., Go, A. S., Arnett, D. K., Blaha, M. J., Cushman, M., … Turner, M. B. (2015). Heart disease and stroke statistics-2015 update: A report from the American Heart Association. *Circulation, 131*(4), e29–322.

Murphy, S. L., Xu, J., Kochanek, K. D., Curtin, S. C., & Arias, E. (2017). Death: Final data for 2015. *National Vital Statistics Reports, 66*(6), 1–75.

National Heart, Lung and Blood Institute (NHLBI). (2009). *Morbidity and mortality: 2009 chart book on cardiovascular, lung and blood diseases*. Bethesda, MD: National Institutes of Health.

Ritchie, H., & Roser, M. (2018). *Causes of death*. Published online. Retrieved from https://ourworldindata.org/causes-of-death

Roth, G. A., Forouzanfar, M. H., Moran, A. E., Barber, R., Nguyen, G., Feigin, V. L., … Murray, C. J. L. (2015). Demographic and epidemiologic drivers of global cardiovascular mortality. *The New England Journal of Medicine, 372*, 1333–1341.

Roth, G. A., Johnson, C., Abajobir, A., Abd-Allah, F., Abera, S. F., Abyu, G., … Murray, C. (2017). Global, regional, and national burden of cardiovascular diseases for 10 causes, 1990 to 2015. *Journal of the American College of Cardiology, 70*(1), 1–25.

Sanderson, J. E., Mayosi, B., Yusuf, S., Reddy, S., Hu, S., Chen, Z., & Timmis, A. (2007). Global burden of cardiovascular disease. *Heart, 93*, 1175.

Sidney, S., Quesenberry, C. P., Jr., Jaffe, M. G., Sorel, M., Nguyen-Huynh, M. N., Kushi, L. H., …, Rana, J. S. (2016). Recent trends in cardiovascular mortality in the United States and public health goals. *Journal of the American Medical Association, 1*(5), 594–599.

Watkins, D. A., Johnson, C. O., Colquhoun, S. M., Karthikeyan, G., Beaton, A., Bukhman, G., … Roth, G. A. (2017). Global, regional and national burden of rheumatic heart disease, 1990–2015. *New England Journal of Medicine, 377*, 713–722.

Weight Control Information Network. (2010). *National Institute of Diabetes and Digestive and Kidney Diseases (NIDDK)*. Bethesda, MD: U.S. National Institutes of Health and Human Services.

World Health Organization. (2005). *Preventing chronic diseases: A vital investment: WHO global report*. Geneva, Switzerland: World Health Organization.

World Health Organization. (2009). *WHO disease and injury country estimates*. Geneva, Switzerland: World Health Organization.

World Health Organization. (2010). *World Health Organization statistical information system (WHOSIS)*. Geneva, Switzerland: World Health Organization.

World Health Organization. (2016). *Global hearts initiative*. Geneva, Switzerland: World Health Organization.

Yusuf, S., Reddy, S., Ôunpuu, S., & Anand, S. (2001). Global burden of cardiovascular diseases: Part I: General considerations, epidemiologic transition, risk factors, and impact of urbanization. *Circulation, 104*, 2746–2753.

CHAPTER 3

Epidemiology of Ischemic (Coronary) Heart Disease

▶ Definition of Ischemic/ Coronary Heart Disease

Ischemic heart disease/coronary heart disease* refers to a deficiency of blood supply to the heart muscle leading to deprivation of oxygen essential for the proper functioning of the myocardium and related heart tissues and structures. About 98% of the time, ischemic heart disease results from atherosclerosis (atherogenesis), a long-term process leading to the development of lipid-laden plaques within blood vessels of the heart and other organs. Such atherosclerotic plaques can cause stenosis (narrowing) and obstruction of the coronary arteries, and they can also rupture, resulting in thrombotic or embolic occlusion of coronary blood vessels. A thrombus refers to the formation of a stationary clot upon rupture of an atherosclerotic plaque within a blood vessel while an embolus refers to a clot that breaks away from its original site of plaque rupture and travels downstream in the blood and occludes a smaller caliber blood vessel.

▶ Sudden Cardiac Death and Myocardial Infarction in Ischemic Heart Disease

Without effective therapy, ischemic heart disease invariably culminates in sudden cardiac death or acute myocardial infarction. These two conditions often occur simultaneously although sudden cardiac death does not necessarily imply that a myocardial infarction was the cause.

Sudden Cardiac Death is a phenomenon in which the heart suddenly and unexpectedly stops beating resulting in loss of blood flow, and without immediate treatment, death occurs within minutes. Technically, the condition is defined as death from cardiac malfunction occurring within 1 hour of symptom onset and loss of consciousness. This catastrophic event accounts for about 50% of deaths from cardiovascular disease in the United States. Clinical and/or pathological evidence of ischemic heart disease is detected in approximately 80% of patients with sudden cardiac death (Chugh et al., 2008; Sara, Eleid, Gulati, & Holmes, 2014).

---

* I note at the outset of this chapter that the terms "ischemic heart disease" and "coronary heart disease" are used synonymously. Because reduction in coronary blood flow is virtually always the cause of the lack of oxygenation (ischemia) of the myocardium, the term "coronary heart disease" is favored by some authors. The terms are thus used interchangeably in the text depending upon which one is used by the authors of the referenced work.

Myocardial Infarction specifically means the death (infarct) of cardiac muscle (myocardium). The vast majority of acute myocardial infarctions (over 95%) are caused by lack of blood flow and depletion of oxygen (ischemia) due to complete occlusion of coronary arteries by the buildup of atherosclerotic plaque with superimposed thrombus (blood clot) (Arbustini et al., 1999; Badimon & Vilahur, 2014). The process of atherosclerosis (called atherogenesis) (Figure 3.3) is discussed in this chapter and the epidemiology of myocardial infarction and sudden cardiac death are discussed in a subsequent chapter.

▶ Global Epidemiology of Ischemic/Coronary Heart Disease

Ischemic heart disease is the leading cause of death and disability worldwide. Of the 17.65 million deaths caused by cardiovascular diseases in 2016, an all-time high of 9.48 million deaths (nearly 54%) were attributable to ischemic heart disease. Ischemic heart disease is currently the leading cause of death in the United States, Canada, Australia, Japan, all countries of Western Europe and Scandinavia, and many countries of South America. In addition, ischemic heart disease claims the most lives in many Eastern and Central European countries, including Russia and the Ukraine, Latin America, the Pacific islands, and most of Asia, including India and Pakistan.

The total number of deaths from ischemic heart disease increased by 19% during the decade, 2006–2016, from 7.96 million deaths in 2006 to 9.48 million deaths in 2016. Nevertheless, during the same time period, age-standardized deaths from ischemic heart disease actually *declined* by 11.6% (from approximately 170 per 100,000 to 150 per 100,000), a reduction largely driven by global improvements in prevention and therapy. This apparent paradox (increasing total deaths and decreasing age-standardized death rates) is primarily due to increasing longevity in the world population resulting in greater numbers of older people who are more susceptible to ischemic heart disease and other forms of cardiovascular disease (Global Burden of Disease 2016 Causes of Death Collaborators, 2017).

Reductions in age-standardized mortality rates of ischemic heart disease are most evident in high- and middle-income nations for both men and women. However, over the past several decades, age-standardized rates for men have remained more than twice that of the rates for women. The marked gender difference in mortality rates is evident from longitudinal data collected and reported by many developed nations such as Finland (**FIGURE 3.1**).

Specific reasons for the "gender gap" in mortality rates of ischemic heart disease are unclear. Cardiovascular diseases including ischemic heart disease develop 7–10 years later in women than men, possibly due to protective "anti-atherosclerotic" effects of high levels of circulating estrogens in premenopausal women. Presumably, coincident with diminished levels of estrogen after menopause, cholesterol levels increase thereby promoting atherosclerosis and the development of ischemic heart disease in postmenopausal women at later ages. By comparison, younger men are more likely than women to have elevated levels of cholesterol, and furthermore, men are more likely to be chronic smokers than women, thereby promoting both atherosclerosis and hypertension, two major risk factors for the development of ischemic heart disease. Notwithstanding, there are several other risk factors that show significant gender differences including the distribution of body fat, glucose tolerance, and response to stress and psychosocial factors.

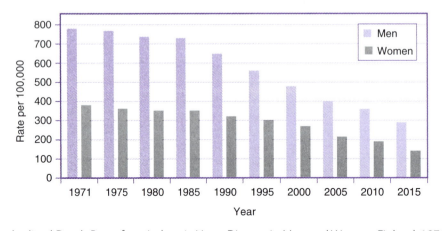

FIGURE 3.1 Age-Standardized Death Rates from Ischemic Heart Disease in Men and Women, Finland, 1971–2015.

Data from Office of Statistics of Finland. (2018). *Ischaemic heart disease still the cause of one in five deaths.* Helsinki: Statistics Finland.

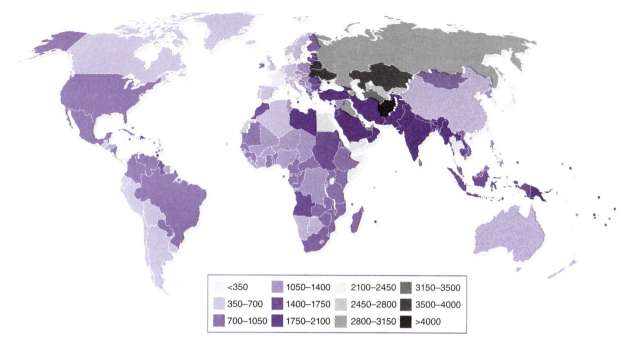

FIGURE 3.2 Disability-Adjusted Life Years (DALY) for Ischemic Heart Disease, 2004.

Data from World Health Organization. (2008). *The global burden of disease: 2004 update*. Geneva: WHO. Available at www.who.int/evidence/bod. Age-standardized DALY from ischemic heart disease by country (per 100,000 inhabitants). Disability-adjusted life years (DALYs) are rates per 100,000 people that combine Years of Life Lost (YLL) due to premature mortality in the population and the Years Lost due to Disability (YLD) for incident nonfatal cases of the disease (DALY = YLL + YLD). One DALY represents the loss of one year of healthy life.

Biological and environmental differences between men and women that influence the risk of developing ischemic heart disease remain to be fully clarified by further research (Appelman, van Rijn, Ten Haaf, Boersma, & Peters, 2015; Mass & Appelman, 2010; Zhao et al., 2017).

Disability from Ischemic Heart Disease

The global pattern of disability-adjusted life years (DALY) lost to ischemic heart disease reflects the highest disease burden in many developing nations of the world including Russia, India, North Africa, and the Middle East (**FIGURE 3.2**). By comparison, lower DALY values are observed in developed nations such as the United States, Canada, Western Europe, Japan, and Australia/New Zealand, where improvements in the healthcare system have produced declines in the mortality and morbidity from ischemic heart disease. Notably, the populations of certain developing countries (e.g., China) have also sustained relatively low rates of ischemic heart disease.

▶ Atherogenesis and Atherosclerosis

Atherosclerosis (atherogenesis) refers to the development of atheromas in the arterial walls of humans and other mammals. Atheromas consist of focal deposits of plaque material that develop just beneath the intima

(the endothelial lining) of arteries. These fibrofatty plaques have a lipid core of cholesterol and cholesterol derivatives covered by a fibrous cap of smooth muscle (Robbins & Cotran, 1979).

Two theories of atherosclerosis have been the subject of long-standing debate among cardiovascular researchers. More than 150 years ago, the famous German pathologist Rudolph Virchow postulated that the accumulation of lipids in arteriolar walls causes atherosclerosis (Virchow, 1856). It is important to note that Virchow also suggested that the disease process involved *inflammation* stimulated by the abnormal subintimal presence of lipids.

Significant evidence supporting the "*lipid hypothesis*" came from a study in 1913 by Nikolai Anitschkow who demonstrated that dietary cholesterol induced the development of atheromatous plaques in the arteries of rabbits (Anitschkow, 1913; Anitschkow & Chatalov, 1913). According to this hypothesis, low-density lipoproteins (LDL) circulating in the blood are oxidized by free radicals to form oxidized LDL that damage the arterial wall and stimulate the influx of macrophages and other immune cells. Lipid-laden macrophages (called foam cells) plus extracellular cholesterol and cholesterol derivatives form the core of the plaque beneath the arterial wall. With enlargement and maturation of the plaque over time, smooth muscle cells are stimulated to grow over the plaque to form a fibrous cap (Duff & McMillan, 1951).

A second hypothesis (often called the "*response to injury hypothesis*") proposes that atherogenesis is an inflammatory disease (Ross & Glomset, 1973, 1976). According to this hypothesis, injury to the endothelial lining of the artery stimulates an inflammatory response resulting in smooth muscle proliferation and, subsequently, infiltration of the wound by macrophages and other inflammatory cells. Without resolution, recursive cycles of chronic inflammation ensue, leading to the release of hydrolytic enzymes, cytokines, chemokines, and growth factors that cause further cellular damage and eventually produce focal areas of cell necrosis. As stated by Ross, "Each characteristic lesion of atherosclerosis represents a different stage in a chronic inflammatory process in the artery; if unabated and excessive, this process will result in an advanced complicated lesion." (Ross, 1999).

A compromise of these two hypotheses put forth by Steinberg and others is that both mechanisms are intricately involved in the genesis of atherosclerotic plaques (e.g., that hypercholesterolemia and inflammation in atherogenesis are *"two sides of the same coin."*) (Steinberg, 2005). This dual hypothesis postulates the following sequence of pathogenesis: (1) hypercholesterolemia (in particular, high LDL) induces adhesion of leukocytes to the arterial endothelium, (2) circulating monocytes and lymphocytes penetrate into the subendothelial space, (3) oxidized LDL accumulates beneath the endothelium, (4) macrophages are attracted to the developing lesion and become engorged with oxidized LDL to form "foam cells," (5) the sustained presence of oxidized LDL and its derivative forms stimulate a vicious cycle of recursive inflammation involving infiltration by macrophages and other immune cells, (6) focal areas of cell necrosis ensue, and (7) smooth muscle cells grow over the lesion producing a fibrous cap. The time sequence of atherogenesis is many years, often decades, first resulting in fibrous streaks in the arterial walls and subsequently progressing to the development of complex atheromas that can obstruct the arterial lumen *per se* or rupture giving rise to thrombotic or embolic occlusion of small caliber arteries (**FIGURE 3.3**).

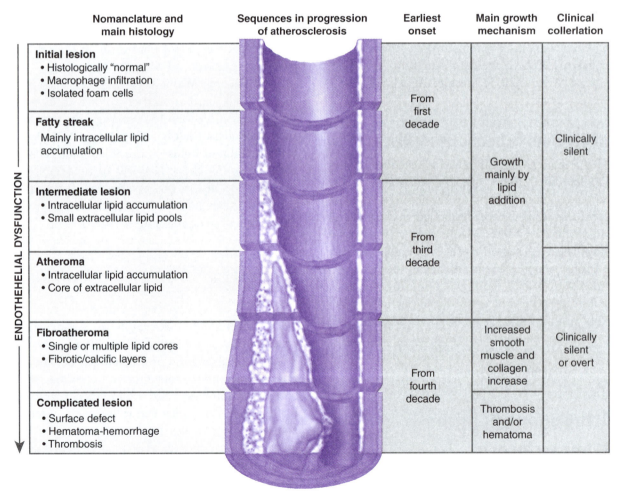

FIGURE 3.3 Progression of Atherogenesis.

Reproduced from Matthews, K. A. (2005). Psychological perspectives on the development of coronary heart disease. *American Psychologist, 60*(8), 783–796.

Other Mechanisms of Ischemic/Coronary Heart Disease

While atherosclerosis is invariably involved in the genesis of ischemic/coronary heart disease, other mechanisms may also play an etiologic role, either independently or in combination with the development of atheromatous plaques. For example, hemodynamic reductions in coronary perfusion may result from conditions that damage the aortic valve and compromise coronary filling, such as syphilis and rheumatic heart disease. Since the metabolic needs of the myocardium are high, hypermetabolic states (e.g., vigorous exercise, hyperthyroidism, pregnancy) may also accentuate ischemic disease. In addition, conditions that diminish the oxygen carrying capacity of the blood (e.g., all forms of anemia) may also contribute to imbalance in the supply and demand of oxygen to the myocardium (Robbins & Cotran, 1979).

Historical Perspectives of the Epidemiology of Ischemic/ Coronary Heart Disease

Prospective epidemiologic investigations conducted in the past half century have contributed significantly to our understanding of the pathogenesis of ischemic/coronary heart disease. These include the Seven Countries Study, the Framingham Study, and MONICA, which are discussed in the following paragraphs.

The Seven Countries Study

The Seven Countries Study conducted by Ancel Keys and colleagues examined the effects of diet in an international prospective cohort of 12,763 men, aged 40–59 years, in 16 population samples from seven different countries (Italy, Greece, former Yugoslavia, the Netherlands, Finland, United States, and Japan). All participants were healthy at the time of study entry. Baseline information was collected during 1958–1964 and vital statistics verified at regular intervals over 25 years of follow-up. Cardiovascular events and other health outcomes were adjudicated and rates and correlations calculated among and within population samples to determine effects of diet and other potential risk factors (Keys, 1970; Keys et al., 1967, 1980). The study was the first to demonstrate that serum cholesterol

is a biomarker of impending coronary heart disease and that the risk increases with intake of saturated fats and decreases with intake of monounsaturated fatty acids (primarily from olive oil). Risk increases were also associated with elevated blood pressure (hypertension), cigarette smoking, sedentary lifestyle, and obesity.

Among the sample populations examined, the cohort from Crete in Greece had the lowest rates of coronary heart disease. The *Mediterranean diet* of this population *"is characterized by abundant plant foods (fruit, vegetables, breads, other forms of cereals, potatoes, beans, nuts, and seeds), fresh fruit as the typical daily dessert,* **olive oil** *as the principal source of fat, dairy products (principally cheese and yogurt), and fish and poultry consumed in low to moderate amounts, zero to four eggs consumed weekly, red meat consumed in low amounts, and wine consumed in low to moderate amounts, normally with meals"* (Keys, 1970). Low rates of coronary heart disease were also observed among Japanese men who typically consume a low-calorie diet high in fish and rice. Populations consuming diets with higher saturated fats from meat and dairy sources and lower monounsaturated fats had higher adjusted rates of coronary heart disease (**FIGURE 3.4**).

The Framingham Study

Since 1948, investigators at Harvard University have been following generations of the residents of Framingham, Massachusetts, to better understand the determinants of heart disease. The initial cohort consisted of 5209 randomly selected members of the adult population of Framingham, 30–62 years of age, who were enrolled for study in 1948. The ongoing study now includes a second generation of 5124 men and

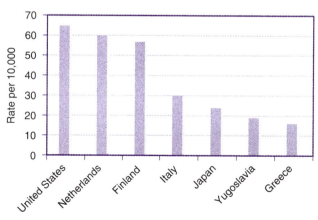

FIGURE 3.4 Annual Incidence of Coronary Heart Disease in the Seven Countries Study.

Data from Keys, A. (1970). *Coronary heart disease in seven countries.* New York, NY: American Heart Association, Monograph No. 29.

women (offspring of the original cohort), a third generation of 4095 men and women, and a new spouse cohort that is currently enrolling subjects.

Since 1950, more than 2000 peer-reviewed scientific articles have been published based upon the Framingham Study. While there have been many research milestones, perhaps the most important finding from the Framingham Study is that coronary heart disease is multifactorial involving both independent effects as well as synergistic interactions of a number of major risk factors including cigarette smoking, hypercholesterolemia, type 2 diabetes mellitus, hypertension, sedentary lifestyle, obesity, dietary factors, and genetic factors. Indeed, a premier accomplishment of Framingham investigators was development of a coronary disease prediction algorithm involving risk factor categories to facilitate accurate risk prediction of coronary heart disease accounting for multiple risk factors. This index is an extremely useful tool for physicians and healthcare workers to instruct patients about their level of risk in order to counsel them on effective preventive and therapeutic interventions.

A series of initial reports based upon the Framingham Study documented significant independent effects of cigarette smoking, hypertension, and hypercholesterolemia in the genesis of ischemic (coronary) heart disease (Dawber & Kannel, 1968; Kannel, Castelli, & McNamara, 1968; Kannel, Castelli, Gordon, & McNamara, 1971; Kannel, Gordon, & Schwartz, 1971). While each of these risk factors independently increases the relative risk of disease by two- to threefold, the interaction of chronic smoking, high blood pressure, and hypercholesterolemia accentuates the risk by more than tenfold in comparison to individuals with no exposure (Levy, 1993). **FIGURE 3.5** depicts the multifactorial nature of ischemic/coronary heart disease culminating in myocardial infarction or stroke.

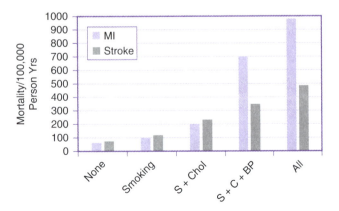

FIGURE 3.5 Synergy of Multiple Risk Factors: MI and Stroke.
Data from Levy, D. (1993). A multifactorial approach to coronary disease risk assessment. *Clinical and Experimental Hypertension*, 15(6), 1077–1086.

The MONICA Project

The MONICA Project (Multinational Monitoring of Trends and Determinants in Cardiovascular Disease) was initiated during the 1980s by the World Health Organization (WHO) in order to monitor the diverse international trends in mortality from cardiovascular disease (CVD) and changes in major CVD risk factors in selected populations. Approximately 15 million men and women aged 35–64 years were targeted for study in 41 MONICA Collaborating Centers around the world. Data collection has been completed after 10 years of follow-up in some population samples and the observed trends in mortality and certain risk factors have been published. MONICA provides a resource for continuing studies of CVD.

Across all sites represented in MONICA, mortality rates from coronary heart disease were, on average, about four times higher for men than women (e.g., the median annual mortality rate was 200 per 100,000 for men compared to 50 per 100,000 for women). Among men, relatively high annual mortality rates (>300 per 100,000) were observed in population samples from Finland, Poland, the United Kingdom, and Russia and low rates were observed in populations of China, France, Switzerland, and Italy. Among women, high rates were observed in the United Kingdom, Poland, and Russia (>90 per 100,000) and low rates in Spain, France, Italy, and China (Tunstall-Pedoe, Kuulasmaa, Tolonen, Davidson, & Mendis, 2003).

Over 10 years of follow-up, the age-adjusted mortality from coronary heart disease declined annually by 2.7% in men and 2.1% in women, although there was wide variability among sites. Correspondingly, systolic blood pressure decreased in men and women, cigarette smoking decreased in men but not women, total cholesterol declined slightly in men and women, and survival following coronary events improved in most of the populations sampled. Nevertheless, there was a disturbing upward trend in the overall prevalence of obesity, particularly among men (Evans et al., 2001; Tunstall-Pedoe et al., 1999, 2003).

▶ Risk Factors for Ischemic/ Coronary Heart Disease

Major risk factors for ischemic heart disease have been called the "four horsemen of the apocalypse" (Harris, 1994). They include cigarette smoking, hypertension, elevated cholesterol, and type 2 diabetes mellitus (Grundy et al., 1998). Cholesterol measures are divisible into various fractions (e.g., high-density lipoprotein

TABLE 3.1 Selected Risk Factors for Ischemic Heart Disease

- Modifiable
  Dyslipidemia, Hypertension, Smoking, Type 2 Diabetes Mellitus, Inflammation

- Nonmodifiable
  Genetics, Increasing Age, Male Gender, Female Menopause

- Contributing Factors and Biomarkers
  Obesity, Sedentary Lifestyle, Type A Personality
  Elevated Cholesterol and LDL Cholesterol
  Elevated C-reactive Protein
  Hyperinsulinemia
  Elevated Homocysteine
  Elevated Renin

[HDL] cholesterol, and LDL cholesterol). Recently, a fifth risk factor, elevated C-reactive protein, which appears to be a valid measure of vascular inflammation, has been tested and verified as having significant predictive value for cardiovascular disease including ischemic/coronary heart disease. **TABLE 3.1** presents a brief listing of important risk factors and biomarkers.

Cholesterol and Ischemic/Coronary Heart Disease

Serum cholesterol has consistently proven to be a valid independent biomarker of impending ischemic heart disease. Early results for men enrolled in the Seven Countries Study suggested that serum cholesterol is linearly related to mortality from coronary heart disease across widely divergent cultures (Keys, 1970; Verschuren et al., 1995).

The Framingham Study provides convincing evidence of the relationship. Lloyd-Jones and colleagues examined the lifetime risk of developing coronary heart disease among 3269 men and 4019 women. Estimates of cumulative risk to age 80 years for individuals with baseline serum cholesterol levels at age 40 years of less than 200 mg/dL, 200–239 mg/dL, and 240 mg/dL or greater were 31%, 43%, and 57% for men and 15%, 26%, and 33% for women. The corresponding 10-year cumulative risks were 3%, 5%, and 12% for men and 1%, 2%, and 5% for women, respectively (Lloyd-Jones et al., 2003). Furthermore, the cumulative risk was inversely related to HDL cholesterol.

Stamler and colleagues (Stamler, Wentworth, & Neaton, 1986; Stamler et al., 1999, 2000) examined the relationship of baseline serum cholesterol to coronary heart disease in three U.S. cohorts of young men and five U.S. cohorts of middle-aged men and observed significant dose responses in mortality from coronary heart disease with increasing serum cholesterol in each cohort. For example, in the large Multiple Risk Factor Intervention Trial (MRFIT) involving a cohort of 69,205 young men aged 35–39 years at baseline, the 16-year mortality rate due to coronary heart disease increased from 2.3 per 1000 for serum cholesterol less than 160 mg/dL to 27.3 per 1000 for serum cholesterol of 280 mg/dL or greater (adjusted relative risk = 8.1, Stamler et al., 2000). Findings from the entire MRFIT cohort of 356,222 men aged 35–57 years at baseline and followed more than 25 years show that the mortality from coronary heart disease rises continuously with serum cholesterol level from a reference value of 160 mg/dL irrespective of age and ethnicity and after adjustment for other risk factors such as smoking, diabetes, and hypertension (Stamler & Neaton, 2008).

Clinical Trials of Statins, Cholesterol, and Coronary Heart Disease

In addition to the epidemiologic investigations that initially established elevated blood cholesterol as a risk factor for coronary heart disease, the results of many large clinical trials have provided definitive evidence that reducing cholesterol either by nonpharmacologic methods or by pharmaceutical medications (statins) leads to a significant reduction in the risk. In particular, statins that lower blood cholesterol have been found to significantly reduce the risk of developing coronary heart disease (Bradford et al., 1991; Downs et al., 1998; Lipid Research Clinics Program, 1984; Strandberg, Lehto, Pyörälä, Kesäniemi, & Oksa, 1997) as well as showing profound therapeutic effects in the prevention of recurrent disease (Nissen et al., 2006; Sever et al., 2005). Cholesterol guidelines based upon a consensus statement from the National Cholesterol Education Program (1993) are shown in **TABLE 3.2.**

Blood Pressure and Ischemic/Coronary Heart Disease

It is well known that elevations in blood pressure increase the risk of developing ischemic/coronary heart disease. Consistent findings have been reported for diverse populations in many studies including the Seven Countries Study and the Framingham Study and based on meta-analyses of data from multiple investigations.

TABLE 3.2 National Cholesterol Education Program (NCEP)

Total Cholesterol	
<200 mg/dL	Desirable
201–239 mg/dL	Borderline Risk
>239 mg/dL	High Risk

LDL Cholesterol	
130 mg/dL	Desirable
131–159 mg/dL	Borderline Risk
>159 mg/dL	High Risk

In an early prospective study conducted during 1956–1960, investigators in the United Kingdom examined blood pressure and blood lipids as predictors of ischemic heart disease in a sample of 687 bus drivers and male conductors working on London Transport's central buses. While higher incidence rates were associated with several factors including age, family history, smoking, and obesity, the predominant predictive factors were "high systolic blood pressure" and "elevated plasma cholesterol," each of which was associated with more than a threefold increase in the incidence (Morris, Kaga, Pattison, Gardner, & Raffle, 1966).

In a landmark study, Kannel and colleagues examined the relation of blood pressure to coronary heart disease among 2282 men and 2845 women in the population sample from Framingham, Massachusetts. Blood pressures were measured at baseline and individuals (who were initially free of coronary disease) were followed over a 14-year period to determine new coronary events. Baseline measures were used to stratify individuals as hypertensive (>160/95 mm Hg), borderline hypertensive (>140/90 mm Hg), or normotensive (<140/90 mm Hg). As shown in **FIGURE 3.6**, the risk of coronary heart disease increased with advancing blood pressure for both men and women at all ages of entry into the study (Kannel, Schwartz, & McNamara, 1969; Kannel, 1996).

Using data from six population samples of the Seven Countries Study, van den Hoogen and colleagues examined associations of systolic and diastolic blood pressure with long-term mortality from coronary heart disease. Blood pressures were measured at baseline in 12,031 men initially free of coronary

disease and followed over 25 years. Results were consistent for the diverse populations under study (United States, Northern Europe, Inland Europe, Southern Europe, Serbia, and Japan) showing a relative risk of 1.28 for each incremental increase of 10 mm Hg in systolic blood pressure or 5 mm Hg in diastolic blood pressure (van den Hoogen et al., 2000).

In a meta-analysis of diastolic blood pressure, stroke, and coronary heart disease involving nine major prospective observational studies and 420,000 individuals followed for an average of 10 years, Mac-Mahon et al. observed a linear dose response in the risk of coronary heart disease with increasing diastolic blood pressure (**FIGURE 3.7**).

Cigarette Smoking and Ischemic/Coronary Heart Disease

Cigarette smoking is not only the dominant cause of lung cancer, chronic bronchitis, and emphysema, but addiction to the smoking habit is also one of the major

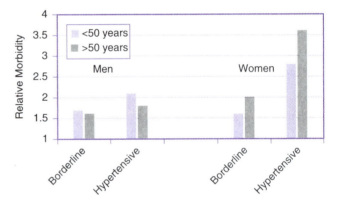

FIGURE 3.6 Risk of Coronary Heart Disease and Blood Pressure, Framingham Study.
Data from Kannel, W. B., Schwartz, M. J., & McNamara, P. M. (1969). Blood pressure and risk of coronary heart disease: The Framingham study. *Diseases of the Chest, 56*(1), 43–52.

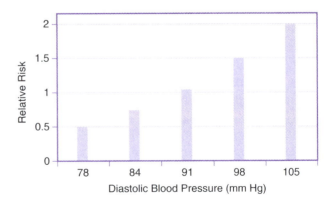

FIGURE 3.7 Coronary Heart Disease Risk by Diastolic BP Level.
Data from MacMahon, S., Peto, R., Collins, R., Godwin, J., Cutler, J., Sorlie, P., … Stamler, J. (1990). Blood pressure, stroke, and coronary heart disease. Part 1, prolonged differences in blood pressure: Prospective observational studies corrected for the regression dilution bias. *Lancet, 335*(8692), 765–774.

causes of ischemic/coronary heart disease. Many epidemiologic studies have examined the relationship of smoking and coronary heart disease in diverse populations throughout the world including China, India, Canada, Sweden, Japan, Switzerland, China, United Kingdom, and the United States. In total, these studies represent more than 30 million person-years of observation, and despite the marked socioeconomic, genetic, and environmental differences in the populations sampled, the findings are remarkably consistent in demonstrating two- to fourfold increases in the mortality from coronary heart disease for chronic smokers compared to nonsmokers (Reports of the Surgeon General, 1983, 1988, 2004).

Results from three early prospective studies, two in the United States and one in United Kingdom, provided strong evidence supporting the etiologic link between cigarette smoking and the development of coronary heart disease.

In 1951, a prospective study of smoking and cause-specific mortality was initiated in cohorts of British physicians (6194 women and 34,440 men). After more than 20 years of follow-up, the investigators concluded that cigarette smoking causes lung cancer, chronic obstructive lung disease (emphysema and chronic bronchitis), and heart disease in both men and women (Doll, Gray, Hafner, & Peto, 1980; Doll & Peto, 1976). The relative mortality estimates for ischemic heart disease by level of smoking are shown in **FIGURE 3.8.** Clearly, the dose response in mortality rates with increasing number of cigarettes smoked per day supports a causal relationship.

In 1954, the United States Public Health Service initiated a prospective study of a cohort of 198,820 male veterans to examine relationships of smoking and other risk factors with chronic diseases including coronary heart disease (Dorn, 1959; Rogot & Murray, 1980). Also in 1954, the American Cancer Society initiated a similar prospective study among a sample of 187,783 men, aged 50–69 years (Hammond, 1960). The results of these two investigations were remarkably similar in demonstrating a dose–response relationship between the level of cigarette smoking and mortality due to coronary heart disease (**FIGURE 3.9**).

Evaluation of two other cohorts provided important confirmation of the causal effect of smoking in the genesis of coronary heart disease. The Framingham Study examined the incidence of coronary heart disease among 2282 middle-aged men by smoking status. After 10 years of follow-up, the relative risk of developing coronary heart disease was twofold higher among men who smoked up to 20 cigarettes per day and threefold higher among men who smoked more than 20 cigarettes per day compared to nonsmokers (Kannel, 1964). Similar risk increases were observed among cigarette smokers in a cohort of 1838 men from Albany, New York (Doyle, Dawber, Kannel, Kinch, & Kahn, 1964).

Risk reductions in coronary heart disease after smoking cessation provide further evidence supporting causality (Report of the Surgeon General, 1990). In a meta-analysis of 20 prospective studies of patients with a diagnosis of coronary heart disease, there was a 36% reduction in the relative risk of mortality for those who quit smoking compared to those who continued to smoke (Critchley & Capewell, 2004). Furthermore, the risk reductions following smoking cessation were

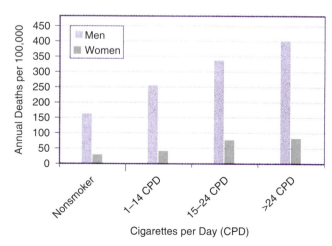

FIGURE 3.8 Smoking and Mortality from Ischemic Heart Disease, British Physicians Study. Rates are for Individuals Aged 65 Years or Younger.

Data from Doll, R., & Peto, R. (1976). Mortality in relation to smoking: 20 years' observations on male British doctors. *British Medical Journal, 2*(6051),1525–1536; Doll, R., Gray, R., Hafner, B., & Peto, R. (1980). Mortality in relation to smoking: 22 years' observations on female British doctors. *British Medical Journal, 280*(6219), 967–971.

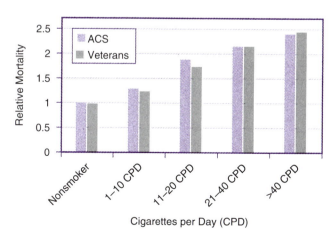

FIGURE 3.9 Mortality from Coronary Heart Disease by Level of Smoking: Two U.S. Cohorts.

Data from Dorn, H. F. (1959). Tobacco consumption and mortality from cancer and other diseases. *Public Health Reports, 74,* 581–593; Hammond, E. C. (1960). Smoking in relationship to heart disease. *American Journal of Public Health and the Nations Health, 50*(3 pt 2), 20–26; Rogot, E., & Murray, J. L. (1980). Smoking and causes of death among U.S. veterans, 16 years of observation. *Public Health Reports, 95*(3), 213–222.

consistent regardless of differences between studies in age, gender, country, and time period. Within 2 years of cessation, the risk is reduced by about 50% and after 10–15 years of cessation, the risk returns to normal.

In addition to the direct effects of active cigarette smoking, passive smoking also appears to increase the risk. In a meta-analysis of 10 cohort and 8 case–control studies, nonsmokers exposed to environmental tobacco smoke had a 25% increase in the relative risk of coronary heart disease (RR = 1.25) compared to nonsmokers with no exposure (He et al., 1999). The relative risk estimates were consistent for cohort studies (RR = 1.21) and case–control studies (RR = 1.51) and for men (RR = 1.22) and women (RR = 1.24). Exposure to the highest level of environmental tobacco smoke (from more than 20 cigarettes per day) was associated with the greatest increase in risk (RR = 1.31) consistent with a dose–response relationship.

There are multiple biological mechanisms by which cigarette smoking and nicotine addiction elevate the risk of ischemic/coronary heart disease. Nicotine itself is a powerful vasoconstrictor that elevates blood pressure and causes hypertension. As shown in **FIGURE 3.10**, the first cigarette of the day induces sharp increases in both systolic and diastolic blood pressure (Gropelli, Giorgi, Omboni, Parati, & Manchia, 1992).

Tobacco carcinogens, reactive oxygen species (ROS), and other constituents and derivatives of cigarette smoke are highly inflammatory to blood vessels, and appear to be cofactors in atherogenesis (Howard et al., 1998). Smoking has also been found to elevate serum cholesterol, possibly through effects on liver metabolism (Muscat, Harris, Haley, & Wynder, 1991) (**FIGURE 3.11**). Finally, chronic smokers typically develop severe chronic lung diseases such as emphysema and chronic bronchitis, and such conditions compromise the oxygenation of hemoglobin, thereby intensifying ischemic conditions in the myocardium and other tissues.

Diabetes and Ischemic/Coronary Heart Disease

Coronary heart disease often follows the diagnosis of type 2 diabetes, particularly in individuals with uncontrolled hyperglycemia and hyperinsulinemia. In the Framingham Study, the risk of developing coronary heart disease was increased nearly threefold in diabetic men and women (Kannel, 1990; Kannel & McGee, 1979) (**FIGURE 3.12**). Many other studies have reported similar findings. For example, in the Atherosclerosis

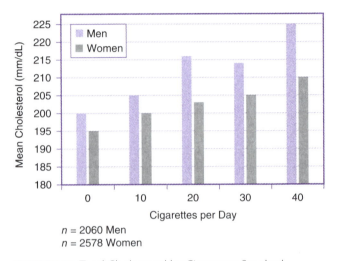

n = 2060 Men
n = 2578 Women

FIGURE 3.11 Total Cholesterol by Cigarettes Smoked.

Data from Muscat, J. E., Harris, R. E., Haley, N. J., & Wynder, E. L. (1991). Cigarette smoking and plasma cholesterol. *American Heart Journal, 121*(1 Pt 1), 141–147.

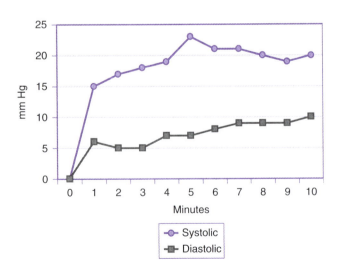

FIGURE 3.10 Change in Blood Pressure after the First Cigarette of the Day.

Data from Gropelli, A., Giorgi, D. M. A., Omboni, S., Parati, G., & Manchia, G. (1992). Persistent blood pressure increase induced by heavy smoking. *Journal of Hypertension, 10*, 495–499.

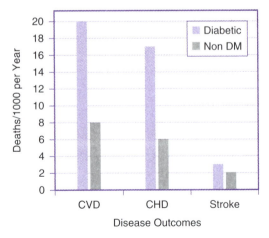

FIGURE 3.12 CVD Mortality by Diabetic Status, The Framingham Study.

CVD = cardiovascular diseases, CHD = coronary heart disease, DM = diabetes mellitus.

Data from Kannel, W. B., D'Agostino, R. B., Wilson, P. W. F., Belanger, A. J., & Gagnon, D. R. (1990). Diabetes, fibrinogen, and risk of cardiovascular disease: The Framingham experience. *American Heart Journal, 120*, 672–676.

Risk in Communities (ARIC) Study of 13,446 individuals from four U.S. communities, the adjusted relative mortality from coronary heart disease for diabetics compared to nondiabetics was 3.45 for women and 2.52 for men (Folsom et al., 1997). In a meta-analysis of 16 prospective cohort studies involving more than 75,000 individuals, the summary relative mortality due to coronary heart disease for diabetics compared to nondiabetics was 2.58 for women and 1.85 for men (Lee, Cheung, Cape, & Zinman, 2000).

Type 2 diabetes mellitus results when insulin fails to stimulate cellular uptake of glucose resulting in hyperglycemia and hyperinsulinemia. In patients with long-term hyperglycemia, nonenzymatic reactions between sugars and proteins form advanced glycosylated end products (AGE) that may accumulate in the walls of blood vessels and heighten the process of atherogenesis (Kilhovd, Berg, Birkeland, Thorsby, & Hanssen, 1999; Kiuchi et al., 2001). Hyperinsulinemia has also been observed to increase the risk in some (not all) studies. The Paris Prospective Study examined insulin levels in 7164 men aged 43–54 years. After more than 10 years of follow-up, the mortality rate due to coronary heart disease was increased by threefold among individuals with the highest levels of fasting glucose (Eschwege et al., 1985). In the Helsinki Policemen Study of 970 men 34–64 years of age and free of coronary disease at baseline, individuals with insulin levels in the highest quintile had triple the risk of suffering a major coronary event (e.g., myocardial infarct) compared to individuals in the lowest quintile over 22 years of follow-up (Pyörälä, Miettinen, Laakso, & Pyörälä, 1998). In a study of 91 cases and 105 controls from the Quebec Cardiovascular Study, investigators demonstrated an independent effect of baseline hyperinsulinemia whereby the odds of developing ischemic heart disease increased 1.6-fold for each standard deviation increase in the insulin concentration. Nevertheless, the biological mechanism by which hyperinsulinemia increases the risk is controversial and may involve interactions with endocrine factors, visceral obesity, and lipid abnormalities (Després et al., 1996).

Inflammation, C-Reactive Protein, Lipoprotein-Associated Phospholipase A2 and Ischemic/Coronary Heart Disease

Atherogenesis (atherosclerosis) is a long-term disease process that causes the development of atheromatous plaques in blood vessels. When plaque buildup and/ or rupture occlude coronary arteries that nourish the myocardium, the end result is ischemic/coronary heart disease, often culminating in myocardial infarction.

Since atherogenesis has been described as a progressive inflammatory disease (Ross, 1999), it is perhaps not surprising that a blood marker of inflammation has been consistently linked to the risk of developing coronary heart disease.

Multiple prospective studies have demonstrated that small elevations in blood levels of the acute reactive inflammatory biomarker, C-reactive protein (CRP), accurately predict increasing risk of coronary heart disease (Cushman et al., 2005; Koenig et al., 1999; Pai et al., 2004; Ridker, Buring, Cook, & Rifai, 2000; Ridker, Glynn, & Hennekens, 1998; Ridker, Nennekens, Buring, & Rifai, 2003; Toss, Lindahl, Siegbahn, & Wallentin, 1997). In fact, some studies suggest that CRP may be a better predictor of impending cardiovascular disease than serum cholesterol (Ridker, Rifai, Rose, Buring, & Cook, 2002). Predictive levels of CRP and corresponding relative risks for cardiovascular events (myocardial infarction or stroke) are shown in **FIGURE 3.13**.

CRP is a pentraxin protein that was previously thought to be an acute phase reactant in the innate immune response to acute inflammation or infection. In acute inflammatory conditions, 100-fold to 10,000-fold increases above baseline levels are measurable in the blood. Only recently has the link between relatively small elevations in CRP and increasing risk of coronary heart disease been observed (Ridker et al., 1998). CRP apparently has multiple functions including opsonization of bacteria and damaged cells leading to their phagocytosis by macrophages and modulation of the complement system (Marnell, Mold, & Du Clos, 2005). In addition to having predictive value

FIGURE 3.13 CRP & Cardiovascular Risk: Women's Health Study & Health Professionals Follow-up Study.

Data from Ridker, P. M., Rifai, N., Rose, L., Buring, J. E., & Cook, N. R. (2002). Comparison of C-reactive protein and low-density lipoprotein cholesterol levels in the prediction of first cardiovascular events. *New England Journal of Medicine, 347*, 1557–1565; Pai, J. K., Pischon, T., Ma, J., Manson, J. E., Hankinson, S. E., Joshipura, K., . . . Rimm, E. B. (2004). Inflammatory markers and the risk of coronary heart disease in men and women. *New England Journal of Medicine, 351*(25), 2599–2610.

for impending coronary heart disease, increasing levels of blood CRP have been observed in association with aging (Hung, Knuiman, Divitini, Davis, & Beilby, 2008), smoking (Bazzano, He, Muntner, Vupputuri, & Whelton, 2003), hypertension (Sung et al., 2003), type 2 diabetes (Ishikawa, Kayaba, Gotoh, Nakamura, & Kajii, 2007), and obesity (Barinas-Mitchell, Cushman, Meilahn, Tracy, & Kuller, 2001).

Lipoprotein-Associated Phospholipase A2 is an enzyme released by inflammatory cells in the development of atherosclerotic plaque within blood vessels. This enzyme specifically induces the recruitment of inflammatory monocytes and promotes their transformation into macrophages and foam cells. The result is thinning of the fibrous cap of atherosclerotic plaque that predisposes to plaque rupture and the occurrence of myocardial infarction, stroke, and other cardiovascular events. Elevated blood levels of Lipoprotein-Associated Phospholipase A2 in the upper quantile have been found to approximately double the risk of cardiovascular events. Testing this enzyme is therefore useful in identifying and managing patients at high risk (Corson, Jones, & Davidson, 2008; Packard et al., 2000).

Hyperhomocysteinemia and Ischemic/Coronary Heart Disease

Hyperhomocysteinemia (elevated homocysteine in the blood) has recently emerged as a potentially modifiable independent risk factor for atherosclerosis and atherothrombosis involving the coronary and peripheral circulation. In a comprehensive meta-analysis of 57 published studies (3 cohort studies, 12 nested case–control studies, and 42 case–control studies) involving 5518 cases with coronary heart disease and 11,068 controls without disease, the summary odds ratio for a 5 μmol/L increase in homocysteine concentration was 1.06 for prospective studies, 1.23 for nested case-control studies, and 1.70 for case–control studies (Ford et al., 2002). The heterogeneity of estimates between the different types of studies has been attributed to the inclusion of subjects with and without prior cardiovascular disease, and some investigators have suggested that homocysteine is most valuable as a biomarker in high-risk subjects or a prognostic indicator for the progression of preexisting cardiovascular disease (De Bree, Verschuren, Kromhout, Mennen, & Blom, 2002). However, in a subsequent meta-analysis of 26 prospective studies involving only subjects without known disease and selected to be of fair to good quality, each 5 μmol/L increase in homocysteine level was found to increase the risk of coronary heart disease by approximately 20%, independently of traditional disease risk factors (Humphrey, Fu, Rogers, Freeman, & Helfand,

2008). Nevertheless, it is noteworthy that reduction of homocysteine through intake of B vitamins has not consistently been found to prevent coronary heart disease or to have therapeutic benefit (Bønaa et al., 2006; Ebbing et al., 2008; Toole et al., 2004).

Elevations in plasma homocysteine are generally caused by enzymatic defects or vitamin B deficiencies (B12, folate) involved in pathways of homocysteine metabolism. The atherogenic propensity associated with hyperhomocysteinemia has been linked to impaired endothelial function at several levels, including reduced nitric oxide synthesis, enhanced oxidative vascular injury, and increased vascular smooth muscle cell proliferation (Welch & Loscalzo, 1998).

Apolipoproteins and Ischemic/Coronary Heart Disease

Apolipoproteins are proteins that bind to lipids (fats). They form lipoproteins that transport and redistribute dietary fats and cholesterol through the bloodstream to various tissues and cells of the body (Mahley, Innerarity, Rall, & Weisgraber, 1985). There are six basic types of apolipoproteins and multiple subtypes, all of which are coded by specific genes (Deeb et al., 1986).

Blood levels of specific types of apolipoproteins and lipoproteins can influence the risk of developing coronary heart disease. For example, certain isoforms of apolipoprotein A (ApoA) complex with low-density lipoprotein particles to form lipoprotein(a), which appears to influence the risk of coronary heart disease. In a meta-analysis of 27 studies involving 5436 deaths or nonfatal myocardial infarctions due to coronary heart disease, individuals with lipoprotein(a) levels in the upper tertile had 1.6 times greater risk than individuals with levels in the lowest tertile (Danesh, Collins, & Peto, 2000).

One ApoA isoform, ApoA1, is the major surface component of HDL and is primarily responsible for efflux of cholesterol from tissues to the liver for excretion. High levels of ApoA1 have therefore been found to be cardioprotective in association with removal of cholesterol from arteries whereas low levels increase the risk. In a case–control study of 3510 acute myocardial infarction patients in U.K. hospitals and 9805 controls, individuals ApoA1 levels in the lowest tertile had a 2.3-fold increase in the relative risk compared to individuals with levels in the highest tertile (Parish et al., 2009). Furthermore, dysfunctional mutant forms of apoA1 have been found to increase the risk of coronary heart disease (Singh, Singh, Gaur, & Kaur, 2007).

Isoforms of apolipoprotein B (ApoB) are the major surface components of LDL that transport cholesterol to target tissues. Two ApoB isoforms are detectable in plasma: ApoB100, which is synthesized in the liver, and ApoB48, which is synthesized in the small intestine (ApoB48 has 48% homology with ApoB100). The liver isoform, ApoB100, is an integral component of very-low-density lipoprotein (VLDL), LDL, and intermediate-density lipoprotein (IDL), all of which transport cholesterol in the blood to target tissues and cells. The level of ApoB100 therefore reflects cholesterol-carrying capacity, and has been found to be an accurate biomarker of coronary heart disease (McQueen et al., 2008).

Individuals with high levels of ApoB are at increased risk for the development of atheromatous plaques and subsequent coronary heart disease. In the U.K. case–control study of acute myocardial infarction by Parish and colleagues, individuals with ApoB levels in the highest tertile had a 2.7-fold increase in the risk compared to individuals with levels in the lowest tertile (Parish et al., 2009).

Recent epidemiologic investigations have found the ratio of ApoB to ApoA1 to be a better predictor of coronary heart disease than either biomarker *per se*. In a nested case–control study of 869 incident cases with fatal or nonfatal coronary heart disease and 1511 controls without disease ascertained from a large European cohort, individuals with ApoB/ApoA1 ratios in the highest quartile had a 2.6-fold increase in the risk (van der Steeg et al., 2007). In a prospective investigation of 9231 adults from the Danish general population who were asymptomatic at baseline and followed for 8 years, women and men with ApoB in the upper versus the lower tertile had hazard ratios for ischemic heart disease of 1.8 and 1.9, respectively (Benn, Nordestgaard, Jensen, & Tybjaerg-Hansen, 2007). Similar results were reported by Parish and colleagues in their case–control investigation of acute myocardial infarction in which individuals with ApoB/ApoA1 ratios in the highest tertile had a 3.8-fold increase in the risk (Parish et al., 2009).

INTERHEART is a large international case–control study of acute myocardial infarction involving 15,152 incident cases and 14,820 gender- and age-matched controls from 262 participating centers in 52 countries throughout Africa, Asia, Australia, Europe, the Middle East, and North and South America (Yusuf et al., 2004). Results of the INTERHEART study showed that the ApoB100/ApoA1 ratio was a better predictor than either individual biomarker *per se* and, in fact, was the strongest risk factor for acute myocardial infarction among all those measured. The relative risk for individuals with ApoB100/ApoA1 ratios in the highest quintile was 3.25 after adjustment for all other risk factors (McQueen et al., 2008). Results

of these recent studies indicate that ApoB and ApoA1 and their ratio may predict impending coronary heart disease even better than HDL and LDL cholesterol.

Other Molecular Factors in the Pathogenesis of Ischemic/Coronary Heart Disease

Many other molecular factors are undoubtedly involved in determining the ultimate disposition of patients suffering from ischemic heart disease. Indeed, the vascular response to ischemia is a dynamic process that is contingent upon multiple factors with complex interactions. Often, the patency of blood vessels impacted by atherosclerotic plaque or thrombotic/embolic material depends upon the balance between factors that regulate vasoconstriction versus vasodilatation. Such factors are derived not only from cells of the arterial wall (the endothelium), but also from circulating platelets and other elements of the bloodstream (Waller, 1989).

Vasoconstrictive factors such as angiotensin II, endothelin, and prostaglandin E2 are balanced by vasodilatory factors such as nitric oxide, serotonin, and prostacyclin. Platelet activation, aggregation, and clotting are modulated by adenosine diphosphate (ADP), serotonin, and thromboxane A2. Acetylcholine from adrenergic nerves stimulates endothelial nitric oxide synthesis and vasodilatation. The kidneys are instrumental in regulation of vascular tone and rapidly respond to changes in blood flow and blood pressure. Low perfusion stimulates the kidneys to secrete renin, which converts angiotensinogen to a more active form, angiotensin I. Subsequently, angiotensin I is converted to the powerful vasoconstrictor, angiotensin II, by angiotensin-converting enzyme (ACE) in the lungs.

The acute nature of catastrophic cardiovascular events such as heart attack and stroke makes it difficult to accurately quantify biological effects of these molecular factors in the human system. Novel techniques combining molecular biology with epidemiologic methods will be required in order to fully elucidate the exact nature of these mechanisms.

▶ Prevention of Ischemic/ Coronary Heart Disease

Ischemic/coronary heart disease is influenced by multiple interactive factors including tobacco addiction, hypertension, dyslipidemia, insulin resistance, glucose intolerance, vascular inflammation, physical inactivity, and obesity. These individual factors rarely occur in isolation and the degree of hazard depends on the number of risk factors present in a given individual. Fortunately, most of these risk factors are modifiable through lifestyle choices (e.g., abstinence from tobacco use, regular aerobic physical exercise, weight control, and consumption of a *heart-healthy* diet (Anand & Yusuf, 2011; Sanderson et al., 2007).

It is, however, readily acknowledged that much controversy exists regarding the most efficacious heart-healthy diet. Perhaps the key reason for the controversy is that 80%–90% of the total cholesterol within the human body is synthesized internally as opposed to being consumed. Since cell structure relies on cholesterol-laden lipid membranes to separate and organize intracellular water, proteins, and nucleic acids, virtually all cells in the body (and particularly liver cells) are fully capable of cholesterol biosynthesis. Thus, modulation of cholesterol, a key factor in atherogenesis, is primarily regulated by biosynthetic and metabolic pathways rather than dietary intake.

Advocates of the Mediterranean diet point to the low rates of coronary heart disease in populations of the coastal regions of southern Italy, Crete, and Greece (Keys, 1970). The Mediterranean diet is characterized by abundant plant foods (fruit, vegetables, whole grain breads, other forms of cereals, potatoes, beans, nuts, and seeds), fresh fruit as the typical daily dessert, olive oil as the principal source of fat, dairy products (principally cheese and yogurt), fish and poultry consumed in low to moderate amounts, zero to four eggs consumed weekly, red meat consumed in low amounts, and wine consumed in low to moderate amounts, normally with meals. In a meta-analysis of 12 prospective studies with a total of 1,574,299 subjects followed for up to 18 years, greater adherence to a Mediterranean diet was associated with significant improvement in health status and significant reductions in overall mortality (9%), mortality from cardiovascular diseases (9%), cancer mortality (6%), and incidence rates of Parkinson's disease and Alzheimer's disease (13%) (Sofi, Cesari, Abbate, Gensini, & Casini, 2008).

Associations of the various types of dietary fats (saturated, polyunsaturated, and monounsaturated) and atherosclerosis are complex, and there is hot debate as to which types and what levels are beneficial, neutral, or detrimental to heart health. The United States Department of Agriculture (USDA) in its food pyramid promotes a low-fat diet, based largely on its view that fat in the diet is atherogenic (USDA, 2010). The American Heart Association, the American Diabetes Association, and the National Cholesterol Education Program make similar recommendations. In contrast, other investigators recommend a shift to higher levels of monounsaturated and certain polyunsaturated fatty acids (PUFA) substituted for saturated fats in the diet.

Recent evidence supporting the concept that substituting PUFA for saturated fat in the diet is cardioprotective comes from a meta-analysis of eight randomized clinical trials involving 13,614 subjects randomized to receive either high- or low-dietary PUFA. After an average follow-up period of 4.25 years, 1042 subjects developed coronary heart disease and the energy intake from PUFA averaged 14.9% of total calories in the intervention group compared to 5% in the control group. Overall, the risk in the intervention group was reduced by 19% compared to the control group and the risk reduction in coronary heart disease was estimated to be 10% per each 5% *increase* in energy from PUFA (Mozaffarian, Micha, & Wallace, 2010). Furthermore, increasing consumption of PUFA has been found to lower HDL cholesterol (Lewington et al., 2007) and may also improve insulin resistance (Salmeron et al., 2001; Summers et al., 2002) and reduce systemic inflammation (De Caterina, Liao, & Libby, 2000; Ferrucci et al., 2006; Pischon et al., 2003).

It is generally accepted that omega-3 fatty acids are beneficial PUFA whereas trans-fatty acids should be avoided (Willett, Sacks, & Trichopoulous, 1995). Some investigators also advocate lowering the ratio of omega-6 PUFA (linoleic acid) to omega-3 PUFA (linolenic acid) in order to maximize protection against cardiovascular disease and other chronic diseases (Simopoulos, 2008).

Increasingly in developed nations, physicians are recommending daily intake of low-dose 81 mg aspirin to reduce the risk of thrombotic cardiovascular events. The epidemiologic evidence supports the judicious use of low-dose aspirin for the chemoprevention of both myocardial infarction and stroke. Current guidelines recommend using low-dose aspirin in adults at higher risk and over the age of 50 years with the caveat that even low-dose aspirin is contraindicated in individuals with known allergies, bleeding diathesis, platelet disorders, and active peptic ulcer disease (Lauer, 2002).

Many randomized clinical investigations have focused on the chemopreventive value of statin drugs in counteracting atherogenesis and reducing the risk of coronary heart disease. In one such trial conducted during a 5-year period in a sample population in Scotland, daily administration of a particular statin (pravastatin) reduced the incidence of coronary death or myocardial infarction by 24% (Ford et al., 2007). Subsequent meta-analyses have confirmed the chemopreventive value of statins against coronary heart disease in *subjects irrespective of the presence of established cardiovascular risk factors.* Meta-analysis of 10 trials enrolling 70,388 men and women *with established cardiovascular risk factors such as diabetes,* showed that statin use reduced the incidence of major coronary events by 30% and cerebrovascular events by 19% (Brugts et al., 2009). A meta-analysis of 20 trials enrolling 63,899 individuals *at relatively low risk* found overall risk reductions of 23% for myocardial infarction, 12% for stroke, and 11% for any cardiovascular-related death (Mills et al., 2008). Statins are now routinely prescribed to lower cholesterol and prevent atherogenesis.

The association of estrogen replacement therapy (ERT) or estrogen plus progesterone therapy and the risk of developing coronary heart disease has been examined in case–control studies, cohort studies, and more recently in randomized placebo-controlled clinical trials. While risk reductions in coronary heart disease were consistently observed in the case–control and cohort studies (Barrett-Connor & Grady, 1998), three randomized clinical trials found just the opposite—that ERT with or without progesterone *increases* the risk (Anderson et al., 2004; Hulley et al., 1998; Rossouw, Anderson, Prentice, 2002). The discrepant results of the observational epidemiologic studies versus the randomized clinical trials have stimulated much debate regarding the risk versus benefit of ERT in postmenopausal women, and controversy still rages as to whether ERT confers cardiovascular benefit or harm (Stevenson, 2009).

Prevention of coronary heart disease as well as all other diseases depends upon the early detection of treatable antecedent conditions through regular physical checkups. Effective anticholesterolemic, antihypertensive, and antidiabetic medications are readily available to maintain serum cholesterol, blood pressure, and blood glucose within normal limits. Sodium (salt) restriction (less than six grams of salt per day) is also important for blood pressure control. Weight reduction programs incorporating healthy nutrition and regular exercise regimes have proven successful in reducing obesity and reaching optimal weight.

In summary, keys to the prevention of coronary heart disease include: (1) education of the general public to provide a better understanding of the widespread and multifactorial nature of the disease, (2) promotion of simultaneously instituting multiple preventive and treatment strategies as early in life as possible, and (3) adopting aggressive preventive strategies before people become symptomatic or suffer a major catastrophic cardiovascular event.

References

Anand, S. S., & Yusuf, S. (2011). Stemming the global tsunami of cardiovascular disease. *Lancet, 377*(9765), 529–532.

Anderson, G. L., Limacher, M., Assaf, A. R., Bassford, T., Beresford, S. A., Black, H., … Women's Health Initiative Writing Group. (2004). Effects of conjugated equine estrogen in postmenopausal women with hysterectomy: The Women's Health Initiative randomized controlled trial. *JAMA, 291*(14), 1701–1712.

Anitschkow, N. N. (1913). Über die Veränderungen der Kaninchenaorta bei experimenteller Cholesterinsteatose. *Beitrage Zur Pathologischen Anatomie, 56,* 379–404.

Anitschkow, N. N., & Chatalov, S. (1913). Über experimentelle Cholesterinsteatose und ihre Bedeutung für die Entstehung einiger pathologischer Prozesse. *Zentralblatt Allgemeine Pathologie, 24,* 1–9.

Appelman, Y., van Rijn, B. B., Ten Haaf, M. E., Boersma, E., & Peters, S. A. (2015). Sex differences in cardiovascular risk factors and disease prevention. *Atherosclerosis, 241*(1), 211–218.

Arbustini, E., Dal Bello, B., Morbini, P., Burke, A. P., Bocciarelli, M., Specchia, G., & Virmani, R. (1999). Plaque erosion is a major substrate for coronary thrombosis in acute myocardial infarction. *Heart, 82,* 269–272.

Badimon, L., & Vilahur, G. (2014). Thrombosis formation on atherosclerotic lesions and plaque rupture. *Journal of Internal Medicine, 276*(6), 618–362.

Barinas-Mitchell, E., Cushman, M., Meilahn, E. N., Tracy, R. P., & Kuller, L. H. (2001). Serum levels of C-reactive protein are associated with obesity, weight gain and hormone replacement therapy in healthy postmenopausal women. *American Journal of Epidemiology, 153*(11), 1094–1101.

Barrett-Connor, E., & Grady, D. (1998). Hormone replacement therapy, heart disease, and other considerations. *Annual Review of Public Health, 19,* 55–72.

Bazzano, L. A., He, J., Muntner, P., Vupputuri, S., & Whelton, P. K. (2003). Relationship between cigarette smoking and novel risk factors for cardiovascular disease in the United States. *Annuals of Internal Medicine, 138*(11), 891–897.

Benn, M., Nordestgaard, B. G., Jensen, G. B., & Tybjaerg-Hansen, A. (2007). Improving prediction of ischemic cardiovascular disease in the general population using apolipoprotein B: The Copenhagen City Heart Study. *Arteriosclerosis Thrombosis Vascular Biology, 27*(3), 661–670.

Bønaa, K. H., Njølstad, I., Ueland, P. M., Schirmer, H., Tverdal, A., Steigen, T., … Rasmussen, K. (2006). Homocysteine lowering and cardiovascular events after acute myocardial infarction. *New England Journal of Medicine, 354,* 1578–1588.

Bradford, R. H., Shear, C. L., Chremos, A. N., Dujovne, C., Downton, M., Franklin, F. A., … Langendorfer, A. (1991). Expanded clinical evaluation of Lovastatin (EXCEL) study results. I. Efficacy in modifying plasma lipoproteins and adverse event profile in 8,245 patients with moderate hypercholesterolemia. *Archives of Internal Medicine, 151*(1), 43–49.

Brugts, J. J., Yetgin, T., Hoeks, S. E., Gotto, A. M., Shepherd, J., Westendorp, R. G. J., … van Domburg, R. (2009). The benefits of statins in people without established cardiovascular disease but with cardiovascular risk factors: Meta-analysis of randomised controlled trials. *BMJ, 338*, b2376.

Chugh, S. S., Reinier, K., Teodorescu, C., Evanado, A., Kehr, E., Al Samara, M., … Jui, J. (2008). Epidemiology of sudden cardiac death: Clinical and research implications. *Progress in Cardiovascular Diseases, 51*(3), 213–228.

Corson, M. A., Jones, P. H., & Davidson, M. H. (2008). Review of the evidence for the clinical utility of Lipoprotein Associated Phospholipase A2 as a cardiovascular risk marker. *American Journal of Cardiology, 101*(Suppl.), 41F–50F.

Critchley, J. A., & Capewell, S. (2004). Smoking cessation for the secondary prevention of coronary heart disease. *Cochrane Database of Systematic Reviews* 2004, Issue 1. Art. No.: CD003041.

Cushman, M., Arnold, A. M., Psaty, B. M., Manolio, T. A., Kuller, L. H., & Burke, G. L. (2005). C-reactive protein and the 10-year incidence of coronary heart disease in older men and women. *Circulation, 112*, 25–31.

Danesh, J., Collins, R., & Peto, R. (2000). Lipoprotein(a) and coronary heart disease. Meta-analysis of prospective studies. *Circulation, 102*(10), 1082–1085.

Dawber, T. R., & Kannel, W. B. (1968). The early diagnosis of coronary heart disease. In C. L. E. H. Sharp & H. Keen (Eds.), *Presymptomatic detection and early diagnosis: A critical appraisal* (pp. 257–281). London: Pitman Medical.

De Bree, A., Verschuren, W. M. M., Kromhout, D., Mennen, L. I., & Blom, H. J. (2002). Homocysteine and coronary heart disease: The importance of a distinction between low and high risk subjects. *International Journal of Epidemiology, 31*, 1268–1272.

De Caterina, R., Liao, J. K., & Libby, P. (2000). Fatty acid modulation of endothelial activation. *American Journal of Clinical Nutrition, 71*, 213S–223S.

Deeb, S., Failor, A., Brown, B. G., Brunzell, J. D., Albers, J. J., & Motulsky, A. G. (1986). Molecular genetics of apolipoproteins and coronary heart disease. *Cold Spring Harbor Symposia Quantitative Biology, 51*(Pt 1), 403–409.

Després, J. P., Lamarche, B., Mauriège, P., Cantin, B., Dagenais, G. R., Moorjani, S., & Lupien, P. J. (1996). Hyperinsulinemia as an independent risk factor for ischemic heart disease. *New England Journal of Medicine, 334*, 952–957.

Doll, R., & Peto, R. (1976). Mortality in relation to smoking: 20 years' observations on male British doctors. *British Medical Journal, 2*(6051),1525–1536.

Doll, R., Gray, R., Hafner, B., & Peto, R. (1980). Mortality in relation to smoking: 22 years' observations on female British doctors. *British Medical Journal, 280*(6219), 967–971.

Dorn, H. F. (1959). Tobacco consumption and mortality from cancer and other diseases. *Public Health Reports, 74*, 581–593.

Downs, J. R., Clearfield, M., Weis, S., Whitney, E., Shapiro, D. R., Beere, P. A., … AFCAPS/TexCAPS Research Group. (1998). Primary prevention of acute coronary events with Lovastatin in men and women with average cholesterol levels—results of AFCAPS/TexCAPS. *JAMA, 279*(20), 1615–1622.

Doyle, J. T., Dawber, T. R., Kannel, W. B., Kinch, S. H., & Kahn, H. A. (1964). The relationship of cigarette smoking to coronary heart disease: The second report of the combined experience of the Albany, NY, and Framingham, Mass, studies. *JAMA, 190*(10), 886–890.

Duff, G. L., & McMillan, G. C. (1951). Pathology of atherosclerosis. *American Journal of Medicine, 11*(1), 92–108.

Ebbing, M., Bleie, Ø., Ueland, P. M., Nordrehaug, J. E., Nilsen, D. W., Vollset, S. E., … Nygård, O. (2008). Mortality and cardiovascular events in patients treated with homocysteine-lowering B

vitamins after coronary angiography: A randomized controlled trial. *JAMA, 300*, 795–804.

Eschwege, E., Richard, J. L., Thibult, N., Ducimetière, P., Warnet, J. M., Claude, J. R., & Rosselin, G. E. (1985). Coronary heart disease mortality in relation with diabetes, blood glucose and plasma insulin levels. The Paris Prospective Study, ten years later. *Hormone and Metabolic Research Supplement, 15*, 41–46.

Evans, A., Tolonen, H., Hense, H. W., Ferrario, M., Sans, S., Kuulasmaa, K., & WHO Project. (2001). Trends in coronary risk factors in the WHO MONICA Project. *International Journal of Epidemiology, 30*, S35–S40.

Ferrucci, L., Cherubini, A., Bandinelli, S., Bartali, B., Corsi, A., Lauretani, F., … Guralnik, J. M. (2006). Relationship of plasma polyunsaturated fatty acids to circulating inflammatory markers. *Journal of Clinical Endocrinology and Metabolism, 91*, 439–446.

Folsom, A. R., Szklo, M., Stevens, J., Liao, F., Smith, R., & Eckfeldt, J. H. (1997). A prospective study of coronary heart disease in relation to fasting insulin, glucose, and diabetes: The Atherosclerosis Risk in Communities (ARIC) Study. *Diabetes Care, 20*, 935–942.

Ford, E. S., Smith, S. J., Stroup, D. F., Steinberg, K. K., Mueller, P. W., & Thacker, S. B. (2002). Homocyst(e)ine and cardiovascular disease: A systematic review of the evidence with special emphasis on case-control studies and nested case-control studies. *International Journal of Epidemiology, 31*, 59–70.

Ford, I., Murray, H., Packard, C. J., Shepherd, J., Macfarlane, P. W., Cobbe, S. M., & West of Scotland Coronary Prevention Study Group. (2007). Long-term follow-up of the West of Scotland Coronary Prevention Study. *New England Journal of Medicine, 357*, 1477–1486.

Global Burden of Disease 2016 Causes of Death Collaborators. (2017). Global, regional, and national under-5 mortality, adult mortality, age-specific mortality, and life expectancy, 1970–2016: A systematic analysis for the Global Burden of Disease Study, 2016. *Lancet, 390*, 1084–1150.

Gropelli, A., Giorgi, D. M. A., Omboni, S., Parati, G., & Manchia, G. (1992). Persistent blood pressure increase induced by heavy smoking. *Journal of Hypertension, 10*, 495–499.

Grundy, S. M., Balady, G. J., Criqui, M. H., Fletcher, G., Greenland, P., Hiratzka, L. F., … Ockene, I. S. (1998). Primary prevention of coronary heart disease: Guidance from Framingham: A statement for healthcare professionals from the AHA Task Force on Risk Reduction. *Circulation, 97*, 1876–1887.

Hammond, E. C. (1960). Smoking in relationship to heart disease. *American Journal of Public Health and the Nations Health, 50*(3 pt 2), 20–26.

Harris, R. E. (1994). *Approaches to the prevention and treatment of hypertension through lifestyle modification*. National Bureau of Information on Coronary Disease. Norwalk, CT: Logical Communications, Inc.

He, J., Vupputuri, S., Allen, K., Prerost, M. R., Hughes, J., & Whelton, P. K. (1999). Passive smoking and the risk of coronary heart disease: A meta-analysis of epidemiologic studies. *New England Journal of Medicine, 340*, 920–926.

Howard, G., Wagenknecht, L. E., Burke, G. L., Diez-Roux, A., Evans, G. W., McGovern, P., … ARIC investigators. (1998). Cigarette smoking and progression of atherosclerosis: The Atherosclerosis Risk in Communities (ARIC) Study. *JAMA, 279*, 119–124.

Hulley, S., Grady, D., Bush, T., Furberg, C., Herrington, D., Riggs, B., Vittinghoff, E., & Heart and Estrogen/Progestin Replacement Study (HERS). (1998). Randomized trial of estrogen plus progestin for secondary prevention of coronary heart disease in postmenopausal women: Heart and Estrogen/progestin Replacement Study (HERS) Research Group. *JAMA, 280*, 605–613.

Humphrey, L. L., Fu, R., Rogers, K., Freeman, M., & Helfand, M. (2008). Homocysteine level and coronary heart disease incidence: A systematic review and meta-analysis. *Mayo Clinic Proceedings, 83*(11), 1203–1212.

Hung, J., Knuiman, M. W., Divitini, M. L., Davis, T., & Beilby, J. P. (2008). Prevalence and risk factor correlates of elevated C-reactive protein in an adult Australian population. *American Journal of Cardiology, 101*, 193–198.

Ishikawa, S., Kayaba, K., Gotoh, T., Nakamura, Y., & Kajii, E. (2007). Metabolic syndrome and C-reactive protein in the general population. *Circulation Journal, 72*, 26–31.

Kannel, W. B. (1964). Cigarette smoking and coronary heart disease. *Annals Internal Medicine, 60*, 1103–1106.

Kannel, W. B. (1996). Blood pressure as a cardiovascular risk factor: Prevention and treatment. *JAMA, 275*(20), 1571–1576.

Kannel, W. B., & McGee, D. L. (1979). Diabetes and cardiovascular disease. The Framingham study. *JAMA, 241*(19), 2035–2038.

Kannel, W. B., Castelli, W. P., & McNamara, P. M. (1968). Cigarette smoking and risk of coronary heart disease. Epidemiologic clues to pathogenesis. The Framingham Study. *National Cancer Institute Monographs, 28*, 9–20.

Kannel, W. B., Castelli, W. P., Gordon, T., & McNamara, P. M. (1971). Serum cholesterol, lipoproteins, and the risk of coronary heart disease. The Framingham study. *Annals Internal Medicine, 74*(1), 1–12.

Kannel, W. B., D'Agostino, R. B., Wilson, P. W. F., Belanger, A. J., & Gagnon, D. R. (1990). Diabetes, fibrinogen, and risk of cardiovascular disease: The Framingham experience. *American Heart Journal, 120*, 672–676.

Kannel, W. B., Gordon, T., & Schwartz, M. J. (1971). Systolic versus diastolic blood pressure and risk of coronary heart disease. The Framingham study. *American Journal of Cardiology, 27*(4), 335–346.

Kannel, W. B., Schwartz, M. J., & McNamara, P. M. (1969). Blood pressure and risk of coronary heart disease: The Framingham study. *Diseases of the Chest, 56*(1), 43–52.

Keys, A. (1970). *Coronary heart disease in seven countries.* New York, NY: American Heart Association, Monograph No. 29.

Keys, A., Aravanis, C., Blackburn, H., Buzina, R., Djordjević, B. S., Dontas, A. S., … Van Buchem, F. S. P. (1980). *Seven countries. A multivariate analysis of death and coronary heart disease* (pp. 1–381). Cambridge, MA and London: Harvard University Press.

Keys, A., Aravanis, C., Blackburn, H. W., Van Buchem, F. S., Buzina, R., Djordjevic, B. D., … Taylor, H. L.(1966). Epidemiologic studies related to coronary heart disease: Characteristics of men aged 40–59 in seven countries. *Acta Medica Scandinavica, 180*(Suppl. to vol. 460), 1–392.

Kilhovd, B. K., Berg, T. J., Birkeland, K. I., Thorsby, P., & Hanssen, K. F. (1999). Serum levels of advanced glycation end products are increased in patients with type 2 diabetes and coronary heart disease. *Diabetes Care, 22*(9), 1543–1548.

Kiuchi, K., Nejima, J., Takano, T., Ohta, M., Hashimoto, H., & Baxter, G. (2001). Increased serum concentrations of advanced glycation end products: A marker of coronary artery disease activity in type 2 diabetic patients. *Heart, 85*(1), 87–91.

Koenig, W., Sund, M., Fröhlich, M., Fischer, H. G., Lowel, H., Doring, A., … Pepys, M. B. (1999). C-reactive protein, a sensitive marker of systemic inflammation, predicts future risk of coronary heart disease in initially healthy middle-aged men. Results from the MONICA-Augsburg cohort study 1984–92. *Circulation, 99*, 237–242.

Lauer, M. S. (2002). Aspirin for primary prevention of coronary events. *New England Journal of Medicine, 346*(19), 1468–1474.

Lee, W. L., Cheung, A. G., Cape, D., & Zinman, B. (2000). Impact of diabetes on coronary disease in women and men: A meta-analysis of prospective studies. *Diabetes Care, 23*, 962–968.

Levy, D. (1993). A multifactorial approach to coronary disease risk assessment. *Clinical and Experimental Hypertension, 15*(6), 1077–1086.

Lewington, S., Whitlock, G., Clarke, R., Sherliker, P., Emberson, J., Halsey, J. … Collins, R. (2007). Blood cholesterol and vascular mortality by age, sex, and blood pressure: A meta-analysis of individual data from 61 prospective studies with 55,000 vascular deaths. *Lancet, 370*, 1829–1839.

Lipid Research Clinics Program. (1984). The lipid research clinics coronary primary prevention trial results I. Reduction in incidence of coronary heart disease. *Journal of American Medicine Association, 251*(3), 351–364.

Lloyd-Jones, D. M., Wilson, P. W. F., Larson, M. G., Leip, E., Beiser, A., D'agostino, R. B., … Levy, D. (2003). Lifetime risk of coronary heart disease by cholesterol levels at selected ages. *Arch Internal Medicine, 163*, 1966–1972.

Maas, A. H. E. M., & Appelman, Y. E. A. (2010). Gender difference in coronary heart disease. *Netherlands Heart Journal, 18*(12), 598–602.

MacMahon, S., Peto, R., Collins, R., Godwin, J., Cutler, J., Sorlie, P., … Stamler, J. (1990). Blood pressure, stroke, and coronary heart disease Part 1, prolonged differences in blood pressure: Prospective observational studies corrected for the regression dilution bias. *Lancet, 335*(8692), 765–774.

Mahley, R. W., Innerarity, T.L., Rall, S. C., & Weisgraber, K. H. (1985). Plasma lipoproteins: Apolipoprotein structure and function. *Journal of. Lipid Research, 25*(12),1277–1294.

Marnell, L., Mold, C., & Du Clos, T. W. (2005). C-reactive protein: Ligands, receptors and role in inflammation. *Clinical Immunology, 117*, 104–111.

McQueen, M. J., Hawken, S., Wang, X., Ounpuu, S., Sniderman, A., Probstfield, J., … Kazmi, K. (2008). Lipids, lipoproteins, and apolipoproteins as risk markers of myocardial infarction in 52 countries (the INTERHEART study): A case-control study. *Lancet, 372*(9634), 224–233.

Mills, E. J., Rachlis, B., Wu, P., Devereaux, P. J., Arora, P., & Perri, D. (2008). Primary prevention of cardiovascular mortality and events with statin treatments a network meta-analysis involving more than 65,000 patients. *Journal of American College of Cardiology, 52*, 1769–1781.

Morris, J. N., Kaga, A., Pattison, D. C., Gardner, M. J., & Raffle, P. A. B. (1966). Incidence and prediction of ischemic heart disease in London busmen. *Lancet*, Sep 10, 553–559.

Mozaffarian, D., Micha, R., & Wallace, S. (2010). Effects on coronary heart disease of increasing polyunsaturated fat in place of saturated fat: A systematic review and meta-analysis of randomized controlled trials. *PLoS Medicine, 7*(3), e1000252.

Muscat, J. E., Harris, R. E., Haley, N. J., & Wynder, E. L. (1991). Cigarette smoking and plasma cholesterol. *American Heart Journal, 121*(1 Pt 1), 141–147.

Nissen, S. E., Nicholls, S. J., Sipahi, I., Libby, P., Raichlen, J. S., Ballantyne, C. M., … Schoenhagen, P. (2006). Effect of very high-intensity statin therapy on regression of coronary atherosclerosis: The ASTEROID trial (PDF). *JAMA, 295*(13), 1556–1565.

Office of Statistics of Finland. (2018). *Ischaemic heart disease still the cause of one in five deaths.* Helsinki: Statistics Finland.

Packard, C. J., O'Reilly, D. S., Caslake, M. J., McMahan, A. D., Ford, I., Cooney, J., … West of Scotland Coronary Prevention Study

Group. (2000). Lipoprotein-associated phospholipase A2 as an independent predictor of coronary heart disease. *New England Journal of Medicine,* 2000(343), 1148–1155.

Pai, J. K., Pischon, T., Ma, J., Manson, J. E., Hankinson, S. E., Joshipura, K., … Rimm, E. B. (2004). Inflammatory markers and the risk of coronary heart disease in men and women. *New England Journal of Medicine, 351*(25), 2599–2610.

Parish, S., Peto, R., Palmer, A., Clarke, R., Lewington, S., Offer, A., … Collins, R. (2009). The joint effects of apolipoprotein B, apolipoprotein A1, LDL cholesterol, and HDL cholesterol on risk: 3510 cases of acute myocardial infarction and 9805 controls. *European Heart Journal, 30*(17), 2137–2146.

Pischon, T., Hankinson, S. E., Hotamisligil, G. S., Rifai, N., Willett, W. C., & Rimm, E. B. (2003). Habitual dietary intake of n-3 and n-6 fatty acids in relation to inflammatory markers among U.S. men and women. *Circulation, 108,* 155–160.

Pyörälä, M., Miettinen, H., Laakso, M., & Pyörälä, K. (1998). Hyperinsulinemia predicts coronary heart disease risk in healthy middle-aged men: The 22-year follow-up results of the Helsinki Policemen Study. *Circulation, 98,* 398–404.

Report of the Surgeon General. (1983). *The health consequences of smoking: Cardiovascular disease.* The Reports of the Surgeon General, 1983: U.S. Department of Health and Human Services (DHHS). Publication No. (PHS) 84-50204.

Report of the Surgeon General. (1988). *The health consequences of smoking: Nicotine addiction.* A report of the Surgeon General. DHHS pub. No. 88-8406.

Report of the Surgeon General. (1990). *The health benefits of smoking cessation. A report of the surgeon general.* Atlanta: U.S. Department of Health and Human Services, Public Health Service, Centers for Disease Control, National Center for Chronic Disease Prevention and Health Promotion, Office on Smoking and Health. DHHS Publication No. (CDC) 90-8416.

Report of the Surgeon General. (2004). *The health consequences of smoking: What it means to you.* Atlanta: U.S. Department of Health and Human Services, Public Health Service, Centers for Disease Control, National Center for Chronic Disease Prevention and Health Promotion, Office on Smoking and Health. DHHS Publication No. (CDC) 90–8416.

Ridker, P. M., Buring, J. E., Cook, N. R., & Rifai, N. (2003). C-reactive protein, the metabolic syndrome, and risk of incident cardiovascular events. *Circulation, 107,* 391–397.

Ridker, P. M., Glynn, R. J., & Hennekens, C. H. (1998). C-reactive protein adds to the predictive values of total and HDL cholesterol in determining risk of first myocardial infarction. *Circulation, 97,* 2007–2011.

Ridker, P. M., Nennekens, C. H., Buring, J. E., & Rifai, N. (2000). C-reactive protein and other markers of inflammation in the prediction of cardiovascular disease in women. *New England Journal of Medicine, 3342*(12), 836–843.

Ridker, P. M., Rifai, N., Rose, L., Buring, J. E., & Cook, N. R. (2002). Comparison of C-reactive protein and low-density lipoprotein cholesterol levels in the prediction of first cardiovascular events. *New England Journal of Medicine, 347,* 1557–1565.

Robbins, S. L., & Cotran, R. S. (1979). *Pathologic basis of disease* (2nd ed.). Philadelphia, WB: Saunders Company.

Rogot, E., & Murray, J. L. (1980). Smoking and causes of death among U.S. veterans, 16 years of observation. *Public Health Reports, 95*(3), 213–222.

Ross, R. (1999). Atherosclerosis—An inflammatory disease. *New England Journal of Medicine, 340,* 115–126.

Ross, R., & Glomset, J. A. (1973). Atherosclerosis and the arterial smooth muscle cell: Proliferation of smooth muscle is a key event in the genesis of the lesions of atherosclerosis. *Science, 180,* 1332–1339.

Ross, R., & Glomset, J. A. (1976). The pathogenesis of atherosclerosis. *New England Journal of Medicine, 295,* 369–377.

Rossouw, J. E., Anderson, G. L., Prentice, R. L., & Women' Health Initiative Writing Group. (2002). Risks and benefits of estrogen plus progestin in healthy postmenopausal women: Principal results From the Women's Health Initiative randomized controlled trial. *JAMA, 288*(3), 321–333.

Salmeron, J., Hu, F. B., Manson, J. E., Stampfer, M. J., Colditz, G. A., Rimm, E. B., & Willett, W. C. (2001). Dietary fat intake and risk of type 2 diabetes in women. *American Journal of Clinical Nutrition, 73,* 1019–1026.

Sanderson, J. E., Mayosi, B., Yusuf, S., Reddy, S., Hu, S., Chen, Z., & Timmis, A. (2007). Global burden of cardiovascular disease. *Heart, 93*(10), 1175.

Sara, J. D., Eleid, M. F., Gulati, R., & Holmes, D. R. Jr. (2014). Sudden cardiac death from the perspective of coronary artery disease. *Mayo Clinical Proceedings, 89*(12), 1685–1698.

Sever, P. S., Poulter, N. R., Dahlöf, B., Wedel, H., Collins, R., Beevers, G., … Mehlsen, J. (2005). Reduction in cardiovascular events with atorvastatin in 2,532 patients with type 2 diabetes: Anglo-Scandinavian Cardiac Outcomes Trial—lipid-lowering arm (ASCOT-LLA). *Diabetes Care, 28*(5), 1151–1157.

Simopoulos, A. P. (2008). The importance of the omega-6/omega-3 fatty acid ratio in cardiovascular disease and other chronic diseases. *Experimental Biology and Medicine* (Maywood), *233,* 674–688.

Singh, P., Singh, M., Gaur, S., & Kaur, T. (2007). The ApoAI-CIII-AIV gene cluster and its relation to lipid levels in type 2 diabetes mellitus and coronary heart disease: Determination of a novel susceptible haplotype. *Diabetes and Vascular Diseases Research, 4*(2), 124–129.

Sofi, F., Cesari, F., Abbate, R., Gensini, G. F., & Casini, A. (2008). Adherence to Mediterranean diet and health status: Meta-analysis. *BMJ (Clinical Research ed.), 337,* a1344.

Stamler, J., Daviglus, M. L., Garside, D. B., Dyer, A. R., Greenland, P., & Neaton, J. D. (2000). Relationship of baseline serum cholesterol levels in 3 large cohorts of younger men to long-term coronary, cardiovascular, and all-cause mortality and to longevity. *JAMA, 284,* 311–318.

Stamler, J., & Neaton, J. D. (2008). The Multiple Risk Factor Intervention Trial (MRFIT)—Importance then and now. *JAMA, 300*(11), 1343–1345.

Stamler, J., Stamler, R., Neaton, J. D., Wentworth, D., Daviglus, M. L., Garside, D., … Greenland, P. (1999). Low-risk factor profile and long-term cardiovascular and noncardiovascular mortality and life expectancy: Findings for 5 large cohorts of young adult and middle-aged men and women. *JAMA, 282,* 2012–2018.

Stamler, J., Wentworth, D., Neaton, J. D., & MRFIT Research Group. (1986). Is relationship between serum cholesterol and risk of premature death from coronary heart disease continuous and graded? Findings in 356,222 primary screenees of the Multiple Risk Factor Intervention Trial (MRFIT). *JAMA, 256*(20), 2823–2828.

Steinberg, D. (2005). Hypercholesterolemia and inflammation in atherogenesis: Two sides of the same coin. *Molecular Nutrition Food Research, 49,* 995–998.

Stevenson, J. C. (2009). Hormone replacement therapy and cardiovascular disease revisited. *Menopause International, 15,* 55–57.

Strandberg, T. E., Lehto, S., Pyörälä, K., Kesäniemi, A., & Oksa, H. (1997). Cholesterol lowering after participation in the

Scandinavian Simvastatin Survival Study (4S) in Finland. *European Heart Journal, 18*(11), 1725–1727.

Summary of the second report of the National Cholesterol Education Program (NCEP). (1993). Expert Panel on Detection, Evaluation, and Treatment of High Blood Cholesterol in Adults (Adult Treatment Panel II). *JAMA, 269*, 3015–3023.

Summers, L. K., Fielding, B. A., Bradshaw, H. A., Ilic, V., Beysen, C., Clark, M. L., ... Frayn, K. N. (2002). Substituting dietary saturated fat with polyunsaturated fat changes abdominal fat distribution and improves insulin sensitivity. *Diabetologia, 45*, 369–377.

Sung, K. C., Suh, J. Y., Kim, B. S., Kang, J. H., Kim, H., Lee, M. H., ... Kim, S. W. (2003). High sensitivity C-reactive protein as an independent risk factor for essential hypertension. *American Journal of Hypertension, 16*, 429–433.

Toole, J. F., Malinow, M. R., Chambless, L. E., Spence, J. D., Pettigrew, L. C., Howard, V. J., ... Stampfer, M. (2004). Lowering homocysteine in patients with ischemic stroke to prevent recurrent stroke, myocardial infarction, and death: The Vitamin Intervention for Stroke Prevention (VISP) randomized controlled trial. *JAMA, 291*, 565–575.

Toss, H., Lindahl, B., Siegbahn, A., & Wallentin, L. (1997). Prognostic influence of increased fibrinogen and C-reactive protein levels in unstable coronary artery disease. *Circulation, 96*, 4204–4210.

Tunstall-Pedoe, H., Kuulasmaa, K., Mähönen, M., Tolonen, H., Ruokokoski, E., & Amouyel, P. (1999). Contribution of trends in survival and coronary-event rates to changes in coronary heart disease mortality: 10-year results from 37 WHO MONICA project populations. Monitoring trends and determinants in cardiovascular disease. *Lancet, 353*(9164), 1547–1557.

Tunstall-Pedoe, H., Kuulasmaa, K., Tolonen, H., Davidson, M., Mendis, S., ... Toša Zikic, M. (2003). *MONICA monograph and multimedia sourcebook.* Geneva, Switzerland: World Health Organization.

U.S. Department of Agriculture. (2010). MyPyramid.gov. Washington, DC: USDA.

van den Hoogen, P. C. W., Feskens, E. J. M., Nagelkerke, N. J. D., Menotti, A., Nissinen, A., Kromhout, D., & The Seven Countries Study Research Group. (2000). The relation between blood pressure and mortality due to coronary heart disease among men in different parts of the world. *New England Journal of Medicine, 342*(1), 1–8.

van der Steeg, W. A., Boekholdt, S. M., Stein, E. A., El-Harchaoui, K., Stroes, E. S., Sandhu, M. S., ... Kastelein, J. J. (2007). Role of the Apolipoprotein B–Apolipoprotein A-1 ratio in cardiovascular risk assessment: A case–control analysis in EPIC-Norfolk. *Annals Internal Medicine, 146*, 640–648.

Verschuren, W. M., Jacobs, D. R., Bloemberg, B. P., Kromhout, D., Menotti, A., Aravanis, C., ... Karvonen, M. J. (1995). Serum total cholesterol and long-term coronary heart disease mortality in different cultures. Twenty-five-year follow-up of the seven countries study. *JAMA, 274*(2), 131–136.

Virchow, R. (1856). Phlogose und Thrombose im Gefässystem. In: *Gesammelte Abhandlungen zur wissenschaftlichen Medizin.* Germany: Staatsdruckerei Frankfurt.

Waller, B. F. (1989). Atherosclerotic and nonatherosclerotic coronary artery factors in acute myocardial infarction. In C. J. Pepine (ed.), *Acute myocardial infarction* (pp. 29–104). Philadelphia, PA: FA Davis.

Welch, G. N., & Loscalzo, J. (1998). Homocysteine and atherothrombosis. *New England Journal of Medicine, 338*, 1042–1050.

Willett, W. C., Sacks, F., & Trichopoulous, A. (1995). Mediterranean diet pyramid: A cultural model for healthy eating. *American Journal of Clinical Nutrition, 61*(6 Suppl.), 1402S–1406S.

Yusuf, S., Hawken, S., Ounpuu, S., Dans, T., Avezum, A., Lanas, F., ... Lisheng, L. (2004). Effect of potentially modifiable risk factors associated with myocardial infarction in 52 countries (the INTERHEART study): Case-control study. *Lancet, 364*(9438), 937–952.

Zhao, M, Vaartjes, I., Graham, I., Grobbee, D., Spiering, W., Klipstein-Grobusch, K., ... Peters, S. A. (2017). Sex differences in risk factor management of coronary heart disease across three regions. *Heart, 103*, 1587–1594.

CHAPTER 4

Epidemiology of Myocardial Infarction

▶ Function of the Heart

The heart is an extraordinary electrochemical muscular organ that sustains human life by efficiently pumping blood through the circulatory system of the body. The normal heart weighs approximately 250–300 g in adult women and 300–350 g in adult men. The heart consists primarily of striated skeletal muscle called myocardium. The myocardium is specially designed to facilitate rapid flux of sodium and potassium ions between myocardial cells and interstitial fluid that is critical for the polarization and depolarization of contracting cardiac muscle fibers (Kumar, Abbas, & Aster, 2017).

The human heart efficiently pumps approximately 5 L of blood through the vascular circulatory system. It pulsates at 70 beats per minute, more than 100,000 times per day without fail over a normal lifespan of more than 80 years. Each heartbeat pumps approximately 60–70 mL of blood into the aorta. Thus, on average, red blood cells cycle about once per minute or 1440 times per day.

Anatomically, the heart is divided into four chambers: The right atrium that receives deoxygenated blood from the superior and inferior vena cava and delivers it to the right ventricle; the right ventricle that receives blood from the right atrium and pumps it through the low-pressure pulmonary circulation where carbon dioxide is exchanged for oxygen in the hemoglobin of the red blood cells; the left

atrium that receives newly oxygenated blood from the pulmonary arteries and delivers it to the left ventricle; and the left ventricle that pumps blood into the aorta for distribution and delivery to all tissues of the body (**FIGURE 4.1**).

Four valves regulate blood flow into and out of the heart chambers: The tricuspid valve that controls blood flow from the right atrium into the right ventricle; the pulmonary valve that controls blood flow from the right atrium into the pulmonary circulation; the mitral valve that regulates blood flow from the left atrium into the left ventricle; and the aortic valve that regulates blood flow from the left ventricle into the aorta (Figure 4.1). The normal two-stage "lub dub" heart sound is due to closure of the atrial valves (closure of the tricuspid and mitral valves causes the "lub" sound) followed by closure of the ventricular valves (closure of the pulmonary and aortic valves causes the "dub" sound).

The regular heartbeat is controlled by electrical impulses synchronously transmitted from the SA node to the AV node (**FIGURE 4.2**). The bundle of His and the Purkinje system of specialized muscle fibers distribute the impulse to the interventricular septum and the left and right ventricles of the myocardium. Depolarization (change of membrane potential from positive to negative) of the atrial myocardium causes the right and left atria to contract first, followed by depolarization and contraction of the right and left ventricles. Sequential contraction of the atria followed

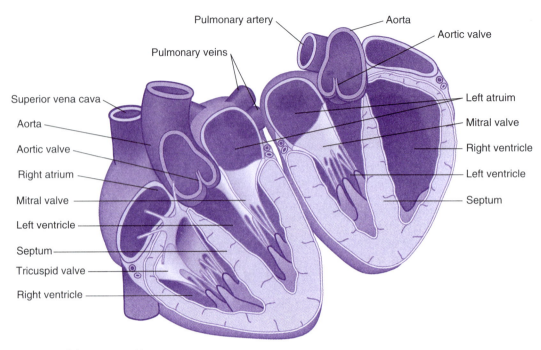

FIGURE 4.1 Structure of the Human Heart.

FIGURE 4.2 Conducting System of the Human Heart.

by the ventricles facilitates efficient blood perfusion through the lungs and the systemic circulation. Each pulsation of the human heart lasts about eight-tenths of 1 second, about half of which is a quiescent period that allows the heart muscle to rest between beats.

The heart is nourished by coronary arteries with a characteristic distribution (**FIGURE 4.3**). The left anterior descending coronary artery supplies most of the apex of the heart and portions of the left and right ventricles, as well as the interventricular septum. The

right coronary artery supplies much of the remaining myocardium, whereas the left circumflex branch supplies a relatively small portion of the left ventricle. Supportive coronary blood flow is supplied by numerous capillaries as well as small anastomotic channels between vessels (Kumar et al., 2017).

The *vagus nerve* (the 10 of 12 paired cranial nerves) innervates the human heart and helps to modulate the heart rate. The right branch of the vagus nerve innervates the sinoatrial (SA) node and the left branch

FIGURE 4.3 Left and Right Coronary Arteries, Human Heart.

innervates the atrioventricular (AV) node. Cholinergic neurotransmitters (acetylcholine) released by the vagus nerve lower the heart rate and cause vasodilatation whereas adrenergic neurotransmitters (epinephrine or adrenaline) secreted by the adrenal glands stimulate the heart to beat faster and cause vasoconstriction. Cholinergic neurotransmitters such as acetylcholine modulate cell function by activating specific G-protein-coupled cell membrane receptors (e.g., nicotinic and muscarinic receptors) whereas adrenergic neurotransmitters such as epinephrine activate a different class of G-protein coupled cell membrane receptors (a and b receptors) (Hoffman & Lefkowitz, 1982; Rosenbaum, Rasmussen, & Kobilka, 2009).

▶ Clinical Parameters of Myocardial Infarction (Heart Attack)

Myocardial infarction (MI), commonly known as a heart attack, is the interruption of blood supply to part of the heart causing a portion of the myocardium to die. Myocardial infarcts are most commonly due to occlusion (blockage) of a coronary artery caused by atherosclerosis or following the rupture of a vulnerable atherosclerotic plaque. The resulting ischemia

(restriction in blood supply) and oxygen shortage, if left untreated for a sufficient period of time, can cause *infarction* of the myocardium and often results in death of the patient.

MI presents with sudden chest pain typically radiating to the left arm or left side of the neck in combination with shortness of breath, nausea, vomiting, heart palpitations, sweating, and anxiety. Approximately 25% of MIs occur without warning (e.g., in the absence of prior chest pain or other symptoms). More often, the onset of MI is gradual over several minutes providing time for emergency treatment. The diagnosis of MI is inferred by electrocardiogram abnormalities and confirmed by elevated blood biomarkers of myocardial necrosis such as creatine kinase and troponin (National Heart, Lung and Blood Institute, 2006). Patients with two subtypes of acute MIs have been identified based upon electrocardiography: Those with elevation of the ST segment of the cardiac rhythm (STEMI) and those without ST elevation (non-STEMI). Elevation of the ST segment indicates thrombotic occlusion of a coronary artery and requires immediate reperfusion therapy with antithrombolytic drugs or percutaneous coronary intervention (Alpert, Thygesen, Antman, & Bassand, 2000). A coronary angiogram allows visualization of narrowing or obstruction of the heart vessels for the immediate institution of potentially lifesaving measures (e.g., angioplasty).

▶ Global Mortality and Morbidity Due to Myocardial Infarctions

Of the 17.9 million deaths caused by cardiovascular diseases in 2016, approximately 85% (15.2 million) were caused by heart attacks (8.9 million) and strokes (6.3 million) (Global Burden of Disease 2016 Causes of Death Collaborators, 2017; WHO, 2017). More than 75% of these deaths occurred in low-income and middle-income countries where education on prevention and access to effective therapy and emergency services are lacking (Mackay & Mensah, 2004; Mendis, Puska, & Norrving, 2011).

The clinical presentation of MI varies from a minor infarct to a life-threatening infarct of substantial and critical segments of the myocardium and sudden death. Those who survive an initial MI are vulnerable to repeat MIs. Currently, the diagnosis of MI involves detection of a significant abrupt rise in cardiac biomarkers in a patient with ischemic heart disease. Such diagnostic criteria are often not available for patients who suffer fatal or nonfatal events out of hospital or in hospitals without facilities to measure diagnostic biomarkers (Mendis et al., 2011).

Current data suggest that each year more than 5.5 million deaths from heart attacks occur in the populations of developing nations at relatively early ages (median age ≈ 50 years). The remaining 2 million deaths from heart attacks occur at later ages in populations of developed nations (median age ≈ 65 years). In addition to the deaths from MIs, more than 5 million people survive these attacks every year, the majority in developed nations where emergency care is available (**FIGURE 4.4**).

The *Disability-Adjusted Life Years* (DALY = YLL + YDL) is a combined measure of the years of life lost due to premature death (YLL) plus the years of healthy life lost due to severe disability (YDL). Estimated DALY arising due to fatal and nonfatal MIs are presented together with coronary heart disease by income level of nations in **FIGURE 4.5**. The world pattern of DALY from MIs is similar to that for ischemic/coronary heart disease reflecting the huge impact of atherosclerosis and the global epidemiologic transition from infectious/parasitic diseases to chronic diseases. High DALY are evident in populous developing nations such as India, Russia, and Egypt compared to low DALY in the developed nations of North America, Western Europe, South America, China, Japan, Australia, and New Zealand. High DALY are also

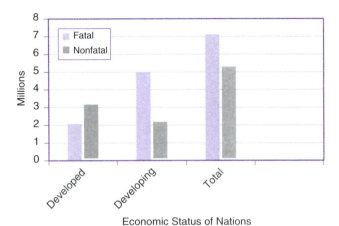

FIGURE 4.4 Fatal and Nonfatal Myocardial Infarctions, World Population, 2009.

Countries are grouped by national annual income per capita: Developed Nations > $10,065, Developing Nations < $10,065.

Data from WHO. (2010). *World health statistics 2010*. Geneva, Switzerland: World Health Organization Statistical Information System (WHOSIS).

apparent in the populations of poverty-stricken countries of central Africa such as Sudan, Chad, Ethiopia, and Nigeria. Populations of these nations are not only prone to coronary heart disease and MIs, but they also suffer a heavy burden of death and disability from malnutrition plus infectious/parasitic diseases causing life-threatening diarrhea, malaria, HIV/AIDS, and tuberculosis.

▶ Time Trends in Myocardial Infarction Rates

Several prospective investigations have noted marked declines in the incidence rates of MIs in the populations of developed nations. In the U.S. Framingham community-based cohort of 9824 men and women aged 40–89 years followed for up to four decades, incidence rates of acute MI diagnosed by electrocardiogram declined by approximately 50% with similar declines in case fatality rates from 1960 to 1999 (Parikh et al., 2009). These declines were attributed primarily to better control of blood pressure, reduced blood levels of cholesterol, and reduced rates of cigarette smoking among participants. Paradoxically, a slight *increase* was noted in the incidence of MIs diagnosed among hospitalized patients, perhaps reflecting increasing use of more sensitive biochemical markers of myocardial necrosis in the diagnosis of MI.

In the international MONICA (Multinational Monitoring Trends and Determinants in Cardiovascular Disease) Project, analysis of 37 sample populations from 21 countries after 10 years of follow-up showed average annual declines in coronary heart disease

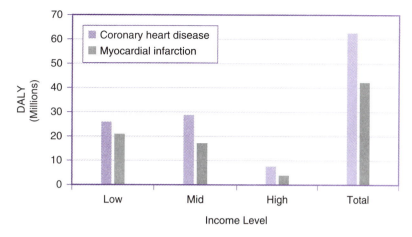

FIGURE 4.5 Global DALY for Coronary Heart Disease and Myocardial Infarction Stratified by Income Level of Nations, 2009.

Countries are grouped by national annual income per capita: Low < $826, Middle: $826–$10,065, High > $10,065.

Data from WHO. (2010). *World health statistics 2010.* Geneva, Switzerland: World Health Organization Statistical Information System (WHOSIS).

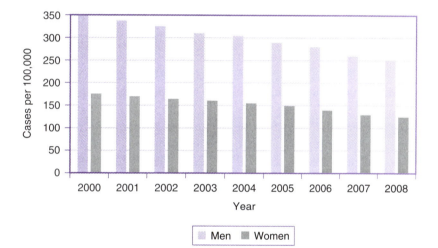

FIGURE 4.6 Incidence of Nonfatal Myocardial Infarction, United States, 2000–2008.

Data from Reynolds, K., Go, A. S., Leong, T. K., Boudreau, D. M., Cassidy-Bushrow, A. E., Fortmann, S. P., . . . Sidney, S. (2017). Trends in incidence of hospitalized acute myocardial infarction in the Cardiovascular Research Network (CVRN). *The American Journal of Medicine, 130,* 317–327.

mortality of 4% in both men and women and average annual declines in coronary events (nonfatal MI or coronary death) of 2.1% for men and 1.4% for women (Tunstall-Pedoe et al., 1994, 1999). The MONICA investigators attributed the majority of the decline in mortality to factors leading to reduced rates of coronary events rather than improved survival.

In the Atherosclerosis Risk in Communities (ARIC) Study, trends in mortality due to coronary heart disease and the incidence of MI among 352,481 adults from four U.S. communities were examined from 1987 to 1994 on the basis of a review of 3023 deaths due to coronary heart disease and 8572 hospitalizations for MI. During this time period, mortality due to coronary heart disease declined by 28% in men and 31% in women. These reductions were accompanied by declines in case fatality rates and rates of recurrent MI as well as improved survival among cases. The ARIC investigators attributed

these findings to primary prevention and reductions in risk factors plus improvements in the treatment of coronary heart disease (Rosamond et al., 1998, 2012). Similar to the Framingham Study, the ARIC Study also found no evidence of a decline in the incidence of MI among hospitalized patients in a cohort examined during 1986–1994, neither in men or women; and in fact, the incidence rates actually increased in certain years (**FIGURE 4.6**, Rosamond et al., 2012).

As pointed out by Levy and Thom, the paradox is explainable in that more sensitive diagnostic tests were routinely implemented during 1990–2000 for hospitalized patients with chest pain, possibly shifting the diagnosis of angina pectoris to MI in some patients, thereby increasing the incidence of MI (Levy & Thom, 1998).

Dramatic shifts occurred in the detection of acute MI around the turn of the 20th century. In particular, the measurement of troponin, a precise marker of myocardial necrosis in hospitalized patients increased to nearly 100% during the period 1996–2001, and as a consequence, detection of small infarcts increased thereby increasing the incidence of acute MI. Following the universal incorporation of more precise methods of detection (e.g., the measurement of troponin), the incidence of acute MI stabilized and subsequently declined. For example, in the ARIC Study, the incidence of acute MI during 1997–2008 declined by 3.8% per year in men and 3.5% per year in women (Rosamond et al., 2012).

Investigators of the *United States Cardiovascular Research Network* also observed a significant declining trend in the incidence of acute MI among hospitalized patients during the first decade of the 20th century. Among hospitalized patients in 13 healthcare programs, 125,435 cases of acute MI were observed during 2000–2008. Overall, the incidence of acute MI declined by 27%, from 230 per 100,000 in 2000 to 169 per 100,000 in 2008. Case fatality rates within 30 days of hospitalization also declined, from 5.7% in 2000 to 3.5% in 2008. These declining trends were similar for men and women although the annual incidence rates for men were consistently double that for women (e.g., 250 versus 125 per 100,000 in 2008). Declines in the incidence of acute MI reflect effects of increasing awareness, prevention and control of cardiovascular disease risk factors in recent decades (Reynolds et al., 2017).

National statistics from the U.S. National Heart, Lung and Blood Institute confirm that marked declines have occurred in mortality and case fatality due to acute MI during the past several decades (Levy & Thom, 1998; National Heart, Lung and Blood Institute, 2009). During the 35-year period from 1970 to 2005, both mortality and case fatality due to acute MI declined by more than 70% (**FIGURE 4.7**).

▶ Risk Factors for Myocardial Infarction

Since ischemic/coronary heart disease is the root cause of most MIs, certain primary risk factors are synonymous including tobacco addiction, hypertension, hyperglycemia (elevated blood glucose), hypercholesterolemia (elevated blood cholesterol), and chronic inflammation. Nevertheless, the abrupt nature of a heart attack also involves other factors.

Heart attack rates are higher in association with intense exertion, either from psychological stress or vigorous physical exercise, especially if the exertion is more intense than usual (Siscovick, Weiss, Fletcher, & Lasky, 1984). Quantitatively, periods of intense exercise and subsequent recovery are associated with an approximate sixfold higher MI rate (compared with other more relaxed time frames) for people who are physically very fit. For those in poor physical condition, the rate differential is over 35-fold higher (Mittleman et al., 1993; Willich et al., 1993). Mechanistically, it is suggested that the spiking of blood pressure on extreme physical/psychological exertion may increase the shear stress on atheromas and the likelihood of plaque rupture (Curfman, 1993). The investigators stress that these findings should not be an impediment to regular aerobic exercise (at least three times weekly for 30 minutes or more) as recommended by the American Heart Association.

Acute severe infection, such as pneumonia, can trigger MI. In a study using within-person comparisons, 20,486 individuals with a first MI and 19,063 individuals with a first stroke were examined. The risk for MI increased fivefold and the risk for stroke increased threefold within a 3-day period after diagnosis of a systemic respiratory tract infection. Furthermore, transient risk increases were also observed following urinary tract infections and the risk estimates for recurrent MI or

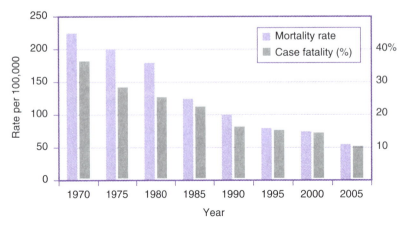

FIGURE 4.7 Decline in Mortality and Case Fatality due to Myocardial Infarction, United States, 1970–2005.

Data from the National Center for Health Statistics, National Vital Statistics Reports. (2009). *Case fatality estimates are for individuals over the age of 65 years.* National Heart, Lung and Blood Institute.

stroke subsequent to infection were similar to those for first events. There was no increase in the risk of MI or stroke in the period after influenza, tetanus, or pneumococcal vaccination. The finding that different infectious processes of different organ systems are associated with a significant transient increase in the risk of cardiovascular events lends strong support to the concept that systemic inflammation itself alters the probability of the occurrence of a vascular event (Smeeth et al., 2004).

A more controversial link is that between *Chlamydophila pneumoniae* infection and atherosclerosis. In a nested case–control study of 103 patients who suffered sudden cardiac death or a nonfatal MI compared to matched controls from the Helsinki Heart Study, the odds ratios (ORs) were elevated more than twofold among individuals with antibodies to *Chlamydophila pneumoniae* (Saikku et al., 1992). While this intracellular organism has been demonstrated in atherosclerotic plaques, evidence is inconclusive as to whether it can be considered a causative factor. Treatment with antibiotics in patients with proven atherosclerosis has not demonstrated a decreased risk of heart attacks or other coronary vascular diseases (Andraws, Berger, & Brown, 2005).

It is well known that the frequency of heart attacks is increased in the early morning hours upon awakening (Beamer et al., 1987; Muller et al., 1985). Some investigators theorize that this high-risk time period may be related to the circadian variation in cortisol production affecting the concentrations of various cytokines and other mediators of inflammation (Fantidis et al., 2002). Other factors potentially underlying this phenomenon include smoking the first cigarette of the day, exercising vigorously, and/or conducting other activities that spike blood pressure in the early morning hours.

Major epidemiologic studies of ischemic/coronary heart disease have elucidated and quantified several individual risk factors and stressed the importance of their multifactorial interactions. These and other selected investigations relevant to the risk of MI are discussed in the following paragraphs.

▶ The INTERHEART Study of Acute Myocardial Infarction

Foremost among the studies of MI is the INTERHEART Study. INTERHEART is a standardized case–control study that screened all patients admitted to the coronary care unit or equivalent cardiology ward for a first (nonfatal) MI at 262 participating centers in 52 countries throughout Africa, Asia, Australia, Europe, the Middle East, and North and South America (Yusuf et al., 2004).

Cases were identified using standardized definitions and enrolled within 24 hours of symptom onset. Matching controls were recruited, resulting in a total of 15,152 incident cases of acute MI and 14,820 controls matched by age (±5 years) and sex but with no history of heart disease. A study questionnaire, translated into 11 languages, was used to collect data on demographic factors (country of origin, first language), socioeconomic status (education, occupation, income), lifestyle (tobacco use, physical activity, dietary patterns), and personal and family history of cardiovascular disease and risk factors (self-reported diabetes and hypertension). Components of the questionnaire were compiled with previously validated questions included in studies of risk factors for cardiovascular disease. Questionnaires were administered by trained staff before the patients left the hospital. Data on medications (prehospital, inhospital, and discharge) and interventions were abstracted from medical charts. Standard physical measurements were recorded in duplicate by the same examiner on each participant: Height, weight, waist and hip circumference, and heart rate. A 20 mL sample of nonfasting blood was drawn from each individual and was frozen and stored for biochemical analyses, including total cholesterol, high-density lipoprotein–cholesterol, apolipoproteins B (ApoB), and A1 (ApoA1). The strength of associations between various risk factors and acute MI was estimated by OR. The investigators calculated the variation in associations according to geographic region, ethnic origin, gender, and age in order to quantify the impact of each risk factor alone and in combination by the Population Attributable Risk (PAR). For comparison of prevalence across distinct subgroups (e.g., by region, country, or ethnic group), potential differences in age structure of the populations were accounted for by direct standardization of the frequencies to the overall INTERHEART age distribution with a five-level age-stratification factor (<45, 46–55, 56–65, 66–70, >70). Final analyses were carried out for 12,461 cases and 9459 controls (Yusuf et al., 2004).

Results of INTERHEART

The mean age for the first presentation of acute MI was 8–10 years younger in men than women worldwide and 10 years younger in Africa, the Middle East, and South Asia compared with other regions of the world. The study identified nine easily measured risk factors accounting for >90% of the risk of acute MI: *Smoking, lipids, hypertension, diabetes, obesity, diet, physical activity, alcohol consumption, and psychosocial factors.* ORs estimated from the study are shown in **TABLE 4.1** (Yusuf et al., 2004).

TABLE 4.1 INTERHEART Study Results

Factor	Controls (%)	Cases (%)	OR
ApoB/ApoA1	20.0	34.5	3.25
Smoking	26.8	45.2	2.97
Diabetes	7.5	18.5	2.37
High BP	21.9	39.0	1.91
Obesity	33.3	56.3	1.62
Stress	9.4	23.6	2.67
Fruit & vegetable diet	42.2	36.8	0.71
Exercise	19.3	14.3	0.86
Alcohol	24.5	24.0	0.91

Data from Yusuf, S., Hawken, S., Ounpuu, S., Dans, T., Avezum, A., Lanas, F., … INTERHEART Study Investigators. (2004). Effect of potentially modifiable risk factors associated with myocardial infarction in 52 countries (the INTERHEART study): Case-control study. *Lancet, 364*(9438), 937–952.

The strongest risk factor detected was the ApoB/ApoA1 ratio. ApoB is the primary apolipoprotein of low-density lipoproteins (LDLs or bad cholesterol) in plasma, which is responsible for carrying cholesterol from the liver to tissues. ApoA1 is the major protein component of high-density lipoprotein (HDL or good cholesterol) in plasma. This protein promotes cholesterol efflux from tissues to the liver for excretion. The relative risk for individuals with ApoB/ApoA1 ratios in the highest quintile was 3.25 after adjustment for all other risk factors (McQueen et al., 2008).

The PAR takes into consideration both the OR and prevalence of a risk factor to estimate the fraction of the risk that can be attributed to that particular risk factor. Based on the INTERHEART results, 50% of acute MIs are attributable to the ApoB/ApoA1 ratio and 36% to current smoking. Thus, these two risk factors, the ApoB/ApoA1 ratio and smoking, account for about two-thirds of the risk for developing an acute MI in the world population. Five factors (smoking, lipids, hypertension, diabetes, and obesity) accounted for about 80% of the PAR. For all nine risk factors combined, the PAR was significantly greater in younger than in older individuals, but consistent in men and women (90% and 94%, respectively). Abdominal obesity was found to be a stronger risk factor than body mass index (BMI), a result that prompted the investigators to recommend that measurement of waist-to-hip ratio should replace BMI as the preferred indicator of obesity. Finally, the 10-year younger mean age for the first presentation of acute MI in Africa, the Middle East, and South Asia compared with other regions of the world implies the onset of an oncoming epidemic and predicts a large increase in cardiovascular disease in these regions in the coming years (Yusuf et al., 2004).

▶ Seven Countries Study of Myocardial Infarction

The Seven Countries Study conducted by Ancel Keys and colleagues examined the effects of diet in an international prospective cohort of 12,763 men, aged 40–59 years, in 16 population samples from seven different countries (Italy, Greece, former Yugoslavia, the Netherlands, Finland, United States, and Japan). The study was the first to demonstrate that serum cholesterol is a biomarker of impending coronary heart disease and that the risk increases with intake of saturated fats and decreases with intake of monounsaturated fatty acids (primarily from olive oil). Risk increases were also associated with elevated blood pressure (hypertension), cigarette smoking, sedentary lifestyle, and obesity. The investigation elucidated the preventive effects of the Mediterranean diet consisting primarily of daily intake of fruits, vegetables, whole grains, olive oil, fish, and poultry (Keys, 1970; Keys et al., 1967, 1980).

▸ Framingham Study of Myocardial Infarction

Since 1948, investigators at Harvard University have been following generations of the residents of Framingham, Massachusetts, to better understand the determinants of heart disease. The initial cohort consisted of 5209 randomly selected members of the adult population of Framingham, 30–62 years of age, who were enrolled for study in 1948. The ongoing study now includes a second generation of 5124 men and women (offspring of the original cohort). A series of initial reports based upon the Framingham Study documented significant independent effects of cigarette smoking, hypertension, hyperglycemia, and hypercholesterolemia in the genesis of ischemic/coronary heart disease and MI (Dawber & Kannel, 1968; Kannel, 1964, 1996; Kannel, Castelli, Gordon, & McNamara, 1971; Kannel, Castelli, & McNamara, 1968; Kannel, D'Agostino, Wilson, Belanger, & Gagnon, 1990; Kannel, Gordon, & Schwartz, 1971; Kannel & McGee, 1979; Kannel, Schwartz, & McNamara, 1969). While each of these risk factors independently increases the relative risk of disease by two- to threefold, the interaction of chronic smoking, high blood pressure, hyperglycemia, and hypercholesterolemia accentuates the risk by more than tenfold in comparison to individuals with no exposure (Levy, 1993; Wilson et al., 1998).

Many other epidemiologic investigations have provided consistent evidence confirming the cause and effect relationship of these factors and their synergistic interactions in the pathogenesis of MI as well as declining trends in mortality and morbidity rates due to coronary heart disease and MI with reductions in these risk factors in past decades. These include the MONICA Project (Tunstall-Pedoe et al., 1994, 1999); the ARIC Study (Rosamond et al., 1998); the Copenhagen City Heart Study I and II (Jensen, Nyboe, Appleyard, & Schnohr, 1991; Nyboe, Jensen, Appleyard, & Schnohr, 1989); the Minnesota Heart Survey (McGovern, Jacobs, & Shahar, 2001); the Worcester Heart Attack Study (Goldberg, Gore, Alpert, & Dalen, 1986; Goldberg, Yarzebski, Lessard, & Gore, 1999); the Corpus Christi Study (Nichaman, Wear, Goff, & Labarthe, 1993); and the Olmstead County Study (Roger et al., 2002).

The sampling design utilized in some U.S. investigations has facilitated comparisons by ethnicity of subpopulations. In the ARIC Study, African American women and men had, respectively, 50% and 80% higher case fatality rates from MI or coronary heart disease than Caucasian Americans (White et al., 1999); and in the Corpus Christi Study, Mexican American women and men had 60% and 30% higher rates of hospitalization due to MI than non-Hispanic Americans (Goff et al., 1997; Nichaman et al., 1993).

In general, all of these studies provide consistent evidence that most risk factors for atherosclerosis and MI are similar. Factors in common include tobacco addiction, diabetes and hyperglycemia (elevated blood glucose), hypercholesterolemia and hyperlipidemia (especially high LDL cholesterol coupled with low high-density lipoprotein cholesterol), high blood triglycerides, high blood pressure, high C-reactive protein (a measure of inflammation), family history of ischemic heart disease, obesity (BMI of 30 or more), increased waist-to-hip ratio, age, male gender, hyperhomocysteinemia, persistent high stress, and alcohol abuse. It is stressed that these risk factors are not mutually exclusive and often cluster together in the same individual to synergistically increase the risk of developing a MI.

▸ Primary Prevention of Myocardial Infarction

Since many of its risk factors are modifiable, MI is preventable (Kuller, Neaton, Caggiula, & Falvo-Gerard, 1980; Manson et al., 1992; Stamler, Wentworth, & Neaton, 1986). Primary prevention is the reciprocal of exposure to proven risk factors. Avoid tobacco, eat a heart-healthy diet, maintain blood pressure, blood glucose, and blood lipids (cholesterol) within normal limits, exercise daily, and maintain optimal weight for height.

A key component of prevention for all individuals is to have regular (annual) physical checkups to detect elevations in blood pressure, blood glucose, serum cholesterol, or other irregularities. Effective antihypertensive and antidiabetic medications are readily available to maintain blood pressure and blood glucose within normal limits. Sodium (salt) restriction (less than 6 g of salt per day) is also important for blood pressure control. Weight reduction programs incorporating healthy nutrition and regular exercise regimes have proven successful in reducing obesity and reaching optimal weight.

TABLE 4.2 elaborates guidelines for the prevention of cardiovascular disease (including MI) according to the American Heart Association. In the paragraphs that follow, the epidemiologic evidence regarding several selected factors (dietary fat, aspirin, statins, and estrogen replacement therapy) is discussed.

TABLE 4.2 Lifestyle Modification and Cardiovascular Disease

- Avoid tobacco
- Maintain serum cholesterol within normal limits
- Maintain blood glucose within normal limits
- Maintain blood pressure within normal limits
- Weight control (Ideal body weight)
- Sodium reduction (<6 g salt daily)
- Exercise regularly (Aerobic)
- Reduce fat intake (<30% calories)
- Alcohol (<1 oz daily)
- Maintain potassium, calcium, magnesium

Data from Manson, J. E., Tosteson, H., Ridker, P. M., Satterfield, S., Hebert, P., O'Connor, G. T., … Hennekens, C. H. (1992). The primary prevention of myocardial infarction. *The New England Journal of Medicine, 326*(21), 1406–1416; Mackay, J., & Mensah, G. (2004). *Atlas of heart disease and stroke*. Geneva, Switzerland: World Health Organization.

Dietary Fat and Myocardial Infarction

There is much controversy as to what constitutes a *heart-healthy* diet. The *Mediterranean diet* has been championed by many investigators as the most prudent *heart-healthy* diet. Such a diet is characterized by abundant plant foods (fruit, vegetables, whole grain breads, other forms of cereals, potatoes, beans, nuts, and seeds), fresh fruit as the typical daily dessert, olive oil as the principal source of fat, dairy products (principally cheese and yogurt), and fish and poultry consumed in low to moderate amounts. Notably, in a meta-analysis of 12 prospective studies with a total of 1,574,299 subjects followed for up to 18 years, greater adherence to the *Mediterranean diet* was associated with significant improvement in health status and significant reductions in overall mortality (9%), mortality from cardiovascular diseases (9%), cancer mortality (6%), and incidence rates of Parkinson's disease and Alzheimer's disease (13%) (Sofi, Cesari, Abbate, Gensini, & Casini, 2008).

Dietary transition from saturated fats to polyunsaturated fatty acids (PUFA) has been advocated by some investigators, and it is generally accepted that omega-3 fatty acids are beneficial PUFA whereas transfatty acids should be avoided (Willett, Sacks, &

Trichopoulous, 1995). Recent evidence supporting the concept that substituting PUFA for saturated fat in the diet is cardioprotective comes from a meta-analysis of eight randomized clinical trials involving 13,614 subjects randomized to receive either high- or low-dietary PUFA. After an average follow-up period of 4.25 years, 1042 subjects developed coronary heart disease (MI or death from coronary heart disease) and the energy intake from PUFA averaged 14.9% of total calories in the intervention group compared to 5% in the control group. Overall, the risk in the intervention group was reduced by 19% compared to the control group and the risk reduction in coronary heart disease was estimated to be 10% per each 5% *increase* in energy from PUFA (Mozaffarian, Micha, & Wallace, 2010).

Increasing consumption of PUFA has been found to lower high-density lipoprotein cholesterol (Lewington et al., 2007) and may also improve insulin resistance (Salmeron et al., 2001; Summers et al., 2002) and reduce systemic inflammation (De Caterina, Liao, & Libby, 2000; Ferrucci et al., 2006; Pischon et al., 2003). Furthermore, specific types of PUFA may offer greater cardioprotection than others (e.g., omega-3 linolenic acid versus omega-6 linoleic acid) and some investigators advocate lowering the ratio of omega-6 PUFA to omega-3 PUFA in order to maximize protection against MI and other forms of cardiovascular disease (Simopoulos, 2008).

Aspirin and Myocardial Infarction

The use of low dose (81 mg) aspirin for the primary prevention of MI has been examined in numerous studies involving men and women of various cultures. A meta-analysis of four randomized clinical trials found that daily intake confers a reduction of 30% in the rate of MI and a 15% reduction in the rate of developing any cardiovascular disease (Sanmuganathan, Ghahramani, Jackson, Wallis, & Ramsay, 2001). The authors concluded that the benefit exceeded the risk of gastrointestinal hemorrhage for individuals with a coronary event risk of at least 1.5% per year whereas aspirin had limited value for individuals at lesser risk levels. Ten-year risk can be accurately predicted by the *Framingham Coronary Heart Disease Risk Score Algorithm* (D'Agostino, Grundy, Sullivan, & Wilson, 2001). Current guidelines recommend chemoprevention of MI using low-dose aspirin in adults at higher risk and over the age of 50 years with the caveat that even low-dose aspirin is contraindicated in individuals with known allergies, bleeding diathesis, platelet disorders, and active peptic ulcer disease (Lauer, 2002).

Statins and Myocardial Infarction

The role of statins in reducing serum cholesterol thereby counteracting atherogenesis and reducing the risk of coronary heart disease including MI and strokes has been confirmed in a number of randomized clinical trials. In a meta-analysis of 10 studies involving 70,388 subjects *with known cardiovascular risk factors such as diabetes at baseline*, daily statin intake reduced the incidence of major coronary events (MI or coronary death) by 30% (Brugts et al., 2009). In a meta-analysis of 20 studies enrolling 63,899 subjects at relatively low risk, daily statin intake reduced the incidence of MI by 23% (Mills et al., 2008). In addition to lowering serum cholesterol (and particularly LDL cholesterol), statins may also exert a stabilizing influence on evolving atheromatous plaques thereby diminishing their propensity to rupture and cause a MI (Ray & Cannon, 2005). Based on these results, the prescription of statins is now routine in developed countries as an effective chemopreventive strategy to reduce the risk of MI and other cardiovascular events.

Estrogen Replacement Therapy and Myocardial Infarction

Estrogen is a powerful hormone that has significant physiological effects related to cardiovascular health. During the premenopausal years during which women produce estrogens via the ovarian axis, cholesterol levels in women average about 10 mg/dL less than men of corresponding age. Correspondingly, women have lower rates of MIs and other cardiovascular events than men up until about age 65 years, presumably as a consequence of endogenous estrogen biosynthesis as well as many other factors.

Recent molecular studies suggest that estrogen produces vasodilatation through signal transduction of estrogen receptors in the arterial endothelium resulting in biosynthesis of nitric oxide (Mendelsohn & Karas, 1999). Estrogen replacement therapy (ERT) has been found to lower LDL (bad) cholesterol and elevate HDL (good) cholesterol, but is also associated with elevations in triglycerides (Espeland et al., 1998).

ERT is often prescribed to counteract hot flashes and other symptoms of menopause. Administration of estrogen and progesterone is often combined to mimic the female menstrual cycle as a form of hormone replacement therapy (HRT). Millions of women in the United States and throughout the world have received ERT or HRT. Many epidemiologic investigations have focused on the potential role of ERT/HRT in reducing the risk of thrombotic cardiovascular

events such as heart attack and stroke. Several meta-analyses of these investigations show good consistency of results and suggest that ERT/HRT for 5 years or more reduces the risk of coronary heart disease (MI or sudden cardiovascular death) by 35%–50% (Bush, 1990; Grady et al., 1992; Stampfer & Colditz, 1991). Meta-analysis of 25 studies published before 1997 found similar risk reductions for either ERT (30%) or HRT (34%). Albeit, ERT/HRT also appears to increase the risk of developing endometrial cancer and breast cancer (Barrett-Connor & Grady, 1998).

The consistently observed cardioprotective effects of ERT/HRT in observational (nonrandomized) epidemiologic investigations prompted the study of ERT/HRT in randomized clinical trials. Surprisingly, two large placebo-controlled randomized clinical trials, the Heart and Estrogen/Progestin Replacement Study (HERS) and the Women's Health Initiative (WHI), found that ERT/HRT *increased rather than decreased* the risk of thrombotic cardiovascular events (Anderson et al., 2004; Hulley et al., 1998; Rossouw et al., 2002). The discrepant results of the observational epidemiologic studies versus the randomized clinical trials have stimulated much debate regarding the risk versus benefit of ERT/HRT in postmenopausal women.

The Heart and Estrogen/Progestin Replacement Study (HERS) was specifically designed to test the hypothesis that treatment with 0.625 mg/day conjugated equine estrogen (CEE) plus 2.5 mg/day medroxyprogesterone acetate (MPA) would reduce the combined incidence of nonfatal MI and/or death from coronary heart disease compared to placebo in postmenopausal women *with prior history of MI, coronary revascularization, or angiographic evidence of coronary heart disease*. A total of 2763 postmenopausal women (age less than 80 years) consented for enrollment and were randomized for study, 1380 women to the treatment (HRT) arm and 1383 women to the placebo arm. After an average of 4.1 years of follow-up, there was no difference in the primary outcome of nonfatal myocardial and/or coronary death between the hormone and placebo arms. However, a post hoc time-trend analysis revealed a significant 52% increase in cardiovascular events (42.5 events/1000 person-years versus 28.0 events/1000 person-years) during the first year in the HRT group compared with placebo, with a nonsignificant trend toward fewer events in the treatment arm compared with placebo in later years (23.0/1000 person-years versus 34.4/1000 person-years) (Hulley et al., 1998).

WHI was initiated by the National Institutes of Health (NIH) in 1991 (Michels, 2006). The objective of this women's health research initiative was to conduct medical research into some of the major health problems of older women. In particular, randomized controlled trials were designed and funded that address cardiovascular disease, cancer, and osteoporosis. Two of the randomized interventions in WHI involved hormone replacement, a randomized double-blinded placebo-controlled trial of ERT (estrogen replacement alone) versus placebo, and a randomized double-blinded placebo-controlled trial of HRT (estrogen plus progestin) versus placebo.

In the HRT versus placebo clinical trial, 8506 women received equine estrogen plus progestin (MPA) and 8102 received placebo. After an average follow-up of 5.2 years, *the Data Safety and Monitoring Board* recommended termination of the trial due to increased hazards. Observed hazard ratios (HR) were significantly increased for multiple events: Coronary heart disease (HR = 1.29), breast cancer (HR = 1.26), stroke (HR = 1.41), pulmonary embolism (HR = 2.1), and total cardiovascular disease (HR = 1.22) (Rossouw et al., 2002).

In the ERT versus placebo clinical trial, 10,739 postmenopausal women, aged 50–79 years, with prior hysterectomy, were randomized to receive either equine estrogen (*n* = 5310) or placebo (*n* = 5429). This trial was terminated after 6.8 years of average follow-up due to significantly HR for multiple events of interest: Stroke (HR = 1.39), pulmonary embolism (HR = 1.34), and total cardiovascular disease (HR = 1.12) (Anderson et al., 2004).

The results of these three randomized clinical trials argue against the use of either ERT or HRT for alleged cardioprotection in either healthy postmenopausal women or those with a prior history of MI or other forms of coronary heart disease. Obviously, advocates of the administration of exogenous hormones to postmenopausal women can no longer point to a favorable risk versus benefit ratio (Writing Group for WHI, 2002).

It is important to note that subsequent analyses of the WHI trial data sets with stratification by age found that women aged 50–59 years or those who began taking ERT/HRT within 5 years of menopause had lower rates of coronary heart disease compared to women of similar age who received placebo (Manson et al., 2003). Nevertheless, controversy still rages as to whether ERT/HRT has cardiovascular benefit or risk in postmenopausal women (Stevenson, 2009).

Selective Cyclooxygenase-2 (COX-2) Inhibitors and Myocardial Infarction

Nonsteroidal anti-inflammatory drugs (NSAIDs) such as aspirin, ibuprofen, and naproxen relieve pain and inflammation by inhibiting the chief rate-limiting enzymes of prostaglandin biosynthesis: Cyclooxygenase-1 and -2 (COX-1 and COX-2). Both COX-1 and COX-2 convert arachidonic acid and certain other fatty acids into prostaglandins. The prostaglandins are short-acting long-chain hydrocarbon molecules that have a bewildering array of cellular effects. The primary inflammatory prostaglandin, PGE-2, is essential for modulating the inflammatory response of the innate immune system.

The cyclooxygenase enzymes, COX-1 and COX-2, are encoded by two separate genes with substantial homology. However, COX-1 continually synthesizes low levels of prostaglandins in most tissues whereas COX-2 is normally silent unless it is induced by inflammatory stimuli. Induction of COX-2 increases the biosynthesis of PGE-2 by 10- to 100-fold in inflamed tissues and so initiates the inflammatory cycle (e.g., vasodilatation, edema and influx of monocytes, macrophages, and lymphocytes of the immune system).

General NSAIDs such as aspirin and ibuprofen nonselectively inhibit both COX-1 and COX-2, and since COX-1 inhibition can lead to gastric irritation and peptic ulcers in some individuals, the development of drugs that selectively inhibit COX-2 became a priority for the pharmaceutical industry. Two such drugs, rofecoxib (Vioxx) produced by Merck and celecoxib (Celebrex) produced by Pfizer, were approved for prescriptive use in 1998 and soon captured a substantial share of the market for arthritis therapy. Both drugs were widely prescribed among patients with arthritic conditions and proved effective in relieving their pain and inflammation.

But the early success of the selective COX-2 inhibitors soon diminished as post-marketing studies appeared in the literature documenting increased rates of thrombotic cardiovascular events, particularly heart attacks, among rofecoxib users (Bombardier et al., 2000). And in dramatic fashion, the results of a double-blinded placebo-controlled randomized clinical trial designed to test rofecoxib for the chemoprevention of colonic polyps revealed a twofold increase in thrombotic cardiovascular events (including MI and stroke) among participants receiving 25 mg of rofecoxib daily (Bresalier et al., 2005). As a consequence of these findings, in September of 2004, Merck removed rofecoxib (Vioxx) from the world market.

Due to concern about a potential adverse cardiovascular class effect of COX-2 inhibitors, the Pfizer COX-2 blocker, celecoxib (Celebrex), has come under extreme scrutiny by the scientific and medical communities (as well as the general public). One highly publicized randomized clinical trial designed to test celecoxib for the chemoprevention of colonic polyps found 2.3-fold and 3.4-fold increases in the composite cardiovascular end point of death from cardiovascular causes, MI, stroke, or heart failure among participants receiving daily dosages of 200 mg or 400 mg of celecoxib, respectively (Solomon et al., 2005).

Subsequent to this activity, many investigators have queried available databases to examine the cardiovascular risk of both rofecoxib and celecoxib. Notably, differential effects have been noted for celecoxib compared to rofecoxib. In a meta-analysis of each drug based upon published observational studies, an adverse effect of rofecoxib was confirmed (RR = 2.19 for cardiovascular events, predominantly MI) *but not for celecoxib* (RR = 1.06) (McGettigan & Henry, 2006). Furthermore, results of a more comprehensive meta-analysis of celecoxib including 73 published studies also failed to find an effect of celecoxib (Harris, 2009). As shown in **FIGURE 4.8**, this investigation included data from 39 short-term randomized clinical trials, 26 observational case–control and cohort studies, and eight long-term randomized clinical trials. From this analysis, the composite estimate of relative risk for celecoxib and thrombotic cardiovascular events (primarily MI and stroke) was slightly less than unity (RR = 0.98) and the test for heterogeneity did not approach statistical significance. Finally, results of a large randomized clinical trial of 24,000 patients who required daily intake of nonsteroidal anti-inflammatory drugs for osteoarthritis or rheumatoid arthritis revealed that celecoxib was associated with *fewer* adverse cardiovascular events than conventional agents such as ibuprofen and naproxen (Nissen et al., 2016). Thus, based upon the totality of

available evidence from randomized clinical trials and observational studies, celecoxib taken at standard dosages shows no association with thrombotic cardiovascular risk.

Secondary Prevention of Myocardial Infarction

The risk of a recurrent MI decreases with strict blood pressure management, antiplatelet therapy, regulation of cholesterol and blood glucose, and lifestyle changes: Chiefly smoking cessation, regular exercise, limitation of alcohol consumption, and modification of diet. In regard to smoking cessation, counseling should be provided to the patient and family, along with pharmacologic therapy (including nicotine replacement) and formal smoking-cessation programs as appropriate. Counseling on physical activity and weight reduction is also advisable, and all patients recovering from MI should be encouraged to exercise for a minimum of 30 minutes, preferably daily but at least three or four times per week (walking, jogging, cycling, or other aerobic activity). Consensus statements on the secondary prevention of MI (with ST elevation) have recently been updated by the American College of Cardiology and the American Heart Association (Antman et al., 2004).

Dietary therapy low in saturated fat, salt, and cholesterol (less than 7% of total calories as saturated fat and less than 200 mg/d cholesterol) should be started after recovery from the initial MI and upon hospital discharge. In addition, evidence from randomized

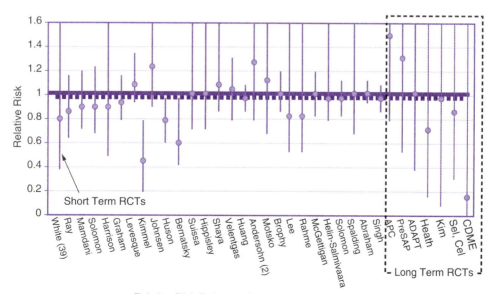

FIGURE 4.8 Meta-analysis of Celecoxib (Celebrex) and Cardiovascular Disease.

Reproduced from Harris, R. E. (2009). Cyclooxygenase-2 (COX-2) blockade in the chemoprevention of cancers of the colon, breast, prostate and lung. *Inflammopharmacology, 17*, 55–67.

clinical trials shows benefit with increased consumption of omega-3-PUFA. The *GISSA Prevenzione Trial (Gruppo Italiano per lo Studio della Sopravvivenza nell'Infarto)*, a randomized trial of 11,324 Italian patients surviving MI, found that addition of omega-3 PUFA reduced the relative risk of coronary death, nonfatal MI, or stroke by 10% (GISSA Prevenzione Trial Investigators, 1999). Total caloric intake should also be balanced with energy output to achieve and maintain a healthy weight.

Blood pressure management using angiotensin-converting enzyme (ACE) inhibiting agents following MI has proven extremely effective in reducing the recurrence risk in several randomized clinical trials. In a randomized placebo-controlled double-blinded trial of 2231 heart failure patients conducted in the United States, those patients who received the ACE-inhibitor, captopril ($n = 1115$), had 25% less recurrent MIs and 37% fewer deaths from cardiovascular events compared to patients receiving placebo ($n = 1116$) after 42 months average follow-up (Pfeffer et al., 1992).

In addition to antihypertensive medications, sustained therapy for heart arrhythmias using β-adrenergic-antagonist therapy (β-blockers) has also been shown to decrease mortality and morbidity and improve symptoms of cardiac ischemia in certain patients who have survived heart attacks (Yusuf, Peto, Lewis, Collins, & Sleight, 1985). Furthermore, compared with other modalities, routine administration of β-adrenergic-antagonist therapy has a relatively favorable cost-effectiveness ratio (Goldman, Sia, Cook, Rutherford, & Weinstein, 1988; Goldman, Weinstein, Goldman, & Williams, 1991).

Statin therapy has also proven to be beneficial in reducing the risk of subsequent cardiovascular events or death following MI. In a large double-blinded placebo-controlled randomized clinical trial involving 3086 patients from centers in Europe, North and South America, and Australia, administration of a statin reduced the incidence of the composite end point (death, nonfatal acute MI, cardiac arrest with resuscitation, or recurrent myocardial ischemia) by 16% (Schwartz et al., 2001). Statin therapy administered to reduce even average cholesterol levels has proven beneficial and cost-effective for men and women who have suffered a first MI (Goldman et al., 1988; Sacks et al., 1996).

Antiplatelet therapy with low-dose aspirin or other antithrombolytic agent (e.g., clopidogrel) has been shown in several studies to reduce the recurrence risk (Peters et al., 2003). On the basis of 12 randomized trials involving 18,788 patients with prior MI, the Antithrombotic Trialists' Collaboration (2002) reported a 25% reduction in the risk of recurrent infarction, stroke, or vascular death in patients receiving prolonged antiplatelet therapy (36 fewer events for every 1000 patients treated). No antiplatelet therapy has proved superior to aspirin in this population, and daily doses of aspirin between 80 and 325 mg appear to be effective (Sagar & Smyth, 1999). Further justification for the use of statins, β-blockers, ACE inhibitors, and antiplatelet drugs to prevent recurrence/death after a first MI comes from a large observational study conducted in the United States (Setoguchi et al., 2008). Using data derived from pharmacy assistance programs and Medicare in New Jersey and Pennsylvania between 1995 and 2004, investigators examined temporal trends in mortality after hospitalization for acute MI in 21,484 community-dwelling elderly patients (average age 80 years) who survived at least 30 days after discharge. Results showed that after adjusting for patient demographics, comorbidities, duration of hospitalization, patterns of previous health service use, and clustering of patients within hospitals, the mortality after MI decreased significantly by approximately 3% per year. These findings and that from other national and international investigations (Pilote, Lavoie, Ho, & Eisenberg, 2000; Swedberg et al., 1992) support the value of implementing proven secondary prevention medications for patients who survive the initial peril of MI. Summarizing, there is a large and expanding body of scientific evidence that has validated the importance of using established secondary prevention therapies (aspirin, clopidogrel, statins, β-blockers, and ACE inhibitors) either alone or in combination in reducing long-term risk of death and recurrent MI in patients with prior coronary heart disease (Gutstein & Fuster, 1998; Moe & Wong, 2010).

Emergency Services for Acute Myocardial Infarction

Immediate action based upon symptoms of an impending MI can prove lifesaving. Ventricular defibrillation can reinstitute the heartbeat in cardiac arrest, and rapid treatment can prevent sustained ischemic damage to the myocardium. Advanced paramedical services include preliminary electrocardiography and administration of oxygen, nitroglycerin, and antithrombotic agents (aspirin) as appropriate. Reperfusion techniques (e.g., thrombolytic therapy, percutaneous coronary intervention [PCI], or bypass surgery) are central to the modern treatment of acute MI (Antman et al., 2004).

References

Alpert, J. S., Thygesen, K., Antman, E., & Bassand, J. P. (2000). Myocardial infarction redefined—a consensus document of The Joint European Society of Cardiology/American College of Cardiology Committee for the redefinition of myocardial infarction. *Journal of the American College of Cardiology, 36*(3), 959–969.

Anderson, G. L., Limacher, M., Assaf, A. R., Bassford, T., Beresford, S. A., Black, H., … Wassertheil-Smoller, S. (2004). Effects of conjugated equine estrogen in postmenopausal women with hysterectomy: The Women's health initiative randomized controlled trial. *JAMA, 291*(14), 1701–1712.

Andraws, R., Berger, J. S., & Brown, D. L. (2005). Effects of antibiotic therapy on outcomes of patients with coronary artery disease: A metaanalysis of randomized controlled trials. *JAMA, 293*(21), 2641–2467.

Antithrombotic Trialists' Collaboration. (2002). Collaborative meta-analysis of randomised trials of antiplatelet therapy for prevention of death, myocardial infarction, and stroke in high risk patients. *BMJ, 324*, 71–86.

Antman, E. M., Anbe, D. T., Armstrong, P. W., Bates, E. R., Green, L. A., Hand, M., … Smith, S. C. Jr. (2004). ACC/AHA guidelines for the management of patients with ST-elevation myocardial infarction—executive summary. A report of the American College of Cardiology/American Heart Association Task Force on Practice Guidelines (Writing Committee to revise the 1999 guidelines for the management of patients with acute myocardial infarction). *Journal of the American College of Cardiology, 44*(3), 671–719.

Barrett-Connor, E., & Grady, D. (1998). Hormone replacement therapy, heart disease, and other considerations. *Annual Review of Public Health, 19*, 55–72.

Beamer, A. D., Lee, T. H., Cook, E. F., Brand, D. A., Rouan, G. W., Weisberg, M. C., … Goldman, L. (1987). Diagnostic implications for myocardial ischemia of the circadian variation of the onset of chest pain. *American Journal of Cardiology, 60*(13), 998–1002.

Bombardier, C., Laine, L., Reicin, A., Shapiro, D., Burgos-Vargas, R., Davis, B., … VIGOR Study Group. (2000). Comparison of upper gastrointestinal toxicity of rofecoxib and naproxen in patients with rheumatoid arthritis. VIGOR study group. *The New England Journal of Medicine, 343*(21), 1520–1528.

Bresalier, R., Sandler, R., Quan, H., Bolognese, J. A., Oxenius, B., Horgan, K., … Adenomatous Polyp Prevention on Vioxx (APPROVe) trial investigators. (2005). Cardiovascular events associated with rofecoxib in a colorectal adenoma chemoprevention trial. *The New England Journal of Medicine, 352*(11), 1092–1102.

Brugts, J. J., Yetgin, T., Hoeks, S. E., Gotto, A. M., Shepherd, J., Westendorp, R. G., … Deckers, J. W. (2009). The benefits of statins in people without established cardiovascular disease but with cardiovascular risk factors: Meta-analysis of randomized controlled trials. *BMJ, 338*, b2376.

Bush, T. L. (1990). The epidemiology of cardiovascular disease in postmenopausal women. *Annals of the New York Academy of Sciences, 592*, 263–271.

Curfman, G. D. (1993). Is exercise beneficial—or hazardous—to your heart? *The New England Journal of Medicine, 329*, 1730–1731.

D'Agostino, R. B. Sr., Grundy, S., Sullivan, L. M., & Wilson, P. (2001). Validation of the Framingham coronary heart disease prediction scores: Results of a multiple ethnic groups investigation. *JAMA, 286*, 180–187.

Dawber, T. R., & Kannel, W. B. (1968). The early diagnosis of coronary heart disease. In C. L. E. H. Sharp, & H. Keen (Eds.), *Presymptomatic detection and early diagnosis: A critical appraisal* (pp. 257–281). London: Pitman Medical.

De Caterina, R., Liao, J. K., & Libby, P. (2000). Fatty acid modulation of endothelial activation. *The American Journal of Clinical Nutrition, 71*, 213S–223S.

Espeland, M. A., Marcovina, S. M., Miller, V., Wood, P. D., Wasilauskas, C., Sherwin, R., … Bush, T. L. (1998). Effect of postmenopausal hormone therapy on lipoprotein(a) concentration: PEPI investigators: Postmenopausal Estrogen/Progestin Interventions. *Circulation, 97*, 979–986.

Fantidis, P., Perez De Prada, T., Fernandez-Ortiz, A., Carcia-Touchard, A., Alfonso, F., Sabaté, M., … Macaya, C. (2002). Morning cortisol production in coronary heart disease patients. *European Journal of Clinical Investigation, 32*(5), 304–308.

Ferrucci, L., Cherubini, A., Bandinelli, S., Bartali, B., Corsi, A., Lauretani, F., … Guralnik, J. M. (2006). Relationship of plasma polyunsaturated fatty acids to circulating inflammatory markers. *The Journal of Clinical Endocrinology & Metabolism, 91*, 439–446.

GISSA Prevenzione Trial Investigators. (1999). Dietary supplementation with n-3 polyunsaturated fatty acids and vitamin E after myocardial infarction: Results of the GISSI-Prevenzione trial. Gruppo Italiano per lo Studio della Sopravvivenza nell'Infarto miocardico. *Lancet, 354*(9177), 447–455.

Global Burden of Disease 2016 Causes of Death Collaborators. (2017). Global, regional, and national under-5 mortality, adult mortality, age-specific mortality, and life expectancy, 1970–2016: A systematic analysis for the Global Burden of Disease Study, 2016. *Lancet, 390*, 1084–1150.

Goff, D. C., Nichaman, M. Z., Chan, W., Ramsey, D. J., Labarthe, D. R., & Ortiz, C. (1997). Greater incidence of hospitalized myocardial infarction among Mexican Americans than non-Hispanic whites. The Corpus Christi Heart Project, 1988–1992. *Circulation, 95*(6), 1433–1440.

Goldberg, R. J., Gore, J. M., Alpert, J. S., & Dalen, J. E. (1986). Recent changes in attack and survival rates of acute myocardial infarction (1975 through 1981). The Worcester heart attack study. *JAMA, 255*(20), 2774–2779.

Goldberg, R. J., Yarzebski, J., Lessard, D., & Gore, J. M. (1999). A two-decades (1975–1995) long experience in the incidence, in-hospital and long-term case-fatality rates of acute myocardial infarction: A community-wide perspective. *Journal of the American College of Cardiology, 33*(6), 1533–1539.

Goldman, L., Sia, S. T., Cook, E. F., Rutherford, J. D., & Weinstein, M. C. (1988). Costs and effectiveness of routine therapy with long-term beta-adrenergic antagonists after acute myocardial infarction. *The New England Journal of Medicine, 319*, 152–157.

Goldman, L., Weinstein, M. C., Goldman, P. A., & Williams, L. W. (1991). Cost-effectiveness of HMG-CoA reductase inhibition for primary and secondary prevention of coronary heart disease. *JAMA, 265*, 1145–1151.

Grady, D., Rubin, S. M., Petitti, D. B., Fox, C. S., Black, D., Ettinger, B., … Cummings, S. R. (1992). Hormone therapy to prevent disease and prolong life in postmenopausal women. *Annals of Internal Medicine, 117*, 1016–1037.

Gutstein, D. E., & Fuster, V. (1998). Pathophysiologic bases for adjunctive therapies in the treatment and secondary prevention of acute myocardial infarction. *Clinical Cardiology, 21*, 161–168.

Harris, R. E. (2009). Cyclooxygenase-2 (COX-2) blockade in the chemoprevention of cancers of the colon, breast, prostate and lung. *Inflammopharmacology, 17*, 55–67.

Hoffman, B. B., & Lefkowitz, R. J. (1982). Adrenergic receptors in the heart. *Annual Review of Physiology, 44*, 475–484.

Hulley, S., Grady, D., Bush, T., Furberg, C., Herrington, D., Riggs, B., ... Vittinghoff, E. (1998). Randomized trial of estrogen plus progestin for secondary prevention of coronary heart disease in postmenopausal women: Heart and Estrogen/progestin Replacement Study (HERS) Research Group. *JAMA, 280*, 605–613.

Jensen, G., Nyboe, J., Appleyard, M., & Schnohr, P. (1991). Risk factors for acute myocardial infarction in Copenhagen, II: Smoking, alcohol intake, physical activity, obesity, oral contraception, diabetes, lipids, and blood pressure. *European Heart Journal, 12*(3), 298–308.

Kannel, W. B. (1964). Cigarette smoking and coronary heart disease. *Annals of Internal Medicine, 60*, 1103–1106.

Kannel, W. B., Castelli, W. P., & McNamara, P. M. (1968). Cigarette smoking and risk of coronary heart disease. Epidemiologic clues to pathogenesis. The Framingham Study. *National Cancer Institute Monograph, 28*, 9–20.

Kannel, W. B., Schwartz, M. J., & McNamara, P. M. (1969). Blood pressure and risk of coronary heart disease: The Framingham study. *Diseases of the Chest, 56*(1), 43–52.

Kannel, W. B., Gordon, T., & Schwartz, M. J. (1971). Systolic versus diastolic blood pressure and risk of coronary heart disease. The Framingham study. *American Journal of Cardiology, 27*(4), 335–346.

Kannel, W. B., Castelli, W. P., Gordon, T., & McNamara, P. M. (1971). Serum cholesterol, lipoproteins, and the risk of coronary heart disease. The Framingham study. *Annals of Internal Medicine, 74*(1), 1–12.

Kannel, W. B., & McGee, D. L. (1979). Diabetes and cardiovascular disease. The Framingham study. *JAMA, 241*(19), 2035–2038.

Kannel, W. B., D'Agostino, R. B., Wilson, P. W. F., Belanger, A. J., & Gagnon, D. R. (1990). Diabetes, fibrinogen, and risk of cardiovascular disease: The Framingham experience. *American Heart Journal, 120*, 672–676.

Kannel, W. B. (1996). Blood pressure as a cardiovascular risk factor: Prevention and treatment. *JAMA, 275*(20), 1571–1576.

Keys, A., Aravanis, C., Blackburn, H. W., Van Buchem, F. S., Buzina, R., Djordjević, B. D., ... Taylor, H. L. (1967). Epidemiologic studies related to coronary heart disease: Characteristics of men aged 40–59 in seven countries. *Acta Medica Scandinavica, Supplementum, 460*, 1–392.

Keys, A. (1970). *Coronary heart disease in seven countries.* New York, NY: American Heart Association, Monograph No. 29.

Keys, A., Aravanis, C., Blackburn, H., Buzina, R., Djordjevic, B. S., Dontas, A. S., ... Van Buchem, F. S. P. (1980). *Seven countries. A multivariate analysis of death and coronary heart disease* (pp. 1–381). Cambridge, MA and London: Harvard University Press.

Kuller, L., Neaton, J., Caggiula, A., & Falvo-Gerard, L. (1980). Primary prevention of heart attacks: The multiple risk factor intervention trial. *American Journal of Epidemiology, 112*(2), 185–199.

Kumar, V., Abbas, A. K., & Aster, J. C. (2017). *Robbins and cotran pathologic basis of disease* (10th ed.). Amsterdam, Netherlands: Elsevier.

Lauer, M. S. (2002). Aspirin for primary prevention of coronary events. *The New England Journal of Medicine, 346*(19), 1468–1474.

Levy, D. (1993). A multifactorial approach to coronary disease risk assessment. *Clinical and Experimental Hypertension, 15*(6), 1077–1086.

Levy, D., & Thom, T. J. (1998). Death rates from coronary disease—progress and a puzzling paradox. *The New England Journal of Medicine, 339*, 915–917.

Lewington, S., Whitlock, G., Clarke, R., Sherliker, P., Emberson, J., Halsey, J., ... Collins, R. (2007). Blood cholesterol and vascular mortality by age, sex, and blood pressure: A meta-analysis of individual data from 61 prospective studies with 55,000 vascular deaths. *Lancet, 370*, 1829–1839.

Mackay, J., & Mensah, G. (2004). *Atlas of heart disease and stroke.* Geneva, Switzerland: World Health Organization.

Manson, J. E., Tosteson, H., Ridker, P. M., Satterfield, S., Hebert, P., O'Connor, G. T., ... Hennekens, C. H. (1992). The primary prevention of myocardial infarction. *The New England Journal of Medicine, 326*(21), 1406–1416.

Manson, J. E., Hsia, P. H. J., Johnson, K. C., Rossouw, J. E., Assaf, A. R., Lasser, N. L., ... Women's Health Initiative Investigators (2003). Estrogen plus progestin and the risk of coronary heart disease. *The New England Journal of Medicine, 349*(6), 523–534.

McGettigan, P., & Henry, D. (2006). Cardiovascular risk and inhibition of cyclooxygenase: A systematic review of the observational studies of selective and nonselective inhibitors of cyclooxygenase 2. *JAMA, 296*(13), 1633–1644.

McGovern, P. G., Jacobs, D. R. Jr., Shahar, E., et al. (2001). Trends in acute coronary heart disease mortality, morbidity, and medical care from 1985 through 1997: The Minnesota heart survey. *Circulation, 104*(1), 19–24.

McQueen, M. J., Hawken, S., Wang, X., Ounpuu, S., Sniderman, A., Probstfield, J., ... Yusuf, S. (2008). Lipids, lipoproteins, and apolipoproteins as risk markers of myocardial infarction in 52 countries (the INTERHEART study): A case-control study. *Lancet, 372*(9634), 224–233.

Mendelsohn, M. E., & Karas, R. H. (1999). The protective effects of estrogen on the cardiovascular system. *The New England Journal of Medicine, 340*, 1801–1811.

Mendis, S., Puska, P., Norrving, B. (2011). In S. Mendis, P. Puska, B. Norrving (Eds.), *Global Atlas on cardiovascular disease prevention and control.* Geneva, Switzerland: World Health Organization, World Heart Federation, World Stroke Organization.

Mendis, S., Thygesen, K., Kuulasmaa, K., Giampaoli, S., Mähönen, M., Ngu Blackett, K., ... Lisheng, L. (2011). World Health Organization definition of myocardial infarction: 2008-09 revision. *International Journal of Epidemiology, 40*(1), 139–146.

Michels, K. B. (2006). The women's health initiative—curse or blessing? *International Journal of Epidemiology, 35*(4), 814–816.

Mills, E. J., Rachlis, B., Wu, P., Devereaux, P. J., Arora, P., & Perri, D. (2008). Primary prevention of cardiovascular mortality and events with statin treatments: A network metaanalysis involving more than 65,000 patients. *Journal of the American College of Cardiology, 52*(22), 1769–1781.

Mittleman, M. A., Maclure, M., Tofler, G. H., Sherwood, J. B., Goldberg, R. J., & Muller, J. E. (1993). Triggering of acute myocardial infarction by heavy physical exertion—protection against triggering by regular exertion. *The New England Journal of Medicine, 329*, 1677–1683.

Moe, K. T., & Wong, P. (2010). Current trends in diagnostic biomarkers of acute coronary syndrome. *Annals of the Academy of Medicine of Singapore, 39*(3), 210–215.

Mozaffarian, D., Micha, R., & Wallace, S. (2010). Effects on coronary heart disease of increasing polyunsaturated fat in place of saturated fat: A systematic review and meta-analysis of randomized controlled trials. *PLoS Medicine, 7*(3), e1000252.

Muller, J. E., Stone, P. H., Turi, Z. G., Rutherford, J. D., Czeisler, C. A., Parker, C., … Braunwald, E. (1985). Circadian variation in the frequency of onset of acute myocardial infarction. *The New England Journal of Medicine, 313*(21), 1315–1322.

National Heart, Lung and Blood Institute. (2006). *Heart attack warning signs.* Bethesda, MD: National Institutes of Health.

National Heart, Lung and Blood Institute. (2009). *Morbidity and mortality: 2009. Chartbook on cardiovascular, lung, and blood diseases.* Bethesda, MD: National Institutes of Health.

Nichaman, M. Z., Wear, M. L., Goff, D. C., Jr., & Labarthe, D. R. (1993). Hospitalization rates for myocardial infarction among Mexican-Americans and non-Hispanic whites. The Corpus Christi Heart Project. *Annals of Epidemiology, 3*(1), 42–48.

Nissen, S. E., Yeomans, N. D., Solomon, D. H., Lüscher, T. F., Libby, P., Husni, M. E., … Lincoff, A. M. (2016). Cardiovascular safety of celecoxib, naproxen, or ibuprofen for arthritis. *The New England Journal of Medicine, 325*(26), 2519–2529.

Nyboe, J., Jensen, G., Appleyard, M., & Schnohr, P. (1989). Risk factors for acute myocardial infarction in Copenhagen. I: Hereditary, educational and socioeconomic factors. Copenhagen City Heart Study. *European Heart Journal, 10*(10), 910–916.

Parikh, N. I., Gona, P., Larson, M. G., Fox, C. S., Benjamin, E. J., Murabito, J. M., … Levy, D. (2009). Long-term trends in myocardial infarction incidence and case fatality in the National Heart, Lung, and Blood Institute's Framingham Heart Study. *Circulation, 119*, 1203–1210.

Peters, R. J., Mehta, S. R., Fox, K. A., Zhao, F., Lewis, B. S., Kopecky, S. L., … Yusuf, S. (2003). Effects of aspirin dose when used alone or in combination with clopidogrel in patients with acute coronary syndromes: Observations from the Clopidogrel in Unstable angina to prevent Recurrent Events (CURE) study. *Circulation, 108*(14), 1682–1687.

Pfeffer, M. A., Braunwald, E., Moye, L. A., Basta, L., Brown, E. J., Cuddy, T. E., … Morton Hawkins, C. (1992). Effect of captopril on mortality and morbidity in patients with left ventricular dysfunction after myocardial infarction. Results of the survival and ventricular enlargement trial. The SAVE Investigators. *The New England Journal of Medicine, 327*(10), 669–677.

Pilote, L., Lavoie, F., Ho, V., & Eisenberg, M. J. (2000). Changes in the treatment and outcomes of acute myocardial infarction in Quebec, 1988–1995. *CMAJ, 163*, 31–36.

Pischon, T., Hankinson, S. E., Hotamisligil, G. S., Rifai, N., Willett, W. C., & Rimm, E. B. (2003). Habitual dietary intake of n-3 and n-6 fatty acids in relation to inflammatory markers among U.S. men and women. *Circulation, 108*, 155–160.

Ray, K. K., & Cannon, C. P. (2005). The potential relevance of the multiple lipid-independent (pleiotropic) effects of statins in the management of acute coronary syndromes. *Journal of the American College of Cardiology, 46*(8), 1425–1433.

Reynolds, K., Go, A. S., Leong, T. K., Boudreau, D. M., Cassidy-Bushrow, A. E., Fortmann, S. P., … Sidney, S. (2017). Trends in incidence of hospitalized acute myocardial infarction in the Cardiovascular Research Network (CVRN). *The American Journal of Medicine, 130*, 317–327.

Roger, V. L., Killian, J., Henkel, M., Weston, S. A., Goraya, T. Y., Yawn, B. P., … Jacobsen, S. J. (2002). Coronary disease surveillance in Olmsted County objectives and methodology. *Journal of Clinical Epidemiology, 55*(6), 593–601.

Rosamond, W. D., Chambless, L. E., Folsom, A. R., Cooper, L. S., Conwill, D. E., Clegg, L., … Wang, C. H. (1998). Trends in the incidence of myocardial infarction and in mortality due to coronary heart disease, 1987–1994. *The New England Journal of Medicine, 339*, 861–867.

Rosamond, W. D., Chambless, L. E., Heiss, G., Mosley, T. H., Coresh, J., Whitsel, E., … Folsom, A. R. (2012). Twenty-two year trends in incidence of myocardial infarction, CHD mortality, and case-fatality in four U.S. communities, 1987–2008. *Circulation, 125*(15), 1848–1857.

Rosamond, W. D., Chambless, L. E., Heiss, G., Mosley, T. H., Coresh, J., Whitsel, E., … Folsom, A. R. (2012). Twenty-two-year trends in incidence of myocardial infarction, coronary heart disease mortality, and case fatality in 4 US communities, 1987–2008. *Circulation, 125*(15), 1848–1857.

Rosenbaum, D. M., Rasmussen, S. G. F., & Kobilka, B. K. (2009). The structure and function of G-protein-coupled receptors. *Nature, 459*(7245), 356–363.

Rossouw, J. E., Anderson, G. L., Prentice, R. L., LaCroix, A. Z., Kooperberg, C., Stefanick, M. L., … Ockene, J. (2002). Risks and benefits of estrogen plus progestin in healthy postmenopausal women: Principal results from the Women's Health Initiative randomized controlled trial. *JAMA, 288*(3), 321–333.

Sacks, F. M., Pfeffer, M. A., Moye, L. A., Rouleau, J. L., Rutherford, J. D., Cole, T. G., … Braunwald, E. (1996). The effect of pravastatin on coronary events after myocardial infarction in patients with average cholesterol levels. Cholesterol and Recurrent Events Trial investigators. *The New England Journal of Medicine, 335*(14), 1001–1009.

Sagar, A., & Smyth, M. R. (1999). A comparative bioavailability study of different aspirin formulations using on-line multidimensional chromatography. *Journal of Pharmaceutical and Biomedical Analysis, 21*, 383–392.

Saikku, P., Leinonen, M., Tenkanen, L., Linnanmäki, E., Ekman, M. R., Manninen, V., … Huttunen, J. K. (1992). Chronic *Chlamydia pneumoniae* infection as a risk factor for coronary heart disease in the Helsinki Heart Study. *Annals of Internal Medicine, 116*(4), 273–278.

Salmeron, J., Hu, F. B., Manson, J. E., Stampfer, M. J., Colditz, G. A., Rimm, E. B., … Willett, W. C. (2001). Dietary fat intake and risk of type 2 diabetes in women. *The American Journal of Clinical Nutrition, 73*, 1019–1026.

Sanmuganathan, P. S., Ghahramani, P., Jackson, P. R., Wallis, E. J., & Ramsay, L. E. (2001). Aspirin for primary prevention of coronary heart disease: Safety and absolute benefit related to coronary risk derived from meta-analysis of randomised trials. *Heart, 85*, 265–271.

Schwartz, G. G., Olsson, A. G., Ezekowitz, M. D., Ganz, P., Oliver, M. F., Waters, D., … Stern, T. (2001). Effects of atorvastatin on early recurrent ischemic events in acute coronary syndromes: The MIRACL study: A randomized controlled trial. *JAMA, 285*, 1711–1718.

Setoguchi, S., Glynn, R. J., Avorn, J., Mittleman, M. A., Levin, R., & Winkelmayer, W. C. (2008). Improvements in long-term mortality after myocardial infarction and increased use of cardiovascular drugs after discharge: A 10-year trend analysis. *Journal of the American College of Cardiology, 51*, 1247–1254.

Simopoulos, A. P. (2008). The importance of the omega-6/omega-3 fatty acid ratio in cardiovascular disease and other chronic diseases. *Experimental Biology and Medicine* (Maywood), *233*, 674–688.

Siscovick, D. S., Weiss, N. S., Fletcher, R. H., & Lasky, T. (1984). The incidence of primary cardiac arrest during vigorous exercise. *The New England Journal of Medicine, 311*, 874–877.

Smeeth, L., Thomas, S. L., Hall, A. J., Hubbgard, R., Farrington, P., & Vallance, P. (2004). Risk of myocardial infarction and stroke after acute infection or vaccination. *The New England Journal of Medicine, 351*, 2611–2618.

Sofi, F., Cesari, F., Abbate, R., Gensini, G. F., & Casini, A. (2008). Adherence to Mediterranean diet and health status: Meta-analysis. *BMJ* (Clinical research ed.), *337*, a1344.

Solomon, S., McMurray, J., Pfeffer, M., Wittes, J., Fowler, R., Finn, P., ... Adenoma Prevention with Celecoxib (APC) Study Investigators. (2005). Cardiovascular risk associated with celecoxib in a clinical trial for colorectal adenoma prevention. *The New England Journal of Medicine, 352*(11), 1071–1080.

Stamler, J., Wentworth, D., & Neaton, J. D. (1986). Is relationship between serum cholesterol and risk of premature death from coronary heart disease continuous and graded? Findings in 356,222 primary screenees of the Multiple Risk Factor Intervention Trial (MRFIT). *JAMA, 256*(20), 2823–2828.

Stampfer, M. J., & Colditz, G. A. (1991). Estrogen replacement therapy and coronary heart disease: A quantitative assessment of the epidemiologic evidence. *Preventive Medicine, 1*, 47–63.

Stevenson, J. C. (2009). Hormone replacement therapy and cardiovascular disease revisited. *Menopause International, 15*, 55–57.

Summers, L. K., Fielding, B. A., Bradshaw, H. A., Ilic, V., Beysen, C., Clark, M. L., ... Frayn, K. N. (2002). Substituting dietary saturated fat with polyunsaturated fat changes abdominal fat distribution and improves insulin sensitivity. *Diabetologia, 45*, 369–377.

Swedberg, K., Held, P., Kjekshus, J., Rasmussen, K., Ryden, L., & Wedel, H. (1992). Effects of the early administration of enalapril on mortality in patients with acute myocardial infarction. Results of the Cooperative New Scandinavian Enalapril Survival Study II (CONSENSUS II). *The New England Journal of Medicine, 327*, 678–684.

Tunstall-Pedoe, H., Kuulasmaa, K., Amouyel, P., Arveiler, D., Rajakangas, A. M., & Pajak, A. (1994). Myocardial infarction and coronary deaths in the World Health Organization MONICA Project: Registration procedures, event rates, and case-fatality rates in 38 populations from 21 countries in four continents. *Circulation, 90*, 583–612.

Tunstall-Pedoe, H., Kuulasmaa, K., Mähönen, M., Tolonen, H., Ruokokoski, E., & Amouyel, P. (1999). Contribution of trends in survival and coronary-event rates to changes in coronary heart disease mortality: 10-year results from 37 WHO MONICA project populations. Monitoring trends and determinants in cardiovascular disease. *Lancet, 353*(9164), 1547–1557.

White, A. D., Rosamond, W. D., Chambless, L. E., Thomas, N., Conwill, D., Cooper, L. S., ... Folsom, A. R. (1999). Sex and race differences in short-term prognosis after acute coronary heart disease events: The Atherosclerosis Risk In Communities (ARIC) study. *American Heart Journal, 138*(3 Pt 1), 540–548.

Willett, W. C., Sacks, F., & Trichopoulous, A. (1995). Mediterranean diet pyramid: A cultural model for healthy eating. *The American Journal of Clinical Nutrition, 61*(6 Suppl.), 1402S–1406S.

Willich, S. N., Lewis, M., Lowel, H., Arntz, H. R., Schubert, F., & Schroder, R. (1993). Physical exertion as a trigger of acute myocardial infarction. *The New England Journal of Medicine, 329*, 1684–1690.

Wilson, P. W., D'Agostino, R. B., Levy, D., Belanger, A. M., Silbershatz, H., & Kannel, W. B. (1998). Prediction of coronary heart disease using risk factor categories. *Circulation, 97*(18), 1837–1847.

World Health Organization. (2017). *Cardiovascular disease.* Geneva, Switzerland: World Health Organization.

Writing Group for the Women's Health Initiative Investigators. (2002). Risks and benefits of estrogen plus progestin in healthy postmenopausal women: Principal results from the Women's Health Initiative randomized controlled trial. *JAMA, 288*(3), 321–333.

Yusuf, S., Peto, R., Lewis, J., Collins, R., & Sleight, P. (1985). Beta blockade during and after myocardial infarction: An overview of the randomized trials. *Progress in Cardiovascular Diseases, 27*(5), 335–371.

Yusuf, S., Hawken, S., Ounpuu, S., Dans, T., Avezum, A., Lanas, F., ... INTERHEART Study Investigators. (2004). Effect of potentially modifiable risk factors associated with myocardial infarction in 52 countries (the INTERHEART study): Case-control study. *Lancet, 364*(9438), 937–952.

© Andrew Brookes/Getty Images

Epidemiology of Sudden Cardiac Death

▶ Introduction

Sudden cardiac death (SCD) is a catastrophic terminal event that can strike without warning at any age. SCDs account for more than one-third of all deaths from cardiovascular disease, which is the leading cause of death worldwide.

▶ Definition of Sudden Cardiac Death

The success of any epidemiologic study is contingent upon the accurate definition of the disease or outcome under investigation. *Sudden cardiac arrest* (SCA) explicitly refers to the abrupt loss of heart function and its ability to pump blood because of interruption of the electrical conduction system of the heart. Without the normal rhythmic transmission of electrical impulses to the myocardium, the heart is unable to pump blood to the brain thereby causing loss of consciousness, and without immediate treatment, the terminal result is SCD. The current definition of SCD is witnessed cardiac death within 1 hour of the loss of consciousness due to SCA, or unwitnessed cardiac death within 24 hours of being seen alive and well (Myerburg, 2002; Myerburg & Castellanos, 2007).

▶ Determining the Causes of Sudden Cardiac Death

Since SCD is unexpected, approximately two-thirds of all cases occur "*out-of hospital*" or are "*dead-on-arrival*" at the Emergency Room, and approximately 50% of these cases are unwitnessed (Zheng, Croft, Giles, & Mensah, 2001). As a consequence, the determination of the exact cause of SCD is an inexact process. Assignment of the cause of death must be inferred from the description of symptoms by witnesses, medical history of decedents, clinical signs and tests conducted post-mortem, and autopsy results.

Deaths that meet the criteria for SCD involve dysfunctional activity of the electrical conducting system of the heart resulting in abrupt and lethal cardiac arrhythmias. In studies of cardiac arrest wherein advanced life support was administered within minutes by trained emergency medical personnel, approximately 75% of cases manifested ventricular fibrillation or ventricular tachycardia whereas 25% had pulseless electrical activity or asystole (the total absence of electrical activity) (Cobb, Fahrenbruch, Olsufka, & Copass, 2002; Mehra, 2007).

Age Distribution and Causes of Sudden Cardiac Death

The most common conditions of the heart that predispose to SCA and death are ischemic heart disease and myocardial infarction. Nevertheless, there are many other potential causes such as cardiomyopathy, myocarditis, heart failure, and drug or alcohol intoxication. Furthermore, non-cardiac causes of sudden death such as *sudden infant death syndrome* (SIDS), pulmonary embolism, stroke, and aortic aneurysm must be ruled out to determine a sudden death of cardiac origin. The causes of SCD differ in men and women and by age, race, and ethnicity (**TABLE 5.1**). The age-specific rates of SCD show an early peak in children and adolescents and a much higher peak among older adults (**FIGURE 5.1**) (Adabag, Luepker, Roger, & Gersh, 2010; Chugh et al., 2008).

Causes of Sudden Cardiac Death in Adults

The majority of SCD cases (~97%) occur in adults over 35 years of age. In Western populations, approximately 80%–90% of adult male cases and 50%–60% of adult female cases involve ischemic heart disease, often in conjunction with acute myocardial infarction and/or myocardial scarring from a prior myocardial infarction. Other significant causes of SCD in adults include congestive heart failure, atrial fibrillation, and certain types

TABLE 5.1 Causes of Sudden Cardiac Death in Men, Women, Children and Adolescents

Causes of SCD	Men (%)	Women (%)	Children & Adolescents (%)
Ischemic heart disease	70–90	50–60	5–10
Acute MI	60–70	40–50	1–5
Old fibrotic MI	10–20	10–20	1–5
Congestive heart failure	10–20	20–30	
Atrial fibrillation	10–20	10–20	
Cardiomyopathy	1–5	1–5	40–50
Myocarditis	1–5	1–5	15–25
Congenital/inherited heart disease	<1	<1	20–30

Data from Chugh, S. S., Reinier, K., Teodorescu, C., Evanado, A., Kehr, E., Samara, M. A., . . . Jui, J. (2008). Epidemiology of sudden cardiac death: Clinical and research implications. *Progress in Cardiovascular Diseases, 51*(3), 213–228; Adabag, A. S., Luepker, R. V., Roger, V. L., & Gersh, B. J. (2010). Sudden cardiac death: Epidemiology and risk factors. *Nature Reviews Cardiology, 7*(4), 216–225.

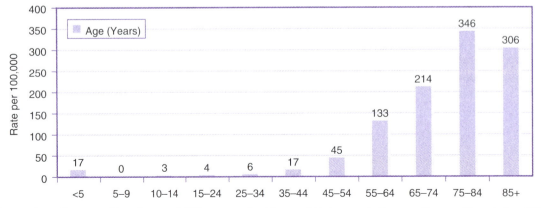

FIGURE 5.1 Age-Specific Annual Incidence of SCD among Residents of Multnomah County, Oregon (*Population 660,486*).

Data from Chugh, S. S., Reinier, K., Teodorescu, C., Evanado, A., Kehr, E., Samara, M. A., . . . Jui, J. (2008). Epidemiology of sudden cardiac death: Clinical and research implications. *Progress in Cardiovascular Diseases, 51*(3), 213–228.

of cardiomyopathy (Table 5.1). Because of the strong association of SCD with ischemic heart disease and myocardial infarction, there is some confusion about the distinction between these three conditions (Chugh et al., 2008; Hayashi, Shimizu, & Albert, 2015).

▶ Ischemic Heart Disease, Myocardial Infarction, and Sudden Cardiac Death

The symptoms and physiology of SCA and SCD are often the sequela of ischemic heart disease and myocardial infarction. Autopsy studies of adult cases of SCD show that up to 90% of men and 60% of women had severe underlying ischemic heart disease and about 60% of adult cases showed signs of acute myocardial infarction or fibrosis from pre-existing myocardial infarction (Adabag, Peterson, et al., 2010; Davies, 1992; Farb et al., 1995).

SCA specifically refers to dysfunction of the electrical conductance system of the heart with sudden and unexpected loss of consciousness and rapid demise, most often before emergency services arrive on the scene. Classically, SCD is preceded by ventricular tachycardia and ventricular fibrillation followed by asystole and total loss of ventricular function.

Ischemic heart disease, by definition, refers to the occlusion of coronary arteries by atherosclerotic plaque and diminished blood flow to the myocardium. As an example of the chain of events involving ischemic heart disease and acute myocardial infarction that could trigger SCD, total occlusion of the left main coronary artery due to a ruptured atherosclerotic plaque could abruptly interrupt the Purkinje electrical conductance pathway of the heart thereby causing an acute myocardial infarction, ventricular tachycardia, and sudden death.

In contrast to SCA and SCD, acute myocardial infarction refers to the infarct (death) of myocardial tissue with characteristic symptoms such as angina pectoris (chest pain), shortness of breath, and rapid heart rate *but without loss of consciousness*. The majority of myocardial infarctions are caused by the occlusion of coronary arteries by atherosclerotic plaque, or embolic clots emanating from a ruptured plaque. Patients with ischemic heart disease who suddenly die from an acute myocardial infarction constitute a large subset of SCDs. Prior myocardial infarction and significant scarring of the myocardium also increases the likelihood of abrupt onset of ventricular tachycardia and SCD (Kuller et al., 1973; Kannel et al., 1987; Davies, 1992; Farb et al., 1995; Virmani, Kolodgie, Burke, Farb, & Schwartz, 2000).

▶ Heart Failure and Sudden Cardiac Death

According to the American Heart Association, heart failure is *"a complex clinical syndrome that can result from any structural or functional cardiac disorder that impairs the ability of the ventricle to fill or eject blood."* With aging of the populations in developed nations, the prevalence of heart failure has dramatically increased. In the United States, more than 7 million Americans have heart failure and more than 300,000 of these patients die annually. Of all deaths in patients with heart failure, 40%–50% are classified as SCD. The presence of heart failure can significantly alter the electrical conducting system of the heart predisposing to sudden lethal arrhythmias and SCD (Tomaselli & Zipes, 2004).

▶ Atrial Fibrillation and Sudden Cardiac Death

Atrial fibrillation (AF) is the most common type of heart arrhythmia affecting more than 33 million people worldwide (Chugh et al., 2014). Chronic AF significantly increases the risk of stroke, heart failure, all-cause mortality, and SCD. Several observational cohort studies show a significant increase in SCD rates among AF patients. For example, in the *Atherosclerosis Risk in Communities* cohort of 15,439 participants, patients with AF were at 2.5-fold greater risk of SCD than those without AF (Chen et al., 2013). Two recently completed randomized clinical trials of AF patients who received different anticoagulant therapies provide confirmation of the high risk of SCD associated with AF. In the *Randomized Evaluation of Long-Term Anticoagulant Therapy* study of warfarin versus dabigatran, SCD accounted for 305 (22%) of the 1371 deaths observed (Marijon et al., 2013), and in the *ENGAGE* study of warfarin versus edoxaban, SCD accounted for 749 (32%) of the 2349 deaths observed (Eisen et al., 2016). In a population-based case control study from the *Oregon Sudden Unexpected Death* Study, the findings suggested that AF in combination with congestive heart failure may amplify the risk of SCD (Piccini & Daubert, 2014; Reinier et al., 2014).

▶ Cardiomyopathy among Adults

Certain cardiomyopathies occur in adults in association with lethal arrhythmia and SCD.

Cardiomyopathies are most commonly detected among the elderly although they can manifest (albeit rarely) early in life. Rates are variable and are high in certain populations. In the Japanese population, 30%–35% of SCD cases are caused by cardiomyopathies compared to 10%–15% of cases in Western populations (Hayashi et al., 2015).

Hypertrophic cardiomyopathy classically refers to progressive enlargement and thickening of the left ventricle. This form of cardiomyopathy is usually caused by the inheritance of mutated genes that disrupt the formation of proteins needed for the normal development and function of myocytes (heart muscle cells). Disease progression is associated with necrosis of myocytes, fibrosis, and scarring of the myocardium, pathologies that increase the likelihood of heart failure, life-threatening arrhythmias, and SCD. Symptoms may manifest early or late in life and are exacerbated by vigorous exercise (Stroumpoulis, Pantazopoulos, & Xanthos, 2010).

Dilated cardiomyopathy is a progressive disease in which the heart chambers become dilated, the ventricular walls become thinned and stretched, and the pumping action of the ventricles declines. Causes of this form of cardiomyopathy are heterogeneous and include alcoholic cardiomyopathy, diabetic cardiomyopathy, viral myocarditis, exposure to certain drugs (cocaine, amphetamines) and chemotherapeutic agents (doxorubicin), and genetic predisposition (Luk, Ahn, Soor, & Butany, 2009).

Arrhythmogenic right ventricular cardiomyopathy is a heritable disease of heart muscle that results in fibro-fatty replacement of the right ventricle. This cardiomyopathy is one of the leading causes of SCD in young adults and athletes. Molecular, genetic and pathologic studies of cases reveal the presence of defective desmosomes that regulate cell-adhesion of myocytes in the myocardium. Several mutations in genes encoding desmosomal proteins have been identified that cause this form of arrhythmia (Corrado, Link, & Calkins, 2017; Marcus et al., 1982).

▶ Causes of Sudden Cardiac Death in Children and Adolescents

SCD in children and adolescents is a *rare* catastrophic event and the causes are markedly different from adults. Three types of conditions cause more than 90% of these cases: Cardiomyopathy (40%–50%), congenital or inherited anomalies (20%–30%), and myocarditis (15%–25%) (Table 5.1). It is noteworthy that approximately 25% of cases in young people occur during sports activities.

Cardiomyopathy

The most common cardiomyopathy observed in cases of SCD among children and adolescents is *hypertrophic cardiomyopathy* in which a portion of the heart (usually the left ventricle) becomes thickened and enlarged. This anomaly is caused by heritable genetic mutations associated with abnormalities in the development of proteins essential for the contraction of sarcomeres (functional units of striated muscle) in the heart. Hypertrophic cardiomyopathy as well as other pathological conditions of the myocardium can abruptly induce lethal arrhythmias, particularly with strenuous exercise in young athletes (Gajewski & Saul, 2010; Maron et al., 1996).

▶ Connective Tissue Disease

Connective tissue diseases are a group of chronic inflammatory diseases that can cause cardiac fibrosis (scarring), conduction defects, arrhythmia, and in some cases, SCD. Certain connective tissue disorders such as systemic sclerosis, systemic lupus erythematosus, and Sjögren's syndrome have an autoimmune etiology, whereas others such as Marfan syndrome and Ehlers–Danlos syndrome are heritable genetic disorders (Lazzerini et al., 2006; Murphy-Ryan, Psychogios, & Lindor, 2010).

Marfan syndrome is an autosomal dominant genetic disorder of connective tissue that affects multiple organ systems. This syndrome is caused by mutations in the *fibrillin-1* gene leading to abnormal development of microfibrils that provide structural support to connective tissue throughout the body, including the heart. Sudden death in individuals with Marfan syndrome is most commonly the result of acute aortic dissection; nevertheless, cases of SCD due to lethal cardiac arrhythmias have also been observed. Pregnancy, exercise, and trauma have been found to heighten the risk of SCD in individuals with Marfan syndrome (Byard, 2006).

▶ Congenital and Inherited Anomalies of the Heart

Congenital and inherited anomalies that increase the risk of SCD include coronary artery anomalies and rare forms of arrhythmias such as Long QT syndrome, Short QT syndrome, Brugada syndrome, and Wolff–Parkinson–White syndrome (Gajewski & Saul, 2010).

Long and Short QT syndromes are autosomal dominant hereditary disorders of electrical channels in which affected individuals have abnormally long or short QT-intervals and propensity to develop potentially lethal ventricular arrhythmias. In these syndromes, mutations in genes that regulate the sodium potassium pump cause dysregulation of action potentials and abnormalities of heart rhythm that heighten the risk of SCD (Tse, Chan, Kenug, & Yan, 2017).

Myocarditis

Myocarditis refers to infection of the myocardium by viruses (Coxsackie B virus, enterovirus, adenovirus, influenza), bacteria (streptococci, meningococci, clostridia), or other microbes (fungi, plasmodia, filaria). Acute myocarditis occurs primarily in children and adolescents and is characterized by focal areas of inflammation, necrosis (death) of myocytes, and infiltrates of lymphocytes and other immune cells. Chronic myocarditis is more common in young adults and typically involves segmental fibrosis (scarring) and inflammation of the myocardium. Acute or chronic myocarditis can trigger an immune response to the infecting agent that interrupts the electrical conducting system of the heart to cause a potentially lethal cardiac arrhythmia (Fontaine, Fornes, & Fontaliran, 2001; Babu-Narayan et al., 2007; Drory et al., 1991).

Valvular Heart Disease

Rheumatic fever is a sequela to infection of the tonsils and pharynx by Group A β-*hemolytic streptococcus* bacteria. The condition is most common in young children, ages 5–15 years, particularly those living in countries with little access to antibiotics for the treatment of throat infections. Untreated infections can spread throughout the body and immune responses to the bacteria can cause severe inflammation and tissue damage, particularly in the joints and the heart valves resulting in *rheumatic heart disease*. Rheumatic heart disease remains a major cause of morbidity and mortality in developing countries and was responsible for more than 300,000 deaths in 2016. The vast majority (~85%) of these deaths occurred in populations living in underdeveloped regions of India, Southeast Asia, and sub-Saharan Africa (Talawar & Gupta, 2016). Furthermore, there are reports of SCD accounting for significant mortality in patients with rheumatic heart disease. In contrast, rheumatic fever and rheumatic heart disease are rare in developed countries such as the United States, Canada, Australia, Japan, Western Europe, and Scandinavia,

due in large part to improved hygienic conditions, better nutrition and the widespread use of antibiotics and other anti-microbial agents to treat infections (Celermajer, Chow, Marijon, Anstey, & Woo, 2012).

▶ Trauma

An unusual cause of SCD is *commotio cordis* which is due to non-penetrating chest wall impact in individuals with a normal heart. These cases are due to the timing of chest wall impact (e.g., by a baseball) within the repolarization phase of the cardiac cycle. The majority of cases occur in young athletes (Maron, Gohman, Kyle, Estes, & Link, 1996; Maron et al., 2002).

▶ Overall Mortality (Incidence) of Sudden Cardiac Death

It should be noted that for SCD or for any other type of death, the incidence rate is the same as the mortality rate. Thus, reported annual incidence rates of SCD should be interpreted in the same way as reported annual mortality rates of SCD. Estimates of incidence and mortality are rates for populations as opposed to *case fatality rates* that are death rates for cases with a specific type of disease.

The *Oregon Sudden Unexpected Death Study* was designed to identify cases of SCD in Multnomah County, Oregon, which includes the Portland metropolitan area, population 660,000. The estimated annual incidence of SCD in the study was 53 per 100,000 (Chugh et al., 2008). A similar annual estimate (52 per 100,000) was obtained from a study of a large cohort (population 414,277) in western Ireland. Nevertheless, prospective studies of prospective cohorts in Canada, the United States, the Netherlands, Japan, and China have observed wide variation in incidence rates of SCD ranging from 30 to 100 cases per 100,000 (Adabag, Luepker, Roger, & Gersh, 2010; de Vreede-Swagemakers et al., 1997; Hua et al., 2009; Maruyama et al., 2012; Nichol et al., 2008).

Based on recently reported annual incidence rates of SCD and using an average age-adjusted rate of 70 per 100,000, the estimated number of SCDs per year in the current United States population of 325.7 million ranges from 195,000 to 270,000 with an average value of about 230,000 cases. Using the same estimates for the current world population of 7.55 billion, the projected global number of SCDs ranges from 4.5 to 6.3 million with an average value of 5.3 million, approximately 30% of all 17.65 million cardiovascular deaths.

▶ Declining Trends in Sudden Cardiac Death

Declining trends in the incidence of SCD have been observed in several cohort studies. For example, in the Framingham Heart Study, the incidence of SCD declined by 46% (from 185 to 100 per 100,000) during the 50-year period from 1950 to 1999 coincident with a 57% decline (from 470 to 200 per 100,000) in death rates from coronary heart disease over the same time period (Fox, Evans, Larson, Kannel, & Levy, 2004).

A similar trend was observed in the Rotterdam Study that assessed SCD incidence among adults over the age of 45 years in the Ommoord district of Rotterdam, the Netherlands, during 1990–2010. During two decades of observation, the age-gender-adjusted annual incidence of SCD declined by 55%, from 470 to 210 per 100,000 (Niemeijer et al., 2015).

Likewise, in a population-based longitudinal study conducted in Japan, the age-gender-adjusted incidence of SCD declined from 76 per 100,000 during 1981–1985 to 36.8 per 100,000 in 2001–2005, an overall reduction of 53% for the 25-year follow-up period of the study (**FIGURE 5.2**). Coincident with this reduction, the incidence of coronary heart disease decreased from 98 per 100,000 to 58 per 100,000, a reduction of 42% over the same time. Regarding other risk factors, the prevalence of heavy drinking and current smoking declined significantly in men, hypertension decreased slightly in both men and women, but the prevalence of diabetes more than doubled in men and women (Maruyama et al., 2012).

In the long-standing study of cardiovascular diseases in the Olmstead County cohort in Minnesota, the annual incidence of SCD declined from 110 to 50 per 100,000 during 1995–2009, a reduction of 55%. During this same period, the annual incidence of myocardial infarction declined nearly 50% from 150 to 80 per 100,000, and the prevalence of current smoking declined from 20% to 15%. Nevertheless, the prevalence of other cardiovascular risk factors (e.g., obesity, diabetes mellitus, hypertension, hypercholesterolemia) either increased or did not change (Hurt et al., 2012).

Trends in SCD mortality rates among children and young adults also appear to be on the decline in many populations. Based on a death certificate study of more than 1.42 million subjects aged 1–34 years in the United States conducted during 1999–2015, a total of 31,492 SCDs were identified. During the study period, the annual incidence of SCD declined from 1.48 to 1.13 per 100,000, a reduction of 24%. Nevertheless, there were disparities by age and racial groups (e.g., significantly higher rates were observed for African American subjects and young adults aged 26–34 years) (El-Assaad, Al-Kindi, & Aziz, 2017).

Despite these declining trends in SCD mortality rates, some studies suggest that SCD risk may not be declining in young adults. For example, a recent study of SCD in Australia observed overall reductions in annual SCD incidence of 17% in men and a 31% in women during 1997–2010. However, reductions were only observed for adults over 55 years of age and not for younger men and women. Additional studies are needed to confirm this finding (Feng et al., 2017).

▶ Risk Factors and Predisposing Conditions for Sudden Cardiac Death in Adults

SCD is the catastrophic termination of chronic processes that damage the heart. The principal predisposing condition for SCD is ischemic heart disease which is present in approximately 80% of adult cases. Other conditions of the heart that increase the risk are acute myocardial infarction, fibrosis from pre-existing myocardial infarction, chronic heart failure, AF, and cardiomyopathy. Certain extra-cardiac diseases also increase SCD risk, the main ones being chronic hypertension and type 2 diabetes mellitus.

FIGURE 5.2 Trends in the Annual Incidence of Sudden Cardiac Death in Japan, 1981–2005.

Data from Maruyama, M., Ohira, T., Imano, H., Kitamura, A., Kiyama, M., Okada, T., ... Iso, H. (2012). Trends in sudden cardiac death and its risk factors in Japan from 1981 to 2005: The Circulatory Risk in Communities Study (CIRCS). *British Medical Journal Open, 2*, e000573.

Increased blood levels of biomarkers for predisposing conditions also increase the risk of SCD. They include low density lipoprotein cholesterol, C reactive protein (CRP, a systemic measure of inflammation), and lipoprotein-associated phospholipase A2.

Behavioral risk factors for SCD and its predisposing conditions include chronic smoking, obesity, sedentary lifestyle, chronic alcohol abuse, unhealthy diet (diet high in fat, calories and salt), abuse of opiates and other drugs, and chronic stress.

Certain risk factors such as age, gender, and genetic predisposition are irrevocable. For example, women have lower risk than men during the premenopausal years, but during their postmenopausal years, differences in the rates of heart disease (including SCD) for men and women tend to dissipate with age.

Cardiomyopathies are often genetically determined and may not be detected until symptoms appear late in life. The diagnosis of cardiomyopathy typically requires advanced imaging of the heart for detection of structural anomalies or electrocardiogram to detect irregular heart rhythm.

Predisposing conditions and risk factors for SCD may independently cause SCD, but more often they combine to form a "web of causation" of the event. The presence of multiple causative factors and the potential for interaction and risk modification make it extremely difficult to predict which individuals are at highest risk for SCD. Furthermore, assessment of SCD risk must also take into consideration specific "triggers" of cardiac arrest and death.

▶ The Trigger-Substrate Hypothesis of Sudden Cardiac Death

SCD may involve a predisposing condition (substrate) and an environmental trigger that incites a lethal arrhythmia of the heart. Potential triggers include time of day, strenuous physical activity, alcohol excess, sexual intercourse, outbreaks of anger, and/or situations of high stress. For example, vigorous physical activity might trigger the rupture of atherosclerotic plaque in an individual with ischemic heart disease causing embolic occlusion of coronary arteries, acute myocardial infarction, and lethal arrhythmia. In support of this hypothesis, rates of acute myocardial infarction, stroke, and SCD have been found to show prominent peaks in the morning hours after awakening, which may be due to heightened stimulation of the sympathetic nervous system triggered by stress and/or physical activity (Willich, Maclure, Mittleman, Arntz, & Muller, 1993).

Nevertheless, some studies have failed to find strong evidence that vigorous physical activity serves as a trigger for SCD. For example, in the *Oregon Sudden Unexpected Death Study*, among 304 subjects who experienced cardiac arrest, 17% were sleeping, 63% reported light physical activity, 13% moderate activity, 5% strenuous activity, and 2% were engaged in sexual activity during or just prior to the event. Thus, the vast majority of cases (80%) were either asleep or performing light physical activity during the episode. The investigators concluded that physical activity has less importance than the presence of substrate conditions in causing SCA and suggested that additional studies are needed to identify individuals at high risk for SCD (Chugh et al., 2008).

▶ Surviving "Out-of-Hospital" Sudden Cardiac Arrest

Survival of "out-of-hospital" SCD is low, less than 5% in the United States and other developed countries, and less than 1% in underdeveloped countries. Several programs have been implemented to improve survival from out-of-hospital SCA. Results suggest that early administration of cardiopulmonary resuscitation (CPR) and in particular, shock therapy (defibrillation), have a significant life-saving impact in persons who manifest SCA (Caffrey, Willoughby, Pepe, & Becker, 2002).

During 2005–2007, investigators in Japan conducted a nationwide study of whether dissemination of automated external defibrillators in public places could improve survival among patients who had out-of-hospital cardiac arrest. The study included a total of 12,631 cases who had an arrest that was of cardiac origin and that was witnessed by bystanders. Among these cases, 462 (3.7%) received immediate shock therapy administered by laypersons using the public defibrillators. Among patients receiving early defibrillation, 31.6% were alive after 1 month with minimal neurological impairment compared to only 14% who did not receive early defibrillation (Kitamura et al., 2010).

In 2004, the United States Centers for Disease Control (CDC) established the *Cardiac Arrest Registry to Enhance Survival* (CARES) program in order to find ways to improve survival among patients who suffer out-of-hospital SCA. Among 31,689 SCA cases observed over the initial 5 years of the program, the overall survival rate was only 9.6%. Among patients who received CPR administered by a bystander, survival was slightly better (11.2%) than those who did not receive CPR (7.0%). Notably, among 2087 patients with detectable heart sounds who received either CPR or shock therapy from a bystander using a public automated external defibrillator, survival increased three-fold to 33.7% (McNally et al., 2011).

The *Minnesota Resuscitation Consortium* was established in 2011 to provide standardized, evidence-based resuscitation, and post-resuscitation care to the population of Minnesota. During 2011–2014, 5192 cases of SCA occurred in participating counties. Among 2637 patients with detectable heart sounds who received CPR and/or shock therapy, survival was 38% compared to only 14% overall (Adabag et al., 2017).

▶ Prevention of Sudden Cardiac Arrest and Death

Multiple risk factors and pre-existing heart diseases contribute to the "web of causation" of SCD. Prevention therefore requires a multifaceted approach including risk-factor reduction, drug therapies, cardiac procedures, widespread education on life-saving techniques such as CPR, and implementation of new approaches such as public use of automated external defibrillators (Sotoodehnia, Zivin, Bardy, & Siscovick, 2001; Zipes & Wellens, 1998).

Despite these efforts, SCD continues to be a major public health challenge. This is largely because the majority of SCDs occur unexpectedly and "out-of-hospital" in individuals without high-risk profiles or previously diagnosed heart disease. In cases of SCA, death will occur within a few minutes unless appropriate resuscitation measures are implemented. Recently, the American Heart Association recommended 10 measures for the prevention of SCD among individuals at high SCD risk (**TABLE 5.2**). Notwithstanding, these guidelines primarily pertain to those individuals with specific heart conditions (heart failure, prior myocardial infarction, ventricular arrhythmia), a strong family history of heart disease, or those who have already survived a cardiac

---

TABLE 5.2 Ten Recommended Measures to Reduce Sudden Cardiac Death

Recommendations to Prevent SCD by the American Heart Association, 2016

1. Smoking cessation intervention in patients who suffered SCA, have a life-threatening ventricular arrhythmia, or are at risk of SCD.

2. Screening for family history of SCD.

3. Screening for asymptomatic left ventricular dysfunction among individuals who have a strong family history of cardiomyopathy and SCD.

4. Referring for *CPR* and *automated external defibrillator* (AED) education those family members of patients who are hospitalized with known heart conditions that increase the risk of SCA.

5. Use of *implantable cardioverter defibrillators* (ICDs) for prevention of SCD in patients with heart failure and reduced ejection fraction who have expected survival at least 1 year.

6. Use of guideline-directed medical therapy for prevention of SCD in patients with heart failure and reduced ejection fraction.

7. Use of guideline-directed medical therapy for prevention of SCD in patients with heart attack and reduced ejection fraction.

8. Documenting the absence of reversible causes of ventricular tachycardia/ventricular fibrillation cardiac arrest and/or sustained ventricular tachycardia before a secondary-prevention ICD is placed.

9. Counseling eligible patients about an ICD.

10. Counseling first-degree relatives of survivors of SCA associated with an inheritable condition about the need for screening for the inheritable condition.

arrest. For example, patients with certain conditions may require *implantable cardioverter defibrillators* or guideline-directed medications (Al-Khatib et al., 2017). Further progress will depend on the development of improved methods to identify those persons who are most susceptible and targeting them for enhanced monitoring and intervention (Albert & Ruskin, 2001; Sotoodehnia et al., 2001).

References

Adabag, A. S., Luepker, R. V., Roger, V. L., & Gersh, B. J. (2010). Sudden cardiac death: Epidemiology and risk factors. *Nature Reviews Cardiology, 7*(4), 216–225.

Adabag, A. S., Peterson, G., Apple, F. S., Titus, J., King, R., & Luepker, R. V. (2010). Etiology of sudden death in the community: Results of anatomical, metabolic, and genetic evaluation. *American Heart Journal, 159*(1), 33–39.

Adabag, S., Hodgson, L., Garcia, S., Anand, V., Frascone, R., Conterato, M., … Yannopoulos, D. (2017). Outcomes of sudden cardiac arrest in a state-wide integrated resuscitation program: Results from the Minnesota Resuscitation Consortium. *Resuscitation, 110*, 95–100.

Albert, C. M., & Ruskin, J. N. (2001). Risk stratifiers for sudden cardiac death (SCD) in the community: Primary prevention of SCD. *Cardiovascular Research, 50*(2), 186–196.

Al-Khatib, S. M., Yancy, C. W., Solis, P., Becker, L., Benjamin, E. J., Carrillo, R. G., … Varosy, P. D. (2017). 2016 AHA/ACC clinical performance and quality measures for prevention of sudden cardiac death: A report of the American College of Cardiology/American Heart Association Task Force on Performance Measures. *Circulation: Cardiovascular Quality and Outcomes, 10*, e000022.

Babu-Narayan, S. V., McCarthy, K. P., Ho, S. Y., Magee, A. G., Kilner, P. J., & Sheppard, M. N. (2007). Myocarditis and sudden cardiac death in the young. *Circulation, 116*, e122–e125.

Byard, R. W. (2006). Sudden and unexpected death in Marfan syndrome. In M. Tsokos (Ed.), *Forensic pathology reviews* (Vol. 4). Totowa, NJ: Humana Press.

Caffrey, S. L., Willoughby, P. J., Pepe, P. E., & Becker, L. B. (2002). Public use of automated external defibrillators. *New England Journal of Medicine, 347*, 1242–1247.

Celermajer, D. S., Chow, C. K., Marijon, E., Anstey, N. M., & Woo, K. S. (2012). Cardiovascular disease in the developing world: Prevalences, patterns, and the potential of early disease detection. *Journal of the American College of Cardiology, 60*(14), 1207–1216.

Chen, L. Y., Sotoodehnia, N., Bůžková, P., Lopez, F. L., Yee, L. M., Heckbert, S. R., … Alonso, A. (2013). Atrial fibrillation and the risk of sudden cardiac death: The Atherosclerosis Risk in Communities study and Cardiovascular Health Study. *JAMA Internal Medicine, 173*, 29–35.

Chugh, S. S., Havmoeller, R., Narayanan, K., Singh, D., Rienstra, M., Benjamin, E. J., …. Murray, C. J. (2014). Worldwide epidemiology of atrial fibrillation: A global burden of disease 2010 study. *Circulation, 129*, 837–847.

Chugh, S. S., Reinier, K., Teodorescu, C., Evanado, A., Kehr, E., Samara, M. A., … Jui, J. (2008). Epidemiology of sudden cardiac death: Clinical and research implications. *Progress in Cardiovascular Diseases, 51*(3), 213–228.

Cobb, L. A., Fahrenbruch, C. E., Olsufka, M., & Copass, M. K. (2002). Changing incidence of out-of-hospital ventricular fibrillation, 1980–2000. *Journal of the American Medical Association, 28*, 3008–3013.

Corrado, D., Link, M. S., & Calkins, H. (2017). Arrhythmogenic right ventricular cardiomyopathy. *New England Journal of Medicine, 376*, 61–72.

Davies, M. J. (1992). Anatomic features in victims of sudden coronary death: Coronary artery pathology. *Circulation, 85*(2 Suppl.), 19–24.

de Vreede-Swagemakers, J. J., Gorgels, A. P., Dubois-Arbouw, W. I., van Ree, J. W., Daemen, M. J., Houben, L. G., & Wellens, H. J. (1997). Out-of-hospital cardiac arrest in the 1990's: A population-based study in the Maastricht area on incidence, characteristics and survival. *Journal of the American College of Cardiology, 30*(6), 1500–1505.

Drory, Y., Turetz, Y., Hiss, Y., Lev, B., Fisman, E. Z., Pines, A., & Kramer, M. R. (1991). Sudden unexpected death in persons <40 years of age. *American Journal of Cardiology, 68*, 1388–1392.

Eisen, A., Ruff, C. T., Braunwald, E., Nordio, F., Corbalán, R., Dalby, A., … Giugliano, R. P. (2016). Sudden cardiac death in patients with atrial fibrillation: Insights from the ENGAGE AF-TIMI 48 Trial. *Journal of the American Heart Association, 5*, e003735.

El-Assaad, I., Al-Kindi, S. G., & Aziz, P. F. (2017). Trends of out-of-hospital sudden cardiac death among children and young adults. *Pediatrics, 140*(6), 1438.

Farb, A., Tang, A. L., Burke, A. P., Sessums, L., Liang, Y., & Virmani, R. (1995). Sudden coronary death: Frequency of active coronary lesions, inactive coronary lesions, and myocardial infarction. *Circulation, 92*, 1701–1709.

Feng, J. L., Nedkoff, L., Knuiman, M., Semsarian, C., Ingles, J., Briffa, T., & Hickling, S. (2017). Temporal trends in sudden cardiac death from 1997 to 2010: A data linkage study. *Heart Lung & Circulation, 26*(8), 808–816.

Fontaine, G., Fornes, P., & Fontaliran, F. (2001). Myocarditis as a cause of sudden death. *Circulation, 103*, e12.

Fox, C. S., Evans, J. C., Larson, M. G., Kannel, W. B., & Levy, D. (2004). Temporal trends in coronary heart disease mortality and sudden cardiac death from 1950 to 1999: The Framingham Heart Study. *Circulation, 110*, 522–527.

Gajewski, K. K., & Saul, J. P. (2010). Sudden cardiac death in children and adolescents (excluding Sudden Infant Death Syndrome). *Annals of Pediatric Cardiology, 3*(2), 107–112.

Hayashi, M., Shimizu, W., & Albert, C. M. (2015). The spectrum of epidemiology underlying sudden cardiac death. *Circulation Research, 116*(12), 1887–1906.

Hua, W., Zhang, L. F., Wu, Y. F., Liu, X. Q., Guo, D. S., Zhou, H. L., … Zhang, S. (2009). Incidence of sudden cardiac death in China: Analysis of 4 regional populations. *Journal of the American College of Cardiology, 54*, 1110–1118.

Hurt, R. D., Weston, S. A., Ebbert, J. O., McNallan, S. M., Croghan, I. T., Schroeder, D. R., & Roger, V. L. (2012). Myocardial infarction and sudden cardiac death in Olmsted County, Minnesota, before and after smoke-free workplace laws. *Archives of Internal Medicine, 172*(21), 1635–1641.

Kannel, W. B., Cupples, L. A., & D'Agostino, R. B. (1987). Sudden death risk in overt coronary heart disease: The Framingham Study. *American Heart Journal, 113*(3), 799–804.

Kitamura, T., Iwami, T., Kawamura, T., Nagao, K., Tanaka, H., & Hiraide, A. (2010). Nationwide public-access defibrillation in Japan. *New England Journal of Medicine, 362*, 994–1004.

Kuller, L. H., Cooper, M., Perper, J., & Fisher, R. (1973). Myocardial infarction and sudden death in an urban community. *Bulletin of the New York Academy of Medicine, 49*, 532–543.

Lazzerini, P. E., Capecchi, P. L., Guideri, F., Acampa, M., Galeazzi, M., & Laghi Pasini, F. (2006). Connective tissue diseases and cardiac rhythm disorders: An overview. *Autoimmunity Reviews, 5*(5), 306–313.

Luk, A., Ahn, E., Soor, G. S., & Butany, J. (2009). Dilated cardiomyopathy: A review. *Journal of Clinical Pathology, 62*, 219–225.

Marcus, F. I., Fontaine, G. H., Guiraudon, G., Frank, R., Laurenceau, J. L., Malergue, C., & Grosgogeat, Y. (1982). Right ventricular dysplasia: A report of 24 adult cases. *Circulation, 65*, 384–398.

Marijon, E., Le Heuzey, J.-Y., Connolly, S., Yang, S., Pogue, J., Brueckmann, M., … Yusuf, S. (2013). Causes of death and influencing factors in patients with atrial fibrillation: A competing-risk analysis from the randomized evaluation of long-term anticoagulant therapy study. *Circulation, 128*, 2192–2201.

Maron, B. J., Gohman, T. E., Kyle, S. B., Estes, N. A., & Link, M. S. (2002). Clinical profile and spectrum of commotio cordis. *Journal of the American Medical Association, 287*, 1142–1146.

Maron, B. J., Shirani, J., Poliac, L. C., Mathenge, R., Roberts, W. C., & Mueller, F. O. (1996). Sudden death in young competitive athletes: Clinical, demographic, and pathological profiles. *Journal of the American Medical Association, 276*(3), 199–204.

Maruyama, M., Ohira, T., Imano, H., Kitamura, A., Kiyama, M., Okada, T., … Iso, H. (2012). Trends in sudden cardiac death and its risk factors in Japan from 1981 to 2005: The Circulatory Risk in Communities Study (CIRCS). *British Medical Journal Open, 2*, e000573.

McNally, B., Robb, R., Mehta, M., Vellano, K., Valderrama, A. L., Yoon, P. W., … Kellermann, A. (2011). Out-of-Hospital cardiac arrest surveillance—Cardiac arrest registry to enhance survival (CARES), United States, October 1, 2005–December 31, 2010. *Morbidity and Mortality Weekly Report, Surveillance Summaries, 60*(8), 1–19.

Mehra, R. (2007). Global public health problem of sudden cardiac death. *Journal of Electrocardiology, 40*(6 Suppl.), S118–S122.

Murphy-Ryan, M., Psychogios, A., & Lindor, N. M. (2010). Hereditary disorders of connective tissue: A guide to the emerging differential diagnosis. *Genetics in Medicine, 12*, 344–354.

Myerburg, R. J. (2002). Scientific gaps in the prediction and prevention of sudden cardiac death. *Journal of Cardiovascular Electrophysiology, 13*, 709–723.

Myerburg, R., & Castellanos, A. (2007). In P. Libby, R. O. Bonow, D. L. Mann, & D. P. Zipes (Eds.), *Braunwald's heart disease. A textbook of cardiovascular medicine* (8th ed., pp. 933–974). Philadelphia, PA: Saunders.

Nichol, G. H., Thomas, E., Callaway, C. W., Hedges, J., Powell, J. L., Aufderheide, T. P., … Stiell, I. (2008). Regional variation in out-of-hospital cardiac arrest incidence and outcome. *Journal of the American Medical Association, 300*(12), 1423–1431.

Niemeijer, M. N., van den Berg, M. E., Leening, M. J. G., Hofman, A., Franco, O. H., Deckers, J. W., … Eijgelsheim, M. (2015). Declining incidence of sudden cardiac death from 1990–2010 in a general middle-aged and elderly population: The Rotterdam Study. *Heart Rhythm, 12*(1), 123–129.

Piccini, J. P., & Daubert, J. P. (2014). Atrial fibrillation and sudden cardiac death. Is heart failure the middleman? *JACC: Heart Failure, 2*(3), 228–229.

Reinier, K., Marijon, E., Uy-Evanado, A., Teodorescu, C., Narayanan, K., Chugh, H., … Chugh, S. S. (2014). The association between atrial fibrillation and sudden cardiac death: The relevance of heart failure. *JACC Heart Failure, 2*(3), 221–227.

Sotoodehnia, N., Zivin, A., Bardy, G. H., & Siscovick, D. S. (2001). Reducing mortality from sudden cardiac death in the community: Lessons from epidemiology and clinical applications research. *Cardiovascular Research, 50*(2), 197–209.

Stroumpoulis, K. I., Pantazopoulos, I. N., & Xanthos, T. T. (2010). Hypertrophic cardiomyopathy and sudden cardiac death. *World Journal of Cardiology, 2*(9), 289–298.

Talwar, K. K., & Gupta, A. (2016). Predictors of mortality in chronic rheumatic heart disease. *Indian Journal of Medical Research, 144*(3), 311–313.

Tomaselli, G. F., & Zipes, D. P. (2004). What causes sudden death in heart failure? *Circulation Research, 95*, 754–763.

Tse, G., Chan, Y. W. F., Kenug, W., & Yan, B. P. (2017). Electrophysiological mechanisms of long and short QT syndromes. *IJC Heart & Vasculature, 14*, 8–13.

Virmani, R., Kolodgie, F. D., Burke, A. P., Farb, A., & Schwartz, S. M. (2000). Lessons from sudden coronary death: A comprehensive morphological classification scheme for atherosclerotic lesions. *Arteriosclerosis, Thrombosis, and Vascular Biology, 20*, 1262–1275.

Willich, S. N., Maclure, M., Mittleman, M., Arntz, H. R., & Muller, J. E. (1993). Sudden cardiac death. Support for a role of triggering in causation. *Circulation, 87*, 1442–1450.

Zheng, Z.-J., Croft, J. B., Giles, W. H., & Mensah, G. A. (2001) Sudden cardiac death in the United States, 1989 to 1998. *Circulation, 104*, 2158–2163.

Zipes, D. P., & Wellens, H. J. J. (1998). Sudden cardiac death. *Circulation, 98*, 2334–235.

© Andrew Brookes/Getty Images

CHAPTER 6

Epidemiology of Stroke (Cerebral Infarction)

▶ Ischemic and Hemorrhagic Strokes

A stroke or cerebral infarction is the rapidly developing loss of brain function due to interruption of the cerebral blood supply and necrosis of neurons in part of the brain. Strokes are diagnosed based on clinical symptoms (e.g., the degree and specificity of acute loss of brain function) plus imaging techniques such as computed tomography (CT) scans and magnetic resonance imaging (MRI). The traditional definition of stroke published by the World Health Organization in 1978 is "a neurological deficit of cerebrovascular cause that persists beyond 24 hours or is interrupted by death within 24 hours." The time frame of 24 hours divides stroke from transient ischemic attack (TIA), the latter referring to a milder form of ischemia in which all neurological symptoms resolve within 24 hours.

Strokes are pathologically categorized into two major types: Ischemic strokes and hemorrhagic strokes. Ischemic strokes are those that are caused by interruption of the cerebral blood supply without bleeding whereas hemorrhagic strokes involve rupture of a cerebral blood vessel and leakage of blood into the brain. Approximately 85% of strokes are classified as ischemic and the remainder (about 15%) are hemorrhagic. Hemorrhagic strokes are often further subdivided into intracerebral hemorrhage and subarachnoid hemorrhage. Intracerebral hemorrhage accounts for about 10% of all strokes. This subtype involves the leakage of blood from cerebral vessels directly into the brain. Subarachnoid hemorrhage accounts for about 5% of all strokes and involves the leakage of blood into the subarachnoid space between the arachnoid membrane and the pia mater at the periphery of the brain (Donnan, Fisher, Macleod, & Davis, 2008).

Hippocrates (460–370 BC) first described the sudden paralysis characteristic of an ischemic stroke (Thompson, 1996). Ischemia (lack of oxygen) of brain tissue rapidly develops when one of the cerebral arteries is occluded by a thrombus (a blood clot) or embolus (detached fragment of a blood clot) or when a cerebral blood vessel ruptures leading to frank hemorrhage of blood into the brain. Brain tissue ceases to function if deprived of oxygen for more than 60–90 seconds and after approximately 3 hours, will suffer irreversible injury possibly leading to death (infarction) of the tissue. As a result, the affected area of the brain is unable to function, leading to inability to move one or more limbs on one side of the body, inability to understand or formulate speech, or inability to see one side of the visual field.

The postmortem pathologic examination of brains from patients suffering fatal strokes has provided critical information regarding the distribution of cerebral infarction and the distinction between ischemic and hemorrhagic strokes. The famous German pathologist, Rudolph Virchow, is credited with first describing thromboembolism as a major event in the pathogenesis of stroke (Schiller, 1970).

Ischemic strokes are most often caused by occlusive thrombi in larger blood vessels of the brain such as the internal carotid, the upper vertebral, and lower basilar arteries (Fisher, 1975). Occlusive thrombi tend to occur in and around ruptured atheromatous plaques that have developed in the lining (endothelium) of these blood vessels. Emboli that migrate from other sites (e.g., the heart or aorta) and occlude smaller caliber cerebral arteries of the brain can also cause an ischemic stroke.

Various systems have been devised to categorize the subtypes of ischemic stroke based upon clinical symptoms and imaging studies. In one system, the *Trial of Organization 10172 in Acute Stroke Treatment* (TOAST), ischemic strokes are categorized into five specific etiologic subtypes: (1) thrombus or embolus arising from large artery atherosclerosis, (2) cardioembolism, (3) small vessel occlusion (lacunae) associated with diabetes and/or hypertension, (4) other etiology such as coagulopathy (e.g., sickle cell anemia), and (5) undetermined etiology (Adams et al., 1993).

In contrast to ischemic strokes, intracerebral hemorrhagic strokes are more likely to involve embolic occlusion and rupture of smaller cerebral blood vessels. By definition, intracerebral hemorrhagic strokes involve the leakage of blood from cerebral blood vessels directly into the brain. Occlusive emboli are found most frequently at points of arterial bifurcation (branching) or narrowing of the lumens of cerebral blood vessels. Emboli typically arise when a fragment of thrombus is dislodged in the left ventricle of the heart or the aortic arch and travels into a small caliber cerebral artery, often a branch of the middle cerebral artery (Schoene, 1979). Emboli typically arise in the heart as a consequence of atrial fibrillation.

A special subtype of hemorrhagic stroke is caused by subarachnoid hemorrhage. Subarachnoid hemorrhage arises due to leakage of blood from ruptured blood vessels into the subarachnoid space surrounding the brain. Ruptured aneurysms are the cause of 85% of cases of subarachnoid hemorrhage. The collection of blood in the subarachnoid space can cause compression of the brain thereby leading to infarction and stroke. Subarachnoid hemorrhagic strokes have a very high case fatality rate (40%–50%) and frequently occur in young adults (van Gijn, Kerr, & Rinkel, 2007).

Hemorrhagic strokes, especially the subarachnoid hemorrhagic subtype, are usually caused by the rupture of aneurysms which are balloon-like dilatations of the walls of diseased blood vessels. Aneurysms most commonly occur in cerebral arteries (cerebral aneurysm) at the base of the brain (the Circle of Willis) and in the aorta (aortic aneurysm). As the size of an aneurysm increases, there is an increased risk of rupture, which can result in severe hemorrhage, other complications, or even death.

Hemorrhagic strokes injure and destroy neurons due to physical compression of tissue from the expanding hematoma, ischemia due to loss of blood supply, and direct toxic effects of blood on brain tissue and vasculature. Loss of consciousness, headache, and vomiting tend to occur more often in hemorrhagic stroke than in thrombosis because of the increased intracranial pressure from the leaking blood compressing the brain.

Whether a stroke is classified as ischemic or hemorrhagic, the underlying pathogenesis invariably involves the long-term process of atherogenesis (development of atheromatous plaque in blood vessels). Cerebral infarction (stroke) is one of two major culminating events of this process, the other being heart attack (myocardial infarction). Upon rupture of an atheromatous plaque, platelet activation and initiation of the clotting cascade rapidly ensue resulting in formation of a thrombus or embolus and potential occlusion of cerebral blood vessels, ischemia and infarction (death) of neurons, and significant loss of brain function and/or death. Hypertension is also a primary risk factor, particularly for hemorrhagic stroke.

▶ Vascular Network of the Brain

Oxygenated blood from the left heart travels upward through the carotid and vertebral arteries arising from the aortic arch and is distributed to the brain through a complex network of cerebral arteries, arterioles, and capillaries (**FIGURE 6.1**). At the base of the brain, the internal carotid and vertebral arteries join to form the arterial Circle of Willis, an intricate system with branches that nourish many of the internal structures of the brain.

Approximately 15% of the blood ejected by the left ventricle of the heart is jettisoned upwards into the brain. The cerebral arteries deliver oxygenated blood, glucose, and other nutrients to the brain and the cerebral veins carry deoxygenated blood back to the heart, removing carbon dioxide, lactic acid, and other metabolic products. Although the human brain represents only 2% of the total body weight, it consumes 20% of total body oxygen, and 25% of total body energy. The arterial circulation that nourishes the brain consists of hundreds of branching vessels that become progressively smaller at each bifurcation. The tortuous nature of this arterial network predisposes to stenosis (narrowing) due to atherosclerotic plaque and/or acute occlusion of blood flow by a thrombus or embolism, particularly in and around the junctions where larger vessels bifurcate into smaller caliber vessels.

The lining (endothelium) of very small blood vessels (capillaries) of the brain consists of cells with tight junctions that prevent invasion/contamination by bacteria and other substances in the blood. This is the *blood–brain barrier* first identified by the German bacteriologist and Nobel Laureate, Paul Ehrlich, and his student Edwin Goldman in 1909 (Bradbury, 1979).

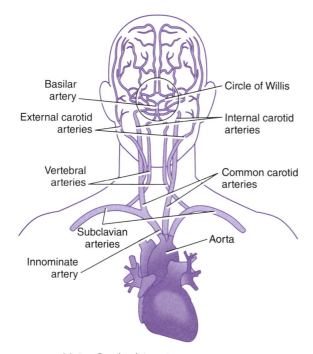

FIGURE 6.1 Major Cerebral Arteries.

▶ Global Mortality of Stroke

In 2015, strokes caused 6.33 million deaths in the world population, approximately 11% of all deaths reported in that year (Roth et al., 2017). Although age-specific incidence and mortality rates of stroke have declined in many developed nations, rates are increasing in developing nations which contain the majority of the world population. As a consequence, the annual number of deaths from stroke has increased by about 1.67 million in the past quarter century (e.g., in the 25-year period between 1990 and 2015, stroke-related deaths increased by 36% from 4.66 million in 1990 to 6.33 million in 2015) (Feigin et al., 2014, 2015; Lopez, Mathers, Ezzati, Jamison, & Murray, 2006; National Heart Lung Blood Institute, 2009; Roth et al., 2017; World Health Organization, 2009, 2010).

Stroke ranks second in overall global mortality behind ischemic heart disease. In the 21st century, these two conditions have caused more than one quarter of all deaths in the world population. Annual stroke mortality rates adjusted for age and gender reflect a wide range from less than 50 deaths per 100,000 in nations of North America, Western Europe, and Australia to greater than 250 deaths per 100,000 in nations of Northern and Central Asia, Eastern Europe, Middle Africa, and the South Pacific (**FIGURE 6.2**). Approximately 85% of the annual deaths from stroke (5.4 million) occur in developing nations where both the incidence and mortality are increasing. The international trends in the mortality from

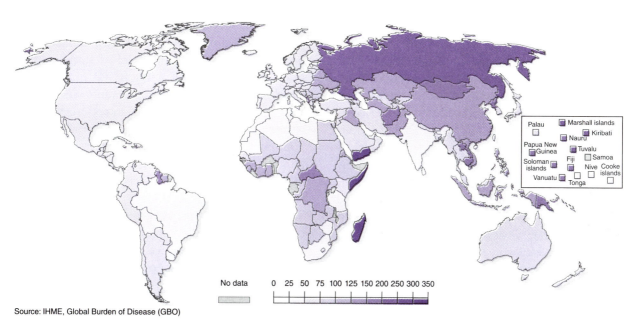

Source: IHME, Global Burden of Disease (GBO)

FIGURE 6.2 Global Mortality from Stroke: 2016.

Data from International Health Metrics and Evaluation (IHME), Global Burden of Disease (GBD); Our World in Data.

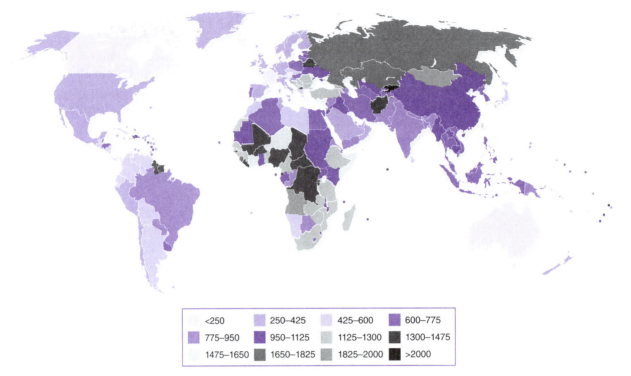

<250	250–425	425–600	600–775
775–950	950–1125	1125–1300	1300–1475
1475–1650	1650–1825	1825–2000	>2000

FIGURE 6.3 Disability-Adjusted Life Years for Cerebrovascular Disease, 2004.

No data were reported for Greenland.

Data from World Health Organization. (2008). *The global burden of disease: 2004 update*. Geneva: WHO. Available at www.who.int/evidence/bod

stroke are similar to that for coronary heart disease and cardiovascular disease.

Strokes cause both death and disability thus creating a dual health burden. A combined measure of disease health burden that takes into account the years of life lost due to premature death (YLL) plus the years lost due to severe disability (YLD) is the Disability-Adjusted Life Years (DALY = YLL + YLD).

National estimates of the DALYs that are lost due to cerebrovascular disease (primarily stroke) are depicted in **FIGURE 6.3** (Johnston, Mendis, & Mathers, 2009; Mackay & Mensah, 2004). The global DALY pattern is quite similar to that for stroke mortality. The DALYs show a wide range from less than 250 years of life lost annually in certain high-income nations (North America, Western Europe, Australia) to levels greater than 2000 in some middle- and low-income nations (Eastern Europe, Russia, and Central Africa). In general, high-income nations have lower DALYs and middle and low-income nations have higher DALYs. In a systematic review of mortality and DALY rates, the national per-capita income was found to be the strongest predictor of stroke mortality and DALY loss even after adjustment for cerebrovascular disease risk factors (Johnston et al., 2009). This pattern reflects earlier onset of both fatal and nonfatal debilitating strokes in nations with inadequate resources to support effective preventive and therapeutic health services.

▶ Decline in Stroke Mortality in Developed Nations

In developed nations, most notably in North America, Japan, and Western Europe, mortality rates from stroke have declined markedly in the past half-century (Feigin, Lawes, Bennett, & Anderson, 2003; Johnston et al., 2009; Murray & Lopez, 1997; Sudlow & Warlow, 1997). The declining mortality trend in the age-adjusted mortality from stroke in the United States is depicted in **FIGURE 6.4**. These declining trends in mortality are largely attributable to primary prevention (avoidance of smoking and maintaining blood pressure, serum cholesterol and blood glucose within normal limits using both nonpharmacologic and pharmacologic methods) plus secondary prevention (treatment of hypertension, hyperlipidemia, and hyperglycemia and use of antithrombotic/antiplatelet therapy [e.g., low-dose aspirin, for individuals with atrial fibrillation]) (Straus, Majumdar, & McAlister, 2002). Evidence supporting the value of each of these preventive modalities is discussed in the section of this chapter on stroke prevention.

Recent data from the United States indicate that the decline in mortality from stroke has stalled and that in certain ethnic groups (e.g., African Americans and Hispanics) the mortality rates have risen about 3% per year since 2013. The reversal in mortality trends

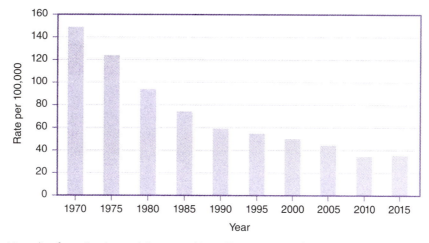

FIGURE 6.4 Decline in Mortality from Stroke and Coronary Heart Disease: United States, 1970–2015.

Data from National Institutes of Health, Center for Health Statistics, 2009; Yang, Q., Ton, X., Schieb, L., Vaughan, A., Gillespie, C., & Wiltz, J. L. (2017). Vital signs: Recent trends in stroke death rates; United States, 2000–2015. *Morbidity and Mortality Weekly Report (MMWR)*, *66*(35), 933–939.

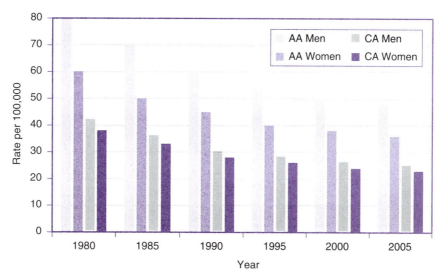

FIGURE 6.5 Stroke Mortality in African Americans and Caucasian Americans: United States, 1980–2005.

Data from US Center for Health Statistics, National Institutes of Health, 2009. The Stroke Belt, USA.

may be related to the increasing prevalence of obesity and chronic hypertension (Yang et al., 2017).

▶ Racial Differences in Stroke Mortality in the United States

Racial disparities in stroke mortality and incidence are similar to that for coronary heart disease with rates being markedly higher among African Americans compared to Caucasian Americans (**FIGURE 6.5**). Various reasons have been proposed to explain this disparity including greater exposure to known risk factors and relatively poor access to both preventive and therapeutic healthcare services. In particular, the high prevalence and inadequate management of

hypertension probably account for much of the excess in stroke mortality among African Americans (Gillum, 1999; Kittner, White, Losonczy, Wolf, & Hebel, 1990).

In 1962, investigators at the Centers for Disease Control and Prevention noted a concentration of high mortality from stroke in certain regions of the southeastern United States (Atlantic coastal plain counties of North Carolina, South Carolina, Georgia, and the Mississippi Delta) (Casper, Wing, Anda, Knowles, & Pollard, 1995). The Stroke Belt in the United States is typically defined to include the states of Alabama, Arkansas, Georgia, Indiana, Kentucky, Louisiana, Mississippi, North Carolina, South Carolina, Tennessee, and Virginia. In 1980, these 11 states had age-adjusted stroke mortality rates more than 10% above the national average (National Heart, Lung and Blood Institute, 1996). Some investigators also include northern Florida as part of the Stroke Belt due to the high mortality from stroke (Siegel, Wolfe, Wilcox, & Deeb, 1992).

Several factors have been proposed to explain the high stroke mortality observed in the Stroke Belt. As discussed in the following section on risk factors, stroke is a catastrophic culminating event of multifactorial disease processes. It is therefore likely that the Stroke Belt reflects a web of causative factors such as hypertension, obesity, smoking, lack of exercise, atherosclerosis-prone diets high in fat and fried foods, and relatively poor access to emergency medical services. One striking feature of the U.S. Stroke Belt is its overlying pattern with U.S. lung cancer mortality (Centers for Disease Control and Prevention, 2004). As shown in **FIGURE 6.6**, the Stroke Belt also has high lung cancer mortality, perhaps reflecting the contribution of smoking to both conditions (Peto et al., 2006).

▶ Risk Factors for Stroke

The INTERSTROKE Study

The INTERSTROKE Study provides an international perspective on the risk factors for stroke (O'Donnell et al., 2010). This investigation was conducted in

parallel with the INTERHEART Study of myocardial infarction during 2007–2010. INTERSTROKE was designed as a standardized case–control study involving 22 countries worldwide. The investigation compared 2337 cases with acute stroke to 3000 controls without stroke that were matched to the cases by age and gender. The findings are summarized in **TABLE 6.1**.

Collectively, 10 risk factors accounted for almost 90% of the population attributable risk for acute stroke in the INTERSTROKE Study. As expected, the strongest risk factor was hypertension (odds ratio = 2.6); nevertheless, several other factors including smoking, abdominal obesity (measured by high waist to hip ratio), hyperlipidemia (measured by high ApoB/ApoA1 ratio), a dietary risk score, and alcohol abuse were also significant risk factors for both ischemic stroke and hemorrhagic stroke (O'Donnell et al., 2010).

The findings of INTERSTROKE provide international confirmation of a number of modifiable stroke risk factors that were first identified and quantified through many previous epidemiologic investigations. Nonmodifiable risk factors for stroke include the aging process (the risk of acute stroke doubles for each decade of life after age 55 years),

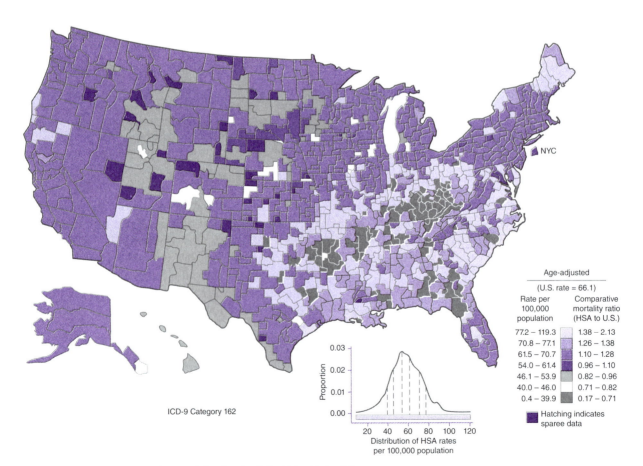

FIGURE 6.6 Lung Cancer Mortality and the Stroke Belt, 2004, United States.
Centers for Disease Control and Prevention, National Center for Health Statistics, United States Department of Health and Human Services, 2004.

TABLE 6.1 Risk Factors for Stroke: INTERSTROKE Study, 2010

Risk Factor	Odds Ratio	Population Attributable Risk (%)
Hypertension	2.6	35
Current smoking	2.1	19
Waist to hip ratio	1.7	26
Unhealthy diet	1.4	19
Regular exercise	0.7	29
Diabetes mellitus	1.4	5
Alcohol abuse	1.5	4
Psychological factors	1.3	5
Cardiac disease	1.5	7
ApoB/ApoA1	1.9	25

Data from O'Donnell, M. J., Xavier, D., Liu, L., Zhang, H., Chin, S. L., Rao-Melacini, P., … INTERSTROKE Investigators. (2010). Risk factors for ischaemic and intracerebral haemorrhagic stroke in 22 countries (the INTERSTROKE study): A case-control study. *Lancet, 376*(9735), 112–123.

gender (men are at higher risk), and hereditary factors (a family history of stroke in one or more first degree relatives [father, mother, sibling] approximately doubles the risk).

Blood Pressure and Stroke

The strongest risk factor for stroke is hypertension, which is clinically definable as systolic blood pressure above 140 mm Hg or diastolic blood pressure above 90 mm Hg. Hypertension is modifiable through both nonpharmacologic modalities as well as by pharmacologic therapy (e.g., taking antihypertensive medications).

Homeostatic regulation of blood pressure is a complex physiological process dependent upon kidney function, vasoactive hormones, the sympathetic and parasympathetic divisions of the autonomic nervous system, the central nervous system, and many lifestyle factors such as diet, exercise, physical condition, body mass, and emotional status. Since hypertension is a powerful risk factor in the development of stroke, the risk factors for stroke and hypertension

are synonymous. These include smoking, high dietary salt, obesity, elevated blood lipids, diabetes mellitus (particularly type 2 diabetes), sedentary life style, drug abuse (cocaine), and certain emotional factors (high stress or depression).

The evidence that blood pressure is a major causative factor in the genesis of strokes is compelling. In an exhaustive meta-analysis involving more than 1 million subjects from 61 prospective studies published in the scientific literature, the rates of stroke mortality were compared according to systolic and diastolic blood pressure at baseline (Lewington et al., 2002). The authors included all prospective observational studies that collected data on blood pressure, blood cholesterol, date of birth (or age), and sex at baseline, and in which cause of death and date of death (or age at death) for all participants during more than 5000 person-years of follow-up were available.

As shown in **FIGURE 6.7**, persons with systolic blood pressure 20 mm Hg less than the reference category (>115 mm Hg) or persons with diastolic blood pressure 10 mm Hg less than the reference category (>75 mm Hg) significantly reduced their risk of death from stroke. Reductions in mortality were somewhat dependent upon age—older individuals (70 years and older) reduced their risk by 30%–50% whereas younger individuals (less than 70 years) reduced their risk by 50%–60% (Lewington et al., 2002). These data, compiled from the existing literature on blood pressure and stroke from prospective investigations, clearly and definitively accentuate the attributes of maintaining blood pressure within normal limits.

Ecological studies are designed to provide estimates of correlations between population-based disease incidence rates (or mortality rates) and exposure rates of potential risk factors. Such correlations do not necessarily imply causality and should be interpreted cautiously as a basis for further etiologic investigations.

Ecological studies show positive correlations between prevalence rates of hypertension and incidence and mortality rates of stroke. In the World Health Organization MONICA Project, blood pressure prevalence estimates for population samples from around the Baltic Sea were found to be positively correlated with the incidence of stroke in men ($r = 0.87$) and women ($r = 0.70$) (Stegmayr et al., 1996); subsequently, a further analysis of MONICA data revealed positive correlations for men ($r = 0.42$) and women ($r = 0.56$) in 18 population samples from widely diverse geographic regions (Stegmayer et al., 1997). These studies prompted an analysis of 16 MONICA population samples that revealed significant negative correlations between frequencies of effective blood pressure control in hypertensive cases and incidence and mortality

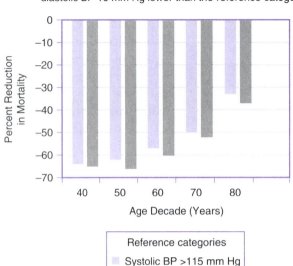

Estimates are for adults of increasing age with systolic BP 20 mm Hg lower or diastolic BP 10 mm Hg lower than the reference categories.

Reference categories
Systolic BP >115 mm Hg
Diastolic BP >75 mm Hg

FIGURE 6.7 Reduction in Stroke Mortality in Adults with Reduced Blood Pressure.

Data from Lewington, S., Clarke, R., Qizilbash, N., Peto, R., Collins, R., & Prospective Studies Collaboration. (2002). Age-specific relevance of usual blood pressure to vascular mortality: A meta-analysis of individual data for one million adults in 61 prospective studies. *Lancet, 360,* 1903–1913.

rates of stroke (Banegas & Pérez-Regadera, 1998; Banegas, Rodriguez-Artalejo, de la Cruz, Guallar-Castillón, & del Rey Calero, 1998). Finally, hypertension and stroke were also positively correlated ($r = 0.78$) in an international study of North American and European nations (Wolf-Maier et al., 2003).

Review and meta-analysis of data from clinical trials provide strong evidence that aggressive treatment of elevated blood pressure using antihypertensive medications significantly reduces the risk of acute stroke. For example, a meta-analysis of 398 such trials found a risk reduction of 21% across all studies with adjustment for interindividual variability in response to different classes of antihypertensive medications (Webb, Fischer, Mehta, & Rothwell, 2010).

In an exploration of three Japanese cohorts containing a total of 27,172 adults aged 40–69 years in successive time periods from 1963 to 1994, the incidence of acute stroke after 10 years of average follow-up showed a significant dose response with increasing blood pressure (BP) and even individuals with suboptimal blood pressure (systolic BP between 130 and 139 mm Hg or diastolic BP between 80 and 89 mm Hg) were at higher risk than individuals with lesser BP (Imano et al., 2009). These findings suggest that the early management of even mild hypertension with antihypertensive medications is beneficial in the primary prevention of acute stroke.

Lowering elevated BP among first stroke victims by antihypertensive medication has also been found to be effective in the prevention of recurrent strokes. In a meta-analysis of 10 clinical trials, administration

of antihypertensive agents to first stroke victims reduced the incidence of recurrent stroke by about 30% (Lakhan & Sapko, 2009).

Cigarette Smoking and Stroke

Smoking has been etiologically linked to stroke in a number of epidemiologic investigations. In an early meta-analysis of data from 32 separate epidemiologic studies (17 cohort studies, 14 case–control studies, and one clinical trial), the summary relative risk of stroke associated with cigarette smoking was 1.5 and there was a significant dose response in risk with number of cigarettes smoked (e.g., the summary estimates of relative risk for daily smokers of 1–10, 11–20, and >20 cigarettes were 1.37, 1.45, and 1.82, respectively) (Shinton & Beevers, 1989). Estimates by subtype also suggested that the risk of subarachnoid hemorrhage associated with smoking (RR = 2.93) was elevated more so than other subtypes of stroke (RR = 1.43). These results are in close agreement with findings of the large international INTERSTROKE case–control study in which heavy smoking also resulted in an approximate twofold increase in the risk of stroke (O'Donnell et al., 2010). Selected prospective cohort studies of smoking and stroke are described in the following paragraphs.

The impact of cigarette smoking on the incidence of stroke was examined in the Framingham Heart Study cohort of 4255 men and women aged 36–68 years and free of symptoms at baseline. During 26 years of follow-up, 459 strokes were detected in the cohort. After adjustment for age, gender, and other risk factors, the relative risk of stroke among heavy smokers (at least two packs per day) was double that of light smokers (less than 10 cigarettes per day). Among individuals who quit smoking during the study, stroke risk decreased to the level of nonsmokers by 5 years after smoking cessation (Wolf, D'Agostino, Kannel, Bonita, & Blanger, 1988).

The Oslo Study was designed as a prospective cohort study of cardiovascular diseases in Norway. The cohort contained 16,173 men aged 40–49 years who were asymptomatic at baseline. After 18 years of follow-up, 85 individuals suffered fatal strokes in the cohort, only four of whom had never smoked. Daily smokers compared to never-smokers had a relative risk of 3.5 and individuals who smoked cigarettes, pipes, and cigars had a relative risk of 6.1. On average, the cases had significantly increased systolic and diastolic BP compared to disease-free individuals (Håheim, Holme, Hjermann, & Leren, 1996).

The British Regional Heart Study was designed as a prospective cohort study to examine risk factors for cardiovascular disease in the United Kingdom. The cohort consisted of 7735 asymptomatic men aged 40–59 years at baseline randomly drawn from 24 British towns during 1978–1980. During 12.5 years of average follow-up, 167 individuals suffered strokes. Current smokers and ex-smokers had relative risks of 3.7 and 1.7, respectively, compared to never-smokers and those who smoked pipes or cigars had a relative risk of 2.2. Individuals who quit smoking reduced their risk significantly after 5 years of smoking cessation (Wannamethee, Shaper, Whincup, & Walker, 1995).

Investigators at Harvard studied smoking and stroke in a prospective cohort of 118,539 asymptomatic women aged 30–55 years at baseline. During 8 years of follow-up, 274 strokes were identified and classified by subtype. Compared to never-smokers, women who smoked 1–24 cigarettes per day had an age-adjusted relative risk of 2.2 for all subtypes of stroke and those who smoked 25 or more cigarettes per day had a relative risk of 3.7. The risk of subarachnoid hemorrhagic stroke among heavy smokers was increased nearly tenfold. These prospective data support a causal relationship between smoking and stroke in women (Colditz et al., 1988).

As a part of the U.S. Physicians' Health Study (a randomized clinical trial designed to determine the value of aspirin and beta-carotene in preventing cardiovascular disease among 22,022 male physicians), associations between smoking and stroke have been examined in ancillary studies. After 10 years of follow-up, 312 individuals suffered nonfatal strokes.

Adjusted relative risks were 1.2 for former smokers, 2.0 for current smokers of less than 20 cigarettes per day, and 2.5 for current smokers of 20 or more cigarettes per day (Robbins, Manson, Lee, Satterfield, & Hennekens, 1994).

In a subsequent investigation of the same cohort of U.S. male physicians, investigators examined the risk of specific subtypes of hemorrhagic stroke (subarachnoid hemorrhage and intracerebral hemorrhage). After nearly 18 years of follow-up, 139 hemorrhagic strokes were identified and subclassified by subtype. Compared to never-smokers, men smoking fewer than 20 cigarettes per day had a relative risk of 1.6 (for all subtypes of hemorrhagic stroke) and men smoking 20 or more cigarettes per day had a relative risk of 2.4. The effects of smoking were similar for subtypes of hemorrhagic strokes (Kurth et al., 2003).

Subarachnoid hemorrhagic strokes arise from the leakage of blood from ruptured blood vessels or aneurysms into the subarachnoid space. These lesions often occur in the Circle of Willis and its branches.

According to a review of 51 studies from 21 countries, the average annual incidence of subarachnoid hemorrhage is 9.1 per 100,000. Rates were highest in Japan and Finland (>20 per 100,000) and lowest in countries of South and Central America (<5 per 100,000) (de Rooij, Linn, van der Plas, Algra, & Rinkel, 2007). Populations at highest risk for subarachnoid hemorrhage have high rates of smoking and hypertension (Stegmayr et al., 1997) and episodic alcohol abuse (Makela et al., 2001).

Feigin and colleagues examined the relationship of smoking to subarachnoid hemorrhage in a meta-analysis of 26 prospective cohort studies involving 306,620 participants in the Asia-Pacific region. This region has active research centers in Japan, China, Taiwan, South Korea, Singapore, and Australia. During a median follow-up of 8.2 years, a total of 236 incident cases of subarachnoid hemorrhage were observed. Current smoking and elevated systolic BP (>140 mm Hg) independently increased the risk of subarachnoid hemorrhage (summary hazard ratios: 2.4 and 2.0, respectively) whereas no significant associations were found for cholesterol, body mass index, or drinking alcohol. For this population, it is estimated that 19% of cases are attributable to systolic BP >140 mm Hg and 29% of cases are attributable to smoking (Feigin et al., 2005).

In summary, the epidemiologic evidence is compelling that smoking accounts for a substantial portion of the morbidity and mortality due to stroke. Mechanistically, tobacco's addictive agent, nicotine, is a potent vasoconstrictor, and smoking the first cigarette of the day causes an abrupt rise in BP (Gropelli,

Giorgi, Omboni, Parati, & Manchia, 1992; Omvik, 1996). Furthermore, numerous molecular studies have demonstrated that various elements of tobacco smoke including nicotine are highly inflammatory to the lining (endothelium) of blood vessels and are etiologically involved in the genesis of atherosclerotic plaque (Surgeon General's Report, 2004).

Alcohol Abuse and Stroke

The effects of alcohol on the cardiovascular system are dependent upon dose. While some observational studies have found that moderate or light consumption of alcoholic beverages confers a slight risk reduction, other studies of heavy consumption have noted an increase in the risk. To clarify the relationship, Reynolds and colleagues conducted a meta-analysis of alcohol and stroke using data from 35 published case–control and cohort studies. Compared to those who never consumed alcohol, individuals consuming more than 60 g (about five drinks) per day had relative risks of 1.6 for any stroke, 1.4 for ischemic stroke, and 2.2 for hemorrhagic stroke. In contrast, those individuals consuming less than 12 g of alcohol daily had a slight risk reduction (RR = 0.83). The results suggest that alcohol abuse significantly increases the risk of stroke whereas light drinking may offer slight protection (Reynolds et al., 2003).

Cocaine, Amphetamines, and Stroke

Ischemic and hemorrhagic strokes occasionally occur in temporal association with the use/abuse of illicit drugs. In a case series of 167 stroke patients entered into the Maryland Stroke Data Bank, data were obtained on drug abuse for 116 cases. Eleven of these stroke patients (9.5%) reported a history of recent drug use, and five of these gave a history of cocaine abuse (Sloan, Kittner, Rigamonti, & Price, 1991).

There is also some evidence that amphetamine use is associated with an increased risk of stroke. In a cross-sectional study of hospital discharge data for young adults treated in Texas hospitals, amphetamine abuse was associated with ischemic stroke (odds ratio = 4.95) and cocaine abuse was associated with both ischemic stroke (OR = 2.03) and hemorrhagic stroke (OR = 2.33). These data suggest the potential danger of stroke with abuse of stimulant drugs (Westover, McBride, & Haley, 2007).

Atrial Fibrillation and Stroke

Atrial fibrillation is the most common cardiac arrhythmia (abnormal heart rhythm). In this condition, the normal electrical impulses that arise in the sinoatrial node of the heart become disorganized leading to fibrillation (quivering) of the heart muscle rather than coordinated contractions. A review and analysis of population-based surveys conducted in the United States revealed that atrial fibrillation increases exponentially with age and that approximately 70% of cases are diagnosed after 65 years of age (**FIGURE 6.8**). The median age of onset was about 75 years of age (Feinberg, Blackshear, Laupacis, Kronmal, & Hart, 1995).

An international team of investigators recently examined the worldwide epidemiology of atrial fibrillation using data from population-based studies published during 1980–2010 from 21 regions of the *Global Burden of Disease* (GBD) Project of the World Health Organization. Estimates of prevalence, incidence, and mortality for atrial fibrillation were obtained for men and women of each region. Based upon prevalence estimates per 100,000 for 2010 (596 for men and 373 for women), the investigators estimated that 33.5 million people in the world population have atrial fibrillation (20.9 million men and 12.6 million women). Global annual age-adjusted incidence rates of atrial fibrillation per 100,000 were, on average, about 35%

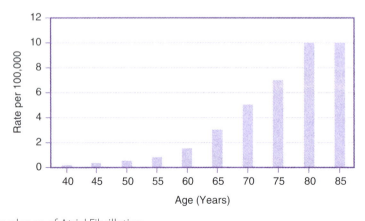

FIGURE 6.8 Age-specific Prevalence of Atrial Fibrillation.

Data from Feinberg, W. M., Blackshear, J. L., Laupacis, A., Kronmal, R., & Hart, R. G. (1995). Prevalence, age distribution, and gender of patients with atrial fibrillation. *Archives of Internal Medicine, 155*, 469–473.

higher in men than women, and rates increased by 28% in men (from 61 to 78) and 36% in women (from 44 to 60) during the 20-year study period. There was significant variation in incidence rates among GBD regions; overall, rates in developing nations were approximately twofold higher in developed nations compared to developing nations. Age-adjusted incidence rates were highest in North America (264 for men and 196 for women) and lowest in the Asia-Pacific region (34 in men and 20 in women). Global mortality due to atrial fibrillation (annual deaths per 100,000) doubled in both men and women during the 20-year study period (average rates in 1990 and 2010 were 0.85 and 1.65 per 100,000, respectively). In 2015, there were 195,300 deaths from atrial fibrillation in the world population, more than double the number reported in 1990. A significant fraction of deaths attributable to atrial fibrillation (~20%) are sudden cardiac deaths. The authors suggest that the current epidemiological data on atrial fibrillation constitutes a global epidemic of this condition with about 5 million new cases being diagnosed each year. Reasons for the increase in global rates of atrial fibrillation include

aging trends in the global population, improved imaging techniques for detection, and increasing exposure to cardiovascular risk factors such as hypertension and atherosclerosis that cause arterial stiffness, diastolic dysfunction, and atrial volume overload (Chugh et al., 2017; Roth et al., 2017).

Chronic atrial fibrillation carries an increased risk of stroke. As depicted in **FIGURE 6.9**, a thrombus in the left ventricular chamber of the heart can be dislodged by atrial fibrillation and migrate into the brain via the internal carotid artery leading to embolic occlusion of a cerebral artery and acute stroke.

Several epidemiologic investigations have found that individuals diagnosed with atrial fibrillation have a markedly increased risk of stroke. **TABLE 6.2** presents relative risk estimates from four separate studies of atrial fibrillation and stroke: Framingham in the United States (Wolf, Abbott, & Kannel, 1991), the Shibata Study in Japan (Nakayama et al., 1997; Tanaka et al., 1985), the Reykjavik Study in Iceland (Onundarson, Thorgeirsson, Jonmundsen, Sigfusson, & Hardarson, 1987), and an investigation in the United Kingdom (Flegel, Shipley, & Rose, 1987).

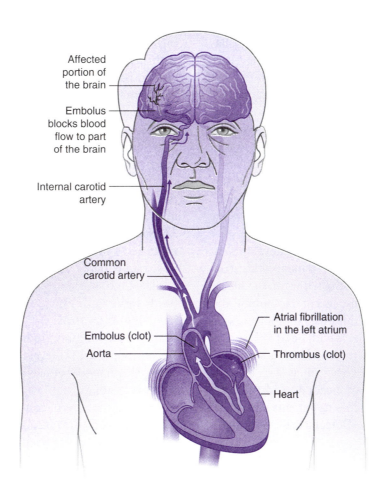

FIGURE 6.9 Genesis of Acute Stroke by Atrial Fibrillation.

TABLE 6.2 Atrial Fibrillation and Risk of Stroke				
		Stroke Rate		
Study Location	Mean Age	AF	No AF	Relative Risk
Framingham, United States	70	4.1	0.74	5.6
Shibata, Japan	65	5.0	0.90	5.6
Reykjavik, Iceland	52	1.6	0.23	7.2
Whitehall, UK	60	1.8	0.26	6.9

AF = Atrial Fibrillation

Stroke Rate = annual percentage of individuals who developed stroke

Source: Data from Wolf, P. A., Abbott, R. D., & Kannel, W. B. (1991). Atrial fibrillation as an independent risk factor for stroke: The Framingham Study. *Stroke, 22,* 983–988; Tanaka, H., Hayashi, M., Date, C., Imai, K., Asada, M., Shoji, H., … Shimada, T. (1985). Epidemiologic studies of stroke in Shibata, a Japanese provincial city: Preliminary report on risk factors for cerebral infarction. *Stroke, 16,* 773–780; Onundarson, P. T., Thorgeirsson, G., Jonmundsen, E., Sigfusson, N., & Hardarson, T. (1987). Chronic atrial fibrillation—Epidemiologic features and 14 year follow-up: A case-control study. *European Heart Journal, 8,* 521–527; Flegel, K. M., Shipley, M. J., & Rose, G. (1987). Risk of stroke in nonrheumatic atrial fibrillation. *Lancet, 1,* 526–529; Halperin, J. L., & Hart, R. G. (1988). Atrial fibrillation and stroke: New ideas, persisting dilemmas. *Stroke, 19,* 937–941.

The data of **TABLE 6.2** reflect greater than fivefold increases in the relative risk of stroke associated with atrial fibrillation for populations of diverse culture living in markedly different environments. Furthermore, some studies suggest that women with atrial fibrillation may be at greater risk than men (e.g., analysis of the Japanese cohort in Shibata after more than 15 years of follow-up revealed a twofold higher stroke risk for women with atrial fibrillation [RR = 10.7] compared to men [RR = 5.2]) (Nakayama et al., 1997). These estimates and data from several other studies suggest that about one in three individuals with atrial fibrillation will experience a stroke during their lifetime (Halperin & Hart, 1988). The value of antithrombotic agents in the prevention atrial fibrillation is discussed below in the section on prevention.

Atrial fibrillation is also linked to the development and progression of heart failure. In patients with atrial fibrillation, impaired filling of the left ventricle during systole may result in diminished cardiac output and heart failure. Reciprocally, diminished blood flow to the coronary arteries in patients with heart failure may cause ischemic damage to the conducting system of the heart resulting in heart arrhythmias such as atrial fibrillation. Clinical trials are needed to identify the best pharmacologic approaches in patients with atrial fibrillation and heart failure (Kotecha & Piccini, 2015).

Blood Lipids and Stroke

The INTERSTROKE investigation of stroke risk factors determined that the lipoprotein ratio of ApoB to ApoA1 was a stronger risk factor for stroke than other measures of lipids such as low-density lipoprotein (LDL) cholesterol or total cholesterol (O'Donnell et al., 2010). Consequently, investigators are continuing to explore the association of certain lipoproteins with the risk of cardiovascular disease including stroke. For example, one lipoprotein that specifically binds low-density (bad) cholesterol is lipoprotein(a). A meta-analysis of 27 prospective studies revealed a significant risk increase (RR = 1.6) in coronary heart disease among persons with elevated lipoprotein(a) levels (Danesh, Collins, & Peto, 2000).

The relationship of lipoprotein(a) to stroke was recently examined in a meta-analysis of 31 epidemiologic (Smolders, Lemmens, & Thijs, 2007). In 23 case–control studies involving 2600 strokes, the mean level of lipoprotein(a) was significantly higher in stroke patients than controls and individuals with higher than normal values were at increased risk (odds ratio: 2.37). In five prospective cohort studies involving 1645 strokes, the incidence of stroke was more frequent among individuals in the highest tertile of lipoprotein(a) levels measured at baseline. The authors conclude that elevated lipoprotein(a) is a risk factor for stroke.

Serum cholesterol continues to be of interest as a biomarker of cardiovascular disease risk and its relationship to stroke has been examined in many epidemiologic investigations. The results of these studies are mixed; some showing increased risk with high levels whereas others have found no association. A team of investigators attempted to clarify the association in a meta-analysis of 45 epidemiologic studies involving 450,000 individuals with 5–30 years of follow-up (average: 16 years) and a total of 7.3 million person-years of observation during which 13,397 participants experienced a stroke. The summary estimates of relative risk from this analysis were null reflecting no association of total blood cholesterol to the risk of stroke (Prospective Studies Collaboration, 1995).

Despite these null results, some investigators have noted rising levels of blood cholesterol in many Asian nations and therefore have continuing concern about potential impending increases in the incidence of stroke and other cardiovascular events. To explore this possibility, a team of investigators examined the association of blood cholesterol with incident coronary heart disease and stroke in the Asia-Pacific region (Asia-Pacific Cohort Studies Collaboration, 2003). Meta-analysis was applied to the combined data from 29 prospective cohorts containing 352,033 individuals from sites in China, Japan, Taiwan, South Korea, Singapore, and Australia. During 2 million person-years of follow-up, 4842 fatalities/events due to cardiovascular disease were recorded. In this investigation, each 1 mmol per liter (38.7 mg per deciliter) increase in total blood cholesterol was associated with a 35% increase in the risk of coronary death and a 25% increase in the risk of fatal or nonfatal ischemic stroke. There was a modest inverse association of cholesterol with hemorrhagic stroke. These results were similar for both Asian and non-Asian cohorts prompting the investigators to suggest that "*rising population-wide levels of cholesterol would be expected to contribute to a substantial increase in the overall burden of cardiovascular diseases in this region*" (Asia-Pacific Cohort Studies Collaboration, 2003).

In view of such disparate results, it appears advisable to continue investigation of the association between cholesterol and the risk of stroke. Since many risk factors are involved in the genesis of all cardiovascular diseases including stroke, careful adjustment for confounding will be necessary to elucidate independent effects.

Diabetes Mellitus and Stroke

The rising incidence of diabetes mellitus in the developed world parallels the rising incidence of obesity. Adult-onset or type 2 diabetes is linked with overeating, metabolic overload, and obesity. The relationship of diabetes to the onset of stroke has been the subject of more than 100 epidemiologic investigations. There is compelling evidence that patients with diabetes mellitus are two to three times more likely to develop stroke than individuals with normal blood glucose;

furthermore, diabetic individuals commonly manifest hypertension, obesity, and hyperlipidemia, which are also independent risk factors for stroke.

In a comprehensive literature review and meta-analysis, investigators of the Emerging Risk Factors Collaboration examined associations of diabetes, fasting blood glucose, and the risk of stroke and other cardiovascular diseases. The analysis of diabetes-related risk was based on 97 studies; 54 of them contributed to the separate analysis of risk associated with fasting blood glucose. Collectively, they provided 8.5 million person-years of follow-up, with a median time to a first vascular event, fatal or nonfatal, of 10.8 years. The hazard ratios (HR) for ischemic stroke and hemorrhagic stroke were both significantly increased, 2.27 and 1.56, respectively. The risk of coronary heart disease was also increased (HR = 2.0). Elevated levels of fasting blood glucose were also associated with increased risk (e.g., levels exceeding 6.0 mmol/L [126 mg/dL]) increased the risk of cardiovascular events by 70%). The investigators point out that the results can be generalized for only those populations of developed high-income nations predominantly represented in the studies. Additional studies are needed to quantify the vascular disease burden attributable to diabetes in low- and middle-income countries (Emerging Risk Factors Collaboration, 2010).

Obesity and Stroke

Obesity is a potentially important risk factor in the web of causation of stroke as well as most other cardiovascular diseases. A team of investigators in Italy and the United Kingdom conducted a systematic review and meta-analysis of prospective studies addressing the relationship of overweight and obesity to the incidence of ischemic and hemorrhagic stroke. Twenty-five studies were included with 2,274,961 participants and 30,757 events. The body mass index (BMI = kg/m^2) was used to define overweight and obesity. The relative risk for ischemic stroke increased by 22% in overweight individuals (BMI between 25 and 30) and by 64% in obese individuals (BMI of 30 or more). The risk for hemorrhagic stroke showed no increase in overweight individuals and the risk increase in obese individuals (24%) did not quite reach statistical significance. The results suggest that any degree of overweight may increase the risk of ischemic stroke (Strazzullo et al., 2010).

Obesity is integral to several important physiological and biological mechanisms that are known to increase the risk of stroke and other cardiovascular outcomes (Poirier et al., 2006). For example, weight gain increases BP and the majority of hypertensive people are either overweight or obese (Stamler, Stamler, Riedlinger, Algera, & Roberts, 1978). In addition, obesity has been found to accelerate atherogenesis in young men (McGill et al., 2002) and is associated with dyslipidemia (Brown et al., 2000). Furthermore, obesity in combination with insulin resistance, type 2 diabetes, and elevated triglycerides defines a complex known as the *metabolic syndrome*, which carries a high risk of myocardial infarction and stroke (Eckel, Grundy, & Zimmet, 2005). Excess adiposity is also associated with increased secretion of inflammatory adipokines that may stimulate atherogenesis (Rost et al., 2001). To summarize, obesity increases BP, insulin resistance, and blood lipids, and promotes inflammation and atherosclerosis, all of which predispose to stroke.

Inflammation, C-Reactive Protein, and Stroke

Atherogenesis is often characterized as an inflammatory disease (Ross, 1999). Indeed, the inflammatory biomarker, C-reactive protein (CRP), has shown value as a valid predictor of impending coronary heart disease (Ridker, Rifai, Rose, Buring, & Cook, 2002).

To clarify the association of CRP with the risk of stroke, investigators in Boston studied the association of plasma CRP levels with the incidence of first ischemic stroke or TIA in the Framingham Study original cohort. The study included 591 men and 871 women (mean age about 70 years) with no history of stroke or TIA during their clinic examination during 1980–1982. The CRP levels were measured using an enzyme immunoassay on previously frozen serum samples. During 12–14 years of follow-up, 196 ischemic strokes and TIAs occurred. Independent of age, men in the highest CRP quartile had a twofold higher risk of ischemic stroke/TIA (RR = 2.0), and women had an almost threefold higher risk (RR = 2.7) compared to those in the lowest quartile. The trend in the risk of stroke with increasing quartiles of CRP was highly significant. After adjustment for smoking, total/HDL cholesterol, systolic BP, and diabetes, the increase in risk across CRP quartiles remained statistically significant for both men and women. The investigators concluded that elevated plasma CRP levels significantly predict the risk of ischemic stroke and TIA in the elderly (Rost et al., 2001).

▶ Prevention of Stroke

As is true for all cardiovascular diseases, stroke is a multifactorial disease; and as a consequence, preventive strategies must be designed to influence multiple factors in order to be successful. Similar to myocardial infarction, stroke is the culminating event of chronic disease processes that interact in a complex web of causation. Pathogenic mechanisms include hypertension, inflammation, atherogenesis, tobacco addiction, insulin resistance, alcohol abuse, obesity, and atrial fibrillation. All of these risk factors are potentially modifiable through appropriate lifestyle choices and/or therapeutic modalities.

Lifestyle decisions believed to have a favorable impact on stroke prevention include avoidance of tobacco use in any form; maintaining optimal body weight (BMI between 20 and 25) through exercise and healthy eating; limiting salt intake to less than 6 g daily; limiting alcohol intake to no more than one drink daily; eating a diet with at least five servings of fruits and vegetables daily; eating fish and other sources of omega-3 polyunsaturated fatty acids on a regular basis (at least twice per week); exercising daily (e.g., brisk walking for 30 minutes); maintaining BP, blood glucose, and blood cholesterol within normal limits through careful monitoring and pharmacologic therapy if needed; chemoprevention of thrombosis with low-dose aspirin; and management of atrial fibrillation, hypertension, diabetes, and hyperlipidemia by appropriate sustained therapeutic care.

Diet and Stroke Prevention

Diet has been studied extensively in the prevention of stroke with mixed results. Ancel Keys and his colleagues found that the Mediterranean diet had the greatest benefit in the prevention of cardiovascular and cerebrovascular diseases including stroke (Keys et al., 1980). Furthermore, several other epidemiologic studies have found that increasing consumption of fruits and vegetables is associated with a decreased risk of stroke. Investigators at St. George University in London conducted a meta-analysis of eight studies consisting of nine independent cohorts in order to more precisely quantify the relationship of stroke and intake of fruits and vegetables (He, Nowson, & MacGregor, 2006). Their analysis included dietary data on 257,551 individuals followed on average for 13 years with detection of 4917 stroke events. Compared to individuals who consumed less than three servings of fruits and vegetables daily, individuals consuming 3–5 servings had an 11% risk reduction and individuals consuming more than five servings had a 26% risk reduction. Estimates were consistent for both ischemic and hemorrhagic stroke and the authors suggest that daily consumption of five or more servings of fruits and vegetables has preventive value.

Various mechanisms have been advanced to explain the beneficial impact of consuming abundant fruits and vegetables in the diet. Fruits and vegetables are rich sources of potassium, folate, fiber, antioxidants (vitamin C, beta-carotene, and flavonoids), and anti-inflammatory agents, all of which appear to have favorable effects in helping to maintain optimal BP, blood lipids, and blood glucose.

Investigators at Harvard examined relationships of certain dietary factors (fish and omega-3 fatty acids) and the risk of stroke in the Nurses' Health Study. This prospective cohort study enrolled women aged 34–59 years who were disease-free at baseline and agreed to complete a food frequency questionnaire and be followed to determine cardiovascular and other disease outcomes. A total of 79,839 eligible women were followed for up to 14 years (1,086,261 person-years) during which 574 incident strokes were detected. Women who ate fish five or more times per week significantly reduced their risk of stroke (RR = 0.48) compared to those who ate none, and there was a significant inverse dose response of decreasing risk with increasing consumption. Furthermore, women consuming high levels of omega-3 polyunsaturated fatty acids also lowered their risk (RR = 0.72). Stratification of the data by stroke subtypes revealed risk reductions for ischemic stroke but not for hemorrhagic stroke (Iso et al., 2001).

Investigators at Boston University conducted a meta-analysis of prospective studies to further examine the association of fish consumption with risk of stroke. Nine cohorts were identified in eight studies that provided relative risk estimates. Compared with individuals who consumed little or no fish, those who consumed fish at least five times per week reduced their risk by 31% (RR = 0.69) and even consumption levels of once per week resulted in a significant protective effect (RR = 0.87). Stratification of data by subtype of stroke revealed significant risk reductions for ischemic stroke but not for hemorrhagic stroke (He et al., 2004).

Fish are the main dietary source of long-chain omega-3 polyunsaturated fatty acids (PUFA), and these compounds have been shown to have favorable effects on BP, arrhythmias, lipid profile, platelet aggregation, and endothelial function (Harris, 1997; Nestel, 1990). One principal mechanism by which fish consumption could benefit the cardiovascular system is reduction of inflammatory prostaglandins. Omega-3 and other complex polyunsaturated fatty acids are not readily transformed into arachidonic acid, the chief substrate of the inflammatory cascade. Intake of fish and other omega-3 polyunsaturated fatty acids could therefore reduce atherogenesis by inhibiting the inflammatory cascade (Dyerberg, Bang, Stoffersen, Moncada, & Vane, 1978).

Salt and Stroke Prevention

The level of salt intake in the diet has significant impact on BP and consequently influences the risk of stroke. Strazzullo, D'Elia, Bakwin-Kandala, and Cappuccio (2009) conducted a comprehensive meta-analysis of 19 independent cohort samples from 13 studies involving 177,025 participants, over 11,000 vascular events and follow-up of 3.5–19 years. They found that high salt intake (greater than 6 g of salt per day) was associated with a 23% increase in the incidence of acute stroke.

Conversely, reduction in salt intake is advisable to reduce BP for stroke protection. Strong evidence for this inverse association comes from the international INTERSALT Study involving 10,172 men and women aged 20–59 years enrolled for study in 52 centers from around the world (Intersalt Cooperative Research Group, 1988). The INTERSALT investigation was specifically designed to examine the relationship between BP and 24-hour urinary excretion of electrolytes (sodium and potassium). Regression analysis revealed a significant linear relationship between sodium excretion and BP whereby each 100 mmol reduction in sodium excretion independently reduced systolic BP by 9 mm Hg. The results of INTERSALT also demonstrated that high urinary potassium is associated with lower (more optimal) BP whereas high body mass and alcohol abuse significantly increase BP.

Anticoagulation Drugs and Stroke Prevention

It has been estimated that one in three individuals who manifest atrial fibrillation will experience a stroke in their lifetime (Halperin & Hart, 1988). Atrial fibrillation is the most frequently diagnosed arrhythmia and in the United States population alone, 2.3 million people are affected. The prevalence of atrial fibrillation increases with age, approaching 10% in people older than 80 years. Management of atrial fibrillation includes many modalities: Pharmacologic therapy aimed to keep patients in sinus rhythm and to control rate, electrical cardioversion, catheter ablation, as well as anticoagulation to prevent thromboembolic disease.

Oral anticoagulants such as warfarin or aspirin have been the mainstay of stroke prevention in patients with atrial fibrillation for more than half a century. A number of randomized clinical trials have been conducted to assess and compare the value of such drugs. In a meta-analysis of data from five completed trials, treatment of atrial fibrillation with warfarin reduced the risk of stroke by 84% in women and

60% in men (the total risk reduction was 68%). By comparison, treatment with aspirin produced lesser effects (15% risk reduction for the 75 mg dosage and 44% reduction for the 325 mg dosage). No increases were noted in the frequency of bleeding episodes for either drug. These findings support the value of anti-thrombotic (warfarin) therapy in stroke prevention for patients with atrial fibrillation (Atrial Fibrillation Investigators, 1994).

Additional studies have been conducted to evaluate the effectiveness and safety of warfarin administration to patients with atrial fibrillation in clinical practice. For example, a U.S. study of 11,526 patients with atrial fibrillation who were treated in usual care settings in Northern California found a 51% reduction in the risk of thromboembolism among those treated with warfarin compared to those not receiving warfarin (Go et al., 2003). Furthermore, several randomized studies have shown that immediate aspirin therapy followed by warfarin therapy is an effective approach for the prevention of recurrence after a first stroke or ischemic attack (Hart, Palacio, & Pearce, 2002).

Statins in Stroke Prevention

As already discussed in this chapter, there is controversy regarding the association of serum cholesterol and stroke. Some studies suggest that elevated levels increase the risk (Asia-Pacific Cohort Studies Collaboration, 2003) whereas others do not (Prospective Studies Collaboration, 1995). Nevertheless, there appears to be consistency of evidence supporting the role of statin use to reduce stroke risk in patients with hyperlipidemia.

Investigators at Leiden University Medical Center in the Netherlands examined HMG-CoA reductase inhibitors[*] and the risk of stroke in a meta-analysis of 13 randomized clinical trials that enrolled 20,438 participants. A total of 181 strokes was observed in patients randomized to treatment with an HMG-CoA reductase inhibitor and 261 strokes in patients randomized to placebo. Treatment with an HMG-CoA reductase inhibitor led to an overall risk reduction of 31% (odds ratio = 0.69) (Blauw, Lagaay, Smelt, & Westendorp, 1997).

More recently, investigators in London conducted a meta-analysis to evaluate the impact of statin therapy on the risk of death in general, and the risk of stroke, specifically, among more than 121,000 study volunteers that participated in 42 clinical research

trials. Among the volunteers taking statin drugs, death from any cause was reduced by 12% and the relative risk of stroke (all types) was reduced by 16%. Risk reductions were proportional to the magnitude of LDL cholesterol reduction achieved after initiation of statin therapy. Furthermore, analysis by subtype of stroke revealed that the risk of only ischemic "non-hemorrhagic" strokes was reduced by statin therapy. Ischemic strokes generally result from atherosclerosis of the carotid arteries and intracerebral arteries that supply the brain with blood. The incidence of "hemorrhagic" strokes, which usually result from poorly controlled high BP, was not reduced by statin therapy (O'Regan, Wu, Arora, Perri, & Mills, 2008).

The combined data suggest that statin therapy prevents ischemic stroke and reinforces the value of cholesterol reduction in reducing the risk of cardiovascular disease. Clearly, judicious administration of statins for cholesterol reduction is a valuable component of multifactorial strategies for the prevention of stroke, myocardial infarction, and other forms of coronary heart disease.

Surgical Intervention

Surgical procedures such as carotid endarterectomy or carotid angioplasty can be used to remove significant atherosclerotic narrowing (stenosis) of the carotid artery (the primary conduit for blood supply to the brain). Evidence of benefit comes from the analysis of pooled data from two randomized clinical trials involving 5893 patients (the European Carotid Surgery Trial and the North American Symptomatic Carotid Endarterectomy Trial). For patients with greater than 50% stenosis of carotid arteries, endarterectomy reduced the 5-year risk of stroke from 20% to 5% (Rothwell, Eliasziw, Gutnikov, Warlow, & Barnett, 2004).

References

Adams, H. P., Bendixen, B. H., Kappelle, L. J., Biller, J., Love, B. B., Gordon, D. L., & Marsh, E. E., 3rd. (1993). Classification of subtype of acute ischemic stroke. Definitions for use in a multicenter clinical trial. TOAST. Trial of Org 10172 in Acute Stroke Treatment. *Stroke, 24*(1), 35–41.

Asia-Pacific Cohort Studies Collaboration. (2003). Cholesterol, coronary heart disease, and stroke in the Asia Pacific region. *International Journal of Epidemiology, 32*, 563–572.

Atrial Fibrillation Investigators. (1994). Risk factors for stroke and efficacy of antithrombotic therapy in atrial fibrillation.

---

[*] The enzyme HMG-CoA reductase (3-hydroxy-3-methyl-glutaryl-CoA reductase) is the rate-limiting enzyme of the mevalonate pathway, the metabolic pathway that produces cholesterol in humans and other mammals. This enzyme is the primary target of the cholesterol-lowering drugs known collectively as the statins.

Analysis of pooled data from five randomized controlled trials. *Archives of Internal Medicine, 154*(13), 1449–1557.

Banegas J. R., & Pérez-Regadera, A. G. (1998). Hypertension control as an indicator of the geographical variation of stroke. *Stroke, 29*, 867–868.

Banegas, J. R., Rodriguez-Artalejo, F., de la Cruz, T. J. J., Guallar-Castillón, P., & del Rey Calero, J. (1998). Blood pressure in Spain: Distribution, awareness, control, and benefits of a reduction in average pressure. *Hypertension, 32*, 998–1002.

Blauw, G. J., Lagaay, M., Smelt, A. H. M., & Westendorp, R. G. J. (1997). A meta-analysis of randomized, placebo-controlled, double-blind trials with HMG-CoA reductase inhibitors. *Stroke, 28*, 946–950.

Bradbury, M. (1979). *The concept of a blood-brain barrier.* New York: John Wiley and Sons Ltd.

Brown, C. D., Higgins, M., Donato, K. A., Rohde, F. C., Garrison, R., Obarzanek, E., … Horan, M. (2000). Body mass index and the prevalence of hypertension and dyslipidemia. *Obesity Research, 8*, 605–619.

Casper, M. L., Wing, S., Anda, R. F., Knowles, M., & Pollard, R. A. (1995). The shifting stroke belt. Changes in the geographic pattern of stroke mortality in the United States, 1962 to 1988. *Stroke, 26*(5), 755–760.

Centers for Disease Control and Prevention. (2004). National Center for Health Statistics, United States Department of Health and Human Services.

Chugh, S. S., Havmoeller, R., Narayanan, K., Singh, D., Rienstra, M., Benjamin, E. J., … Murray, C. J. (2017). Worldwide epidemiology of atrial fibrillation: A Global Burden of Disease 2010 study. *Circulation, 120*(8), 837–847.

Colditz, G. A., Bonita, R., Stampfer, M. J., Willett, W. C., Rosner, B., Speizer, F. E., & Hennekens, C. H. (1988). Cigarette smoking and risk of stroke in middle-aged women. *New England Journal of Medicine, 318*(15), 937–941.

Danesh, J., Collins, R., & Peto, R. (2000). Lipoprotein(a) and coronary heart disease. Meta-analysis of prospective studies. *Circulation, 102*(10), 1082–1085.

de Rooij, N. K., Linn, F. H., van der Plas, J. A., Algra, A., & Rinkel, G. J. (2007). Incidence of subarachnoid haemorrhage: A systematic review with emphasis on region, age, gender and time trends. *Journal of Neurology, Neurosurgery, and Psychiatry, 78*(12), 1365–1372.

Donnan, G. A., Fisher, M., Macleod, M., & Davis, S. M. (2008). Stroke. *Lancet, 371*(9624), 612–1623.

Dyerberg, J., Bang, H. O., Stoffersen, E., Moncada, S., & Vane, J. R. (1978). Eicosapentaenoic acid and prevention of thrombosis and atherosclerosis? *Lancet, 2*, 117–119.

Eckel, R. H., Grundy, S. M., & Zimmet, P. Z. (2005). The metabolic syndrome. *Lancet, 365*, 1415–1428.

Emerging Risk Factors Collaboration. (2010). Diabetes mellitus, fasting blood glucose concentration, and risk of vascular disease: A collaborative meta-analysis of 102 prospective studies. *Lancet, 375*, 2215–2222.

Feigin, V. L., Forouzanfar, M. H., Krishnamurthi, R., Mensah, G. A., Connor, M., Bennett, D. A., …. Global Burden of Diseases, Injuries, and Risk Factors Study 2010 (GBD 2010) and the GBD Stroke Experts Group. (2014). Global and regional burden of stroke during 1990–2010: Findings from the Global Burden of Disease Study 2010. *Lancet, 383*(9913), 245–254.

Feigin, V. L., Krishnamurthi, R., Parmar, P., Norrving, B., Mensah, G. A., Bennett, D. A., … GBD 2013 Stroke Panel Experts Group. (2015). Update on the global burden of ischemic and hemorrhagic stroke in 1990–2013: The GBD 2013 study. *Neuroepidemiology, 45*(3), 161–176.

Feigin, V. L., Lawes, C. M., Bennett, D. A., & Anderson, C. S. (2003). Stroke epidemiology: A review of population-based studies of incidence, prevalence, and case fatality in the late 20th century. *Lancet Neurology, 2*, 43–53.

Feigin, V. L., Parag, V., Lawes, C. M., Rodgers, A., Suh, I., Woodward, M., … Asia Pacific Cohort Studies Collaboration. (2005). Smoking and elevated blood pressure are the most important risk factors for subarachnoid hemorrhage in the Asia-Pacific region: An overview of 26 cohorts involving 306,620 participants. *Stroke, 36*, 1360–1365.

Feinberg, W. M., Blackshear, J. L., Laupacis, A., Kronmal, R., & Hart, R. G. (1995). Prevalence, age distribution, and gender of patients with atrial fibrillation. *Archives of Internal Medicine, 155*, 469–473.

Fisher, C. M. (1975). Anatomy and pathology of the cerebral vasculature. *Modern Concepts in Cerebrovascular Disease, 1*, 41.

Flegel, K. M., Shipley, M. J., & Rose, G. (1987). Risk of stroke in nonrheumatic atrial fibrillation. *Lancet, 1*, 526–529.

Gillum, R. F. (1999). Stroke mortality in blacks: Disturbing trends. *Stroke, 30*, 1711–1715.

Go, A. S., Hylek, E. M., Chang, Y., Phillips, K. A., Henault, L. E., Capra, A. M., … Singer, D. E. (2003). Anticoagulation therapy for stroke prevention in atrial fibrillation: How well do randomized trials translate into clinical practice? *JAMA, 290*(20), 2685–2692.

Gropelli, A., Giorgi, D. M. A., Omboni, S., Parati, G., & Manchia, G. (1992). Persistent blood pressure increase induced by heavy smoking. *Journal of Hypertension, 10*, 495–499.

Håheim, L. L., Holme, I., Hjermann, I., & Leren, P. (1996). Smoking habits and risk of fatal stroke: 18 years follow up of the Oslo Study. *Journal of Epidemiology and Community Health, 50*(6), 621–624.

Halperin, J. L., & Hart, R. G. (1988). Atrial fibrillation and stroke: New ideas, persisting dilemmas. *Stroke, 19*, 937–941.

Harris, W. S. (1997). n-3 fatty acids and serum lipoproteins: Human studies. *The American Journal of Clinical Nutrition, 65*(Suppl. 5), 1645S–1654S.

Hart, R. G., Palacio, S., & Pearce, L. A. (2002). Atrial fibrillation, stroke, and acute antithrombotic therapy: Analysis of randomized clinical trials. *Stroke, 33*, 2722–2727.

He, F. J., Nowson, C. A., & MacGregor, G. A. (2006). Fruit and vegetable consumption and stroke: Meta-analysis of cohort studies. *Lancet, 367*(9507), 320–326.

He, K., Song, Y., Daviglus, M. L., Liu, K., Van Horn, L., Dyer, A. R., … Greenland, P. (2004). Fish consumption and incidence of stroke: A metaanalysis of cohort studies. *Stroke, 35*, 1538–1542.

Imano, H., Kitamura, A., Sato, S., Kiyama, M., Ohira, T., Yamagishi, K., … Shimamoto, T. (2009). Trends for blood pressure and its contribution to stroke incidence in the middle-aged Japanese population: The Circulatory Risk in Communities Study (CIRCS). *Stroke, 40*(5), 1571–1577.

Intersalt Cooperative Research Group. (1988). Intersalt: An international study of electrolyte excretion and blood pressure. Results for 24 hour urinary sodium and potassium excretion. *BMJ, 297*(6644), 319–328.

Iso, H., Rexrode, K. M., Stampfer, M. J., Manson, J. E., Colditz, G. A., Speizer, F. E., & Hennekens, C. H. (2001). Intake of fish and omega-3 fatty acids and risk of stroke in women. *JAMA, 285*, 304–312.

Johnston, S. C., Mendis, S., & Mathers, C. D. (2009). Global variation in stroke burden and mortality: Estimates from monitoring, surveillance, and modelling. *Lancet Neurology, 8*(4), 345–354.

Keys, A., Aravanis, C., Blackburn, H., Buzina, R., Djordjević, B. S., Dontas, A. S., … Van Buchem, F. S. P. (1980). *Seven countries. A multivariate analysis of death and coronary heart disease* (pp. 1–381). Cambridge, MA and London: Harvard University Press.

Kittner, S. J., White, L. R., Losonczy, K. G., Wolf, P. A., & Hebel, J. R. (1990). Black-white differences in stroke incidence in a national sample. The contribution of hypertension and diabetes mellitus. *JAMA, 264*, 1267–1270.

Kotecha, D., & Piccini, J. P. (2015). Atrial fibrillation in heart failure: What should we do? *European Heart Journal, 36*(46), 3250–3257.

Kurth, T., Kase, C. S., Berger, K., Schaeffner, E. S., Buring, J. E., & Gaziano, M. (2003). Smoking and the risk of hemorrhagic stroke in men. *Stroke, 34*, 1151–1155.

Lakhan, S. E., & Sapko, M. (2009). Blood pressure lowering treatment for preventing stroke recurrence: A systematic review and meta-analysis. *International Archives of Medicine, 2*, 30.

Lewington, S., Clarke, R., Qizilbash, N., Peto, R., Collins, R., & Prospective Studies Collaboration. (2002). Age-specific relevance of usual blood pressure to vascular mortality: A meta-analysis of individual data for one million adults in 61 prospective studies. *Lancet, 360*, 1903–1913.

Lopez, A. D., Mathers, C. D., Ezzati, M., Jamison, D. T., & Murray, C. J. (2006). Global and regional burden of disease and risk factors, 2001: Systematic analysis of population health data. *Lancet, 367*, 1747–1757.

Mackay, J., & Mensah, G. (2004). *Atlas of heart disease and stroke.* Geneva, Switzerland: World Health Organization.

Makela, P., Fonager, K., Hibell, B., Nordlund, S., Sabroe, S., & Simpura, J. (2001). Episodic heavy drinking in four Nordic countries: A comparative survey. *Addiction, 96*, 1575–1588.

McGill, H. C., Jr., McMahan, C. A., Herderick, E. E., Zieske, A. W., Malcom, G. T., Tracy, R. E., … Pathobiological Determinants of Atherosclerosis in Youth (PDAY) Research Group. (2002). Obesity accelerates the progression of coronary atherosclerosis in young men. *Circulation, 105*, 2712–2718.

Murray, C. J., & Lopez, A. D. (1997). Mortality by cause for eight regions of the world: Global Burden of Disease Study. *Lancet, 349*(9061), 1269–1276.

Nakayama, T., Date, C., Yokoyama, T., Yoshiike, N., Yamaguchi, M., & Tanaka, H. (1997). A 15.5-year follow-up study of stroke in a Japanese provincial city: The Shibata Study. *Stroke, 28*, 45–52.

National Heart, Lung and Blood Institute. (1996). *Stroke belt initiative.* Bethesda, MD: National Institutes of Health.

National Heart, Lung and Blood Institute. (2009). Fact book fiscal year 2009. Bethesda, MD: Center for Health Statistics, National Institutes of Health.

Nestel, P. J. (1990). Effects of n-3 fatty acids on lipid metabolism. *Annual Review of Nutrition, 10*, 49–167.

O'Donnell, M. J., Xavier, D., Liu, L., Zhang, H., Chin, S. L., Rao-Melacini, P., … INTERSTROKE investigators. (2010). Risk factors for ischaemic and intracerebral haemorrhagic stroke in 22 countries (the INTERSTROKE study): A case-control study. *Lancet, 376*(9735), 112–123.

O'Regan, C., Wu, P., Arora, P., Perri, D., & Mills, E. J. (2008). Statin therapy in stroke prevention: A meta-analysis involving 121,000 patients. *American Journal of Medicine, 121*(1), 24–33.

Omvik, P. (1996). How smoking affects blood pressure. *Blood Press, 5*, 71–77.

Onundarson, P. T., Thorgeirsson, G., Jonmundsen, E., Sigfusson, N., & Hardarson, T. (1987). Chronic atrial fibrillation—Epidemiologic features and 14 year follow-up: A case-control study. *European Heart Journal, 8*, 521–527.

Peto, R., Lopez, A. D., Boreham, J., Thun, M., & Heath, C., Jr. (2006). *Mortality from smoking in developed countries 1950–2000: Indirect estimates from National Vital Statistics.* London: Oxford University Press.

Poirier, P., Giles, T. D., Bray, G. A., Hong, Y., Stern, J. S., Pi-Sunver, X. P., & Eckel, R. H. (2006). Obesity and cardiovascular disease: Pathophysiology, evaluation, and effect of weight loss. Arteriosclerosis, thrombosis, and vascular biology. *Journal of the American Heart Association, 26*, 968–976.

Prospective Studies Collaboration. (1995). Cholesterol, diastolic blood pressure, and stroke: 13,000 strokes in 450,000 people in 45 prospective cohorts. Prospective studies collaboration. *Lancet, 346*(8991–8992), 1647–1653.

Reynolds, K., Lewis, B., Nolen, J. D., Kinney, G. L., Sathya, B., & He, J. (2003). Alcohol consumption and risk of stroke: A meta-analysis. *JAMA, 289*(5), 579–588.

Ridker, P. M., Rifai, N., Rose, L., Buring, J. E., & Cook, N. R. (2002). Comparison of C-reactive protein and low-density lipoprotein cholesterol levels in the prediction of first cardiovascular events. *New England Journal of Medicine, 347*, 1557–1565.

Robbins, A. S., Manson, J. E., Lee, I. M., Satterfield, S., & Hennekens, C. (1994). Cigarette smoking and stroke in a cohort of U.S. male physicians. *Annals of Internal Medicine, 120*(6), 458–462.

Ross, R. (1999). Atherosclerosis—an inflammatory disease. *New England Journal of Medicine, 340*, 115–126.

Rost, N. S., Wolf, P. A., Kase, C. S., Kelly-Hayes, M., Silbershatz, H., Massaro, J. M., … Wilson, P. W. (2001). Plasma concentration of C-reactive protein and risk of ischemic stroke and transient ischemic attack: The Framingham Study. *Stroke, 32*, 2575–2579.

Roth, G. A., Johnson, C., Abajobir, A., Abd-Allah, F., Abera, S. F., Abyu, G., … Murray, C. (2017). Global, regional, and national burden of cardiovascular diseases for 10 causes, 1990 to 2015. *Journal of American College of Cardiology, 70*(1), 26–28.

Rothwell, P. M., Eliasziw, M., Gutnikov, S. A., Warlow, C. P., & Barnett, H. J. (2004). Endarterectomy for symptomatic carotid stenosis in relation to clinical subgroups and timing of surgery. *Lancet, 363*(9413), 915–924.

Schiller, F. (1970). Concepts of stroke before and after Virchow. *Medical History, 14*(2), 115–131.

Schoene, W. C. (1979). The nervous system. In S. L. Robbins, & R. S. Cotran (Eds.), *Pathologic basis of disease* (2nd ed.) (pp. 1530–1598). Philadelphia, PA: WB Saunders Company.

Shinton, R., & Beevers, G. (1989). Meta-analysis of relation between cigarette smoking and stroke. *BMJ, 298*, 789–794.

Siegel, P. Z., Wolfe, L. E., Wilcox, D., & Deeb, L. C. (1992). North Florida is part of the stroke belt. *Public Health Reports, 107*(5), 540–543.

Sloan, M. A., Kittner, S. J., Rigamonti, D., & Price, T. R. (1991). Occurrence of stroke associated with use/abuse of drugs. *Neurology, 41*(9), 1358–1364.

Smolders, B., Lemmens, R., & Thijs, V. (2007). Lipoprotein (a) and stroke: A meta-analysis of observational studies. *Stroke, 38*, 1959–1964.

Stamler, R., Stamler, J., Riedlinger, W. F., Algera, G., & Roberts, R. H. (1978). Weight and blood pressure. Findings in hypertension screening of 1 million Americans. *JAMA, 240*, 1607–1610.

Stegmayr, B., Asplund, K., Kuulasmaa, K., Rajakangas, A. M., Thorvaldsen, P., & Tuomilehto, J. (1997). Stroke incidence and mortality correlated to stroke risk factors in the WHO MONICA Project. An ecological study of 18 populations. *Stroke, 28*, 1367–1374.

Stegmayr, B., Harmsen, P., Rajakangas, A. M., Rastenyté, D., Sarti, C., Thorvaldsen, P., & Tuomilehto, J. (1996). Stroke around the Baltic Sea: Incidence, case fatality and population risk factors in Denmark, Finland, Sweden, and Lithuania. *Cerebrovascular Disease, 6*, 80–88.

Straus, S. E., Majumdar, S. R., & McAlister, F. A. (2002). New evidence for stroke prevention: Scientific review. *JAMA, 288*(11), 1388–1396.

Strazzullo, P., D'Elia, L., Bakwin-Kandala, N., & Cappuccio, F. P. (2009). Salt intake, stroke, and cardiovascular disease: Meta-analysis of prospective studies. *BMJ, 339*, b4567.

Strazzullo, P., D'Elia, L., Cairella, G., Garbagnati, F., Cappuccio, F. P., & Scalfi, L. (2010). Excess body weight and incidence of stroke: Meta-analysis of prospective studies with 2 million participants. *Stroke, 41*, e418–e426.

Sudlow, C. L., & Warlow, C. P. (1997). Comparable studies of the incidence of stroke and its pathological types: Results from an international collaboration. International Stroke Incidence Collaboration. *Stroke, 28*, 491–499.

Surgeon General's Report. (2004). *The health consequences of smoking: A report of the surgeon general.* Washington, DC: Office of the Surgeon General, U.S. Department of Health and Human Services.

Tanaka, H., Hayashi, M., Date, C., Imai, K., Asada, M., Shoji, H., … Shimada, T. (1985). Epidemiologic studies of stroke in Shibata, a Japanese provincial city: Preliminary report on risk factors for cerebral infarction. *Stroke, 16*, 773–780.

Thompson, J. E. (1996). The evolution of surgery for the treatment and prevention of stroke. The Willis Lecture. *Stroke, 27*(8), 1427–1434.

van Gijn, J., Kerr, R. S., & Rinkel, G. J. (2007). Subarachnoid haemorrhage. *Lancet, 369*(9558), 306–318.

Wannamethee, S. G., Shaper, A. G., Whincup, P. H., & Walker, M. (1995). Smoking cessation and the risk of stroke in middle-aged men. *JAMA, 274*(2), 155–160.

Webb, A. J. S., Fischer, U., Mehta, Z., & Rothwell, P. M. (2010). Effects of antihypertensive drug class on interindividual variation in blood pressure and risk of stroke: A systematic review and meta-analysis. *Lancet, 375*(9718), 906–915.

Westover, A. N., McBride, S., & Haley, R. W. (2007). Stroke in young adults who abuse amphetamines or cocaine: A population-based study of hospitalized patients. *Archives of General Psychiatry, 64*(4), 495–502.

Wolf, P. A., Abbott, R. D., & Kannel, W. B. (1991). Atrial fibrillation as an independent risk factor for stroke: The Framingham Study. *Stroke, 22*, 983–988.

Wolf, P. A., D'Agostino, R. B., Kannel, W. B., Bonita, R., & Blanger, A. J. (1988). Cigarette smoking as a risk factor for stroke: The Framingham Study. *JAMA, 259*(7), 1025–1029.

Wolf-Maier, K., Cooper, R. S., Banegas, J. R., Giampaoli, S., Hense, H. W., Joffres, M., … Vescio, F. (2003). Hypertension prevalence and blood pressure levels in 6 European countries, Canada, and the United States. *JAMA, 289*, 2363–2369.

World Health Organization. (1978). *Cerebrovascular disorders* (Offset Publications). Geneva, Switzerland: World Health Organization.

World Health Organization. (2009). *WHO disease and injury country estimates.* Geneva, Switzerland: World Health Organization.

World Health Organization. (2010). World Health Organization Statistical Information System (WHOSIS). Global Health Observatory (GHO), Geneva, Switzerland: World Health Organization, http://www.who.int/GHO/

Yang, Q., Ton, X., Schieb, L., Vaughan, A., Gillespie, C., & Wiltz, J. L. (2017). Vital signs: Recent trends in stroke death rates; United States, 2000–2015. *Morbidity and Mortality Weekly Report (MMWR), 66*(35), 933–939.

CHAPTER 7

Epidemiology of Heart Failure

▶ Introduction

Heart failure (HF) is a major public health crisis afflicting 38 million persons worldwide and 6.5 million in the United States. Despite advances in prevention and therapy, HF continues to plague the world population with high rates of mortality and morbidity.

▶ Definition of Heart Failure

The American Heart Association defines HF as "*a complex clinical syndrome that can result from any structural or functional cardiac disorder that impairs the ability of the ventricle to fill or eject blood.*" The diagnosis of HF is based on the presence of a constellation of symptoms that typically include inappropriate dyspnea (shortness of breath), venous hypertension, and abnormalities of the heart and lungs such as cardiomegaly, arrhythmia, and pulmonary edema. Functional impairments of HF include: (1) the inability of the left ventricle of the heart to pump sufficient blood into the aorta, (2) inability of the right ventricle to pump sufficient blood into the lungs, (3) or both. The two major forms of HF, *Systolic and Diastolic HF*, are discussed below and illustrated in **FIGURE 7.1**.

Diastolic heart failure

Systolic heart failure

FIGURE 7.1 Comparison of Diastolic and Systolic Heart Failure.
Arrows denote direction of blood flow.

Systolic Heart Failure

In "*systolic heart failure*," the myocardium (heart muscle) of the ventricular walls is weakened, the ventricles are dilated, and their contracting power is impaired. The contractive force of the left ventricle is measured by the "*ejection fraction*" which is the fraction (percent) of blood volume pumped out of the heart into the aorta with each contraction. This is usually measured by an echocardiogram. In the normal heart, the left ventricular ejection fraction ranges from 50% to 60% whereas in systolic HF the ejection fraction drops below 50% and often falls below 40%. As the ejection fraction falls and the volume of blood in the left ventricle increases, there is retrograde pooling of blood into the left atrium, the lungs, the right chambers of the heart, and eventually blood vessels throughout the body. Thus, systolic HF typically transforms into "*congestive heart failure* (CHF)" with marked edema and congestion of the heart, lungs, and body. This condition is often preceded by a myocardial infarction (MI) (heart attack) that destroys a significant portion of the myocardium thereby reducing the contractile force of the left ventricle. Systolic HF is also called "*HF with reduced ejection fraction* (HFREF)."

Diastolic Heart Failure

In "*diastolic heart failure*," the ventricular walls are thickened and stiff with less blood volume than normal and though the ventricle pumps out 50% or more of the blood volume, the amount ejected with each contraction is less than normal. In this condition, there is increased resistance to filling of one or both ventricles of the heart and though the ejection fraction may be normal, the volume of blood pumped with each contraction is insufficient to meet the metabolic demands of the body. Diastolic HF is also called "*HF with preserved ejection fraction* (HFPEF)."

Cor Pulmonale and Right-Sided Heart Failure

While about 60% of patients who develop HF manifest impaired left ventricular myocardial function, some cases are due to abnormalities of the right ventricle, the heart valves, the pericardium, or certain metabolic disturbances. A condition known as *cor pulmonale* specifically refers to right ventricular hypertrophy secondary to high blood pressure in the arteries of the lungs (*pulmonary hypertension*). Pulmonary hypertension increases resistance to right ventricular contraction, which over time can damage the right ventricle leading to *right-sided* HF. Pulmonary hypertension has variable causes such as chronic obstructive pulmonary disease (COPD: Emphysema and/or chronic bronchitis), active tuberculosis, or other chronic infectious or obstructive conditions of the lungs. Pulmonary hypertension may also occur subsequent to left-sided HF as a consequence of retrograde pooling of blood resulting in pulmonary edema and hypertension that ultimately damages the right ventricle.

The Framingham Heart Study: Incidence and Prevalence of Heart Failure

The Framingham Heart Study, established in 1948, has provided important epidemiologic data on the prevalence, incidence, secular trends, prognosis, predisposing conditions, and modifiable risk factors of HF. This long-standing prospective cohort study originated with a population-based sample of residents of Framingham, Massachusetts, ages 28–62 years. After four decades of follow-up, 652 persons of 9405 participants had developed CHF. Both the incidence and prevalence of CHF increased exponentially with age (**FIGURES 7.2** and **7.3**). Annual incidence rates by age decile were higher in men peaking in the eighth decade of life at 27 per 1000 in men and 22 per 1000 in women. Conversely, the prevalence rates by age decile were slightly higher in women due to their longer survival. The prevalence of CHF approximately doubled with each decade of life after age 50 approaching 10% in persons 80 or more years of age. Five-year survival of CHF was significantly higher in women than men (38% versus 25%) although 84.5% of cases eventually died of the disease (Ho, Pinsky, Kannel, & Levy, 1993; Kannel & Belanger, 1991; McKee, Castelli, McNamara, & Kannel, 1971).

The overall lifetime risk of CHF was approximately 20% for men and women, and notably, sustained antecedent hypertension approximately doubled the risk. Furthermore, the lifetime risk was lowered significantly by considering only cases *without* an antecedent MI (11.4% in men and 15.4% in women). These results underscore the need for a greater emphasis on prevention of CHF through hypertension control and prevention of MI (Lloyd-Jones et al., 2002).

The Rotterdam Heart Study

The Rotterdam Heart Study is a prospective population-based cohort study of cardiovascular diseases (CVDs),

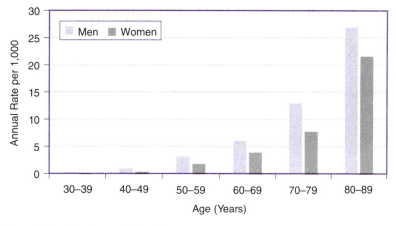

FIGURE 7.2 Incidence of Heart Failure by Age and Gender.

Data from Kannel, W. B., & Belanger, A. J. (1991). Epidemiology of heart failure. *American Heart Journal*, *121*, 951–956; Ho, K. K., Pinsky, J. L., Kannel, W. B., & Levy, D. (1993). The epidemiology of heart failure: The Framingham Study. *Journal of the American College of Cardiology, 22*(4 Suppl. A), 6A–13A.

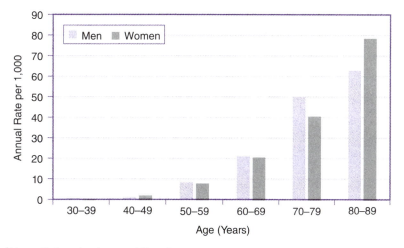

FIGURE 7.3 Prevalence of Heart Failure by Age and Gender.

Data from Kannel, W. B., & Belanger, A. J. (1991). Epidemiology of heart failure. *American Heart Journal*, *121*, 951–956; Ho, K. K., Pinsky, J. L., Kannel, W. B., & Levy, D. (1993). The epidemiology of heart failure: The Framingham Study. *Journal of the American College of Cardiology, 22*(4 Suppl. A), 6A–13A.

including HF, in Ommoord, a suburb of Rotterdam in the Netherlands. The study monitored the incidence and prevalence of HF among 7734 adults aged 55 years or older who were free of disease at baseline over 7.1 years of average follow-up time. Both the incidence and the prevalence of HF increased sharply with age and the lifetime risk of developing HF was slightly higher in men than women (33% versus 29%). Among the 725 incident cases of HF detected in the study, median survival was 2.1 years and only 35% survived 5 years after the initial diagnosis (Bleumink et al., 2004).

▸ United States Trends in Heart Failure

In the United States, the annual age-adjusted incidence of HF has declined slightly since 2000. Estimates from a large cohort of residents of Olmsted County, Minnesota, followed during 1979–2010 showed little temporal change until 2000 after which there was a significant decline in both men and women (**FIGURE 7.4**). During 2000–2010, the overall age-gender-adjusted incidence declined by 37% over the decade (Gerber et al., 2015; Roger et al., 2004).

Despite the decline in the *incidence* of HF over time in the United States, the *prevalence* has increased markedly, particularly among the elderly. During the past half century, the number of living cases of HF has more than quadrupled and nearly 80% of cases are over the age of 75 years. Currently, there are more than 6.5 million Americans living with HF and the prevalence, approximately 2.0%, is continuing to rise with the aging of the population (**FIGURE 7.5**). The increasing prevalence of HF is partially due to the "*epidemiologic transition*" wherein death rates from acute infectious, parasitic and nutritional deficiency diseases that occur early in life have decreased dramatically in the United States as well as most other developed nations resulting in a predominance of geriatric individuals who are predisposed to chronic diseases. Furthermore, patients with HF as well as those with conditions that

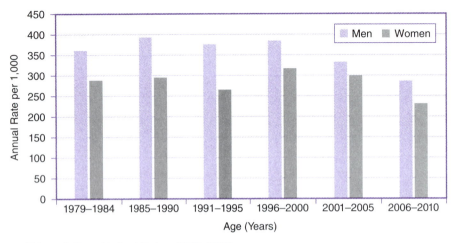

FIGURE 7.4 Incidence of Heart Failure, United States, 1979–2010.

Data from Roger, V. L., Weston, S. A., Redfield, M. M., Hellermann-Homan, J. P., Killian, J., Yawn, B. P., & Jacobsen, S. J. (2004). Trends in heart failure incidence and survival in a community-based population. *JAMA, 292*(3), 344–350; Gerber, Y., Weston, S. A., Redfield, M. M., Chamberlain, A. M., Manemann, S. M., Jiang, R., . . . Roger, V. L. (2015). A Contemporary appraisal of the heart failure epidemic in Olmsted County, Minnesota, 2000–2010. *JAMA Internal Medicine, 175*(6), 996–1004.

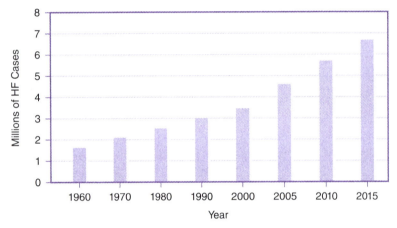

FIGURE 7.5 Prevalent Cases of Heart Failure: United States, 1960–2015.

Data from Benjamin, E. J., Blaha, M. J., Chiuve, S. E., Cushman, M., Das, S. R., Deo, R., . . . Muntner, P. (2017). Heart disease and stroke statistics—2017 update: A report from the American Heart Association. *Circulation, 135*, e146–e603; Go, A. S., Mozaffarian, D., Roger, V. L., Benjamin, E. J., Berry, J. D., Borden, W. B., . . . Turner, M. B. (2013). Heart disease and stroke statistics—2013 update: A report from the American Heart Association. *Circulation 127*(1), e6–e245; Thomas, T., Haase, N., Rosamond, W., Howard, V. J., Rumsfeld, J., Manolio, T., . . . American Heart Association Statistics Committee and Stroke Statistics Subcommittee. (2006). Heart disease and stroke statistics—2006 update. *Circulation, 113*, e85–e151; Fang, J., Mensah, G. A., Croft, J. B., & Keenan, N. L. (2008). Heart failure-related hospitalization in the US, 1979 to 2004. *Journal of the American College of Cardiology, 52*(6), 428–434.

predispose to HF are surviving longer which has sustained the high incidence of HF among the elderly and produced a significant increase in the prevalence of this disease (Benjamin et al., 2017; Fang, Mensah, Croft, & Keenan, 2008; Go et al., 2013; O'Connor, 2017; Roger et al., 2012; Thomas et al., 2006).

▶ The Epidemic of Hospitalizations for Heart Failure

One major consequence of the rising prevalence of HF is the startling increase in the rate of hospitalizations. As shown in **FIGURE 7.6**, the hospitalization rates for CHF have increased more than fourfold for persons 65 years and older and more than twofold for younger adults since 1970 in the United States (National Heart

Lung and Blood Institute, 2009). As pointed out by Dr. Eugene Braunwald, "the prime candidates for the development of heart failure are patients with hypertension in whom death from stroke has been prevented by antihypertensive therapy and survivors of acute MI who have been spared death from arrhythmia" (Braunwald, 1997). Such patients currently account for more than 1 million primary hospital admissions annually and another 2 million patients have HF as a secondary diagnosis. Indeed, almost 50% of HF patients are readmitted within 6 months for recurrent decompensation which has resulted in an epidemic of hospitalizations among HF survivors who now live longer with the disease (O'Connor, 2017; Munir et al., 2017; Roger et al., 2012).

HF is a global pandemic now afflicting nearly 38 million people worldwide. Population-based studies in the United States and Europe have found that while the incidence of HF has remained stable, the

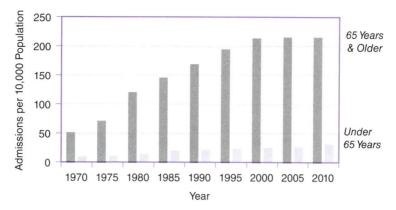

FIGURE 7.6 Hospitalization Rates for Congestive Heart Failure, 1970–2010, United States.

Data from National Heart Lung and Blood Institute (NHLBI, 2009). *Morbidity and mortality; 2009 Chart book on cardiovascular, lung and blood diseases*. Bethesda, MD: National Institutes of Health; Benjamin, E. J., Blaha, M. J., Chiuve, S. E., Cushman, M., Das, S. R., Deo, R., . . . Muntner, P. (2017). Heart disease and stroke statistics—2017 update: A report from the American Heart Association. *Circulation, 135*, e146–e603. Global Trends in Heart Failure.

prevalence is rising due to improved therapy leading to increased survival among patients. Nevertheless, even in developed nations, 20%–40% of HF patients die within 1 year of diagnosis and more than 50% die within 5 years of their first hospital admission for HF (Ponikowski et al., 2012; Savarese & Lund, 2017).

In contrast to developed nations wherein HF develops primarily in geriatric patients subsequent to chronic hypertension, coronary heart disease and/or MI, in *underdeveloped nations* with poor economies and substandard healthcare systems, infectious diseases are responsible for the majority of cases. For example, RHD due to streptococcal infection of the heart valves is a prominent cause of HF in Africa, SE Asia, and the Middle East. Other infectious conditions that predispose to HF in underdeveloped nations include HIV disease, tuberculosis, Chagas' disease (parasitic *Trypanosoma cruzi* infection) and malaria (Bloomfield, Barasa, Doll, & Velazquez, 2013; Celermajer, Chow, Marijon, Anstey, & Woo, 2012; Ponikowski et al., 2012).

Mortality of Heart Failure

Mortality rates among patients with HF are extraordinarily high. Follow-up studies of HF patients diagnosed during 1990–1999 in the Framingham Heart Study, show that approximately 10% of patients died within 30 days of hospitalization, and the estimated mortality rates at 1, 5, and 10 years were 25%, 50%, and 80%, respectively (Levy et al., 2002). Similar estimates were obtained by investigators in the United Kingdom who studied 54,313 HF patients diagnosed during 1998–2012. Overall death rates were 19%, 49%, and 71% at 1, 5, and 10 years, respectively, and did not change over time (Taylor et al., 2017). Annual HF mortality rates per 100,000 in the United States are about 30% higher in men than women (104

versus 80 among Caucasians in 2006) and in a cohort study designed to compare ethnic differences, African Americans had a 25% higher case fatality than Caucasians after 5 years of follow-up. While there is some evidence that survival from HF has improved in recent years with fluid restriction, reduction of dietary salt, and administration of antihypertensive and anti-arrhythmic medications, hospitalizations and readmission rates continue to rise (Bui, Horwich, & Fonarow, 2011; Levy et al., 2002; Loehr, Rosamond, Chang, Folsom, & Chambless, 2008).

Data on HF mortality in low-income nations are sparse and limited to hospitalized patients. A recent analysis of deaths from HF among 240,000 HF patients hospitalized in 31 low- and middle-income countries found an overall in-hospital mortality of 8.3% compared to about 5.3% in European and U.S. hospitals (Callender et al., 2014).

Diseases Predisposing to Heart Failure

Conditions that elevate the risk of HF fall into two broad categories: those that appear late in life in association with chronic diseases versus those that appear much earlier in life in association with acute infectious diseases. HF typically develops as a consequence of a "*web of causation*" of predisposing CVDs and events. Chronic CVDs that elevate the risk of developing HF include long-standing hypertension, coronary (ischemic) heart disease, type 2 diabetes mellitus, valvular heart disease, and heart arrhythmias such as atrial fibrillation (AF) (**FIGURE 7.7**). These conditions are occurring with increasing prevalence, particularly among the elderly populations living in low- and middle-income countries as well as high-income countries (Curtis et al., 2008).

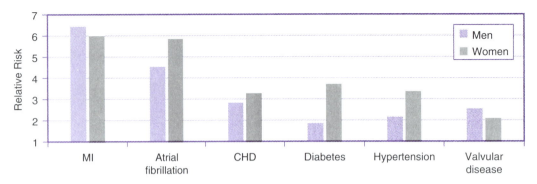

FIGURE 7.7 Congestive Heart Failure: Predisposing Conditions.

Data from Levy, D., Larson, M. G., Vasan, R. S., Kannel, W. B., & Ho, K. K. L. (1996). The progression from hypertension to congestive heart failure. *Journal of the American Medical Association, 275*, 1557–1562; Maisel, W. H., & Stevenson, L. W. (2003). Atrial fibrillation in heart failure: Epidemiology, pathophysiology, and rationale for therapy. *The American Journal of Cardiology, 91*(6), 2–8.

Early evidence showing that pre-existing CVDs independently or in combination cause HF comes from the Framingham Heart Study. Among 578 adults who developed HF in the original Framingham cohort, 76% of men and 79% of women had a medical history of chronic hypertension and 46% of men and 27% of women had a prior diagnosis of coronary (ischemic) heart disease. Furthermore, compared to individuals without diabetes, the risk of HF was 2–3-fold higher in diabetic men and 3–6-fold higher in diabetic women. Other predisposing conditions included *Rheumatic heart disease* (RHD) and cardiomyopathy in 2%–3% of HF cases (Ho et al., 1993; Kannel & Belanger, 1991; Levy, Larson, Vasan, Kannel, & Ho, 1996; Lloyd-Jones et al., 2002).

Acute MI is often a harbinger for the development of HF. Prospective results from the Framingham cohort showed that 52% of male HF cases and 34% of female HF cases had survived an acute MI, and antecedent MI increased the hazard ratio of HF by about six fold (Levy et al., 1996). Many other studies have also observed that HF is a frequent sequela of MI, occurring in about 50% of survivors. In general, the greater the size of the infarct and loss of cardiomyocytes (heart muscle cells) in the left ventricular wall, the higher the risk of developing HF (Wolk, Scheidt, & Killip, 1972).

The association of HF with AF was first noted by Paul Dudley White more than a century ago. AF is present in 13%–27% of patients with HF and may develop prior to, at the same time, or after the diagnosis of HF. Consequently, the etiologic association of AF and HF is complex and in some patients, the two conditions may in fact develop concurrently with one exacerbating the other. Certainly, alteration of the normal heart rhythm may compromise effective atrial and ventricular contractile function thereby facilitating the development of HF; and reciprocally, the failing heart may induce conduction abnormalities that

promote the development of AF. Notably, the presence of both conditions has been found to adversely influence survival (Anter, Jessup, & Callans, 2009; Maisel & Stevenson, 2003).

Thyroid disorders can cause heart arrhythmias, elevation of blood pressure, and AF, all of which predispose to HF. In a large Danish cohort study of thyroid disorders, individuals with hyperthyroidism (elevated thyroxine) had a significant increase in the incidence of HF compared to individuals with normal thyroid function. Thyroid disorders are 5–10 times more common in women and may involve thyroid autoimmune reactions, high or low dietary intake of iodine or goitrogenic agents, and hormonal factors (Selmer et al., 2012, 2014).

Hypertrophy of the right ventricle of the heart and *right-sided HF* can develop as a consequence of *cor pulmonale*. This condition develops due to increased blood pressure of the arteries of the lungs (*pulmonary hypertension*). In response to increased pulmonary vascular resistance, the right ventricle gradually undergoes hypertrophy and dilatation (*cor pulmonale*) which can lead to diminished contractile force and ultimate failure. COPD: Emphysema and/or chronic bronchitis, which is primarily caused by chronic cigarette smoking and/or heightened exposure to air pollution, is the fourth leading cause of death in the world population. In patients with COPD, lung function is impaired and hypoxia, inflammation and loss of capillaries commonly cause vascular remodeling and pulmonary hypertension. This scenario can lead to cor pulmonale and right-sided HF (Chaouat, Naeije, & Weitzenblum, 2008).

In low- and middle-income nations, HF often develops in conjunction with acute infectious processes such as rheumatic fever, HIV disease, tuberculosis, Chagas' disease, and malaria. Among the infectious conditions that can lead to HF, RHD is the most prominent, particularly in underdeveloped regions of the world, such as sub-Saharan Africa, where many populations have little access to modern health care. RHD is a chronic progressive condition caused by recurrent pharyngeal infections by *Group A beta-hemolytic streptococcal bacteria* with invasion of the heart valves. Over time, the heart valves become fibrotic leading to HF and ultimately death. Prevalence rates of RHD detected by echocardiographic screening among school children are particularly high (2%–5%) in sub-Saharan Africa and India (Bloomfield et al., 2013).

Active tuberculosis with invasion of the pericardium (the membranous sac around the heart) by *mycobacteria tuberculosis* is a primary cause of chronic pericardial inflammatory disease in sub-Saharan Africa. Tuberculous pericarditis can transform to CHF and accounts for about 10% of patients hospitalized with HF in this region. This condition is often exacerbated by HIV co-infection in patients residing in sub-Saharan African nations were the rates of both infectious conditions are high. Death rates approach 40% within 1 year of diagnosis if both infectious conditions are present (Mayosi et al., 2008).

Malaria, particularly due to infection by *Falciparum plasmodium*, causes disseminated hemolysis and anemia, which can lead to widespread organ damage including HF. Severe malarial infections may damage the myocardium due to the combined effects of anemia, ischemia, inflammation, and oxidative stress (Marrelli & Brotto, 2016).

Chagas' disease is an infection with *T. cruzi* transmitted by the bite of the reduviid bug (the kissing bug). This infection is endemic in certain regions of Central and South America and causes approximately 12,500 deaths annually; 60% due to sudden cardiac death, 25% due to HF, and 15% due to stroke. The genesis of Chagas cardiomyopathy involves immune-mediated myocardial injury (Rassi Jr, Rassi, & Marin-Neto, 2010).

Nutritional deficiencies can also contribute to the development of HF, not only in underdeveloped nations but also in developed countries. Anemia occurs when the production of erythrocytes (red blood cells) does not keep pace with normal red blood cell loss and the erythrocyte count falls below normal. The most common form of anemia is *iron deficiency anemia* in which there is insufficient iron for erythrocyte production (erythropoiesis). Anemia reduces hemoglobin and oxygen delivery to the myocardium and elevates the risk of coronary (ischemic) heart disease, MI as well as HF. Notably, studies of patients hospitalized for HF in developed nations have found that 30%–60% were anemic (Tang & Katz, 2006).

Beriberi refers to a specific dietary deficiency of thiamine (vitamin B1) associated with right-sided HF. This condition primarily occurs in certain regions of sub-Saharan Africa, India, and SE Asia where the diet is chiefly white rice and devoid of thiamine. In patients with chronic thiamine deficiency, there is enlargement and congestive failure of the right heart in conjunction with disseminated edema throughout the body, a condition known as "*wet beriberi*" (Prinzo, 1999). While beriberi is rarely diagnosed in developed countries where vitamin intake is presumed sufficient, a recent study in a large Canadian hospital found that one-third of patients with CHF manifested thiamine deficiency (Hanninen, Darling, Sole, Barr, & Keith, 2006). Deficiencies of other micronutrients including vitamin D, selenium, and zinc may also play a role in the development of HF and it will be important to investigate the therapeutic value of micronutrient supplementation for HF patients (Newman et al., 2007).

Certain metabolic abnormalities can interrupt the energy requirements of the heart muscle and impair heart function. Disturbances in glucose and lipid metabolism and regulation of intracellular calcium can cause cardiomyopathy by diminishing mitochondrial energy production. Several genetic syndromes have been identified that cause abnormalities of the mitochondrial respiratory chain or result in abnormal deposition of glycogen or lysosomal products in the myocardium and other organs. Such cardiomyopathies are rare and can cause fatal CHF in children (Guertl, Noehammer, & Hoefler, 2000). Chronic conditions that predispose to cardiomyopathy in adults include alcohol abuse (Piano, 2002), hemochromatosis (iron overload) (Sekhri, Sanal, DeLorenzo, Aronow, & Maguire, 2011), sarcoidosis, a multisystem granulomatous disease (Gujja, Rosing, Tripodi, & Shizukuda, 2010), and amyloidosis (the deposition of amyloid in the myocardium) (Liao & Ward, 2017). Furthermore, platelet activation and/or dysfunction may play a role in the thromboembolic complications and/or the progression of HF (Chung & Lip, 2006).

▶ Behavioral Risk Factors for Heart Failure

Behavioral risk factors that predispose to HF are synonymous with the risk factors for the predisposing cardiovascular conditions and events discussed in the above section. Major risk factors in developed countries such as the United States include chronic cigarette smoking, high salt consumption, sedentary lifestyle, unhealthy diet high in fat, sugar, and calories, hypercholesterolemia, obesity, nutritional deficiencies, chronic stress, alcohol abuse, and hyperthyroidism. Nevertheless, in underdeveloped countries where acute infectious diseases and nutritional deficits were once the most common causes of heart disease, there has also been a striking rise in rates of CVDs including HF due to chronic exposures and conditions. It is important to realize that these factors often occur together and synergistically increase the risk (**TABLE 7.1**).

Cigarette smoking is a major risk factor in the development of chronic hypertension due to the potent vasoconstrictive properties of nicotine, the primary addictive agent of tobacco. Systemic hypertension due to increased vascular resistance is a common feature of coronary artery disease, left ventricular hypertrophy, and *left-sided* HF. Hypertension also causes AF and

markedly elevates the risk of MI which in turn predisposes to HF. Chronic smokers are also at high risk for the development of COPD and pulmonary hypertension, which can precipitate *cor pulmonale* and *right-sided* HF.

Diets high in fat, sugar, and calories are primarily responsible for the global pandemic of obesity. Obesity is a powerful risk factor for the development of type 2 diabetes mellitus, a condition that markedly increases the risk of developing all forms of CVDs including HF. There is also a strong graded relationship between obesity and hypertension. As body mass increases, the added pressure on the arterial walls increases vascular resistance and blood pressure rises (Kenchaiah et al., 2002).

Westernized diets high in fat and calories are primarily responsible for the high rates of

TABLE 7.1 Behavioral Risk Factors for Heart Failure

Risk Factor	Predisposing Chain of Events in Heart Failure
Smoking	Hypertension, coronary heart disease, atrial fibrillation, MI COPD, pulmonary hypertension, *cor pulmonale*
Diet high in fat, sugar, calories	Obesity, diabetes, hypertension, hypercholesterolemia, atherosclerosis, coronary heart disease, atrial fibrillation, MI
High salt intake	Hypertension, atrial fibrillation, MI
Sedentary lifestyle	Obesity, diabetes, hypertension, coronary heart disease, atrial fibrillation, MI
Chronic stress	Depression, hypertension, atrial fibrillation, MI
Alcohol abuse, toxins	Hypertension, cardiotoxicity, cardiomyopathy
Infection	
Beta-Streptococcus	Rheumatic heart disease, valvular disease
Mycobacterium TB	Tuberculosis, pericarditis, myocarditis
Plasmodium malariae	Malaria, anemia, ischemic heart disease
T. cruzi	Chagas disease, cardiomyopathy
Nutritional Deficiency	
Thiamine	Wet beriberi, cardiomyopathy
Iron	Anemia, ischemic heart disease

hypercholesterolemia, atherosclerosis, and coronary heart disease in elderly populations of developed nations. When atherosclerotic plaques rupture, the resulting thromboembolus can totally occlude key coronary arteries and cause a myocardial infarct. Damage to the heart by myocardial infarct is the strongest risk factor for subsequent HF.

Sedentary lifestyle and lack of exercise are independent risk factors for the development of HF. Many studies have observed that regular physical activity reduces the risk of obesity, hypertension, coronary heart disease, diabetes and MI; and reciprocally, lack of exercise increases the risk of all of these conditions that predispose to HF (Young et al., 2014).

High salt consumption is another of the major risk factors for the development of chronic hypertension, AF, and subsequent HF. Average salt consumption in developed countries such as the United States average about 9 g per day which translates to 3600 mg of sodium. Sustained daily levels above 6 g of salt (2300 mg of sodium) elevate the risk of hypertension by 2–4-fold compared to levels below 3.5 g (1500 mg of sodium). One mechanism by which salt elevates blood pressure involves greater fluid retention with high sodium intake which increases blood volume and vascular resistance (Rusinaru et al., 2012).

Chronic stress and depression elevate the risk of all CVDs including HF. In a recent meta-analysis, clinically significant depression was present in 21% of all patients, and the prevalence increased to more than 40% among HF patients with end-stage disease. Furthermore, mortality was twofold higher among HF patients with depression compared to those without depression (Rutledge, Reis, Linke, Greenberg, & Mills, 2006). Recent studies suggest that chronic psychological stress activates the sympathetic nervous system by inducing sustained release of cortisol and norepinephrine (adrenaline) from the adrenal glands resulting in elevation of blood pressure, increased serum levels of cholesterol and glucose, and promotion of atherogenesis (Grippo & Johnson, 2002).

Alcohol abuse is a major risk factor for toxin-induced cardiomyopathy. While moderate daily intake of alcoholic beverages may be beneficial to the cardiovascular system, long-term high intake may severely damage the myocardium resulting in dilated cardiomyopathy and HF. There is also a historic overlap between chronic alcoholism and thiamine deficiency which may synergistically elevate the risk of HF (Piano, 2002).

Populations living in regions of the world where chronic infectious diseases such as tuberculosis,

HIV, and malaria are endemic and malnutrition and nutritional deficiencies are common have recently experienced marked increases in the rates of CVD including HF. Currently, approximately 80% of the 17 million annual deaths due to CVD occur in low- and middle-income countries. In sub-Saharan Africa, the prevalence of hypertension is nearly 50% in adults over 25 years of age, and annual CVD mortality rates are higher than in the developed world ranging from 300 to 600 deaths per 100,000. Individuals in the developing world are therefore at "*double jeopardy*" for developing heart disease, not only due to infectious diseases and malnutrition, but also from persisting uncontrolled hypertension and other chronic CVD risk factors. It is imperative that the prevention, detection, management, and control of hypertension and other chronic CVD risk factors be given high priority. There is obviously a critical need for effective health education programs to prevent smoking, reduce dietary salt, promote healthy diets and physical exercise to combat obesity, and advocate healthy psychosocial lifestyles in order to curb the emerging epidemic of heart disease in the developing world (Dunlay et al., 2009; Cappuccio & Miller, 2016).

▶ Race and Gender Differences in Heart Failure

Several studies have focused on differences in the rates of HF by race and gender and according to the type of HF. In general, men have higher incidence and mortality rates than women and African Americans have higher rates than Caucasians.

In the initial Framingham Heart Study, incidence rates in men were 30%–40% higher than women at all ages. Likewise, mortality rates among male patients were approximately 20% higher than female patients (Ho et al., 1993; Levy et al., 2002; Mahmood & Wang, 2013; McKee et al., 1971).

In the cohort study of residents of Olmstead County, Minnesota, the annual incidence of HF during 1979–2000 was 31% higher in men than women (378 versus 289 per 100,000) and the age-adjusted mortality after the diagnosis of HF was 33% higher in men than women (Roger et al., 2004).

In the *Atherosclerosis Risk in Communities* (ARIC) study, age-adjusted incidence rates per 1000 person years varied markedly by gender and race. Rates per 1000 person years were more than twofold higher in African-American women than Caucasians

(8.1 versus 3.4) and 50% higher in African-American men than Caucasians (9.1 versus 6.0). Case fatality was also higher in African Americans than Caucasians (e.g. 23.7 versus 20.2% after 5 years). These rate differences were attributable to greater exposure to multiple risk factors (cholesterol, smoking, dietary salt) and higher rates of predisposing conditions (obesity, diabetes, hypertension, left ventricular hypertrophy, and coronary heart disease) in African Americans (Loehr et al., 2008).

Heart Failure and Ejection Fractions

At the time of diagnosis, patients with HF are routinely categorized according to the ejection fraction of the left ventricle as measured by echocardiology. It is standard practice to dichotomize patients into two groups: Those with ejection fractions less than 40% (HF with reduced ejection fraction or HFREF) versus those with ejection fractions above 50% (HF with preserved ejection fraction or HFPEF). Systolic HF in which the left ventricle is weak and dilated is associated with HFREF, and diastolic HF in which the left ventricle is thickened and fibrotic is associated with HFPEF (Figure 7.1). Some investigators have advised development of a third category of patients with ejection fractions between 40% and 50% (Lam, Donal, Kraigher-Krainer, & Vasan, 2011).

Recent studies suggest that the relative frequencies of new (incident) cases of HFREF and HFPEF are approximately equal; however, the *prevalence* of HFPEF appears to be increasing faster than HFREF. In the *Organized Program to Initiate Lifesaving Treatment in Hospitalized Patients with Heart Failure* (OPTIMIZE) study, 20,118 patients with left ventricular systolic disease were compared to 21,149 patients with preserved systolic function. The majority of patients with preserved systolic function were elderly women with pre-existing hypertension and/or AF, whereas those with systolic disease were more likely to be men with hypertension, prior coronary (ischemic) heart disease, and/or MI (Fonarow et al., 2007).

Similar findings were observed by investigators of the *Japanese Cardiac Registry of Heart Failure in Cardiology* (JCARE-CARD), a national prospective registry database of hospitalized HF patients in which 985 patients with HFREF were compared to 429 patients with HFPEF. In this investigation, the majority of HFPEF patients were women in their 70s with hypertension and non-ischemic conditions such as AF or anemia, whereas most patients with HFREF were men in their 60s with hypertension and coronary (ischemic) heart disease and/or MI. In all of the recent studies comparing HFREF to HFPEF, reported mortality estimates remain high for all categories of HF and effective case-specific management strategies are yet to be established (Lam et al., 2011; Pandey et al., 2018; Tsutsui, Tsuchihashi-Makaya, & Kinugawa, 2010).

Primary Prevention of Heart Failure

The key to effective primary prevention of disease is early education and widespread dissemination of knowledge regarding how to avoid major risk factors. The American Heart Association tracks seven key health factors and behaviors that increase the risk of developing CVD including HF. For primary prevention, "*Life's Simple 7*" are basic guidelines to avoid developing CVD. These guidelines include avoidance of smoking, regular physical activity, eating a healthy diet with daily intake of fruits and vegetables and less than 6 grams of salt, maintaining ideal body weight (BMI of 25 or less), and controlling serum cholesterol, blood pressure, and blood sugar within normal limits. Implementation of these guidelines early in life is instrumental for an effective program of primary CVD prevention (Benjamin et al., 2017).

Secondary Prevention of Heart Failure

Effective secondary prevention of CVD and HF involves a multifactorial approach to early detection and intervention. Secondary prevention therefore includes multifaceted population screening for the early detection of elevated blood pressure, cholesterol and glucose so that both non-pharmacologic and pharmacologic measures can be instituted to return levels of these factors to within normal limits. Major attention must also be given to identifying and revising unhealthy dietary and exercise patterns in order to lessen adiposity. Recent studies also underscore the importance of diagnosing and effectively treating major depressive disorders that chronically elevate stress and deregulate neurochemical pathways that have significant negative impact on the cardiovascular system (Dhar & Barton, 2016).

There is increasing interest in the value of biomarkers for the early detection of impending HF. One such biomarker is C-reactive protein (CRP), a pentraxin protein that is synthesized in the liver in response to a variety of inflammatory cytokines. Levels of CRP increase rapidly in response to inflammation, infection, and trauma. The function of CRP is to opsonize (target) damaged or necrotic cells for destruction by complement and macrophages of the innate immune system. Elevated levels of CRP have been found to portend HF in elderly individuals and adverse outcomes in HF patients (Braunwald, 2008).

Other biomarkers that are associated with the development of HF include stress-related neurohormones such as norepinephrine and cortisol that activate the sympathetic nervous system, reactive oxygen species that are formed by oxidative stress and myofibrillar proteins (cardiac troponins) that are released by injured myocytes. Currently, biomarkers that are the gold standard in determining diagnosis and prognosis of HF are B-type natriuretic peptides (BNP) that are secreted by damaged cardiomyocytes in response to overexpression of the renin–angiotensin–aldosterone system and elevated blood pressure (Gaggin & Januzzi, 2013).

▶ Therapy and Tertiary Prevention for Patients with Heart Failure

Fluid retention and congestion are hallmarks of HF, and they are associated with both severe symptoms and poor outcomes. Dietary sodium and fluid restrictions should therefore be implemented in all patients with CHF. Limiting patients to 2 g/day of dietary sodium and 2 L/day of fluid lessens congestion and decreases the need for diuretics. The skillful use of diuretic therapy remains fundamental to the successful management of HF. Other effective measures include smoking cessation, restricted alcohol intake, judicious use of antihypertensive and diabetic medications, weight loss to achieve ideal weight, and carefully monitored aerobic exercise (Ellison & Felker, 2017).

References

Anter, E., Jessup, M., & Callans, D. J. (2009). Atrial fibrillation and heart failure. *Circulation, 119*, 2516–2525.

Benjamin, E. J., Blaha, M. J., Chiuve, S. E., Cushman, M., Das, S. R., Deo, R., … Muntner, P. (2017). Heart disease and stroke statistics—2017 update: A report from the American Heart Association. *Circulation, 135*, e146–e603.

Bleumink, G. S., Knetsch, A. M., Sturkenboom, M. C. J. M., Straus, S. M. J. M., Hofman, A., Deckers, J. W., … Stricker, B. H. C. (2004). Quantifying the heart failure epidemic: Prevalence, incidence rate, lifetime risk and prognosis of heart failure: The Rotterdam Study. *European Heart Journal, 25*(18), 1614–1619.

Bloomfield, G. S., Barasa, F. A., Doll, J. A., & Velazquez, E. J. (2013). Heart failure in sub-Saharan Africa. *Current Cardiology Reviews, 9*(2), 157–173.

Braunwald, E. (1997). Shattuck lecture–cardiovascular medicine at the turn of the millennium: Triumphs, concerns, and opportunities. *New England Journal of Medicine, 337*(19), 1360–1369.

Braunwald, E. (2008). Biomarkers in heart failure. *New England Journal of Medicine, 358*, 2148–2159.

Bui, A. L., Horwich, T. B., & Fonarow, G. C. (2011). Epidemiology and risk profile of heart failure. *Nature Reviews Cardiology, 8*(1), 30–41.

Callender, T., Woodward, M., Roth, G., Farzadfar, F., Lemarie, J.-C., Gicquel, S., … Rahimi, K. (2014). Heart failure care in low- and middle-income countries: A systematic review and meta-analysis. *PLoS Med, 11*(8), e1001699.

Cappuccio, F. P., & Miller, M. A. (2016). Cardiovascular disease and hypertension in sub-Saharan Africa: Burden, risk and interventions. *Internal Emergency Medicine, 11*, 299–305.

Celermajer, D. S., Chow, C. K., Marijon, E., Anstey, N. M., & Woo, K. S. (2012). Cardiovascular disease in the developing world: Prevalences, patterns, and the potential of early disease detection. *Journal of American College of Cardiology, 60*(13), 1207–1216.

Chaouat, A., Naeije, R., & Weitzenblum, E. (2008). Pulmonary hypertension in COPD. *European Respiratory Journal, 32*(5), 1371–1385.

Chung, I., & Lip, G. Y. H. (2006). Platelets and heart failure. *European Heart Journal, 27*(22), 2623–2631.

Curtis, L. H., Whellan, D. J., Hammill, B. G., Hernandez, A. F., Anstrom, K. J., Shea, A. M., & Schulman, K. A. (2008). Incidence and prevalence of heart failure in elderly persons, 1994–2003. *Archives of Internal Medicine, 168*, 418–424.

Dhar, A. K., & Barton, D. A. (2016). Depression and the link with cardiovascular disease. *Front Psychiatry, 7*, 33.

Dunlay, S. M., Weston, S. A., Jacobsen, S. J., & Roger, V. L. (2009). Risk factors for heart failure: A population-based case-control study. *American Journal of Medicine, 122*(11), 1023–1028.

Ellison, D. H., & Felker, G. M. (2017). Diuretic treatment in heart failure. *New England Journal of Medicine, 377*, 1964–1975.

Fang, J., Mensah, G. A., Croft, J. B., & Keenan, N. L. (2008). Heart failure-related hospitalization in the U.S., 1979 to 2004. *Journal of the American College of Cardiology, 52*(6), 428–434.

Fonarow, G. C., Stough, W. G., Abraham, W. T., Albert, N. M., Gheorghiade, M., Greenberg, B. H., … Young, J. B. (2007). Characteristics, treatments, and outcomes of patients with preserved systolic function hospitalized for heart failure: A report from the OPTIMIZE-HF Registry. *Journal of the American College of Cardiology, 50*(8), 768–777.

Gaggin, H. K., & Januzzi, J. L. (2013). Biomarkers and diagnostics in heart failure. *Biochimica et Biophysica Acta (BBA)–Molecular Basis of Disease, 1832*(12), 2442–2450.

Gerber, Y., Weston, S. A., Redfield, M. M., Chamberlain, A. M., Manemann, S. M., Jiang, R., … Roger, V. L. (2015). A contemporary appraisal of the heart failure epidemic in Olmsted County, Minnesota, 2000–2010. *JAMA Internal Medicine, 175*(6), 996–1004.

Go, A. S., Mozaffarian, D., Roger, V. L., Benjamin, E. J., Berry, J. D., Borden, W. B., … Turner, M. B. (2013). Heart disease and stroke statistics—2013 update: A report from the American Heart Association. *Circulation, 127*(1), e6–e245.

Grippo, A. J., & Johnson, A. K. (2002). Biological mechanisms in the relationship between depression and heart disease. *Neuroscience & Biobehavioral Reviews, 26*(8), 941–962.

Guertl, B., Noehammer, C, & Hoefler, G. (2000). Metabolic cardiomyopathies. *International Journal of Experimental Pathology, 81*(6), 349–372.

Gujja, P., Rosing, D. R., Tripodi, D. J., & Shizukuda, Y. (2010). Iron overload cardiomyopathy, better understanding of an increasing disorder. *Journal of the American College of Cardiology, 56*(13), 1001–1012.

Hanninen, S. A., Darling, P. B., Sole, M. J., Barr, A., & Keith, M. E. (2006). The prevalence of thiamin deficiency in hospitalized patients with congestive heart failure. *Journal of the American College of Cardiology, 47*(2), 354–361.

Ho, K. K., Pinsky, J. L., Kannel, W. B., & Levy, D. (1993). The epidemiology of heart failure: The Framingham Study. *Journal of the American College of Cardiology, 22*(4 Suppl. A), 6A–13A.

Kannel, W. B., & Belanger, A. J. (1991). Epidemiology of heart failure. *American Heart Journal, 121*, 951–956.

Kenchaiah, S., Evans, J. C., Levy, D., Wilson, P. W., Benjamin, E. J., Larson, M. G., … Vasan, R. S. (2002). Obesity and the risk of heart failure. *New England Journal of Medicine, 347*(5), 305–313.

Lam, C. S. P., Donal, E., Kraigher-Krainer, E., & Vasan, R. S. (2011). Epidemiology and clinical course of heart failure with preserved ejection fraction. *European Journal of Heart Failure, 13*(1), 18–28.

Levy, D., Kenchaiah, S., Larson, M. G., Benjamin, E. J., Kupka, M. J., Ho, K. K. L., & Murabito, J. M. (2002). Long-term trends in the incidence of and survival with heart failure. *New England Journal of Medicine, 347*, 1397–1402.

Levy, D., Larson, M. G., Vasan, R. S., Kannel, W. B., & Ho, K. K. L. (1996). The progression from hypertension to congestive heart failure. *Journal of the American Medical Association, 275*, 1557–1562.

Liao, R., & Ward, J. E. (2017). Amyloid cardiomyopathy: Disease on the rise. *Circulation Research, 120*, 1865–1867.

Lloyd-Jones, D. M., Larson, M. G., Leip, E. P., Beiser, A., D'Agostino, R. B., Kannel, W. B., … Levy, D. (2002). Lifetime risk for developing congestive heart failure: The Framingham Heart Study. *Circulation, 106*, 3068–3072.

Loehr, L. R., Rosamond, W. D., Chang, P. P., Folsom, A. R., & Chambless, L. E. (2008). Heart failure incidence and survival (from the Atherosclerosis Risk in Communities study). *American Journal of Cardiology, 101*, 1016–1022.

Maisel, W. H., & Stevenson, L. W. (2003). Atrial fibrillation in heart failure: Epidemiology, pathophysiology, and rationale for therapy. *The American Journal of Cardiology, 91*(6), 2–8.

Mahmood, S. S., & Wang, T. J. (2013). The epidemiology of congestive heart failure: The Framingham Heart Study perspective. *Global Heart, 8*(1), 77–82.

Marrelli, M. T., & Brotto, M. (2016). The effect of malaria and anti-malarial drugs on skeletal and cardiac muscles. *Malaria Journal, 15*, 524.

Mayosi, B. M., Wiysonge, C. S., Ntsekhe, M., Gumedze, F., Volmink, J. A., Maartens, G., … Commerford, P. J. (2008). Mortality in patients treated for tuberculous pericarditis in sub-Saharan Africa. *South African Medical Journal, 98*(1), 36–40.

McKee, P. A., Castelli, W. P., McNamara, P. M., & Kannel, W. B. (1971). The natural history of congestive heart failure: The Framingham Study. *New England Journal of Medicine, 285*, 1441–1446.

Munir, M. B., Sharbaugh, M. S., Thoma, F. W., Nisar, M. U., Kamran, A. S., Althouse, A. D., & Saba, S. (2017). Trends in hospitalization for congestive heart failure, 1996–2009. *Clinical Cardiology, 40*(2), 109–119.

National Heart, Lung and Blood Institute. (2009). *Fact book fiscal year 2009.* Bethesda, MD: Center for Health Statistics, National Institutes of Health.

Newman, K. P., Bhattachary, S. K., Munir, A., Davis, R. C., Soberman, J. E., & Ramanathan, K. B. (2007). Macro- and micronutrients in patients with congestive heart failure, particularly African-Americans. *Vascular Health Risk Management, 3*(5), 743–747.

O'Connor, C. M. (2017). High heart failure readmission rates: Is it the health system's fault? *JACC: Heart Failure, 5*(5), 393.

Pandey, A., Omar, W., Ayers, C., LaMonte, M., Klein, L., Allen, N., … Berry, J. D. (2018). Sex and race differences in lifetime risk of heart failure with preserved ejection fraction and heart failure with reduced ejection fraction. *Circulation, 137*(17), 1814–1823.

Piano, M. R. (2002). Alcoholic cardiomyopathy: Incidence, clinical characteristics, and pathophysiology. *Chest, 121*(5), 1638–1650.

Ponikowski, P., Ander, S. D., Al Habib, K. F., Cowie, M. R., Force, T. L., Hu, S., … Filippatos, G. (2012). Heart failure: Preventing disease and death worldwide. *European Society of Cardiology, 1*(1), 4–25. Oxford PharmaGenesis, U.K.

Prinzo, Z. W. (1999). *Thiamine deficiency and it prevention and control in major emergencies.* Geneva, Switzerland: World Health Organization, Department of Nutrition for Health and Development, 99.13.

Rassi, Jr A., Rassi, A., & Marin-Neto, J. A. (2010). Chagas disease. *The Lancet, 375*(9723), 1388–1402.

Roger, V. L., Go, A. S., Lloyd-Jones, D. M., Benjamin, E. J., Berry, J. D., Borden, W. B., … on behalf of the American Heart Association Statistics Committee and Stroke Statistics Subcommittee. (2012). Heart disease and stroke statistics-2012 update. *Circulation, 125*, e2–e220.

Roger, V. L., Weston, S. A., Redfield, M. M., Hellermann-Homan, J. P., Killian, J., Yawn, B. P., & Jacobsen, S. J. (2004). Trends in heart failure incidence and survival in a community-based population. *Journal of the American Medical Association, 292*(3), 344–350.

Rusinaru, D., Tribouilloy, C., Berry, C., Richards, A. M., Whalley, G. A., Earle, N., … MAGGIC Investigators. (2012). Relationship of serum sodium concentration to mortality in a wide spectrum of heart failure patients with preserved and with reduced ejection fraction: An individual patient data meta-analysis: Meta-Analysis Global Group in Chronic heart failure (MAGGIC). *European Journal of Heart Failure, 14,* 1139–1146.

Rutledge, T., Reis, V. A., Linke, S. E., Greenberg, B. H., & Mills, P. J. (2006). Depression in heart failure: A meta-analytic review of prevalence, intervention effects, and associations with clinical outcomes. *Journal of the American College of Cardiology, 48*(8), 1527–1537.

Savarese, G., & Lund, L. H. (2017). Global public health burden of heart failure. *Cardiac Failure Review, 3*(1), 7–11.

Sekhri, V., Sanal, S., DeLorenzo, L. J., Aronow, W. S., & Maguire, G. P. (2011). Cardiac sarcoidosis: A comprehensive review. *Archives of Medical Science, 7*(4), 546–554.

Selmer, C., Olesen, J. B., Hansen, M. L., Lindhardsen, J., Olsen, A. M. S., Madsen, J. C., … Gislason, G. H. (2012). The spectrum of thyroid disease and risk of new onset atrial fibrillation: A large population cohort study. *British Medical Journal, 345,* e7895.

Selmer, C., Olesen, J. B., Hansen, M. L., von Kappelgaard, L. M., Madsen, J. C., Hansen, P. R., … Gislason, G. H. (2014). Subclinical and overt thyroid dysfunction and risk of all-cause mortality and cardiovascular events: A large population

study. *Journal of Clinical Endocrinology & Metabolism, 99*(7), 2372–2382.

Tang, Y. D., & Katz, S. D. (2006). Anemia in chronic heart failure. *Circulation, 113,* 2454–2461.

Taylor, C. J., Ryan, R., Nichols, L., Gale, N., Hobbs, F. D. R., & Marshall, T. (2017). Survival following a diagnosis of heart failure in primary care. *Family Practice, 34*(2), 161–168.

Thomas, T., Haase, N., Rosamond, W., Howard, V. J., Rumsfeld, J., Manolio, T., … American Heart Association Statistics Committee and Stroke Statistics Subcommittee. (2006). Heart disease and stroke statistics—2006 update. *Circulation, 113,* e85–e151.

Tsutsui, H., Tsuchihashi-Makaya, M., & Kinugawa, S. (2010). Clinical characteristics and outcomes of heart failure with preserved ejection fraction: Lessons from epidemiological studies. *Journal of Cardiology, 5*(1), 13–22.

Wolk, M. J., Scheidt, S., & Killip, T. (1972). Heart failure complicating acute myocardial infarction. *Circulation, 45,* 1125–1138.

Young, D. R., Reynolds, K., Sidell, M., Brar, S., Ghai, N. R., Sternfeld, B., … Quinn, V. P. (2014). Effects of physical activity and sedentary time on the risk of heart failure. *Circulation: Heart Failure, 7,* 21–27.

CHAPTER 8

Epidemiology of Aortic Aneurysm and Dissection

▶ Introduction

Aneurysms of the aorta are divisible into two major categories: Thoracic (above the diaphragm) and abdominal (below the diaphragm). Either type is defined as dilatation or outpouching of the aorta with a diameter that is 50% greater than normal. Thoracic aneurysms are further divided into those of the ascending aorta (70%), the aortic arch (10%), and the descending aorta (20%). Abdominal aneurysms can be categorized into those above and below the renal arteries. The majority of abdominal aortic aneurysms develop below the renal arteries. **FIGURE 8.1** shows the anatomic distribution of thoracic and abdominal aortic aneurysms.

▶ Pathogenesis of Aortic Aneurysm, Dissection, and Rupture

The wall of the aorta consists of three layers: The innermost layer, the *tunica intima*, consists of the endothelium (simple squamous epithelium) surrounded by a connective tissue basement membrane with elastic fibers (the internal elastic membrane). The middle layer, the *tunica media*, is primarily smooth muscle and is usually the thickest layer. The *tunica media* is surrounded by the external elastic membrane. The outer layer, the *tunica adventitia*, consists primarily of fibroblasts. True aneurysms involve dilatation of all three layers of the arterial wall.

▶ Thoracic Versus Abdominal Aortic Aneurysms

The pathogenesis of thoracic aortic aneurysms is mixed and differs from that of abdominal aortic aneurysms. Thoracic aneurysms of the ascending aorta are characterized by damage to the smooth muscle cells of the tunica media whereas thoracic aneurysms of the descending aorta and abdominal aortic aneurysms involve atherosclerotic damage to both the tunica intima and tunica media (Vapnik et al., 2016).

The characteristic pathologic finding in thoracic aneurysms of the ascending aorta is *cystic medial necrosis*. This refers to degeneration and fragmentation of elastic fibers, loss of smooth muscle cells, and accumulation of basophilic ground substance in the tunica media of the arterial wall. Thoracic aortic aneurysms are characterized by *acute aortic dissection* due to blood traversing along the lamellar planes of the weakened tunica media and the formation of blood-filled channels within the aortic wall. Blood reaches the tunica media through a tear in the tunica intima at high pressure points in the ascending aorta or the aortic arch (White, Broder, Mando-Vandrick, Wendell, & Crowe, 2013).

FIGURE 8.1 Anatomic Distribution of Aortic Aneurysms.

In contrast to the aneurysms of the ascending aorta, thoracic aneurysms of the descending aorta and abdominal aortic aneurysms are associated with severe atherosclerosis and the development of atheromas beneath the tunica intima causing thinning and destruction of the tunica media. Abdominal aortic aneurysms are often filled with thrombus (clotted blood) that produce emboli that invariably lodge in smaller vessels of the lower extremities to cause obstruction and *peripheral artery disease* (PAD) (Isselbacher, 2014). Models of pathogenesis for thoracic and abdominal aortic aneurysms are shown in **FIGURE 8.2**.

▶ Aortic Dissection or Rupture

Acute aortic dissection and/or rupture are the most common life-threatening disorders affecting the aorta. The vast majority (about 95%) of aortic aneurysms develop without symptoms over a span of several years. Aneurysms are most often diagnosed incidentally on careful review of chest X-rays, or when they are complicated by dissection or rupture with the sudden onset of severe pain (Akin & Nienaber, 2014; Thrumurthy, Karthikesalingam, Patterson, Holt, & Thompson, 2011).

A team of international investigators examined clinical data from a large case series of 464 patients with acute aortic dissections enrolled from 12 referral centers in six countries from 1996 to 1998. The referral centers were all members of the *International Registry*

of Aortic Dissections (IRAD). The data included the presenting history, physical findings, management, and mortality as well as physician review of hospital records. Among all 464 cases, 289 (62%) involved the ascending aorta and the aortic arch and 175 (38%) occurred in the descending thoracic aorta. Among all cases, 65% were male, 72% had a history of hypertension, 31% had a history of atherosclerosis, 18% had prior cardiac surgery, and only 16% had a known aortic aneurysm. Approximately 5% of cases had Marfan's syndrome (a heritable connective tissue disorder) and the average age at onset in these cases was early (35 years). Female patients were older on average (68 versus 61 years) and had a higher mortality rate than males (34% versus 24%). Onset was typically heralded by the abrupt occurrence of acute chest pain and, in more than 11% of cases, congestive heart failure, or stroke were present at the time of onset. Among patients with dissection of the descending thoracic aorta, 122 of 174 evaluable cases (70%) presented with hypertension whereas in those with dissection of the ascending aorta or the arch of the aorta, only 99 of 277 cases (36%) presented with hypertension (Hagan et al., 2000).

Aortic aneurysms become more prone to dissection or rupture as they grow and expand. In a study of 304 cases followed by serial imaging conducted at Yale University, aneurysms of the aorta expanded by about 1 mm per year and the risk of rupture or dissection increased more than 5-fold when the diameter exceeded 6 cm compared to 4 cm or less.

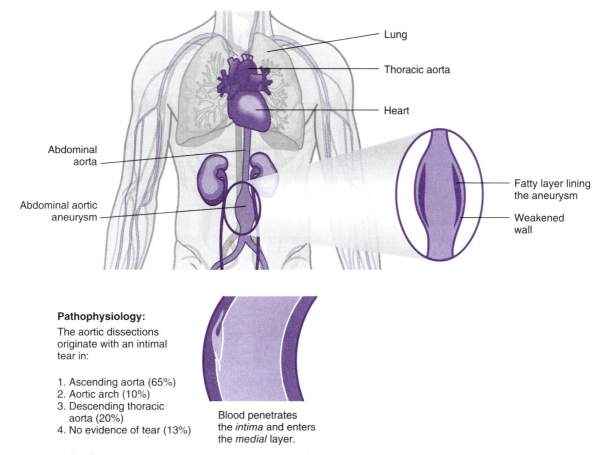

Pathophysiology:
The aortic dissections originate with an intimal tear in:

1. Ascending aorta (65%)
2. Aortic arch (10%)
3. Descending thoracic aorta (20%)
4. No evidence of tear (13%)

Blood penetrates the *intima* and enters the *medial* layer.

FIGURE 8.2 Models of Pathogenesis: Thoracic Versus Abdominal Aortic Aneurysms.

The rate of rupture or dissection in aneurysms exceeding 6 cm was 7% per year with 12% mortality (Davies et al., 2002).

Once an aortic aneurysm reaches a critical diameter (approximately 6 cm), the vessel cannot distend further and a transient rise in blood pressure to around 200 mm Hg during stress or exertion can exceed the arterial wall strength and trigger aortic dissection or rupture. The immediate mortality rate in aortic dissection/rupture is approximately 1% per hour over the first several hours after onset, making early diagnosis and treatment critical for survival (Booher & Eagle, 2011; Elefteriades, 2008; Goldfinger et al., 2014; Isselbacher, 2005).

▶ Incidence of Thoracic Aortic Aneurysm and Dissection

Population-based registries such as those in Scandinavian countries provide critical information on the prevalence, incidence, and survival of chronic diseases. A recent report provides estimates of the annual incidence of thoracic aortic aneurysms from a long-term study of the Swedish population. The study identified 14,229 individuals with thoracic aortic aneurysm or dissection in the Swedish population of approximately 8.7 million from 1987 to 2002. Over the 16-year time span of the study, the incidence of thoracic aortic disease rose by 52% in men and by 28% in women to reach 16.3 per 100,000 per year and 9.1 per 100,000 per year, respectively (**FIGURE 8.3**). The investigators attributed the increase in incidence to improved diagnostic imaging and better case ascertainment. Operations for aneurysm repair increased 15-fold in women and 7-fold in men, and 30-day mortality of surgically treated patients declined from 25% to 13% during the study period (Olsson, Thelin, Ståhle, Ekbom, & Granath, 2006).

▶ Trends in Mortality from Aortic Aneurysm and Dissection

A team of investigators reviewed data from the *Global Burden of Disease* database to estimate global and

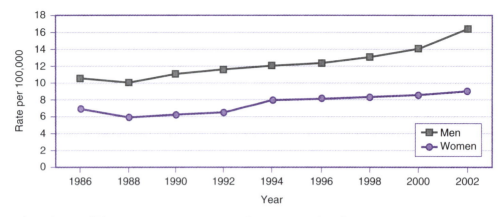

FIGURE 8.3 Annual Incidence of Thoracic Aortic Aneurysm or Dissection in Sweden, 1987–2002.

Data from Olsson, C., Thelin, S., Ståhle, E., Ekbom, A., & Granath, F. (2006). Thoracic aortic aneurysm and dissection: Increasing prevalence and improved outcomes reported in a nationwide population-based study of more than 14,000 cases from 1987 to 2002. *Circulation, 114*(24), 2611–2618.

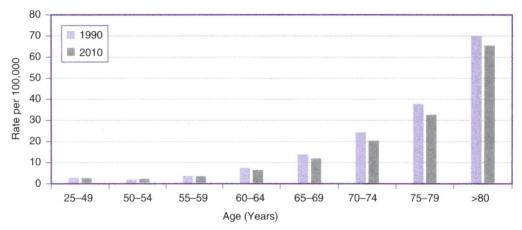

FIGURE 8.4 Global Age-Specific Mortality from Aortic Aneurysms, 1990 Versus 2010.

Data from Sampson, U. K. A., Norman, P. E., Fowkes, F. G. R., Aboyans, V., Song, Y., Harrell, F. E., Jr., … Criqui, M. H. (2014). Global and regional burden of aortic dissection and aneurysms: Mortality trends in 21 world regions, 1990 to 2010. *Global Heart, 9*(1), 171–180.

regional mortality from aortic dissections and aortic aneurysms. Data were compiled for 21 regions in 1990 and 2010, and rates were estimated by age, gender, and region. Mortality rates were variable ranging from high values of 8 per 100,000 in Australasia and Western Europe to low values of less than 1 per 100,000 in many underdeveloped countries where reporting is less reliable. Overall, men had higher annual aortic aneurysm death rates than women: 3.1 versus 2.1 per 100,000. **FIGURE 8.4** compares age-specific mortality rates for 1990 and 2010 using the combined data of the 21 regions. On average, there was a 16% reduction in the age-specific mortality rates over the 20-year span of the study (Sampson et al., 2014).

Investigators at the University of Leicester in Great Britain recently studied the trends in mortality from thoracic aortic aneurysms and aortic dissections reported during 1994–2010 by 18 member nations of the World Health Organization. Across all populations, the annual mortality from thoracic aortic aneurysms declined by 5%–10% in men and 3%–6% in

women and mortality from aortic dissection declined by 2%–3% in men and 1%–2% in women. Nevertheless, there was heterogeneity of trends among populations (e.g., significant *decreases* in mortality were observed in 13 of the 18 member nations whereas significant *increases* were observed in four nations: Japan, Romania, Denmark, and Hungary). The mortality rates observed in different populations were positively correlated with blood pressure and blood cholesterol and negatively correlated with body mass index. Furthermore, improved imaging techniques, increased awareness, and timely intervention using improved surgical techniques for aortic repair have also had a favorable impact (Isselbacher, 2014; Sidloff et al., 2014).

According to recent data from the Global Burden of Disease study 2015, the age-standardized global death rate for aortic aneurysms, dissections, and ruptures was 2.6 per 100,000 in 2013, which represents a 15% median decline since 1990. Nevertheless, because of the aging of populations in reporting nations, the actual number of deaths increased from 99,600 in 1990 to 168,200 deaths in 2015 (Benjamin et al., 2018; Roth et al., 2017).

▶ Gender Differences in Prevalence of Thoracic Aneurysms

Multiple investigations have demonstrated that men are at greater risk than women for the development of aortic aneurysms whereas data on aortic dissections is limited. Gender differences in the age-specific frequencies of acute aortic dissections were therefore examined among 1078 patients ascertained during 1996–2001 in the *International Registry of Acute Aortic Dissection*. Across all ages, men developed aortic dissections about twice as often as women (68% versus 32%). However, as shown in **FIGURE 8.5**, the male predominance was most striking at young ages, with men outnumbering women by 4:1 at ages less than 50. With increasing age, the gender difference lessened, and among those older than 75, men and women were equally represented. On average, women were about 7 years older than men at the time of aortic dissection (67 versus 60 years of age) (Nienaber et al., 2004).

The 7- to 10-year average delay in the onset of cardiovascular diseases in women compared to men has been attributed to protective effects of relatively high levels of circulating endogenous estrogens in premenopausal women. With the onset of menopause and the depletion of ovarian estrogens, rates of cardiovascular disease increase among women and become similar to the rates in men. This pattern is consistent for all forms of cardiovascular diseases including aortic aneurysms, dissections, and ruptures.

One explanation that has been advanced to explain the gender difference in cardiovascular

disease pertains to the balance of estrogens and androgens in women versus men. During the premenopausal years, women have lower average blood levels of LDL cholesterol and total cholesterol compared to men, presumably because of the anticholesterolemic effects of estrogen. After menopause, female levels of cholesterol rise considerably in conjunction with the lower levels of estrogen (Maas & Appelman, 2010). In regard to aneurysms of the descending aorta, the vast majority involve atherosclerosis and the formation of atheromatous plaque in the aortic wall. It is therefore plausible that the male preponderance of aortic aneurysms at earlier ages compared to women may be at least partially due to gender differences in the changing balance of estrogens and androgens that influence atherosclerosis throughout the lifespan.

▶ Causes and Risk Factors of Aortic Aneurysms

Multiple conditions and risk factors predispose to the development of aortic aneurysms. In particular, cardiovascular risk factors such as coronary artery disease, smoking, hypertension, diabetes, and hyperlipidemia have been implicated as elevating the risk for aneurysms of the descending aorta and the abdominal aorta *but not the ascending thoracic aorta*. Other conditions and risk factors for aortic aneurysms include congenital anomalies, heritable connective tissue disorders, certain infectious diseases, trauma, weight lifting, and the use of certain drugs. These are discussed in the following sections.

Cardiovascular Risk Factors and Abdominal Aortic Aneurysm

Investigators at China Medical University in Shenyang conducted a meta-analysis to estimate trends

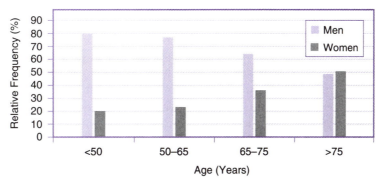

FIGURE 8.5 Frequency of Males Versus Females with Acute Aortic Dissections by Age.

Data from Nienaber, C. A., Fattori, R., Mehta, R. H., Richartz, B. M., Evangelista, A., Petzsch, M., ... Bossone, E. (2004). Gender related differences in acute aortic dissection. *Circulation, 109*(24), 3014–3021.

in the prevalence and odds ratios for risk factors of *abdominal aortic aneurysms* at least 3 cm in diameter. Their analysis included data from 56 reports and included studies conducted in America, Europe, Australia, and Asia. The overall prevalence of abdominal aneurysms in adults 55 years or older was 4.8% and the prevalence was 3.8 times higher in men than women (6% in men and 1.6% in women). Asia had the lowest prevalence (0.5%) and Australia the highest (6.7%). Odds ratios were highest for claudication/PAD (OR = 3.0), smoking (OR = 2.1), and coronary artery disease (OR = 1.8) whereas there was only a modest effect of hypertension (OR = 1.3) (Li et al., 2013).

Investigators at University Hospital in Lausanne, Switzerland conducted a meta-analysis of risk factors for *abdominal aortic aneurysms* among patients 60 years or older. Their analysis of 14 cross-sectional studies found significant associations with male gender (OR = 5.7), smoking (OR = 2.4), history of myocardial infarction (OR = 2.3), and peripheral vascular disease (OR = 2.5). Hypertension was only weakly associated with abdominal aortic aneurysm (OR = 1.3) and there was no association with diabetes (Cornuz, Sidoti Pinto, Tevaearai, & Egger, 2004).

Findings of these meta-analyses provide strong evidence that several major pre-existing cardiovascular conditions (ischemic/coronary heart disease, myocardial infarction, smoking and PAD) markedly elevate the risk of developing abdominal aortic aneurysms. All of these conditions are linked to atherosclerotic disease as the dominant etiology in the pathogenesis of aneurysms of the descending and abdominal aorta.

Atherosclerosis Versus Genetics: Thoracic Aortic Aneurysms

Investigators in the Massachusetts General Hospital Thoracic Aortic Center at Harvard recently reported the results of a prospective study of patients with thoracic aneurysms monitored by computerized tomography and magnetic resonance imaging during 1992–2013. The study included 844 patients with thoracic aortic aneurysms that were at least 4 cm in diameter at the time of detection. Two distinct pathological patterns emerged. Among 628 aneurysms of the ascending aorta, 572 (91%) developed *without* atherosclerotic changes, whereas the majority of aneurysms involving the descending

aorta (88%) showed the presence of atheromas. Compared to cases with aneurysms of the descending aorta, those with aneurysms of the ascending aorta were younger, less likely to be women, and less likely to have diabetes mellitus, hypertension, or a history of smoking. Approximately one-third of cases with aneurysms of the ascending aorta had bicuspid aortic valves or TGFβ vasculopathies. Notably, 101 (41%) of the 244 cases with aneurysms involving the descending thoracic aorta also developed abdominal aortic aneurysms. Follow-up of all cases revealed that hypertension and atherosclerosis were significant independent predictors of adverse events such as aortic dissection, aortic rupture, aortic repair, or death. These findings suggest that aneurysms of the ascending thoracic aorta are more likely to have a genetic or congenital basis whereas aneurysms of the descending thoracic aorta are primarily due to atherosclerosis (Vapnik et al., 2016).

Bicuspid Aortic Valve and Ascending Thoracic Aortic Aneurysm

Bicuspid aortic valve is the most common of all congenital heart valve anomalies with a prevalence of approximately 1%–2% in the general population and a male predominance of approximately 3:1. This anomaly is often present in certain genetic syndromes such as Turner syndrome wherein females have a single X chromosome. Patients with bicuspid aortic valve are at increased risk for the development of thoracic ascending aneurysms and aortic dissections. As shown in **FIGURE 8.6**, the aortic valve is normally tricuspid with three equal size cusps in order to equalize the pressure dynamics of blood outflow from the left ventricle of the heart. In contrast, the bicuspid aortic valve has cusps of unequal size and is prone to incomplete closure resulting in aortic stenosis and/or aortic insufficiency accompanied by hemodynamic derangements including abnormal flow turbulence and increased stroke volume. These conditions beget progressive dilatation of the ascending aorta, decreased thickness of the vessel walls, increased wall tension, and severe degeneration, or loss of elastic fibers in the tunica media. Over time, progression of these processes can ultimately result in aortic aneurysm, aortic dissection, and death (Isselbacher, 2005; Losenno, Goodman, & Chu, 2012; van de Pol, Kurakula, DeRuiter, & Goumans, 2017).

FIGURE 8.6 Tricuspid and Bicuspid Aortic Valves.

Connective Tissue Disorders and Thoracic Aortic Aneurysms

Several connective tissue disorders that have a genetic basis increase the risk of thoracic aortic aneurysms. The most prominent of these are Marfan's syndrome, Ehler–Danlos syndrome, and Loeys–Dietz syndrome, all of which show autosomal dominant patterns of inheritance. These syndromes are caused by heritable genetic mutations that alter the development of connective tissues that are critical to the integrity of the arterial wall. For example, in Marfan's syndrome, one or more genes that regulate fibrillin biosynthesis are mutated resulting in abnormal elastic fibers and smooth muscle cells of the medial layer of the arterial wall (Cooper, Walsh, Sadat, Hayes, & Boyle, 2009).

Infection and Aortic Aneurysm

An *infected aortic aneurysm* is a localized dilatation of the aorta that becomes infected. Such infections are rare and more likely to occur in individuals who are immunocompromised (e.g., those with HIV disease, recipients of organ transplants, or individuals with immune deficiencies). *Staphylococcus* and *Salmonella* bacteria have the greatest affinity for the vessel wall and are most likely to cause infected aneurysms. Nevertheless, many other organisms have been cultured from infected aneurysms including *Streptococcus*, *Pseudomonas*, and *Mycobacterium tuberculosis*. Patients with atherosclerosis are at greatest risk of developing an infected aortic aneurysm. Although infected aneurysms are relatively uncommon (1%–2% of cases), they are life-threatening due to the high rate of arterial rupture (Kim, 2010; Laohapensang, Rutherford, & Arworn, 2010).

Prior to the development and use of antibiotics, thoracic aortic aneurysms were most often attributable to *tertiary syphilis*. Though syphilis has virtually disappeared in developed nations since the advent of antibiotics, cases of thoracic aortic aneurysms involving tertiary syphilis are still occasionally reported in developing nations. In the development of a syphilitic aneurysm, the invasion of the aortic wall by *Treponema pallidum* destroys the *vasa vasorum* (the network of small blood vessels in the arterial wall) which causes necrosis of the elastic fibers and connective tissue in the tunica adventitia. Without treatment, the case-fatality rate of syphilitic aneurysm approaches 80% due to the high rate of rupture (Paulo, Cascarejo, & Vouga, 2012).

Peripheral Artery Disease and Abdominal Aortic Aneurysms

PAD is occlusion of the arterial vessels that supply blood to the lower extremities. This condition is attributable to the development of atherosclerotic

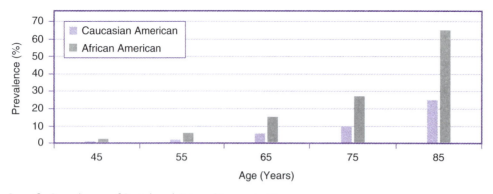

FIGURE 8.7 Age-Specific Prevalence of Peripheral Artery Disease in Men.

Data from Allison, M. A., Ho, E., Denenberg, J. O., Langer, R. D., Newman, A. B., Fabsitz, R. R., & Criqui, M. H. (2007). Ethnic-specific prevalence of peripheral arterial disease in the United States. *American Journal of Preventive Medicine*, 32, 328–333.

plaque and/or atherosclerotic thromboemboli of the affected blood vessels. Clinically, PAD is characterized by intermittent claudication (calf pain) when walking that is relieved by rest. The standard diagnostic test for PAD is measurement of systolic blood pressures in the arms and ankles and calculating the ankle brachial index (ABI) as the ratio of these blood pressures (e.g., ABI = ankle blood pressure/brachial artery blood pressure). The standard cutoff for diagnosing PAD is ABI < 0.90 (Criqui & Aboyans, 2015).

PAD is uncommon before the age of 50 years but thereafter the prevalence rises sharply (e.g., in Caucasian Americans, the prevalence exceeds 20% after 80 years of age). However, there are significant ethnic differences in the prevalence of PAD; for example, age-specific prevalence estimates for African Americans are approximately double that for Caucasian Americans (**FIGURE 8.7**). The markedly higher prevalence of PAD among African American men and women is primarily due to their greater exposure to the risk factors for atherosclerotic conditions (Allison et al., 2007; Criqui & Aboyans, 2015).

Investigators at the University of Edinburgh in the United Kingdom examined data from 34 community-based studies to estimate recent trends in the global prevalence of PAD and associated risk factors. They estimated that in 2010, 202 million people in the world population were living with PAD, compared to 164 million in 2000, an increase of approximately 23% for the decade of study. Significant risk factors included prior history of cardiovascular disease (OR = 2.3), hypertension (OR = 1.6), current smoking (OR = 2.1), former smoking (OR = 1.9), diabetes (OR = 1.7), elevated C-reactive protein (OR = 1.7), elevated cholesterol (OR = 1.2), and increasing age decile (OR = 1.4). Results suggest that due to the increasing numbers of elderly people in many populations of the world, the global burden of PAD is rising (Fowkes et al., 2013).

Nearly all abdominal aortic aneurysms develop from atheromas of the arterial wall, and they are often filled with thrombus (clotted blood) which can break off and travel downstream to lodge in small vessels of the extremities. Thromboembolic occlusion of the popliteal arteries proximal to the calf muscles is a major cause of ischemia, intermittent claudication, and PAD. In a study conducted in Spain, 151 (13%) of 1166 patients with PAD had abdominal aortic aneurysms detected by abdominal ultrasound. The prevalence rose to 17% for male PAD patients over the age of 75 years (Barba, Estallo, Rodríguez, & Baquer de Céniga, 2005). The presence of PAD is often a harbinger for an abdominal aortic aneurysm.

▶ Mortality from Peripheral Artery Disease

Aside from mortality due to PAD-associated conditions such as dissection or rupture of abdominal aortic aneurysms, PAD can also be a direct cause of death. For example, severely occlusive PAD can cause tissue necrosis requiring foot or leg amputation, and if untreated, tissue necrosis can cause life-threatening gangrene and sepsis. During 2015, 52,500 deaths in the world population were attributed to PAD. The southern sub-Saharan region of Africa, where there is limited access to antibiotics and advanced surgical techniques, had the highest mortality rates (3 per 100,000) (Roth et al., 2017).

▶ Other Risk Factors for Aortic Aneurysm, Dissection, and Rupture

Weightlifting and the use of certain drugs (e.g., cocaine and amphetamines) have been linked to aortic dissection and rupture, perhaps because of acute hemodynamic stress and spikes in blood pressure that occur during these activities. Patients with pheochromocytoma (a rare tumor of the adrenal glands that secretes catecholamines) are also prone to marked fluctuations in blood pressure and heart rate that may trigger aortic dissection or rupture. Finally, aortic dissection/rupture may also complicate inflammatory conditions of the aorta such as aortitis, most commonly giant cell arteritis (Braverman, 2010; Goran, 2008).

▶ Prevention and Screening

Aneurysms of the descending thoracic aorta and the abdominal aorta are predominantly caused by chronic atherosclerotic damage to arterial walls. Guidelines for the primary prevention of descending aortic aneurysms, dissection, and rupture are therefore similar to those for ischemic heart disease. The objective is to reduce exposure to factors known to initiate and promote atherosclerosis in blood vessels. The major recommendations are to avoid cigarette smoking and the use of any tobacco product, eat a healthy diet, maintain normal weight for height, exercise daily, control blood pressure, blood glucose, blood cholesterol, and C-reactive protein within normal limits, and refrain from abusing alcohol or other drugs with hemodynamic impact.

It is important to identify those individuals with genetic conditions and/or congenital anomalies that elevate the risk of aortic aneurysm development. Among such individuals, noninvasive serial imaging by ultrasonography to detect small aneurysms may be advisable. Among older adults, the results of four large randomized clinical trials showed that a one-time screening for abdominal aortic aneurysms significantly reduced mortality among men aged 65–75 years who had a history of smoking (LeFevre, 2014). For patients with small aneurysms, medical therapy with agents that regulate the heart rhythm and reduce blood pressure can be administered to reduce the rate of aneurysm growth. Referral for surgical repair is based on aneurysm diameter, location, and etiology (Goldfinger et al., 2014).

References

Akin, I., & Nienaber, C. A. (2014). Interventional treatment strategies of thoracic aortic pathologies. *European Review for Medical and Pharmacological Sciences, 18*(17), 2562–2574.

Allison, M. A., Ho, E., Denenberg, J. O., Langer, R. D., Newman, A. B., Fabsitz, R. R., & Criqui, M. H. (2007). Ethnic-specific prevalence of peripheral arterial disease in the United States. *American Journal of Preventive Medicine, 32*, 328–333.

Barba, A., Estallo, L., Rodríguez, L., & Baquer de Céniga, M. V. (2005). Detection of abdominal aortic aneurysm in patients with peripheral artery disease. *European Journal of Vascular and Endovascular Surgery, 30*(5), 504–508.

Benjamin, E. J., Virani, S. S., Callaway, C. W., Chamberlain, A. M., Chang, A. R., Cheng, S. … Muntner, P. (2018). Heart disease and stroke statistics-2018 update: A report from the American Heart Association. *Circulation*, 2018. 10.1161/CIR.0000000000000558

Booher, A. M., & Eagle, K. A. (2011). Diagnosis and management issues in thoracic aortic aneurysm. *American Heart Journal, 162*(1), 37–46.

Braverman, A. C. (2010). Acute aortic dissection: Clinician update. *Circulation, 122*(2), 184–188.

Cooper, D. G., Walsh, S. R., Sadat, U., Hayes, P. D., & Boyle, J. R. (2009). Treating the thoracic aorta in Marfan syndrome: Surgery or TEVAR? *Journal of Endovascular Therapy, 16*(1), 60–70.

Cornuz, J., Sidoti Pinto, C., Tevaearai, H., & Egger, M. (2004). Risk factors for asymptomatic abdominal aortic aneurysm: Systematic review and meta-analysis of population-based screening studies. *European Journal of Public Health, 14*, 343–349.

Criqui, M. H., & Aboyans, V. (2015). Epidemiology of peripheral artery disease. *Circulation Research, 116*(9), 1509–1526.

Davies, R. R., Goldstein, L. J., Coady, M. A., Tittle, S. L., Rizzo, J. A., Kopf, G. S., & Elefteriades, J. A. (2002). Yearly rupture or dissection rates for thoracic aortic aneurysms: Simple prediction based on size. *The Annals of Thoracic Surgery, 73*(1), 17–28.

Elefteriades, J. A. (2008). Thoracic aortic aneurysm: Reading the enemy's playbook. *Current Problems in Cardiology, 33*(5), 203–277.

Fowkes, F. G., Rudan, D., Rudan, I., Aboyans, V., Denenberg, J. O., McDermott, M. M., … Criqui, M. H. (2013). Comparison of global estimates of prevalence and risk factors for peripheral artery disease in 2000 and 2010: A systematic review and analysis. *Lancet, 382* (9901), 1329–1340.

Goldfinger, J. Z., Halperin, J. L., Marin, M. L., Stewart, A. S., Eagle, K. A., & Fuster, V. (2014). Thoracic aortic aneurysm and dissection. *Journal of the American College of Cardiology, 64*(16), 1725–1739.

Goran, K. P., 2008. Pheochromocytomas in aortic dissection patients: Have they been missing or missed? *The American Journal of Emergency Medicine, 26*(5), 626–627.

Hagan, P. G., Nienaber, C. A., Isselbacher, E. M., Bruckman, D., Karavite, D. J., Russman, P. L., … Moore, A. G. (2000). The International Registry of Acute Aortic Dissection (IRAD): New insights into an old disease. *Journal of American Medical Association, 283*(7), 807–903.

Isselbacher, E. M. (2005). Thoracic and abdominal aortic aneurysms. *Circulation, 111*, 816–828.

Isselbacher, E. M. (2014). Trends in thoracic aortic aneurysms and dissection, out of the shadows and into the light. *Circulation, 130*, 2267–2268.

Kim, Y. (2010). Infected aneurysm: Current management. *Annals of Vascular Diseases, 3*(1), 7–15.

Laohapensang, K., Rutherford, R. B., & Arworn, S. (2010). Infected aneurysm. *Annals Vascular Diseases, 3*(1), 16–23.

LeFevre, M. L., on behalf of the U.S. Preventive Services Task Force. (2014). Screening for abdominal aortic aneurysm: U.S. Preventive Services Task Force recommendation statement. *Annals of Internal Medicine, 161*(4), 281–290.

Li, X., Zhao, G., Zhang, J., Duan, Z., & Xin, S. (2013). Prevalence and trends of the abdominal aortic aneurysms epidemic in general population—A meta-analysis. *PLoS One, 8*(12), e81260.

Losenno, K. L., Goodman, R. L., & Chu, M. W. A. (2012). Bicuspid aortic valve disease and ascending aortic aneurysms: Gaps in knowledge. *Cardiology Research and Practice, 2012*(1), 145202, 16 pages.

Maas, A. H. E. M., & Appelman, Y. E. A. (2010). Gender differences in coronary heart disease. *Netherlands Heart Journal, 18*(12), 598–602.

Nienaber, C. A., Fattori, R., Mehta, R. H., Richartz, B. M., Evangelista, A., Petzsch, M., … Bossone, E. (2004). Gender related differences in acute aortic dissection. *Circulation, 109*(24), 3014–3021.

Olsson, C., Thelin, S., Ståhle, E., Ekbom, A., & Granath, F. (2006). Thoracic aortic aneurysm and dissection: Increasing prevalence and improved outcomes reported in a nationwide population-based study of more than 14,000 cases from 1987 to 2002. *Circulation, 114*(24), 2611–2618.

Paulo, N., Cascarejo, J., & Vouga, L. (2012). Syphilitic aneurysm of the ascending aorta. *Interactive Cardiovascular and Thoracic Surgery, 14*(2), 223–225.

Roth, G. A., Johnson, C., Abajobir, A., Abd-Allah, F., Abera, S. F., Abyu, G., … Alla, F. (2017). Global, regional, and national burden of cardiovascular diseases for 10 Causes, 1990 to 2015. *Journal of the American College of Cardiology, 70*(1), 1–25.

Sampson, U. K. A., Norman, P. E., Fowkes, F. G. R., Aboyans, V., Song, Y., Harrell, F. E., Jr., … Criqui, M. H. (2014). Global and regional burden of aortic dissection and aneurysms: Mortality trends in 21 world regions, 1990 to 2010. *Global Heart, 9*(1), 171–180.

Sidloff, D., Choke, E., Stather, P., Bown, M., Thompson, J., & Sayers, R. (2014). Mortality from thoracic aortic diseases and associations with cardiovascular risk factors. *Circulation, 130*, 2287–2294.

Thrumurthy, S. G., Karthikesalingam, A., Patterson, B. O., Holt, P. J., & Thompson, M. M. (2011). The diagnosis and management of aortic dissection. *British Medical Journal, 344*, d8290.

van de Pol, V., Kurakula, K., DeRuiter, M. C., & Goumans, M. J. (2017). Thoracic aortic aneurysm development in patients with bicuspid aortic valve: Hat is the role of endothelial cells? *Frontiers in Physiology, 8*, 938.

Vapnik, J. S., Bum Kim, J., Isselbacher, E. M., Ghoshhajra, B. B., Cheng, Y., Sundt, T. M., … Lindsay, M. E. (2016). Characteristics and outcomes of ascending versus descending thoracic aortic aneurysms. *American Journal of Cardiology, 117*(10), 1683–1690.

White, A., Broder, J., Mando-Vandrick, J., Wendell, J., & Crowe, J. (2013). Acute aortic emergencies-Part 2 aortic dissections. *Advanced Emergency Nursing Journal, 35*(1), 28–52.

© Andrew Brookes/Getty Images

CHAPTER 9

Epidemiology of Venous Thromboembolism and Pulmonary Embolism

▶ Introduction

The venous network of the circulatory system transports deoxygenated blood from the periphery back to the heart. In venous blood, carbon dioxide (CO_2) replaces oxygen (O_2) on the hemoglobin molecules of red blood cells for transport to the lungs where CO_2 is exhaled and O_2 is inhaled.

As with arteries that carry oxygenated blood, the venous walls are comprised of three distinct layers. However, the range of blood pressures in veins (5–10 mm Hg) is much lower than arterial pressures, and the walls of veins are thinner and more distensible than those of the arteries. The *tunica intima*, the innermost layer, consists of the endothelium (simple squamous epithelium) surrounded by a connective tissue basement membrane with elastic fibers (the internal elastic membrane). The middle layer, the *tunica media*, is primarily smooth muscle and is usually the thickest layer; the external elastic membrane surrounds it. The outer layer, the *tunica adventitia*, consists primarily of fibroblasts.

The veins have crescent-shaped bicuspid valves that are spaced at regular intervals. Valves of the venous system are one-way valves that open and rapidly close to prevent retrograde backflow of venous blood (**FIGURE 9.1**). Pulsatile contraction of skeletal muscles in the extremities pump venous blood back to the right atrium of the heart. Venous blood is then pumped into the lungs by the right ventricle where CO_2 is exchanged for O_2.

Veins are generally grouped into two categories. The superficial subcutaneous venous system transports blood from the skin and subcutaneous tissue through small caliber communicating veins into the deep veins. The deep venous system includes the iliac, femoral, popliteal, and deep femoral veins. The deep veins generally run parallel to the corresponding arteries.

▶ Venous Thromboembolism

Venous thrombosis occurs when red blood cells, fibrin, and platelets interact with specific blood proteins called coagulation (clotting) factors to form a thrombus (clot) within an intact vein. In 1856, Rudolf Virchow, the famous German pathologist, proposed a triad of factors that cause venous thrombosis: (1) hypercoagulability, (2) hemodynamic changes (stasis and turbulence), and (3) endothelial injury and/or dysfunction. *Virchow's triad* is fundamental to the pathogenesis of *venous thromboembolism* (VTE) and its two components, *deep vein thrombosis* (DVT) and *pulmonary embolism* (PE). Stasis is the predominant factor in Virchow's triad and when combined with either hypercoagulability or vessel damage, a clot usually forms (Kumar, Hanlin, Glurich, Mazza, & Yale, 2010).

Thrombosis (formation of blood clots) can occur anywhere in the venous circulation. *Superficial venous thrombosis* can occlude blood flow in the superficial veins and is associated with the development of *varicose veins* and/or *thrombophlebitis*. Varicose veins are bulging and contorted superficial veins that are visible just beneath the skin. Thrombophlebitis refers to inflammation within a blood vessel due to an occlusive thrombus.

The term *VTE* refers to the presence of *DVT* complicated by *PE*. DVT occurs in the deep veins of the legs, arms, or pelvis and may cause occlusion of these vessels. PE occurs when a deep vein thrombus breaks loose and is carried to the heart and into the lungs where it lodges to interrupt the pulmonary blood supply. PEs can be life-threatening and are responsible for significant morbidity and mortality. A simplified model of the pathogenesis of VTE is shown in **FIGURE 9.2**.

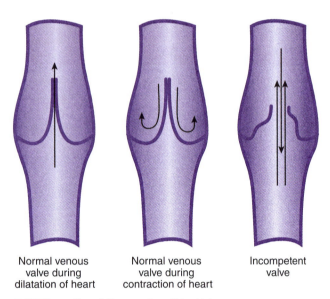

Normal venous valve during dilatation of heart

Normal venous valve during contraction of heart

Incompetent valve

FIGURE 9.1 Blood Flow in One-Way Valves.

What is Deep Vein Thrombosis (DVT)?

A blood clot (thrombus) that forms in a deep vein of the leg or pelvis either partially or totally blocking the flow of blood

What is Pulmonary Embolism (PE)?

A pulmonary embolism is caused when:

① A Deep Vein Thrombosis (blood clot). or part of it, breaks off from the vein

② The break away clot travels through the bloodstream, to the heart and migrates toward the lung

③ The clot blocks a vessel in the lung, interrupting blood supply

Deep vein clot

Break away clot

Deep vein clot

FIGURE 9.2 Venous Thromboembolism.

▶ Incidence of Venous Thromboembolism

VTE is rare in children and adolescents and predominantly manifests late in life. The age-specific annual incidence of VTE increases exponentially with age in both men and women. For example, among residents of Olmstead County, Minnesota, followed during 1966–1990, the annual age-specific VTE rate increased from less than 100 per 100,000 for individuals under 50 years of age to over 900 per 100,000 for those over the age of 80 years (Figure 9.2). Overall, the age-adjusted annual rate was higher in men than women (130 versus 110 per 100,000). Nevertheless, the rates in premenopausal women were slightly higher than men, and after age 85, the rates were similar for men and women. The similar or slightly higher rates in women under 50 years of age compared to men are related to the coagulant effects of high levels of circulating estrogens in premenopausal women (Silverstein et al., 1998) (**FIGURE 9.3**).

Individuals with an initial episode of VTE are at high risk for the development of subsequent episodes. Follow-up of patients in the Olmstead County cohort showed that approximately 30% of cases developed recurrent disease within 10 years of the first diagnosis (Heit et al., 2000).

Other studies have also observed differences in the incidence rates of VTE by age, gender, and ethnicity. Results of three large cohort studies conducted in the United States confirmed that most cases occur among the elderly (e.g., rates were threefold higher in individuals over 65 years of age compared to individuals aged 45–54 years). Overall, men have about 30% higher rates than women, and African Americans have about 40% higher rates than Caucasian Americans. The observed differences appear to be primarily attributable to higher exposure to predisposing conditions

and risk factors for VTE in certain age, gender, and ethnic groups (Cushman et al., 2004; White, Dager, Zhou, & Murin, 2006; Zakai et al., 2014).

Recent estimates of the annual age-adjusted incidence of VTE (which includes DVT and/or PE) were derived for 188 countries from the *Global Burden of Diseases Project Report* plus systematic reviews and studies reported in the literature. The age-adjusted incidence of VTE varied widely from 79 per 100,000 in Hong Kong to 269 per 100,000 in Denmark. The rates tended to be higher in developed nations due to advanced methods of imaging and early detection of thrombotic disease (Wendelboe & Raskob, 2016).

Secular trends have been observed in the incidence of VTE in populations of developed countries. In the United States, a cohort study of 5025 residents of Worcester, Massachusetts, revealed an 82% increase in the annual VTE rate during 25 years of follow-up (from 73 per 100,000 in 1985 to 133 per 100,000 in 2009). The investigators attributed part of the increase to improved diagnostic methods, especially for PE; nevertheless, they also noted that current prevention and treatment strategies are less than optimal (Huang, Goldberg, Anderson, Kiefe, & Spencer, 2014).

▶ Trends in Mortality and Case Fatality from Pulmonary Embolism

Investigators at Emory University in Atlanta, Georgia, analyzed deaths from PE reported on death certificates in the United States during 1979–1998. Among nearly 43 million decedents, 573,000 (1.3%) were attributed to PE. The age-adjusted mortality rates from PE declined by 51% during the 20-year study period, from 191 per million in 1979 to 94 per million in 1998, decreasing by 56% in men and 46% in women. Despite the overall

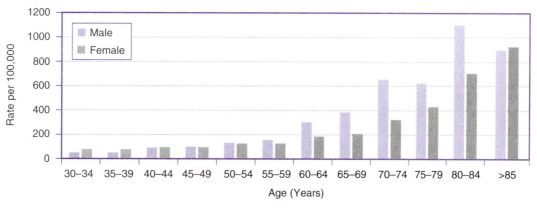

FIGURE 9.3 Annual Age-Specific Incidence of VTE.

Data from Silverstein, M. D., Heit, J. A., Mohr, D. N., Petterson, T. M., O'Fallon, W. M., & Melton, L. J. 3rd (1998). Trends in the incidence of deep vein thrombosis and pulmonary embolism: A 25-year population-based study. *Archives of Internal Medicine, 158*, 585–593.

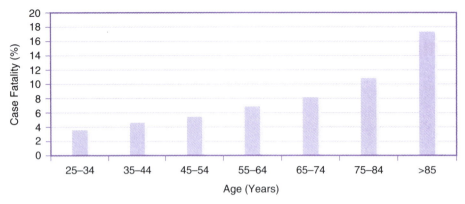

FIGURE 9.4 Age-Specific In-Hospital Case Fatality of Pulmonary Embolism.

Data from Stein, P. D., Kayali, F., & Olson, R. E. (2004). Estimated case fatality rate of pulmonary embolism, 1979 to 1998. *The American Journal of Cardiology, 93*(9), 1197–1199.

decline in mortality, men had 20%–30% higher mortality rates than women, and African Americans had 50% higher mortality rates than Caucasian Americans. The investigators attributed much of the overall reduction in mortality to prevention and reduced incidence rates (Horlander, Mannino, & Leeper, 2003).

PE has a very high case fatality rate. In the Olmstead County cohort, nearly 25% of patients who presented with PE suffered sudden death, and less than 50% of PE patients survived beyond 1 year (Heit et al., 1999).

The in-hospital case fatality rate of PE depends on whether or not patients reach the hospital alive and in stable condition. Investigators at Michigan State University conducted a long-term study of in-hospital fatality rates among PE patients during 1999–2008 using the *United States Nationwide Inpatient Sample*. This sample contains data from 5 to 8 million hospital stays from about 1000 hospitals and is designed to approximate a 20% sample of U.S. nonfederal, short-term hospitals. A total of 2.1 million hospitalized cases of PE were examined and the number of PE cases in the sample increased more than twofold during the 10-year study, from 136,740 in 1999 to 311,620 in 2008. Approximately 96.6% of PE patients were hospitalized in stable condition (not in shock and not ventilator-dependent) compared to only 3.4% in unstable condition (in shock or ventilator-dependent). Most PE patients (72%) had comorbid conditions such as myocardial infarction, heart failure, or stroke. Notably, patients who were hospitalized in stable condition had in-hospital case fatality rates that were markedly lower than patients who were hospitalized in unstable condition. The overall in-hospital case fatality for stable patients was 11% in 1999 and 6% in 2008 whereas patients who were unstable at the time of hospitalization had case fatality rates of 39% in 1999 and 36% in 2008. The 10-year reduction in case fatality for stable patients was more than fourfold

greater than for unstable patients (45% versus 10%). Among stable patients who did not receive therapy with anti-thrombolytic medication, in-hospital survival was slightly improved by inserting a *vena cava filter* designed to remove clots from venous blood (Stein, Matta, Alrifai, & Rahman, 2012).

There are also differences in the case fatality of PE by age and race. Based upon data from the U.S. National Hospital Discharge Survey for the period 1979–1998, in-hospital case fatality rates of PE are nearly five-fold higher in patients 85 years or older compared to patients under the age of 35 years (**FIGURE 9.4**). During this period, African Americans had 43% higher case fatality than Caucasian Americans, whereas the case fatality was similar for men and women of the same ethnicity (Stein, Kayali, & Olson, 2004).

Mortality and case fatality from VTE are significantly increased by comorbid conditions such as cancer. In a Canadian study using healthcare databases of the province of Québec, a total of 91,761 cases of VTE were identified and followed during 2000–2009. The overall age-sex-adjusted annual incidence of VTE was 122 per 100,000 person-years and the case fatality rate at one year was 23%. Notably, the case fatality was markedly higher (53%) for VTE patients with cancer (Tagalakis, Patenaude, Kahn, & Suissa, 2013).

▶ Risk Factors and Predisposing Conditions for Venous Thromboembolism

VTE is a multifactorial disease involving both acquired and genetic factors that predispose to thrombosis. Major predisposing events and conditions include recent hospitalization, recent surgery, immobilization, and cancer. In addition, there are specific behavioral risk factors and genetic conditions that heighten the risk. These are discussed in the following paragraphs.

Investigators at the Mayo clinic used a nested case–control approach to examine the role of exogenous hormone use and other risk factors for venous VTE among female residents of Olmsted County, Minnesota. The study included 726 cases with VTE and 930 controls matched by gender, age, and episodes of medical care. Conditions and risk factors for VTE or PE based on study results for women are listed in **TABLE 9.1**. Risk estimates were exceptionally high for when who had recent major surgery (OR = 19.0) or active cancer (OR = 14.8). Leg paresis among neurological patients, hospitalization for acute illness, nursing home confinement, and trauma or bone fracture independently increased the risk, and changes in the endocrine profile due to pregnancy, oral contraceptive use, or hormone replacement therapy were also significant risk factors among women (Barsoum et al., 2010).

Many other studies have focused on the predisposing conditions and risk factors for VTE. It is important to note that hospitalization and nursing home confinement together account for nearly 60% of primary cases of VTE, and an additional 20% of cases occur in individuals with active cancer (Heit, 2015; Heit, Spencer, & White, 2016).

▶ Exogenous Estrogens and Venous Thromboembolism

The use of oral contraceptive pills and hormone replacement therapy produces a variety of changes in the coagulation system of the blood. The most important effects are related to *increased* levels of procoagulant factors (fibrinogen and prothrombin) and *decreased* levels of anticoagulant factors (Protein S and anti-thrombin) in the clotting cascade. Since hundreds of millions of women use either oral contraceptives or postmenopausal hormone replacement, it is advisable to continue exploration for safer compounds and alternative routes of administration (e.g., transdermal application), particularly for women at high risk for VTE (Rosendaal, Van Hylckama Vlieg, Tanis, & Helmerhorst, 2003; Rosendaal et al., 2002).

▶ Genetic Predisposition to Venous Thromboembolism

Multiple genetic defects have been identified that increase the risk of thrombosis and VTE. For example, *factor V Leiden* is a mutated form of *factor V* of the clotting cascade. Approximately 5% of Caucasians are heterozygous for *factor V Leiden* (they carry one mutated gene and one normal gene). Heterozygous individuals for *factor V Leiden* have a 5–7-fold increase in the risk of VTE (DVT or PE) compared to non-carriers. Thrombotic tendencies in subjects with the *factor V Leiden* mutation are caused by the inability of *activated protein C* to effectively inactivate the clotting factor encoded by the gene (Ornstein & Cushman, 2003).

The presence of *factor V Leiden* also interacts with other risk factors to synergistically increase the risk of VTE. Premenopausal women who carry the *factor V Leiden* mutation and use oral contraceptive pills have a 35-fold increase in VTE risk compared to women of similar age with normal *factor V*. Postmenopausal women with the *factor V Leiden* mutation who use estrogen replacement therapy have a 15-fold higher risk than those without the mutation (Rosendaal et al., 2002, 2003).

Heritable effects have been observed for several antithrombin and other anticoagulant proteins that diminish the risk of thrombosis and for prothrombin and other procoagulant factors that enhance the risk. For example, a study of 22,590 Danish twin pairs

TABLE 9.1 Independent Risk Factors and Conditions for VTE or PE in Women	
Exposure	**Odds Ratio**
Major surgery	19.0
Active cancer	14.6
Leg paresis	6.1
Hospitalization for acute illness	5.1
Nursing home confinement	4.6
Trauma or fracture	4.6
Pregnancy or postpartum	4.2
Oral contraceptives	4.0
Estrogen + progestin therapy	2.5
Estrogen replacement therapy	1.8

Data from Barsoum, M. K., Heit, J. A., Ashrani, A. A., Leibson, C. L., Petterson, T. M., & Bailey, K. R. Is progestin an independent risk factor for incident venous thromboembolism? A population-based case-control study. *Thrombosis Research, 126*(5), 373–378.

revealed significant genetic susceptibility to VTE in males but not females, suggesting that sex-linked clotting disorders may enhance thrombophilia (Larsen et al., 2003). Furthermore, recent investigations suggest that inherited or acquired disorders that predispose to thrombosis (thrombophilia) interact with certain behavioral risk factors such as obesity and tobacco smoking to enhance the risk (Heit, 2015; Heit, Spencer, & White, 2016).

▶ Cardiovascular Risk Factors and Venous Thromboembolism

Investigators at the University of Insubria in Varese, Italy, conducted a meta-analysis of data from 21 case–control and cohort studies to evaluate associations between VTE and traditional risk factors for cardiovascular diseases. Results revealed increased risk estimates for obesity (OR = 2.33), hypertension (OR = 1.51), diabetes mellitus (OR = 1.42), smoking (OR = 1.18), and hypercholesterolemia (OR = 1.16). These findings suggest that exposure to multiple cardiovascular risk factors significantly increase the risk of developing VTE (Ageno, Becattini, Brighton, Selby, & Kamphuisen, 2008).

▶ Prevention of Venous Thromboembolism

VTE is preventable using strategies that inhibit the formation of blood clots. Preventive strategies should therefore target the three factors of Virchow's triad: stasis, vessel injury, and hypercoagulability.

In the community, the risk of stasis in the venous system is increased by lack of exercise and sedentary lifestyle. Regular daily aerobic exercise for 30–60 minutes is therefore essential for prevention (e.g., walking, jogging, biking, and swimming). Long periods of immobilization without exercise should be avoided. Hospitalized patients are at particularly high risk for stasis because they are immobilized and in addition may have multiple other risk factors thereby creating a "web of causation" for thrombosis. Compression stockings, intermittent pneumatic compression devices, leg elevation, and physical therapy should be used routinely, and

anti-thrombolytic prophylaxis should be considered for surgical patients, cancer patients, and patients with hypercoagulable conditions (Holten, 2004).

Vascular damage is the result of injury to the vessel wall that disrupts the endothelium. It should be noted that over half of VTE episodes are preceded by conditions that "*provoke*" blood vessel damage and thrombosis. Provoked VTE is defined as an episode of VTE preceded within 90 days by major trauma, surgery, marked immobility, or associated with active cancer or chemotherapy. Direct or indirect vessel injury may also arise from placement of a central venous catheter, vasculitis, sepsis, and/or hyperhomocysteinemia. All such medical conditions should be appropriately managed to reduce the risk for thrombosis and blood vessel damage. For example, patients with hyperhomocysteinemia require supplemental vitamins (folic acid and vitamin B12) to prevent thrombotic events (den Heijer et al., 1996).

Traumatic injuries are a significant cause of vascular damage that can provoke DVT and/or PE. Accidents do not occur randomly and most are preventable. Mechanisms of traumatic injury include motor vehicle crashes, firearms, falls (particularly by the elderly), fires, burns, drownings, and poisonings. Injury prevention strategies cover a wide variety of approaches including early education and training, enactment and enforcement of legislation and product safety regulations, engineering advances designed to reduce hazards in the environment, and economic incentives to promote healthy lifestyles, and penalties to reduce harmful behaviors (Krimston & Griffiths, 2003).

Abnormalities in platelets as well as in the coagulation and fibrinolytic pathways contribute to hypercoagulability. Individuals with familial or genetic hypercoagulable states (thrombophilia) should be identified and cautioned to avoid other risk factors. Benefits and risks of prophylaxis using antithrombotic agents should be considered on a case-by-case basis (Stevens et al., 2016).

Several traditional risk factors for cardiovascular diseases also increase the risk of developing VTE. Independent effects have been noted for obesity, hypertension, diabetes, smoking, and hypercholesterolemia, and it is therefore important to avoid smoking and maintain body mass, blood pressure, glucose, and cholesterol within normal limits. The key to prevention is a multifaceted approach in order to delimit the web of causation of thrombotic disease.

References

Ageno, W., Becattini, C., Brighton, T., Selby, R., & Kamphuisen, P. W. (2008). Cardiovascular risk factors and venous thromboembolism: A meta-analysis. *Circulation, 117*(1), 93–102.

Barsoum, M. K., Heit, J. A., Ashrani, A. A., Leibson, C. L., Petterson, T. M., & Bailey, K. R. (2010). Is progestin an independent risk factor for incident venous thromboembolism? A population-based case-control study. *Thrombosis Research, 126*(5), 373–378.

Cushman, M., Tsai, A. W., White, R. H., Heckbert, S. R., Rosamond, W. D., Enright, P., & Folsom, A. R. (2004). Deep vein thrombosis and pulmonary embolism in two cohorts: The longitudinal investigation of thromboembolism etiology. *American Journal of Medicine, 117*(1), 19–25.

den Heijer, M., Koster, T., Blom, H. J., Bos, G. M., Briet, E., Reitsma, P. H., … Rosendaal, F. R. (1996). Hyperhomocysteinemia as a risk factor for deep-vein thrombosis. *New England Journal of Medicine, 334*, 759–762.

Heit, J. A. (2015). Epidemiology of venous thromboembolism. *Nature Reviews Cardiology, 12*(8), 464–474.

Heit, J. A., Mohr, D. N., Silverstein, M. D., Petterson, T. M., O'Fallon, W. M., & Melton, L. J., 3rd. (2000). Predictors of recurrence after deep vein thrombosis and pulmonary embolism: A population-based cohort study. *Archives of Internal Medicine, 160*(6), 761–768.

Heit, J. A., Silverstein, M. D., Mohr, D. N., Petterson, T. M., O'Fallon, W. M., & Melton, L. J. 3rd. (1999). Predictors of survival after deep vein thrombosis and pulmonary embolism: A population-based, cohort study. *Archives of Internal Medicine, 159*, 445–453.

Heit, J. A., Spencer, F. A., & White, R. H. (2016). The epidemiology of venous thromboembolism. *Journal of Thrombosis and Thrombolysis, 41*, 3–14.

Holten, K. B. (2004). Preventing VTE in hospitalized patients. *Journal of Family Practice, 53*(1), 38–40.

Horlander, K. T., Mannino, D. M., & Leeper, K. V. (2003). Pulmonary embolism mortality in the United States, 1979–1998: An analysis using multiple-cause mortality data. *Archives of Internal Medicine, 163*, 1711–1717.

Huang, W., Goldberg, R. J., Anderson, F. A., Kiefe, C. I., & Spencer, F. A. (2014). Secular trends in occurrence of acute venous thromboembolism: The Worcester VTE study (1985–2009). *American Journal of Medicine, 127*(9), 829–839.

Krimston, J., & Griffiths, K. (2003). Best practices in injury prevention: The Nicholas Rosecrans Award. *Journal of Emergency Medical Services, 28*, 66–83.

Kumar, D. R., Hanlin, E., Glurich, I., Mazza, J. J., & Yale, S. H. (2010). Virchow's contribution to the understanding of thrombosis and cellular biology. *Clinical Medicine & Research, 8*(3–4), 168–172.

Larsen, T. B., Sørensen, H. T., Skytthe, A., Johnsen, S. P., Vaupel, J. W., & Christensen, K. (2003). Major genetic susceptibility for venous thromboembolism in men: A study of Danish twins. *Epidemiology, 14*(3), 328–332.

Ornstein, D. L., & Cushman, M. (2003). Factor V Leiden. *Circulation, 107*, e94–e97.

Rosendaal, F. R., Van Hylckama Vlieg, A., Tanis, B. C., & Helmerhorst, F. M. (2003). Estrogens, progestogens and thrombosis. *Journal of Thrombosis and Haemostasis, 1*, 1371–1380.

Rosendaal, F. R., Vessey, M., Rumley, A., Daly, E., Woodward, M., Helmerhorst, F. M., & Lowe, G. D. (2002). Hormonal replacement therapy, prothrombotic mutations and the risk of venous thrombosis. *British Journal of Haematology, 116*(4), 851–854.

Silverstein, M. D., Heit, J. A., Mohr, D. N., Petterson, T. M., O'Fallon, W. M., & Melton, L. J. 3rd. (1998). Trends in the incidence of deep vein thrombosis and pulmonary embolism: A 25-year population-based study. *Archives of Internal Medicine, 158*, 585–593.

Stein, P. D., Kayali, F., & Olson, R. E. (2004). Estimated case fatality rate of pulmonary embolism, 1979–1998. *The American Journal of Cardiology, 93*(9), 1197–1199.

Stein, P. D., Matta, F., Alrifai, A., & Rahman, A. (2012). Trends in case fatality rate in pulmonary embolism according to stability and treatment. *Thrombosis Research, 130*(6), 841–846.

Stevens, S. M., Woller, S. C., Bauer, K. A., Kasthuri, R., Cushman, M., Streiff, M., … Douketis, J. D. (2016). Guidance for the evaluation and treatment of hereditary and acquired thrombophilia. *Journal of Thrombosis and Thrombolysis, 41*, 154–164.

Tagalakis, V., Patenaude, V., Kahn, S. R., & Suissa, S. (2013). Incidence of and mortality from venous thromboembolism in a real-world population: The Q-VTE study cohort. *The American Journal of Medicine, 126*(9), 832–839.

Wendelboe, A. M., & Raskob, G. E. (2016). Global burden of thrombosis: Epidemiologic aspects. *Circulation Research, 118*, 1340–1347.

White, R. H., Dager, W. E., Zhou, H., & Murin, S. (2006). Racial and gender differences in the incidence of recurrent venous thromboembolism. *Thrombosis and Haemostasis, 96*(3), 267–273.

Zakai, N. A., McClure, L. A., Judd, S. E., Safford, M. M., Folsom, A. R., Lutsey, P. L., & Cushman, M. (2014). Racial and regional differences in venous thromboembolism in the United States in 3 cohorts. *Circulation, 129*, 1502–1509.

CHAPTER 10

Epidemiology of Hypertension

▶ Introduction

*C*hronic hypertension is a major force in the genesis of cardiovascular disease (CVD). *Hypertensive heart disease* refers to cardiac pathologies that are specifically caused by chronic hypertension, primarily left ventricular hypertrophy and heart failure. Hypertensive heart disease *per se* causes nearly 1 million deaths annually in the world population.

Chronic hypertension is also a significant independent risk factor for nearly all other forms of CVD including ischemic heart disease, myocardial infarction, congestive heart failure, cardiac arrhythmias such as atrial fibrillation, stroke, peripheral artery disease, aortic aneurysm, rupture and dissection, venous thromboembolism, pulmonary embolism, and sudden cardiac death. Furthermore, chronic hypertension synergistically interacts with other CVD risk factors such as smoking, diabetes, hypercholesterolemia, obesity, and chronic inflammation. CVDs that involve chronic hypertension cause more than 17 million deaths annually in the world population (Roth et al., 2017).

▶ Clinical Definition of Hypertension

The following statement from collaborating investigators at the U.S. National Center for Health Statistics, the Centers for Disease Control, Johns Hopkins University, the National Heart, Lung and Blood Institute, and the University of Texas at Houston summarizes important points regarding hypertension (Burt et al., 1995):

> High blood pressure is one of the most important modifiable risk factors for CVD. It is an extremely common finding in the community and a risk factor for myocardial infarction, stroke, congestive heart failure, end-stage renal disease, and peripheral vascular disease. Pharmacological treatment of hypertension has been shown to decrease the risk of CVD complications, including stroke, coronary heart disease, and renal insufficiency. Nonpharmacological intervention provides an effective means to lower blood pressure and has been emphasized increasingly as a useful method for both prevention and treatment of high blood pressure.

The diagnosis of hypertension is made when an individual's blood pressure is chronically elevated above certain threshold levels. Two blood-pressure measurements, systolic and diastolic, are routinely taken during a physical examination. Systolic blood pressure is the arterial pressure (at the level of the brachial artery in the upper arm) during contraction of the heart whereas diastolic blood pressure is the arterial pressure between contractions when the heart is at rest.

For decades, hypertension had been defined as systolic blood pressure equal to or greater than 140 mm Hg or diastolic blood pressure equal to or greater than 90 mm Hg. Nevertheless, there was considerable controversy regarding optimal blood pressure since some studies reported risk increases of certain cardiovascular conditions (e.g., stroke, myocardial infarction, congestive heart failure, arterial aneurysm, and renal failure) at lower levels than 140/90 mm Hg. In 2003, a consensus statement from the *Seventh Report of the Joint National Committee on Prevention, Detection, Evaluation, and Treatment of High Blood Pressure* defined a suboptimal "prehypertensive" category for individuals with systolic levels between 130 and 139 mm Hg or diastolic levels between 80 and 89 mm Hg (Chobanian et al., 2003).

Then on November 13, 2017, a major change in the guidelines defining hypertension was recommended by an expert panel of 21 scientists representing the American College of Cardiology (ACC), the American Heart Association (AHA), and nine other health professional organizations. The major change was lowering the threshold for the diagnosis of hypertension to create two stages of hypertension and eliminating the "prehypertensive" category. According to these new guidelines, Stage 1 hypertension is now defined as systolic blood pressure between 130 and 139 mm Hg or diastolic blood pressure between 80 and 89 mm Hg, and Stage 2 hypertension is defined as systolic blood pressure equal to or greater than 140 mm Hg or diastolic blood pressure equal to or greater than 90 mm Hg. The new guidelines also categorize individuals with systolic pressure between 120 and 129 and diastolic pressure less than 80 mm Hg as having "elevated" blood pressure (Whelton et al., 2017) (**TABLE 10.1**).

Analysis of data from the *National Health and Nutrition Survey* (NHANES) collected during 2011–2014 suggests that application of the new guidelines increases the crude prevalence of hypertension among U.S. adults to 45.6% compared to 31.9% by the old guidelines. According to the authors of this investigation, "the 2017 ACC/AHA hypertension guideline has the potential to increase hypertension awareness, encourage lifestyle modification and focus antihypertensive medication initiation and intensification on U.S. adults with high CVD risk" (Muntner et al., 2017).

The major evidence in support of the change in guidelines for the diagnosis of hypertension came from the *Systolic Blood Pressure Intervention Trial* (SPRINT) conducted in the United States with support from the National Institutes of Health (NIH). In the trial, 9361 adults aged 50 years or older who had systolic blood pressure of 130 mm Hg or higher, were not diabetic, and had elevated 10-year cardiovascular risk (15% or higher based on the Framingham risk index) were randomized into two "target" groups for the reduction of blood pressure. One group (*n* = 4678) received intensive antihypertensive treatment designed to reduce blood pressure below 120 mm Hg whereas the other group (*n* = 4683) received standard therapy designed to maintain blood pressure below 140 mm Hg. Patients enrolled in the study were ascertained from more than 100 clinic sites in the United States. Results after a median follow-up of 3.3 years indicated that intensive therapy designed to lower blood pressure to less than 120 mm Hg reduced cardiovascular events by 25% and reduced the overall risk of death by 27% compared to standard therapy to maintain blood pressure below 140 mm Hg (SPRINT Research Group, 2015).

It is noteworthy that not all health organizations have endorsed these new guidelines. For example, the *American Academy of Family Physicians (AAFP)* did not endorse the new guidelines because of the lack of systematic review of the total body of evidence and failure to address potential harms of treatment-related side effects. For example, patients in SPRINT who received more intensive therapy to lower blood pressure had more serious adverse events (hypotension, syncope, acute kidney injury, or renal failure) than patients who received standard care (AAFP, 2017).

Another issue is assuming the results of clinical trials will be valid in the community. With respect to studies of blood pressure, one must consider whether the condition of patients at the time that blood pressure is measured in a clinical trial is the same as patients measured during a standard visit to a family physician. In clinical trials such as SPRINT, multiple blood pressures are typically taken in patients who are in a non-stressful environment, whereas during a physical examination by a clinician, a quick blood-pressure measurement may be temporarily elevated because the patient is nervous and anxious, a condition known as "white coat or transient hypertension" (Helvaci &

TABLE 10.1 New Classification of Blood Pressure		
Classification	**Systolic Pressure (mm Hg)**	**Diastolic Pressure (mm Hg)**
Normal	<120	<80
Elevated	120–129	<80
Hypertensive (Stage 1)	130–139	80–89
Hypertensive (Stage 2)	≥140	≥90

Data from Whelton, P. K., Carey, R. M., Aronow, W. S., Casey, D. E., Jr, Collins, K. J., Dennison Himmelfarb, C., ... Wright, J. T., Jr. (2017). Guideline for the prevention, detection, evaluation, and management of high blood pressure in adults: Executive summary: A report of the American College of Cardiology/American Heart Association Task Force on Clinical Practice Guidelines. *Hypertension, 71*(6), 1269–1364.

Seyhanli, 2006; Ruxer, Mozdzan, Baranski, Wozniak-Sosnowska, & Markuszewski, 2007).

▶ Global Epidemiology of Hypertension

Epidemiologic studies discussed in this chapter are based on the long-standing definition of hypertension as systolic blood pressure ≥ 140 mm Hg or diastolic blood pressure ≥ 90 mm Hg. This corresponds to "Stage 2 hypertension" according to the new guidelines proposed in 2017 by the American Heart Association and the American College of Cardiology (Table 10.1).

A team of investigators at Tulane University School of Public Health and Tropical Medicine, United States, and the University of Oxford, United Kingdom conducted a comprehensive analysis of worldwide data to assess the global burden of hypertension. They estimated that approximately one-quarter of the world's adult population (more than 1 billion people) manifested hypertension at the turn of the 21st century, and if current trends continue, the prevalence is projected to increase to about 29% (more than 2 billion people) by 2025 (Kearney et al., 2005).

These estimates were based upon a comprehensive analysis of available data on blood pressure from 18 national, 3 multisite, and 9 regional studies. Countries and regions represented in the study included Korea (Kim, Jones, Kim, & Hong, 1994), Taiwan (InterASIA Collaborative Group, 2003; Pan, Chang, Yeh, Hsiao, & Hung, 2001), South Africa (Steyn, Gaziano, Bradshaw, Laubscher, & Fourie, 2001), Cameroon (Mbanya, Minkoulou, Salah, & Balkau, 1998), West Africa (Cooper et al., 1997), Tanzania (Edwards et al., 2000), Zimbabwe (Mufunda et al., 2000), China (Gu et al., 2002), Turkey (Sonmez et al., 1999), Egypt (Ibrahim et al., 1995), Venezuela (Sulbaran, Silva, Calmon, & Vegas, 2000), Paraguay (Ramirez, Pino, Furiasse, Lee, & Fowkes, 1995), Mexico (Arroyo et al., 1999), India (Gupta, Guptha, Gupta, & Prakash, 1995; Gupta & Sharma, 1994; Malhotra, Kumari, Kumar, Jain, & Sharma, 1999; Singh et al., 1997a, 1997b), United States (Burt et al., 1995; Wolz et al., 2000), Canada (Joffres et al., 1997), Spain (Banegas et al., 1998), England (Primatesta, Brookes, & Poulter, 2001), Germany (Thamm, 1999), Greece (Stergiou, Thomopoulou, Skeva, & Mountokalakis, 1999), Italy (Giampaoli et al., 2001), Scandinavian countries near the Baltic Sea (Stegmayr et al., 1996), Australia (Bennett & Magnus, 1994), Japan (Baba et al., 1991), and Slovakia (Riecansky & Egnerova, 1991).

Based upon the pooled data from all these studies, 26.4% of the world's adult population (over the age of 20 years) manifested hypertension (26.6% of men and 26.1% of women). Approximately one-third of hypertensive cases were detected in economically developed countries and the remaining two-thirds in developing countries. Relatively high prevalence levels (exceeding 30%) were observed for men and women combined in Western European and Scandinavian nations (Germany, Italy, Spain, and Sweden), Japan, former socialistic economies (Russia), and nations in Latin America and the Caribbean (Mexico, Paraguay, and Venezuela); moderate levels (between 20% and 30%) were observed in North America (United States and Canada), the Middle East (Egypt and Turkey), sub-Saharan Africa, India, Australia, and China; and low levels (less than 20%) were observed in nations of Southeast Asia (Taiwan, Korea, and Thailand). Populations of urban areas tended to have higher levels than rural areas (e.g., the prevalence of hypertension in rural areas of western India was significantly less than in urban areas [31% versus 22%]). Less-developed nations had a lower overall prevalence of hypertension than economically developed nations (22.9% versus 37.3%). Nevertheless, the authors point out that rates of hypertension are increasing more rapidly in populations of developing nations; and since these populations are larger, the burden of hypertension and related cardiovascular and renal diseases is projected to increase worldwide over the next decade (Kearney et al., 2005).

Though the cumulative prevalence of hypertension was similar for men and women, gender differences were noted in the age-specific prevalence patterns of hypertension (Kearney et al., 2005). As shown in **FIGURE 10.1**, men had the higher prevalence until age 50, after which the prevalence for women was greater. Potential reasons for the age differential in the prevalence of hypertension between men and women include (1) a protective effect of endogenous estrogens in women during the premenopausal years and (2) the effect of increased longevity and survivorship among women in the later decades of life.

▶ Hypertensive Heart Disease

Hypertensive Heart Disease refers to pathological conditions of the heart that are specifically caused by chronically elevated blood pressure. The most prominent of these conditions are left ventricular hypertrophy and heart failure. According to the latest *International Classification of Diseases* (ICD-10), hypertensive heart disease has two subcategories, hypertensive heart disease with or without heart failure, which are distinguishable from ischemic heart disease and other forms of heart disease.

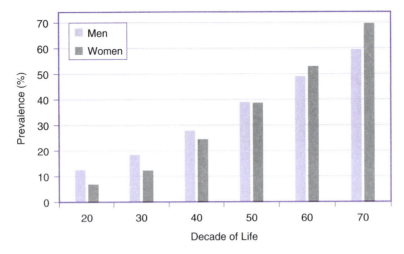

FIGURE 10.1 Age-Specific Prevalence of Hypertension.

Data from Kearney, P. M., Whelton, M., Reynolds, K., Muntner, P., Whelton, P. K., & He, J. (2005). Global burden of hypertension: Analysis of worldwide data. *Lancet 365*(9455), 217–223.

The *Global Burden of Disease 2015* study is a multinational research project designed to estimate incidence, prevalence, and mortality of major diseases for the years 1980–2015 using population-based data from 195 countries. In the study, hypertensive heart disease was defined as symptomatic heart failure due to the direct and long-term effects of hypertension. During 2015, 962,400 deaths were attributed to hypertensive heart disease, a marked increase from the 630,000 deaths reported by the World Health Organization in 1990. Currently, more than 6 million people suffer from hypertensive heart disease in the world population, and the prevalence is highest (about 1.36%) for individuals over 80 years of age (Roth et al., 2017; Wang & Naghavi, 2016).

It is noteworthy that a recent proposal adds ischemia and atrial fibrillation to the profile of conditions that may be classified as hypertensive heart disease. Obviously, adjudication of the exact cause of death is complex and the assigned cause listed on the death certificate may be inaccurate. Furthermore, since high blood pressure is a risk factor for atherosclerosis and multiple other forms of CVD, death rates from hypertensive heart disease provide an incomplete measure of the burden of disease due to high blood pressure (Alegría-Ezquerra, González-Juanatey, & González-Maqueda, 2006).

Atherosclerosis, Hypertension, and Cardiovascular Disease

Atherosclerosis refers to the deposition of lipid-laden atheromatous plaque in arterial walls. As the process progresses over time, arteries become rigid, narrowed, and occluded. Atheromatous plaques may also

rupture producing occlusive thromboembolisms of coronary and/or cerebral arteries resulting in myocardial infarctions and/or strokes.

Atherosclerosis is the major process in the development of ischemic heart disease, the leading cause of death worldwide. Multiple cofactors interact in the process of atherosclerosis including dyslipidemia, glucose intolerance, and hypertension. Epidemiologic investigations and clinical trials provide clear evidence that chronic hypertension is a significant independent risk factor for atherosclerosis, ischemic heart disease, and other forms of CVD, and that reductions in blood pressure decrease the risk of these conditions (Blacher, Levy, Mourad, Safar, & Bakris, 2016; Franklin & Wong, 2013; Kannel, 1995; Law, Morris, & Wald, 2009).

Elevated blood pressure can induce shear-related injury to the endothelial lining of blood vessels and increase oxidative stress and levels of reactive oxygen species (ROS) in the arterial wall. Hypertension-induced endothelial injury, oxidative stress, inflammation, and vascular cell proliferation amplify the atherosclerotic process (Dzau, 1990; Harrison & Gongora, 2009; Touyz & Briones, 2011).

Ecological Patterns of Hypertension

Marked differences have been observed in the prevalence rates of hypertension among populations, even those of highly developed nations. For example, surveys of European populations consistently show higher levels than in North-American populations, a finding based upon combined analysis of national cross-sectional surveys conducted in the 1990s in Germany, Finland, Sweden, England, Spain, Italy, Canada, and

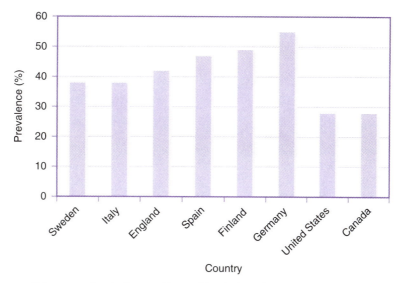

FIGURE 10.2 The Prevalence of Hypertension in Europe Versus North America.

Data from National surveys conducted during the 1990s. Data from Wolf-Maier, K., Cooper, R. S., Banegas, J. R., Giampaoli, S., Hense, H., Joffres, M., ... Vescio, F. (2003). Hypertension and blood pressure levels in 6 European countries, Canada, and the US. *JAMA, 289*, 2363–2369.

the United States (Wolf-Maier et al., 2003). As shown in **FIGURE 10.2**, the prevalence of hypertension in the European populations sampled ranged 38%–55% compared to 28% in the United States and Canada.

In a subsequent study designed to examine the impact of treatment strategies in European versus North-American populations, 66% and 49% of individuals previously diagnosed with severe hypertension (defined as blood pressure > 160/95 mm Hg) in the United States and Canada, respectively, had controlled blood-pressure levels (within normal limits) compared to only 23%–38% of individuals in European populations (Wolf-Maier et al., 2004). The investigators emphasize the need for improved pharmacologic management of high blood pressure to reduce the risk of cardiovascular and renal diseases.

National prevalence rates of hypertension have been found to be highly correlated with mortality and incidence rates of CVDs, particularly stroke. In the World Health Organization MONICA Project, blood pressure prevalence estimates for population samples from around the Baltic Sea showed positive correlations with the incidence rates of stroke in men ($r = 0.87$) and women ($r = 0.70$) (Stegmayr et al., 1996); and subsequently, positive correlations were also observed ($r = 0.42$ for men and $r = 0.56$ for women) in an analysis of 18 MONICA population samples from diverse geographic regions (Stegmayr et al., 1997). These results prompted further analysis of data on 16 population samples from MONICA that demonstrated a negative correlation between the frequency of effective control of blood pressure in individuals with hypertension and the incidence of stroke (Banegas & Pérez-Regadera, 1998). Hypertension and stroke were also positively correlated ($r = 0.78$) in the international

comparison study of North-American and European nations (Wolf-Maier et al., 2004).

▸ Hypertension in the United States Stroke Belt

The Stroke Belt in the United States is comprised of 11 states including Alabama, Arkansas, Georgia, Indiana, Kentucky, Louisiana, Mississippi, North Carolina, South Carolina, Tennessee, and Virginia. In 1980, these 11 states had age-adjusted stroke-mortality rates more than 10% above the national average (National Heart, Lung and Blood Institute, 1996). As shown in **FIGURE 10.3**, 10 of these states are represented in the cluster of states in the southeastern United States with the highest prevalence rates of hypertension (Nwankwo et al., 2011). Obviously, there is significant overlap in the distributions of hypertension and stroke.

▸ Ethnicity and Hypertension in the United States

An interdisciplinary team of U.S. investigators studied hypertension by gender and ethnicity in a cross-sectional survey of 9901 adults in the third U.S. National Health and Nutrition Examination Survey, 1988–1994, NHANES III (Burt et al., 1995). The study included in-home and clinic examinations for the measurement of blood pressure. Based on this survey, 24% of the U.S. adult population was found to be hypertensive (24.7% of men and 23.4% of women). However, there were large differences in

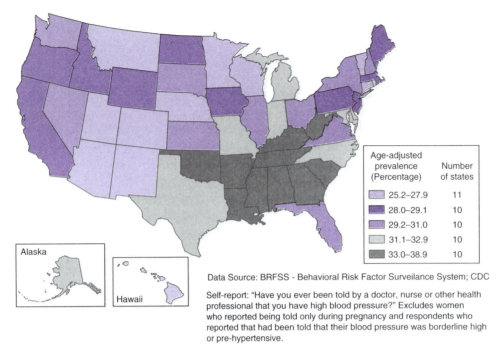

FIGURE 10.3 Hypertension and the Stroke Belt in the United States, 2011.

Reproduced from Nwankwo, T., Yoon, S. S., Burt, V., & Gu, Q. (2013). *Hypertension among adults in the US: National Health and Nutrition Examination Survey, 2011–2012* (NCHS Data Brief, No. 133). Hyattsville, MD: National Center for Health Statistics, Centers for Disease Control and Prevention, U.S. Deptartment of Health and Human Services.

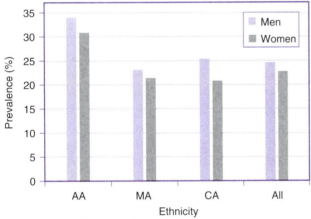

AA = African Americans
MA = Mexican Americans
CA = Caucasian Americans
Estimates are age-adjusted to the 1990 U.S. population

FIGURE 10.4 Prevalence of Hypertension by Ethnicity in the United States: NHANES II Data, 1988–1991.

Data from Burt, V. L., Whelton, P., Roccella, E. J., Brown, C., Cutler, J. A., Higgins, M., ... Labarthe, D. (1995). Prevalence of hypertension in the US adult population. Results from the Third National Health and Nutrition Examination survey, 1988–91. *Hypertension 25*, 305–313.

the age-adjusted prevalence estimates by ethnicity (**FIGURE 10.4**). African Americans had markedly higher levels (32.4%) than Caucasian Americans (23.3%) and Mexican Americans (22.6%).

Various reasons have been proposed to explain the higher predisposition of African Americans to the development of hypertension. Racial differences may be due, at least in part, to genetic differences in the regulation of dietary sodium by the kidneys. Furthermore, *Endothelin*-1, a powerful local vasoconstrictor, appears to be secreted at higher levels in the blood vessels of African Americans compared to other ethnic groups (see the section of this chapter on genetics and hypertension for discussion of these mechanisms).

As shown in Figure 10.4, the age-adjusted prevalence estimates from NHANES III were slightly higher for men than women of each ethnic group, although differences were small. As noted above, women appear to have some protection against the development of hypertension and related vascular conditions during their premenopausal years, which may account for the small differences in the age-adjusted estimates.

Overall, 69% of hypertensive individuals in NHANES III were aware of their condition prior to measurement and 53% were taking an antihypertensive agent. Nevertheless, only 35% of Mexican Americans with high blood pressure were receiving treatment and 25% or less of treated individuals were achieving adequate control of their blood pressure, irrespective of ethnicity.

▶ Time Trends of Hypertension in the United States

A subsequent analysis of NHANES data compared blood-pressure data for samples of U.S. adults aged 18 years or older ascertained during 1988–1994 ($n = 16{,}351$) and approximately 10 years later during

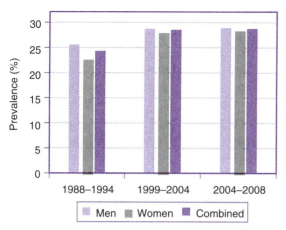

Estimates are age-adjusted to the 2000 U.S. population

FIGURE 10.5 Trends in the Prevalence of Hypertension in the United States, NHANES, 1988–2008.

Data from National Health and Nutrition Survey. Cutler, J. A., Sorlie, P. D., Wolz, M., Thom, T., Fields, L. E., & Roccella, E. J. (2008). Trends in the hypertension prevalence, awareness, treatment, and control rates in United States adults between 1988–1994 and 1999–2004. *Hypertension 52*(5), 818–827; Egan, B. M., Zhao, Y., & Axon, R. N. (2010). US trends in prevalence, awareness, treatment, and control of hypertension, 1988–2008. *JAMA, 303*(20), 2043–2050.

1999–2004 (n = 14,430). Analysis and evaluation of these data focused on changes in blood pressure during the interim and the potential factors responsible (Cutler et al., 2008).

As shown in **FIGURE 10.5**, the age-standardized prevalence of hypertension increased from 24.4% to 28.9% among the U.S. adult population during 1988–1994 to 1999–2004, an increase of 4.5% in the 10-year period. Perhaps surprisingly, a larger increase was observed in women (5.6%) than men (3.2%), and the final prevalence estimates for men and women sampled during 1999–2004 were similar (28.8% for men and 28.5% for women). In regression models, increases in body mass and obesity accounted for a significant fraction of the increase in hypertension, particularly among men. In women, age was the most important factor, presumably because of their greater longevity and the development of hypertension relatively late in life. While individuals of all ethnic groups demonstrated improved awareness, treatment, and control of their blood pressure, nearly 40% of hypertensive individuals were unaware of their condition at the time of measurement and 65% of hypertensive individuals did not achieve adequate blood-pressure control with treatment. The authors point out that these trends are expected to translate into higher rates of cardiovascular and renal diseases in certain U.S. subpopulations (Cutler et al., 2008; Egan, Zhao, & Axon, 2010).

Investigators in the United States are continuing to examine the NHANES databases to assess progress in treating and controlling hypertension. Analysis of blood-pressure data for cross-sectional samples of U.S. adults obtained for successive 2-year intervals during 1999–2016 reveals that the overall prevalence

of hypertension has stabilized at approximately 29%. The proportion of hypertensive patients who were treated and had controlled blood pressure increased to 50.1% during 2004–2008 but then declined slightly to 48.6% in the most recent survey during 2015–2016 (Egan et al., 2010; Fryar, Ostchega, Hales, Zhang, & Kruszon-Moran, 2017).

Time Trends of Hypertension in India

India provides an interesting contrast to developed nations as a model for longitudinal studies of hypertension in a large developing nation with both rural and urban populations. The prevalence rates of severe hypertension (>160/95 mm Hg) have trended upwards in both urban and rural populations of India since the middle of the 20th century, but the levels remained relatively low: less than 15% in urban populations and less than 5% in rural populations (Gupta, 1999; Gupta, AI-Odat, & Gupta, 1996; Gupta & Sharma, 1994; Gupta et al., 1995).

Albeit, surveys of hypertension defined by revised criteria (>140/90 mm Hg) for the period 1995–2002 reflect markedly higher prevalence rates, particularly for urban populations. Pooling of epidemiologic studies shows that hypertension is present in about 25% of urban subjects and 10% of rural subjects in India. Furthermore, prevalence rates exceeding 40% have been observed for both men and women in certain urban populations (Gupta, 2004). The accelerating rates of hypertension and related conditions in India are representative of other developing nations around the globe.

Physiological Control of Blood Pressure

Blood-pressure regulation in the human body is complex and dependent upon multiple factors including cardiac output, total blood volume, blood viscosity, and resistance of blood vessels (arteries) to blood flow. Blood pressure can be numerically expressed as *Blood Pressure = Cardiac Output √Peripheral Resistance.* Consequently, assessment of blood pressure is essential in determining the viability of heart function and the integrity of blood vessels.

Multiple physiological, cellular, and molecular processes are important for maintaining normal blood pressure. In particular, normal kidney function is vital for blood-pressure control and patients with renal disease often develop hypertension due to hyperactivity of the *renin–angiotensin system*. The central nervous system can elicit rapid changes in blood pressure by stimulating the release of epinephrine (adrenaline), a powerful vasoconstrictor, from the adrenal glands in the "*fight or flight*" response to stress or a perceived environmental threat. The autonomic nervous system can also elicit minute to minute changes in blood pressure in response to environmental stimuli through the *baroreceptor reflex* described below. Furthermore, locally acting agents with vasoconstricting or vasodilating effects are important for the maintenance of vascular tone. Regulatory mechanisms of arterial blood pressure are broadly subdivided into *short-term* and *long-term* regulation.

The central nervous system responds rapidly to environmental stimuli by activation of the "*fight or flight*" response. Firing of adrenergic nerve cells and release of epinephrine (adrenaline) into the bloodstream by the adrenal glands immediately increases the heart rate, contracts blood vessels, dilates air passages, and intensifies awareness.

The autonomic nervous system helps regulate *short-term* changes in blood pressure through the *baroreceptor reflex*. The baroreceptor reflex refers to immediate changes in arterial blood pressure in response to signals sent from baroreceptors located in the carotid arteries and the arch of the aorta to the medulla of the brain stem. Stimulus of the heart, arteries, and veins by nerve impulses from the medulla adjust arterial blood pressure by altering the speed and force of contractions of the heart and modulating the resistance of peripheral blood vessels to blood flow by vasoconstriction or vasodilatation.

The *renin–angiotensin system* is primarily responsible for the *long-term* regulation of blood pressure and blood volume. Classically, juxtaglomerular cells in the *kidney* monitor the dynamics of blood flow and in response to low blood pressure and flow secrete the enzyme renin, which in turn cleaves the peptide angiotensinogen converting it into angiotensin I, which is inactive. Angiotensin I is converted to angiotensin II in the *lungs* by angiotensin-converting enzyme (ACE). Angiotensin II is a powerful vasoconstrictor throughout the body and is the main effector molecule of the renin–angiotensin system (Paul, Poyan Mehr, & Kreutz, 2006).

In response to elevated levels of angiotensin II (or potassium) in the blood, the adrenal cortex secretes a steroidal hormone called aldosterone. Aldosterone stimulates retention of sodium and excretion of potassium by the kidney, thereby increasing blood volume and arterial blood pressure.

Aldosterone acts on the distal convoluted tubule and the cortical collecting duct in the kidneys, causing them to reabsorb more sodium and water from the urine in exchange for potassium. Aldosterone also acts on the central nervous system to increase thirst and appetite for salt.

Maintenance of vascular tone is also dependent upon vasoconstrictive and vasodilator substances that are locally secreted by the endothelial cells that line blood vessels. Endothelin-1 is a polypeptide with potent vasoconstrictive activity (Yanagisawa, Kurihara, & Kimura, 1988). This protein rapidly elicits smooth muscle cell contraction and infusion of endothelin-1 in humans increases blood pressure and total peripheral resistance of blood vessels (Haynes, Hand, Johnstone, Padfield, & Webb, 1994).

Nitric oxide is a potent vasodilator that is continuously secreted by endothelial cells of the arterial lining in response to changes in blood pressure and blood flow disturbances. Nitric oxide plays an important role in maintaining normal blood pressure and adequate blood flow and its homeostatic effects are diminished in hypertensive persons. Nitric oxide also inhibits platelet adhesion and aggregation and suppresses migration and proliferation of vascular smooth muscle cells.

▶ Essential Hypertension

Hypertension is divided into two subtypes: *Essential hypertension* and *secondary hypertension*. Most individuals (about 95%) have *essential hypertension*, which means that no specific cause has been identified. Individuals with *secondary hypertension* have a specific underlying cause that has elevated their blood pressure (see discussion of this subtype in the following section).

Essential hypertension develops due to the interaction of multiple factors in a *web of causation*. While exact causes are difficult to establish in the majority of individual patients, the evidence confirming the multifactorial nature of essential hypertension is overwhelming. Two major risk factors stand out: obesity and chronic alcohol abuse. Nevertheless, many other factors undoubtedly contribute to the pathogenesis of essential hypertension including tobacco addiction, excess dietary sodium (salt), low dietary potassium, vitamin D deficiency, excess of certain dietary fats, sedentary lifestyle, psychological factors (stress or depression), and genetic predisposition. Each of these risk factors is discussed in a following section of this chapter.

▶ Secondary Hypertension

Hypertension that develops from a known cause (often a hormonal disorder) is called *secondary hypertension*. Secondary hypertension accounts for only about 5% of all cases of hypertension. Various hormonal disorders are known to cause secondary hypertension (Robbins & Cotran, 1979). Selected disorders are described in the following paragraphs.

Cushing's syndrome is caused by excess circulating cortisol due to either long-term administration of synthetic forms of cortisol (such as prednisone or dexamethasone) or oversecretion of cortisol by the adrenal glands as a result of pituitary-hypothalamic dysfunction. Cortisol has properties like aldosterone and therefore causes sodium retention and increased blood volume leading to hypertension (Whitworth, Brown, Kelly, & Williamson, 1995). The syndrome is also characterized by a variety of other phenotypic abnormalities including truncal obesity, moon facies, diabetes mellitus, osteoporosis, polycythemia, skin striae, and immunosuppression.

Hyperthyroidism often produces an increase in the *systolic blood pressure* by promoting vasoconstriction and accelerating the heart rate and the force of heart contractions. These effects are due to unbridled secretion of thyroid hormones by the thyroid gland that stimulate specific receptors present in the myocardium and vasculature (Brent, 1994). Conversely, *hypothyroidism* occasionally produces an increase in the *diastolic blood pressure*, possibly due to increased resistance in peripheral blood vessels.

Conn's syndrome is due to hypersecretion of aldosterone by the adrenal glands (often by an adrenal adenoma). Elevated aldosterone causes hypertension through effects on the kidney including sodium retention, potassium wasting, and increased blood volume. In Conn's syndrome, there is *decreased* secretion of renin by the kidneys.

Acromegaly (gigantism) is due to excess circulating growth hormone often due to a pituitary adenoma. The association with hypertension is manifest in about 50% of individuals with acromegaly. Growth hormone has been found to have mineralocorticoid activity and excess levels lead to retention of sodium and increased blood volume.

Pheochromocytomas are rare neuroendocrine tumors that usually arise in the adrenal glands. Their overproduction of catecholamines (adrenaline) stimulates the heart and cardiovascular system resulting in severe hypertension in patients with these tumors.

▶ Hypertension of Pregnancy (Preeclampsia)

Hypertension in pregnant women is known as preeclampsia. If untreated, preeclampsia can progress to a life-threatening condition called eclampsia, which is the development of protein in the urine, generalized swelling (edema), and seizures. Preeclampsia occurs in up to 10% of first pregnancies, usually in the third trimester after the 32nd week. Some women develop preeclampsia as early as 20 weeks, although this is rare. The condition is much more common in women who are pregnant for the first time and its frequency drops significantly in second pregnancies. Preeclampsia can also occur up to 6 weeks postpartum (Robbins & Cotran, 1979).

The cause of preeclampsia remains elusive and most likely involves the interaction of multiple variables. Placental ischemia (lack of oxygen) appears to be a common feature. One proposed scenario is that preeclampsia arises from rejection of the placenta by the maternal immune system which in turn leads to compromised placental perfusion and the release of inflammatory, vasoconstrictive, and prothrombotic prostaglandins (Moffett & Hiby, 2007). Glomerular filtration is reduced in the kidneys and there is marked retention of salt and water accompanied by increased irritability of the central nervous system. Vitamin deficiencies, obesity, and gestational diabetes have also been observed in association with preeclampsia (Ilekis, Reddy, & Roberts, 2006).

▶ Risk Factors for Essential Hypertension

Epidemiologic investigations conducted over the past half century have identified and quantified several major risk factors for cardiovascular conditions including hypertension. International collaborations have made many of these studies possible. Pertinent findings from selected studies are presented in the following paragraphs.

Obesity and Hypertension

In the INTERSALT study, the relationship between body mass index, BMI = ht (kg)/wt^2(m), and blood pressure was studied in 10,079 men and women, aged 20–59 years of age, sampled from 52 centers around the world. The BMI was significantly associated with both systolic and diastolic blood pressure, independent of age, alcohol intake, smoking, and sodium and potassium urinary excretion. Based upon regression analysis, each 10 kg increase in body weight increased systolic and diastolic blood pressure by 3 and 2.2 mm Hg, respectively (Dyer & Elliott, 1989). The investigators of INTERSALT estimate that about 30% of cases of hypertension are attributable to obesity (defined as BMI of at least 30 kg/m²) and the attributable risk may be as high as 60% in younger individuals under 45 years of age (Dyer, Elliott, & Shipley, 1990).

Many other epidemiologic studies have revealed a strong graded relationship between obesity and hypertension. Data from the NHANES show the striking linear relationship between BMI and rising blood pressure in the American adult population (Aneja, El-Atat, McFarlane, & Sowers, 2004) (**FIGURE 10.6**). In regression models corrected for age, a BMI gain of 1.7 kg/m² in men or 1.25 kg/m² in women corresponds to an increase in systolic blood pressure of 1 mm Hg (Kissebah & Krakower, 1994).

The Nurses' Health Study involving 82,473 women revealed that a 5-kg weight gain after age 18 was associated with a 60% higher relative risk of developing hypertension (Huang et al., 1998) compared to those women who gained 2 kg or less. Those who gained 25 kg or more increased their risk more than fivefold. Similar increases in blood pressure and the development of hypertension with increasing body mass have been observed in other populations (Wilsgaard, Schirmer, & Arnesen, 2000) as well as in children (He, Ding, Fong, & Karlberg, 2000). In the Framingham cohort, obesity

independently accounted for 78% and 65% of essential hypertension in men and women, respectively (Kannel, Garrison, & Dannenberg, 1993).

Nonpharmacologic reduction in weight has been found to reduce blood pressure. In a meta-analysis of 25 randomized controlled trials published between 1966 and 2002 with a total of 4874 participants, a net weight reduction of 5.1 kg through energy restriction, increased physical activity, or both, reduced systolic blood pressure by 4.4 mm Hg and diastolic blood pressure by 3.6 mm Hg. Greater blood-pressure reductions were observed in subjects who lost more weight. These results provide clear evidence that dietary modification and exercise are effective in reducing both weight and blood pressure (Neter, Stam, Kok, Grobbee, & Geleijnse, 2003).

Various weight reduction medications are now on the market and some have been evaluated in randomized placebo-controlled clinical trials. An international team of investigators recently examined effects of three agents in a meta-analysis. Thirty trials of 1–4 years, duration met the inclusion criteria: 10 evaluated *orlistat* (*n* = 10,631 participants), 10 evaluated *sibutramine* (*n* = 2623 participants), and 4 evaluated *rimonabant* (*n* = 6365 participants). Compared to placebo, significant average weight reductions were observed for each medication: 2.9 kg for orlistat, 4.2 kg for sibutramine, and 4.7 kg for rimonabant. Notably, orlistat and rimonabant also significantly *reduced* blood pressure whereas sibutramine actually *increased* blood pressure. An excess of other adverse events (e.g., gastrointestinal distress and mood disorders) was observed with treatment possibly diminishing the value of these medications (Rucker, Padwal, Li, Cuioni, & Lau, 2007).

The following statement excerpted from a review by Aneja and colleagues (2004) provides a lucid synopsis of the pathogenic link between obesity and hypertension.

> *It is becoming clear that the adipocyte is not merely an inert organ for storage of energy but that it also secretes a host of factors that interact with each other and may result in elevated blood pressure. Of particular importance is the putative role of leptin in the causation of hypertension via an activation of the sympathetic nervous system and a direct effect on the kidneys, resulting in increased sodium reabsorption leading to hypertension. Obesity per se may have structural effects on the kidneys that may perpetuate hypertension, leading to an increased incidence of end-stage renal disease that results in further hypertension. Adipose tissue may elaborate angiotensin from its own local renin-angiotensin*

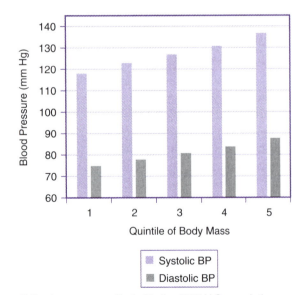

Estimates are age-adjusted to the 2000 U.S. population.

FIGURE 10.6 Body Mass Index and Blood Pressure, United States.

Data from Aneja, A., El-Atat, F., McFarlane, S. I., & Sowers, J. R. (2004). Hypertension and obesity. *Recent Progress in Hormone Research, 59,* 169–205.

system. The distribution of body fat is considered important in the genesis of the obesity-hypertension syndrome, with a predominantly central distribution being particularly ominous. Weight loss is the cornerstone in the management of the obesity-hypertension syndrome. It may be achieved with diet, exercise, medications, and a combination of these measures. Anti-obesity medications that are currently undergoing clinical trials may play a promising role in the management of obesity and may also result in lowering of blood pressure. Anti-hypertensives are considered important components in the holistic approach to the management of this complex problem. (p. 169)

Salt and Hypertension

One of the primary objectives of the international INTERSALT study was to elucidate the relationship between urinary electrolytes and blood pressure. Associations of 24-hour urinary sodium and potassium were explored in more than 10,000 adults from 52 centers worldwide. Regression models indicated that each 100 mmol increase in urinary sodium increased systolic and diastolic blood pressure by 6 and 2.5 mm Hg, respectively. Conversely, each 100 mmol increase in urinary potassium decreased systolic and diastolic blood pressure by 2 and 1 mm Hg, respectively. Adjustment for body mass decreased the magnitude of these estimates by up to 50%. These results support recommendations for a combined approach to the prevention of hypertension including lower sodium and higher potassium intakes plus weight reduction to prevent and control obesity (Dyer, Elliott, Shipley, Stamler, & Stamler, 1994).

Effects of dietary salt reduction on blood pressure have been investigated in several randomized clinical trials. In a recent meta-analysis of trials of 4 or more weeks' duration, 24-hours urinary sodium and blood pressure were examined from 17 trials enrolling 734 hypertensive patients and 11 trials enrolling 2220 normotensive patients. Among hypertensive patients, reducing urinary sodium by 100 mmol per day (equivalent to 6 grams of salt) produced a 7.1 mm Hg decrease in systolic blood pressure. Among normotensive subjects, the corresponding decrease in systolic blood pressure with reduced sodium was 3.6 mm Hg. These results demonstrate the significant impact of salt restriction in reducing blood pressure for both hypertensive and normotensive individuals (He & MacGregor, 2002).

These and many other epidemiologic investigations clearly link chronic excessive salt intake and salt retention to the genesis of hypertension. Nevertheless, the precise mechanisms by which salt retention increases blood pressure and causes hypertension remain unresolved. Much depends on the level of hydration in individual patients. With dehydration, sodium retention in the kidneys leads to hyperosmolality of blood, which may induce osmol receptors that cause vasoconstriction (Brooks, Haywood, & Johnson, 2005). In individuals who are sufficiently hydrated, sodium retention increases blood volume due to osmosis, thus increasing vascular resistance. It has recently been discovered that elevated plasma sodium induces secretion of the adrenocortical hormone, ouabain, which has multiple effects that raise blood pressure (e.g., inhibition of the Na+ pump plus cardiotonic and vasotonic effects) (Blaustein, Zhang, Chen, & Hamilton, 2006).

Alcohol and Hypertension

Alcohol consumption has been linked to the development of hypertension in several epidemiologic investigations. The association was first reported by Lian more than a century ago who found that heavy wine drinking among French servicemen elevated the risk of hypertension (>160/100 mm Hg) by threefold compared to moderate drinking (Lian, 2015).

In a cross-sectional survey conducted in the United States (the *Lipids Research Clinics Prevalence Study*), prevalence relationships between alcohol consumption and systolic and diastolic blood pressure were examined in 2482 men and 2301 women aged 20 years or older sampled from nine North-American populations. In men, the relationship between alcohol and hypertension was linear. Men who consumed 30 mL or more of alcohol per day were 1.5–2 times more likely to have hypertension than nondrinkers. In women, the prevalence relationship between alcohol consumption and hypertension was U-shaped: heavy drinkers and individuals who abstained from alcohol were about twice as likely to have hypertension compared to moderate drinkers. As a possible explanation for the increased prevalence of hypertension among women who reported no alcohol consumption, women in this category had higher levels of obesity than other subgroups. Regression analysis indicated that consuming 30 mL of alcohol per day increased systolic blood pressure by 2–6 mm Hg. Effects of alcohol on blood pressure were independent of age, gender, obesity, smoking, regular exercise, education, and hormone replacement therapy in women (Criqui, Mebane, Wallace, Heiss, & Holdbrook, 1982).

As a part of the INTERSALT study, alcohol intake and blood pressure were studied among 4844 men and 4837 women aged 20–59 years ascertained from 50 centers worldwide. Overall, higher levels of alcohol consumption were associated with higher blood pressures in both men and women. Men who consumed at least 500 mL of alcohol per week had average systolic and diastolic blood pressures that were 4.6 and 3.0 mm Hg higher than nondrinkers, and women who consumed at least 300 mL of alcohol per week had average systolic and diastolic blood pressures that were 3.9 and 3.1 mm Hg higher than nondrinkers. The observed effects of alcohol on blood pressure were independent of body mass and urinary excretion of sodium and potassium. Based on these results, the INTERSALT investigators recommended that individuals at high risk by virtue of their heavy drinking should be targeted for intervention (Marmot et al., 1994).

Since blood pressure is highly labile and subject to acute effects of alcohol and other factors, the influence of time elapsed since last ingestion has come under consideration. In a cross-sectional study, 1089 Brazilian adults from Porto Alegre were studied to assess effects of the time elapsed between the last ingestion of alcohol and the time of blood-pressure measurement. Positive associations were observed between the amount of alcohol consumed, increasing blood pressure, and the presence of hypertension (defined as blood pressure equal to or exceeding 160/95 mm Hg). Compared to nondrinkers, consumption of 30 g of alcohol per day produced average increases of 1.5 and 2.3 mm Hg in systolic and diastolic blood pressure in men, and 2.1 and 3.2 mm Hg in women. The prevalence of hypertension was nearly threefold higher among those ingesting more than 30 g of alcohol per day (odds ratio = 2.9). Furthermore, the time elapsed between the last ingestion of alcohol and time of blood-pressure measurement was independently associated with the prevalence of hypertension (e.g., men who drank alcohol within 13–23 hours of blood-pressure measurement were 2.6 times more likely to be hypertensive compared to those with longer intervals). These results suggest that alcohol has a time-dependent impact on blood pressure that may be related to the level of consumption and drug pharmacology (Moreira, Fuchs, Moraes, Bredemeier, & Duncan, 1998).

In another study designed to examine blood-pressure changes related to patterns of alcohol consumption, current alcohol consumption outside of meals was explored as a risk factor in 2609 men and women from western New York. Notably, individuals who consumed alcohol separately from meals exhibited significantly higher relative risks than those who consumed alcohol during mealtime (Stranges et al.,

2004). This result lends some support to a potential benefit of consuming a small amount of alcohol with meals (Klatsky, 2004).

The U-curve relationship of alcohol consumption and hypertension that has been observed in some studies is a source of controversy in the scientific literature. There appears to be consensus that heavy alcohol consumption increases blood pressure and the risk of hypertension, but the impact of light to moderate consumption is not as clear, with some studies reporting a decline in risk and others not. A team of investigators at Harvard reexamined the question in prospective analysis of 28,848 women from the Women's Health Study and 13,455 men from the Physician's Health Study who were free of hypertension at baseline. During 10.9 and 21.8 years of average follow-up, 8680 women and 6012 men developed hypertension (defined as systolic pressure equal to or exceeding 140 mm Hg or diastolic pressure equal to or exceeding 90 mm Hg). In women, the dose–response pattern was a J-shaped curve wherein light to moderate drinking slightly decreased the risk and heavy drinking or complete abstinence increased the risk. In men, the dose–response curve was linear, reflecting only increasing risk with increasing alcohol intake. The threshold for increased risk emerged at one drink per day for men (RR = 1.26) whereas the threshold for women occurred at three drinks per day (multivariate-adjusted RR = 1.84). Results therefore add to the evidence that heavy alcohol consumption significantly increases the risk of hypertension and lend support to the existence of differential effects of alcohol in men and women (Sesso, Cook, Buring, Manson, & Gaziano, 2008).

Randomized clinical trials have been conducted to examine effects of reducing alcohol intake on blood pressure. In a meta-analysis of 15 randomized controlled trials enrolling 2234 participants consuming 3–6 alcoholic drinks per day, alcohol reduction resulted in significant decreases in average systolic and diastolic blood pressures (3.3 and 2.0 mm Hg, respectively). Greater reductions in blood pressure were noted for individuals with higher blood pressures at baseline. Results support effective intervention to reduce alcohol consumption as an important lifestyle modification for the prevention and treatment of hypertension, particularly among heavy drinkers (Tomson & Lip, 2006; Xin et al., 2001).

Mechanisms by which alcohol increases blood pressure remain under study and have not been resolved (Clark, 1985; Klatsky, 2004). Alcohol metabolism is complex, involving first pass metabolism in the stomach and secondary metabolism in the liver. Compared to men, women have lower average total body water than men, a higher proportion of fat, and lower levels of alcohol-metabolizing enzymes, both in the stomach and in the liver (Frezza et al., 1990). These features are associated with higher blood levels of alcohol in women at comparable amounts of ingestion. Nevertheless, as pointed out already, women appear to have a higher threshold than men for the hypertensive effects of alcohol (e.g., four drinks per day versus one drink per day based on one recent study) (Sesso et al., 2008).

One mechanistic link between alcohol and blood pressure that is of special interest involves the induction of *hypoglycemia* by alcohol consumption. Recent animal studies have shown that alcohol induces redistribution of blood flow within the pancreas, leading to markedly increased insulin secretion by the pancreatic *islets of Langerhans*, thus resulting in lowered blood sugar and hypoglycemia (Huang & Sjöholm, 2007). In 1939, Kraines and Gellhorn reported that hypoglycemia increases the blood pressure in psychiatric patients by stimulating the sympathetic nervous system (Kraines & Gellhorn, 1939). More recent studies have confirmed that hypoglycemia stimulates the sympathetic nervous system as well as the adrenal glands causing release of epinephrine and thereby elevating blood pressure (Feldman-Billard, Massin, Meas, Guillausseau, & Héron, 2010; Sommerfield, Wilkinson, Webb, & Frier, 2007). Thus, it seems likely that alcohol-induced hypoglycemia may be at least partially responsible for the observed increase in blood pressure and hypertension among heavy drinkers.

▶ Tobacco and Hypertension

Multiple epidemiologic investigations have consistently demonstrated that smoking is a key risk factor in the genesis of CVDs including coronary heart disease, myocardial infarction, and stroke. Nevertheless, epidemiologic studies do not provide consistent evidence that smoking increases the risk of developing hypertension. Furthermore, blood pressure measured in the physician's office has been found to be similar for smokers compared to nonsmokers, a paradoxical finding in view of the acute vasoconstrictive impact of nicotine (Gropelli, Giorgi, Omboni, Parati, & Manchia, 1992; Omvik, 1996).

To resolve this paradox, investigators from the Cardiovascular Disease and Hypertension Center at New York Hospital/Cornell Medical Center conducted a case–control study to compare the blood pressures of 59 untreated hypertensive individuals who smoked at least two packs of cigarettes per day (cases) with 118 untreated hypertensive individuals who were nonsmokers (controls). The controls were group-matched to the cases by age, sex, and race. While blood pressures

measured in an office setting were similar, ambulatory measurements of systolic blood pressure taken throughout the day were significantly higher for smokers than nonsmokers (145 versus 140 mm Hg). The average difference in ambulatory systolic blood pressure between smokers and nonsmokers was greatest among individuals over the age of 50 years (153 versus 142 mm Hg). Blood pressure levels returned to normal levels during sleep for both groups (approximately 120/80 mm Hg). These results show that hypertensive smokers have higher ambulatory blood pressure during the waking hours than hypertensive nonsmokers, consistent with their higher risk for the development of CVD (Mann, James, Wang, & Pickering, 1991).

More recently, the causal link between smoking and the development of hypertension has been validated in follow-up studies of normotensive individuals who were assigned a risk score (e.g., the *Framingham Risk Prediction Score*) based on several factors including smoking status. In the Framingham Heart Study, risk scores were determined for 1717 participants 20–69 years of age based upon their age, sex, systolic and diastolic blood pressure, parental history of hypertension, BMI, and cigarette smoking. During 3.8 years of average follow-up time, 726 new cases of hypertension (>140/90 mm Hg) were detected in the cohort. In regression models, risk scores were highly correlated with increasing blood pressure and current smoking was a significant individual predictor of the development of hypertension (Parikh et al., 2008).

Further testing of the *Framingham Risk Prediction Score* was conducted in a European cohort of 2704 London-based civil servants aged 35–68 years. Each participant was evaluated and assigned a risk score based on age, sex, BMI, and smoking status at the beginning of each of three 5-year intervals. A total of 2043 incident cases of hypertension were detected in the three 5-year follow-up data cycles. As in the Framingham cohort, the risk score proved to be a valid tool for the prediction of hypertension in this cohort, and current smoking was the strongest individual predictor of hypertension (Kivimäki et al., 2009).

▶ Insulin Resistance, Diabetes Mellitus, and Hypertension

Diabetes mellitus is a major chronic disease caused by dysfunctional regulation and metabolism of blood glucose. It arises either from (1) inadequate secretion of insulin by cells of the *islets of Langerhans* in the pancreas (type 1 diabetes mellitus) or (2) ineffectiveness of insulin in transporting glucose into cells of the body for energy (type 2 diabetes mellitus). Type 1 diabetes is more common in children and accounts for a relatively small percentage of cases (approximately 5%) whereas type 2 diabetes usually arises in adults and is much more prevalent, accounting for approximately 95% of cases. The epidemiology of diabetes mellitus is covered later.

Type 2 diabetes arises because the cells of the body become resistant to the usual effects of insulin in stimulating glucose uptake for energy. Ineffectual glucose uptake in the presence of insulin is appropriately called "*insulin resistance.*" In type 2 diabetes, since the cells of the body are insulin-resistant, glucose remains in the blood, and blood glucose levels become inordinately high, a condition known as *hyperglycemia.* Furthermore, pancreatic cells may attempt to compensate for high levels of blood glucose by secreting more insulin, a condition known as *hyperinsulinemia.*

The clinical definition of diabetes is when the *fasting blood glucose* (blood glucose measured after 8 hours without food) exceeds 125 mg/dL. Insulin resistance is defined as a *prediabetic* state in which the fasting blood glucose level is between 110 mg/dL and 125 mg/dL. Diabetes and insulin resistance are often confirmed by a *glucose-tolerance test* in which blood glucose levels are measured following an oral-loading dose of glucose. Persistence of elevated blood glucose above 200 mg/dL for more than 2 hours indicates diabetes and a level between 140 mg/dL and 200 mg/dL indicates insulin resistance.

In 1966, Welborn and colleagues studied 19 patients with essential hypertension and found that their plasma-insulin levels were significantly elevated compared to normotensive controls (Welborn, Breckenridge, Rubinstein, Dollery, & Fraser, 1966). This was the first of many investigations that have examined insulin and insulin resistance as risk factors for the development of hypertension. Selected studies of population samples from around the globe are discussed in the following paragraphs.

In the United States, Dr. Gerald Reaven and colleagues assessed insulin levels and other factors in 33 obese women aged 27–77 years of age and found that fasting serum-insulin level was the strongest predictor of systolic and diastolic blood pressure (Lucas, Estigarribia, Darga, & Reaven, 1985). In Israel, Modan and colleagues studied hypertension and glucose intolerance in 2475 adults randomly sampled from a central population registry. They found increased rates of hypertension with impaired glucose-tolerance (rate ratio = 1.48) as well as in patients with type 2 diabetes (rate ratio = 2.26) (Modan et al., 1985).

In Italy, insulin resistance was measured in 13 young adults (mean age = 38) with severe essential hypertension and 11 normotensive control subjects matched by age and weight. Total insulin-induced glucose uptake was markedly impaired among the

hypertensive individuals (3.8 versus 6.3 mg per minute per kg body weight) (Ferrannini et al., 1987). In an Italian case–control study of 41 patients with essential hypertension and 41 normotensive control subjects, 45% of hypertensive patients had abnormal glucose-tolerance tests compared to 10% of normotensive subjects (Zavaroni et al., 1992).

Investigators in Sweden studied relationships of glucose metabolism, insulin resistance, obesity, and hypertension in 143 newly diagnosed hypertensive patients. Insulin resistance and hyperinsulinemia were associated with hypertension in both obese and non-obese individuals compared to normotensive individuals (Pollare, Lithell, & Berne, 1990).

The Insulin Resistance Atherosclerosis Study (IRAS) was designed to prospectively examine insulin resistance and other risk factors for hypertension in U.S. cohorts of differing ethnicities. Participants included 564 non-Hispanic Caucasian Americans, 505 Hispanic Americans, and 403 African Americans aged 40–69 years. Study results reflect increased prevalence rates of hypertension with progressively higher degrees of impaired glucose tolerance for each cohort and across all cohorts: 30% for normal subjects, 39% for prediabetic individuals, and 46% for individuals with type 2 diabetes mellitus (**FIGURE 10.7**). Multivariate regression analysis of nondiabetic subjects revealed independent effects of gender (male), BMI, insulin resistance, and fasting blood glucose on the development of hypertension. Nevertheless, among

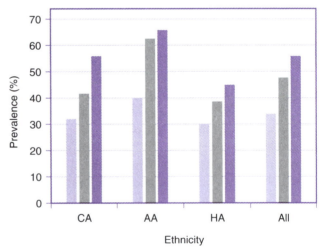

CA = Caucasian American, AA = African American,
HA = Hispanic American, GT = Glucose Tolerance,
DM II = Diabetes Mellitus II

FIGURE 10.7 Prevalence of Hypertension by Glucose Intolerance and Ethnicity.

Data from Saad, M. F., Rewers, M., Selby, J., Howard, G., Jinagouda, S., Fahmi, S., ... Haffner, S. M. (2004). Insulin resistance and hypertension: The Insulin Resistance Atherosclerosis Study. *Hypertension 43*, 1–8.

diabetic subjects, insulin resistance was not a significant predictor of hypertension (Saad et al., 2004).

While these investigations implicate insulin resistance and impaired glucose uptake as significant risk factors in the development of hypertension, not all patients with essential hypertension manifest insulin resistance. Clearly, a significant fraction of hypertensive patients, perhaps up to 50%, manifest hyperinsulinemia and/or insulin resistance; whereas the remaining half does not (Landberg, 1995; Reaven, 1988). The findings demonstrate the complexity of interactions involving glucose regulation and blood pressure, and related physiological mechanisms.

As pointed out by Dr. Gerald Reaven (2003) in his discussion of hypertension, insulin resistance, diabetes, and coronary heart disease:

Hyperglycemia develops in insulin-resistant individuals when they no longer are able to secrete the large amount of insulin necessary to overcome insulin resistance. Similarly, it seems likely that hypertension only develops when some unknown compensatory response (or responses) is no longer able to overcome the metabolic changes associated with insulin resistance and compensatory hyperinsulinemia that favor an increase in blood pressure. (p. 270)

The Metabolic Syndrome (Syndrome X)

Dietary Calcium and Hypertension

The discovery that dietary calcium may influence blood pressure was first reported by McCarron and colleagues in the 1980s (McCarron, 1985). These early studies demonstrated that low dietary calcium was associated with hypertension and that per-capita calcium consumption by adults in the United States was inversely related to the probability of being hypertensive. The initial investigation was a small pilot study comparing 44 normotensive control subjects with 46 cases with essential hypertension. Dietary assessment revealed significantly less daily calcium consumption in the cases compared to controls (668 versus 886 mg) (McCarron, Morris, & Cole, 1982).

Subsequently, several other epidemiologic studies and clinical trials also found an association between low dietary calcium and hypertension, and reciprocally, beneficial effects of supplemental calcium in reducing blood pressure. In a meta-analysis of 40 randomized clinical trials conducted during 1966–2003 and involving a total of 2492 participants, calcium supplementation of 1200 mg per day produced average reductions of 1.86 and 0.99 mm Hg in systolic and diastolic blood pressures, respectively. Greater reductions (1.63 and 1.30 mm Hg) were noted for individuals with low dietary calcium at baseline (<800 mg daily) (van Mierlo et al., 2006). Nevertheless, there was considerable heterogeneity among studies in the response to supplemental calcium, and some studies did not discern an effect (Trumbo & Ellwood, 2007). It has been suggested that lack of adjustment for baseline factors (e.g., levels of dietary calcium, vitamin D, and blood pressures among participants) may be responsible for the heterogeneity of effect among studies (McCarron & Reusser, 1999).

One notable example of a "null study" is the randomized double-blinded placebo-controlled trial of calcium and vitamin D supplementation in the U.S. Women's Health Initiative (WHI). In this study, 36,282 postmenopausal women were randomly assigned to receive 1000 mg of elemental calcium plus 400 international units (IU) of vitamin D daily or placebo in double-blind fashion. Over a median follow-up time of 7 years, there were no significant differences detected in systolic or diastolic blood pressures between the treatment and placebo groups. Furthermore, among 17,122 normotensive women at baseline, the hazard ratio for the incidence of hypertension for the treatment arm of the study was virtually unchanged after 7 years of follow-up (HR = 1.01). Stratified analysis of data according to baseline factors (race, blood pressure, low dietary calcium, and vitamin D) did not reveal effects for subgroups of interest (Margolis et al., 2008). These results provide no evidence that supplemental calcium plus vitamin D reduces blood pressure or the incidence of hypertension in postmenopausal women, regardless of baseline status.

Genetics of Hypertension

Certain genetic syndromes have been found to cause hypertension. As might be expected, the ones best described involve dysfunction of sodium transport in the kidney. Liddle's syndrome is due to a rare mutant gene that causes constitutive activation of the sodium transport channel in the renal tubules of the kidney. Patients with Liddle's syndrome develop severe intractable hypertension at an early age (often during infancy) due to their high sodium retention (Shimkets et al., 1994). Gordon's syndrome is caused by a rare mutant gene that disturbs the sodium-chloride transport channel in the distal renal tubules resulting in enhanced chloride and sodium retention thereby causing hypertension by the third decade of life (Gordon, Geddes, Pawse, & O'Halloran, 1970).

African Americans have higher rates of hypertension than Caucasian Americans (Burt et al., 1995), which has been attributed to their heightened retention of sodium (salt) by the renin–angiotensin system (Luft et al., 1991; Weinberger, 1993). Specific genes encode vital components of the renin–angiotensin system including renin, angiotensinogen, ACE, and angiotensin receptors, and recent genetic association studies have searched for effects of alleles of these genes among relatives with familial hypertension.

In a recent study involving 192 African-American families, single-nucleotide polymorphisms of genes encoding renin and the angiotensin receptor (AGTR-1) were found to be significantly associated with the development of essential hypertension (Zhu et al., 2003). These results take on added significance since the primary effector molecule of the renin–angiotensin system, *angiotensin* II, has been found to increase expression of the gene that encodes endothelin-1, a potent local vasoconstrictive protein secreted by the endothelium of blood vessels (Hong et al., 2004).

Differences in endothelin-1 have been observed in association with the higher rates of hypertension among African Americans compared to other ethnic groups. In a clinical study designed to examine blood levels of endothelin-1 among hypertensive subjects, African-American men and women with hypertension were found to have considerably higher endothelin-1 levels than Caucasians with hypertension (Ergul, Parish, Puett, & Ergul, 1996). In other studies, normotensive African-American men had twofold higher levels than age-matched Caucasian men (Evans, Phillips, Singh, Bauman, & Gulati, 1996) and African-American adolescents had higher levels than Caucasians (Treiber et al., 2000). In view of these findings, the influence of genes that regulate the renin–angiotensin system as well as vasoactive substances within blood vessels may play a role in elevating the susceptibility to hypertension among African Americans.

▶ Prevention of Hypertension

A variety of risk factors, many of which are modifiable, play an interactive role in the development of hypertension including age, race, gender, BMI, excess dietary salt, tobacco addiction, high alcohol intake, dietary potassium and calcium deficiencies, elevated blood levels of cholesterol and glucose, lack of exercise, and psychological factors such as stress and depression (Australian Institute of Health and Welfare, 2011; Whelton, 1994). Intensive nonpharmacological intervention targeting multiple factors is thus essential for the primary prevention of developing high blood pressure (Centers for Disease Control, 2007; Working Group on Primary Prevention of Hypertension, 1993).

Effective intervention to combat hypertension demands incorporation of community-based blood-pressure screening programs to identify those patients with elevated blood pressure (Joint National Committee on Detection, Evaluation, and Treatment of High Blood Pressure, 1993). Pharmacologic therapy for the management of hypertension has proven effective in improving cardiovascular and renal function and reducing the risk of myocardial infarction, stroke, and renal failure (Burt et al., 1995; Collins et al., 1990; Hebert, Moser, Mayer, Glynn, & Hennekens, 1993; Shulman et al., 1989).

Prolonged assessment in which repeated measurements of blood pressure are taken in a relaxed environment provides the most accurate method of detecting a significant rise in blood pressure above normal. According to new guidelines recommended by the AHA, individuals who manifest systolic blood pressure of 120–129 mm Hg have elevated blood pressure. Lifestyle changes are therefore recommended to lower blood pressure before the initiation of prescription–drug therapy. The following guidelines for implementing lifestyle changes are recommended by the British Hypertension Society (**TABLE 10.2**).

TABLE 10.2 Nonpharmacologic Guidelines to Reduce Blood Pressure

- Weight reduction and regular (daily) aerobic exercise
- Reducing dietary sugar
- Reducing sodium (salt) in the diet to less than 6 g
- Additional dietary changes beneficial to reducing blood pressure (e.g., the DASH diet [dietary approaches to stop hypertension], which is rich in fruits and vegetables and low-fat or fat-free dairy products)
- Increasing dietary potassium and calcium
- Abstaining from or discontinuing tobacco use
- Limiting alcohol consumption to one drink daily
- Reducing stress and depression
- Maintaining blood levels of cholesterol and glucose within normal limits

Data from Saad, M. F., Rewers, M., Selby, J., Howard, G., Jinagouda, S., Fahmi, S., ... Haffner, S. M. (2004). Insulin resistance and hypertension: The Insulin Resistance Atherosclerosis Study. *Hypertension 43*, 1–8.

In consideration of nonpharmacologic approaches to blood-pressure control, it is noteworthy that dietary modification has been shown to have significant benefit in reducing blood pressure in hypertensive patients. The *Dietary Approaches to Stop Hypertension (DASH)* study was specifically designed to assess the impact on blood pressure of a *combination diet* rich in fruits, vegetables, and low-fat dairy products with reduced saturated and total fat. The study randomized 459 adults with systolic blood pressure less than 160 mm Hg and diastolic blood pressure between 80 and 95 mm Hg into a treatment arm (*n* = 230) to receive the DASH diet and a control arm (*n* = 229) without dietary modification. At 8 weeks of follow-up, the combination DASH diet reduced systolic and diastolic blood pressures by 5.5 and 3.0 mm Hg, respectively, compared to the control diet. Among participants with more severe hypertension (blood pressure exceeding 140/90 mm Hg), the DASH diet produced even greater reductions in average blood pressure (11.4 and 5.5 mm Hg, respectively). The DASH Study investigators concluded that a diet rich in fruits, vegetables, and low-fat dairy foods with reduced saturated and total fat can substantially lower blood pressure, even in patients with more severe hypertension (Appel et al., 1997).

As discussed in separate chapters of this text, epidemiologic studies provide convincing evidence that hypertension is etiologically linked to the pathogenesis of thromboembolic cardiovascular events such as ischemic heart disease, stroke, and myocardial infarction (Fiebach et al., 1989; MacMahon et al., 1990; Stamler, Stamler, & Neaton, 1993) as well as renal insufficiency and failure (Whelton, Perneger, Klag, & Brancati, 1992). Successful intervention to curb global increases in these conditions will therefore require intensive multifactorial non-pharmacologic strategies targeting the modifiable risk factors of hypertension as well as effective pharmacologic management of blood pressure for hypertensive individuals.

References

Alegría-Ezquerra, E., González-Juanatey, J. R., & González-Maqueda, I. (2006). Hypertensive heart disease: A proposed clinical classification. *Revista Española de Cardiología, 59*(4), 398–399.

American Academy of Family Physicians. (2017). Guidelines developed by external organizations not endorsed by the AAFP. *American Family Physician, 96*(12), 760.

Aneja, A., El-Atat, F., McFarlane, S. I., & Sowers, J. R. (2004). Hypertension and obesity. *Recent Progress in Hormone Research, 59*, 169–205.

Appel, L. J., Moore, T. J., Obarzanek, E., Vollmer, W. M., Svetkey, L. P., Sacks, F. M., ... DASH Collaborative Research Group. (1997). A clinical trial of the effects of dietary patterns on blood pressure. *New England Journal of Medicine, 336*, 1117–1124.

Arroyo, P., Fernandez, A., Loria, A., Kuri-Morales, P., Orozco-Rivadeneyra, S., Olaiz, G., & Tapia-Conyer, R. (1999). Hypertension in urban Mexico: The 1992–93 national survey of chronic diseases. *Journal of Human Hypertension, 13*, 671–675.

Australian Institute of Health and Welfare. (2011). Risk Factor Prevalence Data.

Baba, S., Pan, W. H., Ueshima, H., Ozawa, H., Komachi, Y., Stamler, R., ... Stamler, J. (1991). Blood pressure levels, related factors, and hypertension control status of Japanese and Americans. *Journal of Human Hypertension, 5*, 317–332.

Banegas, J. R., & Pérez-Regadera, A. G. (1998). Hypertension control as an indicator of the geographical variation of stroke. *Stroke, 29*, 867–868.

Banegas, J. R., Rodriguez-Artalejo, F., de la Cruz, T. J. J., Guallar-Castillon, P., Calero, J., & del Rey, C. J. (1998). Blood pressure in Spain: Distribution, awareness, control, and benefits of a reduction in average pressure. *Hypertension, 32*, 998–1002.

Bennett, S. A., & Magnus, P. (1994). Trends in cardiovascular risk factors in Australia. Results from the National Heart Foundation's Risk Factor Prevalence Study, 1980–1989. *The Medical Journal of Australia, 161*, 519–527.

Blacher, J., Levy, B. I., Mourad, J. J., Safar, M. E., & Bakris, G. (2016). From epidemiological transition to modern cardiovascular epidemiology: Hypertension in the 21st century. *Lancet, 388*, 530–532.

Blaustein, M. P., Zhang, J., Chen, L., & Hamilton, B. P. (2006). How does salt retention raise blood pressure? *American Journal of Physiology, Regulatory, Integrative and Comparative Physiology, 290*(3), R514–R523.

Brent, G. A. (1994). Mechanisms of disease: The molecular basis of thyroid hormone action. *New England Journal of Medicine, 331*, 847–853.

Brooks, V. L., Haywood, J. R., & Johnson, A. K. (2005). Translation of salt retention to central activation of the sympathetic nervous system in hypertension. *Clinical and Experimental Pharmacology and Physiology, 32*, 426–432.

Burt, V. L., Whelton, P., Roccella, E. J., Brown, C., Cutler, J. A., Higgins, M., ... Labarthe, D. (1995). Prevalence of hypertension in the US adult population. Results from the Third National Health and Nutrition Examination survey, 1988–91. *Hypertension, 25*, 305–313. https://doi.org/10.1161/01.HYP.25.3.305

Centers for Disease Control. (2007). Division for Heart Disease and Stroke Prevention. Department of Health and Human Services.

Chobanian, A. V., Bakris, G. L., Black, H. R., Cushman, W. C., Green, L. A., Izzo, J. L., Jr., ... National High Blood Pressure Education Program Coordinating Committee. (2003). Seventh report of the Joint National Committee on prevention, detection, evaluation, and treatment of high blood pressure. *Hypertension, 42*(6), 1206–1252.

Clark, L. T. (1985). Alcohol-induced hypertension: Mechanisms, complications, and clinical implications. *Journal of the National Medical Association, 77*(5), 385–389.

Collins, R., Peto, R., MacMahon, S., Hebert, P., Fiebach, N. H., Eberlein, K. A., ... Hennekens, C. H. (1990). Blood pressure, stroke, and coronary heart disease, part II: Short-term reductions in blood pressure: Overview of randomised drug trials in their epidemiological context. *Lancet, 335*, 827–838.

Cooper, R., Rotimi, D., Ataman, S., McGee, D., Osotimehin, B., Kadiri, S., ... Wilks, R. (1997). The prevalence of hypertension in seven populations of West African origin. *American Journal of Public Health, 87,* 160–168.

Criqui, M. H., Mebane, I., Wallace, R. B., Heiss, G., & Holdbrook, M. J. (1982). Multivariate correlates of adult blood pressures in nine North American populations: The lipid research clinics prevalence study. *Preventive Medicine, 11,* 391–402.

Cutler, J. A., Sorlie, P. D., Wolz, M., Thom, T., Fields, L. E., & Roccella, E. J. (2008). Trends in the hypertension prevalence, awareness, treatment, and control rates in United States adults between 1988–1994 and 1999–2004. *Hypertension, 52*(5), 818–827.

Dyer, A. R., & Elliott, P. (1989). The INTERSALT study: Relations of body mass index to blood pressure. INTERSALT Co-operative Research Group. *Journal of Human Hypertension, 3*(5), 299–308.

Dyer, A. R., Elliott, P., & Shipley, M. J. (1990). Body mass index versus height and weight in relation to blood pressure: Findings for the 10,079 persons in the INTERSALT study. *American Journal of Epidemiology, 131,* 589–596.

Dyer, A. R., Elliott, P., Shipley, M., Stamler, R., & Stamler, J. (1994). Body mass index and associations of sodium and potassium with blood pressure in INTERSALT. *Hypertension, 23,* 729–736.

Dzau, V. J. (1990). Atherosclerosis and hypertension: Mechanisms and interrelationships. *Journal of Cardiovascular Pharmacology, 15*(Suppl. 5), S59–S64.

Edwards, R., Unwin, N., Mugus, F., Whiting, D., Rashid, S., Kissima, J., ... Alberti, K. G. (2000). Hypertension prevalence and care in an urban and rural area of Tanzania. *Journal of Hypertension, 18*(2000), 145–152.

Egan, B. M., Zhao, Y., & Axon, R. N. (2010). US trends in prevalence, awareness, treatment, and control of hypertension, 1988–2008. *JAMA, 303*(20), 2043–2050.

Ergul, S., Parish, D. C., Puett, D., & Ergul, A. (1996). Racial differences in plasma endothelin-1 concentrations in individuals with essential hypertension. *Hypertension, 28,* 652–655.

Evans, R. R., Phillips, B. G., Singh, G., Bauman, J. L., & Gulati, A. (1996). Racial and gender differences in endothelin-1. *The American Journal of Cardiology, 78,* 486–488.

Feldman-Billard, S., Massin, P., Meas, T., Guillausseau, P. J., & Héron, E. (2010). Hypoglycemia-induced blood pressure elevation in patients with diabetes. *Archives of Internal Medicine, 170*(9), 829–831.

Ferrannini, E., Buzzigoli, G., Bonadonna, R., Giorico, M. A., Oleggini, M., Graziadei, L., ... Bevilacqua, S. (1987). Insulin resistance in essential hypertension. *New England Journal of Medicine, 317,* 350–357.

Fiebach, N. H., Hebert, P. R., Stampfer, M. J., Colditz, G. A., Willett, W. C., Rosner, B., ... Hennekens, C. H. (1989). A prospective study of high blood pressure and cardiovascular disease in women. *American Journal of Epidemiology, 130,* 646–654. doi:10.1016/j.gheart.2012.12.004. Epub 2013 Mar 15.

Franklin, S. S., & Wong, N. D. (2013). Hypertension and cardiovascular disease: Contributions of the Framingham Heart Study. *Global Heart, 8*(1), 49–57.

Frezza, M., di Padova, C., Pozzato, G., Terpin, M., Baraona, E., & Lieber, C. S. (1990). High blood alcohol levels in women. The role of decreased gastric alcohol dehydrogenase activity and first-pass metabolism. *New England Journal of Medicine, 322*(2), 95–99.

Fryar, C. D., Ostchega, Y., Hales, C. M., Zhang, G., & Kruszon-Moran, D. (2017). *Hypertension prevalence and control among adults: United States, 2015–2016* (NCHS Data Brief, No. 289). Hyattsville, MD: National Center for Health Statistics.

Giampaoli, S., Palmieri, L., Dima, F., Pilotto, L., Vescio, M. F., & Vanuzzo, D. (2001). Socioeconomic aspects and cardiovascular risk factors: Experience at the Cardiovascular Epidemiologic Observatory. *Italian Heart Journal, 2,* 294–302.

Gordon, R., Geddes, R., Pawse, C., & O'Halloran, M. (1970). Hypertension and severe hyperkalaemia associated with suppression of renin and aldosterone and completely reversed by dietary sodium restriction. *Australasian Annals of Medicine, 19*(4), 287–294.

Gropelli, A., Giorgi, D. M. A., Omboni, S., Parati, G., & Manchia, G. (1992). Persistent blood pressure increase induced by heavy smoking. *Journal of Hypertension, 10,* 495–499.

Gu, D., Reynolds, K., Wu, X., Chen, J., Duan, X., Muntner, P., ... The International Collaborative Study of Cardiovascular Disease in ASIA. (2002). Prevalence, awareness, treatment, and control of hypertension in China. *Hypertension, 40,* 920–927.

Gupta, R. (1999). Hypertension in India: Definition, prevalence and evaluation. *Journal of the Indian Medical Association, 97,* 74–80.

Gupta, R. (2004). Trends in hypertension epidemiology in India. *Journal of Human Hypertension, 18,* 73–78.

Gupta, R., AI-Odat, N. A., & Gupta, V. P. (1996). Hypertension epidemiology in India: Meta-analysis of fifty-year prevalence rates and blood pressure trends. *Journal of Human Hypertension, 10,* 465–472.

Gupta, R., Guptha, S., Gupta, V. P., & Prakash, H. (1995). Prevalence and determinants of hypertension in the urban population of Jaipur in western India. *Journal of Hypertension, 13,* 1193–1200.

Gupta, R., & Sharma, A. K. (1994). Prevalence of hypertension and subtypes in an Indian rural population: Clinical and electrocardiographic correlates. *Journal of Human Hypertension, 8,* 823–829.

Harrison, D. G., & Gongora, M. C. (2009). Oxidative stress and hypertension. *Medical Clinics of North America, 93*(3), 621–635.

Haynes, W. G., Hand, M. F., Johnstone, H. A., Padfield, P. L., & Webb, D. J. (1994). Direct and sympathetically mediated venoconstriction in essential hypertension. *Journal of Clinical Investigation, 94,* 1359–1364.

He, F. J., & MacGregor, G. A. (2002). Effect of modest salt reduction on blood pressure: A meta-analysis of randomized trials. Implications for public health. *Journal of Human Hypertension, 16*(11), 761–770.

He, Q., Ding, Z. Y., Fong, D. Y., & Karlberg, J. (2000). Blood pressure is associated with body mass index in both obese and normal children. *Hypertension, 36,* 165–170.

Hebert, P., Moser, M., Mayer, J., Glynn, R. J., & Hennekens, C. H. (1993). Recent evidence on drug therapy of mild to moderate hypertension and decreased risk of coronary heart disease. *Archives of Internal Medicine, 153,* 578–581.

Helvaci, M. R., & Seyhanli, M. (2006). What a high prevalence of white coat hypertension in society. *Internal Medicine, 45*(10), 671–674.

Hong, J. H., Chan, P., Kiu, J. C., Juan, S. H., Huang, M. T., Lin, J. G., & Cheng, T. H. (2004). Angiotensin II induces endothelin-1 gene expression via extracellular signal-related kinase pathway in rat aortic smooth muscle cells. *Cardiovascular Research, 61*(1), 159–168.

Huang, Z., & Sjöholm, Å. (2007). Ethanol acutely stimulates islet blood flow, amplifies insulin secretion, and induces hypoglycemia via nitric oxide and vagally mediated mechanism. *Endocrinology, 149*(1), 232–236.

Huang, Z., Willett, W. C., Manson, J. E., Rosner, B., Stampfer, M. J., Speizer, F. E., & Colditz, G. A. (1998). Body weight, weight change and the risk of hypertension in women. *Annals of Internal Medicine, 128*, 81–88.

Ibrahim, M. M., Rizk, H., Appel, L. J., el Aroussy, W., Helmy, S., Sharaf, Y., … Whelton, P. K. (1995). Hypertension prevalence, awareness, treatment, and control in Egypt. Results from the Egyptian National Hypertension Project (NHP). NHP Investigative Team. *Hypertension, 26*, 886–890.

Ilekis, J. V., Reddy, U. M., & Roberts, J. M. (2006). Review article: Pre-eclampsia—A pressing problem: An executive summary of a National Institute of Child Health and Human Development Workshop. *Reproductive Sciences, 14*(6), 508–523.

InterASIA Collaborative Group. (2003). Cardiovascular risk factor levels in urban and rural Thailand: The International Collaborative Study of Cardiovascular Disease in Asia (InterASIA). *European Journal of Cardiovascular Prevention and Rehabilitation, 10*, 249–257.

Joffres, M. R., Ghadirian, P., Fodor, J. G., Petrasovits, A., Chockalingam, A., & Hamet, P. (1997). Awareness, treatment, and control of hypertension in Canada. *American Journal of Hypertension, 10*, 1097–1102.

Joint National Committee on Detection, Evaluation, and Treatment of High Blood Pressure. (1993). The fifth report of the Joint National Committee on the Detection, Evaluation, and Treatment of High Blood Pressure. *Archives of Internal Medicine, 153*, 154–183.

Kannel, W. B. (1995). Framingham study insights into hypertensive risk of cardiovascular disease. *Hypertension Research, 18*(3), 181–196.

Kannel, W. B., Garrison, R. J., & Dannenberg, A. L. (1993). Secular blood pressure trends in normotensive persons. *American Heart Journal, 12*, 1154–1158.

Kearney, P. M., Whelton, M., Reynolds, K., Muntner, P., Whelton, P. K., & He, J. (2005). Global burden of hypertension: Analysis of worldwide data. *Lancet, 365*(9455), 217–223.

Kim, J. S., Jones, D. W., Kim, S. J., & Hong, Y. P. (1994). Hypertension in Korea: A national survey. *American Journal of Preventive Medicine, 10*, 200–204.

Kissebah, A. H., & Krakower, G. R. (1994). Regional adiposity and morbidity. *Physiological Review, 74*, 761–811.

Kivimäki, M., Batty, D., Singh-Manoux, A., Ferrie, J. E., Tabak, A. G., Jokela, M., … Shipley, M. J. (2009). Validating the Framingham Hypertension Risk Score. *Hypertension, 54*, 496–501.

Klatsky, A. L. (2004). Alcohol-associated hypertension: When one drink makes a difference. *Hypertension, 4*, 805–806.

Kraines, S. H., & Gellhorn, E. (1939). The effects of insulin hypoglycemia on the blood pressure response to oxygen deficiency in man. *American Journal of Psychiatry, 95*(5), 1067–1075.

Landberg, L. (1995). Obesity-related hypertension and the insulin resistance syndrome. *Transactions of the American Clinical and Climatological Association, 106*, 69–76.

Laurent, S. (2004). Guidelines from the British Hypertension Society. *BMJ, 328*, 593–594.

Law, M. R., Morris, K., & Wald, N. J. (2009). Use of blood pressure lowering drugs in the prevention of cardiovascular disease: Meta-analysis of 147 randomised trials in the context of expectations from prospective epidemiological studies. *British Medical Journal, 338*, b1665.

Lian, C. L. (1915). L'alcoolisme, caused hypertension arterielle. *Bulletin de l'Academie de Medicine, 74*, 525–528.

Lucas, C. P., Estigarribia, J. A., Darga, L. L., & Reaven, G. M. (1985). Insulin and blood pressure in obesity. *Hypertension, 7*, 702–706.

Luft, F. C., Miller, J. Z., Grim, C. E., Fineberg, N. S., Christian, J. C., Daugherty, S. A., & Weinberger, M. H. (1991). Salt sensitivity and resistance of blood pressure. Age and race as factors in physiological responses. *Hypertension, 17*(1 Suppl.), I102–I108.

MacMahon, S., Peto, R., Cutler, J., Collins, R., Sorlie, P., Neaton, J., … Stamler, J. (1990). Blood pressure, stroke, and coronary heart disease, part I: Prolonged differences in blood pressure: Prospective observational studies corrected for the regression dilution bias. *Lancet, 335*, 765–774.

Malhotra, P., Kumari, S., Kumar, R., Jain, S., & Sharma, B. K. (1999). Prevalence and determinants of hypertension in an unindustrialized rural population of North India. *Journal of Human Hypertension, 13*, 467–472.

Mann, S. J., James, G. D., Wang, R. S., & Pickering, T. G. (1991). Elevation of ambulatory systolic blood pressure in hypertensive smokers. *JAMA, 265*(17), 2226–2228.

Margolis, K. L., Ray, R. M., Van Horn, L., Manson, J. E., Allison, M. A., Black, H. R., … Women's Health Initiative Investigators. (2008). Effect of calcium and vitamin D supplementation on blood pressure. *Hypertension, 52*, 847–855.

Marmot, M. G., Elliott, P., Shipley, M. J., Dyer, A. R., Ueshima, H. U., Beevers, D. G., … Stamler, J. (1994). Alcohol and blood pressure: The INTERSALT study. *British Medical Journal, 308*, 1263–1267.

Mbanya, J. C., Minkoulou, E. M., Salah, J. N., & Balkau, B. (1998). The prevalence of hypertension in rural and urban Cameroon. *International Journal of Epidemiology, 27*, 181–185.

McCarron, D. A. (1985). Is calcium more important than sodium in the pathogenesis of essential hypertension. *Hypertension, 7*, 607–627.

McCarron, D. A., Morris, C. D., & Cole, C. (1982). Dietary calcium in human hypertension. *Science, 217*(4556), 267–269.

McCarron, D. A., & Reusser, M. E. (1999). Finding consensus in the dietary calcium blood pressure debate. *Journal of the American College of Nutrition, 18*(90005), 398S–405S.

Modan, M., Halkin, H., Almog, S., Lusky, A., Eshkol, A., Shefi, M., … Fuchs, Z. (1985). Hyperinsulinemia: A link between hypertension, obesity and glucose intolerance. *Journal of Clinical Investigation, 75*, 809–817.

Moffett, A., & Hiby, S. E. (2007). How does the maternal immune system contribute to the development of pre-eclampsia? *Placenta, 28*(Suppl. A), S51–S56.

Moreira, L. B., Fuchs, F. D., Moraes, R. S., Bredemeier, M., & Duncan, B. B. (1998). Alcohol intake and blood pressure: The importance of time elapsed since last drink. *Journal of Hypertension, 16*, 175–180.

Mufunda, J., Scott, L. J., Chifamba, J., Matenga, J., Sparks, B., Cooper, R., & Sparks, H. (2000). Correlates of blood pressure in an urban Zimbabwean population and comparison to other populations of African origin. *Journal of Human Hypertension, 14*, 65–73.

Muntner, P., Carey, R. M., Gidding, S., Jones, D. W., Taler, S. J., Wright, J. T., & Whelton, P. K. (2017). Potential U.S. Population Impact of the 2017 American College of Cardiology/American Heart Association High Blood Pressure Guideline. *Journal of the American College of Cardiology, 137*(2), 109–118.

National Heart, Lung and Blood Institute. (1996). *Stroke belt initiative*. Washington, DC: National Institutes of Health.

Neter, J. E., Stam, B. E., Kok, F. J., Grobbee, D. E., & Geleijnse, J. M. (2003). Influence of weight reduction on blood pressure: A meta-analysis of randomized controlled trials. *Hypertension, 42*, 878–884.

Nwankwo, T., Yoon, S. S., Burt, V., & Gu, Q. (2013). *Hypertension among adults in the U.S: National Health and Nutrition Examination Survey, 2011–2012* (NCHS Data Brief, No. 133). Hyattsville, MD: National Center for Health Statistics, Centers for Disease Control and Prevention, U.S. Department of Health and Human Services.

Omvik, P. (1996). How smoking affects blood pressure. *Blood Pressure, 5*(2), 71–77.

Pan, W. H., Chang, H. Y., Yeh, W. T., Hsiao, S. Y., & Hung, Y. T. (2001). Prevalence, awareness, treatment and control of hypertension in Taiwan: Results of Nutrition and Health Survey in Taiwan (NAHSIT) 1993–1996. *Journal of Human Hypertension, 15*, 793–798.

Parikh, N. I., Pencina, M. J., Wang, T. J., Benjamin, E. J., Lanier, K. J., Levy, D., ... Vasan, R. S. (2008). A risk score for predicting near–term incidence of hypertension: The Framingham Heart Study. *Annals of Internal Medicine, 148*(2), 102–110.

Paul, M., Poyan Mehr, A., & Kreutz, R. (2006). Physiology of local renin-angiotensin systems. *Physiological Reviews, 86*(3), 747–803.

Pollare, T., Lithell, H., & Berne, C. (1990). Insulin resistance is a characteristic feature of primary hypertension independent of obesity. *Metabolism, 39*, 167–174.

Primatesta, P., Brookes, M., & Poulter, N. R. (2001). Improved hypertension management and control: Results from the Health Survey for England 1998. *Hypertension, 38*, 827–832.

Ramirez, M. O., Pino, C. T., Furiasse, L. V., Lee, A. J., & Fowkes, F. G. (1995). Paraguayan National Blood Pressure Study: Prevalence of hypertension in the general population. *Journal of Human Hypertension, 9*, 891–897.

Reaven, G. M. (1988). Role of insulin resistance in human disease. *Diabetes, 37*, 1595–1607.

Reaven, G. M. (2003). Insulin resistance, hypertension and coronary heart disease. *Journal of Clinical Hypertension, 5*(4), 269–274.

Riecansky, I., & Egnerova, A. (1991). Cardiovascular program in Slovakia—Results achieved over the years 1978-1989. *Bratislavske Lekarske Listy, 92*, 203–218.

Robbins, S. L., & Cotran, R. S. (1979). *Pathologic basis of disease*. Philadelphia, PA: WB Saunders Company.

Roth, G. A., Johnson, C., Abajobir, A., Abd-Allah, F., Abera, S. F., Abyu, G., ... Murray, C. (2017). Global, regional, and national burden of cardiovascular diseases for 10 Causes, 1990 to 2015. *Journal of the American College of Cardiology, 70*(1), 1–25.

Rucker, D., Padwal, R., Li, S. K., Cuioni, C., & Lau, D. C. W. (2007). Long term pharmacotherapy for obesity and overweight: Updated meta-analysis. *BMJ, 335*, 1194–1199.

Ruxer, J., Mozdzan, M., Baranski, M., Wozniak-Sosnowska, U., & Markuszewski, L. (2007). White coat hypertension in type 2 diabetic patients. *Polskie Archiwum Medycyny Wewnętrznej, 117*(10), 452–456.

Saad, M. F., Rewers, M., Selby, J., Howard, G., Jinagouda, S., Fahmi, S., ... Haffner, S. M. (2004). Insulin resistance and hypertension: The Insulin Resistance Atherosclerosis Study. *Hypertension, 43*, 1–8.

Sesso, H. D., Cook, N. R., Buring, J. E., Manson, J. E., & Gaziano, J. M. (2008). Alcohol consumption and the risk of hypertension in women and men. *Hypertension, 51*, 1080–1087.

Shimkets, R. A., Warnock, D. G., Bositis, C. M., Nelson-Williams, C., Hansson, J. H., Schambelan, M., ... Lifton, R. P. (1994). Liddle's syndrome: Heritable human hypertension caused by mutations in the beta subunit of the epithelial sodium channel. *Cell, 79*(3), 407–414.

Shulman, N. B., Ford, C. E., Hall, W. D., Blaufox, M. D., Simon, D., Langford, H. G., & Schneider, K. A. (1989). Prognostic value of serum creatinine and effect of treatment of hypertension on renal function: Results from the Hypertension Detection and Followup Program. *Hypertension, 13*(Suppl. I), I-80–I-93.

Singh, R. B., Beegom, R., Ghosh, S., Niaz M. A., Rastogi, V., Rastogi, S. S., ... Nangia, S. (1997a). Epidemiological study of hypertension and its determinants in an urban population of North India. *Journal of Human Hypertension, 11*, 679–685.

Singh, R. B., Sharma, J. P., Rastogi, V., Niaz, M. A., & Singh, N. K. (1997b). Prevalence and determinants of hypertension in the Indian social class and heart survey. *Journal of Human Hypertension, 11*, 51–56.

Sommerfield, A. J., Wilkinson, I. B., Webb, D. J., & Frier, B. M. (2007). Vessel wall stiffness in type 1 diabetes and the central hemodynamic effects of acute hypoglycemia. *American Journal of Physiology Endocrinology and Metabolism, 293*(5), E1274–E1279.

Sonmez, H. M., Basak, O., Camci, C., Baltaci, R., Karazeybek, H. S., Yazgan, F., ... Celik, S. C. (1999). The epidemiology of elevated blood pressure as an estimate for hypertension in Aydin, Turkey. *Journal of Human Hypertension, 13*, 399–404.

SPRINT Research Group, Wright, J. T., Jr., Williamson, J. D., Whelton, P. K., Snyder, J. K., Sink, K. M., ... Ambrosius, W. T. (2015). A randomized trial of intensive versus standard blood-pressure control. *New England Journal of Medicine, 373*(22), 2103–2116.

Stamler, J., Stamler, R., & Neaton, J. D. (1993). Blood pressure, systolic and diastolic, and cardiovascular risks: U.S. population data. *Archives of Internal Medicine, 153*, 598–615.

Stegmayr, B., Asplund, K., Kuulasmaa, K., Rajakangas, A., Thorvaldsen, P., & Tuomilehto, J. (1997). Stroke incidence and mortality correlated to stroke risk factors in the WHO MONICA Project: An ecological study of 18 populations. *Stroke, 28*, 1367–1374.

Stegmayr, B., Harmsen, P., Rajakangas, A. M., Rastenyté, D., Sarti, C., Thorvaldsen, P., & Tuomilehto, J. (1996). Stroke around the Baltic Sea: Incidence, case fatality and population risk factors in Denmark, Finland, Sweden and Lithuania. *Cerebrovascular Disease, 6*, 80–88.

Stergiou, G. S., Thomopoulou, G. C., Skeva, I. I., & Mountokalakis, T. D. (1999). Prevalence, awareness, treatment, and control of hypertension in Greece: The Didima study. *American Journal of Hypertension, 12*, 959–965.

Steyn, K., Gaziano, T. A., Bradshaw, D., Laubscher, R., & Fourie, J. (2001). South African Demographic and Health Coordinating Team. Hypertension in South African adults: Results from the demographic and health survey, 1998. *Journal of Hypertension, 19*, 1717–1725.

Stranges, S., Wu, T., Dorn, J. M., Freudenheim, J. L., Muti, P., Farinaro, E., ... Trevisan, M. (2004). Relationship of alcohol drinking pattern to the risk of hypertension: A population-based study. *Hypertension, 44*, 813–819.

Sulbaran, T., Silva, E., Calmon, G., & Vegas, A. (2000). Epidemiologic aspects of arterial hypertension in Maracaibo, Venezuela. *Journal of Human Hypertension, 14,* S6–S9.

Thamm, M. (1999). Blood pressure in Germany: Current status and trends. *Gesundheitswesen, 61,* S90–S93.

Tomson, J., & Lip, G. Y. H. (2006). Alcohol and hypertension: An old relationship revisited. *Alcohol and Alcoholism, 41*(1), 3–4.

Touyz, R. M., & Briones, A. M. (2011). Reactive oxygen species and vascular biology: Implications in human hypertension. *Hypertension Research, 34,* 5–14.

Treiber, F. A., Jackson, R. W., Davis, H., Pollock, J. S., Kapuku, G., Mensah, G. A., & Pollock, D. M. (2000). Racial differences in Endothelin-1 at rest and in response to acute stress in adolescent males. *Hypertension, 35,* 72–725.

Trumbo, P. R., & Ellwood, K. C. (2007). Supplemental calcium and risk reduction of hypertension, pregnancy-induced hypertension, and preeclampsia: An evidence-based review by the US Food and Drug Administration. *Nutrition Reviews, 65,* 78–87.

van Mierlo, L. A., Arends, L. R., Streppel, M. T., Zeegers, M. P., Kok, F. J., Grobbee, D. E., & Geleijnse, J. M. (2006). Blood pressure response to calcium supplementation: A meta-analysis of randomized controlled trials. *Journal of Human Hypertension, 20*(8), 571–580.

Wang, H., Naghavi, M., & GBD 2015 Mortality and Causes of Death Collaborators. (2016). Global, regional, and national life expectancy, all-cause mortality, and cause-specific mortality for 249 causes of death, 1980–2015: A systematic analysis for the Global Burden of Disease Study 2015. *The Lancet, 388*(10053), 1459–1544.

Weinberger, M. H. (1993). Racial differences in renal sodium excretion: Relationship to hypertension. *American Journal of Kidney Diseases, 21*(4), 41–45.

Welborn, T. A., Breckenridge, A., Rubinstein, A. H., Dollery, C. T., & Fraser, T. R. (1966). Serum-insulin in essential hypertension and in peripheral vascular disease. *Lancet, 1,* 1136–1137.

Whelton, P. K. (1994). Epidemiology of hypertension. *Lancet, 334,* 101–106.

Whelton, P. K., Carey, R. M., Aronow, W. S., Casey, D. E., Jr., Collins, K. J., Dennison Himmelfarb, C., … Wright, J. T., Jr. (2017). Guideline for the prevention, detection, evaluation, and management of high blood pressure in adults: Executive summary: A report of the American College of Cardiology/American Heart Association Task Force on Clinical Practice Guidelines. *Hypertension, 71*(6), 1269–1364.

Whelton, P. K., Perneger, T. V., Klag, M. J., & Brancati, F. L. (1992). Epidemiology and prevention of blood pressure-related renal disease. *Journal of Hypertension, 10*(Suppl. 7), S77–S84.

Whitworth, J. A., Brown, M. A., Kelly, J. J., & Williamson, P. M. (1995). Mechanisms of cortisol-induced hypertension in humans. *Steroids, 60*(1), 76–80.

Wilsgaard, T., Schirmer, H., & Arnesen, E. (2000). Impact of body weight on blood pressure with a focus on sex differences: The Tromso Study, 1986–1995. *Archives of Internal Medicine, 160*(18), 2847–2853.

Wolf-Maier, K., Cooper, R. S., Banegas, J. R., Giampaoli, S., Hense, H., Joffres, M., … Vescio, F. (2003). Hypertension and blood pressure levels in 6 European countries, Canada, and the US. *JAMA, 289,* 2363–2369.

Wolf-Maier, K., Cooper, R. S., Kramer, H., Banegas, J. R., Giampaoli, S., Joffres, M. R., … Thamm, M. (2004). Hypertension treatment and control in five European countries, Canada and the United States. *Hypertension, 43,* 10–17.

Wolz, M., Cutler, J., Roccella, E. J., Rohde, F., Thom, T., & Burt, V. (2000). Statement from the National High Blood Pressure Education Program: Prevalence of hypertension. *American Journal of Hypertension, 13,* 103–104.

Working Group on Primary Prevention of Hypertension. (1993). Report of the National High Blood Pressure Education Program Working Group on Primary Prevention of Hypertension. *Archives of Internal Medicine, 153,* 186–208.

Xin, X., He, J., Frontini, M. G., Ogden, L. G., Motsamai, O. I., & Whelton, P. K. (2001). Effects of alcohol reduction on blood pressure. *Hypertension, 38,* 1112–1117.

Yanagisawa, M., Kurihara, H., & Kimura, S. (1988). A novel potent vasoconstrictor peptide produced by vascular endothelial cells. *Nature, 332,* 411–415.

Zavaroni, I., Mazza, S., Dall'Aglio, E., Gasparini, P., Passeri, M., & Reaven, G. M. (1992). Prevalence of hyperinsulinaemia in patients with high blood pressure. *Journal of Internal Medicine, 231,* 235–240.

Zhu, X., Chang, Y. P. C., Yan, D., Weder, A., Cooper, R., Luke, A., … Chakravarti, A. (2003). Associations between hypertension and genes in the renin-angiotensin system. *Hypertension, 41,* 1027–1034.

Epidemiology of Cancer

© Andrew Brookes/Getty Images

CHAPTER 11

Pathogenesis of Cancer

Zachary M. Harris and Randall E. Harris

▶ Biological Basis of Cancer

Cancer is the uncontrolled growth and spread of abnormal cells in the body. Cancers (malignant neoplasms) can arise from virtually any tissue and are usually named by the anatomic site of origin. Examples include breast cancer, prostate cancer, colon cancer, and lung cancer, the four cancers responsible for most cancer deaths in many developed nations such as the United States. Cancer cells can divide continuously, invade other tissues, and spread (metastasize) to other organs through the blood and lymph. These primary features (uncontrolled cell division, invasion of contiguous tissue, and metastasis) distinguish cancerous growths from noncancerous (benign) cellular growths, the latter being self-limiting with no ability to invade tissue or metastasize.

Cancer is further defined according to the cell of origin based on microscopic examination by pathologists. Adenocarcinomas arise from the cuboidal epithelial cells that line the ducts of glandular tissue (e.g., adenocarcinomas of the breast, prostate, colon, or lung). Squamous cell carcinomas arise from the flat pavement cells that cover the skin and line portals of entry or exit in the human body (e.g., squamous cell carcinomas of the oral cavity, upper airways, esophagus, uterine cervix, urinary tract, or anus). Sarcomas arise from connective tissue (fibrosarcoma) or bone (osteosarcoma). Malignant gliomas arise from glial cells that provide vital support to neurons in the central nervous system. Adenocarcinomas, squamous cell carcinomas, sarcomas, and gliomas are solid tumors, as opposed to cancerous growths of immune cells that arise in the bone marrow (leukemias) or the lymph nodes (lymphomas) and circulate in the blood or the lymphatic system.

▶ Evolution of Cancer

Solid cancerous growths (tumors) develop most often from cells of the epithelial lining of organs of the body (e.g., lungs, colon, breast, prostate), and less often from dividing cells of muscle, bone, and the central nervous system. The evolution of solid tumors is thought to be a long-term process spanning many years and often decades.

The hematopoietic (blood) cancers (leukemias, lymphomas) arise from lymphocytes, granulocytes, or other dividing cells of the bone marrow and the lymphatic system. Leukemias and lymphomas develop much more rapidly than solid tumors, perhaps over the span of a few months or even weeks.

▶ Cell Division (Mitosis) and Cancer

Approximately 90% of all cancers are solid tumors that originate in the epithelial lining of various organs of the gastrointestinal tract (oral cavity, esophagus, stomach, liver, pancreas, colon, rectum), the genitourinary tract (kidney, urinary bladder, uterine cervix, vagina), and the reproductive tract (breast, ovary, prostate). Solid tumors called *basal cell carcinomas* can also arise from the stratified (layered) epithelial covering of the skin. Collectively, all epithelial-derived tumors are called *carcinomas*.

In sharp contrast to epithelial-derived carcinomas, only about 8% of malignant neoplasms arise from cells of the immune system (lymphomas and leukemias), less than 2% arise from connective tissues (sarcomas of muscle, bone, and fat), and less than 1% develop in the central nervous system (gliomas and meningiomas). This distinct histologic pattern of cancer appears to be driven to a large extent by the relatively high cell-division rates of epithelial and hematopoietic cell populations compared to connective tissue and the central nervous system. Periods of increased cell division during the life span also increase the likelihood of cancer development; for example, sarcomas of connective tissues arise in conjunction with bursts of cell division in fat and muscle cell populations and the elongation of bones during the early developmental years. Clearly, cancer is more likely to develop in those cell populations with higher rates of cell division. "In general, the greater the replicative activity, the greater the cancer risk" (Robbins & Cotran, 1979).

▶ Cancer and the Cell Cycle

Cancer can be succinctly defined as "deranged cell division." In cancer research, it is thus important to understand fundamental characteristics of the cell-division cycle. In humans, normal cell division is an extraordinarily complex process whereby a progenitor (mother) cell forms two replicate daughter cells. In this remarkable miracle of nature, amino acids are efficiently transformed into millions of proteins and enzymes necessary for DNA replication, chromosomal formation, and reproduction of all the working parts of the newly created cells.

Normal Cell Division and Cell Cycle

The human cell cycle consists of a preparatory phase of nutrient and energy buildup (G1 phase), DNA synthesis and replication of double-stranded DNA (S phase), condensation of DNA into 46 chromosomes and preparation for mitosis (G2 phase), and segregation of chromosomes to create two genetically equivalent daughter cells (mitosis or M phase) (**FIGURE 11.1**). Cytokinesis takes place after the segregation of chromosomes and is the final event in the cell-division cycle. During cytokinesis, the cytoplasm and cytoplasmic organelles (e.g., mitochondria, Golgi apparatus, endoplasmic reticulum, ribosomes, lysosomes) are equally distributed to create two daughter cells with chromosomes, cytoplasm, organelles, nuclear and plasma membranes, and microtubular cytoskeletons that are virtual mirror images.

Progression through the cell cycle is tightly regulated by a family of genes called *cyclins* and the proteins they encode. Cyclins are activated by the docking of hormones, growth factors, and other extracellular

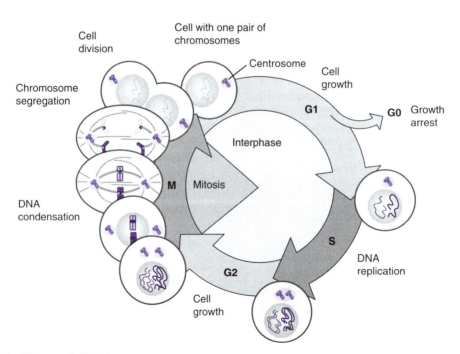

FIGURE 11.1 Model of Human Cell Cycle.

signaling molecules to cell-surface receptors that trigger events inside the cell, a process known as *signal transduction*. Extracellular signaling molecules that modulate cell division include hormones of the endocrine system (e.g., estrogen, progesterone, testosterone, and thyroxine), paracrine factors that act locally (e.g., growth factors, cytokines, and prostaglandins), and autocrine factors released by the cells themselves (e.g., certain interleukins) (Hancock, 2010).

The cyclin proteins bind to cyclin-dependent kinases (CDKs), which modulate the passage of the cell through the sequential phases of the cell-division cycle. The cyclins and CDKs function by phosphorylation of signaling proteins that regulate transcription and translation of genes essential for cell division. Furthermore, inhibitors of CDK encoded by specific genes (e.g., p53, RB, p27, APC, CHEK1, CHEK2) function as *gatekeepers* of error-free DNA synthesis by facilitating repair of any DNA-coding errors that occurred during the S phase of the cell-division cycle (Deninger, 1999).

One very important gatekeeper gene, p53, encodes a protein that checks for errors or damage in newly replicated DNA near the end of the S phase of the cell-division cycle. As shown in the schematic of **FIGURE 11.2**, the p53 protein prompts the enzymatic repair of DNA damage before the cell progresses through the final steps of cell division. If excess DNA damage is detected, the cell undergoes apoptosis (programmed cell death), thereby preventing the proliferation of abnormal cells. In the absence of normal p53 function, cells with DNA damage (or mutations that predispose to cancer development) may continue to grow and divide (Figure 11.2). Because of its important role in eliminating mutant cells and conserving genomic stability, the p53 gene has been deemed the "guardian of the human genome" (Efeyan & Serrano, 2007).

G0 (Functional) Phase of the Cell Cycle

The G0 phase of the cell cycle is the nonreplicating "functional" period of the cell. During G0, newly formed cells undergo differentiation and carry out their designated functions; for example, epithelial cells produce and secrete proteins and glycoproteins, inflammatory cells produce and secrete prostaglandins and cytokines, immune cells produce and secrete antibodies, muscle cells exert contractile energy, skeletal cells provide structural support, fat cells store energy, endocrine cells secrete hormones, endothelial cells maintain blood pressure and water balance, neurons conduct impulses, and so on. The human body consists of trillions of cells that respond synchronously to changes in environmental conditions to maintain internal equilibrium (homeostasis) of life-sustaining functions.

▶ Life Spans of Human Cells

The life spans and G0 phases of different types of cells are highly variable. In recent studies, isotopic (C^{14}) carbon dating has been used to accurately estimate the life spans of different cell types. These investigations

Normal p53

DNA is damaged by heat, radiation, or chemicals

p53 delays cell division and triggers enzymes to repair damaged DNA

p53 monitors daughter cells: those with repaired DNA are allowed to divide (top branch); those with DNA damage beyond repair are marked for destruction (bottom branch).

Abnormal p53

Cancer cell

Mutated p53 allows cells with damaged DNA to divide. Cells with accumulating DNA damage may become cancerous.

FIGURE 11.2 Mechanism of Action of p53 in Cell Division.

confirm the wide range of normal cell life spans; for example, intestinal epithelial cells live only a few days, skin epithelial cells live a few weeks, lymphocytes live for months, macrophages live for years, muscle and fat cells live for decades, and nerve cells (neurons) live for the entire life span of the human host (Spalding, Bhardwaj, Buchholz, Druid, & Frisén, 2005).

▶ Turnover of Human Cells

Populations of cells with relatively short life spans continuously undergo rapid self-renewal and have considerable regenerative capacity. The turnover rate of a given cell population depends on the delicate balance between the rate of programmed cell death (apoptosis) and the rate of cell replacement by cell division (mitosis) of progenitor cells (stem cells). Factors that upset this balance may lead to malignant transformation (Pellettieri & Alvarado, 2007).

Most epithelial cell populations continuously self-renew during adult life and have relatively short turnover times. Under normal physiologic conditions, intestinal epithelium turns over (is replaced) within about 5 days, skin epithelium within about 1 month, and lung epithelium within about 6 months. In general, cell populations that have fast and furious rates of cell turnover are more prone to cancer development than those that turn over more slowly (Blanpain, Horsley, & Fuchs, 2007).

Cells of the immune system are continuously formed from progenitor cells (stem cells) in the bone marrow by a process called *hematopoiesis*. However, mature immune cells ordinarily do not divide unless stimulated by inflammation or infection and have relatively long life spans (months or years). It is during periods of accelerated cell division that cells of the immune system are most likely to undergo malignant transformation.

Throughout the early years of life, and especially during puberty, the cell populations of bone, muscle, and fat show high mitotic rates in conjunction with rapid growth and development, after which cell populations stabilize and cell division subsides. Indeed, cells of mature connective tissues divide infrequently and tend to have long life spans. Fat cells (adipocytes) and muscle cells divide only occasionally to replace about 5% of their respective cell populations every year. Bone undergoes continuous remodeling throughout life whereby old bone is resorbed by cells called osteoclasts and new bone is formed by osteoblasts; however, this process replaces less than 10% of skeletal cells annually. Some cells do not undergo mitotic division and therefore rarely form malignant

neoplasms (e.g., neurons of the central nervous system and cells of cardiac and skeletal muscle) (Spalding et al., 2005).

▶ Evolution of Cancer in the Human Host

In epithelial cell populations, normal cell division is restricted to stem cells that are in contact with the basement membrane. Mitosis of an epithelial stem cell produces one new stem cell, which remains in contact with the basement membrane and therefore retains replicative potential, and one new daughter cell that loses contact with the basement membrane and matures and differentiates into a functional cell. As newly formed daughter cells migrate to higher layers of stratified epithelium, they eventually undergo programmed cell death, which is called *apoptosis*, and are sloughed off at the surface (Marshman, Booth, & Potten, 2002).

The normal pattern of epithelial cell replacement is distinctly different from carcinomas, where the cancer cells divide indefinitely and fail to undergo apoptosis. The evolution of a solid cancerous tumor proceeds through a continuum of steps, wherein cells undergo visible morphological changes of the nucleus and cytoplasm (Holowaty, Miller, Rohan, & To, 1999; Kumar, Abbas, & Aster, 2014). The following paragraphs provide a brief description of the cell types that appear during the evolution of cancer. The progression of normal epithelial cells to invasive cancer is depicted for the epithelium of the uterine cervix in **FIGURE 11.3**.

Dysplasia (Premalignant Lesions)

Dysplasia is a distinct benign growth that arises from the epithelial cells lining various organs. In dysplasia, the cell nucleus becomes prominent, the cytoplasm appears swollen and vacuolated, and the cells exhibit increased rates of cell division and disordered maturation.

Dysplasia invariably precedes the development of cancer, and dysplastic lesions that serve as precursors of cancer can be detected at several anatomic sites. Examples of premalignant lesions include actinic keratosis of the skin, leukoplakia of the oral cavity, Barrett's esophagus, fibrocystic disease with atypia of the breast, adenomatous polyps of the colon, dysplasia of the prostate, and intraepithelial neoplasia of the uterine cervix. Fortunately, all such dysplastic lesions do not have the ability to invade or metastasize and they are curable by surgical excision or other methods of

Partially transformed cell

1 An epithelial cell becomes partially transformed.

Blood vessels

Lymph vessel

2 This cell multiplies, forming a mass of dysplastic cells.

3 These dysplastic cells grow rapidly, forming a localized cancerous tumor.

4 The cancer cells secrete chemicals that allow them access to other tissues, the lymphatic system, and the bloodstream.

Cancer cell secretions

FIGURE 11.3 Progression of Normal Cervical Epithelium to Invasive Cancer.

ablation. Clearly, the early detection and treatment of such lesions is an important component of effective cancer control.

Carcinoma In Situ

When solid cancerous tumors arise, they are at first confined to their original location and have not broken through the basement membranes into surrounding tissues. A confined neoplasm of the epithelial cell layer is thus called *carcinoma in situ (CIS)*. Such in situ lesions represent a defined step in cancer evolution. They exhibit all the features of malignancy except invasiveness and metastasis; namely, the cells of in situ neoplasms manifest unchecked mitosis and proliferation, maturation failure and resistance to death, and disordered organization of the cell population. And yet, the in situ neoplasm is theoretically curable by excision because it has not spread beyond its original location and is contained by the basement membrane.

Invasive Cancer

In contrast to in situ neoplasms, invasive cancers have broken through the basement membrane to spread beyond their original location into contiguous tissues. This is a critical step in the evolution of cancer because surgical excision may no longer be effective as a form of cancer therapy. The breach of the basement membranes by cancer cells requires acquisition of certain new functions (e.g., the secretion of proteolytic enzymes that degrade basement membranes).

Metastatic Cancer

Metastatic disease represents the final step in the evolution of cancer. Cancer cells first invade contiguous tissues, and then spread through lymphatic channels and blood vessels to other anatomic sites. Cancer causes death by metastasizing (spreading) to vital organs such as the liver, brain, and spine. It is within these vital organs that the cancer cells overwhelm the normal cellular constituency, resulting in the collapse of their life-sustaining functions. Early detection prior to the development of invasive cancer and metastasis is therefore vitally important to the successful treatment and survival of cancer patients. The entire process of cancer development often goes unheeded and undetected by the human immune system over a period of many years; hence the term *silent killer* has been aptly applied to describe cancer in its various forms.

▶ Theories of Carcinogenesis

Cancerous growths result from a complex process known collectively as *carcinogenesis*. Although numerous theories of carcinogenesis have been proposed, considerable controversy exists as to which one is correct. Nevertheless, there is reasonable consensus that carcinogenesis is definable as a disease of the genes or a "DNA disease." Although genetic changes are ultimately responsible for the uncontrolled cell division and aberrant growth dynamics that characterize all forms of cancer, this does not imply that cancer-predisposing genetic alterations are heritable. In fact, about 95% of malignant neoplasms arise due to non-heritable genetic alterations acquired during the life span rather than inherited cancer-predisposing genes. Two main theories of carcinogenesis are discussed in

this text: The *somatic mutation theory* and the *epigenetic theory*.

Somatic Mutation Theory of Cancer

Because a variety of genetic (DNA) mutations have been identified through molecular studies of cancerous tissues (Fearon & Vogelstein, 1990), the process of carcinogenesis is considered by many to result from the accumulation of two or more somatic mutations that impact upon control of the cell cycle or other features of neoplastic development (Knudson, 2001). This idea was first proposed in 1953 by Carl Nordling in Sweden, who stated that the cancerous cell contains not one but a number of mutated genes. The occurrence of such accumulations of mutations may be expected to increase according to a certain exponent of age as well as according to the increase of cell proliferation (Nordling, 1953).

In 1971, Alfred Knudson published a study of 48 cases of retinoblastoma, a devastating tumor of the retina that occurs primarily in children under 5 years of age. Based on the time sequence of tumors in these cases, Knudson hypothesized that retinoblastoma arises from two sequential mutational events. In the heritable form, a mutated gene is inherited from one parent and the second occurs in somatic cells of the retina. In the nonheritable form, both mutations occur in somatic cells of the retina (Knudson, 1971). The mutated retinoblastoma gene, Rb1, was later discovered by a team of investigators in Boston (Dryja, Friend, & Weinberg, 1986). The Rb1 gene was the first tumor suppressor-gene ever discovered, and Knudson's two-hit mutation theory of retinoblastoma has been generalized as the *somatic mutation theory of cancer*.

Somatic mutations are base-pair changes in DNA that occur during the human life span in cells of the body, in contrast to mutations that are "inherited" from parents through the germline. The somatic mutation theory of cancer is based on the premise that cancer arises from a single somatic cell and that tumor progression and development involve the accumulation of multiple DNA mutations that occur as the abnormal cells continue to replicate over time. It is postulated (but not proven) that with each successive mutation, the evolving clone of cancer cells acquires new properties that favorably impact tumor growth, invasion of contiguous tissues, and eventually metastasis to other anatomic sites.

Although the somatic mutation theory of cancer is the dominant paradigm of carcinogenesis, the emerging molecular evidence is not entirely consistent with this model. For example, many cancers arise without evidence of accumulating somatic mutations, and studies of precancerous and cancerous tissues often fail to disclose either chromosomal aberrations or mutated tumor–suppressor genes and oncogenes (Soto & Sonnenschein, 2004). Furthermore, mutational events that are identified in cancerous tissues may have occurred late in tumor development as the result of cancer development, rather than being the cause (Lijinsy, 1989; Loeb, Loeb, & Anderson, 2003; Prehn, 1994).

Epigenetic Theory of Cancer

The existing scientific evidence is inconsistent with the hypothesis that cancer always arises from a single "mutated" cell and progresses due to accumulation of subsequent mutations that confer a survival advantage to cancer cells. An alternative hypothesis, the *epigenetic theory of cancer*, proposes that cancer develops due to activation or deactivation of certain genes that have a major impact on mechanisms of cell survival and cell division, *but in the absence of mutations that alter the DNA sequence* (Momparler, 2003; Verma, Maruvada, & Srivastara, 2004). Any process that modifies the expression of genes that control major mechanisms of cancer development (e.g., mitosis, apoptosis, angiogenesis, mutagenesis, immunosuppression, and metastasis) could obviously fuel the process of cancer development.

In the epigenetic theory, there is no change in the underlying base-pair sequence of the DNA; rather, nongenetic factors of the cellular microenvironment cause genes to be expressed differently. Epigenetic programming involves chemical reactions such as the addition or removal of methyl groups (CH_3) or acetyl groups (NH_2) to/from DNA or histones that alter the conformation of the DNA and determine whether genes are expressed or suppressed.

The best-known example of programmed epigenetic changes in human biology is the process of cellular differentiation that occurs during embryogenesis. During embryogenesis, a single fertilized egg with a fixed genotype undergoes continuous mitosis and cell differentiation, leading to cell lineages consisting of billions of cells with extraordinarily diverse phenotypes (e.g., neurons, blood vessels, muscles, bones, epithelium). Cell differentiation produces such phenotypic diversity through programmed activation and inactivation of different sets of genes. Thus, differentiated cells in multicellular organisms express only the genes that are necessary for their own phenotypic activity. Furthermore, once a cell lineage becomes fully differentiated and mature, its inherent epigenetic

pattern of genetic expression is usually preserved over multiple generations of cell division throughout the human life span. Nevertheless, certain molecular factors are capable of disrupting the normal epigenetic phenotype of a cell population, giving rise to mechanisms that initiate and promote the development of malignant tumors. Molecular mechanisms responsible for the genesis of specific forms of cancer are addressed in the next section.

▶ Molecular Mechanisms of Carcinogenesis

Several molecular mechanisms, acting either alone or in combination, are likely responsible for the initiation and promotion of carcinogenesis in a given individual. These mechanisms can be broadly categorized into six distinct groups: *Mutagenesis, mitogenesis, angiogenesis, metastasis, inhibition of apoptosis,* and *immunosuppression* with reduced antineoplastic activity of T and B lymphocytes. A brief overview of each of these mechanisms is given in the following sections. More thorough reviews can be found in the literature (Howe, Subbaramaiah, Brown, & Dannenberg, 2001; Shiff & Rigas, 1999).

Mutagenesis
Germline and Somatic Mutations

Gene mutations can be either inherited from a parent or acquired during a person's lifetime. Mutations that are passed from parent to offspring are called hereditary mutations or *germline mutations* (because they are present in the egg and sperm cells, which are also called germ cells).

Somatic mutations occur in the DNA of individual cells at some time during the life span. Somatic mutations can be caused by environmental factors such as ionizing radiation from the sun or free radical compounds formed by physiologic processes such as lipid peroxidation, or they can result from spontaneous errors that occur during DNA replication in the cell cycle. Acquired mutations in somatic cells (cells other than germ cells) cannot be passed on to the next generation (**FIGURE 11.4**).

Mutations that occur only in an egg or a sperm cell, or those that occur just after fertilization, are called *de novo mutations*. A genetic disorder in which an affected individual has a mutation in every cell but has no family history of the disorder may be attributable to a de novo mutation.

Somatic Mutation
Occurs in nongermline cells
Nonheritable
Mutation present in tumor only

Nonheritable mutation

Germline Mutation
Occurs in egg or sperm
Heritable
Mutation present in all cells of offspring

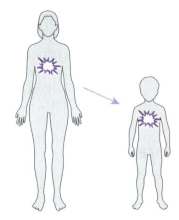

Heritable mutation

FIGURE 11.4 Somatic and Germline Mutations.

Mutations and Cancer

Accumulated mutagenic damage to DNA is believed to contribute substantially to the etiology of cancer; and it is indeed true that hundreds of genetic alterations have been identified that appear to influence carcinogenesis. Nevertheless, the form and timing of genetic alterations that spur the initiation, growth, and development of neoplastic cell populations remain elusive (Ames, Durston, Yamasaki, & Lee, 1973; Armitage & Doll, 1956; Cairns, 1975; Knudson, 1971; Loeb et al., 2003).

Subtypes of Genetic Alterations

Genetic alterations that have been found to influence carcinogenesis are divisible into distinct subtypes. They include (1) subtle base-pair changes that alter gene function, (2) cytogenetically observable alterations in chromosome number (gain or loss of chromosomes) that produce genetic instability, (3) chromosomal translocations that create fusion genes that enhance neoplastic transformation, and (4) gene amplification whereby multiple copies of cancer-promoting genes are overexpressed. It is notable that genetic alterations are a common feature of most forms of cancer but not of normal cell populations (Lengauer, Kinzler, & Vogelstein, 1998).

Causes of Mutagenesis

Mutations may be caused by exposure to both intrinsic and extrinsic factors. Several natural intrinsic physiologic processes generate reactive oxygen species that have mutagenic potential. Chief among them are aerobic respiration (oxidative phosphorylation), anaerobic respiration (glycolysis), lipid peroxidation, and chronic inflammation.

Intrinsic Mutagens

Aerobic respiration (*oxidative phosphorylation*) converts glucose to the high-energy compound adenosine triphosphate (ATP) in the mitochondria of the cytoplasm. The process of oxidative phosphorylation, which involves the flow of high-energy electrons through the electron transport chain, continuously generates DNA-damaging reactive oxygen species such as hydrogen peroxide, superoxide, and hydroxyl radicals. Because mitochondria contain haploid DNA unprotected by histones, mitochondrial DNA is highly vulnerable to oxidative damage mediated by persistent exposure to these compounds (Griffiths, Doudican, Shadel, & Doetsch, 2009).

The *Warburg Effect*, discovered by Otto Warburg and colleagues in 1924, describes the switch from oxidation phosphorylation to anaerobic respiration (glycolysis and lactate fermentation) for energy production in a wide spectrum of cancer cells (Warburg, 1956; Warburg, Posener, & Negelein, 1924). Warburg observed that cancer cells exhibit a high rate of glycolysis even in the presence of oxygen (*aerobic glycolysis*), a process that supplies energy for rapid cancer-cell proliferation (Lunt & Vander Heiden, 2011). Although rapid cell proliferation per se may enhance mutagenesis of nuclear DNA, recent studies suggest that the diminution of reactive oxygen species with transition from oxidative phosphorylation to aerobic glycolysis may actually protect the mitochondrial DNA from damage (Ericson et al., 2012).

It is well known that the oxidative biodegradation of lipids (*lipid peroxidation*) in the human system generates reactive electrophilic compounds that have mutagenic potential. For example, malondialdehyde is a naturally occurring product of lipid peroxidation that is both mutagenic and carcinogenic (Marnett, 1999). Lipid peroxidation of polyunsaturated fatty acids is a self-propagating chain reaction that generates a variety of reactive oxygen species that are capable of interacting with DNA to cause mutations (Burcham, 1998).

Chronic inflammation stimulates the release of reactive oxygen species and reactive nitrogen species, which can interact with DNA to cause mutations. Furthermore, spontaneous breakdown of prostaglandins of the prostaglandin cascade produce the mutagenic agent malondialdehyde, which reacts with DNA under physiological conditions to form DNA adducts. Prolonged chemical exposures, persistent foreign bodies, chronic infection, and obesity are all causes of chronic inflammation (Ferguson, 2010).

The normal process of cell division has an intrinsic form of mutagenesis (Burnett, 1974). With every cell division there is incomplete duplication of the chromosomal tips (called telomeres). Successive cell divisions in a cell lineage therefore result in shortening of DNA until a point is reached where the daughter cells are no longer capable of dividing (called the *Hayflick limit*). This intrinsic mutational event is the basis for the *telomere theory of aging*—namely, as an ever-increasing percentage of cells reach their Hayflick limit and are unable to replicate, the defense, maintenance, and repair mechanisms of the body become increasingly impaired (Hayflick, 1985, 2007).

Extrinsic Mutagens

Exogenous mutagenic factors include ionizing radiation, infectious agents, and certain chemicals found in some foods, beverages, drugs, and complex mixtures such as tobacco smoke and polluted air. Ionizing radiation carries enough kinetic energy to cause breaks and other damage in double-stranded DNA. Sources of ionizing radiation include cosmic rays from the sun, radon decay products from rock, medical X-rays, fallout from nuclear weapons, and discharges of radioactive waste from nuclear reactors. Light from the sun that reaches the earth is primarily nonionizing because ionizing rays are largely filtered out by ozone and other gases in the atmosphere. However, nonionizing ultraviolet rays may also induce DNA mutations by photochemical reactions (Doll, 1995; Gilbert, 2009).

Various infectious agents have strong mutagenic potential, particularly viruses that use the host DNA for replication (e.g., human immunodeficiency virus [HIV], human papillomaviruses [HPVs], hepatitis viruses, Kaposi's sarcoma virus, and Epstein–Barr virus). Such viruses have the ability to incorporate their genomes into human DNA, thereby causing structural changes and modification of gene expression. For example, integrated viral genes may encode proteins that bind to and inactivate the host tumor suppressor-gene products that normally provide checks and balances on the cell cycle and thereby regular cell growth (zur Hausen, 1991). Furthermore, some viruses such as simian virus 40 (SV40) contain *oncogenes* that induce cancerous changes in the host cell (Bocchetta, Miele, Pass, & Carbone, 2003).

Tobacco smoke is a complex mixture of more than 5000 gases and compounds, many of which are carcinogenic and/or mutagenic. Tobacco smoke contains three major classes of mutagenic substances: Polycyclic aromatic hydrocarbons, nitrosamines, and heterocyclic amines. The metabolism of tobacco carcinogens is complex and involves activation versus detoxification by liver enzymes. The carcinogens of tobacco smoke, their uptake and metabolism, and the mechanisms by which they cause DNA mutations and DNA damage have been thoroughly discussed elsewhere (Hecht, 1999).

Food and beverages may also contain mutagenic agents. Notably, thermic reactions during cooking of meat can form mutagenic compounds such as heterocyclic amines and polycyclic aromatic hydrocarbons. Metabolic activation of such compounds by liver enzymes may increase their mutagenic potency. Grains and other foods may be contaminated with molds, fungal organisms, or bacteria that produce toxic substances with mutagenic properties; for example, ingestion of grain contaminated by the mold *Aspergillus flavus* results in exposure to the mycotoxin aflatoxin B1, which is highly mutagenic to hepatocytes. Food preservatives such as sodium nitrite may be metabolized in the stomach to form nitrosamines with mutagenic and carcinogenic properties. Ethanol present in alcoholic beverages has been classified as a human carcinogen by the International Agency for Research on Cancer (IARC). Dioxins with carcinogenic properties have been identified in foods and beverages. Heavy salt intake may damage the gastric epithelium and promote mutagenesis and carcinogenesis. Finally, excessive consumption of omega-6 polyunsaturated fatty acids may promote mutagenesis and carcinogenesis by enhancing chronic activation of the inflammatory cascade and the formation of reactive oxygen species (Sugimura, 2000).

Mitogenesis

Mitogens are factors that stimulate cell division (mitosis). There are a multitude of such factors that are both intrinsic and extrinsic to the human system. Intrinsic mitogens include hormones of the endocrine system and growth factors and cytokines that exert primarily paracrine effects. Whereas *endocrine* factors (hormones) travel through the blood to exert their effects, *paracrine* factors are secreted into the microenvironment near the cell producing them to elicit local cellular responses. A special form of cell signaling involves *autocrine* factors that bind to receptors on the secreting cell to elicit cell division or changes (**FIGURE 11.5**). Hormones can be either steroids or polypeptides, whereas virtually all growth factors and cytokines are polypeptides.

Endocrine Factors

The human endocrine system is highly complex and consists of multiple secreting and responding organs and tissues (e.g., the central nervous system, the hypothalamic-pituitary axis, the thyroid and parathyroid glands, the thymus, the adrenal glands, the lungs, the gastrointestinal tract, the liver, the pancreas, the kidneys, the bone marrow, gonadal organs of the reproductive tract, and the immune system). A few examples of important endocrine factors with mitogenic activity are presented here.

Steroidal hormones (estrogen, progesterone, testosterone, glucocorticoids, vitamin D_3, and retinoids) are all small lipophilic molecules that easily penetrate both the cellular and nuclear membranes to enter the nucleus, where they bind to their respective receptors that are ligand-dependent transcription factors. These ligand–receptor complexes bind to specific DNA response elements in the promoter regions of genes to regulate gene expression and cell division in target cell populations.

Polypeptide hormones secreted by specific endocrine organs travel through the blood bound to carrier proteins and elicit their responses in distant cell populations. Pituitary hormones with mitogenic impact on their target tissues include growth hormone (GH), thyroid-stimulating hormone (TSH), follicular-stimulating hormone (FSH), luteinizing hormone (LH), and adrenocorticotropic hormone (ACTH). Hormones are released from the pituitary under the influence of releasing hormones secreted by the hypothalamus.

Insulin is a polypeptide hormone secreted by the beta cells in the pancreas that regulates carbohydrate and fat metabolism and induces glucose uptake for energy in muscle cells and storage in fat cells. Insulin also can stimulate the proliferation of fat and smooth muscle cells. Compounds with close homology to insulin, *insulin-like growth factors (IGFs)*, are synthesized and secreted by the liver under the influence of pituitary GH. The IGF compounds make up the *IGF axis*, which promotes cell proliferation and the inhibition of cell death (apoptosis) in a variety of tissues (Le Roith, 1997).

Glucagon is a polypeptide hormone secreted by the alpha cells in the pancreas that induces the breakdown of glycogen and release of glucose into the bloodstream by the liver. The effects of glucagon and insulin therefore counterbalance one another in maintaining normal levels of blood glucose. Glucagon and *glucagon-like factors (GLFs)* have been found

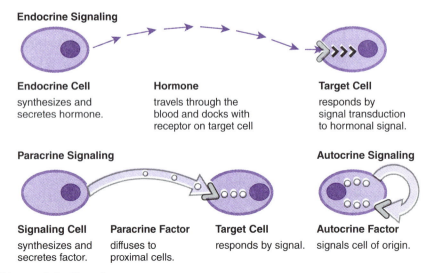

FIGURE 11.5 Types of Intercellular Signaling.

to stimulate the proliferation of intestinal epithelium (Kieffer & Habener, 1999).

Calcitonin and parathyroid hormone are polypeptide hormones synthesized by the thyroid and parathyroid glands, respectively. These hormones coordinate bone remodeling and maintain calcium homeostasis. Calcitonin stimulates bone formation by osteoblasts whereas parathyroid hormone induces bone resorption by osteoclasts (Carter & Schipani, 2006).

Erythropoietin is a hormone that is essential for red blood cell (erythrocyte) production. This glycoprotein is secreted by the kidneys and induces the differentiation and growth of erythrocytes from progenitor cells in the bone marrow.

Paracrine Factors

Several paracrine factors called *growth factors* can also stimulate cell division in certain tissues, particularly sites of wound-healing and inflammation. Examples include epidermal growth factor (EGF), fibroblast growth factor (FGF), transforming growth factors (TGFα and TGFβ), and platelet-derived growth factor (PDGF); there are many others. Each of these mitogens elicits cellular responses through interaction with specific receptor molecules on cell membranes. For example, PDGF induces proliferation of fibroblasts, smooth muscle cells, and monocytes; EGF is mitogenic for fibroblasts and many types of epithelial cells; FGF induces growth and development of blood vessels; and TGFα has mitogenic effects similar to EGF, whereas TGFβ has growth inhibitory effects in many cell populations.

Cytokines are proteins secreted by immune cells that help orchestrate both the induction and effector phases of all immune and inflammatory responses, including cell proliferation, intercellular communication, and cell death. The term *cytokine* is often used specifically to refer to a wide variety of locally acting immunomodulating agents (e.g., interleukins, interferons, tumor necrosis factor) that facilitate the immune response. Nevertheless, certain cytokines effectively spur the proliferation of other cells. For example, specific interleukins secreted by activated T lymphocytes (IL-2 and IL-4) stimulate the clonal expansion of other immune cells in response to viral infection (Dinarello, 2007).

Prostaglandins and *leukotrienes* are short-lived compounds derived from fatty acids that modulate important physiological functions. Prostaglandins, particularly PGE1 and PGE2, are the principal mediators of the inflammatory response, whereas leukotrienes are involved in allergic and asthmatic reactions. Some prostaglandins have potent mitogenic activity in epithelial cell populations; for example, PGE2, the chief prostaglandin of the inflammatory response, stimulates proliferation of the mammary epithelium (Harris, 2007).

Mitogen-Activated Protein Kinase Cascade

Mitogenic hormones and growth factors stimulate cell division by a process known as *signal transduction* in which the mitogen activates specific receptors on the cell membranes of target cells that, in turn, initiate tightly regulated cascades of intracellular signaling by mitogen-activated protein kinases (MAPKs) (**FIGURE 11.6**). Human cells contain multiple MAPK pathways, each consisting of specific cytoplasmic protein kinases that are sequentially phosphorylated. Certain of these protein kinases are translocated into the nucleus, where they induce the expression of genes necessary for cell division. Each MAPK pathway consists of a specific profile of protein kinases that ultimately control cell differentiation, cell proliferation, and cell death in a specific tissue. In humans, more than 500 different protein kinase genes and approximately 50 distinct MAPK cascades have now been identified (Manning, Whyte, Martinez, Hunter, & Sudarsanam, 2002; Pearson et al., 2001).

Extrinsic Factors

In general, any form of cellular injury can result in a mitogenic response by the afflicted tissue. Causative factors of cell injury include microbial infection, physical agents (burns, radiation, trauma), chemical exposures (toxins, caustic substances), ischemia, necrosis, and all types of immunological reactions. All such exposures elicit an immediate inflammatory response of the innate immune system. Although acute inflammation is self-limited and of short duration, chronic inflammation is associated histologically with the persisting presence of immune cells and is nearly always

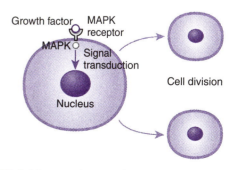

FIGURE 11.6 Mitogen-Activated Protein Kinase (MAPK) Cascade.

accompanied by the proliferation of blood vessels and involved tissues.

Chronic inflammation is maintained by constitutive overexpression of cyclooxygenase-2 (COX-2), which is the rate-limiting enzyme of the prostaglandin cascade. The COX-2 enzyme efficiently catalyzes the conversion of essential dietary fats (principally arachidonic acid and unconjugated linoleic acid) into prostaglandins. Chronic inflammation and continuous overexpression of COX-2 markedly amplify the biosynthesis of PGE-2, which is the chief prostaglandin of the inflammatory cascade. This short-lived intercellular hormone can induce the transcription of specific genes in the nucleus of nearby cells. In particular, PGE-2 has been found to stimulate the transcription of genes that have powerful mitogenic effects (Harris, 2007; Herschman, 2007).

Contact inhibition is a special form of growth control by which cells ordinarily do not divide when in close contact with one another. This phenomenon is regulated by the density of the cell population, the access of cells to nutrients, and protein complexes of beta-catenin and cadherins that control cell-to-cell adhesion. In general, an intact *E-cadherin-catenin complex* maintains normal intercellular adhesion and limits cell division, whereas loss of function of this complex permits or enhances cell proliferation and leads to invasion and metastasis by malignant cells (Wijnhoven, Dinjens, & Pignatelli, 2000).

Angiogenesis

Angiogenesis is a normal and vital physiological process by which new blood vessels develop from pre-existing vessels. *Vascular endothelial growth factor (VEGF)* is a potent stimulant of de novo blood vessel formation (angiogenesis) in a variety of tissues. Once believed to be present only in the endothelial lining of blood vessels, VEGF has now been discovered in virtually all types of cancers. Indeed, the process of angiogenesis is fundamental to the growth, development, and metastatic spread of cancerous tumors (Folkman, 2006; Folkman & Klagsbrun, 1987).

When a tumor outgrows its blood supply, cancer cells secrete VEGF to signal nearby blood vessels, which respond by sprouting new vessels that grow into the tumor (**FIGURE 11.7**). This sprouting process involves the secretion of proteolytic enzymes by the activity is amplified in cancer cells that proliferate indefinitely but is virtually undetectable in normal somatic cells that undergo programmed apoptosis. Maintenance of telomere integrity by telomerase therefore protects cancer cells from apoptosis, and reciprocally, inhibition of telomerase and loss of telomeres elicits an apoptotic response. For this reason, apoptotic factors that selectively target cancer cells may be of value in cancer therapy (Mondello & Scovassi, 2004).

FIGURE 11.7 Angiogenesis Cascade in Tumor Growth and Development.

Suppression of Apoptosis

Apoptosis, or controlled cell death, is an important regulatory mechanism for the maintenance of homeostasis in cell populations. Dysfunctional apoptosis results in immortalization of cells, a key feature of cancer cells. Apoptosis is regulated by an intrinsic pathway that originates inside the cell and an extrinsic pathway that originates outside the cell.

The intrinsic pathway involves mitochondrial release of cytochrome *c* and activation of caspase 9 and other enzymes that destroy the cell. Intrinsic apoptosis is triggered when the expression of two nuclear genes, Bcl-2 and BAX, favors BAX. The extrinsic pathway involves activation of death receptors on the cell membrane by tumor necrosis factors alpha and beta, and other epigenetic factors. This results in activation of caspase 8 and other enzymes that destroy the cell (Lowe & Lin, 2000).

Telomeres are sequences of DNA that cap the ends of eukaryotic chromosomes. In normal cell populations, as mentioned earlier, telomeres are lost from the chromosomal tips with each successive cell division, and eventually cell division ceases and apoptosis occurs. However, in abnormally proliferating cells, a special reverse transcriptase enzyme called *telomerase* replicates the terminal DNA sequence of chromosomes and restores telomeres to the chromosomal tips (**FIGURE 11.8**). Telomerase activity is amplified in cancer cells that proliferate indefinitely but is virtually undetectable in normal somatic cells that undergo programmed apoptosis. Maintenance of telomere integrity by telomerase therefore protects cancer cells from apoptosis, and reciprocally, inhibition of telomerase and loss of telomeres elicits an apoptotic response. For this reason, apoptotic factors that selectively target cancer cells may be of value in cancer therapy (Mondello & Scovassi, 2004).

Metastasis

Metastatic spread of cancer occurs by direct invasion of proximal tissues, lymphatic invasion, and hematogenous dissemination. Epithelial carcinomas develop from cells that are anchored by the basement membrane, a thin collagenous membrane that serves as a mechanical barrier to invasion of underlying tissues by malignant cells. Obviously, a key initial step in the metastatic spread of epithelial tumors is penetration of the basement membrane by cancer cells. Proteolytic enzymes called *matrix metalloproteinases (MMPs)* secreted by cancer cells facilitate penetration of the basement membrane. These zinc-dependent enzymes are important for normal tissue remodeling and repair and are capable of degrading collagen, proteins, and other components of the basement membrane. By secreting MMPs, cancer cells can break through the basement membrane as well as other cell membranes and gain access to underlying tissues, lymphatics, and blood vessels, thereby facilitating cancer metastasis (Deryugina & Quigley, 2006; Itoh & Nagase, 2002) (**FIGURE 11.9**).

The HER-2/neu oncogene is a member of the epidermal growth factor receptor (EGFR) family. It is an important mediator of cancer-cell growth and metastasis. When the HER-2/neu receptor protein is activated, multiple other factors are activated that promote tumor development and metastatic spread of cancer cells. For example, VEGF is secreted to promote the sprouting of new blood vessels (angiogenesis) and MMPs are produced that degrade cell membranes and basement membranes and are thus associated with tumor invasiveness, metastasis, and poor survival. Overexpression of HER-2/neu is now widely used by clinicians as a biomarker of poor prognosis and metastasis for patients with invasive breast cancer, and the HER-2/new

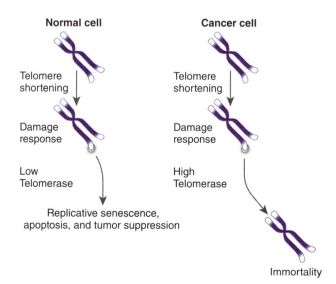

FIGURE 11.8 Telomeres and Apoptosis.

Cancer cells breach the basement membrane, enter the bloodstream, and invade distant tissues by secreting *matrix metalloproteinases* (MMPs) that biodegrade cell membranes.

FIGURE 11.9 Matrix Metalloproteinase (MMP) Activity in Metastatic Cancer.

receptor is a molecular target for breast-cancer therapy (Coussens et al., 1985; Olayioye, 2001).

Immunosuppression

Immunosuppression is a characteristic feature of cancer patients that correlates with disease promotion and progression. Prostaglandins, particularly PGE-2, are important modulators of immunosuppression. Pockaj et al. (2004) found that increased levels of PGE-2 suppress the immunocompetence of helper T-cells and dendritic cells in newly diagnosed breast-cancer patients. Specifically, elevated levels of PGE-2 were associated with reduced secretion of anti-tumor factors by T-cells (interferon gamma, tumor necrosis factor alpha, and interleukins IL-2 and IL-12) and loss of immunocompetence in dendritic cells (reduced secretion of stimulatory molecules, loss of antigen-sensitizing function, reduced phagocytic activity, and lack of maturation potential). Defective T-cell and dendritic cell function due to COX-2–driven PGE-2 biosynthesis is therefore an important mechanism by which tumors evade immunosurveillance.

Inflammogenesis of Cancer

Chronic inflammation can induce untoward epigenetic changes in gene expression leading to cancer development. More than 150 years ago the famous German pathologist, Rudolph Virchow, suggested that chronic inflammation leads to cancer development by increasing uncontrolled cellular proliferation (Balkwill & Mantovani, 2001; Virchow, 1863). Inflammation is the natural response of the immune system to infection, injury, and other forms of irritation. Ordinarily, the inflammatory response is self-limiting and beneficial, resulting in removal of offending factors and restoration of structure and function of the inflamed tissue. Nevertheless, the persistence of inflammatory factors can cause dysregulation of the immune system resulting in chronic inflammation and the development of affiliated conditions such as rheumatoid arthritis, lupus erythematosus, ulcerative colitis, and multiple sclerosis.

Inflammation is regulated by two major classes of compounds (prostaglandins and leukotrienes) that

FIGURE 11.10 Chronic Inflammation and Carcinogenesis.

are secreted by cells of the immune system. These lipid compounds are synthesized from arachidonic acid by the action of two rate-limiting enzymes, cyclooxygenase (COX) and 5-lipoxygenase (LOX). Prostaglandins are derived from the COX pathway and leukotrienes from LOX pathway (Busse, 1998; Ricciotti & FitzGerald, 2011).

Epidemiologic studies have consistently found that regular intake of anti-inflammatory compounds that inhibit COX and/or LOX have significant anticancer effects (Harris, Beebe-Donk, & Alshafie, 2007). Furthermore, molecular studies have linked chronic inflammation and the overexpression of COX and LOX to the development of multiple forms of cancer (Schneider & Pozzi, 2011).

In a recent study, levels of expression of genes encoding the two rate-limiting enzymes of the prostaglandin and leukotriene cascades (COX and LOX) were examined in tumor samples from 1090 women with breast cancer (Kennedy & Harris, 2018). Notably, the mean expression of COX genes ranked above the 99th percentile of all 20,500 genes, and levels of expression of COX and LOX genes were highly correlated with genes that promote all the essential features of carcinogenesis (mutagenesis, mitogenesis, angiogenesis, reduced apoptosis, metastasis, and immunosuppression). The authors suggest that mammary carcinogenesis often evolves as a progressive series of highly specific cellular and molecular changes in response to induction of constitutive overexpression of the prostaglandin and leukotriene cascades in the *inflammogenesis of cancer* (**FIGURE 11.10**).

References

Ames, B. N., Durston, W. E., Yamasaki, E., & Lee, F. D. (1973). Carcinogens are mutagens: A simple test system combining liver homogenates for activation and bacteria for detection. *Proceedings of the National Academy of Sciences of the United States of America, 70*(8), 2281–2285.

Armitage, P., & Doll, R. (1956). The age distribution of cancer and a multi-stage theory of carcinogenesis. *British Journal of Cancer, 8*, 1–12.

Balkwill, F., & Mantovani, A. (2001). Inflammation and cancer: Back to Virchow? *Lancet, 357*, 539–545.

Blanpain, C., Horsley, V., & Fuchs, E. (2007). Epithelial stem cells: Turning over new leaves. *Cell, 128*, 445–458.

Bocchetta, M., Miele, L., Pass, H. I., & Carbone, M. (2003). Notch-1 induction, a novel activity of SV40 required for growth of SV40-transformed human mesothelial cells. *Oncogene, 22*(1), 81–89.

Burcham, P. C. (1998). Genotoxic lipid peroxidation products: Their DNA damaging properties and role in formation of endogenous DNA adducts. *Mutagenesis, 13*(3), 287–305.

Burnett, M. (1974). *Intrinsic mutagenesis.* Lancaster, England: Medical and Technical Publishing Company.

Busse, W. W. (1998). Leukotrienes and inflammation. *American Journal of Respiratory and Critical Care Medicine, 157*(1), 210–218.

Cairns, J. (1975). Mutation selection and the natural history of cancer. *Nature, 255,* 197–200.

Carter, P. H., & Schipani, E. (2006). The roles of parathyroid hormone and calcitonin in bone remodeling: Prospects for novel therapeutics. *Endocrine, Metabolic and Immune Disorders—Drug Targets, 6*(1), 59–76.

Coussens, L., Yang-Feng, T. L., Liao, Y. C., Chen, E., Gray, A., McGrath, J., … Francke, U. (1985). Tyrosine kinase receptor with extensive homology to EGF receptor shares chromosomal location with neu oncogene. *Science, 230*(4730), 1132–1139.

Deninger, P. (1999). Genetic instability in cancer: Caretaker and gatekeeper genes. *Ochsner Journal, 1*(4), 206–209.

Deryugina, E. I., & Quigley, J. P. (2006). Matrix metalloproteinases and tumor metastasis. *Cancer Metastasis Review, 25*(1), 9–34.

Dinarello, C. A. (2007). Historical review of cytokines. *European Journal of Immunology, 37*(Suppl. 1), S34–S45.

Doll, R. (1995). Hazards of ionizing radiation: 100 years of observations on man. *British Journal of Cancer, 72*(6), 1339–1349.

Dryja, T. P., Friend, S., & Weinberg, R. A. (1986). Genetic sequences that predispose to retinoblastoma and osteosarcoma. *Symposium on Fundamental Cancer Research, 39,* 115–119.

Efeyan, A., & Serrano, M. (2007). p53: Guardian of the genome and policeman of the oncogenes. *Cell Cycle, 6*(9), 1006–1010.

Ericson, N. G., Kulawiec, M., Vermulst, M., Sheahan, K., O'Sullivan, J., Salk, J. J., & Bielas, J. H. (2012). Decreased mitochondrial DNA mutagenesis in human colorectal cancer. *PLoS Genetics, 8*(6), e1002689.

Fearon, E. R., & Vogelstein, B. A. (1990). A genetic model for colorectal tumorigenesis. *Cell, 61*(5), 759–767.

Ferguson, L. R. (2010). Chronic inflammation and mutagenesis. *Mutation Research, 690*(1–2), 3–11.

Folkman, J. (2006). Angiogenesis. *Annual Review of Medicine, 57,* 1–18.

Folkman, J., & Klagsbrun, M. (1987). Angiogenic factors. *Science, 235*(4787), 442–447.

Gilbert, E. S. (2009). Ionising radiation and cancer risks: What have we learned from epidemiology? *International Journal of Radiation Biology, 85*(6), 467–482.

Griffiths, L. M., Doudican, N. A., Shadel, G. S., & Doetsch, P. W. (2009). Mitochondrial DNA oxidative damage and mutagenesis in Saccharomyces cerevisiae. *Methods in Molecular Biology, 554,* 267–286.

Hancock, J. T. (2010). *Cell signaling* (3rd ed.). New York, NY: Oxford University Press.

Harris, R. E. (2007). Cyclooxygenase-2 (COX-2) and the inflammogenesis of cancer. *Subcellular Biochemistry, 42,* 63–126.

Harris, R. E., Beebe-Donk, J., & Alshafie, G. A. (2007). Cancer chemoprevention by cyclooxygenase 2 (COX-2) blockade: Results of case control studies. *Subcellular Biochemistry, 42,* 193–212.

Hayflick, L. (1985). The cell biology of aging. *Clinics in Geriatric Medicine, 1*(1), 15–27.

Hayflick, L. (2007). Entropy explains aging, genetic determinism explains longevity, and undefined terminology explains misunderstanding both. *PLoS Genetics, 3*(12), e220.

Hecht, S. S. (1999). Tobacco smoke carcinogens and lung cancer. *Journal of the National Cancer Institute, 91*(14), 1194–1210.

Herschman, H. R. (2002). Historical aspects of COX-2. Cloning and characterization of the cDNA, protein and gene. In R. E. Harris (Ed.), *COX-2 blockade in cancer prevention and therapy* (pp. 13–32). Totowa, NJ: Humana Press.

Holowaty, P., Miller, A. B., Rohan, T., & To, T. (1999). Natural history of dysplasia of the uterine cervix. *Journal of the National Cancer Institute, 91*(3), 252–258.

Howe, L. R., Subbaramaiah, K., Brown, A. M. C., & Dannenberg, A. J. (2001). Cyclooxygenase-2: A target for the prevention and treatment of breast cancer. *Endocrine-Related Cancer, 8,* 97–114.

Itoh, Y., & Nagase, H. (2002). Matrix metalloproteinases in cancer. *Essays in Biochemistry, 38,* 21–36.

Kennedy, B. M., & Harris, R. E. (2018). Cyclooxygenase and lipoxygenase gene expression in the inflammogenesis of breast cancer. *Inflammopharmacology, 26*(4), 909–923.

Kieffer, T. J., & Habener, J. F. (1999). The glucagon-like peptides. *Endocrine Reviews, 20,* 876–913.

Knudson, A. G. (1971). Mutation and cancer: Statistical study of retinoblastoma. *Proceedings of the National Academy of Sciences of the United States of America, 68,* 820–823.

Knudson, A. G. (2001). Two genetic hits (more or less) to cancer. *Nature Review Cancer, 1*(2), 157–162.

Kumar, V., Abbas, A. K., & Aster, J. C. (2014). *Robbins & Cotran pathologic basis of disease* (9th ed.). Philadelphia, PA: Mosby & Saunders.

Lengauer, C., Kinzler, K. W., & Vogelstein, B. (1998). Genetic instabilities in human cancers. *Nature, 396,* 643–649.

Le Roith, D. (1997). Insulin-like growth factors. *New England Journal of Medicine, 336,* 633–640.

Lijinsy, W. (1989). A view of the relation between carcinogenesis and mutagenesis. *Environmental and Molecular Mutagenesis, 14*(Suppl. 16), 78–84.

Loeb, L. A., Loeb, K. R., & Anderson, J. P. (2003). Multiple mutations and cancer. *Proceedings of the National Academy of Sciences of the United States of America, 100,* 776–781.

Lowe, S. W., & Lin, A. W. (2000). Apoptosis in cancer. *Carcinogenesis, 21*(3), 485–495.

Lunt, S. Y., & Vander Heiden, M. G. (2011). Aerobic glycolysis: Meeting the metabolic requirements of cell proliferation. *Annual Review of Cell and Developmental Biology, 27,* 441–464.

Manning, G., Whyte, D. B., Martinez, R., Hunter, T., & Sudarsanam, S. (2002). The protein kinase complement of the human genome. *Science, 298*(5600), 1912–1934.

Marnett, L. J. (1999). Lipid peroxidation-DNA damage by malondialdehyde. *Mutation Research, 424*(102), 83–95.

Marshman, E., Booth, C., & Potten, C. S. (2002). The intestinal epithelial stem cell. *Bioessays, 24,* 91–98.

Momparler, R. L. (2003). Cancer epigenetics. *Oncogene, 22*(42), 6479–6483.

Mondello, C., & Scovassi, A. I. (2004). Telomeres, telomerase, and apoptosis. *Biochemistry and Cell Biology, 82*(4), 498–507.

Nordling, C. O. (1953). A new theory on the cancer-inducing mechanism. *British Journal of Cancer, 7,* 68–72.

Olayioye, M. A. (2001). Update on HER-2 as a target for cancer therapy: Intracellular signaling pathways of ErbB2/HER-2 and family members. *Breast Cancer Research, 3*(6), 385–389.

Pearson, G., Robinson, F., Beers Gibson, T., Xu, B. E., Karandikar, M., Berman, K., & Cobb, M. H. (2001). Mitogen-activated protein (MAP) kinase pathways: Regulation and physiological functions. *Endocrine Review, 22*(2), 153–183.

Pellettieri, J., & Alvarado, A. S. (2007). Cell turnover and adult tissue homeostasis: From humans to planarians. *Annual Review of Genetics, 41*, 83–105.

Pockaj, B. A., Basu, G. D., Pathangey, L. B., Gray, R. J., Hernandez, J. L., Gendler, S. J., & Mukherjee, P. (2004). Reduced T-cell and dendritic cell function is related to cyclooxygenase-2 overexpression and prostaglandin E2 secretion in patients with breast cancer. *Annals of Surgical Oncology, 11*, 328–339.

Prehn, R. T. (1994). Cancers beget mutations versus mutations beget cancers. *Cancer Research, 54*(5), 296–300.

Ricciotti, E., & FitzGerald, G. A. (2011). Prostaglandins and inflammation. *Arteriosclerosis, Thrombosis, and Vascular Biology, 31*(5), 986–1000.

Robbins, S. L., & Cotran, R. S. (1979). Neoplasia. In S. L. Robbins & R. S. Cotran (Eds.), *Pathologic basis of disease* (pp. 141–187). Philadelphia, PA: W. B. Saunders Company.

Schneider, C., & Pozzi, A. (2011). Cyclooxygenases and lipoxygenases in cancer. *Cancer and Metastasis Reviews, 30*, 277–294.

Shiff, S. J., & Rigas, B. (1999). The role of cyclooxygenase inhibition in the antineoplastic effects of nonsteroidal anti-inflammatory drugs (NSAIDs). *Journal of Experimental Medicine, 190*, 445–450.

Soto, A. M., & Sonnenschein, C. (2004). The somatic mutation theory of cancer: Growing problems with the paradigm? *Bioessays, 26*(10), 1097–1107.

Spalding, K. L., Bhardwaj, R. D., Buchholz, B. A., Druid, H., & Frisén, J. (2005). Retrospective birth dating of cells in humans. *Cell, 122*(1), 133–143.

Sugimura, T. (2000). Nutrition and dietary carcinogens. *Carcinogenesis, 21*(3), 387–395.

Verma, M., Maruvada, P., & Srivastara, S. (2004). Epigenetics and cancer. *Critical Reviews in Clinical Laboratory Sciences, 41*, 5–6.

Virchow, R. (1863). Aetiologie der neoplastischen Geschwulst/ Pathogenie der neoplastischen Geschwulste. In *Die Krankhaften Geschwülste* (pp. 57–101). Berlin, Germany: Verlag von August Hirschwald.

Warburg, O. (1956). On the origin of cancer cells. *Science, 123*(3191), 309–314.

Warburg, O., Posener, K., & Negelein, E. (1924). Über den Stoffwechsel der Carcinomzelle. *Biochemische Zeitschrift, 152*, 309–344.

Wijnhoven, B. P. L., Dinjens, W. N. M., & Pignatelli, M. (2000). E-cadherin-catenin cell-cell adhesion complex and human cancer. *British Journal of Surgery, 87*, 992–1005.

zur Hausen, H. (1991). Viruses in human cancers. *Science, 254*(5035), 1167–1173.

© Andrew Brookes/Getty Images

CHAPTER 12

Global Epidemiology of Cancer

▶ Global Burden of Cancer

"There is no term in the entire lexicon of medicine that strikes more terror than the word "cancer," and with considerable justification" (Robbins & Cotran, 1979). That quote from the classic text *Pathologic Basis of Disease* written in 1974 by Stanley L. Robbins and Ramzi S. Cotran still rings true with the writing of this book more than 40 years later. Despite unprecedented medical and public health efforts, many forms of cancer still remain incurable and prematurely strike down millions of people each year. The metastatic spread of cancer to vital organs of the body usually results in massive tissue destruction, loss of life-sustaining functions, and ultimately, the untimely death of the human host.

During the last few decades, global estimates of cancer incidence and mortality have been periodically reported by investigators at the *International Agency for Research on Cancer* (IARC), in Lyon, France, the *World Health Organization* (WHO) in Geneva, Switzerland, and most recently, the *Institute for Health Metrics and Evaluation* (IHME), at the University of Washington in Seattle. In the following sections of this chapter, the most recent global estimates of cancer incidence and mortality are presented for 2018 and global and national trends are discussed based upon reports from IARC, WHO, and IHME. Based on data reported by IARC and WHO, 18.08 million new cases of cancer and 9.56 million cancer deaths occurred in the world population during 2018. These estimates reflect increases of 44% in new cases of cancer and 26% in cancer deaths during the past decade, 2008–2018 (Boyle & Levin, 2008; Ferlay et al., 2010, 2013, 2018).

Among the 18.08 million new cases of cancer diagnosed in 2018, 2.09 million (11.6%) were cancers of the lung. Cancers of the breast (2.09 million), colon and rectum (1.85 million), prostate (1.28 million), stomach (1.03 million), liver (0.84 million), and esophagus (0.57 million) accounted for an additional 42.4% of all new cases.

Lung cancer was by far the deadliest malignancy, causing 1.76 million deaths (18.4% of the total cancer deaths), more than double the number of deaths from any other malignancy. Deaths from colorectal cancer (0.88 million), liver cancer (0.78 million), stomach cancer (0.78 million), breast cancer (0.63 million), esophageal cancer (0.51 million), pancreatic cancer (0.43 million), prostate cancer (0.36 million), cervical cancer (0.31 million), leukemia (0.31 million), and lymphoma (0.25 million) accounted for an additional 55% of the total cancer deaths in 2018. The ratio of mortality to incidence (a crude measure of case fatality) was highest for pancreatic cancer (94%), liver cancer (93%), lung cancer (84%), and esophageal cancer (83%) (Ferlay et al., 2018).

Estimates of disability-adjusted life-years (DALY) measure the years of productive life lost due to premature death and/or disability from disease. During 2008, 170 million DALY were attributed to cancer worldwide (Soerjomataram et al., 2012). By comparison, 213 million DALY were attributed to cancer in 2016, an increase of 25% (Fitzmaurice et al., 2018).

177

Among people of all ages, cancer is the third leading cause of death (behind heart disease and infectious conditions); in people living in economically developed countries such as the United States and Great Britain, cancer has now surpassed heart disease as the leading cause of death in people under the age of 85 years (Ferlay et al., 2010, 2013; Jemal et al., 2011; Thun, DeLancey, Center, Jemal, & Ward, 2010).

▶ Global Burden of Cancer in Men and Women

The global burden of cancer is markedly higher in men than in women. In 2018, the number of cancer deaths among men (5.39 million) was 29% higher than among women (4.17 million). In the same year, the age-standardized cancer incidence in men was 20% higher than in women (218.6 per 100,000 versus 182.6 per 100,000), and the age-standardized cancer mortality in men was 48% higher than in women (122.7 per 100,000 versus 83.1 per 100,000) (Ferlay et al., 2018).

The deadliest cancers differ in men and women. Of the 4.65 million deaths from cancer in men during 2012, nearly 24% (1.1 million) were caused by lung cancer and other malignancies of the respiratory tract (larynx, trachea) and 40% (1.88 million) were caused by malignancies of the gastrointestinal tract (stomach, liver, esophagus, colon/rectum, gallbladder, pancreas,

and oral cavity). An additional 11% of male cancer deaths (0.53 million) were caused by malignancies of the genitourinary tract (prostate, testes, kidneys, bladder), and 7% (0.33 million) were due to lymphomas and leukemias (Ferlay et al., 2013). A similar pattern is evident in the data for 2018; among 5.39 million deaths from cancer in men, approximately 22% of deaths (1.18 million) were caused by lung cancer, 39% (2.1 million) were caused by malignancies of the gastrointestinal tract, 12% (0.62 million) were caused by malignancies of the male genitourinary tract, and 6% (0.32 million) were caused by leukemia or lymphoma (Fitzmaurice et al., 2018; Ferlay et al., 2018) (**FIGURE 12.1**).

Among the 3.55 million women who died from cancer in 2012, breast cancer caused the most deaths (0.52 million), followed closely by lung cancer (0.49 million). Gastrointestinal cancers (stomach, liver, esophagus, colon/rectum, gallbladder, pancreas, and oral cavity) together accounted for 1.20 million deaths, and malignancies of the genitourinary tract (uterus, cervix, and ovaries) caused 0.49 million deaths. Lymphoma and leukemia caused an additional 0.21 million deaths among women worldwide (Ferlay et al., 2013). In 2018, among 4.17 million women who died from cancer, breast cancer caused 0.63 million deaths, lung cancer caused 0.56 million deaths, gastrointestinal cancers caused 1.41 million deaths, malignancies of the female genitourinary tract caused 0.59 million deaths and leukemia and lymphoma caused 0.23 million deaths (**FIGURE 12.2**).

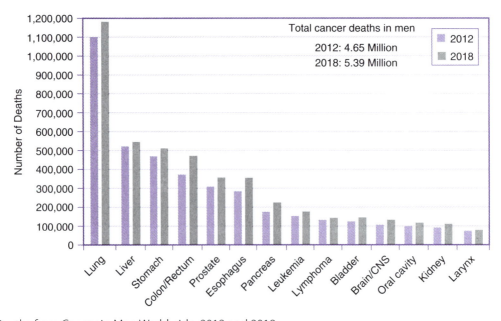

FIGURE 12.1 Deaths from Cancer in Men Worldwide, 2012 and 2018.

Data from Ferlay, J., Shin, H. R., Bray, F., Forman, D., Mathers, C., & Parkin, D. M. (2010). Estimates of worldwide burden of cancer in 2008: GLOBOCAN 2008. *International Journal of Cancer, 127*, 2893–2917; Ferlay, J., Soerjomataram, I., Ervik, M., Dikshit, R., Eser, S., Mathers, C., . . . Bray, F. (2013). *GLOBOCAN 2012 v1.0. Cancer incidence and mortality worldwide: IARC CancerBase No. 11* [Internet]. Lyon, France: International Agency for Research on Cancer; Ferlay, J., Ervik, M., Lam, F., Colombet, M., Mery, L., Piñeros, M., . . . Bray, F. (2018). *Global cancer observatory: Cancer today*. Lyon, France: International Agency for Research on Cancer. Retrieved from https://gco.iarc.fr/today; Fitzmaurice, C., Allen, C., Barber, R. M., Barregard, L., Bhutta, Z. A., Brenner, H., . . . Global Burden of Disease Cancer Collaboration. (2017). Global, regional, and national cancer incidence, mortality, years of life lost, years lived with and disability-adjusted life-years for 32 cancer groups, 1990 to 2015: A systematic analysis for the Global Burden of Disease Study. *JAMA Oncology, 3*(4), 524–548; Fitzmaurice, C., Akinyemiju, T. F., Al Lami, F. H., Alam, T., Alizadeh-Navaei, R., Allen, C., . . . Global Burden of Disease Cancer Collaboration. (2018, June 02). Global, regional, and national cancer incidence, mortality, years of life lost, years lived with disability, and disability-adjusted life-years for 29 cancer groups, 1990 to 2016: A systematic analysis for the Global Burden of Disease Study. *JAMA Oncology*. Online publication. doi:10.1001/jamaoncol.2018.2706.

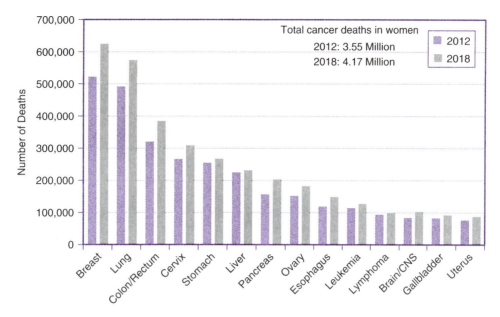

FIGURE 12.2 Deaths from Cancer in Women Worldwide, 2012 and 2018.

Data from Ferlay, J., Shin, H. R., Bray, F., Forman, D., Mathers, C., & Parkin, D. M. (2010). Estimates of worldwide burden of cancer in 2008: GLOBOCAN 2008. *International Journal of Cancer, 127,* 2893–2917; Ferlay, J., Soerjomataram, I., Ervik, M., Dikshit, R., Eser, S., Mathers, C., ... Bray, F. (2013). *GLOBOCAN 2012 v1.0. Cancer incidence and mortality worldwide: IARC CancerBase No. 11* [Internet]. Lyon, France: International Agency for Research on Cancer; Ferlay, J., Ervik, M., Lam, F., Colombet, M., Mery, L., Piñeros, M., ... Bray, F. (2018). *Global cancer observatory: Cancer today.* Lyon, France: International Agency for Research on Cancer. Retrieved from https://gco.iarc.fr/today; Fitzmaurice, C., Allen, C., Barber, R. M., Barregard, L., Bhutta, Z. A., Brenner, H., ... Global Burden of Disease Cancer Collaboration. (2017). Global, regional, and national cancer incidence, mortality, years of life lost, years lived with and disability-adjusted life-years for 32 cancer groups, 1990 to 2015: A systematic analysis for the Global Burden of Disease Study. *JAMA Oncology, 3*(4), 524–548; Fitzmaurice, C., Akinyemiju, T. F., Al Lami, F. H., Alam, T., Alizadeh-Navaei, R., Allen, C., ... Global Burden of Disease Cancer Collaboration. (2018, June 02). Global, regional, and national cancer incidence, mortality, years of life lost, years lived with disability, and disability-adjusted life-years for 29 cancer groups, 1990 to 2016: A systematic analysis for the Global Burden of Disease Study. *JAMA Oncology.* Online publication. doi:10.1001/jamaoncol.2018.2706.

Data from Ferlay, J., Shin, H. R., Bray, F., Forman, D., Mathers, C., & Parkin, D. M. (2010). Estimates of worldwide burden of cancer in 2008: GLOBOCAN 2008. *International Journal of Cancer, 127,* 2893–2917; Ferlay, J., Soerjomataram, I., Ervik, M., Dikshit, R., Eser, S., Mathers, C., ... Bray, F. (2013). *GLOBOCAN 2012 v1.0. Cancer incidence and mortality worldwide: IARC CancerBase No. 11* [Internet]. Lyon, France: International Agency for Research on Cancer; Fitzmaurice, C., Allen, C., Barber, R. M., Barregard, L., Bhutta, Z. A., Brenner, H., ... Global Burden of Disease Cancer Collaboration. (2017). Global, regional, and national cancer incidence, mortality, years of life lost, years lived with disability, and disability-adjusted life-years for 32 cancer groups, 1990 to 2015: A systematic analysis for the Global Burden of Disease Study. *JAMA Oncology, 3*(4), 524–548; Fitzmaurice, C., Akinyemiju, T. F., Al Lami, F. H., Alam, T., Alizadeh-Navaei, R., Allen, C., ... Global Burden of Disease Cancer Collaboration. (2018). Global, regional, and national cancer incidence, mortality, years of life lost, years lived with disability, and disability-adjusted life-years for 29 cancer groups, 1990–2016: A systematic analysis for the Global Burden of Disease Study. *JAMA Oncology.* online publication. doi:10.1001/jamaoncol.2018.2706; Ferlay, J., Ervik, M., Lam, F., Colombet, M., Mery, L., Piñeros, M., ... Bray, F. (2018). *Global cancer observatory: Cancer today.* Lyon, France: International Agency for Research on Cancer. Retrieved from https://gco.iarc.fr/today.

▶ Histological Profile of Global Cancer

Carcinomas arising from epithelial cells lining various anatomic organs make up the vast majority of malignant neoplasms. The site-specific global cancer data for 2012, 2016, and 2018 suggest that more than 90% of new cases were carcinomas; other forms of cancer (leukemias, lymphomas, myelomas, sarcomas, germ-cell tumors, and brain tumors) accounted for the remainder (Ferlay et al., 2013, 2018; Fitzmaurice et al., 2017). This 9 to 1 predominance of carcinomas relative to other forms of cancer reflects the markedly higher rates of cell division in epithelial cell populations compared to other cell populations (e.g., muscle, fat, bone, brain, nervous system, and immune system).

▶ Global Trends in Cancer

Estimated numbers of new cancer cases and deaths from cancer have increased steadily in the 21st century (Boyle & Levin, 2008; Ferlay et al., 2010, 2013, 2018; Fitzmaurice et al., 2018; Parkin, Bray, Ferlay, & Pisani, 2001; WHO, 2004) (**FIGURE 12.3**). During the period 2000–2018, the annual number of new cases increased by nearly 79% (from 10.1 to 18.1 million), and the annual number of cancer deaths increased by 55% (from 6.2 to 9.6 million).

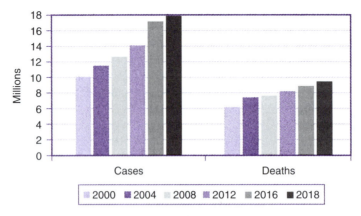

FIGURE 12.3 Global Trends in New Cases of Cancer and Deaths from Cancer During the 21st Century.

Data from Boyle, P., & Levin, B. (Eds.). (2008). *IARC world cancer report*. Lyon, France: International Agency for Research on Cancer (IARC) Publications; Ferlay, J., Shin, H. R., Bray, F., Forman, D., Mathers, C., & Parkin, D. M. (2010). Estimates of worldwide burden of cancer in 2008: GLOBOCAN 2008. *International Journal of Cancer, 127*, 2893–2917; Ferlay, J., Soerjomataram, I., Ervik, M., Dikshit, R., Eser, S., Mathers, C., . . . Bray, F. (2013). *GLOBOCAN 2012 v1.0. Cancer incidence and mortality worldwide: IARC CancerBase No. 11* [Internet]. Lyon, France: International Agency for Research on Cancer; Ferlay, J., Ervik, M., Lam, F., Colombet, M., Mery, L., Piñeros, M., . . . Bray, F. (2018). *Global cancer observatory: Cancer today*. Lyon, France: International Agency for Research on Cancer. Retrieved from https://gco.iarc.fr /today; Parkin, D. M., Bray, F., Ferlay, J., & Pisani, P. (2001). Estimating the world cancer burden: GLOBOCAN 2000. *International Journal of Cancer, 94*, 153–156; World Health Organization. (2004). *Global burden of disease 2004 update*. Geneva, Switzerland: Author; Fitzmaurice, C., Allen, C., Barber, R. M., et al., Global Burden of Disease Cancer Collaboration. (2017). Global, regional, and national cancer incidence, mortality, years of life lost, years lived with disability, and disability-adjusted life-years for 32 cancer groups, 1990 to 2015: A systematic analysis for the Global Burden of Disease Study. *JAMA Oncology, 3*(4), 524–548; Fitzmaurice, C., Akinyemiju, T. F., Al Lami, F. H., et al., Global Burden of Disease Cancer Collaboration. (2018). Global, regional, and national cancer incidence, mortality, years of life lost, years lived with disability, and disability-adjusted life-years for 29 cancer groups, 1990 to 2016: A systematic analysis for the Global Burden of Disease Study. *JAMA Oncology*. Published online June 02, 2018. doi:10.1001/jamaoncol.2018.2706.

METHODOLOGY

Incidence and Mortality

Incidence is the number of new cases arising during a specific period of time in a defined population. *Mortality* is the number of deaths occurring during a defined period of time in a specified population. Incidence and mortality are often expressed as rates per 100,000 persons per year. Incidence and mortality rates can be estimated for specific age groups or exposure groups within populations.

Age-Standardized Cancer Rates

Age-standardization is a technique that adjusts cancer rates for differences in the age distributions of populations being compared. This technique is very useful in examining trends in rates of cancer over time or comparing rates in different populations. This is because the incidence and mortality rates for most cancers increase rapidly with age, so that populations containing a high proportion of old people will tend to have a higher overall (crude) rate than one with mainly young people. Age-standardization adjusts the age-specific rates of populations being compared to the age structure of a reference population. In the direct method of age-standardization, age-specific rates for successive 5-year age intervals (e.g., 0–4, 5–9, 10–14, 15–19, 20–24) are weighted by the age distribution of a standard (reference) population (e.g., the standard world population). The formula for calculating an age-standardized rate from a set of age-specific rates estimated for a population using the age distribution of the world population is

$$ASR(W) = \Sigma rf$$

where r is the age-specific rate and f is the frequency of the world population in the corresponding 5-year age interval (Ahmad et al., 2001; Stewart & Kleihues, 2003).

However, it is important to realize that these startling increases in new cancer cases and deaths from cancer have been driven largely by the growth and aging of the world population. During the time period 2000–2018, the world population increased from 6 to 7.5 billion (~17%) and life expectancy increased from 68 to 71 years (~4%) (World Bank, 2014). Because the majority of malignancies are diagnosed late in life (e.g., 55%–60% of new cases are diagnosed after age 65 years), elderly populations are expected to have higher crude (unadjusted) rates of cancer than younger populations.

Global Trends in Cancer Incidence and Mortality

The age-standardized rates of annual cancer incidence and mortality estimated for the world population during 2000–2018 reflect distinctly different patterns and much smaller changes than the dramatically increased numbers of new cancer cases and cancer deaths (79% and 55%, respectively) observed during the same time period. In men, annual cancer incidence rates increased by 8.3% during 2000–2018 (from 201.9 to 218.6 cases per 100,000), whereas in women,

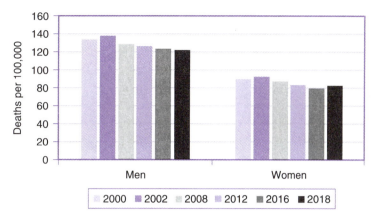

FIGURE 12.4 Global Trends in Age-Standardized Mortality Rates of Cancer for Men and Women During the 21st Century.

Data from Boyle, P., & Levin, B. (Eds.). (2008). *IARC world cancer report*. Lyon, France: International Agency for Research on Cancer (IARC) Publications; Ferlay, J., Shin, H. R., Bray, F., Forman, D., Mathers, C., & Parkin, D. M. (2010). Estimates of worldwide burden of cancer in 2008: GLOBOCAN 2008. *International Journal of Cancer, 127*, 2893–2917; Ferlay, J., Soerjomataram, I., Ervik, M., Dikshit, R., Eser, S., Mathers, C., . . . Bray, F. (2013). *GLOBOCAN 2012 v1.0. Cancer incidence and mortality worldwide: IARC CancerBase No. 11* [Internet]. Lyon, France: International Agency for Research on Cancer; Ferlay, J., Ervik, M., Lam, F., Colombet, M., Mery, L., Piñeros, M., . . . Bray, F. (2018). *Global cancer observatory: Cancer today*. Lyon, France: International Agency for Research on Cancer. Retrieved from https://gco.iarc.fr/today; Parkin, D. M., Bray, F., Ferlay, J., & Pisani, P. (2005). Global cancer statistics, 2002. *CA: A Cancer Journal for Clinicians, 55*, 74–108; Parkin, D. M., Bray, F., Ferlay, J., & Pisani, P. (2001). Estimating the world cancer burden: GLOBOCAN 2000. *International Journal of Cancer, 94*, 153–156.

rates increased by 15.7% (from 157.8 cases to 182.6 cases per 100,000). In contrast, annual cancer mortality rates peaked for both men and women in 2002 and have since declined (from 137.7 to 122.7 deaths per 100,000 in men and from 92.1 to 83.1 deaths per 100,000 in women in during 2002–2012, *decreases* of 11% and 10%, respectively) (**FIGURE 12.4**). In an independent study, the age-adjusted cancer mortality rate for both men and women declined by 14.7% or about 0.9% per year during 2000–2016 (Roser & Ritchie, 2018). The age-standardized rates thus reflect decreasing cancer mortality in the face of slight increases in cancer incidence and marked increases in the numbers of new cases of cancer and cancer deaths in the world population since the turn of the century (Boyle & Levin, 2008; Ferlay et al., 2010, 2013, 2018; Parkin et al., 2001; Parkin, Bray, Ferlay, & Pisani, 2005).

Although the examination of combined data from national registries and surveillance systems is critical in establishing global trends and patterns of cancer, such ecological studies must be supplemented by intensive epidemiologic and molecular investigations of individual forms of malignancy in order to elucidate causation. Indeed, there is considerable variation in the incidence and mortality of different cancers by geographic area of the world, which is a consequence not only of growth and aging of the inherent populations, but also of many other factors such as exposure to causative agents (e.g., tobacco and alcohol), development of predisposing conditions (e.g., obesity, inflammation, infection, and other chronic conditions), and access to screening and health care. For example, overall cancer incidence rates estimated from 45 cancer registries were found to vary by sixfold in men (82 per 100,000 in Algerians to 453 per 100,000 in African Americans) and fourfold in women (80 per

100,000 in Algerians to 302 per 100,000 in Caucasian Americans) (Jemal, Center, DeSantis, & Ward, 2010). Furthermore, incidence and mortality rates of many forms of cancer are decreasing in populations of developed countries such as the United States but are surging in populations of less-developed countries with their adoption of unhealthy lifestyles that increase cancer risk (e.g., addiction to tobacco and alcohol, lack of exercise, chronic exposure to infectious agents, and consumption of diets high in fat and calories) (Jemal et al., 2010; Stewart & Wild, 2014). Factors that increase or decrease cancer risk are discussed in the following sections of this chapter.

▶ Cancer in Developing Versus Developed Nations

Profiles of cancer differ dramatically in developing versus developed nations (Garcia et al., 2007; Jemal et al., 2010, 2011). Among men living in developing nations, the total number of deaths due to either liver cancer or stomach cancer is more than four times higher than in developed nations, reflecting high rates of infection by liver viruses (hepatitis B virus [HBV] and hepatitis C virus [HCV]) and stomach bacteria (e.g., *Helicobacter pylori*), plus contamination of food supplies by molds that produce highly carcinogenic aflatoxins. Reciprocally, deaths from colorectal cancer or prostate cancer occur more frequently in men living in developed nations, partly due to diets high in fat and calories and low in fiber, fruits, and vegetables. Lung cancer, caused predominantly by chronic tobacco smoking, is the leading cause of cancer death in men of developing and developed nations (**FIGURE 12.5**).

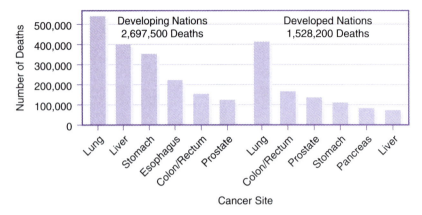

FIGURE 12.5 Deaths from Cancer Among Men in Developing Versus Developed Nations, 2008. Developing nations include populations of Africa, the Caribbean, Central America, South America, Asia (less Japan), and Oceania (Melanesia, Micronesia, and Polynesia). Developed nations include populations of North America, Europe, the Russian Federation, Japan, and Australia/New Zealand.

Data from Jemal, A., Center, M. M., DeSantis, C., & Ward, E. M. (2010). Global patterns of cancer incidence and mortality rates and trends. *Cancer Epidemiology, Biomarkers and Prevention, 19,* 1893–1907; Jemal, A., Bray, F., Center, M. M., Ferlay, J., Ward, E., & Forman, D. (2011). Global cancer statistics. *CA: A Cancer Journal for Clinicians, 61*(2), 69–90.

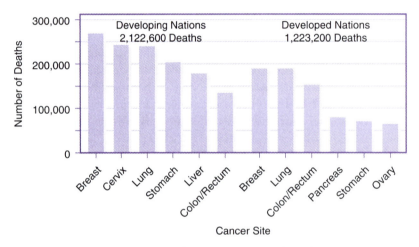

FIGURE 12.6 Deaths from Cancer Among Women in Developing Versus Developed Nations, 2008. *Caption*: Developing nations include populations of Africa, the Caribbean, Central America, South America, Asia (less Japan), and Oceania (Melanesia, Micronesia, and Polynesia). Developed nations include populations of North America, Europe, the Russian Federation, Japan, and Australia/New Zealand.

Data from Jemal, A., Center, M. M., DeSantis, C., & Ward, E. M. (2010). Global patterns of cancer incidence and mortality rates and trends. *Cancer Epidemiology, Biomarkers and Prevention, 19,* 1893–1907; Jemal, A., Bray, F., Center, M. M., Ferlay, J., Ward, E., & Forman, D. (2011). Global cancer statistics. *CA: A Cancer Journal for Clinicians, 61*(2), 69–90.

Breast cancer is the leading cause of death from cancer among women in both developing and developed nations. Among women living in developing nations, cancer of the uterine cervix is the second leading cause of death from cancer, principally due to lack of screening for premalignant dysplastic lesions of the cervical mucosa. Lung cancer causes nearly as many deaths as breast cancer in developed nations, and rising rates of smoking among women worldwide have resulted in increasing numbers of female lung-cancer deaths in all populations. Death from stomach cancer or liver cancer occurs more frequently in developing nations, whereas cancers of the colon and rectum, pancreas, and ovaries cause relatively more deaths in developed nations (**FIGURE 12.6**).

The contrasting patterns of cancer in the populations of developing and developed nations reflect the impact of major differences in lifestyles, environmental exposures, and access to health care. Developing nations are characterized by poverty and as a consequence, large segments of their populations suffer from inadequate nutrition, poor sanitation and hygiene, polluted environments, and lack of access to preventive, diagnostic, and therapeutic healthcare resources. Environmental conditions in impoverished populations favor transmission of infectious diseases that predispose to cancers of the stomach, liver, uterine cervix, and other exposed tissues. Without resources for prevention, screening, and early detection, case fatality rates are high and survival short for all forms of cancer in such populations.

In developed nations, advanced public health systems have been designed and implemented to ensure food and water safety, improve sanitation and personal hygiene, reduce pollution, and provide timely access to health care. Notably, such measures have resulted in higher standards of living and increased life spans in these populations. Nevertheless, the obesity pandemic arising from dietary excesses and sedentary lifestyles has contributed to high rates of cancers of the colon, rectum, pancreas, breast, and prostate in developed nations.

One common theme in both developing and developed nations is the continuing addiction of many people to tobacco smoking. Most disturbingly, the total number of smokers is rising globally, and it is indeed startling that worldwide, more than 1 billion men and women smoke cigarettes. While smoking rates have declined in some developed countries such as the United States and Australia that have instituted antismoking campaigns, smoking bans in public places, and higher cigarette taxes, smoking rates are rising sharply in many populations, especially in low- and middle-income nations where there is virtually no education about the specific health risks of tobacco use. It is estimated that 80% of current smokers live in the developing world, a fact that heralds an impending global epidemic of lung cancer and other tobacco-related diseases (WHO, 2008, 2012). More details on tobacco and cancer appear in a later section of this chapter.

▶ Cancer Mortality in the United States

Despite the declaration of war on cancer by President Richard Nixon in 1971, the number of new cases of cancer and deaths from cancer continues to increase in the United States. Shortly after this presidential declaration, the U.S. National Cancer Institute (NCI) established the Surveillance, Epidemiology, and End Results (SEER) program in order to monitor the impact of cancer in the United States. Data collection by member tumor registries of SEER began January 1, 1973. The SEER program currently collects and publishes cancer incidence and survival data

from 18 population-based cancer registries covering approximately 26% of the U.S. population including all ethnic groups. The SEER registries routinely collect data on patient demographics, primary tumor site, tumor morphology and stage at diagnosis, first course of treatment, and follow-up for vital status. The SEER program is the only comprehensive source of population-based information in the United States that includes stage of cancer at the time of diagnosis and patient survival data (Horner et al., 2009; SEER, 2014).

Based on recent estimates, approximately 1.66 million new cases of invasive cancer are being diagnosed annually in the United States (excluding carcinomas in situ, and basal and squamous cell carcinomas of the skin), and more than 580,000 Americans die from cancer annually (about 1600 people each day). Lung cancer is the leading cause of cancer deaths in both men and women (American Cancer Society, 2018).

FIGURES 12.7 and **12.8** show chronological trends in cancer mortality for U.S. men and women for the period 1930–2015 (American Cancer Society, 2018). Among men, more than half of cancer deaths are due to cancers of the lung and bronchus, prostate, colon, and rectum. Although lung-cancer mortality has declined slightly since about 1990, the male death rates from this malignancy are still more than double that of any other anatomic site. In 1983, prostate cancer surpassed colorectal cancer as the second leading cause of cancer deaths in men. During the past two decades, the mortality rates for both prostate and colorectal cancer show evidence of a gradual decline. Notably, the death rates for cancers of the liver and biliary tract have nearly doubled since 1990, due in part to increasing rates of viral hepatitis and non-alcoholic liver cirrhosis. Mortality rates for other malignancies have remained fairly constant, with the exception of the rates for stomach cancer, which have declined dramatically beginning in about 1930, similar to the pattern for women.

Among women, cancers of the lung and bronchus, breast, and colon and rectum account for more than half of all cancer deaths in the United States. In 1987, lung cancer surpassed breast cancer as the leading cause of cancer death in women. During 1950–2005, lung-cancer mortality among U.S. women increased by more than 600%; and though the rates have declined over the past decade, lung cancer still accounts for about 25% of all female cancer deaths. Breast cancer mortality remained remarkably constant throughout the 20th century but appears to be declining slightly

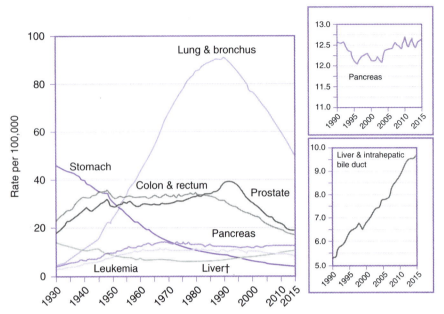

Trends in Cancer Death Rates* Among Males, United States, 1930–2015

*Age-adjusted to the 2000 U.S. standard population. †Includes intrahepatic bile duct, gallbladder, and other biliary.
Note: Due to International Classification of Diseases coding changes, numerator information for colorectal, liver, and lung cancers has changed over time.
Source: National Center for Health Statistics, Centers for Disease Control and Prevention, 2017.

FIGURE 12.7 Trends in Cancer Mortality Among U.S. Men, 1930–2015.

Reprinted from American Cancer Society. (2018). *Cancer facts and figures, 2015*. Atlanta, GA: Author. Retrieved from http://www.cancer.org/research/cancerfactsstatistics/cancerfactsfigures2015/index

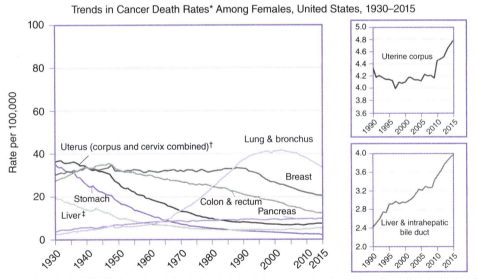

Trends in Cancer Death Rates* Among Females, United States, 1930–2015

*Age-adjusted to the 2000 U.S. standard population. † Uterus includes uterine corpus and uterine cervix combined. ‡Includes intrahepatic bile duct, gallbladder, and other biliary.
Note: Due to International Classification of Diseases coding changes, numerator information for colorectal, liver, lung, and uterine cancers has changed over time.
Source: National Center for Health Statistics, Centers for Disease Control and Prevention, 2017.

FIGURE 12.8 Trends in Cancer Mortality Among U.S. Women, 1930–2015.

Reprinted from American Cancer Society. (2018). *Cancer facts and figures, 2015*. Atlanta, GA: Author. Retrieved from http://www.cancer.org/research/cancerfactsstatistics/cancerfactsfigures2015/index

in recent years. Mortality rates for cervical cancer and stomach cancer steadily declined from high to low levels during the same time period. Colorectal cancer mortality has also gradually declined since the 1950s from rates above 30 per 100,000 to rates now lower than 20 deaths per 100,000. Two increasing trends in mortality are noteworthy; the mortality rates due to

cancers of the liver and biliary tract have increased sharply since 1990, and mortality from cancer of the uterine corpus has risen since 2000 (American Cancer Society, 2018).

The declines in mortality for some forms of cancer in the U.S. population reflect reductions in smoking and other risk factors plus earlier detection and better therapies; however, not all demographic groups have benefited equally. Indeed, cancer mortality and incidence rates vary considerably by race and by gender. In particular, men have about 30% higher cancer death rates than women, and African-American men have the highest death rates from cancers of the lung and bronchus, prostate, and colon and rectum compared to any of the other racial or ethnic groups in the United States.

▶ Epidemiologic Transition of Cancer

The 2014 World Cancer Report released by WHO warns of an impending "tidal wave" of cancer in many populations of the world (Stewart & Wild, 2014). The rising global burden of cancer is a prominent feature of the *epidemiologic transition* whereby chronic diseases are gradually replacing acute diseases in the world population. This phenomenon is undoubtedly a consequence of the improving economic standards of many nations, which has translated into better health and greater longevity for their native populations. But although good health coupled with increasing longevity is generally viewed as beneficial, it is also clear that the epidemiologic transition has produced a concomitant risk of chronic pathogenic processes that are typically manifested later in life. Such is the case for most adult forms of cancer, which are usually diagnosed after years and often decades of growth and development during which there are no detectable clinical symptoms.

FIGURE 12.9 shows the increasing proportion of incident cancers in older versus younger adults since 1980 and the corresponding data for developing versus developed regions of the world. During the period 1980–2010, the proportion of incident

cancers diagnosed among people living in economically developing regions increased from 50% to 65%, and the proportion of new cases diagnosed in people over 65 years of age increased from 35% to 55% (Bray & Moller, 2006; Thun et al., 2010). Clearly, the greatest increases in cancer rates have occurred in the elderly populations of low- and middle-income nations (e.g., the developing regions). Based on the latest available global cancer statistics, approximately 60% of new cancer cases and 70% of all cancer deaths now occur in Africa, Asia, Central America, and South America (Stewart & Wild, 2014). Such populations have a virtual "perfect storm" of increasing longevity coupled with predisposing behavioral factors and conditions that increase cancer risk (e.g., addiction to tobacco and alcohol, unhealthy nutrition, obesity, physical inactivity, and widespread exposure to certain sexually transmitted infectious agents that predispose to malignant transformation).

▶ Web of Causation of Cancer

Most (if not all) cancers are caused by the cumulative effects of multiple causal factors that interact in a *web of causation*. As a consequence, establishing definitive proof of causality and quantifying the contribution of an individual risk factor to causation are challenging. In 1964, in the U.S. Surgeon General's Report to the Nation on Smoking and Lung Cancer, an international panel of imminent scientists formulated the "criteria of judgment" for establishing causality of a disease (U.S. Surgeon General, 1964). In a subsequent paper, British epidemiologist Hill (1965) expounded on these criteria and developed a general framework for establishing causal inference from associations observed in epidemiologic investigations. The criteria of judgment include

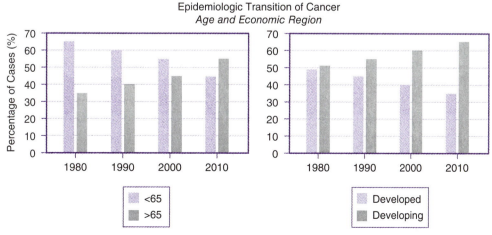

Millions of New Cases: 1980: 6.6, 1990: 8.1, 2000: 10.1, 2010: 13.3

FIGURE 12.9 Relative Frequency of New Cases of Cancer by Age and Economic Region, 1980–2010.

Data from Bray, F., & Moller, B. (2006). Predicting the future burden of cancer. *Nature Reviews Cancer, 6*, 63–74.

(1) consistency of the association across independent studies, (2) strength of the association and dose response of increasing risk with increasing exposure, (3) a temporal relationship between exposure and pathogenesis, (4) biological plausibility of the association, and (5) coherence of the association when the totality of evidence is considered. Fulfillment of these criteria is essential in establishing the causal significance of a risk factor.

Evidence for or against causality of disease by a putative disease-modifying factor may come from different types of epidemiologic investigations. In prospective cohort studies, enrolled individuals are examined and queried at baseline to gather information about exposures and conditions that may influence their cancer risk; these individuals are then followed over time to determine who develops disease and who remains healthy. Such studies provide direct estimates of *relative risk (RR)* for specific factors and conditions. In retrospective case control studies, cases with a specific form of cancer are compared to matched controls without cancer to assess differences in exposure variables. In these studies, risk is quantified by estimating the *odds ratio (OR)* for specific factors and conditions.

Consistency, strength of association, and dose response can be examined simultaneously by a *meta-analysis* of independent epidemiologic studies. Homogeneity of RR estimates and heightened disease risk with increasing exposure (dose response) favor causality. Proof of biological plausibility and establishing the temporal sequence of exposure and pathogenesis rely on laboratory and molecular studies. It is important that such studies reveal a biologically plausible molecular mechanism of pathogenesis associated with exposure to the risk factor. Coherence implies that all evidence "sticks together" and that the proposed causal relationship is supported by the totality of evidence.

In summary, causal inference requires fulfillment of all of the criteria of judgment: observational studies of individuals and populations showing that exposure significantly elevates disease risk, laboratory and molecular studies of exposed human tissues and specimens that reveal a biologically plausible molecular mechanism of pathogenesis, and if available, randomized clinical trials and field trials of prevention and therapy targeting the causal risk factor that effectively reduce disease risk.

METHODOLOGY

Incidence and Relative Risk

The standard measure of effect in a *prospective* epidemiologic study is the relative risk (RR), which quantifies the increase or decrease in the incidence of disease with exposure to a putative disease-modifying factor. Prospective cohort studies are designed to track health outcomes in defined samples of individuals (cohorts) who are disease-free at baseline. Individuals in the cohort are initially classified according to factors that may influence disease risk and are then followed over time to detect new cases of the disease under study. The *RR* is calculated from a prospective cohort study as the ratio of disease incidence among those exposed to a factor to the disease incidence among those not exposed to the factor: $RR = i_e/i_o$, where i_e = the incidence rate with exposure and i_o = the incidence rate without exposure. Estimates of RR are interpreted as follows:

- RR = 1.0 suggests that the factor has no effect.
- RR > 1.0 suggests that the factor increases the risk.
- RR < 1.0 suggests that the factor decreases the risk.

Hazard Ratio

A related measure of risk is the *hazard ratio (HR)*, a parameter that is estimated by regression analysis of prospective data in which the *time to event* from baseline is recorded. Like the RR, HR = 1.0 suggests no effect, HR > 1.0 suggests increased risk, and HR > 1.0 suggests decreased risk. The difference between RR and HR is that the RR is a cumulative measure of risk at a single point in time (usually at the end of the follow-up period) whereas the HR measures the ratio of disease risk among subjects with exposure to a factor compared to subjects without exposure *at any point in time during the entire follow-up period*. Hence, HR = 1.50 indicates that those with exposure are at 50% greater risk than those without exposure *at any point in time during follow-up*, whereas RR = 1.50 indicates that those with exposure are at 50% greater risk than those without exposure *at the end of the follow-up period*.

Odds and Odds Ratio

The standard measure of effect in a retrospective epidemiologic study is the *odds ratio* (OR). The OR is estimated from retrospective case control studies wherein cases with a disease are compared to controls without the disease. In case control studies, it is very important to assemble a sample of controls that are matched to the cases by age, gender, location, and other factors to assure that they have the same opportunity for exposure to putative disease-modifying factors as the cases. The OR is calculated as the ratio of the odds of exposure to a putative disease-modifying factor among cases to the odds of exposure among controls: OR = Exposure odds among cases/Exposure odds among controls. For diseases with low incidence rates, the odds ratio approximates the relative risk (OR ≈ RR). The OR and the RR are interpreted in similar fashion:

- OR = 1.0 suggests that the factor has no effect.
- OR > 1.0 suggests that the factor increases the risk.
- OR > 1.0 suggests that the factor decreases the risk.

Meta-Analysis of Risk Estimates

Meta-analysis is a procedure designed to formally evaluate the consistency of RR estimates from k independent studies and give an unbiased estimate of RR across all studies. Each estimate of RR with its 95% confidence interval (CI) is first converted to ln(RR) with a corresponding variance estimate (v). A combined estimate is then obtained in logarithmic form by weighting individual estimates by $w = 1/v$. The formula for the combined estimate is ln(RR*) = Σw ln(RR)/Σw. This is simply the weighted average of the k logarithmic RR estimates where the weights (w) are the inverse of the corresponding error variances ($w = 1/v$). The combined estimate is given by taking the antilog of ln(RR*), RR* = e^{lnRR*}. A chi square test of heterogeneity called *Cochran's Q test* can be utilized to test for differences among studies. The test statistic for this procedure is

$$Q = \Sigma w(lnRR - lnRR*)^2$$

which is compared to a critical chi square value with $k-1$ degrees of freedom (Borenstein, Hedges, Higgins, & Rothstein, 2009).

Lifestyle and Environment in Cancer Development

British epidemiologists Richard Doll and Richard Peto first quantified the relative contribution of lifestyle and environmental factors to overall cancer mortality (Colditz, Selelrs, & Trapido, 2006; Doll & Peto, 1981). It is notable that only 5%–10% of cancers can be attributed to germline (heritable) genetic defects, whereas the remaining 90%–95% are attributable to environment and lifestyle. **FIGURE 12.10** shows the relative importance of broad classes of environmental and lifestyle factors as percentages of global cancer mortality. Of all cancer-related deaths, approximately 30% are due to chronic tobacco smoking, 30%–35% are due to dietary factors (in particular, the excess consumption of calories resulting in obesity), 15%–20% are due to cancer-causing infectious agents, and 3%–4% are due to alcohol abuse (AACR, 2012).

Various approaches have been used to quantify the impact of lifestyle and environmental factors on the risk of developing various forms of cancer. These include literature reviews, estimates of risk from prospective and retrospective studies, analysis of pooled data, and meta-analysis of published data (Colditz et al., 2006).

One widely used measure of the overall impact of an individual risk factor on a specific disease is the

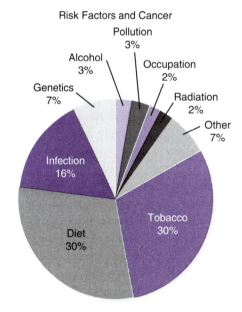

FIGURE 12.10 Lifestyle and Environmental Factors in Cancer Risk.

Data from American Association for Cancer Research. (2012). AACR cancer progress report 2012. *Clinical Cancer Research, 18*, S1–S100.

population attributable risk (also called the *population attributable fraction*). The population attributable risk quantifies the fraction of disease that is due to the presence of a particular risk factor in the population under investigation (e.g., the fraction of lung cancer due to cigarette smoking is about 85%). This parameter can also be thought of as the proportion of cancer cases that could be avoided if exposure to the risk factor was completely eliminated. It is important to remember that such estimates do not account for synergism between multiple factors in disease causation.

A recent investigation examined estimates of the population attributable cancer risk for selected lifestyle and environmental factors in the United Kingdom. Study results suggested that 43% of all incident cancers diagnosed in the U.K. population during 2010 were attributable to 14 major lifestyle and environmental factors. Smoking alone accounted for about 20% of all incident cases, and dietary factors (lack of fruits and vegetables, deficient fiber intake, excess consumption of red and processed meat, and high salt intake) and lack of exercise accounted for an additional 16% of cases (Parkin, Boyd, & Walker, 2011).

▶ Tobacco and Cancer

Tobacco smoking is the most important cancer risk factor. The World Health Organization reports that during the 20th century approximately 50 million people died from tobacco-associated cancers (WHO, 2006, 2008). It is estimated that approximately 50% of regular chronic smokers eventually succumb to tobacco-related cancer, and most die prematurely (International Agency for Cancer Research [IARC], 1986, 2004; Parkin et al., 2005; Peto, Lopez, Boreham, & Thun, 2006; Peto, Lopez, Boreham, Thun, & Heath, 1992; WHO, 2008). Multiple forms of cancer have been linked to chronic exposure of various organs to tobacco smoke, predominantly from smoking cigarettes but also from smoking tobacco in pipes, cigars, and bidis (thin cigarettes consisting of a small amount of tobacco wrapped in the leaf of the *tendu* tree, commonly used in India and South Asia). Tobacco smoking causes about 30% of all cancer deaths, making tobacco smoke the single most lethal source of carcinogens.

▶ 1964 U.S. Surgeon General's Report on Smoking and Health

The 1964 Surgeon General's Report on Smoking and Health was a landmark study that unequivocally linked tobacco to lung cancer, laryngeal cancer, and a number of other severe adverse health outcomes (Terry, 1964). This report was developed by a special committee of experts convened by U.S. Surgeon General Luther Terry to examine the existing evidence on smoking and disease. The report highlighted a number of deleterious health consequences of chronic cigarette smoking. Specifically, the report found that chronic smoking was etiologically linked to lung cancer, laryngeal cancer, chronic bronchitis, emphysema, and coronary heart disease. The 1964 Surgeon General's report and many subsequent reports have had a major impact on public attitudes and policy about smoking in the United States and most other developed nations. In the United States, the percentage of adults who smoke cigarettes has declined from 42% in 1964 to 18% in 2012, a trend that has occurred in the face of continuing concerted efforts by the tobacco industry to promote cigarette smoking and the use of other tobacco products. As a consequence of the declining prevalence of smoking, it is estimated that 8 million premature smoking-related deaths have been prevented in the U.S. population during the past half-century (Holford et al., 2014).

Despite the success of tobacco control in reducing premature deaths in the United States and some developed countries, tobacco use has continued to rise globally resulting in a "tobacco pandemic" that has become one of the greatest public health challenges of all time. Recent survey data compiled from the 193 member nations of WHO revealed the startling statistic that 1 in 3 adults in the world population smoke (**FIGURE 12.11**). An even more disturbing fact is that at least 5.4 million of the 1.1 billion adults who are chronically addicted to the smoking habit die annually from lung cancer and other smoking-related diseases such as heart disease, chronic obstructive pulmonary disease (COPD), stroke, and several other cancers (**FIGURE 12.12**) (WHO, 2006, 2008, 2012).

Compared to individuals who avoid the smoking habit, chronic smokers have a 15–30-fold increased risk of dying from lung cancer (Peto et al., 1992). Worldwide, approximately 85%–90% of lung cancers in both men and women are attributable to cigarette smoking. Chronic tobacco use also markedly increases the risk of cancer development at many other anatomic sites, including the oral cavity, larynx, pharynx, nasal cavity, esophagus, stomach, kidney, urinary bladder, pancreas, liver, and uterine cervix (**FIGURE 12.13**). Smoking has also been implicated in the development of certain types of leukemia, such as acute myelocytic leukemia (Gandini et al., 2008; IARC, 1986; Peto, Lopez, Boreham, & Thun, 2006; Peto, Lopez, Boreham, Thun, & Heath, 1992; Terry, 1964; Vineis et al., 2004; WHO, 2008).

The rise in female smoking prevalence is a critical public health concern. In the United States, more

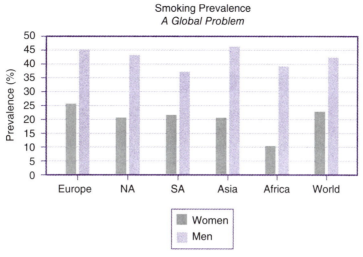

FIGURE 12.11 Global Tobacco Addiction. *Caption*: NA: North America; SA: South America.

Data from World Health Organization. (2008). *WHO report on the global tobacco epidemic, 2008: The MPOWER package.* Geneva, Switzerland: Author.

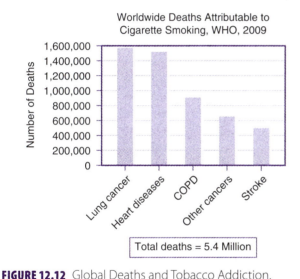

FIGURE 12.12 Global Deaths and Tobacco Addiction.

Data from World Health Organization. (2012). *WHO global report: Mortality attributable to tobacco.* Geneva, Switzerland: Author.

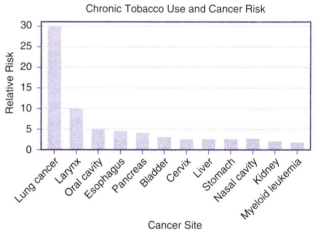

FIGURE 12.13 Relative Risk of Cancer and Chronic Tobacco Smoking.

Data from Peto, R., Lopez, A. D., Boreham, J., Thun, M., & Heath, C. (1992). Mortality from smoking in developed countries: Indirect estimates from national vital statistics. *Lancet, 229,* 1268–1278; Peto, R., Lopez, A. D., Boreham, J., & Thun, M. (2006). *Mortality from smoking in developed countries 1950–2000* (2nd ed.). Geneva, Switzerland: Union for International Cancer Control (UICC).

women now die from smoking-induced lung cancer than from breast cancer, and in some Nordic countries such as Iceland and Denmark, more women than men die from lung cancer. In several European countries, up to 50% of young women are regular smokers, and such high rates will inevitably produce an incredible burden of lung cancer and other smoking-related diseases in women for decades to come (Satcher, 2001).

Cigarette smoke contains three major classes of human carcinogens—polycyclic aromatic hydrocarbons, nitrosamines, and heterocyclic amines—all of which initiate tumors by causing DNA mutations; it also contains a variety of compounds that promote tumor growth and development. The interested reader

is referred to a thorough review of tobacco carcinogenesis that discusses the carcinogens of tobacco smoke, carcinogen uptake and metabolism, and mechanisms by which tobacco carcinogens cause DNA mutations and DNA damage due to the formation of free radicals and reactive oxygen species (Hecht, 1999). Furthermore, cigarette smoke contains powerful stimulants of inflammation and sustained overexpression of inflammatory prostaglandins that upregulate most (if not all) of the molecular mechanisms involved in the genesis and metastasis of malignant neoplasms (Harris, 2007).

Other types of tobacco exposure also have been linked to the development of malignant neoplasms. Pipe and cigar smoking, chewing tobacco, and snuff dipping are all causes of oral cavity cancer, and chronic involuntary (passive) inhalation of tobacco smoke is a risk factor for lung cancer, particularly in women. In counseling individuals about the risk of tobacco use, it is important to keep in mind that tobacco is a major risk factor not only for cancer, but also for a variety of other chronic life-threatening diseases, including cardiovascular disease, myocardial infarction, stroke, chronic bronchitis, emphysema, and asthma.

▶ Diet and Cancer

Only diet rivals tobacco smoke as a cause of cancer, accounting for a comparable number of deaths throughout the world each year. In developed nations, animal (saturated) fat and certain polyunsaturated fatty acids (PUFAs) are associated with cancers of the breast, prostate, and lower gastrointestinal tract (colon and rectum). In developed nations, high-fat diets are linked to the pathogenesis of colorectal cancer, prostate cancer, breast cancer, endometrial cancer, and several other malignancies. In developing nations, diets contaminated by inflammatory and carcinogenic substances often lead to the development of stomach cancer, esophageal cancer, or liver cancer.

The westernized diet of many affluent nations is characterized by the intake of excessive calories from fat, refined carbohydrates, sugar, and animal protein. The westernized diet combined with a sedentary lifestyle can quickly lead to energy imbalance associated with a multitude of chronic diseases such as obesity, type 2 diabetes, cardiovascular disease, arterial hypertension, and cancer. Obesity due to metabolic overload and lack of exercise has been linked to a number of malignancies in the United States and other developed nations. These include colorectal cancer, postmenopausal breast cancer, prostate cancer, endometrial cancer, ovarian cancer, kidney cancer, biliary cancer, and certain forms of esophageal cancer (Calle, Rodriguez, Walker-Thurmond, & Thun, 2003).

Certain types of polyunsaturated fats show differential effects on cancer development. For example, the inflammatory omega-6 PUFA (linoleic acid), which is abundant in the American westernized diet, has been linked to tumor initiation, promotion, and metastasis of colon cancer, breast cancer, endometrial cancer, ovarian cancer, and prostate cancer, whereas the anti-inflammatory omega-3 PUFA (linolenic acid), which is prominent in marine diets, shows antitumor effects.

Gastroesophageal reflux disease (GERD) is a distressing condition of the esophagus that is associated with obesity in the populations of developed nations. In GERD, reflux of stomach acid into the lower esophagus produces morphological changes and dysplasia of the squamous cell lining, a condition known as *Barrett's esophagus*. If left untreated, Barrett's esophagus can progress to invasive esophageal cancer, a highly lethal form of malignancy.

Among non-nutrient food additives, salt is a causal risk factor for stomach cancer, and the decline in stomach cancer mortality throughout the world is largely due to the replacement of salt as a food preservative by refrigeration and other techniques. Nevertheless, many developing nations continue to consume diets high in sodium, thereby resulting in high incidence and mortality rates of stomach cancer.

Aflatoxins are naturally occurring mycotoxins produced by many species of the fungus *Aspergillus*, most notably *Aspergillus flavus* and *Aspergillus parasiticus*. Molds that produce aflatoxins grow on whole grains such as corn, rice, and wheat, as well as on peanuts, almonds, walnuts, sunflower seeds, and spices such as black pepper and coriander. Aflatoxins can contaminate food and food products during processing, storage, or transport when conditions are favorable for mold growth.

Aflatoxin exposure occurs by the ingestion of contaminated foods. On entering the body, aflatoxins are metabolized by the liver into highly carcinogenic epoxides. Chronic exposure to aflatoxins produces liver cancer, a leading cause of death in populations of Southern China, Southeast Asia, and the eastern coastal regions of Africa. Furthermore, aflatoxins and hepatitis viruses (HBV and HCV) interact synergistically in the pathogenesis of liver cancer.

Regular exposure to burning hot beverages, alcohol, and other irritating substances may cause chronic inflammation and the development of dysplastic lesions of the squamous cell lining of the esophagus, a condition known as esophagitis. With continued exposure, such dysplastic changes often progress to esophageal cancer, which is frequently fatal. The practice of ingesting burning hot beverages is commonplace in many cultures of the Far East and the Middle East, where esophageal cancer is a leading cause of cancer death.

Links between diet and cancer may have as much to do with what is *not* in the diet as with what is. For example, low fiber coupled with high fat predisposes to colorectal cancer and perhaps other forms of cancer as well. Many fruits and vegetables contain antioxidants that neutralize free radicals and lessen carcinogenesis, so a lack of fruits and vegetables may contribute to many different types of cancer.

▶ Alcohol and Cancer

Consumption of alcoholic beverages is a major risk factor for malignancies of certain anatomic sites including the oral cavity, the larynx, the esophagus, the liver, and the pancreas. Alcohol abuse in conjunction with chronic cigarette smoking synergistically increases the risk of developing cancer at these anatomic sites. Many epidemiologic studies have also found that regular alcohol consumption independently increases the risk of colon cancer and breast cancer. In 1988, acetaldehyde, the main metabolite of ethanol, was classified as a potent human carcinogen by the International Agency for Research on Cancer and the World Health Organization (IARC & WHO, 1988). More recently, a team of international investigators examined associations between alcohol consumption and cancer risk on a global scale and estimated that 3.6% of all cancers and 3.5% of all cancer deaths are attributable to regular intake of alcoholic beverages (Boffetta, Mashibe, La Vecchia, Zatonski, & Rehm, 2006).

▶ Infection and Cancer

Chronic infections by specific viruses, bacteria, or parasites are responsible for a significant fraction of human cancer (Parkin, 2006). In a recent review and synthesis of global cancer data from 2008, it was estimated that 16.1% of the 12.7 million incident cancers were caused by infectious agents (de Martel et al., 2012).

In developing countries, more than 20% of malignancies and related deaths are caused by infectious agents that cause cervical cancer, liver cancer, stomach cancer, and certain other malignancies. Three pathogens account for a large proportion of the cancer burden in the populations of China, Asia, and Africa: hepatitis viruses (HBV and HCV), which cause liver cancer; sexually transmitted human papillomavirus (HPV) strains 16 and 18, which cause cervical cancer and certain other malignancies; and the food contaminant *H. pylori*, which causes stomach cancer.

In many regions of Central America, Southeast Africa, and India, where HPV infection rates are high and cervical screening programs are nonexistent, cervical cancer ranks first as a cause of cancer death. These populations also have high rates of human immunodeficiency virus (HIV), which predisposes to chronic HPV infection and the development of invasive cervical cancer. Today, more than 80% of all cervical cancer deaths occur in developing countries.

In populations of Eastern and Middle Africa where sexually transmitted diseases (STDs) are rampant, Kaposi's sarcoma due to co-infection by HIV and human herpes virus 8 (HHV-8, also known as Kaposi's sarcoma-associated herpesvirus or KSHV) has become the leading cause of cancer death. In the wetlands of China, India, and the Middle East, parasitic infections by schistosome worms are responsible for high rates of bladder cancer.

In sharp contrast to developing countries, chronic infections account for less than 10% of all malignancies in more developed nations. Stomach cancer has declined in many nations due to replacement of irritating preservatives by refrigeration and ready access to fresh fruits and vegetables and other food products that are free of contamination by *H. pylori*. Early cytological detection of cervical cancer by the Pap test has led to impressive reductions in cervical cancer mortality. Liver cancer rates have also declined in many nations, including China and Thailand, due to effective immunization programs to prevent viral hepatitis and improved storage conditions of staple foods to reduce aflatoxin exposure. Well-designed vaccination programs may prove effective in preventing other cancers arising from known infectious agents; for example, it is likely that vaccination against HBV and high-risk HPV strains may help prevent the development of liver cancer and cervical cancer, respectively.

▶ Global Cancer Prevention and Control

Prevention of disease, including cancer, is often categorized into primary prevention, secondary prevention, and tertiary prevention. Primary prevention refers to avoidance of exposure to disease-causing risk factors. Secondary prevention refers to screening for the detection of antecedent conditions that predispose to disease and are curable by effective treatment or detection of disease at an early stage when effective treatment is likely to restore health. Tertiary prevention involves behavioral changes that limit the progression of disease and improve the quality of life after diagnosis.

A statement from the World Cancer Report, 2008, published by the International Association of Cancer Research (IARC), succinctly captures the essential objectives of effective cancer control:

> *The aim of cancer control is a reduction in both the incidence of the disease and the associated morbidity and mortality, as well as improved life for cancer patients and their families. In addition to substantial*

opportunities for primary prevention, the World Cancer Report also emphasizes the potential of early detection, treatment, and palliative care. It urges all countries to establish comprehensive national cancer control programs, aimed at reducing the incidence of the disease and improving the quality of life for cancer patients and their families. In developing countries in particular, where a large proportion of cancers are detected late in the course of the disease, efforts to achieve earlier diagnosis and delivery of adequate palliative care and pain relief deserve urgent attention. (Boyle & Levin, 2008)

Despite intensive medical and public health efforts, cancer has now surpassed cardiovascular disease as the leading cause of death in people under age 85 years in highly developed nations such as the United States (Parkin et al., 2005). Although some progress has been made in cancer therapy, particularly in the treatment of leukemia in children, conventional methods of surgery, chemotherapy, and radiotherapy have not impacted greatly on the general morbidity and mortality due to many forms of cancer in adults. It is also important to realize that as developing countries succeed in achieving lifestyles similar to Europe, North America, Australia, New Zealand, and Japan, their populations will encounter much higher cancer rates, particularly cancers of the lung, breast, colon, prostate, and other malignancies that tend to appear later in life.

As pointed out by Dr. Moon Chen, Jr., in his review of cancer prevention and control for Asian and Pacific Islander Americans: "In order to achieve the full benefit of cancer prevention, attention must be directed to the unique cultural, linguistic, and behavioral attributes of Asian and Pacific Islander Americans." It is essential that this concept be extended to all target populations. In the words of Dr. Chen: "Effective cancer prevention and control initiatives must incorporate scientific validity, linguistic appropriateness, and cultural competence" (Chen, 1998).

Primary Cancer Prevention

At the core of all cancer prevention and control strategies are the following key elements of primary prevention (see also **TABLE 12.1**):

- Abstinence from tobacco and smoking cessation
- Limiting alcohol intake
- Regular exercise
- Maintaining optimum weight
- Eating a healthy diet with daily fruits and vegetables
- Limiting salt intake
- Practicing safe sex to avoid STDs such as HPV strains 16 and 18 and HIV
- Avoiding exposure to hepatitis viruses such as HBV and HCV
- Vaccination against HPV and HBV
- Avoidance or early treatment of parasitic infections such as schistosomiasis
- Avoiding excessive exposure to sunlight and other sources of radiation such as radon
- Infection control by good personal hygiene and judicious use of antibiotics and antiviral drugs
- Avoiding known chemical carcinogens such as asbestos (occupational hazard), arsenic (water contaminant), aflatoxins (food contaminant), and dioxin (environmental contaminant).

Keep in mind that this list of preventive strategies is far from inclusive and will require continual updating to keep pace with the identification of other carcinogenic factors present in the environment.

Secondary Cancer Prevention

Premalignant lesions and conditions that herald the development of cancer can usually be treated with a much higher likelihood of success than cancer itself. Effective cancer control therefore includes comprehensive cancer screening for the timely diagnosis and effective treatment of cellular lesions that could progress to invasive cancer. Proven screening methodologies with good sensitivity and specificity include mammograms for carcinoma in situ (CIS) of the breast, Papanicolaou (Pap) tests for cervical dysplasia, endoscopies for Barrett's esophagus and stomach ulcers, dental examination for oral leukoplakia, colonoscopy for colorectal adenomas and prostate-specific antigen (PSA), and ultrasound for noninvasive adenocarcinoma of the prostate gland. All of these lesions, if detected early, can be cured by limited surgical resection. Refinements in tissue imaging such as magnetic resonance (MR) and computed tomography (CT) have also led to improvements in the early detection of tumors.

Well-designed population screening programs coupled with skilled surgical excision or ablation of premalignant lesions have already been tremendously successful in reducing the mortality rates of certain cancers in developed nations. Currently, only about half of cancer patients in these populations eventually die from their disease. This differs markedly from developing nations wherein 80% of cancer victims already have late-stage (incurable) tumors when they are diagnosed.

These findings point out the need for development of much better early detection programs in many

TABLE 12.1 Cancer Risk Factors and Preventive Strategies

Risk Factor	Cancer Sites	Prevention
Tobacco use	Lung, pharynx, larynx, uterine cervix, bladder	Abstinence, cessation
Obesity, high fat and high calorie diet, sedentary lifestyle	Breast, prostate, colon, kidney, ovary, lower esophagus	Exercise, weight control, healthy diet with daily fruits and vegetables
Alcohol abuse	Oral cavity, esophagus, pancreas, liver	Limit alcohol intake to one drink or less daily
HPV STI	Uterine cervix, oral cavity, vulva, penis	Avoid exposure, vaccination
Hepatitis virus	Liver and biliary tract	Avoid exposure, vaccination
H. pylori and high salt intake	Stomach	Antibiotics, limit salt intake
Radiation	Skin (melanoma)	Limit sun exposure
Infectious disease	Lymphoma, leukemia	Good personal hygiene, safe sex practices, antibiotics, and antivirals

nations. Such screening modalities must be accurate, safe, inexpensive, and acceptable to the general public. Secondary prevention also mandates regular (annual) physical examinations for identification and treatment of chronic symptomatic medical conditions in individuals with inherent cancer risk factors such as chronic smoking and nicotine addiction, alcohol abuse, COPD, obesity, GERD, and chronic infections such as hepatitis and HIV.

Tertiary Cancer Prevention

Tertiary prevention emphasizes beneficial behavioral changes that limit disease progression and subsequent disability for patients after they have been diagnosed with cancer. Fundamental tertiary preventive practices include smoking cessation, limiting alcohol intake, regular exercise, improved diet, maintenance of optimum weight, and compliance with prescribed treatment regimens. Pain control and palliative care should be implemented when necessary. The ultimate goal of tertiary prevention is to improve the quality of life among cancer survivors and their families.

▶ Cancer Education

Global cancer control polices have been adopted by WHO, IARC, the American Cancer Society (ACS),

the NCI, and many other national and international health organizations. Nevertheless, there is an urgent need for all countries to establish comprehensive national cancer control programs with the objective of reducing cancer incidence and mortality through prevention.

Educational programs should be designed and implemented where they are needed in order to create a high degree of disease awareness regarding the risk factors and early symptoms of cancer and to disseminate accurate information on the cost, safety, and accuracy of cancer screening tests and the availability and effectiveness of cancer treatment modalities. In developing countries in particular, where a large proportion of cancers are detected late in the course of the disease, efforts to achieve earlier diagnosis and delivery of adequate treatment, palliative care, and pain relief deserve immediate attention.

Comprehensive programs of cancer prevention and control must also incorporate effective and carefully evaluated school education programs for early health promotion and disease prevention. Finally, it is imperative that such programs provide continued support of cancer research with particular focus on the molecular biology and molecular genetics of cancer in order to identify etiologic mechanisms of carcinogenesis that translate to effective interventions for the eradication of the disease.

References

Ahmad, O., Boschi-Pinto, C., Lopez, A. D., Murray, C. J. L., Lozano, R., & Inoue, M. (2001). *Age standardization of rates: A new WHO standard*. Geneva, Switzerland: World Health Organization.

American Association for Cancer Research. (2012). AACR cancer progress report 2012. *Clinical Cancer Research, 18,* S1–S100.

American Cancer Society. (2018). *Cancer facts and figures, 2015.* Atlanta, GA: Author. Retrieved from http://www.cancer.org/research/cancerfactsstatistics/cancerfactsfigures2015/index

Boffetta, P., Mashibe, M., La Vecchia, C., Zatonski, W., & Rehm, J. (2006). The burden of cancer attributable to alcohol drinking. *International Journal of Cancer, 119*(4), 884–887.

Borenstein, M., Hedges, L. V., Higgins, J. P. T., & Rothstein, H. R. (2009). *Introduction to meta-analysis.* Hoboken, NJ: John Wiley & Sons.

Boyle, P., & Levin, B. (Eds.). (2008). *IARC world cancer report.* Lyon, France: International Agency for Research on Cancer (IARC) Publications.

Bray, F., & Moller, B. (2006). Predicting the future burden of cancer. *Nature Reviews Cancer, 6,* 63–74.

Calle, E. E., Rodriguez, C., Walker-Thurmond, K., & Thun, M. J. (2003). Overweight, obesity, and mortality from cancer in a prospectively studied cohort of U.S. adults. *New England Journal of Medicine, 348,* 1625–1638.

Chen, M. (1998). Cancer prevention and control among Asian and Pacific Islander Americans. *Cancer, 83*(S8), 1856–1864.

Colditz, G. A., Selelrs, T. A., & Trapido, E. (2006). Epidemiology—identifying the causes and preventability of cancer? *Nature Reviews Cancer, 6,* 75–83.

de Martel, C., Ferlay, J., Franceschi, S., Vignat, J., Bray, F., Forman, D., & Plummer, M. (2012). Global burden of cancers attributable to infections in 2008: A review and synthetic analysis. *Lancet Oncology, 13*(6), 607–615.

Doll, R., & Peto, R. (1981). The causes of cancer: Quantitative estimates of avoidable risks of cancer in the United States today. *Journal of the National Cancer Institute, 66*(6), 1191–1308.

Ferlay, J., Ervik, M., Lam, F., Colombet, M., Mery, L., Piñeros, M., … Bray, F. (2018). *Global cancer observatory: Cancer today.* Lyon, France: International Agency for Research on Cancer. Retrieved from https://gco.iarc.fr/today

Ferlay, J., Shin, H. R., Bray, F., Forman, D., Mathers, C., & Parkin, D. M. (2010). Estimates of worldwide burden of cancer in 2008: GLOBOCAN 2008. *International Journal of Cancer, 127,* 2893–2917.

Ferlay, J., Soerjomataram, I., Ervik, M., Dikshit, R., Eser, S., Mathers, C., … Bray, F. (2013). *GLOBOCAN 2012 v1.0. Cancer incidence and mortality worldwide: IARC CancerBase No. 11* [Internet]. Lyon, France: International Agency for Research on Cancer.

Fitzmaurice, C., Akinyemiju, T. F., Al Lami, F. H., Alam, T., Alizadeh-Navaei, R., Allen, C., … Global Burden of Disease Cancer Collaboration. (2018, June 02). Global, regional, and national cancer incidence, mortality, years of life lost, years lived with disability, and disability-adjusted life-years for 29 cancer groups, 1990 to 2016: A systematic analysis for the Global Burden of Disease Study. *JAMA Oncology.* Online publication. doi:10.1001/jamaoncol.2018.2706.

Fitzmaurice, C., Allen, C., Barber, R. M., Barregard, L., Bhutta, Z. A., Brenner, H., … Global Burden of Disease Cancer Collaboration. (2017). Global, regional, and national cancer incidence, mortality, years of life lost, years lived with disability, and disability-adjusted life-years for 32 cancer groups, 1990 to 2015: A systematic analysis for the Global Burden of Disease Study. *JAMA Oncology, 3*(4), 524–548.

Gandini, S., Botteri, E., Iodice, S., Boniol, M., Lowenfels, A. B., Maisonneuve, P., & Boyle, P. (2008). Tobacco smoking and cancer: A meta-analysis. *International Journal of Cancer, 122*(1), 155–164.

Garcia, M., Jemal, A., Ward, E. M., Center, M. M., Hao, Y., Siegel, R. L., & Thun, M. J. (2007). *Global cancer facts and figures 2007.* Atlanta, GA: American Cancer Society.

Harris, R. E. (2007). Cyclooxygenase 2 (COX-2) and the inflammogenesis of cancer. *Subcellular Biochemistry, 42,* 93–126.

Hecht, S. S. (1999). Tobacco smoke carcinogens and lung cancer. *Journal of the National Cancer Institute, 91*(14), 1194–1210.

Hill, A. B. (1965). The environment and disease: Association or causation? *Proceedings of the Royal Society of Medicine, 58,* 295–300.

Holford, T. R., Meza, R., Warner, K. E., Meernik, C., Jeon, J., Moolgavkar, S. H., & Levy, D. T. (2014). Tobacco control and the reduction in smoking-related premature deaths in the United States, 1964–2012. *Journal of the American Medical Association, 311*(2), 164–171.

Horner, M. J., Ries, L. A. G., Krapcho, M., Neyman, N., Aminou, R., Howlader, N., … Edwards, B. K. (Eds.). (2009). *SEER cancer statistics review, 1975–2006.* Bethesda, MD: National Cancer Institute.

International Agency for Research on Cancer. (1986). *Tobacco smoking. IARC monographs on the evaluation of carcinogenic risks to humans* (Vol. 38). Lyon, France: Author.

International Agency for Research on Cancer. (2004). *Tobacco smoke and involuntary smoking. IARC monographs on the evaluation of carcinogenic risks to humans* (Vol. 83). Lyon, France: Author.

International Agency for Research on Cancer and World Health Organization. (1988). *Alcohol drinking* (Vol. 44). Lyon, France: Author.

Jemal, A., Bray, F., Center, M. M., Ferlay, J., Ward, E., & Forman, D. (2011). Global cancer statistics. *CA: A Cancer Journal for Clinicians, 61*(2), 69–90.

Jemal, A., Center, M. M., DeSantis, C., & Ward, E. M. (2010). Global patterns of cancer incidence and mortality rates and trends. *Cancer Epidemiology, Biomarkers and Prevention, 19,* 1893–1907.

Parkin, D. M. (2006). The global health burden of infection-associated cancers in the year 2002. *International Journal of Cancer, 118*(12), 3030–3044.

Parkin, D. M., Boyd, L., & Walker, L. C. (2011). The fraction of cancer attributable to lifestyle and environmental factors in the U.K. in 2010. Summary and conclusions. *British Journal of Cancer, 105*(S2), S77–S81.

Parkin, D. M., Bray, F., Ferlay, J., & Pisani, P. (2001). Estimating the world cancer burden: GLOBOCAN 2000. *International Journal of Cancer, 94,* 153–156.

Parkin, D. M., Bray, F., Ferlay, J., & Pisani, P. (2005). Global cancer statistics, 2002. *CA: A Cancer Journal for Clinicians, 55,* 74–108.

Peto, R., Lopez, A. D., Boreham, J., & Thun, M. (2006). *Mortality from smoking in developed countries 1950–2000* (2nd ed.). Geneva, Switzerland: International Union Against Cancer (UICC).

Peto, R., Lopez, A. D., Boreham, J., Thun, M., & Heath, C. (1992). Mortality from smoking in developed countries: Indirect estimates from national vital statistics. *Lancet, 229,* 1268–1278.

Robbins, S. L., & Cotran, R. S. (1979). *Pathologic basis of disease* (2nd ed.). Philadelphia, PA: W. B. Saunders.

Roser, M., & Ritchie, H. (2018). Cancer. Published online at *OurWorldInData.org*. Retrieved from https://ourworldindata.org/cancer

Satcher, D. (2001). *Women and smoking: A report of the surgeon general*. Atlanta, GA: Office on Smoking and Health, Centers for Disease Control and Prevention.

Soerjomataram, I., Lortet-Tieulent, J., Parkin, D. M., Ferlay, J., Mathers, C., Forman, D., & Bray, F. (2012). Global burden of cancer in 2008: A systematic analysis of disability-adjusted life-years in 12 world regions. *Lancet, 380*(9856), 1840–1850.

Stewart, B. W., & Kleihues, P. (Eds.). (2003). *IARC world cancer report 2003*. Lyon, France: International Agency for Research on Cancer (IARC) Publications.

Stewart, B. W., & Wild, C. P. (Eds.). (2014). *IARC world cancer report 2014*. Lyon, France: International Agency for Research on Cancer (IARC) Publications.

Surveillance, Epidemiology, and End Results Program. (2014). *Overview of the SEER Program*. Bethesda, MD: National Cancer Institute. Retrieved from http://seer.cancer.gov

Terry, L. (1964). *Smoking and health: Report of the advisory committee to the surgeon general of the Public Health Service*. Washington, DC: U.S. Department of Health, Education and Welfare.

Thun, M. J., DeLancey, J. O., Center, M. M., Jemal, A., & Ward, E. M. (2010). The global burden of cancer: Priorities for prevention. *Carcinogenesis, 31*(1), 100–110.

U.S. Surgeon General. (1964). *Smoking and health*. Washington, DC: U.S. Department of Health, Education, and Welfare.

Vineis, P., Alavanja, M., Buffler, P., Fontham, E., Franceschi, S., Gao, Y. T., … Doll, R. (2004). Tobacco and cancer: Recent epidemiological evidence. *Journal of the National Cancer Institute, 96*(2), 99–106.

World Bank. (2014). *World bank open data*. Washington, DC: World Bank Group. Retrieved from http://data.worldbank.org/data-catalog/world-development-indicators

World Health Organization. (2004). *Global burden of disease 2004 update*. Geneva, Switzerland: Author.

World Health Organization. (2006). *Cancer*. Geneva, Switzerland: Author.

World Health Organization. (2008). *WHO report on the global tobacco epidemic, 2008: The MPOWER package*. Geneva, Switzerland: Author.

World Health Organization. (2012). *WHO global report: Mortality attributable to tobacco*. Geneva, Switzerland: Author.

CHAPTER 13

Epidemiology of Lung Cancer

▶ Anatomy and Function of the Lungs

The human lungs are paired organs that perform the cardinal function of exchanging carbon dioxide in the blood for oxygen in inspired air. The left lung is divided into two lobes and the right lung into three lobes. Together, they contain approximately 1500 miles of airways and 300–500 million alveoli where the carbon dioxide and oxygen exchange occurs. The total surface area of adult human lungs is approximately 70 m² (roughly the same area as one side of a tennis court). If all the capillary vessels that envelop the alveoli were unwound and laid end to end, they would extend for more than 600 miles.

Inspired air is conducted into the lungs through the trachea, the bronchi, and the bronchioles (**FIGURE 13.1**). This *conducting zone* is not involved in gas exchange and is reinforced with cartilage to maintain patency for the inhalation and exhalation of air. Its function is to warm the inspired air to 98.6°F (37°C) and humidify the air. Small projections known as *cilia* effectively cleanse inspired air by wave-like motions that propel foreign material back into the larger bronchi and trachea, where the cough reflex completes the expulsion. Furthermore, mucus-secreting cells and immune cells line the airways and help protect the lungs by trapping viruses, bacteria, pollen, dust, and other foreign material.

Exchange of gases occurs in the *respiratory zone*, which consists of respiratory bronchioles, the alveolar ducts, and the alveoli (Figure 13.1). The alveolar epithelium is a continuous layer of cells consisting of two principal cell types: type I pneumocytes that cover 95% of the alveolar surface and granular type II pneumocytes that secrete pulmonary surfactant (the major lubricant in the lungs) and that are involved in repairing damage to the alveoli. Type I pneumocytes interface with the endothelial cells lining the pulmonary capillaries to facilitate the diffusion of carbon dioxide and oxygen across the alveolar–capillary membrane.

Total lung capacity ranges between 4 and 6 L and is contingent upon age, height, weight, and gender. On average, females have 20%–25% less capacity than males. The typical adult resting respiratory rate is 10–20 breaths per minute, and with each breath about 500 mL of air is exchanged (the tidal volume). Nevertheless, the lungs have a tremendous reserve volume, and the amount of air that can be exchanged by *forced* inspiration and expiration is about 4 L (the vital capacity). The average human breathes approximately 11,000 L of air containing 2.31 L of oxygen per day (Kumar, Abbas, & Aster, 2014; Weinberger, 2004).

▶ Global Burden of Lung Cancer

Based on data published by the *International Agency for Research on Cancer* (IARC) and the *World Health Organization* (WHO), lung cancer caused 1.76 million deaths in 2018 (1.18 million in men and 576,000 in women), more than double that of any other form

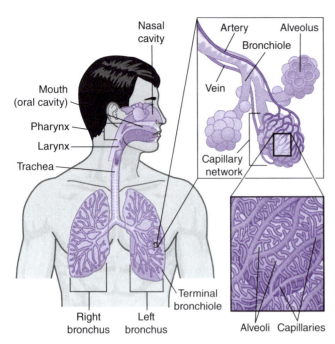

FIGURE 13.1 Diagram of Human Lungs and Alveoli.

of cancer. In the same year, over 2.09 million new cases of lung cancer were diagnosed (1.37 million in men and 725,000 in women), an overall increase of 29.8% since 2008. Nearly 90% of lung cancer patients die from the disease, most within only a few months of diagnosis. Even in developed countries, 25%–30% of all cancer deaths are due to lung cancer. More people die from lung cancer than breast cancer, prostate cancer, and colon cancer combined (Boyle & Levin, 2008; Ferlay et al., 2010, 2013, 2018).

▶ Global Lung Cancer Incidence and Mortality

Despite the increasing numbers of lung cancer cases and deaths worldwide, the age-adjusted rates of incidence and mortality are declining in men and have stabilized in women. For example, the age-adjusted incidence for men declined from approximately 48 per 100,000 in 2005 to 31.5 per 100,000 in 2018, and the rates for women decreased from 17 per 100,000 to 14.6 per 100,000 during the same time period. Clearly, the aging and growth of the world population are the primary forces driving the increased numbers of lung cancer cases and deaths worldwide (Ferlay et al., 2018; Fitzmaurice et al., 2017, 2018).

The death toll from lung cancer in the 20th century exceeded 25 million, and already in the 21st century, 25 million more people have died from lung cancer. Based on the current trajectory of smoking patterns around the globe, it is estimated that 250 million people will die from lung cancer and other smoking-related cancers in the 21st century (Proctor, 2001).

Tobacco smoking is the dominant etiologic factor of lung cancer and is responsible for approximately 87% of cases. The highest rates of lung cancer therefore occur in nations with the highest prevalence rates of chronic smoking such as North America, Europe, and China (**FIGURE 13.2**) (Ferlay et al., 2018). However, in evaluating the global lung cancer incidence and mortality maps in Figure 13.2, it must be kept in mind that lung cancer develops over a long period of time, perhaps decades from initiation until diagnosis. The world lung cancer mortality rates of today are therefore the consequence of many years of past smoking exposure. Indeed, young people throughout the world are taking up the smoking habit with alarming alacrity (greater than 50% in populous countries such as China, India, and Russia), and unless reversed, this unfortunate trend will have devastating health consequences in generations to come. A particularly disturbing global trend is the rising prevalence of chronic smoking among women, which has produced sharp increases in lung cancer incidence and mortality rates among women. For example, the prevalence of smoking among adult women in the United States increased from about 6% in 1924 to 30% by 1980, which caused a 600% increase in lung cancer mortality among U.S. women during the last half of the 20th century (Satcher, 2001). The following statement from officials of the American Cancer Society succinctly describes the global marketing expansion of tobacco throughout the world by the tobacco industry: "Globally, the data are very clear in indicating that the tobacco epidemic has now expanded to and become more focused in the world's low-and middle-income countries, due largely to the expansion of the multinational tobacco industry's marketing efforts in Eastern Europe, Asia, Africa, and Latin America" (Glynn, Seffrin, Brawley, Grey, & Ross, 2010, p. 51).

Notably, the world's most populous country, China, is also the largest producer of tobacco and has the greatest number of smokers. The Chinese tobacco industry produces 42% of the world's cigarettes, and in China's population of 1.35 billion, there are 350 million people who smoke, which accounts for one-third of all smokers on the planet. Approximately 60% of Chinese men smoke and 4% of Chinese women. Recent estimates suggest that 1.3 million of the 5.4 million people in the world who die annually of smoking-related diseases are Chinese (Li, 2012).

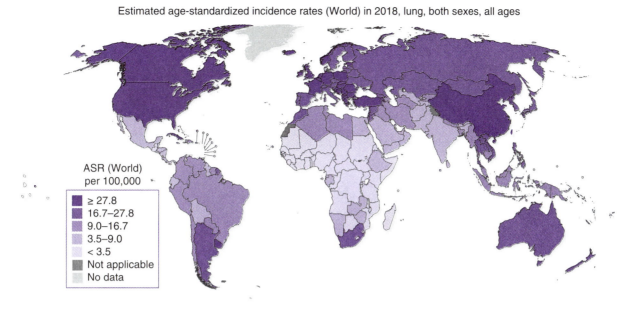

Estimated age-standardized incidence rates (World) in 2018, lung, both sexes, all ages

ASR (World)
per 100,000

≥ 27.8
16.7–27.8
9.0–16.7
3.5–9.0
< 3.5
Not applicable
No data

Estimated age-standardized mortality rates (World) in 2018, lung, both sexes, all ages

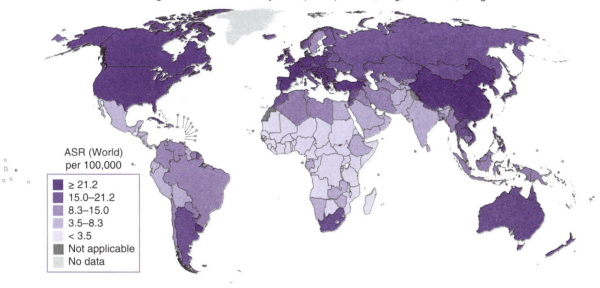

ASR (World)
per 100,000

≥ 21.2
15.0–21.2
8.3–15.0
3.5–8.3
< 3.5
Not applicable
No data

FIGURE 13.2 Global Incidence and Mortality Rates of Lung Cancer, 2018. *Caption*: ASR: Rates per 100,000 are Age-standardized to the World Population, 2000–2025.

Reproduced from Ferlay, J., Ervik, M., Lam, F., Colombet, M., Mery, L., Piñeros, M., ... Bray, F. (2018). *Global cancer observatory: Cancer today*. Lyon, France: International Agency for Research on Cancer. Retrieved from https://gco.iarc.fr/today

▶ Cigarette Smoking and Lung Cancer

The dominant risk factor for lung cancer is cigarette smoking. Early epidemiologic studies by Ernst Wynder and Evarts Graham in the United States and Richard Doll and Bradford Hill in Great Britain clearly demonstrated the etiologic link between cigarette smoking and cancer of the lung (Doll & Hill, 1950; Wynder & Graham, 1950). As shown by the data published by Wynder and Graham in 1950, lung cancer risk steadily rises with increasing smoking intensity; for example,

compared to people who have never smoked, the odds of developing lung cancer is 30-fold higher in women and 50-fold higher in men who smoke at least two packs of cigarettes per day (**FIGURE 13.3**).

Since the pioneering studies of Wynder and Graham in the United States and Doll and Hill in Great Britain, hundreds of subsequent investigations have confirmed the causal role of tobacco smoking in the genesis of lung cancer. A landmark study was the 1964 Surgeon General's Report on Smoking and Health, which provided unequivocal evidence that chronic cigarette smoking causes lung cancer. In a pooled analysis of seven prospective studies cited

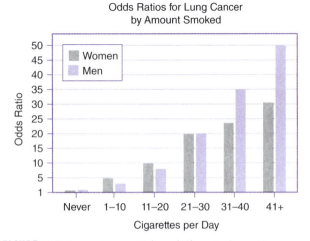

FIGURE 13.3 Lung Cancer Risk and Chronic Cigarette Smoking.

Data from Wynder, E. L., & Graham, E. A. (1950). Tobacco smoking as a possible etiologic factor in bronchiogenic carcinoma. *Journal of the American Medical Association*, 143, 329–336.

in the report, lung cancer mortality among chronic smokers was 11-fold higher than for nonsmokers, and the mortality ratio increased progressively with the amount of smoking. For example, lung cancer mortality among those who smoked two or more packs per day was more than 20-fold higher than for nonsmokers. Similar results were noted for nine case control studies cited in the report (Terry, 1964).

In a recent voluminous investigation of the epidemiologic evidence on smoking and lung cancer, 16,616 estimates of risk ascertained from 287 studies conducted between 1950 and 2000 were examined by meta-analysis. The overall risk of developing any histologic type of lung cancer was markedly elevated in current smokers compared to nonsmokers (relative risk [RR] = 8.4), and the risk for squamous cell carcinoma (RR = 16.9) was higher than for adenocarcinoma (RR = 4.2). The data showed increasing risk with various measures of exposure including increasing amount smoked, duration of smoking, tar level, and earlier age of starting to smoke, and decreasing risk with duration of smoking cessation. Risk increases were noted for ever smoking, current smoking, and ex-smoking; for smoking pipes and cigars; and for all types of cigarettes studied. Significant risk increases were evident for men and women, in younger and older subjects, in all continents studied, and in prospective and retrospective studies. The causal association was clearly evident for each of the major histological types of lung cancer studied, being stronger for squamous and small cell carcinoma, intermediate for large cell carcinoma, and weakest for adenocarcinoma (Lee, Forey, & Coombs, 2012). Similar results of meta-analyses have been reported by several other investigators, underscoring the dominant causal

role of exposure to tobacco smoke in the development of cancer of the human lung (Gandini et al., 2008; Khuder, 2001; Vineis et al., 2004).

▶ Cigarette Smoking and Lung Cancer Mortality in the United States

The cause and effect pattern of smoking and lung cancer is clearly visible on examination of ecologic time trend data in the United States (American Cancer Society, 2014) (**FIGURE 13.4**). In the early years of the 20th century, lung cancer occurred infrequently and was considered a reportable disease in most medical research journals (Wynder & Stellman, 1977). As shown in the figure, the rates began to increase after the advent of cigarette smoking in the 1930s, and thereafter lung cancer incidence and mortality continually climbed, reaching epidemic proportions during mid-century and overwhelming other forms of cancer as the leading cause of cancer death. Note the close parallelism of lung cancer mortality and cigarette use in the United States that has persisted since 1930. The time interval between the exposure curve and the mortality curve reflects an approximate average development time of 20 years or more for lung carcinogenesis (American Cancer Society, 2011). In recent years, annual incidence rates of lung cancer in the U.S. population have declined slightly (2.6% in men and 1.1% in women during 2005–2009). This encouraging trend reflects some success in the

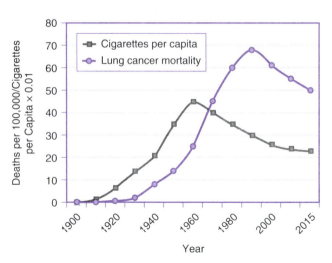

FIGURE 13.4 Lung Cancer Mortality and Cigarettes Per Capita, United States.

Data from American Cancer Society. (2014). *Cancer facts and figures 2014*. Atlanta, GA: Author. Retrieved from http://www .cancer.org/research/cancerfactsstatistics/cancerfactsfigures2014/index (annual mortality rates are the averages for men and women); American Lung Association. (2011). *Trends in tobacco use*. Chicago, IL: Author. Retrieved from http://www.lung.org /finding-cures/our-research/trend-reports/Tobacco-Trend-Report.pdf (annual cigarettes per capita × 0.01).

prevention and control of tobacco use (Henley et al., 2014). Nevertheless, during 2012, more than 160,000 people died from lung cancer (88,000 men and 73,000 women) in the U.S. population, which exceeded the total number of deaths from the next four most deadly cancers (colorectal cancer, breast cancer, pancreatic cancer, and prostate cancer caused a total of 157,000 deaths).

▶ Smoking and Histologic Changes in Lung Tissues

An important confirmatory study of the role of cigarette smoking in the development of lung cancer was published in 1961 by Oscar Auerbach and colleagues. The investigation presented the results of microscopic examination of lung specimens taken at autopsy from 402 men, 63 who died from lung cancer and 339 who died from causes other than lung cancer at the Veterans Administration Hospital in East Orange, New Jersey. For each autopsy case, data on smoking history were ascertained from the family and the frequencies of histological changes observed in smokers and nonsmokers were compared. The *Auerbach protocol* involved histological examination of specimens taken from 208 anatomic sites of each tracheobronchial tree. Results were based on the microscopic examination of 20,665 randomized and coded slides, which clearly showed that the frequency and severity of cellular alterations in the lungs were directly related to the intensity and duration of cigarette smoking by the patient. Lung tissues from smoking cases had significantly higher frequencies of carcinoma in situ, squamous metaplasia, hyperplasia, and loss of cilia than lung tissues from nonsmoking patients. Furthermore, the frequency of lesions increased with the level of smoking. For example, among 65 men who never smoked regularly, 16.8% of 3324 specimens showed at least one histological change in the epithelium, whereas one or more epithelial changes were found in 98.0% of the 13,689 specimens from 274 men who regularly smoked cigarettes and died of causes other than lung cancer and in 99.8% of the 2784 specimens from 63 men who died of lung cancer. Most notably, the frequency of carcinoma in situ was 0% in nonsmokers, 20% in those who smoked less than one pack of cigarettes per day, 48% in those who smoked 1–2 packs per day, 75% in those who smoked more than two packs of cigarettes per day, and 83% in those who died from lung cancer. Based on these results, the investigators concluded the following: "In our

opinion the histologic evidence from this study greatly strengthens the already overwhelming body of epidemiologic evidence that cigarette smoking is a major factor in the causation of bronchogenic carcinoma" (Auerbach, Stout, Hammond, & Garfinkel, 1961, p. 267).

▶ Transition of Lung Cancer Cell Types

Major changes have occurred in the profile of histologic cell types of lung cancer being diagnosed during the past several decades. Specifically, rates of adenocarcinoma of the lung have increased dramatically with corresponding decreases in squamous cell and small (oat) cell carcinoma. The most striking change is the proportion of pulmonary adenocarcinoma compared to squamous cell carcinoma among men and women with lung cancer. During the period 1975–2010, the odds of pulmonary adenocarcinoma to squamous cell carcinoma increased from 0.5 to 1.5 in men with lung cancer and from 1.2 to 2.7 in women with lung cancer. Clearly, pulmonary adenocarcinomas have replaced squamous cell carcinomas as the predominant histologic cell type of lung cancer (**FIGURE 13.5**) (National Cancer Institute, 2014; Meza, Meernik, Jeon, & Cote, 2015).

Concurrent with the changing histologic profile of lung cancer, the composition of U.S. cigarettes has also changed dramatically in recent decades. Filtered brands now dominate the market and currently comprise over 85% of all cigarettes manufactured in the United States. This trend is reflected by decreases in the average tar and nicotine yields per cigarette. Among smokers in the United States, about 96% of women and 92% of men smoke filter cigarettes. Despite this transition to "low-yield" cigarettes, smokers tend to inhale deeper and compensate

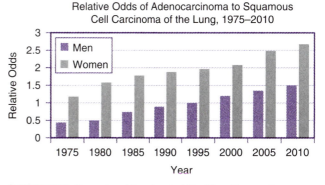

FIGURE 13.5 Changing Histological Profile of Lung Cancer.

Data from Meza, R., Meernik, C., Jeon, J., & Cote, M. L. (2015). Lung cancer incidence trends by gender, race and histology in the United States, 1973–2010. *PLoS One, 10*(3), e0121323.

by smoking more cigarettes, which may account for the drastic increase in lung adenocarcinoma among cigarette smokers in recent years (Augustine, Harris, & Wynder, 1989). As pointed out by Wynder and Muscat (1995):

> Smokers of low-yield (filtered) cigarettes compensate for the low delivery of nicotine by inhaling the smoke more deeply and by smoking more intensely; such smokers may be taking up to 5 puffs/min with puff volumes up to 55 mL. Under these conditions, the peripheral lung is exposed to increased amounts of smoke carcinogens that are suspected to lead to lung adenocarcinoma. (p. 143)

There is also evidence from epidemiologic studies that women have a greater predisposition to smoking-induced lung carcinogenesis than men (Harris, Zang, Anderson, & Wynder, 1993; Risch et al., 1993; Zang & Wynder, 1992). The results of these studies indicate that the risk of lung cancer, particularly adenocarcinoma, is approximately twofold higher in women who smoke than in men of the same age who smoke the same amount. Although it has been suggested that the greater susceptibility of women may relate to estrogens or estrogen receptors in the lung epithelium, the biological basis of the observed differential gender predisposition to tobacco carcinogenesis remains to be clarified.

▶ Cigarette Smoking and Lung Cancer Histology

A team of international investigators recently explored associations of smoking with the major histologic cell types of lung cancer using one of the largest epidemiologic datasets on lung cancer ever assembled. The dataset included 13,169 lung cancer cases and 16,010 controls ascertained from the SYNERGY database of eight European case control studies in 11 European countries and one case control study in Canada during 1985–2005. Controls were frequency-matched to the cases by age, gender, and location. Lung cancer risks were quantified by estimating odds ratios for squamous cell carcinoma, small cell carcinoma, and adenocarcinoma of the lung. Although all histologic types of lung cancer were strongly associated with smoking, the risk estimates were markedly higher for squamous cell and small cell carcinomas compared to adenocarcinomas. As shown in **FIGURE 13.6**, among men and women who smoked 30 or more cigarettes daily, the odds of developing either squamous cell carcinoma or small cell

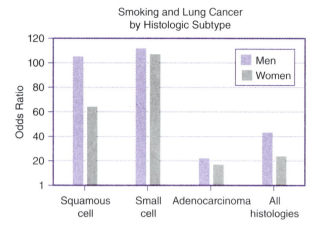

FIGURE 13.6 Odds Ratios for Chronic Smoking by Histologic Subtype of Lung Cancer. *Caption*: Average Level of Current Smoking: 30 or More Cigarettes per Day.

Data from Pesch, B., Kendzia, B., Gustavsson, P., Jöckel, K. H., Johnen, G., Pohlabeln, H., . . . Brüning, T. (2012). Cigarette smoking and lung cancer—relative risk estimates for the major histological types from a pooled analysis of case–control studies. *International Journal of Cancer, 131*(5), 1210–1219.

carcinoma were four to five times higher than the odds of developing adenocarcinoma. There were also differences in the histologic profile of lung cancer in men and women and among smokers versus nonsmokers. Among men, most tumors (53%) were squamous cell carcinomas, 20% were small cell carcinomas, and 27% were adenocarcinomas. Among women, most tumors (50%) were adenocarcinomas, 28% were squamous cell carcinomas, and 22% were small cell carcinomas. Notably, among 889 cases who reported no smoking history, pulmonary adenocarcinoma was the leading subtype (58% and 70% in men and women, respectively). The authors suggest their findings of steeper dose–response gradients in the risk of squamous cell carcinoma and small cell carcinoma compared to adenocarcinoma with increasing exposure to tobacco smoke "may reflect different response pathways of the lung depending on the exposure to pulmonary carcinogens and the extent of tissue damage" (Pesch et al., 2012). Nevertheless, the two- to fourfold higher relative frequencies of nonsmokers among cases of pulmonary adenocarcinoma likely contributed to odds ratios of smaller magnitude than for other subtypes.

▶ Tobacco Carcinogenesis

Tobacco smoke is a complex mixture of more than 5000 gases and compounds, many of which are carcinogenic (Rodgman & Perfetti, 2009). While nicotine is the addictive component of tobacco smoke, multiple carcinogens are also present with the potential to induce cancer-causing mutations in critical genes. Three major classes of carcinogens are present in tobacco smoke:

polycyclic aromatic hydrocarbons (PAHs), nitrosamines, and heterocyclic amines (National Toxicology Program, 2005). The metabolism of carcinogens is complex, involving activation versus detoxification by liver enzymes. The carcinogens of tobacco smoke, their uptake and metabolism, and mechanisms by which they cause DNA mutations and DNA damage have been thoroughly reviewed elsewhere (Hecht, 1999).

In addition to the carcinogens of tobacco smoke, multiple other chemical compounds are present that are highly inflammatory to lung tissue. One of the most damaging and inflammatory of the substances in tobacco smoke is the tobacco residue called *tar*. Tar is the common name given to the particulate matter of tobacco smoke, minus the nicotine and water content. Essentially, tar is a complex mixture of thousands of compounds resulting from the combustion of tobacco and tobacco resins. It is estimated that the lungs of a chronic smoker of 20 or more cigarettes per day for 40 years are exposed to 8–10 kg of tar (Harris et al., 1993). Tar is by nature a sticky substance that is difficult, if not impossible, for the lungs to clear. Adherence to the cilia slows their wave-like motions and eventually stifles their ability to cleanse the airways. With the accumulation of tar in the smoker's lungs, chronic inflammation is inevitable, which in turn stimulates the critical mechanisms of cancer development: mutagenesis, mitogenesis, angiogenesis, inhibition of apoptosis, immunosuppression, and eventually metastasis (Harris, 2007).

▶ Chronic Obstructive Pulmonary Disease and Lung Cancer

Chronic obstructive pulmonary disease (COPD) is recognized as a chronic obstructive inflammatory condition of the lungs. Multiple studies have established a strong link between COPD and cancer of the lung (Raviv, Hawkins, DeCamp, & Kalhan, 2011). The dominant risk factor for both lung cancer and COPD is chronic tobacco smoking. Furthermore, the impaired lung function of COPD patients may also increase their lung cancer risk.

Swedish investigators studied the association of COPD and lung cancer in a large cohort of individuals ($n = 176,997$) for whom spirometry measurements were available at baseline. The stage of COPD was determined using spirometric measures of lung function. During 1971–2001, 834 incident cases of lung cancer were detected in the cohort through linkage with the Swedish National Cancer Registry. As shown

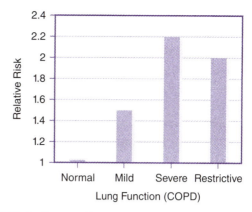

FIGURE 13.7 Chronic Obstructive Pulmonary Disease (COPD) and Lung Cancer.

Data from Purdue, M. P., Gold, L., Järvholm, B., Alavanja, M. C. R., Ward, M. H., & Vermeulen, R. (2007). Impaired lung function and lung cancer incidence in a cohort of Swedish construction workers. *Thorax, 62,* 51–56.

in **FIGURE 13.7**, the relative risk of lung cancer is significantly increased in patients with COPD, and more severe disease accentuates the risk (Purdue et al., 2007).

COPD independently causes nearly 3 million deaths annually in the world population. Overall, COPD ranks fifth in cause-specific mortality and is projected to climb even higher in the coming years. The clear majority of deaths from COPD (nearly 90%) occur in developing countries. In developed countries, COPD currently ranks third in mortality, behind only cardiovascular disease and cancer (WHO, 2008a, 2008b, 2009).

COPD refers to the presence of either of two conditions, emphysema or chronic bronchitis, which may exist simultaneously or separately in a given individual. The diagnosis of COPD is initially suggested by chronic repeated episodes of dyspnea (shortness of breath), wheezing, and coughing with or without mucous production.

In emphysema uncompromised by chronic bronchitis, the patient is typically barrel-chested and dyspneic with obviously prolonged expiration due to air trapping in the lungs. Significant weight loss is a common presenting symptom. Such patients remain well oxygenated and are thus referred to as "pink puffers." Pathologically, the lungs are characterized by permanent enlargement of the air spaces distal to the terminal bronchioles accompanied by significant destruction of the alveolar walls (Weinberger, 2004).

Chronic bronchitis is clinically defined as persistent cough with sputum production for at least 3 months in at least 2 consecutive years. This condition in its pure form involves chronic bacterial or viral infection and inflammation of the lungs. Patients characteristically are obese and may be cyanotic and hypercapnic due to lack of oxygen and excess carbon dioxide in the blood, respectively. Due to the bluish tinge of skin and lips from cyanosis and fluid retention from congestive right heart failure (cor pulmonale), such patients are referred to as "blue bloaters."

The diagnosis of COPD is confirmed using spirometry, a test that measures the ratio of the forced expiratory volume of air in 1 second by the patient (FEV1) to the forced vital capacity of the lungs (FVC). Ratios less than 0.70 are diagnostic of COPD. Radiographic images of the lungs may aid in the diagnosis, and biopsy specimens are sometimes ascertained to microscopically assess the degree of alveolar destruction in emphysema.

It is important to realize that emphysema and chronic bronchitis are often superimposed in the same patient. Indeed, the coexistence of both conditions in the same individual is the rule rather than the exception. However, chronic bronchitis is diagnosed according to clinical parameters (productive cough for 3 months in 2 consecutive years). Consequently, chronic bronchitis is easier to diagnose, giving rise to higher prevalence rates. Nevertheless, pathologic studies of biopsy specimens from COPD patients with late stage disease invariably reflect the presence of components of both emphysema and chronic bronchitis (Weinberger, 2004).

Most COPD cases are caused by chronic exposure to the thousands of noxious chemicals in tobacco smoke and the deposition of tobacco residue (tar) in the lungs (Marsh, Aldington, Shirtcliffe, Weatherall, & Beasley, 2006). Chronic pulmonary inflammation ensues with the influx of inflammatory cells leading to the pathologic changes characteristic of both emphysema and chronic bronchitis. Sustained recursive injury to the pulmonary epithelium coupled with impaired mucociliary clearance of tobacco carcinogens and inflammatory agents may serve to accelerate malignant transformation.

▶ Lung Cancer Risk Factors Other Than Tobacco

Factors that are synergistic with cigarette smoking in heightening the risk of lung cancer include exposure to asbestos fibers, inhalation of decay products of radon gas, and certain chemical exposures related to specific occupations (e.g., arsenic, cadmium, lead, dioxins). Other factors such as genetic predisposition and diet may also modify the risk of lung cancer. In particular, exposures that lead to chronic inflammation in lung tissues have been found to increase the risk.

Radon Gas and Lung Cancer

Radon is a colorless and odorless gas generated by the breakdown of radioactive radium, the decay product of uranium that is found in rocks and soil of the Earth's crust. Radiation decay products can reach the lungs by inhalation, where they are capable of ionizing DNA to produce mutations that could lead to carcinogenesis and the development of lung cancer. In an early ecological study of lung cancer in Maine, estimates of radon levels in domestic water supplies were found to be significantly correlated with county rates of lung cancer across the state (Hess, Weiffenbach, & Norton, 1983). In several studies of uranium miners, exposure to radon particles appeared to increase the risk of lung cancer (Hornung & Meinhardt, 1987; Samet & Hornung, 1990).

Evidence supporting an etiologic link between radon and lung cancer was strengthened by results of the Iowa Radon Study, which evaluated residential exposures among women and found a significant dose response in lung cancer risk with cumulative radon exposures exceeding 4 picocuries per liter (Field et al., 2000). In 1994, the U.S. Environmental Protection Agency (EPA) issued a warning that radon *could be* the second most frequent cause of lung cancer after cigarette smoking, responsible for up to 21,000 lung cancer deaths per year in the United States (Lubin et al., 1994). Nevertheless, the EPA estimates are based on linear extrapolation of high radon exposure in miners to much lower levels of exposure. Currently, the totality of scientific evidence suggests that radon exposure poses an independent risk, albeit small compared to that of tobacco. Furthermore, although not proven, chronic exposure to both tobacco smoke and radon could synergistically elevate the risk of lung cancer. Radon levels vary greatly by locality and the composition of the underlying soil and rocks. This makes the accurate evaluation of individuals' radon exposure extremely difficult; studies sufficiently powered to detect effects of low levels of exposure and interactions are lacking.

Asbestos and Lung Cancer (Mesothelioma)

Asbestos exposure causes mesothelioma, a malignancy of the pleura surrounding the lungs and lining other anatomic organs (e.g., the heart, abdomen, and peritoneal cavity). Approximately 75%–80% of mesotheliomas develop in the pleura of the lungs, 10%–20% in the pleura lining of the peritoneal cavity, and less than 5% develop in the pleura of other organs such as the heart. Worldwide during 2018, mesothelioma was diagnosed in 30,443 individuals (21,662 men and 8781 women) and caused 25,576 deaths (18,332 in men and 7244 in women). Global annual age-adjusted mortality rates of this malignancy are low (0.4 per 100,000 in men and 0.1 per 100,000 in women) (Ferlay et al., 2018).

In the United States, the annual incidence rate during 1975–2015 was 0.99 per 100,000 (1.84 per 100,000 in men and 0.39 per 100,000 in women). Malignant mesothelioma is very aggressive and highly lethal with 5-year survival rates of less than 10% (Noone et al., 2018). Reported annual rates of mesothelioma are highest in Australia and Great Britain (~3 per 100,000). The average time from asbestos exposure to the diagnosis of mesothelioma is approximately 40 years, and most cases (~75%) are diagnosed among elderly individuals 65 years or older. Various occupations have been found to increase the exposure to asbestos (e.g., mining, shipbuilding, carpentry, and plumbing) and elevate the risk of mesothelioma development. Globally, exposure to asbestos is increasing and the burden of mesothelioma is expected to rise in the 21st century (Robinson, 2012).

The etiologic link between lung cancer and asbestos exposure is well established through the studies of Selikoff and colleagues (Selikoff, Hammond, & Churg, 1968). Inhaled asbestos fibers migrate to the periphery of the lung where they become entrapped and cause recursive inflammatory insult and carcinogenesis. Asbestos exposure has been found to significantly increase the risk of cancer of the lung and pleura (mesothelioma) in both men and women (Berry, Newhouse, & Turok, 1972). Furthermore, some investigators have observed a synergistic multiplicative effect between tobacco smoking and asbestos exposure in the development of lung cancer (**FIGURE 13.8**). In a longitudinal study of smoking and asbestos exposure in a cohort of male asbestos insulation workers in the United States and Canada, smoking alone increased the death rate from lung cancer

by 10-fold and asbestos alone increased the rate by fivefold, whereas the combination of asbestos exposure and smoking increased the rate by more than 50-fold compared to subjects with neither exposure (Hammond, Selikoff, & Seidman, 1979). However, there is considerable controversy as to whether the impact of both factors fits an additive model or a multiplicative model (Liddell, 2001). In a meta-analysis of 18 epidemiologic studies that reported relative risk estimates for smoking alone, asbestos alone, and exposure to both factors, the overall estimates of lung cancer risk were RR = 5.5 for smoking, RR = 3.1 for asbestos exposure, and RR = 13.7 for combined exposure, which approximates a simple multiplicative model of synergism slightly better than an additive model (Wraith & Mengersen, 2008).

In developed countries such as Great Britain and the United States, where asbestos has traditionally been widely used in construction and building, asbestos exposure is estimated to account for 2%–3% of lung cancer deaths. Several global committees have reviewed the cancer-causing potential of common occupational substances such as asbestos. For example, IARC and the International Union Against Cancer (IUCC) have identified many workplace materials, including asbestos, that are possible lung carcinogens (McCulloch & Tweedale, 2008).

Wood Smoke and Lung Cancer

Wood smoke contains a mixture of harmful chemical substances in the form of gases and particulate matter such as carbon monoxide, ozone, nitrous oxides, sulfur dioxide, volatile organic compounds, dioxin, potential carcinogens, and inhalable particles. Certain of these compounds, such as benzo(a)pyrene and other PAHs are not only irritating and toxic, but also potent carcinogens. It has been estimated that residential wood combustion may account for up to 75% of the exposure to particle-associated organics and account for a significant fraction (up to 20%) of the cancer risk in the upper respiratory tract of nonsmokers (Lewtas, Lewis, Zweidinger, Stevens, & Cupitt, 1992).

Exposure to wood smoke may increase the risk of lung cancer via a mechanism like that of tobacco. Delgado et al. (2005) studied blood samples from patients with and without lung cancer and found that wood smoke exposure in nonsmokers significantly increased the expression of genes that control cell division such as p53, like the effects of tobacco exposure. Based on results, they suggested that wood smoke exposure is a possible risk factor for the development of lung cancer in nonsmokers.

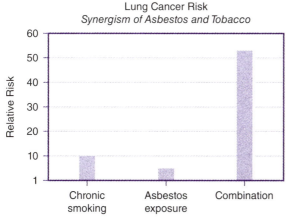

FIGURE 13.8 Asbestos Exposure, Smoking, and the Risk of Lung Cancer.

Data from Hammond, E. C., Selikoff, I. J., & Seidman, H. (1979). Asbestos exposure, cigarette smoking and death rates. *Annals of the New York Academy of Sciences, 330*(1), 473–490.

Air Pollution and Lung Cancer

The role of air pollution in the genesis of lung cancer was examined in a prospective cohort study of more than 1 million American men and women conducted by investigators at the American Cancer Society. Air pollution was measured as the concentration of particulate matter in ambient air. Study results showed that each 1% increase in the concentration of particles in the air produced a 14% increase in the risk of developing a lung cancer (Krewski et al., 2005; Pope et al., 2002). Lung cancer risk was highest for inhalation of ultrafine particles (less than 2.5 μm in diameter) that penetrate further into the lungs (Valavanidis, Fiotakis, & Vlachogianni, 2008).

Dioxins and Lung Cancer

Dioxins and structurally related dioxin-like compounds are environmentally and biologically persistent and induce a spectrum of disease processes. Dioxins are produced by industrial processes, including incineration, chlorine bleaching of paper and pulp, and the manufacture of some pesticides, herbicides, and fungicides. Dioxin is readily absorbed by sediments and soils and persists for decades. Common sources of dioxin included backyard burning of trash, wood stoves, wood-fired commercial boilers, municipal waste incinerators, and pulp and paper mill discharges. Humans are exposed through diet and close proximity to contaminated environments.

In a follow-up study of the population of Seveso, Italy, which was exposed to dioxin after an industrial accident that occurred in 1976, lung cancer mortality among men in high-exposure zones was significantly increased (RR = 1.3, 95% confidence interval [CI] = 1.0 – 1.7) (Bertazzi et al., 2001). Dioxins are metabolized by liver enzymes CYP-1A1 and CYP-1B1 into compounds with carcinogenic potential in lung cells and other tissues (MacPherson, Lo, Ahmed, Pansoy, & Matthews, 2009). Results support continued evaluation of dioxin as a lung carcinogen and underscore the need to also study interactions with tobacco and other risk factors.

Arsenic and Lung Cancer

Arsenic occurs naturally in soil and bedrock and is also used in pressure-treated wood and as an ingredient in pesticides. Long-term exposure to low levels of arsenic in drinking water has been linked to human health risks associated with cancer at multiple sites including the lung, bladder, and skin. DiPaolo and Casto (1979) first demonstrated the malignant transformation of mammalian cells by inorganic arsenic. Subsequently, many other studies have confirmed that arsenic exposure is both mutagenic and carcinogenic in humans (Barrett, Lamb, Wang, & Lee, 1989; Roy & Saha, 2002).

In a 50-year study of a population exposed to arsenic-contaminated drinking water in Chile, Marshall et al. (2007) found that toxic arsenic exposure greatly increased lung cancer risk when exposure occurred in utero or early in life. The investigators stated that "the impact of arsenic in drinking water on this large population is without precedent for environmental causes of human cancer, and it points to the public health priority of ensuring that arsenic concentrations in drinking water are controlled worldwide" (p. 927).

Environmental Tobacco Smoke and Lung Cancer

Over the last several years, much research has focused on the dangers of exposure to environmental tobacco smoke (ETS) or secondhand smoke. Such exposure is also known as passive smoking or involuntary smoking due to breathing in the tobacco smoke from nearby smokers.

Secondhand tobacco smoke arises from the dilution of sidestream smoke from smoldering cigarettes and from the residues of mainstream smoke exhaled by active smokers. More than 4000 chemicals have been identified in ETS and many of them are carcinogenic, including arsenic, benzene, beryllium, cadmium, nickel, chromium, ethylene oxide, polonium, and dioxin (National Toxicology Program, 2005). Furthermore, the ETS inhaled by nonsmokers has higher levels of nitrosamines and smaller particle sizes, leading to easier deposition within the bronchial tree. Specifically, smaller ETS particles are more likely to reach and be held in the lungs, where they dissolve more readily than larger particles. Therefore, the pattern of deposition of smoke particles in the respiratory tract differs between active and passive smokers.

It is estimated that approximately one-third of lung cancer in nonsmokers results from passive exposure to secondhand cigarette smoke (IARC, 2004; U.S. Environmental Protection Agency [EPA], 1992). Furthermore, ETS has been found to increase the risk of developing heart disease and myocardial infarction in adults and is also linked to various conditions in children, including sudden infant death syndrome, ear infections, and asthmatic attacks. Clearly, there is no safe level of exposure to ETS (U.S. Department of Health and Human Services [DHHS], 2006).

Within the United States, many state and local governments have passed laws prohibiting smoking in public facilities such as schools, hospitals, airports, and bus terminals. Increasingly, state and local governments are also requiring private workplaces, including restaurants and bars, to be smoke-free. At the national level, several laws restricting smoking have also been passed; for example, federal U.S. law bans smoking on domestic airline flights, most international flights, and interstate buses and trains, and in federal buildings and facilities. Internationally, several nations, including France, Ireland, New Zealand, Norway, and Uruguay, have also implemented laws requiring workplaces, bars, and restaurants to be smoke-free (DHHS, 2000, 2006).

Diet and Lung Cancer

For many years, an unresolved puzzle that has faced epidemiologists is the discrepant lung cancer rates in Japan versus the United States. Even though the prevalence of chronic cigarette smoking among Japanese men is approximately twice that of U.S. men, their lung cancer rates are substantially lower. For example, an early international case control study of smoking and lung cancer in Japan and the United States found that the relative risk of lung cancer development among chronic smokers is 10-fold higher in U.S. men compared to Japanese men (Wynder, Taioli, & Fujita, 1992). This phenomenon is known as the *Japanese smoking paradox.*

Although considerable research has addressed potential causes of the Japanese smoking paradox, a completely satisfactory explanation has not been forthcoming. Wynder and colleagues suggested that several factors may be involved: Japanese smokers are exposed to lower concentrations of carcinogens in their cigarettes (tobacco blends used in formulating cigarettes differ in the United States and Japan, and most Japanese cigarettes are made with charcoal filters that more effectively filter out nitrates and nitrosamines); Japanese men begin smoking at a later age than U.S. men (2–3 years on average); Japanese men consume less alcohol than U.S. men; and perhaps most importantly, the Japanese consume markedly less fat in their diet compared to Americans. Each of these factors could contribute to enhanced protection against carcinogenesis by tobacco smoke among Japanese compared to U.S. smokers (Stellman et al., 2001; Takahashi et al., 2008; Wynder et al., 1992).

Another important dietary difference between Japan and the United States is in fish consumption. Japan has one of the highest annual levels of fish consumption in the world (70 kg per capita), which is more than fourfold higher than the U.S. level (16 kg per capita) (EPA, 2002; Josupeit, 1996). To examine the role of diet in lung cancer development, Takezaki and colleagues conducted a case control study within Japan and found that consumption of cooked or raw fish reduced the risk of lung cancer in both men and women by about 50%. Eating fresh fish provides an excellent source of complex polyunsaturated fatty acids that are known to have potent anti-inflammatory effects, so it is possible that regular fish consumption by Japanese smokers inhibits or delays lung carcinogenesis by tobacco smoke (Takezaki et al., 2001).

Viruses and Lung Cancer

It is well known that chronic lung infections due to certain viruses cause lung cancer in animals; for example, the Jaagsiekte Sheep Retrovirus (JSRV) causes pulmonary adenocarcinoma in sheep (Leroux et al., 2007). However, the role of viral infections in human lung cancer development has not been definitively proven. Certain viruses have been implicated in lung carcinogenesis by virtue of their presence in lung cancer specimens (e.g., human papillomavirus strains, John Cunningham [JC] virus, simian virus 40 [SV40], BK virus, and cytomegalovirus have been found in cancerous lung tissues) (Cheng et al., 2001; Giuliani et al., 2007). However, it is highly likely that an acute viral infection present at the time of lung cancer diagnosis is an effect of the lowered susceptibility of such patients rather than the cause of a protracted course of carcinogenesis over many years.

Genetics and Lung Cancer

Sir Ronald Aylmer Fisher, the renowned "father of statistics," invented many of the maximum likelihood statistical methods that are still being used in hypothesis testing and the analysis of data. He also founded the field of quantitative genetics, developed methods for genetic linkage analysis, and proposed the concept of additive genetic variance for genes with small effects. Despite his genius for statistics and genetics, Fisher strongly opposed the conclusions of Ernst Wynder, Richard Doll, and Bradford Hill in the early 1950s that smoking caused lung cancer. Fisher compared the correlations in their papers to the "import of apples and the rise of divorce" in order to show that "correlation does not prove causation." In his view, the cause of lung cancer was largely attributable to genetic factors. However, his analysis of the causal association between lung cancer and smoking was flawed by an unwillingness to examine the entire body of available evidence that clearly demonstrated the etiologic link between cigarette smoking and cancer of the lung (Cornfield et al., 1959). It has also been pointed out that Dr. Fisher was employed as a consultant by the tobacco firms and that he himself was a smoker, thereby raising the specter of bias and casting huge doubt on the value of his arguments against the early epidemiologic findings (Stolley, 1991).

In recent years, linkage studies of multigenerational familial aggregations of lung cancer and genome-wide association studies (GWAS) have identified several genetic polymorphisms and mutant forms of genes that regulate key mechanisms of lung carcinogenesis. Most of these candidate genes modify effects of exposure to tobacco smoke, thereby increasing the susceptibility or resistance to tobacco carcinogenesis. Effects have been observed for genes that regulate the cell cycle and cell division (K-ras, p53, p16), genes that control DNA repair enzymes (BER, NER), genes that control the inflammatory cascade and cellular response to the plethora of highly inflammatory elements in tobacco smoke (COX-2), and genes that modulate phase I and phase II liver enzymes (CYP-1A1, CYP-1B1) resulting in heightened activation or dysfunctional metabolism of carcinogenic compounds in tobacco smoke, including PAHs, nitrosamines, and aromatic amines (Aviel-Ronen, Blackhall, Shepherd, & Tsao, 2006; Schwartz, Prysak, Bock, & Cote, 2007). Tobacco smoke may also stimulate epigenetic events that induce or suppress gene expression without changing the DNA base-pair sequence, such as DNA methylation, histone deacetylation, and phosphorylation, and these changes in gene expression may in turn influence susceptibility to lung carcinogenesis.

Cyclooxygenase-2 (COX-2), Inflammation, and Lung Cancer

More than a century ago, the German pathologist Rudolf Virchow (Virchow, 1863) suggested that chronic inflammation leads to cancer development by increasing cellular proliferation. In 1989, an inducible enzyme called cyclooxygenase-2 (COX-2) that initiates the inflammatory cascade was discovered in the laboratories of Dr. Phil Needleman at Monsanto Corporation in St. Louis, Missouri (Fu, Masferrer, Seibert, Raz, & Needleman, 1990; Masferrer, Zweifel, Seibert, & Needleman, 1990; Raz, Wyche, & Needleman, 1989). In 1991, the human version of the COX-2 gene was cloned in the laboratories of Dr. Harvey Herschman at UCLA (Fletcher, Kujubu, Perrin, & Herschman, 1992). Several investigators working in different laboratories were instrumental in the discovery and ultimate cloning of COX-2 (Herschman, 2002).

The COX-2 gene is normally silent in noninflamed tissues, but when stimulated by inflammatory factors (such as those found in tobacco smoke),

COX-2 transcription is triggered, leading to the enzymatic conversion of arachidonic acid into molecules called prostaglandins that are highly inflammatory. Discovery of the inducible COX-2 gene that initiates the inflammatory cascade rekindled interest in the causal link between inflammation and cancer.

Since discovery of the inducible COX-2 gene, a huge volume of cohesive scientific evidence from molecular, animal, and human investigations supports the hypothesis that continuous aberrant induction of COX-2 and up-regulation of the prostaglandin cascade by chronic exposure to a wide variety of inflammatory agents promotes the development of cancer, including cancer of the lung. Indeed, there is evidence that chronic exposure to many highly inflammatory constituents of cigarette smoke plays a significant role in lung carcinogenesis, and reciprocally, that blockade of the process has strong potential for cancer prevention and therapy (Harris, 2002, 2007; Harris, Beebe-Donk, & Alshafie, 2007).

▶ Lung Cancer Diagnosis, Treatment, and Survival

Despite intensive medical efforts involving surgical resection, chemotherapy, and radiation therapy, the survival of patients with pathologically confirmed lung cancer has remained dismally low for decades (**FIGURE 13.9**). The primary reason for the failure of treatment protocols to improve survival is the lack of early detection of lung tumors. Standard chest X-rays and most other imaging techniques have shown little value in detecting lung tumors prior to their invasion of the blood, lymphatics, contiguous tissue, and more distant anatomic sites.

One relatively new imaging technique, low-dose helical computerized tomography (CT), was recently evaluated in a large multicenter screening program involving 31,567 asymptomatic men and women 40 years of age or older, all of whom were at risk for lung cancer because of a history of cigarette smoking or other environmental exposures. Results demonstrated identification of 412 (85%) of 484 lung cancer cases with small clinical stage I lesions having a projected 10-year survival rate of 85% (Henschke et al., 2006). However, other centers were not able to replicate this result (Bach et al., 2007), and a subsequent meta-analysis of data from 15 studies did not establish that low-dose CT reduced mortality from lung cancer (Yau, Lock, & Rodrigues, 2007).

To resolve the issue, the U.S. National Cancer Institute launched a large randomized National Lung Screening Trial (NLST) comparing the effects of

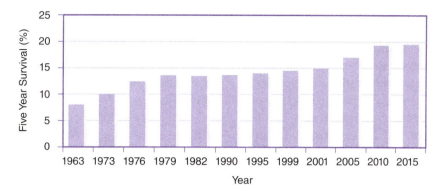

FIGURE 13.9 Trend in 5-Year Lung Cancer Survival, 1960–2015, United States.

Data from Noone, A. M., Howlader, N., Krapcho, M., Miller, D., Brest, A., Yu, M., … Cronin, K. A. (2018). *SEER cancer statistics review, 1975–2015*. Bethesda, MD: National Cancer Institute.

low-dose helical CT and chest X-ray for the early detection and treatment of lung cancer. A total of 53,454 persons ages 55–74 years who were at high risk for lung cancer due to current heavy smoking were enrolled in the trial during 2002–2004. Of these, 26,722 subjects were randomized to the arm receiving screening by low-dose helical CT and 26,732 were randomized to the arm receiving screening by chest X-ray. During the follow-up period (2002–2009), 1060 lung cancers were detected in the low-dose CT group (645 cases per 100,000 person-years) versus 941 lung cancers in the X-ray group (572 cases per 100,000), and there was a 20% reduction in mortality in subjects screened by helical low-dose CT compared to chest X-ray. A major issue with both forms of screening was the high false positive rate (96.4% in the low-dose CT group and 94.5% in the X-ray group). The NLST investigators concluded that low-dose helical CT was effective in reducing lung cancer mortality among heavy smokers but cautioned against its routine use until additional studies rigorously examine methods to reduce the high false positive rate and cost versus benefit of such screening (National Lung Screening Trial Research Team, 2011).

▶ Primary Prevention of Lung Cancer

The primary prevention of lung cancer depends to a large extent on the prevention of cigarette smoking among adolescents and young adults. The National Cancer Institute (NCI), the National Heart, Lung and Blood Institute (NHLBI), and many other public health agencies have developed presentations and other resources designed to disseminate accurate information to elementary-age schoolchildren on the dangers of implementing the smoking habit. Such programs appear to have had some beneficial impact in reducing prevalence rates of smoking in adolescents

from 30%–40% to 20%–25% in the United States over the past 20 years. Paradoxically, the tobacco industry has also sponsored tobacco prevention programs for children. Nevertheless, most efforts by the tobacco industry are intended to diminish media interventions for tobacco control and oppose national, state, and county tobacco control ballot initiatives and referenda (National Cancer Institute, 2008).

In June 2009, the U.S. Senate approved bill H.R. 1256/S.982, known as the Family Smoking Prevention and Tobacco Control Act. The new law grants the U.S. Food and Drug Administration (FDA) the authority to regulate tobacco products by eliminating tobacco marketing to children, requiring health warnings and a complete listing of contents on the packaging of cigarettes and other tobacco products, and requiring changes in tobacco products, such as removal or reduction of harmful ingredients. Despite these public health efforts, a huge segment of the world population continues to smoke, as evidenced by recent WHO data suggesting that 1 in 3 adults continues to smoke (WHO, 2008b). Because of this addictive habit, 5.4 million people are dying annually from tobacco-related diseases such as lung cancer, heart disease, stroke, COPD, and other forms of cancer (see Figures 13.3 and 13.4 earlier in the chapter).

▶ Nonsteroidal Anti-inflammatory Drugs and Lung Cancer

In 1988, Richard Peto and colleagues reported the results of a randomized prospective study of daily aspirin use among 5139 British physicians. The study was designed to determine if 500 mg aspirin daily would reduce the incidence of and mortality from stroke, myocardial infarction, or other vascular conditions. In the study, 3429 of the enrolled subjects were randomly assigned to receive aspirin and 1710 were randomly assigned to avoid taking any aspirin or aspirin products. After 6 years of follow-up, the results provided little evidence of protective benefit of aspirin against vascular diseases; however, the observed death rate from lung cancer was 7.4 per 10,000 person-years in the group treated with aspirin and 11.6 per 10,000 person-years in the control group (relative mortality = 0.64) (Peto et al., 1988). Many subsequent investigations have also observed significant protective effects of aspirin and other nonsteroidal anti-inflammatory drugs (NSAIDs) against the development of lung cancer. For example, in a case control study of lung cancer and NSAIDs, Harris and colleagues observed a risk reduction of 60% (OR = 0.40) with use of selective COX-2 inhibitors, and comparable risk reductions with regular use of ibuprofen (odds ratio [OR] = 0.40) or aspirin (OR = 0.53). Notably, the comparison group in the study consisted of controls who smoked but did not have lung cancer (Harris et al., 2007). In a meta-analysis of 18 studies of lung cancer and NSAIDs, the combined relative risk estimate for regular NSAID use was RR = 0.72 with no evidence of heterogeneity among studies (Harris, 2009).

▶ Smoking Cessation and Lung Cancer

The 1990 Report of the U.S. Surgeon General is devoted to the health benefits of smoking cessation.

Smoking cessation has major and immediate health benefits for men and women of all ages. Though there is typically a small weight gain with smoking cessation with some adverse psychological impact, the health benefits of smoking cessation far exceed any risks.

On average, former smokers live longer than continuing smokers, and the benefits of quitting extend to those who quit at older ages. For example, persons who quit smoking before age 50 have one-half the risk of dying in the next 15 years compared to continuing smokers. Furthermore, women who stop smoking before or early during pregnancy reduce their risk of having a low-birth-weight baby.

Smoking cessation reduces the risk of heart attack and stroke by 50% within the first year after quitting and also rapidly improves pulmonary function in patients with established COPD by reducing respiratory symptoms such as cough, sputum production, and wheezing, and enhancing immune defense mechanisms against respiratory infections such as bronchitis and pneumonia.

Sustained smoking cessation produces a gradual decrease in the risk of developing lung cancer as well as other tobacco-related cancers (Higgins & Wynder, 1988). Paradoxically, there is a slight increase in the risk of lung cancer diagnosis within the first few years after quitting smoking, which is apparently related to the modified growth characteristics of existing lung tumors that enhance their detection (**FIGURE 13.10**).

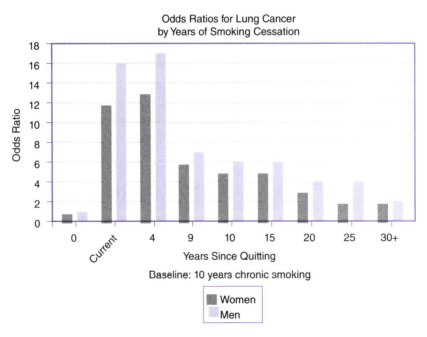

FIGURE 13.10 Smoking Cessation and Lung Cancer Risk.

Data from Higgins, I. T., & Wynder, E. L. (1988). Reduction in risk of lung cancer among ex-smokers with particular reference to histologic type. *Cancer, 62*, 2397–2401.

Electronic Cigarettes (E-cigarettes)

The electronic cigarette (e-cigarette) is a battery-powered device designed to simulate cigarette smoking. The device heats a liquid solution containing nicotine and flavoring and the vapor is inhaled into the lungs to deliver nicotine to the blood. These delivery systems have gained popularity as substitutes for cigarettes and possible aids for smoking cessation. Nevertheless, a recent study suggests that e-cigarette use (known as *vaping*) causes an immediate increase in airway resistance (Vardavas et al., 2011). It is well known that pyrolysis of nicotine produces formaldehyde, acetaldehyde, and a variety of other heterocyclic amines and PAHs with carcinogenic potential. Furthermore, endogenous metabolism of nicotine by liver enzymes produces carcinogenic nitrosamines (Hecht, 1999; Hecht, Adams, & Hoffmann, 1983). Nicotine itself is a powerful vasoconstrictor with mood-altering effects, and the absorption, distribution, metabolism, and excretion of nicotine and related compounds is complex and highly variable from individual to individual (Hukkanen, Jacob, & Benowitz, 2005). Given these concerns, it is important that e-cigarettes be regulated, and their health effects carefully monitored, because there is currently very little scientific evidence on their efficacy for smoking cessation and they are likely to have adverse long-term health effects (Etter, Bullen, Flouris, Laugesen, & Eissenberg, 2011).

References

American Cancer Society. (2014). *Cancer facts and figures 2014*. Atlanta, GA: Author. Retrieved from www.cancer.org/research/cancerfactsstatistics/cancerfactsfigures2014/index

American Lung Association. (2011). *Trends in tobacco use*. Chicago, IL: Author. Retrieved from www.lung.org/finding-cures/our-research/trend-reports/Tobacco-Trend-Report.pdf

Auerbach, O., Stout, A. P., Hammond, E. C., & Garfinkel, L. (1961). Changes in bronchial epithelium in relation to cigarette smoking and in relation to lung cancer. *New England Journal of Medicine, 265*, 253–267.

Augustine, A., Harris, R. E., & Wynder, E. L. (1989). Compensation as a risk factor for lung cancer in smokers who switch from nonfilter to filter cigarettes. *American Journal of Public Health, 79*(2), 188–191.

Aviel-Ronen, S., Blackhall, F. H., Shepherd, F. A., & Tsao, M. S. (2006). K-ras mutations in non-small-cell lung carcinoma: A review. *Clinical Lung Cancer, 8*(1), 30–38.

Bach, P. B., Jett, J. R., Pastorino, U., Tockman, M. S., Swensen, S. J., & Begg, C. B. (2007). Computed tomography screening and lung cancer outcomes. *Journal of the American Medical Association, 297*, 953–961.

Barrett, J. C., Lamb, P. W., Wang, T. C., & Lee, T. C. (1989). Mechanisms of arsenic-induced cell transformation. *Biological Trace Element Research, 21*, 421–429.

Berry, G., Newhouse, M. L., & Turok, M. (1972). Combined effect of asbestos and smoking on mortality from lung cancer and mesothelioma in factory workers. *Lancet, 2*, 476–479.

Bertazzi, P. A., Consonni, D., Bachetti, S., Rubagotti, M., Baccarelli, A., Zocchetti, C., & Pesatori, A. C. (2001). Health effects of dioxin exposure: A 20-year mortality study. *American Journal of Epidemiology, 153*(11), 1031–1044.

Boyle, P., & Levin, B. (Eds.). (2008). *IARC world cancer report*. Lyon, France: International Agency for Research on Cancer (IARC) Publications.

Cheng, Y. W., Chiou, H. L., Sheu, G. T., Hsieh, L. L., Chen, J. T., Chen, C. Y.,... Lee, H. (2001). The association of human papillomavirus 16/18 infection with lung cancer among nonsmoking Taiwanese women. *Cancer Research, 61*(7), 2799–2803.

Cornfield, J., Haenszel, W., Hammond, E. C., Lilienfeld, A. M., Shimkin, M. B., & Wynder, E. L. (1959). Smoking and lung cancer: Recent evidence and a discussion of some questions. *Journal of the National Cancer Institute, 22*, 173–203.

Delgado, J., Martinez, L. M., Sanchez, T. T., Ramirez, A., Iturria, C., & Gonzalez-Avila, G. (2005). Lung cancer pathogenesis associated with wood smoke exposure. *Chest, 128*, 124–131.

DiPaolo, J. A., & Casto, B. C. (1979). Quantitative studies of in vitro morphological transformation of Syrian hamster cells by inorganic metal salts. *Cancer Research, 39*(3), 1008–1013.

Doll, R., & Hill, A. B. (1950). Smoking and carcinoma of the lung. Preliminary report. *British Medical Journal, 2*, 739–748.

Etter, J.-F., Bullen, C., Flouris, A. D., Laugesen, M., & Eissenberg, T. (2011). Electronic nicotine delivery systems: A research agenda. *Tobacco Control, 20*, 243–248.

Ferlay, J., Ervik, M., Lam, F., Colombet, M., Mery, L., Piñeros, M., … Bray, F. (2018). *Global cancer observatory: Cancer today*. Lyon, France: International Agency for Research on Cancer. Retrieved from https://gco.iarc.fr/today

Ferlay, J., Shin, H.-R., Bray, F., Forman, D., Mathers, C., & Parkin, D. M. (2010). Estimates of worldwide burden of cancer in 2008: GLOBOCAN 2008. *International Journal of Cancer, 127*(12), 2893–2917.

Ferlay, J., Soerjomataram, I., Ervik, M., Dikshit, R., Eser, S., Mathers, C., … Bray, F. (2013). *GLOBOCAN 2012 v1.0. Cancer incidence and mortality worldwide: IARC CancerBase No. 11*. Lyon, France: International Agency for Research on Cancer. Retrieved from http://globocan.iarc.fr

Field, R. W., Steck, D. J., Smith, B. J., Brus, C. P., Fisher, E. L., Neuberger, J. S., … Lynch, C. F. (2000). Residential radon gas and lung cancer: The Iowa Radon Lung Cancer Study. *American Journal of Epidemiology, 151*, 1091–1152.

Fitzmaurice, C., Akinyemiju, T. F., Al Lami, F. H., Alam, T., Alizadeh-Navaei, R., Allen, C., … Global Burden of Disease Cancer Collaboration. (2018, June 02). Global, regional, and national cancer incidence, mortality, years of life lost, years lived with disability, and disability-adjusted life-years for 29 cancer groups, 1990–2016: A systematic analysis for the Global Burden of Disease Study. *JAMA Oncology*. Online publication. doi:10.1001/jamaoncol.2018.2706.

Fitzmaurice, C., Allen, C., Barber, R. M., Barregard, L., Bhutta, Z. A., Brenner, H., … Global Burden of Disease Cancer Collaboration. (2017). Global, regional, and national cancer incidence, mortality, years of life lost, years lived with disability, and disability-adjusted life-years for 32 cancer groups, 1990–2015: A systematic analysis for the Global Burden of Disease Study. *JAMA Oncology, 3*(4), 524–548.

Fletcher, B. S., Kujubu, D. A., Perrin, D. M., & Herschman, H. R. (1992). Structure of the mitogen-inducible TIS10 gene and demonstration that the TIS10-encoded protein is a functional prostaglandin G/H synthase. *Journal of Biological Chemistry, 267*, 4338–4344.

Fu, J., Masferrer, J. L., Seibert, K., Raz, A., & Needleman, P. (1990). The induction and suppression of prostaglandin H2 synthase (cyclooxygenase) in human monocytes. *Journal of Biological Chemistry, 265*, 16737–16740.

Gandini, S., Botteri, E., Iodice, S., Boniol, M., Lowenfels, A. B., Maisonneuve, P., & Boyle, P. (2008). Tobacco smoking and cancer: A meta-analysis. *International Journal of Cancer, 122*(1), 155–164.

Giuliani, L., Jaxmar, T., Casadio, C., Gariglio, M., Manna, A., D'Antonio, D., … Ciotti, M. (2007). Detection of oncogenic viruses (SV40, BKV, JCV, HCMV, HPV) and p53 codon 72 polymorphism in lung carcinoma. *Lung Cancer, 57*(3), 273–281.

Glynn, T., Seffrin, J. R., Brawley, O. W., Grey, N., & Ross, H. (2010). The globalization of tobacco use: 21 challenges for the 21st century. *CA: A Cancer Journal for Clinicians, 60*, 50–61.

Hammond, E. C., Selikoff, I. J., & Seidman, H. (1979). Asbestos exposure, cigarette smoking and death rates. *Annals of the New York Academy of Sciences, 330*(1), 473–490.

Harris, R. E. (2002). COX-2 blockade in cancer prevention and therapy: Widening the scope of impact. In: R. E. Harris (Ed.), *COX-2 blockade in cancer prevention and therapy* (pp. 341–365). Totowa, NJ: Humana Press.

Harris, R. E. (2007). COX-2 and the inflammogenesis of cancer. *Subcellular Biochemistry, 42*, 193–212.

Harris, R. E. (2009). Cyclooxygenase-2 (COX-2) blockade in the chemoprevention of cancers of the colon, breast, prostate, and lung. *Inflammopharmacology, 17*, 1–13.

Harris, R. E., Beebe-Donk, J., & Alshafie, G. A. (2007). Reduced risk of human lung cancer by selective cyclooxygenase-2 (COX-2) blockade: Results of a case control study. *International Journal of Biological Sciences, 3*(5), 328–334.

Harris, R. E., Zang, E. A., Anderson, J. I., & Wynder, E. L. (1993). Race and sex differences in lung cancer risk associated with cigarette smoking. *International Journal of Epidemiology, 22*(4), 592–599.

Hecht, S. S. (1999). Tobacco smoke carcinogens and lung cancer. *Journal of the National Cancer Institute, 91*(14), 1194–1210.

Hecht, S. S., Adams, J. D., & Hoffmann, D. (1983). Tobacco-specific nitrosamines in tobacco and tobacco smoke. *IARC Scientific Publications, 45*, 93–101.

Henley, S. J., Richards, R. B., Underwood, J. M., Eheman, C. R., Plescia, M., & McAfee, T. A. (2014). Lung cancer incidence trends among men and women—United States, 2005–2009. *Mortality and Morbidity Weekly Report, 63*(1), 1–5.

Henschke, C. I., Yankelevitz, D. F., Libby, D. M., Pasmantier, M. W., Smith, J. P., Meittinen, O. S., & The International Early Lung Cancer Action Program Investigators. (2006). Survival of patients with stage I lung cancer. *New England Journal of Medicine, 355*(17), 1763–1771.

Herschman, H. R. (2002). Historical aspects of COX-2. In R. E. Harris (Ed.), *COX-2 blockade in cancer prevention and therapy* (pp. 13–32). Totowa, NJ: Humana Press.

Hess, C. T., Weiffenbach, C. V., & Norton, S. A. (1983). Environmental radon and cancer correlations in Maine. *Health Physics, 45*(2), 339–348.

Higgins, I. T., & Wynder, E. L. (1988). Reduction in risk of lung cancer among ex-smokers with particular reference to histologic type. *Cancer, 62*, 2397–2401.

Hornung, R. W., & Meinhardt, T. J. (1987). Quantitative risk assessment of lung cancer in U.S. uranium miners. *Health Physics, 52*(4), 417–430.

Hukkanen, J., Jacob, P., III, & Benowitz, N. L. (2005). Metabolism and disposition kinetics of nicotine. *Pharmacological Reviews, 57*(1), 79–115.

International Agency for Research on Cancer. (2004). *Tobacco smoke and involuntary smoking* (Vol. 83). IARC Monographs on the Evaluation of Carcinogenic Risks to Humans. Lyon, France: Author.

Josupeit, H. (1996). *Global overview on fish consumption. Marketing of aquaculture products. Zaragoza, CIHEAM, Options Méditerranéennes*, No. 17, pp. 9–23. Retrieved from http://om.ciheam.org/om/pdf/c17/96605669.pdf

Khuder, S. A. (2001). Effect of cigarette smoking on major histological types of lung cancer: A meta-analysis. *Lung Cancer, 31*(2–3), 139–148.

Krewski, D., Burnett, R., Jerrett, M., Pope, C. A., Rainham, D., Calle, E., … Thun, M. (2005). Mortality and long-term exposure to ambient air pollution: Ongoing analyses based on the American Cancer Society cohort. *Journal of Toxicology and Environmental Health, 68*(13–14), 1093–1099.

Kumar, V., Abbas, A. K., & Aster, J. C. (2014). *Robbins and Cotran pathologic basis of disease* (9th ed.). Philadelphia, PA: Mosby & Saunders.

Lee, P. N., Forey, B. A., & Coombs, K. J. (2012). Systematic review with meta-analysis of the epidemiologic evidence in the 1900s relating smoking to lung cancer. *BMC Cancer, 12*, 385.

Leroux, C., Girard, N., Cottin, V., Greenland, T., Mornex, J. F., & Archer, F. (2007). Jaagsiekte sheep retrovirus (JSRV): From virus to lung cancer in sheep. *Veterinary Research, 38*(2), 211–228.

Lewtas, J., Lewis, C., Zweidinger, R., Stevens, R., & Cupitt, L. (1992). Sources of genotoxicity and cancer risk in ambient air. Review. *Pharmacogenetics, 2*(6), 288–296.

Li, C. (2012). The political mapping of China's tobacco industry and anti-smoking campaign. In L. John (Ed.), *Thornton China Center Monograph Series* (No. 5). Washington, DC: Brookings Institution.

Liddell, F. D. K. (2001). The interaction of asbestos and smoking in lung cancer. *Annals of Occupational Hygiene, 45*(5), 341–356.

Lubin, J. H., Boice, J. D., Edling, C., Hornung, R. W., Howe, G., & Kunz, E. (1994). *Radon and lung cancer risk: A joint analysis of 11 underground miner studies*. NIH publication No. 94–3644. Rockville, MD: National Institutes of Health.

MacPherson, L., Lo, R., Ahmed, S., Pansoy, A., & Matthews, J. (2009). Activation function 2 mediates dioxin-induced recruitment of estrogen receptor alpha to CYP1A1 and CYP1B1. *Biochemical and Biophysical Research Communications, 385*(2), 263–268.

Marsh, S., Aldington, S., Shirtcliffe, P., Weatherall, M., & Beasley, R. (2006). Smoking and COPD: What really are the risks? *European Respiratory Journal, 28*, 883–884.

Marshall, G., Ferreccio, C., Yua, Y., Bates, M. N., Steinmaus, C., Selvin, S.,... Smith, A. H. (2007). Fifty-year study of lung and bladder cancer mortality in Chile related to arsenic in drinking water. *Journal of the National Cancer Institute, 99*(12), 920–928.

Masferrer, J. L., Zweifel, B. S., Seibert, K., & Needleman, P. (1990). Selective regulation of cellular cyclooxygenase by dexamethasone and endotoxin in mice. *Journal of Clinical Investigation, 86*, 1375–1379.

McCulloch, J., & Tweedale, G. (2008). The challenge of mesothelioma and Irving J. Selikoff. In J. McCulloch & G. Tweedale (Eds.), *Defending the indefensible: The global asbestos industry and its fight for survival* (pp. 84–118). Oxford, U.K.: Oxford University Press.

Meza, R., Meernik, C., Jeon, J., & Cote, M. L. (2015). Lung cancer incidence trends by gender, race and histology in the United States, 1973–2010. *PLoS One, 10*(3), e0121323.

National Cancer Institute. (2008). *Tobacco monograph 19: The role of the media in promoting and reducing tobacco use.* Washington, DC: U.S. Department of Health and Human Services, National Institutes of Health.

National Cancer Institute. (2014). *Cancer statistics. Lung and bronchus. Surveillance, epidemiology, and end results program.* Retrieved from http://seer.cancer.gov/faststats

National Lung Screening Trial Research Team. (2011). Reduced lung-cancer mortality with low-dose computed tomographic screening. *New England Journal of Medicine, 365*, 395–409.

National Toxicology Program. (2005). *Report on carcinogens* (11th ed.). Research Triangle Park, NC: Author.

Noone, A. M., Howlader, N., Krapcho, M., Miller, D., Brest, A., Yu, M., ... Cronin, K. A. (2018). *SEER cancer statistics review, 1975–2015.* Bethesda, MD: National Cancer Institute.

Pesch, B., Kendzia, B., Gustavsson, P., Jöckel, K. H., Johnen, G., Pohlabeln, H., ... Brüning, T. (2012). Cigarette smoking and lung cancer—Relative risk estimates for the major histological types from a pooled analysis of case–control studies. *International Journal of Cancer, 131*(5), 1210–1219.

Peto, R., Gray, R., Collins, R., Wheatley, K., Hennekens, C., Jamrozik, K.,... Norton, S. (1988). Randomised trial of prophylactic daily aspirin in British male doctors. *British Medical Journal (Clinical Research Edition), 296*(6618), 313–316.

Pope, C. A., III, Burnett, R. T., Thun, M. J., Calle, E. E., Krewski, D., Ito, K., & Thurston, G. D. (2002). Lung cancer, cardiopulmonary mortality, and long-term exposure to fine particulate air pollution. *Journal of the American Medical Association, 287*(9), 1132–1141.

Proctor, R. N. (2001). Tobacco and the global lung cancer epidemic. *Nature Reviews Cancer, 1*, 82–86.

Purdue, M. P., Gold, L., Järvholm, B., Alavanja, M. C. R., Ward, M. H., & Vermeulen, R. (2007). Impaired lung function and lung cancer incidence in a cohort of Swedish construction workers. *Thorax, 62*, 51–56.

Raviv, S., Hawkins, K. A., DeCamp, M. M., & Kalhan, R. (2011). Lung cancer in chronic obstructive pulmonary disease. *American Journal of Respiratory and Critical Care Medicine, 183*(9), 1138–1146.

Raz, A., Wyche, A., & Needleman, P. (1989). Temporal and pharmacologic division of fibroblast cyclooxygenase expression into transcriptional and translational phases. *Proceedings of the National Academy of Sciences of the United States of America, 86*, 1657–1661.

Risch, H. A., Howe, G. A., Jain, M., Burch, J. D., Holowaty, E. J., & Miller, A. B. (1993). Are female smokers at higher risk than male smokers? A case-control analysis by histologic type. *American Journal of Epidemiology, 138*(5), 281–293.

Robinson, B. M. (2012). Malignant pleural mesothelioma: An epidemiological perspective. *Annals of Cardiothoracic Surgery, 9*(4), 491–496.

Rodgman, A., & Perfetti, T. A. (2009). *The chemical components of tobacco and tobacco smoke.* London, England: CRC Press.

Roy, P., & Saha, A. (2002). Metabolism and toxicity of arsenic: A human carcinogen. *Current Science, 82*(1), 38–45.

Samet, J. M., & Hornung, R. W. (1990). Review of radon and lung cancer risk. *Risk Analysis, 10*(1), 65–75.

Satcher, D. (2001). *Women and smoking: A report of the surgeon general.* Atlanta, GA: Centers for Disease Control and Prevention.

Schwartz, A. G., Prysak, G. M., Bock, C. H., & Cote, M. L. (2007). The molecular epidemiology of lung cancer. *Carcinogenesis, 28*(3), 507–518.

Selikoff, I. J., Hammond, E. C., & Churg, J. (1968). Asbestos exposure, smoking and neoplasia. *Journal of the American Medical Association, 204*, 104–110.

Stellman, S. D., Takezaki, T., Wang, L., Chen, Y., Citron, M. L., Djordjevic, M. V., ... Aoki, K. (2001). Smoking and lung cancer risk in American and Japanese men: An international case-control study. *Cancer Epidemiology, Biomarkers and Prevention, 10*, 1193–1199.

Stolley, P. D. (1991). When genius errs: R. A. Fisher and the lung cancer controversy. *American Journal of Epidemiology, 133*(5), 416–425.

Takahashi, I., Matsuzaka, M., Umeda, T., Yamai, K., Nishimura, M., Danjo, K., ... Nakaji, S. (2008). Differences in the influence of tobacco smoking on lung cancer between Japan and the USA: Possible explanations for the "smoking paradox" in Japan. *Public Health, 122*(9), 891–896.

Takezaki, T., Hirose, K., Inoue, M., Hamajima, N., Yatabe, Y., Mitsudomi, T., ... Tajima, K. (2001). Dietary factors and lung cancer risk in Japanese: With special reference to fish consumption and adenocarcinomas. *British Journal of Cancer, 84*(9), 1199–1206.

Terry, L. (1964). *Smoking and health: Report of the Advisory Committee to the Surgeon General of the Public Health Service.* Washington, DC: U.S. Department of Health, Education and Welfare.

U.S. Department of Health and Human Services. (2000). *Healthy people 2010: Understanding and improving health* (2nd ed.). Washington, DC: U.S. Government Printing Office.

U.S. Department of Health and Human Services. (2006). *The health consequences of involuntary exposure to tobacco smoke: A report of the surgeon general.* Rockville, MD: Author.

U.S. Environmental Protection Agency. (1992). *Respiratory health effects of passive smoking (also known as exposure to secondhand smoke or environmental tobacco smoke—ETS).* Washington, DC: Author.

U.S. Environmental Protection Agency. (2002). *Estimated per capita fish consumption in the United States.* Washington, DC: Author.

Valavanidis, A., Fiotakis, K., & Vlachogianni, T. (2008). Airborne particulate matter and human health: Toxicological assessment and importance of size and composition of particles for oxidative damage and carcinogenic mechanisms. *Journal of Environmental Science and Health Part C, Environmental Carcinogenesis and Ecotoxicology Reviews, 26*(4), 339–362.

Vardavas, C. I., Anagnostopoulos, N., Kougias, M., Evangelopoulou, V., Connolly, G. N., & Behrakis, P. K. (2011). Short-term pulmonary effects of using an electronic cigarette:

Impact on respiratory flow resistance, impedance, and exhaled nitric oxide. *Chest, 141*(6), 1400–1406.

Vineis, P., Alavanja, M., Buffler, P., Fontham, E., Franceschi, S., Gao, Y. T., … Doll, R. (2004). Tobacco and cancer: Recent epidemiological evidence. *Journal of the National Cancer Institute, 96*(2), 99–106.

Virchow, R. (1863). Aetiologie der neoplastischen Geschwulst/Pathogenie der neoplastischen Geschwulste. In *Die Krankhaften Geschwulste* (pp. 57–101). Berlin: Verlag von August Hirschwald.

Weinberger, S. E. (2004). *Principles of pulmonary medicine* (4th ed.). Philadelphia, PA: W. B. Saunders.

World Health Organization. (2008a). *The global burden of disease: Update 2004*. Geneva, Switzerland: Author.

World Health Organization. (2008b). *WHO report on the global tobacco epidemic, 2008: The MPOWER package*. Geneva, Switzerland: Author.

World Health Organization. (2009). *WHO report on the global tobacco epidemic, 2009*. Geneva, Switzerland: Author.

Wraith, D. Y., & Mengersen, K. (2008). A Bayesian approach to assess interaction between known risk factors: The risk of lung cancer from exposure to asbestos and smoking. *Statistical Methods in Medical Research, 17*, 171.

Wynder, E. L., & Graham, E. A. (1950). Tobacco smoking as a possible etiologic factor in bronchiogenic carcinoma. *Journal of the American Medical Association, 143*, 329–336.

Wynder, E. L., & Muscat, J. E. (1995). The changing epidemiology of smoking and lung cancer histology. *Environmental Health Perspectives, 103*(Suppl. 8), 143–148.

Wynder, E. L., & Stellman, S. D. (1977). The comparative epidemiology of tobacco-related cancers. *Cancer Research, 37*, 4608–4622.

Wynder, E. L., Taioli, E., & Fujita, Y. (1992). Ecologic study of lung cancer risk factors in the U.S. and Japan, with special reference to smoking and diet. *Japanese Journal of Cancer Research, 83*, 418–423.

Yau, G., Lock, M., & Rodrigues, G. (2007). Systematic review of baseline low-dose CT lung cancer screening. *Lung Cancer, 58*(2), 161–170.

Zang, E. A., & Wynder, E. L. (1992). Cumulative tar exposure. A new index for estimating lung cancer risk among cigarette smokers. *Cancer, 70*(1), 69–76.

© Andrew Brookes/Getty Images

CHAPTER 14

Epidemiology of Laryngeal Cancer

▶ Anatomy of the Larynx

The larynx has three anatomic divisions: the supraglottis, glottis, and subglottis. The supraglottis consists of the epiglottis, the false vocal cords, the ventricles, and the aryepiglottic folds. The glottis includes the true vocal cords and the anterior commissure. The subglottis is located below the vocal cords and extends approximately 5 mm into the trachea (Fried & Ferlito, 2009). Some epidemiologic studies of laryngeal cancer have subdivided laryngeal tumors into those arising in the supraglottis and those arising in the glottis (**FIGURE 14.1**).

▶ Histology

Virtually all malignancies of the vocal cords are squamous cell carcinomas. Of these, 75% arise from the true vocal cords (glottis), and the remainder arise from other laryngeal sites.

▶ Global Epidemiology

Cancer of the larynx is diagnosed approximately *seven times* more often in men than in women. Globally in 2018, laryngeal cancer was diagnosed in 154,977 men and 22,445 women and caused 81,806 deaths in men and 12,965 deaths in women. Among

men, cancer of the larynx comprised approximately 1.6% of all cancers and was responsible for 1.5% of all cancer deaths, whereas among women this malignancy accounted for only about 0.3% of all cancers and cancer deaths (Ferlay et al., 2018).

Global age-adjusted incidence and mortality rates for laryngeal cancer in 2018 were more than sixfold higher in men than women. The annual age-adjusted incidence was 3.6 per 100,000 in men and 0.5 per 100,000 in women during 2018, and the annual age-adjusted mortality was 1.9 per 100,000 in men and 0.3 per 100,000 in women (Ferlay et al., 2018).

The incidence and mortality rates of laryngeal cancer are highest in populations with the highest rates of chronic tobacco smoking and alcohol abuse. In particular, male populations characterized by heavy smoking and drinking (Cuba, Poland, Hungary, Romania, Turkey, Turkmenistan, Kazakhstan, Croatia, Russian Federation, Spain, Italy, Portugal, Brazil) have incidence rates that are 4–7 times higher than the average global rate of 1.9 per 100,000 (**FIGURE 14.2**).

▶ Laryngeal Cancer in the United States

The annual incidence of laryngeal cancer has declined by about 40% in the United States since

FIGURE 14.1 Anatomy of the Larynx.

1990. This trend has occurred concurrent with sharp declines in the prevalence of cigarette smoking in U.S. men and women. During 1980–2011, the prevalence of smokers decreased by 40% in men (from 35% to 21%) and by 43% in women (from 30% to 17%). Although the relative declines are similar by gender, the data continue to reflect a four- to fivefold excess of incident cases in men compared to women (Noone et al., 2018) (**FIGURE 14.3**).

▶ Age at Diagnosis of Laryngeal Cancer

Most cases (~97%) of laryngeal cancer are diagnosed after the age of 45 years. The peak years of onset are between 55 and 75 years of age, during which time about 58% of cases are diagnosed (**FIGURE 14.4**). Nevertheless, certain subtypes of laryngeal cancer are being diagnosed at earlier ages; for example, those related to human papillomavirus (HPV) infection manifest on average about 4 years earlier than those associated with tobacco and alcohol (Gillison et al., 2000).

▶ Risk Factors for Laryngeal Cancer

Tobacco and Laryngeal Cancer

Chronic cigarette smoking markedly increases the risk of developing laryngeal cancer, particularly in combination with chronic alcohol consumption. The risk increases with increasing duration and intensity of exposure to each factor. Cigarette smoking is the dominant independent risk factor.

In 1956, Wynder and colleagues conducted a case–control study of 209 cases of laryngeal cancer and matched controls ascertained primarily from Memorial Sloan Kettering Hospital in New York. They noted that nearly all cases (99.5%) reported a history of chronic tobacco smoking, and many reported excessive regular consumption of alcoholic beverages. Derived odds ratios (ORs) from their study show a dose response in risk with increasing intensity of chronic cigarette smoking (OR = 2.7 for about one pack per day and OR = 5.2 for at least two packs per day) (Wynder, Bross, & Day, 1956).

Estimated age-standardized incidence rates (World) in 2018, larynx, males, all ages

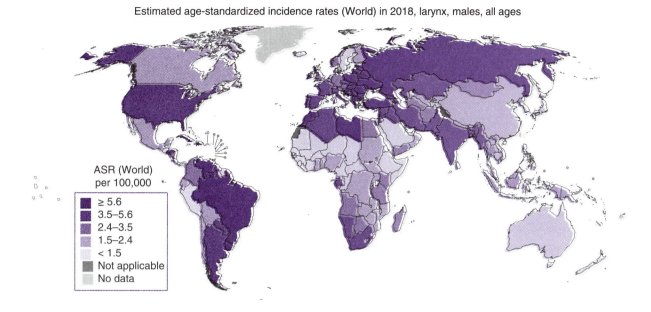

Estimated age-standardized mortality rates (World) in 2018, larynx, males, all ages

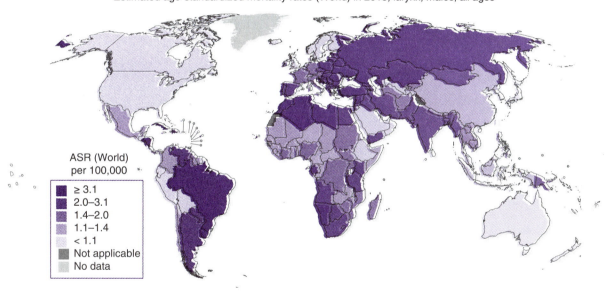

FIGURE 14.2 Global Incidence and Mortality Rates of Laryngeal Cancer in Men, 2018.

Reproduced from Ferlay, J., Ervik, M., Lam, F., Colombet, M., Mery, L., Piñeros, M., … Bray, F. (2018). *Global cancer observatory: Cancer today*. Lyon, France: International Agency for Research on Cancer. Retrieved from https://gco.iarc.fr/today

In 1964, the U.S. Surgeon General Report on Smoking and Health presented data comparing the death rates from cancer and other causes from seven large prospective cohort studies of men in the United States, Great Britain, and Canada. This landmark report provided overwhelming evidence that smoking increases mortality from lung cancer, laryngeal cancer, oral cavity cancer, esophageal cancer, stomach cancer, bladder cancer, chronic bronchitis, emphysema, and heart disease. The estimated mortality from laryngeal cancer among chronic smokers was 5.4 times the expected rate, suggesting a cause and effect relationship (Terry, 1964).

In 1970, Auerbach and colleagues reported the results of microscopic examination of formalin-fixed laryngeal tissues from 942 men who were autopsied at the Veterans Administration Hospital in East Orange, New Jersey. These men died of causes unrelated to

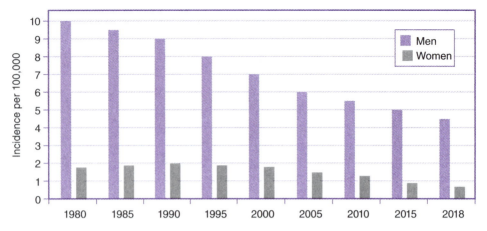

FIGURE 14.3 Incidence of Laryngeal Cancer in Men and Women, United States, 1980–2015. *Caption*: Annual incidence rates per 100,000 are adjusted to the 2000 U.S. population.

Data from Noone, A. M., Howlader, N., Krapcho, M., Miller, D., Brest, A., Yu, M., ... Cronin, K. A. (2018). *SEER cancer statistics review, 1975–2015*. Bethesda, MD: National Cancer Institute.

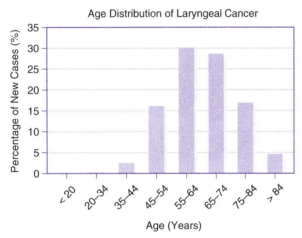

FIGURE 14.4 New Cases of Laryngeal Cancer by Age, United States: 2006–2010.

Data from National Cancer Institute. (2011, 2017). *Surveillance epidemiology, and end results*. SEER Stat Fact Sheets.

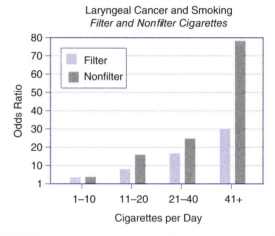

FIGURE 14.5 Cigarette Smoking and Laryngeal Cancer Risk.

Data from Wynder, E. L., Covey, L. S., Mabuchi, K. M., & Mushinski, M. (1976). Environmental factors in cancer of the larynx, a second look. *Cancer, 38*, 1591–1601.

laryngeal cancer. Data on smoking habits of the decedents were collected from spouses or next of kin. Cellular atypia was observed in 99% of laryngeal specimens from smokers compared to 25% of specimens from nonsmokers, and carcinoma in situ was present in 16% of specimens from smokers but was not observed among specimens from nonsmokers. The most significant histological change associated with smoking was "the occurrence of cells with atypical nuclei which are infrequent in nonsmokers, always found in cigarette smokers and increase in numbers with amount of cigarette smoking" (Auerbach, Hammond, & Garfinkel, 1970). These histological findings provided strong pathological evidence that exposure to tobacco smoke is in the causal pathway of the development of laryngeal cancer.

In 1976, Wynder and colleagues conducted a second hospital-based case–control study of laryngeal

cancer designed to examine the effects of smoking filter or nonfilter cigarettes and alcohol consumption. The study compared the smoking and drinking habits of 258 men and 56 women with laryngeal cancer to 516 men and 168 women with other conditions group-matched to the cases by gender, age, and year of interview. Results demonstrated a dramatic dose response of risk with increasing smoking of either filter or nonfilter cigarettes. Among men, chronic smoking at least two packs per day of filter cigarettes for 10 years or more produced a 30-fold risk increase, and smoking two packs per day of nonfilter cigarettes increased the risk nearly 80-fold compared to never-smokers (**FIGURE 14.5**). The investigation also showed that heavy alcohol consumption (seven or more drinks daily) increased the risk by about threefold, and that the cancer risk in former smokers began to decline after about 6 years of smoking cessation. This investigation also found risk increases among pipe and cigar smokers and greater than additive effects for the combined use of tobacco and alcohol (Wynder, Covey, Mabuchi, & Mushinski, 1976).

Several subsequent studies have confirmed the causal role of tobacco smoking in the development of laryngeal cancer. In an important prospective cohort study, 34,439 male British physicians were followed for 50 years (1951–2001) to determine cause-specific mortality rates for cigarette smokers versus nonsmokers. The results revealed a striking dose response in combined mortality from cancers of the mouth, pharynx, and larynx with increasing smoking intensity (**FIGURE 14.6**). Compared to individuals who avoided the smoking habit, heavy smokers were found to have an approximately 11-fold increased risk of dying from a malignancy of the upper aerodigestive tract (Doll, Peto, Boreham, & Sutherland, 2004).

In 1986, a working group of the *International Agency for Research on Cancer* (IARC) found a 10-fold increase in the average risk of developing laryngeal cancer among tobacco smokers versus nonsmokers. This study examined data from 30 studies (25 case–control and 5 cohort studies) and found risk increases for tobacco smoking in various forms, including cigarettes, pipes, cigars, and bidis (tobacco wrapped in the leaf of the tendu tree) (IARC, 1986).

Several investigators have conducted meta-analyses of published data on cigarette smoking and laryngeal cancer. The combined data reflect a strong overall effect of tobacco smoking and a significant dose response in the risk with increased amount of smoking (Ansary-Moghaddam, Huxley, Lam, & Woodward, 2009; Gandini et al., 2008; Peto, Lopez, Boreham, Thun, & Heath, 1992, 1994; Peto, Lopez,

Boreham, & Thun 2006; Vineis et al., 2004; Zeka, Gore, & Kriebel, 2003).

In a meta-analysis of 10 studies that used current smoking as the measure of exposure, current smokers were seven times more likely to develop laryngeal cancer than never-smokers (Gandini et al., 2008). In a meta-analysis of 15 studies that reported risk estimates for either fatal or nonfatal laryngeal cancer, the combined estimated risk among chronic smokers was increased by ninefold compared to nonsmokers (Ansary-Moghaddam et al., 2009).

Alcohol and Laryngeal Cancer

Alcohol consumption is also an independent risk factor for laryngeal cancer, but it has a weaker impact than smoking. A meta-analysis of 20 studies of alcohol and laryngeal cancer revealed an approximate four-fold increase in risk among heavy drinkers (100 g of ethanol per day) compared to nondrinkers, as well as a significant dose response of risk with increasing levels of consumption (**FIGURE 14.7**) (Corrao, Bagnardi, Zambon, & La Vecchia, 2004).

Tobacco and Alcohol: Laryngeal Cancer

Wynder and colleagues first examined the synergism of tobacco and alcohol in the genesis of laryngeal cancer. Their case–control study found independent increases in risk for heavy smoking (OR = 7.0) and chronic alcohol abuse (OR = 3.3), as well as a risk increase among individuals with both risk factors consistent with a multiplicative model (OR = 22.1) (Wynder et al., 1976).

As shown in Figure 14.2, incidence rates of laryngeal cancer in certain populations of Central and Eastern Europe are among the highest in the world. Because these populations have high rates of cigarette

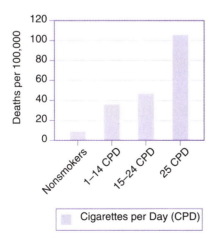

FIGURE 14.6 Annual Mortality from Cancers of the Oral Cavity, Pharynx, and Larynx in Men by Amount Smoked.

Data from Doll, R., Peto, R., Boreham, J., & Sutherland, I. (2004). Mortality in relation to smoking: 50 years' observation on male British doctors. *British Medical Journal, 328*(7455), 1519.

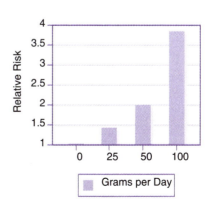

FIGURE 14.7 Alcohol Consumption and Risk of Laryngeal Cancer.

Data from Corrao, G., Bagnardi, V., Zambon, A., & La Vecchia, C. (2004). A meta-analysis of alcohol consumption and the risk of 15 diseases. *Preventive Medicine, 38*(5), 613–619.

smoking and consumption of alcoholic beverages, an international team of investigators conducted a large multicenter case–control study, the Central and Eastern Europe Study, to explore the independent effects and interactions of tobacco and alcohol in the development of laryngeal cancer. During 2000–2002, 384 incident cases and 918 controls frequency-matched by age, gender, and location of residence were ascertained from medical centers in Bucharest (Romania), Budapest (Hungary), Lodz (Poland), Moscow (Russia), and Banksa Bystrika (Slovakia). Dose responses in laryngeal cancer risk by various measures, including cigarette smoking and alcohol consumption, were estimated. Compared to nonsmokers, 20 pack years of cigarette smoking increased laryngeal cancer risk by threefold, and 40 pack years of smoking increased the risk by nearly eightfold. Alcohol consumption in the absence of smoking also increased the risk compared to nondrinkers: The relative risk (RR) was 1.56 for those consuming 20–29 g of alcohol daily and 1.85 for those consuming 40 or more grams of alcohol daily. Interactions of cigarette smoking and alcohol consumption were examined that revealed the presence of multiplicative rather than additive effects; for example, individuals who had smoked or consumed alcoholic beverages for 40 or more years were 14 times more likely to develop laryngeal cancer than those with neither exposure. The investigators estimated that 87% of cases of laryngeal cancer were attributable to tobacco smoking, with a substantial fraction (39%) attributable to the combination of smoking and drinking (Hashibe et al., 2007).

Meta-analysis has also been used to characterize the independent and interactive effects of tobacco and alcohol in the development of laryngeal cancer. In a meta-analysis of 14 studies published between 1966 and 2001 that reported risk estimates for both factors alone and in combination, the effects of smoking and drinking were found to be multiplicative on the RR scale. As shown in **FIGURE 14.8** , the estimated risk increases for heavy smoking alone (RR = 7.7) and heavy drinking alone (RR = 4.5) when multiplied together yield a close approximation to the 35-fold risk increase for high exposure to both cigarette smoking and alcohol consumption (Zeka et al., 2003).

Human Papillomavirus and Laryngeal Cancer

Recent studies suggest that chronic infection of laryngeal tissues by certain strains of HPV increases the risk of neoplastic development. Infection by low-risk HPV strains such as HPV-6 and HPV-11 are predominantly found in benign (noncancerous) papillomas

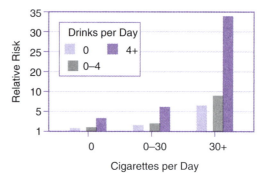

FIGURE 14.8 Risk of Laryngeal Cancer: Synergism of Tobacco and Alcohol.

Data from Zeka, A., Gore, R., & Kriebel, D. (2003). Effects of alcohol and tobacco on aerodigestive cancer risk: A meta-regression analysis. *Cancer Causes and Control, 14*, 897–906.

whereas high-risk strains such as HPV-16 and HPV-18 are characteristic of squamous cell carcinomas.

The link between HPV and the development of squamous cell neoplasms of the larynx and other tissues of the upper aerodigestive tract came from the clinical observation that children of mothers who manifested genital condylomata acuminata (genital warts) occasionally developed juvenile laryngeal papillomas (Quick, Faras, & Krzyzek, 1978). Subsequently, laryngeal papillomas were found to contain HPV-6 and/or HPV-11, the same HPV strains that cause genital condylomata acuminata (Franceschi, Munoz, Bosch, Snijders, & Walboomers, 1996; Gissmann et al., 1983).

Using DNA hybridization techniques, investigators at the Long Island Jewish Medical Center in New York detected HPV-16 DNA in six patients with verrucous carcinoma of the larynx. This form of laryngeal cancer is a variant of squamous cell carcinoma with a papillary wart-like appearance (Abramson, Brandsma, Steinberg, & Winkler, 1985; Brandsma, Steinberg, Abramson, & Winkler, 1986).

The early investigations of HPV in papillomas and verrucous carcinomas of the larynx prompted many subsequent molecular studies of cancer development related to HPV infection in tissues of the larynx as well as other anatomic sites of the upper aerodigestive tract (Maden et al., 1992; Schwartz et al., 1998). Gillison and colleagues tested for HPV in fresh frozen tumor specimens from 253 patients with newly diagnosed or recurrent squamous cell carcinomas of the head and neck using reverse transcriptase polymerase chain reaction (RT PCR) assays. Smoking and drinking histories were also recorded for each case. The RT PCR assays detected HPV in 62 (25%) of the 253 cases and HPV-16 was present in 56 (90%) of the positive cases. Among the 86 cases with laryngeal cancer, 16 (19%) of the cases were positive for HPV. Notably, cases with HPV-positive tumors were *less likely* to be heavy smokers or heavy drinkers than cases with HPV-negative tumors (Gillison et al., 2000).

A team of Scandinavian investigators conducted a nested case–control study of head and neck cancer using serum samples from a cohort of 900,000 individuals living in Norway, Finland, and Sweden. Serum samples were tested for selected strains of HPV among 292 cases with squamous cell carcinoma of the head and neck and 1568 controls matched on age, gender, and time of serum collection. Blood samples were collected, on average, 9.4 years prior to cancer diagnosis. Antibodies against HPV strains were detected by enzyme-linked immunosorbent assay (ELISA). ORs were adjusted for serum cotinine levels (a metabolite of nicotine and a biochemical marker of exposure to tobacco smoke). The study compared 76 patients with laryngeal cancer to 411 matched controls. The overall results revealed that HPV-16 seropositive individuals were 2.2 times more likely to develop squamous cell carcinoma of the head and neck than seronegative individuals, and stratification by anatomic site revealed that HPV-16 infection significantly increased the risk of laryngeal cancer (OR = 2.4). Analysis of 160 tumor specimens using RT PCR revealed that 50% of the oropharyngeal tumors contained HPV-16. These data suggest that HPV-16 infection detectable several years prior to diagnosis heightens the risk of developing squamous cell carcinoma of the larynx and other anatomic sites of the upper aerodigestive tract, including the tongue (OR = 2.7), the oral cavity (OR = 3.6), the oropharynx (OR = 14.4), and the paranasal sinuses (OR = 3.4) (Mork et al., 2001).

Hobbs and colleagues conducted a meta-analysis of case–control studies of HPV-16 infection and cancers of the head and neck with stratification by anatomic site within the upper aerodigestive tract. Twenty studies that identified site-specific head and neck cancer were identified, eight of which reported data on HPV-16 and cancer of the larynx. Significant associations were found between HPV-16 and squamous cell carcinoma at several anatomic sites, but the risk increases were greater for the tonsils (OR = 15.1) and the oropharynx (OR = 4.3) than for the oral cavity (OR = 2.0) and the larynx (OR = 2.0). Results of the investigation suggested that the methodology for detection of HPV infection, ELISA versus RT PCR analysis, was a source of heterogeneity among studies (Hobbs et al., 2006).

A team of investigators in Beijing, China, used meta-analysis to examine the role of HPV infection in the development of squamous cell carcinoma of the larynx. Among 55 eligible studies, the overall HPV prevalence in laryngeal cancer tissues was 28.0% and, most notably, 26.6% were infected with HPV-16, HPV-18, or other high-risk strains. Data from 12 case–control studies were utilized to estimate summary ORs for HPV-16 (OR = 6.1) and HPV-18 (OR = 4.2). The investigators concluded that HPV infection, especially HPV-16 infection, significantly increases the risk of developing laryngeal cancer (Li et al., 2013).

The evidence clearly suggests there is a subset of laryngeal cancers that develop due to infection by HPV-16 and possibly other oncogenic strains of HPV. Cases with HPV-16-positive squamous cell carcinomas of the larynx or other tissues of the upper aerodigestive tract are characterized by high promiscuity consistent with heightened sexual transmission of the virus. Such cases tend to be diagnosed at younger ages than those with tumors arising from exposure to tobacco and alcohol.

Other Risk Factors for Laryngeal Cancer

Several other risk factors have been linked to the development of laryngeal cancer. Laryngeal tumors occasionally arise after incidental radiation exposure either by X-rays taken of the throat early in life or radiotherapy for malignancies of the head and neck (Glanz, 1976; Miyahara, Sato, & Yoshino, 1998). In a follow-up study of 109 patients whose first primary laryngeal cancer was treated by irradiation, eight patients developed a second primary laryngeal cancer in the previously irradiated area after 7–15 years (Martin, Glanz, & Kleinsasser, 1979).

Familial aggregations of laryngeal cancer have been observed, suggesting that some individuals may be genetically susceptible. In a study conducted at the Pomeranian Medical University in Poland, 44 (5.8%) of 753 index cases (probands) with laryngeal cancer reported at least one first-degree relative with laryngeal cancer. Pooled analysis of data from 15 case–control studies involving 2464 probands with laryngeal cancer showed a doubling of the risk in individuals with a family history in one or more first-degree relatives (Negri et al., 2009).

Various medical conditions have been found to increase the risk of laryngeal cancer. These include gastroesophageal reflux disease (GERD), immunosuppression either due to HIV disease or organ transplant, and a previous primary malignancy of the head or neck (Qadeer, Colabianchi, & Vaezi, 2005). Certain environmental exposures may also increase the risk, including chronic exposure to coal dust, wood dust, and asbestos (Muscat & Wynder, 1992). There is also some evidence that certain dietary factors may play a role in the development of laryngeal cancer. Specifically, modest risk increases have been observed among individuals with high intakes of processed meats (De Stefani et al., 1987, 2012; Levi, Pasche, Lucchini, Besetti, & La Vecchia, 2004).

▸ Primary Prevention of Laryngeal Cancer

It is estimated that over 90% of laryngeal cancers are preventable by avoidance of tobacco and alcohol. Because tobacco and alcohol independently and synergistically increase the risk, it is obviously important to avoid exposure to both risk factors. Recent epidemiologic evidence suggests that certain strains of HPV are involved in the genesis of a subset of laryngeal carcinomas as well as several other malignancies (e.g., oropharyngeal, genital, and anal cancers). Avoidance of exposure through safe sexual practices and/or vaccination against oncogenic HPV strains is therefore critical for the primary prevention of all HPV-related malignancies, including laryngeal cancer (D'Souza & Dempsey, 2011).

References

Abramson, A. L., Brandsma, J., Steinberg, B., & Winkler, B. (1985). Verrucous carcinoma of the larynx: Possible human papillomavirus etiology. *Archives of Otolaryngology, 111*, 709–715.

Ansary-Moghaddam, A., Huxley, R. R., Lam, T. H., & Woodward, M. (2009). Risk of upper aerodigestive tract cancer associated with smoking with and without concurrent alcohol consumption. *Mount Sinai Journal of Medicine, 76*, 392–403.

Auerbach, O., Hammond, E. C., & Garfinkel, L. (1970). Histologic changes in the larynx in relation to smoking habits. *Cancer, 25*(1), 92–104.

Brandsma, J. L., Steinberg, B. M., Abramson, A. L., & Winkler, B. (1986). Presence of human papillomavirus type 16 related sequences in verrucous carcinoma of the larynx. *Cancer Research, 46*, 2185–2188.

Corrao, G., Bagnardi, V., Zambon, A., & La Vecchia, C. (2004). A meta-analysis of alcohol consumption and the risk of 15 diseases. *Preventive Medicine, 38*(5), 613–619.

De Stefani, D., Boffetta, P., Ronco, A. L., Deneo-Pellegrini, H., Correa, P., Acosta, G., … Silva, C. (2012). Processed meat consumption and risk of cancer: A multisite case-control study in Uruguay. *British Journal of Cancer, 107*, 1584–1588.

De Stefani, E., Correa, P., Oreggia, F., Leiva, J., Rivero, S., Fernandez, G., … Fontham, E. (1987). Risk factors for laryngeal cancer. *Cancer, 60*, 3087–3091.

Doll, R., Peto, R., Boreham, J., & Sutherland, I. (2004). Mortality in relation to smoking: 50 years' observation on male British doctors. *British Medical Journal, 328*(7455), 1519.

D'Souza, G., & Dempsey, A. (2011). The role of HPV in head and neck cancer and review of the HPV vaccine. *Preventive Medicine, 52*(1), S5–S11.

Ferlay, J., Ervik, M., Lam, F., Colombet, M., Mery, L., Piñeros, M., … Bray, F. (2018). *Global cancer observatory: Cancer today*. Lyon, France: International Agency for Research on Cancer. Retrieved from https://gco.iarc.fr/today

Ferlay, J., Soerjomataram, I., Ervik, M., Dikshit, R., Eser, S., Mathers, C., … Bray, F. (2013). *GLOBOCAN 2012 v1.0, cancer incidence and mortality worldwide: IARC CancerBase No. 11 [Internet]*. Lyon, France: International Agency for Research on Cancer. Retrieved from http://globocan.iarc.fr

Fitzmaurice, C., Akinyemiju, T. F., Al Lami, F. H., Alam, T., Alizadeh-Navaei, R., Allen, C., … Global Burden of Disease Cancer Collaboration. (2018). Global, regional, and national cancer incidence, mortality, years of life lost, years lived with disability, and disability-adjusted life-years for 29 cancer groups, 1990–2016: A systematic analysis for the global burden of disease study. *JAMA Oncology*. doi:10.1001/jamaoncol.2018.2706.

Fitzmaurice, C., Allen, C., Barber, R. M., Barregard, L., Bhutta, Z. A., Brenner, H., … Global Burden of Disease Cancer Collaboration. (2017). Global, regional, and national cancer incidence, mortality, years of life lost, years lived with disability, and disability-adjusted life-years for 32 cancer groups, 1990–2015: A systematic analysis for the Global Burden of Disease Study. *JAMA Oncology, 3*(4), 524–548.

Franceschi, S., Munoz, N., Bosch, X. F., Snijders, P. J. F., & Walboomers, J. M. M. (1996). Human papillomavirus and cancer of the upper aerodigestive tract: A review of epidemiological and experimental evidence. *Cancer Epidemiology Biomarkers and Prevention, 5*, 567–575.

Fried, M. P., & Ferlito, A. (2009). *The larynx* (3rd ed.). San Diego, CA: Plural.

Gandini, S., Botteri, E., Iodice, S., Boniol, M., Lowenfels, A. B., Maisonneuve, P., & Boyle, P. (2008). Tobacco smoking and cancer: A meta-analysis. *International Journal of Cancer, 122*(1), 155–164.

Gillison, M. L., Koch, W. M., Capone, R. B., Spafford, M., Westra, W. H., Li, W., … Sidransky, D. (2000). Evidence for a causal association between human papillomavirus and a subset of head and neck cancers. *Journal of the National Cancer Institute, 92*, 709–720.

Gissmann, L., Wolnik, L., Ikenberg, H., Koldovsky, U., Schnurch, H. G., & Zur Hausen, H. (1983). Human papillomavirus types six and 11 DNA sequences in genital and laryngeal papillomas and in some cervical cancer. *Proceedings of the National Academy of Sciences of the United States of America, 80*, 560–563.

Glanz, H. (1976). Late recurrence or radiation induced cancer of the larynx. *Clinical Otolaryngology and Allied Sciences, 1*(2), 123–129.

Hashibe, M., Boffetta, P., Zaridze, D., Shangina, O., Szeszenia-Dabrowska, N., Mates, D., … Brennan, P. (2007). Contribution of tobacco and alcohol to the high rates of squamous cell carcinoma of the supraglottis and glottis in Central Europe. *American Journal of Epidemiology, 165*(7), 814–820.

Hobbs, C. G. L., Sterne, J. A. C., Bailey, M., Heyderman, R. S., Birchall, M. A., & Thomas, S. J. (2006). Human papillomavirus and head and neck cancer: A systematic review and meta-analysis. *Clinical Otolaryngology, 31*(4), 259–266.

International Agency for Research on Cancer. (1986). Tobacco smoking. *IARC monograph evaluating carcinogenic risk of chemicals to humans* (Vol. 38, pp. 1–421).

Levi, F., Pasche, C., Lucchini, F., Besetti, C., & La Vecchia, C. (2004). Processed meat and the risk of selected digestive tract and laryngeal neoplasms in Switzerland. *Annals of Oncology, 15*(2), 346–349.

Li, X., Gao, L., Li, H., Gao, J., Yang, Y., Zhou, F., … Jin, Q. (2013). Human papillomavirus infection and laryngeal cancer risk: A systematic review and meta-analysis. *Journal of Infectious Diseases, 207*(3), 479–488.

Maden, C., Beckmann, A. M., Thomas, D. B., McKnight, B., Sherman, K. J., Ashley, R. L., … Daling, J. R. (1992). Human papillomaviruses, herpes simplex viruses, and the risk of oral cancer in men. *American Journal of Epidemiology, 135*(10), 1093–1102.

Martin, G., Glanz, H., & Kleinsasser, O. (1979). Ionising rays and laryngeal carcinomas. *Laryngologie, Rhinologie, Otologie, 58*(3), 187–195.

Miyahara, H., Sato, T., & Yoshino, K. (1998). Radiation-induced cancers of the head and neck region. *Acta Otolaryngolica, 533*(Suppl.), 60–64.

Mork, J., Lie, A. K., Glattre, E., Hallmans, G., Jellum, E., Koskela, P., … Dillner, J. (2001). Human papillomavirus infection as a risk factor for squamous-cell carcinoma of the head and neck. *New England Journal of Medicine, 344*(15), 1125–1131.

Muscat, J. E., & Wynder, E. L. (1992). Tobacco, alcohol, asbestos, and occupational risk factors for laryngeal cancer. *Cancer, 69*(9), 2244–2251.

Negri, E., Boffetta, P., Berthiller, J., Curado, M. P., Dal Maso, L., Daudt, A. W., … Hashibe, M. (2009). Family history of cancer: Pooled analysis in the international head and neck cancer epidemiology consortium. *International Journal of Cancer, 124*(2), 394–401.

Noone, A. M., Howlader, N., Krapcho, M., Miller, D., Brest, A., Yu, M., … Cronin, K. A. (2018). *SEER cancer statistics review, 1975–2015*. Bethesda, MD: National Cancer Institute.

Peto, R., Lopez, A. D., Boreham, J., & Thun, M. J. (2006). *Mortality from smoking in developed countries 1950–2000* (2nd ed.). Geneva, Switzerland: International Union Against Cancer (UICC).

Peto, R., Lopez, A. D., Boreham, J., Thun, M., & Heath, C. Jr. (1992). Mortality from tobacco in developed countries: Indirect estimation from national vital statistics. *Lancet, 339*, 1268–1278.

Peto, R., Lopez, A. D., Boreham, J., Thun, M., & Heath, C. Jr. (1994). *Mortality from smoking in developed countries 1950–2000*. Oxford, U.K.: Oxford University Press.

Qadeer, M. A., Colabianchi, N., & Vaezi, M. F. (2005). Is GERD a risk factor for laryngeal cancer? *Laryngoscope, 115*(3), 486–491.

Quick, C. A., Faras, A., & Krzyzek, R. (1978). The etiology of laryngeal papillomatosis. *Laryngoscope, 88*, 1789–1795.

Schwartz, S. M., Daling, J. R., Doody, D. R., Wipf, G. C., Carter, J. J., Madeleine, M. M., … Galloway, D. A. (1998). Oral cancer risk in relation to sexual history and evidence of human papillomavirus infection. *Journal of the National Cancer Institute, 90*, 1626–1636.

Terry, L. (1964). *Smoking and health: Report of the advisory committee to the surgeon general of the public health service*. Washington, DC: U.S. Department of Health, Education, and Welfare.

Vineis, P., Alavanja, M., Buffler, P., Fontham, E., Franceschi, S., Gao, Y. T., … Doll, R. (2004). Tobacco and cancer: Recent epidemiological evidence. *Journal of the National Cancer Institute, 96*(2), 99–106.

Wynder, E. L., Bross, I. J., & Day, E. (1956). A study of environmental factors in cancer of the larynx. *Cancer, 9*, 86–110.

Wynder, E. L., Covey, L. S., Mabuchi, K. M., & Mushinski, M. (1976). Environmental factors in cancer of the larynx, a second look. *Cancer, 38*, 1591–1601.

Zeka, A., Gore, R., & Kriebel, D. (2003). Effects of alcohol and tobacco on aerodigestive cancer risk: A meta-regression analysis. *Cancer Causes and Control, 14*, 897–906.

CHAPTER 15

Epidemiology of Cancers of the Lip, Oral Cavity, and Pharynx

▶ Anatomy of the Oral Cavity

The oral cavity (or mouth) is the initial portion of the alimentary canal. The digestive process begins when food enters the oral cavity and is mechanically masticated by chewing, moistened by saliva, and undergoes reactions with salivary enzymes to initiate chemical digestion. Anatomic structures of the oral cavity include the lips, teeth, hard and soft palate, upper and lower gingiva (or gums), tongue, uvula, tonsils, and pharynx. The pharynx is a channel situated behind the oral cavity and beneath the nasal cavity that extends to the level of the larynx. The oropharynx is continuous with the back of the oral cavity, extending from the soft palate to the epiglottis. A closely related structure is the nasopharynx, a channel that connects the nasal cavity and paranasal sinuses to the upper portion of the oropharynx. The laryngopharynx (also called the hypopharynx) is the portion of the pharynx between the oropharynx and the larynx (**FIGURE 15.1**). The oral cavity and pharynx are lined by stratified squamous epithelium.

Global Epidemiology of Oral Cavity and Lip Cancer

During 2018, malignancies of the oral cavity and lip caused 177,384 deaths in the world population (119,693 in men and 57,691 in women). In the same year, 354,864 new cases of oral cavity and lip cancer were diagnosed (246,420 in men and 108,444 in women), an overall increase of 34.8% during the last decade, 2008–2018. Cancers of the oral cavity and lip constitute approximately 2.0% of all malignant neoplasms and account for about 1.9% of cancer deaths in the human population (Boyle & Levin, 2008; Bray et al., 2018; Ferlay et al., 2010, 2013, 2018).

Global age-adjusted incidence and mortality rates for cancers of the oral cavity and lip in 2018 were more than twofold higher in men than women. The annual age-adjusted incidence was 5.8 per 100,000 in men and 2.3 per 100,000 in women during 2018, and the annual age-adjusted mortality was 2.8 per 100,000 in men and 1.2 per 100,000 in women (Bray et al., 2018; Ferlay et al., 2018).

Globally, more than 60% of oral cavity malignancies occur in the populations of developing nations and nearly two-thirds of cases occur in men; however, the incidence and male-to-female ratio vary considerably according to the risk factors in specific populations. In most populations, there is a predominance of male cases due primarily to the higher prevalence of chronic tobacco and alcohol exposure among men; nevertheless, the changing patterns of exposure to certain risk factors, particularly sexually transmitted infection of the oral cavity by human papillomaviruses (HPVs), have markedly reduced the rate differences in men and women in certain populations (American Cancer Society, 2007).

Global patterns of incidence and mortality rates of oral cavity and lip cancer in 2018 are shown in **FIGURE 15.2** . High incidence rates were observed in

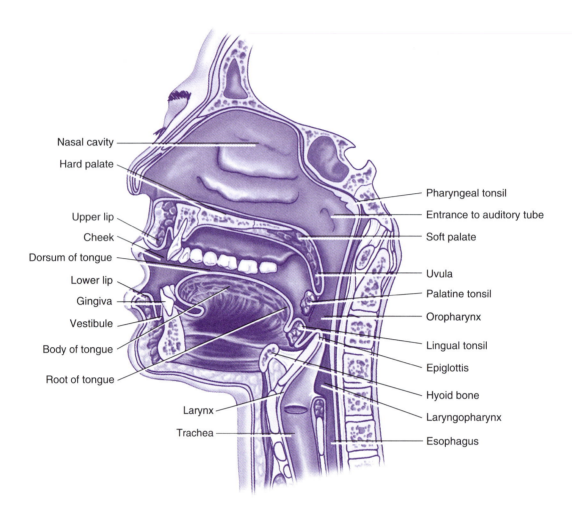

FIGURE 15.1 Anatomy of the Oral Cavity.

developing nations such as India, Pakistan, Bangladesh, and Papua New Guinea in Melanesia. The region with the highest incidence in the world is Patpua New Guinea (27.5 per 100,000 in men and 15.1 per 100,000 in women). In these populations, it is customary for both men and women to chew a mixture of tobacco, areca nut, and betel leaf called "betel quid," which has potent carcinogenic properties (Parkin, Bray, Ferlay, & Pisani, 2005). Also, in certain rural populations of Southern India, *reverse smoking* of tobacco rolled into cigars (called chutta) is particularly popular among women and can lead to the development of cancer of the hard palate. Reverse smoking refers to holding the lighted end of the cigar inside the mouth (Gupta, Mehta, & Pindborg, 1984).

The 2018 incidence rates of oral cavity and lip cancer were also high in several developed nations, including the United States, Canada, Great Britain, Brazil, Spain, France, Germany, Austria, Norway, Denmark, and the Russian Federation. Rates were particularly high in men of Eastern Europe (8.0 per 100,000), presumably due to high rates of chronic smoking and alcohol abuse. The high incidence rate in Australia and New Zealand (9.4 per 100,000) is partially due to lip cancer caused by solar irradiation.

The 2018 mortality rates from oral cavity and lip cancer were higher in developing nations than in developed nations, e.g., 5.0 per 100,000 compared to 1.5 per 100,000 in males. This difference likely reflects the higher prevalence of specific risk factors in less developed nations, most often the chronic exposure of the oral mucosa to both tobacco and alcohol (Bray et al., 2018).

▶ Premalignant Lesions of the Oral Cavity

Cancer of the oral cavity may begin as a dysplastic lesion such as leukoplakia (a white patch) or erythroplakia (a red patch) or any other sore that fails to heal and persists in the mouth for a matter of weeks. Leukoplakia and erythroplakia are caused by chronic exposure to tobacco, alcohol, certain HPV strains (e.g., HPV-16), *Candida albicans* (particularly in immunosuppressed individuals with human immunodeficiency virus

Estimated age-standardized incidence rates (World) in 2018, lip, oral cavity, both sexes, all ages

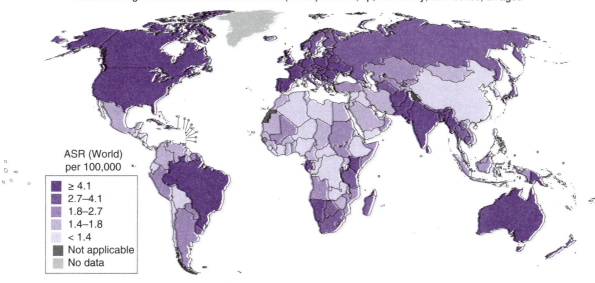

Estimated age-standardized mortality rates (World) in 2018, lip, oral cavity, both sexes, all ages

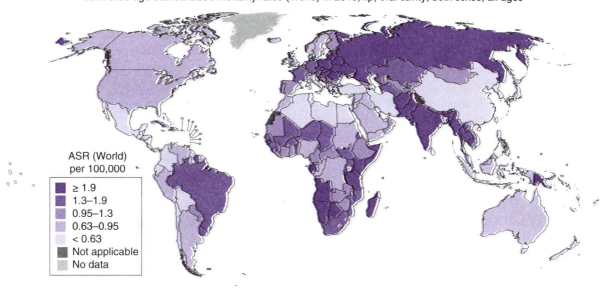

FIGURE 15.2 Global Incidence and Mortality Rates of Cancer of the Lip and Oral Cavity, 2018.

Caption: ASR: Rates per 100,000 are age-standardized to the world population, 2000–2025.

Reproduced with permission from Ferlay, J., Ervik, M., Lam, F., Colombet, M., Mery, L., Piñeros, M., ... Bray, F. (2018). *Global cancer observatory: Cancer today*. Lyon, France: International Agency for Research on Cancer. Retrieved from https://gco.iarc.fr/today

[HIV]), or any combination of these exposures, all of which are risk factors for the development of oral cavity cancer. These lesions usually precede the diagnosis of invasive cancer by 5–10 years. Progression of precancerous lesions to invasive oral cavity cancer can thus be interrupted by their early detection and complete surgical excision. Regular dental care and careful visual inspection of the oral cavity for such lesions are obviously paramount for cancer prevention.

Histology of Oral Cavity Cancer

The vast majority (~90%) of malignancies arising in the oral cavity are squamous cell carcinomas. An additional 5% are adenocarcinomas arising from the salivary glands within the mouth (Shklar, 1979). In a large series of 14,253 cases of oral cavity cancer, 38% developed in the lower lip, 22% in the tongue, 17% in the floor of the mouth, and the remaining 23% at other locations within the oral cavity (Krolls & Hoffman, 1976).

▶ Oral Cavity Cancer Risk Factors

Oral cavity neoplasms are typically diagnosed between the ages of 40 and 70 years and predominate in men. (The male-to-female ratio is 2:1.) In general, the risk factors for oral cavity cancer include conditions that chronically irritate and inflame the gums, tongue, oral mucosa, and lips. The major risk factors are chronic alcohol consumption, chronic cigarette smoking, and chronic infection of the oral cavity by oncogenic strains of HPV. Other risk factors include chronic marijuana smoking, chronic use of smokeless tobacco (snuff and chewing tobacco), poor dental hygiene, and antecedent nutritional deficiencies in iron, vitamin B, and vitamin C (La Vecchia, Tavani, Franceschi, Levi, & Negri, 1997). Immunosuppression due to HIV infection has also been found to increase the risk (Beachler & D'Souza, 2013).

The pathogenesis of oral cavity cancer has recently been linked to infection by certain strains of sexually transmitted HPV. In particular, strains of HPV known to cause cervical cancer (e.g., HPV-16) also profoundly increase the risk of malignant transformation when they infect the oral cavity. As discussed later in this chapter, oropharyngeal cancers that are HPV-positive have a distinctly different risk profile than those that are HPV-negative (Gillison et al., 2008).

Though grouped with other malignancies of the oral cavity, lip cancers comprise another distinct subset of malignancies with their own profile of risk factors. Fair-skinned individuals who are chronically exposed to solar ultraviolet radiation are at increased risk of developing lip cancer (Johnson, Jayasekara, & Amarasinghe, 2011; National Cancer Institute, 2014).

Synergism of Alcohol and Tobacco in Oral Cavity Cancer

The two well-established major risk factors predisposing to oral cavity cancer are alcohol and tobacco. Many independent studies have shown elevated risk in heavy drinkers and heavy smokers (or users of smokeless tobacco) and strongly indicate a synergistic effect between these two risk factors in promoting squamous cell carcinoma of the oral cavity. As an example, an epidemiologic investigation by Blot and colleagues (1988) determined that chronic smoking and drinking had independent ORs of 5.8 and 7.4, respectively, whereas the OR for the combination of chronic smoking and drinking increased the OR more than 35-fold, reflecting a multiplicative synergistic effect (Blot et al., 1988) **(FIGURE 15.3**). Epidemiologic studies in developed countries also suggest that long-term use of alcohol-containing mouthwash is a risk factor. Constant exposure to these alcohol-containing rinses, even in the absence of smoking and drinking, is associated with a significant increase in the risk of developing oral cancer (Kabat & Wynder, 1989).

Although it is well known that tobacco smoke and tobacco juice contain powerful carcinogens and

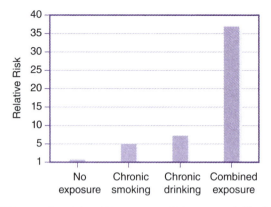

FIGURE 15.3 Combined Exposure to Tobacco and Alcohol Synergistically Increase the Risk of Oral Cavity Cancer.

Data from Blot, W. J., McLaughlin, J. K., Winn, D. M., Austin, D. F., Greenberg, R. S., Preston-Martin, S., ... Fraumeni, J. F. (1988). Smoking and drinking in relation to oral and pharyngeal cancer. *Cancer Research, 48*, 3282–3287; Kabat, G. C., & Wynder, E. L. (1989). Type of alcoholic beverage and oral cancer. *International Journal of Cancer, 43*, 190–194.

inflammatory substances that are linked to carcinogenesis, the mechanism by which alcohol promotes oral cavity cancer remains elusive. Animal studies do not clearly indicate that pure alcohol acts as a direct carcinogen; rather, the studies seem to indicate that alcohol may promote the transport of other carcinogens through the cell membrane either as a solvent or by acting on the cell membrane directly (Seitz & Stickel, 2007).

Though alcohol per se is not carcinogenic, *acetaldehyde*, the major product of alcohol metabolism, is classified as a human carcinogen. In the liver, the enzyme *alcohol dehydrogenase* oxidizes ethanol (alcohol) to form acetaldehyde, which is then oxidized by *acetaldehyde dehydrogenase* to produce *acetic acid* for excretion. Notably, microflora of the saliva can also produce acetaldehyde from ethanol and furthermore, many alcoholic beverages contain acetaldehyde (Homann, Jousimies-Somer, Jokelainen, Heine, & Salaspuro, 1997). Thus, sustained acetaldehyde exposure is likely to play a mechanistic role in the malignant transformation of the oral mucosa (Salaspuro, 2009).

Other possible mechanisms include the induction of microsomal enzymes in the liver that promote the formation of polycyclic aromatic hydrocarbons and/or benzopyrene, interference with DNA repair mechanisms, and epigenetic effects on DNA methylation resulting in epigenetic deregulation of tumor suppressor genes (Poschl & Seitz, 2004). Furthermore, alcohol may be a vehicle for the induction of contaminating carcinogens into the oral cavity (i.e., various alcoholic beverages may contain nitroso compounds, phenols, or a variety of polycyclic aromatic hydrocarbons). Chronic alcohol consumption may also promote nutritional deficiency simply by substituting empty calories and reducing the dietary consumption of important micronutrients and minerals such as vitamins A and

B, and iron. Heavy alcohol consumption coupled with poor nutrition may therefore result in immunosuppression, which may also increase the predisposition to oral cavity cancer (Testino & Borro, 2009).

HPV and Oral Cavity Cancer

It has been shown that chronic infection with high-risk strains of HPV (e.g., HPV-16) is an independent risk factor for the development of oral cavity cancer (D'Souza et al., 2007; Gillison et al., 2000, 2008; La Vecchia et al., 1997).

Maden and colleagues conducted an early case–control study to investigate the potential role of HPV infection in the development of squamous cell carcinoma of the oral cavity. They compared HPV seropositivity and other risk factors, principally tobacco and alcohol use, in 131 male cases of oral cancer to 136 controls that were frequency-matched to the cases by age and location of residence. Seropositivity for HPV was based on reverse transcription polymerase chain reaction (RT PCR) assays of tumor specimens in the cases and oral mucosal specimens in the controls. Odds ratios (ORs) were estimated with adjustment for age, cigarette smoking, and alcohol consumption. Results revealed increases in the risk associated with seropositivity for HPV-6 (OR = 2.9) and HPV-16 (OR = 6.2) (Maden et al., 1992).

Schwartz and colleagues used similar methodology to investigate the potential role of HPV infection in the development of malignancies of the oral cavity. They conducted a case–control study of 284 patients with squamous cell carcinomas of the head and neck and 477 control subjects from the general population similar in age and gender to the cases. Serum samples were tested for the presence of HPV-16 antibodies and tumor specimens from the cases, and samples of the oral mucosa from the control subjects were tested for HPV DNA. Data were also collected on the patients' history of cigarette smoking and alcohol consumption. Among 248 tumor specimens, 64 (26%) were positive for HPV and 43 (67%) of the 64 HPV-positive strains were positive for a high-risk HPV strain. Overall, 16.5% of cases (41 of 248) were positive for HPV-16, a strain that is oncogenic in other tissues such as the uterine cervix. Positivity for HPV-16 increased the risk of developing squamous cell carcinoma of the oral cavity nearly sevenfold (OR = 6.8). This association was not confounded by age, gender, cigarette smoking, or alcohol consumption. The investigators concluded that HPV-16 may contribute to the development of some oral squamous cell carcinomas, possibly in combination with cigarette smoking (Schwartz et al., 1998).

Gillison and colleagues tested for HPV in fresh frozen tumor specimens from 253 patients with newly diagnosed or recurrent squamous cell carcinomas using PCR-based assays. Smoking and drinking histories were also recorded for each case. The PCR assays detected HPV in 62 (25%) of the 253 cases, and HPV-16 was present in 56 (90%) of the positive cases. Notably, cases with HPV-positive tumors were *less likely* to be heavy smokers or heavy drinkers than cases with HPV-negative tumors (Gillison et al., 2000).

Mork and colleagues conducted a nested case–control study of head and neck cancer using serum samples from a cohort of 900,000 individuals living in Norway, Finland, and Sweden. Serum samples were tested for selected strains of HPV among 292 cases with squamous cell carcinoma of the head and neck and 1568 controls matched on age, gender, and time of serum collection. Blood samples were collected, on average, 9.4 years prior to cancer diagnosis. ORs were adjusted for serum cotinine levels (a metabolite of nicotine and biochemical marker of exposure to tobacco smoke). Results revealed that HPV-16-seropositive individuals were 2.2 times more likely to develop squamous cell carcinoma of the head and neck than seronegative individuals. Analysis of 160 tumor specimens using RT PCR revealed that 50% of the oropharyngeal tumors contained HPV-16. Anatomic stratification of the data revealed that HPV-16 increased the risk of cancer development at multiple sites, including the oral cavity (OR = 3.6), the tongue (OR = 2.8), the oropharynx (OR = 14.2), the paranasal sinuses (OR = 3.4), and the larynx (OR = 2.2). These data suggest that HPV-16 infection detectable several years prior to diagnosis significantly heightens the risk of developing squamous cell carcinoma at multiple anatomic sites of the upper aerodigestive tract (Mork et al., 2001).

In a hospital-based case–control study conducted in Baltimore, Gillison and colleagues studied 100 cases with squamous cell carcinoma of the head and neck and 200 control patients without cancer matched to the cases by age, gender, and location. The investigators examined mucosal specimens for serum antibodies to the L1 capsid protein of HPV-16 and its oncogenic proteins (E6 and E7). They also collected data on sexual practices, tobacco smoking, alcohol consumption, and other potential risk factors. Results showed that oral infection by HPV-16 increased the risk more than 14-fold, and seropositivity for the HPV-16 L1 capsid protein increased the risk more than 32-fold compared to seronegative individuals. Strikingly, seropositivity for E6 and/or E7 increased the risk nearly

60-fold. Analysis by PCR detected HPV-16 DNA in 72% of tumor specimens and HPV-16 E6 and/or E7 proteins in 64% of specimens. Sexual activity conducive to HPV exposure also increased the risk (e.g., more than 25 lifetime vaginal-sex partners or more than 5 oral-sex partners more than tripled the risk). Heavy tobacco and alcohol use also increased the risk of oropharyngeal cancer *but primarily among cases without exposure to HPV-16* (D'Souza et al., 2007).

These findings clearly show that the demographic profile of HPV-16–infected patients who develop oral cavity cancer differs markedly from that of patients whose cancer developed from chronic exposure to tobacco and alcohol. In the latter group, the disease is typically diagnosed after age 60, the ratio of African Americans to Caucasians is 2:1, and the ratio of men to women is nearly 3:1. In HPV-16–related disease, chronic exposure to tobacco and alcohol may be absent, the age at diagnosis is much earlier (age 20–50 years), the male-to-female ratio is close to 1:1, and tumors are most likely to develop on the tonsils and base of the tongue (Gillison et al., 2008). Most notably, HPV-16 and HPV-18 are the same viruses responsible for the vast majority of cervical cancers, and HPV is the most common sexually transmitted infection in the United States and elsewhere. Furthermore, infection by high-risk HPV strains is preventable by vaccination (Kenter et al., 2009).

Malignant Transformation by HPV

Oncogenic strains of HPV appear to cause malignant transformation of the oral mucosa in much the same way as in the cervix. The viral DNA integrates into human DNA in the nuclei of healthy cells and uses the cellular machinery to produce two harmful proteins, E6 and E7. These bind to, and shut down, two important tumor suppressor proteins, p53 and pRb. Active pRb prevents excessive cell growth; without it, cells proliferate unchecked. Active p53 arrests the cell division cycle when DNA is damaged, and then either activates DNA repair or initiates cell death. Without p53, a cell replicates wildly even if it has DNA damage (Gillison et al., 2008).

Synergism of HPV and Marijuana in Oral Cavity Cancer

Gillison and colleagues conducted a case–control investigation to explore potential differences in the risk factors for HPV-16–positive and HPV-16–negative oral cavity malignancies (Gillison et al., 2008). Their study compared 240 cases with squamous cell carcinomas of the head and neck with 322 matched controls without

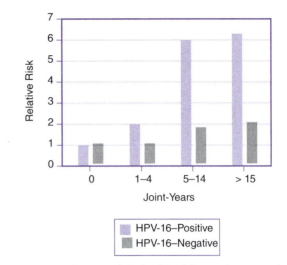

FIGURE 15.4 Relative Risk (RR) of Oral Cavity Cancer with Increasing Joint-Years of Marijuana Smoking in HPV-16–Positive and HPV-16–Negative Squamous Cell Carcinoma of the Head and Neck.

Data from Gillison, M. L., D'Souza, G., Wester, W., Sugar, E., Ziao, W., Begum, S., & Vascidi, R. (2008). Distinct risk factor profiles for human papillomavirus type 16–positive and human papillomavirus type 16–negative head and neck cancers. *Journal of the National Cancer Institute, 100*(6), 407–420

cancer ascertained at the Johns Hopkins Hospital in Baltimore during 2000–2006. Among tumor specimens taken from the 240 cases, 92 (38%) were found to be positive for HPV-16 utilizing *in situ hybridization* methodology. Results revealed marked differences in the risk factors for HPV-16–positive versus HPV-16–negative cases. Sexual behavior (number of oral-sex partners) was strongly associated with HPV-16–positive cases, whereas tobacco use, alcohol use, and poor oral hygiene were associated with HPV-16–negative cases. Surprisingly, use of tobacco and/or alcohol had no effect on the risk of developing HPV-16–negative cancer. An interesting finding was the association of marijuana smoking with cancer risk. The association of marijuana smoking was more pronounced among HPV-16–positive cases than HPV-negative cases, suggesting the possibility of synergism between cannabis and viral exposure (**FIGURE 15.4**).

HIV and Oral Cavity Cancer

The North American AIDS Cohort Collaboration on Research and Design (NA-ACCORD) was created as a part of the International Epidemiologic Databases to Evaluate AIDS (IeDEA) initiative. Investigators with NA-ACCORD are currently monitoring health outcomes among more than 90,000 patients, the majority of whom are HIV-positive, from more than 50 sites throughout the United States and Canada. Recently, investigators with NA-ACCORD examined incidence rates of oral cavity and pharyngeal cancer among 51,151 HIV-positive people in 14 cohorts across North

America during the period 2006–2010. Age-adjusted rates among HIV-positive individuals were compared with rates for the Surveillance, Epidemiology, and End Results (SEER) population during the same period. Results revealed that the annual incidence rate of oral cavity and pharyngeal cancer in HIV-positive individuals was nearly double the rate in the general population (30.1 per 100,000 versus 15.9 per 100,000). The investigators also noted an approximate twofold increase in the incidence of these malignancies among older HIV-positive individuals with a low CD4 count (below 350 helper T lymphocytes per microliter of blood). Notably, all incident cases observed in the HIV-positive cohort were chronic cigarette smokers. These findings suggest that immunosuppression due to HIV infection may increase susceptibility to carcinogenesis in tissues of the oral cavity and pharynx, particularly among smokers (Beachler & D'Souza, 2013).

Lip Cancer and Solar Radiation

Lip cancers account for 30%–40% of all malignancies of the oral cavity. These tumors are predominately squamous cell carcinomas that arise in the lower lip following chronic and excessive exposure to solar ultraviolet radiation. Incidence rates of lip cancer and other forms of skin cancer are highest in Caucasian populations residing in regions with high levels of solar radiation (Johnson et al., 2011).

Ozone (O_3) is an unstable oxygen molecule that effectively filters ultraviolet radiation in the stratosphere (the atmosphere 10–50 km above the Earth). In recent decades, significant thinning of the ozone layer has been noted, particularly over the Earth's polar regions. Ozone depletion is caused by increased levels of chlorofluorocarbons, bromofluorocarbons, and other man-made chemicals that dissociate into reactive molecules at the Earth's surface. These molecules are transported into the stratosphere where they destroy ozone by catalytic reactions (Jones, 1987). The largest "ozone hole" ever recorded was imaged by the U.S. National Aeronautics and Space Administration (NASA) over Antarctica in 2006 (Carlowicz & Lindsey, 2009). Notably, Caucasian populations of Australia and New Zealand who live in closest proximity to the Antarctic ozone hole have the highest rates of lip cancer and skin cancer in the world (Anderson, Wilmouth, Smith, & Sayres, 2012; Moore, Allister, Roder, Pierce, & Wilson, 2001; Moore, Johnson, Pierce, & Wilson, 1999; Narayanan, Saladi, & Fox, 2010; Staples et al., 2006). Epidemiologic data on lip cancer collected by the South Australian Central Cancer Registry during 1977–1996 revealed age-standardized annual incidence rates of 15 per 100,000 in men and 4 per 100,000 in women,

whereas the rates observed for the same time period in the U.S. population of Connecticut were less than 1 per 100,000 for both men and women (Moore et al., 2001; Morse, Pendrys, Neely, & Psoter, 1999).

Global recognition of ozone destruction by chlorofluorocarbons and bromofluorocarbons led to the Montreal Protocol of 1989, which banned the production of ozone-depleting chemicals. Predictive models of ozone depletion by man-made substances suggest that ozone depletion and heightened solar radiation will continue to increase over many decades (Carlowicz, 2009).

Cancer of the lip most often develops in the epithelium of the vermillion, a transition zone between the inner labial mucosa and the outer skin of the lower lip (Molnar, Ronay, & Tapolcsanyi, 1974). The lower lip is 5–10 times more likely to be affected owing to its greater exposure to sunlight. In a recent 25-year retrospective study of 2152 patients from Western Australia with lip cancer, 81% occurred on the lower lip and over 75% developed in men (Abreu, Kruger, & Tennant, 2009). The risk of lip cancer is inversely related to the level of skin pigmentation (i.e., fair-skinned people have the highest risk and dark-skinned individuals the lowest). Chronic abuse of tobacco (particularly pipe and cigar smoking), chronic alcohol abuse, and certain viral infections (e.g., HPV-16) have also been found to increase the risk (Maruccia et al., 2012; Moore et al., 1999; Perea-Milla et al., 2003).

Recent studies indicate that lip cancer occurs at markedly increased rates after organ transplantation and exposure to immunosuppressive drugs. In a population-based nationwide cohort of 8162 kidney transplant recipients, squamous cell lip cancer was diagnosed in 203 patients during periods of receiving immunosuppressive drugs at rates 41 times higher than expected in men and 72 times higher than expected in women (van Leeuwen et al., 2009).

Lip cancer and other forms of skin cancer can be prevented by using sunscreen, avoiding sunburn, limiting other sources of radiation (e.g., tanning salons), and wearing protective clothing, sunglasses, and hats. Most lip cancers are squamous cell carcinomas that have potential for metastatic spread. Nevertheless, because of their highly visible location, most lip cancers are detected and excised at an early stage and mortality rates are quite low (Stebbins & Hanke, 2014).

Other Risk Factors for Oral Cavity Cancer

Plummer–Vinson syndrome (iron deficiency anemia, dysphagia, and atrophy of the oral cavity mucosa) is associated with predisposition to oral cavity cancer. Other conditions that may be associated with oral cavity neoplasms include sprue (malabsorption of wheat germ) and scurvy (deficiency in vitamin C).

Rare malignant neoplasms of the oral cavity include cancers of the salivary glands, including the parotid glands and submandibular glands. These are typically glandular carcinomas with mixed histologic features. A salivary gland carcinoma mixed with marked lymphocytic invasion is called a Warthin's tumor. The risk of salivary gland cancer is increased by ionizing radiation (e.g., in atomic bomb survivors and after radiotherapy) (Boukheris, Curtis, Land, & Dores, 2009), but other risk factors have not been identified.

Malignant melanomas may also present initially in the oral cavity. Risk factors for oral cavity malignant melanomas include certain genetic syndromes, such as Peutz–Jeghers syndrome and Addison's disease, both of which lead to melanotic pigmentation of the oral cavity mucosa (Boardman et al., 1998).

▶ Cancer of the Oropharynx and Laryngopharynx

During 2018, 173,495 new cases were diagnosed, and 85,989 individuals died from cancer of the oropharynx or laryngopharynx in the world population. Approximately 82% of the new cases and deaths occurred in men (141,968 new cases and 71,531 deaths). Cancers of the oropharynx and laryngopharynx constitute approximately 0.9% of all malignant neoplasms and account for about 0.9% of cancer deaths in the human population. The global age-adjusted mortality rate in 2018 was approximately threefold higher in men than in women (1.7 per 100,000 versus 0.6 per 100,000) (Bray et al., 2018; Ferlay et al., 2010, 2013, 2018).

Pathologic and epidemiologic features of malignancies of the oropharynx and laryngopharynx are similar to oral cavity cancer. Tumors arising in these tissues are predominantly squamous cell carcinomas. The global distributions of incidence and mortality rates are similar to the patterns for oral cavity cancer in Figure 15.2.

Neoplasms of the oropharynx and laryngopharynx are typically diagnosed in the elderly and occur more often in men than women. The major risk factors are tobacco smoking, alcohol consumption, and infection by oncogenic strains of HPV (e.g., HPV-16 and HPV-18). Minor risk factors include marijuana smoking; nutritional deficits of iron, vitamin B, and vitamin C; and chronic use of smokeless tobacco (La Vecchia et al., 1997). Immunosuppression due to HIV infection also increases carcinogenesis in tissues of the oral cavity and pharynx (Beachler & D'Souza, 2013).

▶ Cancer of the Nasopharynx

During 2018, 129,079 new cases were diagnosed, and 72,987 individuals died from cancer of the nasopharynx in the world population. Approximately 73% of the new cases and deaths occurred in men (93,416 new cases and 54,280 deaths). Cancer of the nasopharynx constitutes approximately 0.7% of all malignant neoplasms and accounts for about 0.8% of cancer deaths in the human population. The global age-adjusted death rate in 2018 was more than threefold higher in men than in women (1.3 per 100,000 versus 0.4 per 100,000) (Bray et al., 2018; Ferlay et al., 2010, 2013, 2018).

FIGURE 15.5 shows the global patterns of incidence and mortality rates of nasopharyngeal cancer in 2018. Nasopharyngeal carcinoma is rare in most regions of the world, and the low-risk populations in these regions had annual incidence rates less than 1 per 100,000. In contrast, markedly higher rates are evident for the populations of China, the nations of Southeast Asia, and the islands of Oceania. The highest incidence and mortality rates reported in 2018 were in men of Malaysia (9.5 and 5.7 per 100,000) and Indonesia (10.5 and 7.2 per 100,000) (Bray et al., 2018; Ferlay et al., 2018).

Certain populations within nations have very high rates of nasopharyngeal carcinoma. High-risk populations include the Cantonese of Southern China, Hong Kong, and Taiwan; the Inuits (Eskimos) in Greenland and Alaska; the Vietnamese in North Vietnam; and the Arabians of North Africa. Within these populations, several major risk factors for nasopharyngeal carcinoma have been identified.

Histology of Nasopharyngeal Cancer

Malignancies of the nasopharynx are predominantly squamous cell carcinomas that arise from the squamous epithelial lining of the organ. Nasopharyngeal carcinoma has been classified into three distinct histologic types: keratinizing squamous cell carcinoma (Type I) and nonkeratinizing squamous cell carcinoma (Types II and III). Nonkeratinizing malignancies are further classified as either differentiated (Type II) or undifferentiated (Type III). The nonkeratinized Type II and Type III malignancies constitute nearly all the nasopharyngeal carcinomas in high-risk populations, whereas the keratinized Type I malignancies predominate in low-risk populations. The age-specific incidence of Type I malignancies of the nasopharynx increases exponentially with age beginning at about 50 years of age, whereas the age-specific incidence of Types II and III malignancies peaks at about age 50 years and then declines.

Estimated age-standardized incidence rates (World) in 2018, nasopharynx, both sexes, all ages

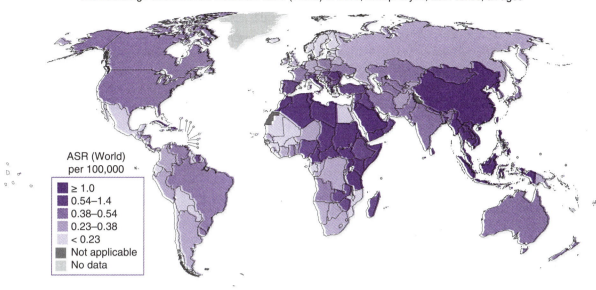

ASR (World)
per 100,000

■ ≥ 1.0
■ 0.54–1.4
■ 0.38–0.54
■ 0.23–0.38
□ < 0.23
■ Not applicable
□ No data

Estimated age-standardized mortality rates (World) in 2018, nasopharynx, both sexes, all ages

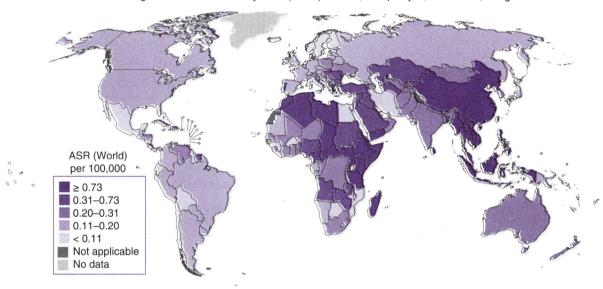

ASR (World)
per 100,000

■ ≥ 0.73
■ 0.31–0.73
■ 0.20–0.31
■ 0.11–0.20
□ < 0.11
■ Not applicable
□ No data

FIGURE 15.5 Global Incidence and Mortality Rates of Nasopharyngeal Cancer, 2018.

Caption: ASR: Rates per 100,000 are age-standardized to the world population, 2000–2025.

Reproduced with permission from Ferlay, J., Ervik, M., Lam, F., Colombet, M., Mery, L., Piñeros, M., ... Bray, F. (2018). *Global cancer observatory: Cancer today*. Lyon, France: International Agency for Research on Cancer. Retrieved from https://gco.iarc.fr/today

Risk Factors for Nasopharyngeal Carcinoma

Nasopharyngeal carcinoma is influenced by a web of causation that includes certain dietary factors, tobacco smoking, alcohol intake, and viral infection. The risk factors are discussed in the following sections.

Dietary Factors and Nasopharyngeal Carcinoma

In 1971, John Ho, a radiation oncologist in Hong Kong, postulated that intake of Cantonese-style salted fish may contribute to the development of nasopharyngeal carcinoma (Ho, 1971). His hypothesis was subsequently confirmed by the results of several case–control studies. For example, an international team of investigators examined the effects of salted foods and other dietary factors in a study of 282 cases of nasopharyngeal carcinoma ascertained from medical centers in Malaysia and an equal number of age- and gender-matched disease-free controls from the general population. Compared to nonconsumers, individuals consuming salted fish at least weekly increased their risk of developing laryngeal carcinoma by more than fourfold (OR = 4.4). Risk increases were also noted for heavy consumption of other salted foods (leafy vegetables, roots, and eggs) as well as alcoholic beverages. Conversely, individuals who regularly consumed fresh fruits and vegetables lowered their risk (Armstrong et al., 1998). The carcinogenic potential of salt-preserved fish is supported by experiments in laboratory rats, which develop malignant nasal and nasopharyngeal tumors after salted fish consumption (Zheng, Luo, Christensson, & Drettner, 1994).

Jeannel and colleagues examined the effects of diet in a study of 80 cases of nasopharyngeal carcinoma ascertained from the Institute Salah Azaiz in Tunisia and 160 disease-free controls matched on age, gender, and place of residence. Compared to nonconsumers, those who regularly consumed pickled vegetables, quaddid (dried mutton in oil), harissa (a very spicy condiment), salted anchovies, or pickled olives were found to be at increased risk (Jeannel et al., 1990).

Tobacco Smoking and Nasopharyngeal Carcinoma

Several epidemiologic studies have noted that chronic tobacco smoking elevates the risk of developing nasopharyngeal carcinoma. In Taiwan, exposure to tobacco and alcohol was studied in 375 cases with histologically confirmed nasopharyngeal carcinoma and 327 healthy community controls matched to the cases on gender, age, and residence. Compared to nonsmokers, those who smoked 25 or more years had a modest increase in risk (OR = 1.7). Consumption of alcoholic beverages had no influence on the risk in this sample of cases and controls from a high-risk population (Cheng et al., 1999). These results are characteristic of several case–control studies conducted in high-risk populations: A modest risk increase in chronic smokers, but no effect associated with ingestion of alcohol at any level (Yu & Yuan, 2002).

Alcohol Consumption and Nasopharyngeal Carcinoma

Although studies of alcohol and nasopharyngeal carcinoma have been uniformly null in high-risk populations, investigations conducted in low-risk populations do find effects of alcohol. Investigators in the United States studied 231 cases of nasopharyngeal carcinoma ascertained from population registries in Washington, Detroit, Connecticut, Iowa, and Utah and 246 disease-free controls matched to the cases on age, gender, and residence. Compared to nonsmokers, individuals who smoked more than 60 pack-years had a sixfold increase in risk (OR = 6.5). Compared to nondrinkers, individuals who reported the heaviest alcohol consumption (21 or more drinks per week)

had a threefold increase in risk (OR = 2.9). The magnitude of risk estimates increased for persons 50 years of age or older, suggesting that a large fraction of elderly cases of nasopharyngeal carcinoma arise due to chronic smoking and alcohol intake (Vaughan et al., 1996).

Formaldehyde and Nasopharyngeal Carcinoma

In 1986, a team of U.S. investigators reported the results of a historical cohort study of mortality among 27,561 workers employed in 10 facilities where there was heavy occupational exposure to formaldehyde. Although overall cancer mortality was not influenced by formaldehyde exposure, the mortality due to nasopharyngeal cancer was significantly increased (Blair et al., 1986). In a subsequent analysis of this same cohort, formaldehyde exposure increased the standardized mortality ratio (SMR) for nasopharyngeal cancer by more than twofold (SMR = 2.1) (Hauptmann, Lubin, Stewart, Hayes, & Blair, 2004). In 2006, the International Agency for Research on Cancer (IARC) classified formaldehyde as carcinogenic to humans (IARC, 2006). Nevertheless, a recent meta-analysis revealed significant heterogeneity among published estimates of risk due to inclusion of a single plant in Connecticut with an unexplained cluster of nasopharyngeal cancers, thereby diminishing support for a causal relationship between formaldehyde exposure and nasopharyngeal cancer (Blanchard, Mundt, Mundt, & Montgomery, 2010).

Other occupational exposures have also been examined, including exposure to wood dust, wood solvents, cotton dust, combustion products, agrichemicals, and pesticides. Of these, exposure to wood dust shows the greatest consistency as a risk factor among studies (Chang & Adami, 2006; Vaughan & Davis, 1991).

Epstein–Barr Virus and Nasopharyngeal Carcinoma

Epstein–Barr virus (EBV) is a herpes virus containing double-stranded DNA that infects 90%–95% of the world population. In Hong Kong, EBV infects 80% of children by the age of 5 years, 90% by the age of 8 years, and almost 100% by the age of 10 years without causing symptoms. In London, EBV infection usually occurs during the teenage years and can cause infectious mononucleosis (Kangro et al., 1994). Transmission occurs through contact with contaminated saliva. The virus initially infects the epithelium of the nasal cavity, the nasopharynx, and the oropharynx, after which it spreads into B lymphocytes.

In infected individuals, EBV persists throughout life as a latent virus in resting memory B lymphocytes. In this state, EBV is dormant and replicates together with the chromosomal DNA of host cells. Latency results in limited expression of EBV genes and concealment from host immunity. Reactivation of EBV is triggered when memory B cells differentiate into plasma cells in response to specific antigenic stimuli (e.g., infection by other microbes). Reactivation leads to replication of viral DNA, assembly and budding of virions from infected cells, and dissemination to other tissues (Draborg, Duus, & Houen, 2013).

Involvement of EBV in the genesis of nasopharyngeal carcinoma was suspected as early as 1966 when cases were found to express antibodies against EBV. Later studies revealed that patients with nasopharyngeal cancer had elevated IgG and IgA antibody titers specific for the viral capsid, viral nuclear antigens, and viral DNA. Viral DNA, RNA, and gene products have also been detected in the tumor cells of most patients. Notably, the titers of IgA antibodies precede the development of nasopharyngeal carcinoma by several years and correlate with tumor burden, remission, and recurrence. The totality of evidence clearly indicates a causal role of EBV infection in the development of nasopharyngeal carcinoma. However, EBV infection alone is not a sufficient cause of nasopharyngeal carcinoma because virtually all adults worldwide are infected, yet only a small fraction develops the malignancy. Therefore, it is apparent that environmental and/or genetic cofactors also contribute to carcinogenesis (Chang & Adami, 2006; Yu & Yuan, 2002).

Immunosuppression and Inflammation in Nasopharyngeal Carcinoma

Immunosuppressive and inflammatory conditions have been found to increase the risk of developing nasopharyngeal carcinoma. In a follow-up study of a large cohort of patients with HIV/AIDS in the United States, the incidence of nasopharyngeal carcinoma was elevated more than twofold compared to the general population (Shebl, Bhatia, & Engels, 2009).

Using data from a registry of national health insurance claims, investigators in Taiwan examined incidence rates of cancer in patients with inflammatory myopathies. A startling finding was a 66-fold increase in the incidence of nasopharyngeal carcinoma among 1059 patients with dermatomyositis compared to the general Taiwanese population (Huang et al., 2009). Dermatomyositis is a rare, systemic autoimmune disease characterized by a distinct skin rash, and inflammation and weakness of skeletal muscles. Some cases of this condition have been linked to reactivation

of latent EBV and other viral or bacterial infections (Callen & Wortmann, 2006).

Genetic Predisposition to Nasopharyngeal Carcinoma

Familial clustering of nasopharyngeal carcinoma has been demonstrated in several studies. Compared to individuals without a family history of nasopharyngeal carcinoma, subjects with an affected first-degree relative (parent, sibling, or child) have a 4- to 10-fold elevation in risk. Notably, certain alleles of the human leukocyte antigen (HLA) locus have been identified that appear to modify genetic susceptibility (Burt et al., 1996). In a meta-analysis of studies in Southern Chinese populations, HLA-A2, -B14, and -B46 were found to be associated with increases in risk, whereas HLA-A11, -B13, and -B22 were associated with decreases in risk (Goldsmith, West, & Morton, 2002).

Molecular studies of nasopharyngeal tumors have revealed a variety of genomic abnormalities, including loss of heterozygosity, chromosomal gains and losses, and epigenetic modification of tumor suppressor genes and oncogenes. Nevertheless, additional studies will be needed to elucidate specific genetic factors that are related to carcinogenesis of the nasopharynx.

Carcinogenesis in the Nasopharynx

Nearly all humans are infected with latent EBV, so carcinogenesis may involve an immunocompromised human host who is predisposed to the reactivation of latent EBV and dissemination of the virus to produce an active EBV infection of the nasopharyngeal epithelium. Active infection of the nasopharynx in combination with exposure to tobacco carcinogens, nitrosamines from salted fish, or other irritating/inflammatory agents may induce DNA damage, episomal changes, and viral integration into the chromosomes of epithelial cells. The expression of specific viral genes might also disable tumor suppressor genes or amplify tumor oncogenes that spur mechanisms of carcinogenesis such as increased cell replication, dysregulation of apoptosis, angiogenesis, and metastasis (Raab-Traub, 2002).

Prevention of Nasopharyngeal Carcinoma

Specific strategies for the primary prevention of nasopharyngeal carcinoma are speculative. However, avoiding regular intake of salt-preserved fish or other foods, tobacco, and regular intake of any substance that causes irritation/inflammation in the upper alimentary canal; limiting alcohol consumption; and increasing regular intake of fresh fruit and vegetables may lower the risk.

References

Abreu, L., Kruger, E., & Tennant, M. (2009). Lip cancer in Western Australia, 1982–2006: A 25-year retrospective epidemiological study. *Australian Dental Journal, 54*, 130–135.

Anderson, J. G., Wilmouth, D. M., Smith, J. B., & Sayres, D. S. (2012). UV dosage levels in summer: Increased risk of ozone loss from convectively injected water vapor. *Science, 337*(6096), 835–839.

Armstrong, R. W., Imrey, P. B., Lye, M. S., Armstrong, M. J., Yu, M. C., & Sani, S. (1998). Nasopharyngeal carcinoma in Malaysian Chinese; salted fish and other dietary exposures. *International Journal of Cancer, 77*, 228–235.

Beachler, D. C., & D'Souza, G. (2013). Oral HPV infection and head and neck cancers in HIV-infected individuals. *Current Opinion in Oncology, 25*(5), 503–510.

Blair, A., Stewart, P., O'Berg, M., Gaffey, W., Walrath, J., Ward, J., … Cubit, D. (1986). Mortality among industrial workers exposed to formaldehyde. *Journal of the National Cancer Institute, 76*(6), 1071–1084.

Blanchard, A. M., Mundt, K. A., Mundt, D. J., & Montgomery, R. R. (2010). Epidemiological studies of formaldehyde exposure and risk of leukemia and nasopharyngeal cancer: A meta-analysis. *Critical Reviews in Toxicology, 40*(2), 85–100.

Blot, W. J., McLaughlin, J. K., Winn, D. M., Austin, D. F., Greenberg, R. S., Preston-Martin, S., … Fraumeni, J. F. (1988). Smoking and drinking in relation to oral and pharyngeal cancer. *Cancer Research, 48*, 3282–3287.

Boardman, L. A., Thibodeau, S. N., Schaid, D. J., Lindor, N. M., McDonnell, S. K., Bugart, L. J., … Hartmann, L. C. (1998). Increased risk for cancer in patients with the Peutz-Jeghers syndrome. *Annals of Internal Medicine, 128*(11), 896–899.

Boukheris, H., Curtis, R. E., Land, C. E., & Dores, G. M. (2009). Incidence of carcinoma of the major salivary glands according to the WHO classification, 1992 to 2006: A population-based study in the United States. *Cancer Epidemiology, Biomarkers and Prevention, 18*, 2899–2906.

Boyle, P., & Levin, B. (Eds.). (2008). *IARC world cancer report.* Lyon, France: International Agency for Research on Cancer (IARC) Publications.

Bray, F., Ferlay, J., Soerjomataram, I., Siegel, R. L., Torre, L. A., & Jemal, A. (2018). Global cancer statistics 2018: GLOBOCAN estimates of incidence and mortality worldwide for 36 cancers in 185 countries. *CA: A Cancer Journal for Clinicians, 68*(6), 394–424.

Burt, R. D., Vaughan, T. L., McKnight, B., Davis, S., Beckmann, A. M., Smith, A. G., … Berwick, M. (1996). Associations between human leukocyte antigen type and nasopharyngeal carcinoma in Caucasians in the United States. *Cancer Epidemiology, Biomarkers and Prevention, 5*, 879–887.

Callen, J. P., & Wortmann, R. L. (2006). Dermatomyositis. *Clinics in Dermatology, 24*(5), 363–373.

Carlowicz, M. (2009). Climate change and atmospheric circulation will make for uneven ozone recovery. Retrieved from http://www.nasa.gov/topics/earth/features/ozone_recovery.html

Carlowicz, M., & Lindsey, R. (2009). *Earth observatory: The world we avoided by protecting the ozone layer.* Greenbelt, MD: Earth Observatory, Goddard Space Flight Center, NASA.

Chang, E. T., & Adami, H.-O. (2006). The enigmatic epidemiology of nasopharyngeal carcinoma. *Cancer Epidemiology, Biomarkers and Prevention, 15*, 1765–1777.

Cheng, Y. J., Hildesheim, A., Hsu, M. M., Chen, I. H., Brinton, L. A., Levine, P. H., … Yang, C. S. (1999). Cigarette smoking, alcohol consumption and risk of nasopharyngeal carcinoma in Taiwan. *Cancer Causes & Control, 10*(3), 201–207.

Draborg, A. H., Duus, K., & Houen, G. (2013). Epstein-Barr virus in systemic autoimmune diseases. *Clinical and Developmental Immunology, 2013*. Retrieved from http://www.hindawi.com/journals/jir/2013/535738

D'Souza, G., Kreimer, A. R., Viscidi, R., Pawlita, M., Fakhry, C., Koch, W. M., … Gillison, M. L. (2007). Case-control study of human papillomavirus and oropharyngeal cancer. *New England Journal of Medicine, 356*(19), 1944–1956.

Ferlay, J., Ervik, M., Lam, F., Colombet, M., Mery, L., Piñeros, M., … Bray, F. (2018). *Global cancer observatory: Cancer today.* Lyon, France: International Agency for Research on Cancer. Retrieved from https://gco.iarc.fr/today

Ferlay, J., Shin, H.-R., Bray, F., Forman, D., Mathers, C., & Parkin, D. M. (2010). Estimates of worldwide burden of cancer in 2008: GLOBOCAN 2008. *International Journal of Cancer, 127*(12), 2893–2917.

Ferlay, J., Soerjomataram, I., Ervik, M., Dikshit, R., Eser, S., Mathers, C., … Bray, F. (2013). *GLOBOCAN 2012 v1.0, cancer incidence and mortality worldwide: IARC CancerBase No. 11.* Lyon, France: International Agency for Research on Cancer. Retrieved from http://globocan.iarc.fr

Gillison, M. L., D'Souza, G., Wester, W., Sugar, E., Ziao, W., Begum, S., & Vascidi, R. (2008). Distinct risk factor profiles for human papillomavirus type 16–positive and human papillomavirus type 16–negative head and neck cancers. *Journal of the National Cancer Institute, 100*(6), 407–420.

Gillison, M. L., Koch, W. M., Capone, R. B., Spafford, M., Westra, W. H., Wu, L., … Sidransky, D. (2000). Evidence for a causal association between human papillomavirus and a subset of head and neck cancers. *Journal of the National Cancer Institute, 92*, 709–720.

Goldsmith, D. B., West, T. M., & Morton, R. (2002). HLA associations with nasopharyngeal carcinoma in Southern Chinese: A meta-analysis. *Clinical Otolaryngology, 27*, 61–67.

Gupta, P. C., Mehta, F. S., & Pindborg, J. J. (1984). Mortality among reverse chutta smokers in south India. *British Medical Journal (Clinical Research Edition), 289*(6449), 865–866.

Hauptmann, M., Lubin, J. H., Stewart, P. A., Hayes, R. B., & Blair, A. (2004). Mortality from solid cancers among workers in formaldehyde industries. *American Journal of Epidemiology, 59*(12), 1117–1130.

Ho, J. H. C. (1971). Genetic and environmental factors in nasopharyngeal carcinoma. In W. Nakahara, K. Nishioka, T. Hirayama, & Y. Ito (Eds.), *Recent advances in human tumor virology and immunology* (pp. 275–295). Tokyo, Japan: University of Tokyo Press.

Homann, N., Jousimies-Somer, H., Jokelainen, K., Heine, R., & Salaspuro, M. (1997). High acetaldehyde levels in saliva after ethanol consumption: Methodological aspects and pathogenetic implications. *Carcinogenesis, 18*(9), 1739–1743.

Huang, Y. L., Chen, Y. J., Lin, M. W., Wu, C. Y., Liu, P. C., Chen, T. J., … Liu, H. N. (2009). Malignancies associated with dermatomyositis and polymyositis in Taiwan: A nationwide population-based study. *British Journal of Dermatology, 161*(4), 854–860.

International Agency for Research on Cancer (IARC). (2006). Formaldehyde, 2-butoxyethanol and 1-tert-butoxypropan-2-ol. *IARC Monographs on the Evaluation of Carcinogenic Risks, 88*, 39–325.

Jeannel, D., Hubert, A., De Vathaire, F., Ellouz, R., Camoun, M., Ben Salem, M., ... De-Thi, G. (1990). Diet, living conditions and nasopharyngeal carcinoma in Tunisia—A case control study. *International Journal of Cancer, 46*, 421–425.

Johnson, N. W., Jayasekara, P., & Amarasinghe, A. A. H. K. (2011). Squamous cell carcinoma and precursor lesions of the oral cavity: Epidemiology and aetiology. *Periodontology, 2000, 57*, 19–37.

Jones, R. R. (1987). Ozone depletion and cancer risk. *Lancet, 330*(8556), 443–446.

Kabat, G. C., & Wynder, E. L. (1989). Type of alcoholic beverage and oral cancer. *International Journal of Cancer, 43*, 190–194.

Kangro, H. O., Osman, H. K., Lau, Y. L., Heath, R. B., Yeung, C. Y., & Ng, M. H. (1994). Seroprevalence of antibodies to human herpes viruses in England and Hong Kong. *Journal of Medical Virology, 43*, 91–96.

Kenter, G. G., Welters, M. J., Valentijn, A. R., Lowik, M. J. G., Berends-van der Meer, D. M. A., Vloon, A. P. G., ... Melief, C. J. M. (2009). Vaccination against HPV-16 oncoproteins for vulvar intraepithelial neoplasia. *New England Journal of Medicine, 361*, 1838–1847.

Krolls, S. O., & Hoffman, S. (1976). Squamous cell carcinoma of the oral soft tissues: A statistical analysis of 14,253 cases by age, sex and race of patients. *Journal of the American Dental Association, 92*, 571–574.

La Vecchia, C., Tavani, A., Franceschi, S., Levi, F., & Negri, M. (1997). Epidemiology and prevention of oral cancer. *Oral Oncology, 33*(5), 302–312.

Maden, C., Beckmann, A. M., Thomas, D. B., McKnight, B., Sherman, K. J., Ashley, R. L., ... Daling, J. R. (1992). Human papillomaviruses, herpes simplex viruses, and the risk of oral cancer in men. *American Journal of Epidemiology, 135*(10), 1093–1102.

Maruccia, M., Onesti, M. G., Parisi, E., Cigna, A., Toccola, A., & Scuder, N. (2012). Lip cancer: A 10-year retrospective epidemiological study. *Anticancer Research, 32*(4), 1543–1546.

Molnar, L., Ronay, P., & Tapolcsanyi, L. (1974). Carcinoma of the lip. Analysis of the material of 25 years. *Oncology, 29*, 101–121.

Moore, S., Johnson, N., Pierce, A., & Wilson, D. (1999). The epidemiology of lip cancer: A review of global incidence and aetiology. *Oral Disease, 5*(3), 185–195.

Moore, S. R., Allister, J., Roder, D., Pierce, A. M., & Wilson, D. F. (2001). Lip cancer in South Australia, 1977–1996. *Pathology, 33*(2), 167–171.

Mork, J., Lie, A. K., Glattre, E., Clark, S., Hallmans, G., Jellum, E., ... Dillner, J. (2001). Human papillomavirus infection as a risk factor for squamous-cell carcinoma of the head and neck. *New England Journal of Medicine, 344*, 1125–1131.

Morse, D. E., Pendrys, D. G., Neely, A. L., & Psoter, W. J. (1999). Trends in the incidence of lip, oral, and pharyngeal cancer: Connecticut, 1935–1994. *Oral Oncology, 35*(1), 1–8.

Narayanan, D. L., Saladi, R. N., & Fox, J. L. (2010). Ultraviolet radiation and skin cancer. *International Journal of Dermatology, 49*(9), 978–986.

National Cancer Institute. (2014). Oral cancer. National Institutes of Health. Retrieved from http://www.cancer.gov/cancertopics/types/oral

Parkin, M. D., Bray, F., Ferlay, J., & Pisani, P. (2005). Global cancer statistics, 2002. *CA: A Cancer Journal for Clinicians, 55*, 74–108.

Perea-Milla López, E., Miñarro-Del Moral, R. M., Martínez-García, C., Zanetti, R., Rosso, S., Serrano, S., ... Redondo, M. (2003). Lifestyles, environmental and phenotypic factors associated with lip cancer: A case-control study in southern Spain. *British Journal of Cancer, 88*, 1702–1707.

Poschl, G., & Seitz, H. K. (2004). Alcohol and cancer. *Alcohol, 39*, 155–165.

Raab-Traub, N. (2002). Epstein-Barr virus in the pathogenesis of NPC. *Seminars in Cancer Biology, 2*(6), 431–441.

Salaspuro, M. (2009). Acetaldehyde as a common denominator and cumulative carcinogen in digestive tract cancers. *Scandinavian Journal of Gastroenterology, 44*(8), 912–925.

Schwartz, S. M., Daling, J. R., Doody, D. R., Wipf, G. C., Carter, J. J., Madeleine, M. M., ... Galloway, D. A. (1998). Oral cancer risk in relation to sexual history and evidence of human papillomavirus infection. *Journal of the National Cancer Institute, 90*, 1626–1636.

Seitz, H. K., & Stickel, F. (2007). Molecular mechanisms of alcohol-mediated carcinogenesis. *Nature Reviews Cancer, 7*, 599–612.

Shebl, F. M., Bhatia, K., & Engels, E. A. (2009). Salivary gland and nasopharyngeal cancers in individuals with acquired immunodeficiency syndrome in United States. *International Journal of Cancer, 126*(10), 2503–2508.

Shklar, G. (1979). The oral cavity, jaws, and salivary glands. In S. L. Robbins & R. S. Cotran (Eds.), *Pathologic basis of disease* (pp. 886–917). Philadelphia, PA: W. B. Saunders.

Staples, M. P., Elwood, M., Burton, R. C., Williams, J. L., Marks, R., & Giles, G. G. (2006). Non-melanoma skin cancer in Australia: The 2002 national survey and trends since 1985. *Medical Journal of Australia, 184*(1), 6–10.

Stebbins, W., & Hanke, C. W. (2014). *Lip cancer: Not uncommon, often overlooked*. New York, NY: Skin Cancer Foundation.

Testino, G., & Borro, P. (2009). Carcinogenesis and alcohol. *Mediterranean Journal of Nutrition and Metabolism, 2*, 89–91.

van Leeuwen, M. T., Grulich, A. E., McDonald, S. P., McCredie, M. R., Amin J., Stewart, J. H., ... Vajdic, C. M. (2009). Immunosuppression and other risk factors for lip cancer after kidney transplantation. *Cancer Epidemiology Biomarkers & Prevention, 18*(2), 561–569.

Vaughan, T. L., & Davis, S. (1991). Wood dust exposure and squamous cell cancer of the upper respiratory tract. *American Journal of Epidemiology, 133*(5), 560–564.

Vaughan, T. L., Shapiro, J. A., Burt, R. D., Sanson, G. M., Berwick, M., Lynch, C. F., & Lyon, J. L. (1996). Nasopharyngeal cancer in a low-risk population: Defining risk factor by histological type. *Cancer Epidemiology, Biomarkers and Prevention, 5*, 587–593.

Yu, M. C., & Yuan, J. M. (2002). Epidemiology of nasopharyngeal carcinoma. *Seminars in Cancer Biology, 12*(6), 421–429.

Zheng, X., Luo, Y., Christensson, B., & Drettner, B. (1994). Induction of nasal and nasopharyngeal tumours in Sprague-Dawley rats fed with Chinese salted fish. *Acta Otolaryngolica, 114*, 98–104.

CHAPTER 16

Epidemiology of Esophageal Cancer

▶ Anatomy and Function of the Esophagus

The esophagus is a muscular tube that transports saliva, food, and liquids from the mouth to the stomach. In the human adult, the esophagus is about 20 cm (8 in.) long. The organ is lined by stratified squamous epithelium. The upper esophageal sphincter, which is located just below the pharynx, allows passage of food and liquids during swallowing. The lower esophageal sphincter, located at the junction of the lower esophagus with the stomach, regulates the passage of food and liquids into the stomach. Just before entering the stomach the esophagus passes through the diaphragm (see **FIGURE 16.1**) (Kumar, Abbas, & Aster, 2014).

▶ Global Epidemiology of Esophageal Cancer

During 2018, 572,034 new cases of esophageal cancer were diagnosed in the world population (399,699 in men and 172,335 in women), and 508,585 people died from this malignancy (357,190 men and 151,395 women). Approximately 70% of cases and deaths were male, and the global age-adjusted annual mortality rate was nearly threefold higher in men than in women (8.3 per 100,000 versus 3.0 per 100,000) (Bray et al., 2018). The annual number of deaths increased by 25% during the decade, 2008–2018, and esophageal cancer

now accounts for 5.3% of all cancer deaths, making it the sixth leading cause of death from cancer. Despite increases in the annual number of cases and deaths, the global age-adjusted incidence and mortality rates of esophageal cancer declined during the last decade

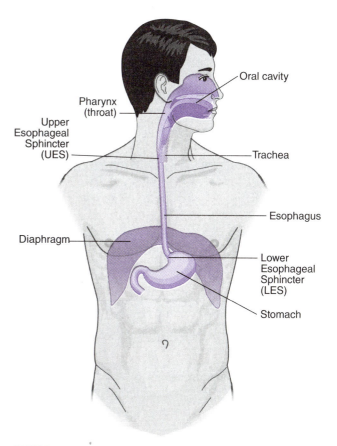

FIGURE 16.1 Anatomy of the Human Esophagus.

239

(by approximately 4% in men and 13% in women). Thus, as with many other chronic diseases, the rising global burden of esophageal cancer is largely due to the aging and growth of the world population (Bray et al., 2018; Ferlay et al., 2010, 2013, 2018).

About 80% of all new cases of esophageal cancer reported during 2008–2018 occurred in less-developed regions of the world. In the populations of these regions, more than 90% of esophageal cancer cases were squamous cell carcinomas. In contrast, the majority of cases in developed regions of the world were adenocarcinomas. As discussed in later sections of this chapter, these two histological cell types of esophageal cancer, squamous cell carcinoma and adenocarcinoma, have different profiles of risk factors (Bray et al., 2018; Ferlay et al., 2013).

Once diagnosed, invasive cancer of the esophagus does not respond well to treatment and has very poor survival rates (only 16% of cases in the United States and 10% of cases in Europe survive at least 5 years). As a consequence, esophageal cancer has a very high ratio of mortality to incidence (~0.88) (American Cancer Society, 2007; Ferlay et al., 2010, 2013, 2018; Parkin, Bray, Ferlay, & Pisani, 2005).

Esophageal cancer displays some of the most striking international epidemiologic characteristics of all diseases (**FIGURE 16.2**). During 2018 as in past years, the highest incidence and mortality rates were observed

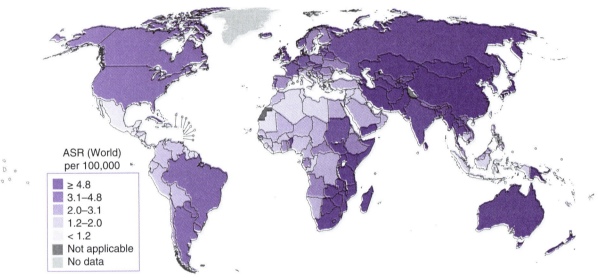

Estimated age-standardized incidence rates (World) in 2018, oesophagus, both sexes, all ages

ASR (World) per 100,000

- ≥ 4.8
- 3.1–4.8
- 2.0–3.1
- 1.2–2.0
- < 1.2
- Not applicable
- No data

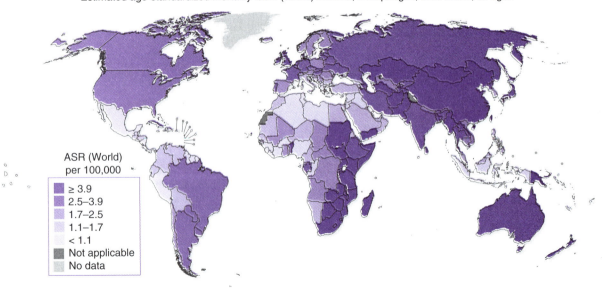

Estimated age-standardized mortality rates (World) in 2018, oesophagus, both sexes, all ages

ASR (World) per 100,000

- ≥ 3.9
- 2.5–3.9
- 1.7–2.5
- 1.1–1.7
- < 1.1
- Not applicable
- No data

FIGURE 16.2 Global Incidence and Mortality Rates of Esophageal Cancer, 2018.

Caption: ASR: Incidence rates per 100,000 are age-standardized to the world population, 2000–2025.

Reproduced with permission from Ferlay, J., Ervik, M., Lam, F., Colombet, M., Mery, L., Piñeros, M., ... Bray, F. (2018). *Global cancer observatory: Cancer today.* Lyon, France: International Agency for Research on Cancer. Retrieved from https://gco.iarc.fr/today

in nations along the East coast of Africa (Kenya, Tanzania, Malawi, Zimbabwe, and South Africa) and in nations of the *Asian esophageal cancer belt* that extends from Northern Iran across North-Central Asia and China (Ferlay et al., 2018; McCormack et al., 2017; Parkin, 2004). In certain high-risk populations of these regions (e.g., Northern Iran and rural areas of China), inordinately high annual rates of squamous cell carcinomas of the esophagus exceeding 100 per 100,000 have been observed in both men and women (Day, 1975; Lin et al., 2017). As discussed in greater detail below, the clustering of multiple risk factors (e.g., alcohol abuse, chronic tobacco smoking, dietary deficiencies, and genetic predisposition) may be primarily responsible for the persistently high rates of esophageal cancer in some populations.

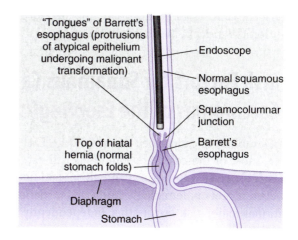

FIGURE 16.3 Barrett's Esophagus.

▶ Pathogenesis of Esophageal Cancer

Esophageal cancer is usually diagnosed during the sixth or seventh decade of life. Male cases far outnumber female cases in most regions; for example, the male-to-female ratio is 7:1 in Eastern Europe. Historically, the majority of esophageal tumors have been squamous cell carcinomas arising from the squamous cell epithelium in the middle or upper third of the esophagus. However, in recent decades, there has been a marked increase in the incidence of adenocarcinomas of the lower esophagus near the gastroesophageal junction, particularly among men of the United States, the United Kingdom, and other developed nations (Eslick, 2009). Indeed, adenocarcinomas of the lower esophagus are now diagnosed more often than squamous cell carcinomas in the United States, the United Kingdom, and Western European nations (Umar & Fleischer, 2008).

Adenocarcinomas of the lower esophagus arise by a sequence of metaplastic and dysplastic changes in the esophageal epithelium known as Barrett's esophagus (Barrett, 1957). Such changes are due to chronic gastroesophageal reflux of acidic stomach fluid into the normally basic environment of the lower esophagus (**FIGURE 16.3**). Barrett's esophagus is a premalignant lesion that must be aggressively treated to halt its progression to invasive esophageal cancer, a condition that is life-threatening. Effective screening strategies have been proposed for high-risk populations using endoscopy with mucosal iodine staining and biopsy to identify severe dysplastic lesions and carcinomas in situ that are curable by radical mucosectomy (Dong, Tank, Li, & Wang, 2002).

TABLE 16.1 Esophageal Cancer Epidemiology		
Characteristic	**Squamous Cell Carcinoma**	**Adenocarcinoma**
Age (years)	60–70	50–60
Anatomic site	Middle and upper	Lower
Risk factors	Alcohol and tobacco	Alcohol and tobacco
	Betel quid	GE reflux (GERD)
	Mycotic contamination	Obesity
	Nutritional deficits	Hiatal hernia
	Hot beverages	Asthma

GE, gastroesophageal junction; GERD, gastroesophageal reflux disease.

▶ Risk Factors for Esophageal Cancer

The risk factors for esophageal cancer differ according to histologic subtype (squamous cell carcinoma versus adenocarcinoma) and anatomic location in the esophagus (**TABLE 16.1**). Among the environmental risk factors for both histologic types, chronic alcoholism and cigarette smoking contribute most heavily to the development of esophageal cancer. This malignancy is 25 times more common among heavy drinkers than among controls. Habitual smokers of cigarettes also have a six- to sevenfold increased frequency of esophageal cancer after adjustment for alcohol consumption (Wynder & Mabuchi, 1973).

▶ Risk Factors for Squamous Cell Carcinomas of the Esophagus

In the esophageal cancer belt of the Middle East and China, most of the cases are squamous cell carcinomas that are related to tobacco and alcohol addiction. However, recent epidemiologic studies have identified additional major risk factors that independently and synergistically elevate the risk. In northern Iran and other populations in the Middle East and India, the cultural practice of consuming steaming hot black tea at temperatures exceeding 70°C (158°F) beginning early in life coupled with nutritional deficiencies in essential vitamins (beta carotene, folate, vitamin C, and vitamin E) are associated with the extraordinarily high rates observed (Islami et al., 2009).

Epidemiologic investigations conducted in the high-risk populations of northern China have also identified multiple factors other than tobacco and alcohol that synergistically enhance the development of squamous cell carcinoma of the esophagus (Yang, 1980). The web of causative factors includes mycotic (fungal) contamination of food and water, fungal conversion of secondary amines and nitrites to potent carcinogens (nitrosamines), fungal toxins (aflatoxins), and nutritional deficiencies in certain vitamins and minerals (selenium, molybdenum) (Chu & Li, 1994).

In Africa, the observed high rates of squamous cell esophageal cancer, particularly in men, are attributed to a web of causative risk factors involving chronic smoking and alcohol consumption, diets poor in fresh fruits and vegetables, and consumption of foods contaminated with *Fusarium verticillioides* (Day, 1975; Dlamini & Bhoola, 2005). During the 20th century there was a gradual transition of the staple diet of South Africa from sorghum to maize (corn), which was associated with the rising rates of this malignancy. Fusarium fungi grow readily on maize, producing fumonisins that reduce nitrates to nitrites and produce nitrosamines that may induce and promote esophageal carcinogenesis (Hendricks & Parker, 2008).

▶ Risk Factors for Barrett's Esophagus and Esophageal Adenocarcinoma

As noted previously, Barrett's esophagus is a premalignant lesion that develops proximal to the gastroesophageal junction, primarily due to reflux of acidic stomach fluid into the lower esophagus. If left untreated, Barrett's esophagus can progress through a sequence of cellular metaplastic and dysplastic changes leading to the development of invasive adenocarcinoma of the esophagus. Patients with Barrett's esophagus have a 30- to 125-fold increased risk of developing invasive adenocarcinoma of the esophagus compared to the general population (Umar & Fleischer, 2008; Yousef et al., 2008). Barrett's esophagus develops in approximately 10% of individuals with long-standing gastroesophageal reflux disease (GERD). Major risk factors for GERD include obesity, hiatal hernia, pregnancy, smoking, alcohol abuse, and asthma (Wong & Fitzgerald, 2005).

The bacterium *Helicobacter pylorus* is a common contaminant of the stomach that can cause stomach ulcers and gastric adenocarcinoma. Gastric infection by *H. pylori* can be treated with antibiotics plus proton pump-inhibiting drugs to counteract excessive secretion of stomach acid. Paradoxically, people who have had such treatment to rid the stomach of *H. pylori* are more prone to develop adenocarcinoma of the esophagus. The biological explanation is that certain strains of *H. pylori* reduce stomach acid, which makes the stomach fluids less harmful to the esophagus (in people with reflux). Thus, *H. pylorus* infection, although causing precancerous and cancerous lesions in the stomach, may actually protect against the development of Barrett's esophagus and esophageal cancer (Blaser & Atherton, 2004; Delaney & McColl, 2005).

▶ Genetic Risk Factors for Esophageal Cancer

Genetic polymorphisms of certain tumor suppressor genes that modulate cell division may also contribute to the genesis of esophageal cancer. Bani-Hani et al. (2000) found genetic polymorphisms in cyclin D1 and p53 that increased the risk by sixfold and threefold, respectively, and Reid et al. (2001) observed a 16-fold increase in the risk of esophageal cancer with loss of heterozygosity in p53.

Genetic syndromes involving malformations in esophageal structure also increase the risk of developing cancer of the esophagus. Achalasia due to dysfunction of the gastrointestinal sphincter interrupts the passage of food from the esophagus into the stomach and elevates the risk of esophageal cancer by 15-fold. Plummer–Vinson syndrome consists of iron deficiency anemia coupled with muscle atrophy, dysphagia, and the formation of esophageal rings or webs in the upper esophagus. This syndrome is associated with the development of squamous cell carcinomas proximal to the upper esophageal webs (Wynder, Hultberg, Jacobsson, & Bross, 1957).

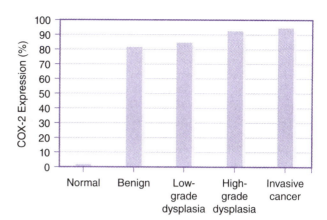

FIGURE 16.4 COX-2 in Progression of Barrett's Esophagus to Cancer.

Data from Harris, R. E. (2007). COX-2 and the inflammogenesis of cancer. *Subcellular Biochemistry, 42,* 193–212.

Prevention of Esophageal Cancer

The primary prevention of esophageal cancer obviously involves avoiding exposure of the esophagus to alcohol, tobacco, boiling hot beverages, and other caustic substances. In developing nations, intake of moldy grains and other foods or beverages fermented from moldy grain should be avoided. International efforts are now being directed to the obesity pandemic in order to reduce the burden of obesity-related diseases.

Multiple epidemiologic studies have examined the potential role of aspirin and other nonsteroidal anti-inflammatory drugs (NSAIDs) in the prevention of esophageal cancer. In a recent meta-analysis of these studies, Corley, Kerlikowske, Verma, and Buffler (2003) determined that regular use of NSAIDs was associated with a 40% reduction in the risk of esophageal cancer. The NSAIDs are known to reduce inflammation by inhibiting the cyclo-oxygenase enzymes, COX-1 and COX-2, that are responsible for the synthesis of prostaglandins of the inflammatory cascade. It is therefore notable that the inducible inflammatory gene COX-2, which is silent in normal esophageal mucosa, becomes markedly overexpressed throughout the progression of Barrett's esophagus to esophageal cancer (Harris, 2007) (**FIGURE 16.4**).

In high-risk populations, endoscopic screening for Barrett's esophagus or other dysplastic changes in the esophageal mucosa coupled with ablative treatment has proven effective in preventing the development of esophageal cancer (Dong et al., 2002; Spechler, 2001). Treatments found effective include administration of proton pump inhibitors (Yeh, Gerson, & Triadafilopoulos, 2003) and ablation by radiofrequency energy (Shaheen et al., 2009). Patients with Barrett's esophagus or other premalignant lesions should thus seek immediate treatment to prevent progression to esophageal cancer.

References

American Cancer Society. (2007). *Global cancer facts and figures, 2007.* Atlanta, GA: Author.

Bani-Hani, K., Martin, I. G., Hardie, L. J., Mapstone, N., Briggs, J. A., Forman, D., & Wild, C. P. (2000). Prospective study of cyclin D1 overexpression in Barrett's esophagus: Association with increased risk of adenocarcinoma. *Journal of the National Cancer Institute, 92,* 1316–1321.

Barrett, N. (1957). The lower esophagus lined by columnar epithelium. *Surgery, 41*(6), 881–894.

Blaser, M. J., & Atherton, J. C. (2004). *Helicobacter pylori* persistence: Biology and disease. *Journal of Clinical Investigation, 113,* 321–333.

Bray, F., Ferlay, J., Soerjomataram, I., Siegel, R. L., Torre, L. A., & Jemal, A. (2018). Global cancer statistics 2018: GLOBOCAN estimates of incidence and mortality worldwide for 36 cancers in 185 countries. *CA: A Cancer Journal for Clinicians, 68*(6), 394–424.

Chu, F. S., & Li, G. Y. (1994). Simultaneous occurrence of fumonisin B1 and other mycotoxins in moldy corn collected from the People's Republic of China in regions with high incidences of esophageal cancer. *Applied and Environmental Microbiology, 60*(3), 847–852.

Corley, D. A., Kerlikowske, K., Verma, R., & Buffler, P. (2003). Protective association of aspirin/NSAIDs and esophageal cancer: A systematic review and meta-analysis. *Gastroenterology, 124,* 47–56.

Day, N. E. (1975). Some aspects of the epidemiology of esophageal cancer. *Cancer Research, 35,* 3304–3307.

Delaney, B., & McColl, K. (2005). *Helicobacter pylori* and gastro-oesophageal reflux disease. *Alimentary Pharmacology and Therapeutics, 22*(Suppl. 1), 32–40.

Dlamini, Z., & Bhoola, K. (2005). Esophageal cancer in African blacks of Kwazulu Natal, South Africa: An epidemiological brief. *Ethnicity and Disease, 15*(4), 786–789.

Dong, Z., Tank, P., Li, L., & Wang, G. (2002). The strategy for esophageal cancer control in high-risk areas of China. *Japanese Journal of Clinical Oncology, 32,* 10–12.

Eslick, G. D. (2009). Epidemiology of esophageal cancer. *Gastroenterology Clinics, 38*(1), 17–25.

Ferlay, J., Ervik, M., Lam, F., Colombet, M., Mery, L., Piñeros, M., … Bray, F. (2018). *Global cancer observatory: Cancer today.* Lyon, France: International Agency for Research on Cancer. Retrieved from https://gco.iarc.fr/today

Ferlay, J., Shin, H.-R., Bray, F., Forman, D., Mathers, C., & Parkin, D. M. (2010). Estimates of worldwide burden of cancer in 2008: GLOBOCAN 2008. *International Journal of Cancer, 127*(12), 2893–2917.

Ferlay, J., Soerjomataram, I., Ervik, M., Dikshit, R., Eser, S., Mathers, C., … Bray, F. (2013). *GLOBOCAN 2012 v1.0, cancer incidence and mortality worldwide: IARC CancerBase No. 11* [Internet]. Lyon, France: International Agency for Research on Cancer. Retrieved from http://globocan.iarc.fr

Harris, R. E. (2007). COX-2 and the inflammogenesis of cancer. *Subcellular Biochemistry, 42*, 193–212.

Hendricks, D., & Parker, M. I. (2008). Oesophageal cancer in Africa. *International Union of Biochemistry and Molecular Biology Life, 53*(4–5), 263–268.

Islami, F., Pourshams, A., Nasrollahzadeh, D., Kamangar, F., Fahimi, S., Shakeri, R., … Boffetta, P. (2009). Tea drinking habits and oesophageal cancer in a high risk area in Northern Iran: Population based case-control study. *British Medical Journal, 338*, b929.

Kumar, V., Abbas, A. K., & Aster, J. C. (2014). *Robbins and Cotran pathologic basis of disease* (9th ed.). Philadelphia, PA: Mosby & Saunders.

Lin, Y., Totsuka, Y., Shan, B., Wang, C., Wei, W., Qiao, Y., … He, Y. (2017). Esophageal cancer in high-risk areas of China: Research progress and challenges. *Annals of Epidemiology, 27*(3), 215–221.

McCormack, V. A., Menya, D., Munishi, M. O., Dzamalala, C., Gasmelseed, N., Leon Roux, M., … Schüz, J. (2017). Informing etiologic research priorities for squamous cell esophageal cancer in Africa: A review of setting-specific exposures to known and putative risk factors. *International Journal of Cancer, 140*(2), 259–271.

Parkin, D. M. (2004). International variation. *Oncogene, 23*, 6329–6340.

Parkin, M. D., Bray, F., Ferlay, J., & Pisani, P. (2005). Global cancer statistics, 2002. *CA: A Cancer Journal for Clinicians, 55*, 74–108.

Reid, B. J., Prevo, L. J., Galipeau, P. C., Sanchez, C. A., Longton, G., Levine, D. S., & Rabinovitch, P. S. (2001). Predictors of progression in Barrett's esophagus II: Baseline 17p (p53) loss of heterozygosity identifies a patient subset at increased risk for neoplastic progression. *American Journal of Gastroenterology, 96*, 2839–2848.

Shaheen, N. J., Sharma, P., Overholt, B., Wolfsen, H. C., Sampliner, R. E., Wang, K. K., … Lightdale, C. J. (2009). Radiofrequency ablation in Barrett's esophagus with dysplasia. *New England Journal of Medicine, 360*, 2277–2288.

Spechler, S. J. (2001). Screening and surveillance for complications related to gastroesophageal reflux disease. *American Journal of Medicine, 111*(Suppl. 8A), 130–136.

Umar, S. B., & Fleischer, D. E. (2008). Esophageal cancer: Epidemiology, pathogenesis and prevention. *Nature Reviews Clinical Practice Gastroenterology and Hepatology, 5*, 517–526.

Wong, A., & Fitzgerald, R. C. (2005). Epidemiologic risk factors for Barrett's esophagus and associated adenocarcinoma. *Clinical Gastroenterology and Hepatology, 3*(1), 1–10.

Wynder, E. L., Hultberg, S., Jacobsson, F., & Bross, I. J. (1957). Environmental factors in cancer of the upper alimentary tract. A Swedish study with special reference to Plummer–Vinson (Paterson-Kelly) syndrome. *Cancer, 10*, 470–482.

Wynder, E. L., & Mabuchi, K. (1973). Etiological and environmental factors in esophageal cancer. *Journal of the American Medical Association, 226*, 1546–1548.

Yang, C. S. (1980). Research on esophageal cancer in China: A review. *Cancer Research, 40*, 2633–2644.

Yeh, R. W., Gerson, L. B., & Triadafilopoulos, G. (2003). Efficacy of esomeprazole in controlling reflux symptoms, intraesophageal, and intragastric pH in patients with Barrett's esophagus. *Diseases of the Esophagus, 16*(3), 193–198.

Yousef, F., Cardwell, C., Cantwell, M. M., Galway, K., Johnston, B. T., & Murray, L. (2008). The incidence of esophageal cancer and high-grade dysplasia in Barrett's esophagus: A systematic review and meta-analysis. *American Journal of Epidemiology, 168*(3), 237–249.

CHAPTER 17

Epidemiology of Stomach Cancer

▶ Anatomy and Function of the Stomach

The stomach is a hollow muscular organ juxtaposed between the esophagus and the duodenum with a resting volume ranging from 45 to 75 mL in the human adult. The stomach is lined by specialized epithelium that secretes proteases (enzymes that digest protein) and hydrochloric acid. The acidic nature of the stomach inhibits bacterial growth and facilitates the correct acid environment for activation of the enzymes secreted by the gastric epithelium. The stomach lining is folded into rugae to allow expansion and contraction. On expansion, the stomach easily holds 1 L of food. The outer stomach wall consists of three layers of striated smooth muscle innervated by branches of the vagus nerve. Bolus (masticated food) entering the stomach at the gastroesophageal sphincter is churned by muscular contractions of the stomach wall (called peristalsis). Chyme (partially digested food) passes from the stomach through the pyloric sphincter into the duodenum of the small intestine where the extraction of nutrients begins (see **FIGURE 17.1**) (Kumar, Abbas, & Aster, 2014).

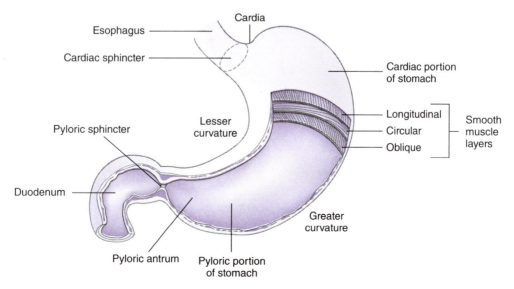

FIGURE 17.1 Anatomy of the Stomach.

▶ Global Epidemiology of Stomach Cancer

Stomach cancer is the fifth most commonly diagnosed malignancy worldwide and the second leading cause of cancer death, ranking behind only lung cancer. During 2018, 1,033,701 new cases were diagnosed (683,754 in men and 349,947 in women), and 782,685 persons died from stomach cancer (513,555 men and 269,130 women). Global age-adjusted annual mortality rates were more than twofold higher in men than in women (11.7 per 100,000 versus 5.2 per 100,000).

Overall, the annual number of deaths increased by 6.1% and the annual number of new cases increased by 4.6% during the last decade, 2008–2018. Nevertheless, the annual mortality rate declined by 18% in men and 25% in women during the same period (Bray et al., 2018; Ferlay et al., 2010).

Global patterns of the incidence and mortality rates of stomach cancer in 2018 are shown in **FIGURE 17.2**. About 70% of the cases and deaths occurred in developing countries (more than half in China and Eastern Asia). Mongolia had the highest annual mortality rate (25 per 100,000) and mortality rates were also high in China (17.5 per 100,000), the Russian Federation (10.8

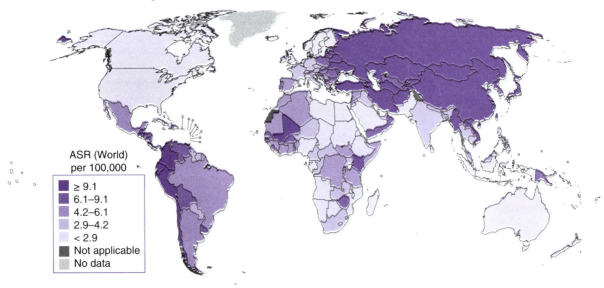

FIGURE 17.2 Global Incidence and Mortality Rates of Stomach Cancer, 2018.

Caption: ASR: Rates per 100,000 are age-standardized to the world population, 2000–2025.

Reproduced with permission from Ferlay, J., Ervik, M., Lam, F., Colombet, M., Mery, L., Piñeros, M., ... Bray, F. (2018). *Global cancer observatory: Cancer today.* Lyon, France: International Agency for Research on Cancer. Retrieved from https://gco.iarc.fr/today

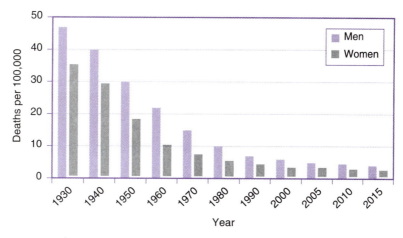

FIGURE 17.3 Stomach Cancer Mortality Rates in the United States, 1930–2015.

Caption: Mortality rates are age-adjusted to the U.S. population of 2000.

Data from American Cancer Society. (2009). *Cancer statistics*. Atlanta, GA: Author; Noone, A. M., Howlader, N., Krapcho, M., Miller, D., Brest, A., Yu, M., . . . Cronin, K. A. (2018). *SEER cancer statistics review, 1975–2015*. Bethesda, MD: National Cancer Institute.

per 100,000), and in nations of Eastern Asia, Eastern Europe, and the Andean regions of South America. In Africa, the highest mortality was observed in the nation of Mali (12.3 per 100,000). Among developed nations, the Republic of Korea (South Korea) had the highest incidence of stomach cancer (39.6 per 100,000) and the incidence was also high in Japan (27.5 per 100,000). The observed global patterns of stomach cancer rates in 2018 were similar to those of 2008 and 2012 (Bray et al., 2018; Ferlay et al., 2010, 2013, 2018).

Globally, the number of individuals who develop stomach cancer continues to rise; however, incidence and mortality rates in most developed countries as well as many developing countries are trending downward due to improved food preservation and sanitation by refrigeration. Nevertheless, even if current downward trends in the incidence and mortality of stomach cancer continue, the growth of the world population combined with increasing longevity will likely result in a net increase in the overall number of gastric cancers diagnosed and deaths from this malignancy for several decades to come (Brenner, Rothenbacher, & Arndt, 2009; Forman & Burley, 2006).

Mortality rates of stomach cancer are declining worldwide, and in many nations the declines have been dramatic (Ferlay et al., 2010, 2013, 2018). In the United States, death rates from stomach cancer have declined by nearly 90% in men and women since 1930 (Jernal et al., 2005; Noone et al., 2009) (**FIGURE 17.3**).

A similar pattern has emerged in Japan, the nation with the highest stomach cancer mortality in the world in 1950 (nearly 100 deaths per 100,000 in men) (**FIGURE 17.4**). Since then, mortality rates from stomach cancer have declined by nearly 70% in Japanese men and 90% in Japanese women (Inoue & Tsugane, 2005;

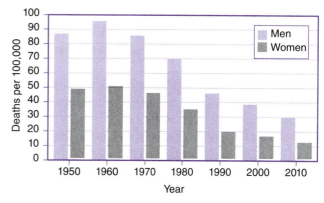

FIGURE 17.4 Stomach Cancer Mortality Rates in Japan, 1950–2010.

Caption: Mortality rates are age-adjusted to the Japanese population of 1985.

Data from Inoue, M., & Tsugane, S. (2005). Epidemiology of gastric cancer in Japan. *Postgraduate Medical Journal, 81*, 419–424.

Tajima, Kuroishi, & Oshima, 2004). In Switzerland and neighboring European countries, stomach cancer mortality has fallen by 60% within one generation (Crew & Neuget, 2006).

▶ Stomach Cancer Prevention: Epidemiology of an Unplanned Triumph

Howson, Hiyama, and Wynder (1986) described the decline in stomach cancer incidence and mortality among developed countries within the past 50 years as the "epidemiology of an unplanned triumph." The major reason for the decline in stomach cancer in developed countries is the rapid and widespread escalation of refrigeration since 1900. Expansion of industrial refrigeration has meant fresher produce for the consumer and, in turn, has resulted in higher per capita intake of vitamins A, C, and E, which protect against gastric carcinogenesis. Furthermore, the increase in refrigeration has reduced the need for salting and pickling, two traditional means of food preservation associated with increased gastric cancer risk.

Considerable experimental evidence suggests that high salt concentration enhances gastric carcinogenesis. High salt consumption damages the stomach mucosa and can induce severe gastritis, heightening the predisposition to nitrosamines and other carcinogens. Chronic atrophic gastritis and its associated lesion, intestinal metaplasia, are the precursor conditions most closely linked to increased gastric cancer risk (Joosens et al., 1996).

Due to the widespread use of refrigeration, fish and meat can be readily preserved without salting. Reductions in the incidence and mortality rates are therefore particularly impressive in Nordic countries in which fish consumption is traditionally high (e.g., Iceland). In populations that still prefer salty food (e.g., Portugal and Brazil [salted cod, bacalao], Japan and Korea [salted pickles and salad]), stomach cancer rates remain high but have also declined significantly in recent years (Howson et al., 1986).

Another important reason for the reduction in stomach cancer mortality is that improved food sanitation through better techniques of processing, handling, and refrigeration has reduced exposure to the infectious microbe *Helicobacter pylorus*, particularly among children. This bacterium is known to cause chronic stomach inflammation, and bacterial infiltrates of the organism are commonly found associated with gastric adenocarcinoma and its precursor lesions. Studies combining methods of epidemiology and microbiology clearly suggest that *H. pylorus* should be considered as a major causal factor of gastric carcinoma (Kelley & Duggan, 2003).

An additional factor contributing to the declining rates of stomach cancer is the availability in many countries of fresh fruits and vegetables throughout the year. Technological advances in production, storage, packaging, and transportation over the past several decades have facilitated the global transport of fresh produce to consumers in a timely manner at affordable prices (Huang & Huang, 2004). There is considerable evidence suggesting that diets high in fruits and vegetables and low in salt, nitrites, and starch reduce the risk of developing stomach cancer (Bertuccio et al., 2013; Campbell, Sloan, & Kreiger, 2008).

Certain nitroso-compounds are carcinogenic in animal models and can induce glandular stomach adenocarcinomas resembling human gastric cancer.

Conceivably, nitrosamides can be formed in the human stomach through an interaction between nitrite and suitable substrates. From 1925 to 1981, the content of nitrates and nitrites in cured meats in the United States decreased by 75% while gastric cancer mortality rates declined by two-thirds (Howson et al., 1986).

Cigarette smoking and other forms of tobacco addiction are also significant risk factors for the development of stomach cancer. A recent comprehensive review and meta-analysis of the available data found a twofold increase in the risk of stomach cancer among male chronic smokers (Ladeiras-Lopes et al., 2008). There is also consistent evidence that tobacco addiction in combination with chronic alcohol consumption synergistically heightens the risk by fivefold (Sjödahl et al., 2007).

Ecological studies have shown an inverse association between gastric cancer risk and socioeconomic status. These observations led to the hypothesis that high carbohydrate intake at an early age predisposes to increased gastric cancer risk. However, intracountry and time-trend comparisons have shown little association between carbohydrate intake and gastric cancer risk (Larsson, Bergkvist, & Wolk, 2006). Some studies suggest that the dietary glycemic load, a measure of the impact of total carbohydrate intake on blood sugar, is linked to the risk of stomach cancer (Augustin, Gallus, Negri, & La Vecchia, 2004); however, other studies do not support the view that a high starch diet and related measures such as the glycemic index or glycemic load enhance predisposition to gastric carcinoma (Lazarevic, Nagomi, & Jermic, 2009).

▶ *Helicobacter pylorus* and Stomach Cancer

In 1984, two Australian scientists, Drs. Barry J. Marshall and J. Robin Warren, made the remarkable discovery that a bacterium naturally inhabits the strong acid environment in the stomachs of patients with gastritis and stomach ulcers (Marshall & Warren, 1984). The bacterium was named *H. pylorus* due to its spiraled flagella that make it highly motile and able to avoid the severe acidity of the stomach fluids. In recognition of this remarkable discovery, Marshall and Warren were awarded the 2005 Nobel Prize for Medicine and Physiology.

Subsequent investigations have found that *H. pylorus* contaminates the stomachs of approximately 50% of humans (Pounder & Ng, 1995). The bacterium appears to be readily transmitted by oral–oral and oral–fecal routes, and infection is associated with conditions of poor sanitation (Brown, 2000).

Persistent colonization of the stomach by *H. pylori* results in chronic gastritis, an inflammatory condition of the stomach lining. The severity of the inflammation underlies the genesis of *H. pylori*-related diseases, including peptic ulcer, duodenal ulcer, and stomach cancer (Shiotani & Graham, 2002). Specifically, certain strains of *H. pylorus* that are seropositive for the CagA antigen are highly inflammatory and carcinogenic and are often present in specimens of gastric ulcers and gastric carcinomas (National Institutes of Health, 1994). Molecular epidemiologic studies have determined that severe chronic atrophic gastritis due to infection by CagA-positive strains of *H. pylorus* increases the risk of gastric cancer by more than 10-fold (Palli et al., 2007). Perhaps the most compelling evidence supporting *H. pylorus* as the major etiologic factor in the genesis of gastric cancer comes from a prospective study of 1526 Japanese participants in which gastric cancers developed in 2.9% of infected individuals and in none of the noninfected individuals (Uemura et al., 2001). A model of gastric carcinogenesis involving the progression of inflammatory *H. pylorus* infection to gastric ulceration and cancer is shown in **FIGURE 17.5**.

It is also important to realize that chronic *H. pylorus* infection interacts synergistically with other factors in the progression of carcinogenesis in the gastric mucosa. Such interactions are particularly evident in certain regions of China and Mongolia where consumption of salted and smoked foods is commonplace and conditions are ideal for the transmission of *H. pylorus* infections (e.g., crowded living conditions, family size, sharing a bedroom, low socioeconomic status, low educational level, poor sanitation, and infrequent hand washing) (Yang, 2006). High rates of smoking and alcohol consumption further exacerbate the risk. This web of causative factors is responsible for the high rates of stomach cancer in China and the staggering fact that more than 50% of stomach cancer deaths worldwide occur in this region.

Interactions involving multiple strains of *H. pylorus* and other infectious and parasitic agents have also been

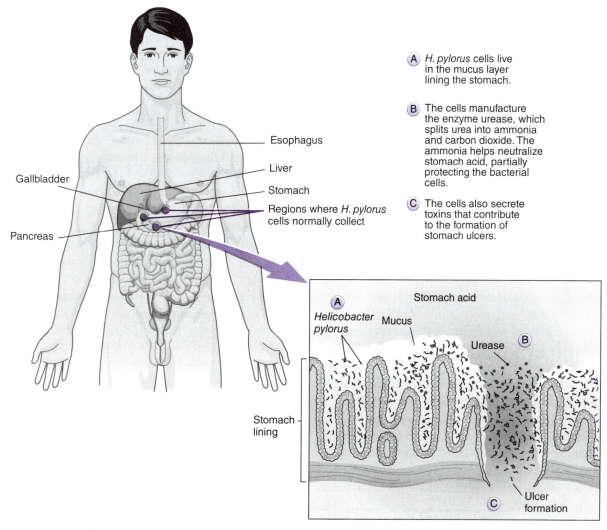

(A) *H. pylorus* cells live in the mucus layer lining the stomach.

(B) The cells manufacture the enzyme urease, which splits urea into ammonia and carbon dioxide. The ammonia helps neutralize stomach acid, partially protecting the bacterial cells.

(C) The cells also secrete toxins that contribute to the formation of stomach ulcers.

FIGURE 17.5 Model of *Helicobacter pylorus* Infection in Gastric Carcinogenesis.

explored. For example, certain regions of Africa with high rates of stomach cancer (e.g., Mali and Zaire) are also prone to multiple gastrointestinal infections and mosquito-borne malarial infections that could further compromise host immunity, thereby promoting more severe *H. pylorus* infections (Blaser, 1993; Blaser & Atherton, 2004).

Gastric carcinogenesis is thus a multifactorial, multistep process, in which chronic inflammation due to *H. pylorus* infection is most often the major determinant. Indeed, any factor or condition that causes chronic tissue damage and a persisting cycle of inflammation, necrosis, and regeneration carries an increased cancer risk. Examples of the "inflammogenesis of cancer" are present throughout the gastrointestinal tract (e.g., consumption of very hot beverages and squamous cell carcinoma of the esophagus, gastroesophageal reflux of stomach acid and adenocarcinoma of the esophagus, chronic gastritis induced by *H. pylorus* infection and stomach cancer, Crohn's disease and cancer of the small intestine, ulcerative colitis, and colon cancer) (Harris, 2007).

Histologic and Anatomic Subtypes of Stomach Cancer

More than 90% of gastric cancers are adenocarcinomas, which are divisible pathologically and anatomically into two subtypes: (1) poorly differentiated or *diffuse* adenocarcinomas arising near the cardia (just distal to the gastroesophageal junction) and (2) well-differentiated or *intestinal* adenocarcinomas that arise elsewhere in the corpus of the stomach (noncardia adenocarcinomas) (Crew & Neuget, 2006).

Well-differentiated (intestinal) noncardia adenocarcinomas of the stomach are thought to develop primarily as a consequence of environmental factors such as chronic *H. pylorus* infection, particularly due to CagA-positive strains, resulting in chronic severe atrophic gastritis that progresses to invasive cancer. Synergism of *H. pylorus* with other environmental factors including high salt diets, nutritional deficits, and chronic tobacco and alcohol exposure can exacerbate the risk. The noncardia intestinal subtype of gastric cancer predominates in high-risk regions of the world, and its rates have declined dramatically in many developed nations, primarily due to refrigeration replacing salt preservation of fish and meat, better access to fresh fruits and vegetables, improved sanitation, reductions in tobacco and alcohol addiction, and effective antibiotic therapy for *H. pylorus* infections.

In contrast to the decline in noncardia intestinal gastric cancer, the rates of diffuse gastric adenocarcinomas arising near the cardia are increasing in many developed nations, particularly among Caucasian males. The increasing incidence of the diffuse type of adenocarcinomas arising near the cardia of the stomach is related to obesity and other conditions that predispose to gastroesophageal reflux disease (GERD) and Barrett's esophagus (Crew & Neuget, 2006). It has been hypothesized that ablation of colonization of the stomach by *H. pylorus* has accentuated the development of these conditions in some developed populations (Blaser & Atherton, 2004).

Genetic Predisposition to Stomach Cancer

Evidence for a genetic predisposition to gastric cancer comes from both epidemiologic studies and reports of multigenerational pedigrees with excess cases of gastric cancer among relatives. Systematic case–control and cohort analyses of gastric cancer patients have shown that the risk of gastric cancer in first-degree relatives of index cases (probands) is increased two- to threefold.

Mutations, polymorphisms, and epigenetic changes in the expression of certain genes have been implicated in gastric carcinogenesis, particularly for the diffuse type of adenocarcinoma that arises in the cardia near the gastroesophageal junction. Familial clusters of hereditary diffuse gastric carcinoma have been discovered. Such families manifest key germline mutations in the CDH1 gene that encodes E-cadherin, an important calcium-dependent cell adhesion molecule (Lynch, Grady, Suriano, & Huntsman, 2005).

Excess cases of gastric cancer have also been observed in families with the adenomatous polyposis coli (APC) gene, which predisposes to familial adenomatous polyposis (FAP), and in families with hereditary nonpolyposis colorectal cancer (also called the Lynch syndrome), which is due to mutated mismatch DNA repair genes (Lynch et al., 2005). Other genetic and familial factors are also known to influence gastric cancer risk. Blood group A has been reported to be more prevalent among gastric cancer cases than among controls and appears to be associated with the development of the diffuse type of disease. Patients with pernicious anemia are also at increased risk for the development of gastric cancer. Pernicious anemia is due to the lack of intrinsic factor and failure to absorb vitamin B_{12} (Bevan & Houlston, 1999).

▶ Prevention of Stomach Cancer

Present knowledge suggests that gastric carcinoma is caused by interactions among carcinogens and inflammatory factors derived from chronic *H. pylorus* infection, nitrate/nitrite-rich diets, and gastric mucosa irritation, and damage by salt or other factors such as tobacco and alcohol. Salt restriction (less than 6 g per day), avoidance of processed meats, abstinence from tobacco, and limitation of alcohol intake are all important for prevention and control.

Notably, infection by the bacterium *H. pylorus* causes chronic stomach inflammation that can initiate and promote cancerous lesions. Elimination of the bacterium through antibiotic therapy is therefore paramount for the prevention and control of gastric cancer. For example, a recent intervention study in high-risk rural populations in the province of Nariño in the Andes Mountains of Colombia demonstrated that administration of antibiotics for *H. pylorus* produced regression of precancerous gastric lesions (Correa et al., 2000). In the same study, supplemental administration of vitamin C or beta carotene also showed benefit, suggesting that both disease initiation and progression may be counteracted by sufficient year-round ingestion of fresh fruits and vegetables.

References

Ahmedin, J., Murray, T., Ward, E., Samuels, A., Tiwari, R. C., Ghafoor, A., … Thun, J. M. (2005). Cancer statistics, 2005. *CA Cancer Journal for Clinicians, 55,* 10–30.

Augustin, L. S. A., Gallus, S., Negri, E., & La Vecchia, C. (2004). Glycemic index, glycemic load and risk of gastric cancer. *Annals of Oncology, 15*(4), 581–584.

Bertuccio, P., Rosato, V., Andreano, A., Ferraroni, M., Decarli, A., Edefonti, V., & La Vecchia, C. (2013). Dietary patterns and gastric cancer risk: A systematic review and meta-analysis. *Annals of Oncology, 24,* 1450–1458.

Bevan, S., & Houlston, R. S. (1999). Genetic predisposition to gastric cancer. *Quarterly Journal of Medicine, 92,* 5–10.

Blaser, M. J. (1993). Malaria and the natural history of *Helicobacter pylori* infection [letter]. *Lancet, 342,* 551.

Blaser, M. J., & Atherton, J. C. (2004). *Helicobacter pylori* persistence: Biology and disease. *Journal of Clinical Investigation, 113,* 321–333.

Bray, F., Ferlay, J., Soerjomataram, I., Siegel, R. L., Torre, L. A., & Jemal, A. (2018). Global cancer statistics 2018: GLOBOCAN estimates of incidence and mortality worldwide for 36 cancers in 185 countries. *CA: A Cancer Journal for Clinicians, 68*(6), 394–424.

Brenner, H., Rothenbacher, D., & Arndt, V. (2009). Epidemiology of stomach cancer. In M. Verma (Ed., pp. 467–477), *Cancer epidemiology. Methods in molecular biology* (Vol. 472, pp. 467–477). Totowa, NJ: Humana Press.

Brown, L. M. (2000). *Helicobacter pylori*: Epidemiology and routes of transmission. *Epidemiology Review, 22*(2), 283–297.

Campbell, P., Sloan, M., & Kreiger, N. (2008). Dietary patterns and risk of incident gastric adenocarcinoma. *American Journal of Epidemiology, 167,* 295–304.

Correa, P., Fontham, E. T. H., Bravo, J. C., Bravo, L. E., Ruiz, B., Zarama, G., … Mera, R. (2000). Chemoprevention of gastric dysplasia: Randomized trial of antioxidant supplements and anti-*Helicobacter pylori* therapy. *Journal of the National Cancer Institute, 92*(23), 1881–1888.

Crew, K. D., & Neuget, A. I. (2006). Epidemiology of gastric cancer. *World Journal of Gastroenterology, 12*(3), 354–362.

Ferlay, J., Ervik, M., Lam, F., Colombet, M., Mery, L., Piñeros, M., … Bray, F. (2018). *Global cancer observatory: Cancer today*. Lyon, France: International Agency for Research on Cancer. Retrieved from https://gco.iarc.fr/today

Ferlay, J., Shin, H.-R., Bray, F., Forman, D., Mathers, C., & Parkin, D. M. (2010). Estimates of worldwide burden of cancer in 2008: GLOBOCAN 2008. *International Journal of Cancer, 127*(12), 2893–2917.

Ferlay, J., Soerjomataram, I., Ervik, M., Dikshit, R., Eser, S., Mathers, C., … Bray, F. (2013). *GLOBOCAN 2012 v1.0. Cancer incidence and mortality worldwide: IARC CancerBase No. 11* [Internet]. Lyon, France: International Agency for Research on Cancer. Retrieved from http://globocan.iarc.fr

Forman, D., & Burley, V. J. (2006). Gastric cancer: Global pattern of the disease and an overview of environmental risk factors. *Best Practice & Research Clinical Gastroenterology, 20*(4), 633–649.

Harris, R. E. (2007). Cyclooxygenase 2 (COX-2) and the inflammogenesis of cancer. *Subcellular Biochemistry, 42,* 93–126.

Howson, C. P., Hiyama, T., & Wynder, E. L. (1986). The decline in gastric cancer: Epidemiology of an unplanned triumph. *Epidemiology Reviews, 8,* 1–27.

Huang, S., & Huang, K. (2007). Increased U.S. imports of fresh fruits and vegetables. *A Report from the Economic Research Service, FTS-328-01.* Washington, DC: United States Department of Agriculture. Retrieved from http://www.ers.usda.gov/media/187841/fts32801_1_.pdf

Inoue, M., & Tsugane, S. (2005). Epidemiology of gastric cancer in Japan. *Postgraduate Medical Journal, 81,* 419–424.

Jernal, A., Murray, T., Ward, E., Samuels, A., Tiwari, R. C., Ghafoor, A., … Thun, J. M. (2005). Cancer statistics, 2005. *CA Cancer Journal for Clinicians, 55,* 10–30.

Joosens, J. V., Hill, M. J., Elliott, P., Stamler, R., Stamler, J., Lesaffre, E., … Kesteloot, H. (1996). Dietary salt, nitrate and stomach cancer mortality in 24 countries. *International Journal of Epidemiology, 25*(3), 494–504.

Kelley, J. R., & Duggan, J. M. (2003). Gastric cancer epidemiology and risk factors. *Journal of Clinical Epidemiology, 56,* 1–9.

Kumar, V., Abbas, A. K., & Aster, J. C. (2014). *Robbins and cotran pathologic basis of disease* (9th ed.). Philadelphia, PA: Mosby & Saunders.

Ladeiras-Lopes, R., Pereira, A. K., Nogueira, A., Pinheiro-Torres, T., Pinto, I., Santos-Pereira, R., & Lunet, N. (2008). Smoking and gastric cancer: Systematic review and meta-analysis of cohort studies. *Cancer Causes and Control, 7,* 689–701.

Larsson, S. C., Bergkvist, L., & Wolk, A. (2006). Glycemic load, glycemic index and carbohydrate intake in relation to risk of stomach cancer: A prospective study. *International Journal of Cancer, 188*(12), 3167–3169.

Lazarevic, K., Nagomi, A., & Jermic, M. (2009). Carbohydrate intake, glycemic index, glycemic load and risk of gastric cancer. *Central European Journal of Public Health, 17*(2), 75–78.

Lynch, H. T., Grady, W., Suriano, G., & Huntsman, D. (2005). Gastric cancer: New genetic developments. *Journal of Surgical Oncology, 90*(3), 114–133.

Marshall, B. J., & Warren, J. R. (1984). Unidentified curved bacilli in the stomach of patients with gastritis and peptic ulceration. *Lancet, 1*(8390), 1311–1315.

National Institutes of Health. (1994). NIH consensus statement: *Helicobacter pylori* in peptic ulcer disease. NIH consensus development panel on *Helicobacter pylori* in peptic ulcer disease. *Journal of the American Medical Association, 272*(1), 65–69.

Noone, A. M., Howlader, N., Krapcho, M., Miller, D., Brest, A., Yu, M., … Cronin, K. A. (2018). *SEER cancer statistics review, 1975–2015.* Bethesda, MD: National Cancer Institute.

Palli, D., Masala, G., Del Giudice, G., Plebani, M., Basso, D., Berti, D., … Gonzalez, C. A. (2007). CagA+ *Helicobacter pylori* infection and gastric cancer risk in the EPIC-EURGAST study. *International Journal of Cancer, 120*(4), 859–867.

Pounder, R. E., & Ng, D. (1995). The prevalence of *Helicobacter pylori* infection in different countries. *Alimentary Pharmacology and Therapeutics, 9*(Suppl. 2), 33–39.

Shiotani, A., & Graham, D. Y. (2002). Pathogenesis and therapy of gastric and duodenal ulcer disease. *Medical Clinics of North America, 86*(6), 1447–1466.

Sjödahl, K., Lu, Y., Nilsen, T. I., Ye, W., Hveem, K., Vatten, L., & Lagergren, J. (2007). Smoking and alcohol drinking in relation to risk of gastric cancer: A population-based, prospective cohort study. *International Journal of Cancer, 120*(1), 128–132.

Tajima, K., Kuroishi, T., & Oshima, A. (Eds.). (2004). *Monograph on cancer research, No. 51. Cancer mortality and morbidity statistics. Japan and the world.* Tokyo, Japan: Japanese Cancer Association/Karger.

Uemura, N., Okamoto, S., Yamamoto, S., Matsumura, N., Yamaguchi, S., Yamakido, M., … Schlemper, R. J. (2001). *Helicobacter pylori* infection and the development of gastric cancer. *New England Journal of Medicine, 345,* 784–789.

Yang, L. (2006). Incidence and mortality of gastric cancer in China. *World Journal of Gastroenterology, 12*(1), 17–20.

© Andrew Brookes/Getty Images

Epidemiology of Colorectal Cancer

▶ Global Epidemiology of Colorectal Cancer

During 2018, colorectal (large bowel) cancer was diagnosed in 1,800,977 individuals and caused 861,663 deaths in the world population. In that year, 1,006,019 new cases were detected in men and 794,958 new cases in women, and colorectal cancer caused 8.8% of all cancer deaths in men (474,606 deaths) and 9.3% in women (387,057 deaths). During the decade, 2008–2018, the annual number of cases of colorectal cancer in the world population increased by 46% and the number of deaths from this malignancy increased by 42% (Bray et al., 2018).

The incidence rates of colorectal cancer in 2018 were more than threefold higher in developed countries than in developing countries (30.3 versus 8.4 per 100,000 in men and 20.9 versus 5.9 per 100,000 in women). Likewise, the mortality rates were more than twofold higher in developed versus developing countries (12.8 versus 5.7 per 100,000 in men and 8.5 versus 3.8 per 100,000 in women). The global age-adjusted incidence was 47% higher in men than in women (23.1 versus 15.7 per 100,000), and the mortality from colorectal cancer was 51% higher in men than in women (10.6 versus 7.0 per 100,000) (Bray et al., 2018; Ferlay et al., 2010).

FIGURE 18.1 depicts the extreme international variability in colorectal cancer incidence and mortality rates in 2018. Colorectal cancer is the second most frequently diagnosed malignancy in affluent societies but remains relatively uncommon in many developing countries. Regions with high incidence and mortality rates include North America, Northern and Western Europe, Northern Asia (Russia), Australia and New Zealand, and the southernmost nations of South America. Low rates were observed in the nations of Central Africa, Central America, and Southern Asia. Nevertheless, colorectal cancer incidence rates are increasing in economically transitioning countries. For example, the current age-adjusted annual incidence and mortality rates in China (23.7 per 100,000 and 10.9 per 100,000, respectively) are comparable to the rates in developed countries such as the United States (25.6 per 100,000 and 8.2 per 100,000) (Bray et al., 2018; Center & Jemal, 2009; Ferlay et al., 2010, 2013, 2018; Garcia et al., 2007). Five-year survival rates following the diagnosis of colorectal cancer also show wide international variability ranging from 30% in India to 65% in the United States (Parkin, Bray, Ferlay, & Pisani, 2005).

▶ Pathogenesis of Colorectal Cancer

As with most other solid cancerous tumors, colorectal cancer evolves over a period of years and even decades. Approximately 65%–70% of large bowel cancers develop in the descending sigmoid colon and rectum and the remainder develop in the transverse and ascending portions of the colon (**FIGURE 18.2**). More than 95% of

Estimated age-standardized incidence rates (World), colorectum, both sexes, all ages

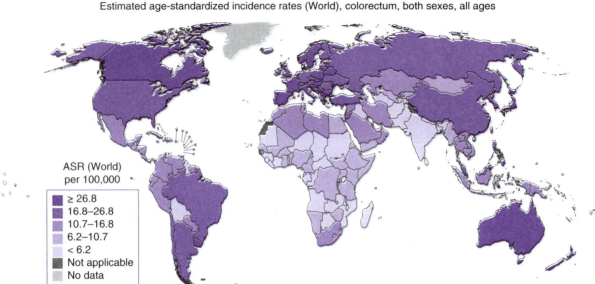

Estimated age-standardized mortality rates (World) in 2018, colorectum, both sexes, all ages

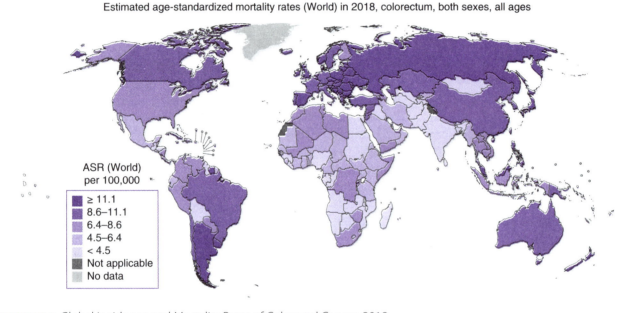

FIGURE 18.1 Global Incidence and Mortality Rates of Colorectal Cancer, 2018.

Caption: ASR: Rates per 100,000 are age-standardized to the world population, 2000–2025.

Reproduced with permission from Ferlay, J., Ervik, M., Lam, F., Colombet, M., Mery, L., Piñeros, M., ... Bray, F. (2018). *Global cancer observatory: Cancer today*. Lyon, France: International Agency for Research on Cancer. Retrieved from https://gco.iarc.fr/today

colorectal cancers are adenocarcinomas, and many of them secrete mucin. Carcinomas of the sigmoid colon and rectum often grow in an annular fashion producing a so-called "napkin-ring" constriction and obstruction of the bowel. Carcinomas of the ascending colon tend to extend along the bowel wall and are much less likely to cause obstruction. Colorectal cancer often develops as a sequential series of steps beginning with focal dysplasia and hyperplasia of the epithelial lining and progressing to the formation of adenomatous and villous polyps, carcinoma in situ, and ultimately invasive cancer (Kumar, Abbas, Fausto, & Astor, 2009). It is notable that colon carcinogenesis invariably progresses in the presence of inflammation (Harris, 2007).

▶ Risk Factors for Colorectal Cancer

Comprehensive scientific evidence suggests that colorectal cancer is largely influenced by several lifestyle factors. The risk of colorectal cancer development is increased by diets high in fat and low in fiber, sedentary lifestyle, obesity, alcohol and tobacco addiction, and deficiencies in vitamin D, calcium, and possibly selenium. Genetic syndromes involving mutant mismatch repair genes and tumor suppressor genes account for only a small percentage of cases. The following sections discuss each of these risk factors individually.

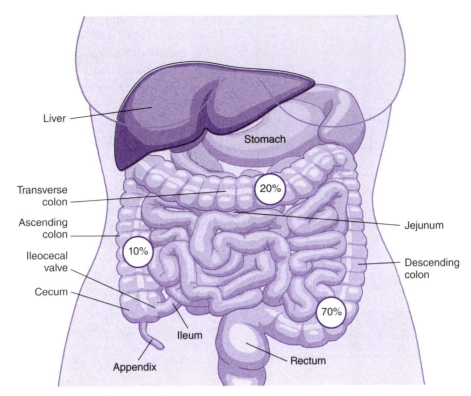

FIGURE 18.2 Anatomic Distribution of Colorectal Cancer.

Dietary Fat and Colorectal Cancer

The wide geographic variation in the rates of colorectal cancer is most likely a consequence of differences in diet. Wynder and colleagues initially postulated that colon cancer development is linked to high intake of dietary fat that upsets the balance of gut flora (Wynder, Kajitani, Ishikawa, Dodo, & Takano, 1969). This hypothesis was based on the historic low rates of colorectal cancer in Japan compared to high rates in the United States corresponding to their low- and high-fat diets, respectively. Many subsequent epidemiologic investigations have consistently found that the risk of colorectal cancer increases with high intake of saturated fat and animal fat and reciprocally, that the risk is reduced with increased intake of fish and fish oil (Boyle & Langman, 2000; Lipkin, Reddy, Newmark, & Lamprecht, 1999). For example, Willett and colleagues found that U.S. women who ate beef, pork, or lamb daily had a 2.5-fold higher risk compared to women reporting little consumption (Willett, Stampfer, Colditz, Rosner, & Speizer, 1990). In an investigation conducted in 24 European nations, increasing the intake of omega-3 fatty acids from fish and fish oil conferred significant protection against colon cancer development, even in populations consuming diets high in total fats (Caygill & Hill, 1995). Animal studies are in general agreement with the epidemiologic evidence in finding that a high amount of omega-6 fatty acids from beef, corn oil, or lard in the diet enhances chemically induced tumor development in laboratory animals, and reciprocally that increasing the intake of omega-3 fatty acids from fish, fish oil, and olive oil decreases carcinogenesis (Reddy & Maeura, 1984).

Marked increases in the rates of colorectal cancer in some countries have also been linked to higher levels of fat intake. A striking example is the Japanese population wherein rates have risen more than fourfold in the past 50 years in close parallel with the increase in per capita fat calories (**FIGURE 18.3**). Furthermore, in studies of migrants from low-risk to high-risk regions, the rates of colon cancer show dramatic increases after a single generation, suggesting that the risk for tumor development in the large bowel increases rapidly with transition to a high-fat diet (Matsumura, 2001; Noone et al., 2018; Wynder, Fujita, Harris, Hirayama, & Hiyama, 1991; Yu, Harris, Gao, Gao, & Wynder, 1991).

Mechanistically, it is theorized that diets high in fat promote secretion of bile acids from the liver and biliary tree. These bile acids are dehydrogenated by anaerobic bacteria of the colon (clostridia and bacteroides) to form the carcinogenic metabolites deoxycholic acid and lithocholic acid. In addition, diets high in fat typically contain sterols that have mitogenic activity. A key high-risk enzyme is β-glucuronidase, which is responsible for hydrolysis of sterol conjugates so that they may be recirculated (Lipkin et al., 1999).

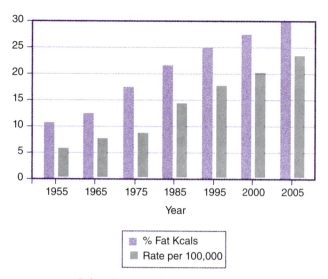

FIGURE 18.3 Colon Cancer Mortality and Dietary Fat in Japan: 1955–2005.

Caption: Annual mortality rates are age-adjusted to the Japanese population of 2000.

Data from Center for Cancer Control and Information Services. (2010). *Cancer statistics in Japan.* Tokyo, Japan: National Cancer Center; Matsumura, Y. (2001). Emerging trends of nutrition: Transition and trade-offs. Nutrition trends in Japan. *Asia Pacific Journal of Clinical Nutrition, 10*(Suppl.), S40–S47; Wynder, E. L., Fujita, Y., Harris, R. E., Hirayama, T., & Hiyama, T. (1991). Comparative epidemiology of cancer between the United States and Japan: A second look. *Cancer, 67*(3), 746–763.

Dietary Fiber and Colorectal Cancer

Burkitt (1971) is primarily responsible for formulating the high-fat/low-fiber hypothesis of colon cancer. This hypothesis is based on the low incidence of colon cancer and other intestinal diseases in the African countries where Burkitt conducted his surgical practice. In populations consuming a high-fiber, low-fat diet, Burkitt observed virtually none of the large bowel diseases that are commonplace in westernized societies such as hemorrhoids, diverticulosis, diverticulitis, ulcerative colitis, Crohn's disease, and colorectal cancer. His recommendations for prevention of colon cancer specify high levels of fiber intake throughout life (40 g of fiber daily with a high proportion of bran) (Burkitt, 1973; Burkitt, Walker, & Painter, 1974).

Although many early epidemiologic investigations consistently supported the "Burkitt hypothesis" that high fiber intake reduces the risk of colorectal cancer (Greenwald, Lanza, & Eddy, 1987; Levin & Dozois, 1991; Trock, Lanza, & Greenwald, 1990), some more recent epidemiologic investigations have failed to show protective effects of dietary fiber (Fuchs et al., 1999; Nakaji et al., 2001). A pooled analysis of 13 prospective cohort studies determined that the age-adjusted relative risk (RR) of colorectal cancer was significantly reduced by high intake of fiber (RR = 0.84), but also found that adjustment for a large profile of other factors dissipated the effect (Park et al., 2005). On the other hand, Howe and colleagues conducted a meta-analysis of 13 case–control studies and found that the highest level of fiber intake reduced the risk of colorectal cancer by 50% (Howe et al.,

1992). Furthermore, results from the large European Prospective Investigation into Cancer and Nutrition (EPIC) show that colon cancer risk declines by about 9% per quintile increase in fiber intake (multivariate adjusted RR = 0.58 for the highest versus lowest quintile) (Bingham et al., 2005, 2010). It is important to note that in most of these studies, particularly those that did not show protection, the type of fiber was not considered, and the highest level of fiber consumption was far below the 40-g daily threshold recommended by Denis Burkitt.

Several preclinical trials also have examined the impact of dietary fiber in animal models of colorectal carcinogenesis. The results suggest that colorectal protection depends on the type and level of fiber and that wheat bran inhibits tumor development more consistently than other sources of fiber (Reddy, 1995). The totality of evidence from studies of colon cancer in animals and humans remains compatible with Burkitt's original hypothesis that diets high in fiber, particularly wheat bran fiber, provide significant protection against the development of colorectal cancer.

Protective mechanisms of fiber within the large bowel can be broadly divided into those from soluble and insoluble fiber. Increasing the level of insoluble fiber increases fecal bulk, thereby reducing transit time and diluting the concentration of toxic and carcinogenic compounds. Soluble fiber binds to bile acids and bile salts that may irritate the colorectal mucosa; furthermore, soluble fiber is fermented to single-chain fatty acids such as butyrate that maintain homeostasis of cell proliferation and apoptosis (Anderson et al., 2009; Wong, de Souza, Kendall, Emam, & Jenkins, 2006).

Alcohol, Tobacco, and Colorectal Cancer

Chronic alcohol abuse is etiologically linked to colorectal carcinogenesis (Cho et al., 2004; Mizoue et al., 2008; Su & Arab, 2004). Analysis of data from the National Health and Nutrition Examination Survey (NHANES) in the United States showed a 70% increase in colorectal cancer among individuals who consumed one or more servings of alcoholic beverages daily (Su & Arab, 2004). In a pooled analysis of eight prospective cohort studies performed in five countries, Cho and colleagues (2004) found that the risk increased by 40% at the highest level of alcohol consumption (>45 g of alcohol daily). Mizoue and colleagues analyzed data from five Japanese studies and estimated that one-quarter of all colorectal cancers in Japan are attributable to alcohol consumption above 23 g daily (Mizoue et al., 2008).

Chronic tobacco addiction has also been linked to colorectal cancer development. The epidemiologic evidence shows that chronic smokers have a two- to threefold increased incidence of premalignant adenomas of the colon compared to nonsmokers (Giovannucci, 2001). In a meta-analysis of 106 studies, Botteri et al. (2008) concluded that smoking significantly increases both the incidence and mortality of colorectal cancer. The existing evidence therefore supports the addition of colorectal cancer to the list of tobacco-associated malignancies.

Various mechanisms may be responsible for the effects of alcohol and tobacco on colorectal carcinogenesis. One mechanism involves the combination of chronic alcohol consumption and folate deficiency. As ethanol enters the large bowel, it is metabolized into acetaldehyde by anaerobic microbes; acetaldehyde, in turn, rapidly degrades folate. Because folate is essential for normal DNA synthesis and repair, its rapid degradation by acetaldehyde could readily lead to DNA instability and carcinogenesis in the colorectal mucosa (Duthie, 1999; Homann, Tillonen, & Salaspuro, 2000).

Alcohol consumption may also delay peristalsis in the large bowel and increase transit time and exposure to carcinogens and other toxic substances. Carcinogens from tobacco can reach the colorectal mucosa through the gastrointestinal tract or the circulatory system and may accentuate mutagenesis, inflammation, and carcinogenesis, particularly in the distal colon (Zisman, Nickolov, Brand, Gorchow, & Roy, 2006). There is also speculation that tobacco and alcohol may synergistically heighten the risk of colorectal cancer.

Vitamin D, Calcium, and Colorectal Cancer

As initially noted by Garland and Garland (1980), there is a gradient of colorectal cancer rates with latitude (i.e., the rates become higher in populations that are more distant from the equator). On careful examination, the current patterns of global colorectal cancer incidence and mortality reflect a similar gradient (see Figure 18.1). This observation has given rise to the hypothesis that colon cancer development may be related to the lack of vitamin D due to decreased exposure to sunlight in populations more distant from the equator. Activated vitamin D is necessary for the absorption of dietary calcium, an important mineral for the maintenance of physiologic homeostasis in the human body, particularly the regulation and control of cell division and the cell cycle in proliferating cell populations such as the colorectal mucosa.

Higher levels of vitamin D and calcium intake have been found to reduce the risk of colorectal cancer in several epidemiologic studies (Gorham et al., 2005). For example, the relationship of vitamin D and cancer mortality was examined in the Third National Health and Nutrition Examination Survey (NHANES III). Baseline levels of serum 25-hydroxylated vitamin D were measured in 16,818 participants aged 17 years or older with follow-up from 1988 to 2000. Although there was no overall effect on cancer mortality, individuals with serum vitamin D levels of 80 nmol/L or higher at baseline experienced a 72% reduction in colorectal cancer mortality compared to individuals with levels lower than 50 nmol/L (Freedman, Looker, Chang, & Graubard, 2007).

Despite the beneficial impact of vitamin D and calcium observed in epidemiologic studies, a randomized clinical trial involving postmenopausal women of the Women's Health Initiative (WHI) failed to show any benefit. In this study, daily supplementation of calcium and vitamin D for 7 years had no effect on the incidence of colorectal cancer. The long latency associated with the development of colorectal cancer and the limited 7-year duration of the trial may have contributed to this null finding (Wactawski-Wende, Morley Kotchen, & Anderson, 2006).

Insulin, Insulin-Like Growth Factors, and Colorectal Cancer

High levels of circulating insulin and insulin-like growth factors (IGFs) have been found to increase the risk of developing colorectal cancer (Giovannucci, 2007). Insulin is secreted by the beta cells in the islets of Langerhans of the pancreas and is the chief hormone that regulates blood glucose. The IGFs are polypeptide hormones that share sequence homology with insulin. They are synthesized in the liver and other organs in response to growth hormone from the pituitary gland. Although the main function of IGF is to regulate human growth and development, it also stimulates cell proliferation and angiogenesis and inhibits apoptosis in the colorectal mucosa.

Individuals who manifest clinical conditions associated with high levels of insulin and IGF-1 such as type 2 diabetes mellitus, the metabolic syndrome, and acromegaly are at increased risk for the development of colorectal cancer. Furthermore, phenotypic and lifestyle factors associated with hyperinsulinemia (physical inactivity, high body mass index, central adiposity) and high IGF-1 levels (tall stature), as well as dietary patterns that stimulate insulin resistance or secretion, including high consumption of sucrose, various sources of starch, a high glycemic index, and high intake of certain types of fat, also increase the risk (Giovannucci, 2001, 2007; Giovannucci, Colditz, Stampfer, & Willett, 1996; Terry, Miller, & Rohan, 2002). It is clear that components of the IGF axis (IGF-1, IGF-2, IGF cell membrane receptors, and binding molecules) constitute an important molecular interface with exposures that initiate and promote colorectal carcinogenesis.

Ulcerative Colitis, Crohn's Disease, and Colorectal Cancer

Chronic inflammatory conditions of the intestinal tract also predispose to the development of colorectal cancer. Ulcerative colitis is characterized by chronic inflammation and ulceration of the epithelial lining of the colon plus other extra-colonic lesions. The primary site of attack is usually in the descending (left) colon. About 1% of colorectal cancer patients have a history of chronic ulcerative colitis. The risk of developing colorectal cancer varies inversely with the age of onset of the colitis and directly with the extent of colonic involvement and the duration of active disease. It is estimated that 40%–50% of individuals with long-standing ulcerative colitis eventually develop colon cancer (Kumar et al., 2009).

Crohn's disease, a granulomatous inflammatory condition of the intestinal tract, also increases the risk of colorectal cancer development, but to a lesser extent than ulcerative colitis. Many investigators have noted many similarities in ulcerative colitis and Crohn's disease. Both diseases appear to have an autoimmune basis and are characterized by similar alterations in the IGF axis (Street et al., 2004). Quite possibly these conditions represent different immune and tissue responses to one or more highly inflammatory etiologic factors.

Genetics of Colorectal Cancer

The investigation of a large multigenerational kindred by Aldred Scott Warthin in the early 1900s identified a hereditary form of colorectal cancer. Warthin documented 33 relatives with colorectal cancer or endometrial cancer among 70 members of the pedigree. Hereditary nonpolyposis colorectal cancer (HNPCC) was later named the *Lynch syndrome* after Henry T. Lynch, who documented two large kindreds with this autosomal-dominant syndrome (Lynch, Shaw, Magnuson, Larsen, & Krush, 1966). Lynch and colleagues initially designated HNPCC as the cancer family syndrome (Lynch, Guirgis, Lynch, & Harris, 1977; Lynch, Lynch, & Harris, 1977).

The cause of HNPCC is an inherited (germline) mutation in at least one of a set of genes that normally repair DNA, the mismatch repair genes. In 1993 the first of the HNPCC genes (MSH2) was discovered on chromosome 2 by a team of international investigators (Aaltonen et al., 1993). Soon after, MLH1 was

discovered on chromosome 3 (Aaltonen et al., 1994). It was determined that mutations in these two genes accounted for 90% of the known HNPCC families. Carriers of either mutant gene have a lifetime colon cancer risk approaching 100%. The Lynch syndrome accounts for a small percentage of all colorectal cancer cases, perhaps 1%–3%.

In 1951, Eldron J. Gardner published a report of a large Utah family containing many relatives with diffuse polyps of the colon and intestinal tract and multiple relatives with colorectal cancer (Gardner, 1951). Gardner's syndrome is a rare familial form of familial adenomatous polyposis (FAP) characterized by the presence of multiple polyps in the colon together with tumors outside the colon. In Gardner's syndrome, the extracolonic tumors may include osteomas of the skull, thyroid cancer, epidermoid cysts, fibromas, sebaceous cysts, and desmoid tumors.

FAP and Gardner's syndrome are caused by an autosomal-dominant germline mutation in the adenomatous polyposis coli (APC) gene located on chromosome 5q21 (band q21 on chromosome 5) (Leppert et al., 1987). The APC gene is a *tumor suppressor gene* that regulates cell adhesion, cell migration, and apoptosis in the colorectal epithelium. Mutations of the APC gene inactivate its protein function, leading to initiation and promotion of colorectal carcinogenesis. Inactivation of both copies of the APC is required to initiate polyp development (Fearon, 2011).

The countless polyps in the colon of FAP patients predispose to the development of colon cancer with 100% probability unless the colon is removed. The onset of polyps occurs during the teenage years, and the average age at diagnosis of colon cancer is 35–40 years. Polyps can also grow in the stomach, duodenum, spleen, kidneys, liver, mesentery, and small bowel. In a small number of cases, polyps have also appeared in the cerebellum. Extracolonic cancers related to FAP commonly appear in the thyroid, liver, and kidneys.

Cooking Methods and Colorectal Cancer

Certain cooking methods can lead to carcinogenic compounds that reach the large bowel. For example, heterocyclic amines are formed on the surface of high-protein foods such as meat or fish on exposure to high-temperature cooking processes such as frying or boiling, and particularly charcoal broiling. Furthermore, mutagens other than heterocyclic amines in meats cooked at high temperature (e.g., pyridines and quinoxalines) may also play a role in increasing the risk of distal adenomas and colorectal tumors (Wu et al., 2006).

Nonsteroidal Anti-inflammatory Drugs (NSAIDs): Chemoprevention of Colorectal Cancer

The results of many epidemiologic studies provide strong evidence that regular intake of nonsteroidal anti-inflammatory drugs (NSAIDs) such as aspirin and ibuprofen reduces the risk of colorectal cancer development. In a meta-analysis of the published estimates, significant risk reductions were observed in 28 of 32 studies, and regular use of NSAIDs produced a 43% reduction in the risk (**FIGURE 18.4**) (Harris, 2009). In randomized clinical trials, regular aspirin use also has been found to decrease the risk of colonic adenomas, the precursors of most colon cancers (Baron et al., 2003).

Molecular studies show that inflammatory biomarkers are often expressed throughout the progression of colorectal carcinogenesis. Most impressive is the overexpression of the inducible cyclooxygenase-2 (COX-2) enzyme, which is responsible for prostaglandin biosynthesis in the inflammatory cascade (Harris, 2007).

In a case–control study of colon cancer, Harris and colleagues compared the effects of over-the-counter NSAIDs with prescription drugs that selectively inhibit COX-2. Their results suggest that both over-the-counter NSAIDs and selective COX-2 inhibitors produce significant reductions in the risk of colon cancer, underscoring their strong potential for colon cancer chemoprevention (Harris, Beebe-Donk, & Alshafie, 2008).

Exogenous Estrogens and Colorectal Cancer

Although postmenopausal hormone replacement therapy (HRT) has been found to increase the risk of developing cardiovascular disease, breast cancer, and endometrial cancer, there is consistent evidence from epidemiologic studies that HRT *reduces* the risk of colorectal cancer (MacLennan, MacLennan, & Ryan, 1991). A meta-analysis of 18 studies determined that current HRT use resulted in a 34% decrease in the risk (Nelson, Humphrey, Nygren, Teutsch, & Allen, 2002). This finding is supported by the results of a randomized clinical trial in the Women's Health Initiative (WHI) in which the incidence of colorectal cancer was 44% less in women receiving HRT (estrogen plus progesterone) compared to those receiving a placebo (Chlebowski et al., 2004).

Risk Factor Differences: Colon Cancer and Rectal Cancer

Malignancies of the colon and rectum are discussed together as colorectal cancer in this chapter. While these tumors share a number of clinical features and risk factors and their global patterns are similar, they exhibit some notable epidemiological and genetic differences. For example, in a study of women in the United States, family history was a stronger risk factor and physical activity had a greater protective effect for colon cancer than for rectal cancer (Wei et al., 2004). Colon cancer is also more common and has higher mortality than rectal cancer, particularly in men. In 2018, the global age-adjusted incidence of colon cancer was 13.1 per 100,000 in men and 10.1 per 100,000 in women, whereas the incidence of rectal cancer was 10.0 per 100,000 in men and 5.6 per 100,000 in women. Likewise, global mortality rates for colon cancer (6.5 and 4.2 per 100,000 in men and women, respectively) were higher than the corresponding rates for rectal cancer (4.2 and 2.4 per 100,000) (Bray et al., 2018).

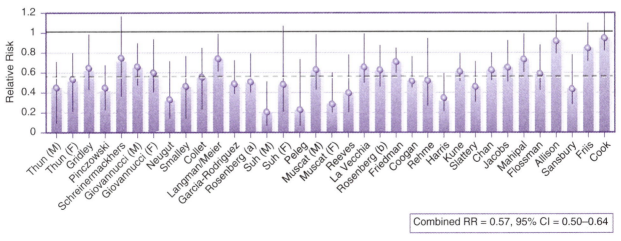

FIGURE 18.4 Colon Cancer and NSAIDs.

Caption: Note: Investigators are cited in the figure; M & F denote studies of males or females; a and b denote separate studies by same investigator.

Data from Harris, R. E. (2009). Cyclooxygenase-2 (COX-2) blockade in the chemoprevention of cancers of the colon, breast, prostate, and lung. *Inflammopharmacology, 17,* 1–13.

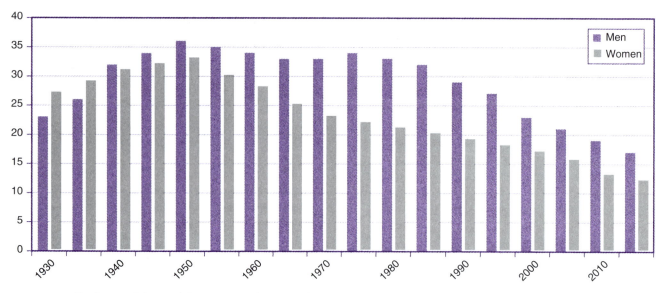

FIGURE 18.5 Decline in Colorectal Cancer Mortality, United States, 1930–2015.

Data from Garcia, M., Jemal, A., Ward, E. M., Center, M. M., Hao, Y., Siegel, R. L., & Thun, M. J. (2007). *Global cancer facts and figures, 2007*. Atlanta, GA: American Cancer Society. Retrieved from http://www.cancer.org/acs/groups/content/@nho/documents/document /globalfactsandfigures2007rev2p.pdf; Noone, A. M., Howlader, N., Krapcho, M., Miller, D., Brest, A., Yu, M., . . . Cronin, K. A. (2018). *SEER cancer statistics review, 1975–2015*. Bethesda, MD: National Cancer Institute.

In addition, recent genetic studies have identified different mutations associated with colon and rectal carcinogenesis; e.g., colon malignancies have a higher frequency of mutations of K-ras and other genes that disrupt control of cell division, while rectal malignancies are more likely to have only mutations of the APC gene that cause development of adenomatous polyps (Frattini et al., 2004). These findings suggest the need for future investigations that take into account genetic mutations and risk factor differences by anatomic subsite within the large bowel.

▶ Screening for Colorectal Cancer

In recent decades, rates of colorectal cancer have gradually increased in populations of developing nations in association with their transition to diets with higher fat and lower fiber content and lifestyle changes that heighten predisposition. In contrast, colorectal mortality rates have gradually declined in highly developed nations such as the United States (Garcia et al., 2007).

The declining trends in colorectal cancer death rates differ for U.S. men and women (**FIGURE 18.5**). In women, rates began to decline in the mid-20th century and have decreased by more than 60%. In men, rates began to decline during 1970–1980 and have decreased by about 45%. Several factors may have contributed to these declines, including greater awareness, increased screening, more efficacious treatment, improvement in diet, reduction in risk factors, and possibly greater use of chemopreventive agents such as NSAIDs. It is notable that these declines have occurred in the face of concurrent epidemics of obesity and related conditions such as type 2 diabetes.

A recent study suggests that the declining pattern of colorectal mortality in the United States is most compatible with a relatively large contribution from screening and a smaller but demonstrable impact of risk factor reductions and improved treatments (Edwards et al., 2009). Colonoscopy has gained greater acceptance in the general population and is the most reliable method of screening for the early detection of adenomatous polyps and cancer of the large bowel. In addition, visual determination of the exact location and size of existing tumors is an invaluable tool in planning and implementing definitive surgical resection. Colonoscopic imaging coupled with effective surgery has produced 5-year survival rates greater than 90% for patients whose tumors have not progressed beyond the bowel wall (National Cancer Institute, 2007).

References

Aaltonen, L. A., Peltomiki, P., Leach, F. S., Sistonen, P., Pylkkanen, L., Mecklin, J. P., . . . de la Chapelle, A. (1993). Clues to the pathogenesis of familial colorectal cancer. *Science, 260,* 812–816.

Aaltonen, L. A., Peltomiki, P., Mecklin, J. P., Jirvinen, H., Jass, J. R., Green, J. S., . . . de la Chapelle, A. (1994). Replication errors in benign and malignant tumors from hereditary nonpolyposis colorectal cancer patients. *Cancer Research, 54,* 1645–1648.

Anderson, J. W., Baird, P., Davis, R. H., Ferreri, S., Knudtson, M., Koraym, A., … Williams, C. L. (2009). Health benefits of dietary fiber. *Nutrition Review, 67*(4), 188–205.

Baron, J. A., Cole, B. F., Sandler, R. S., Haile, R. W., Ahnen, D., Bresalier, R., … van Stolk, R. U. (2003). A randomized trial of aspirin to prevent colorectal adenomas. *New England Journal of Medicine, 348*, 891–899.

Bingham, S. A., Day, N. E., Luben, R., Ferrari, P., Slimani, N., Norat, T., … Riboli, E. (2010). Dietary fibre in food and protection against colorectal cancer in the European Prospective Investigation into Cancer and Nutrition (EPIC): An observational study. *Lancet, 361*, 1496–1501.

Bingham, S. A., Norat, T., Moskal, A., Ferrari, P., Slimani, N., Clavel-Chapelon, F., … Riboli, E. (2005). Is the association with fiber from foods in colorectal cancer confounded by folate intake? *Cancer Epidemiology, Biomarkers and Prevention, 14*, 1552–1556.

Botteri, E., Iodice, S., Bagnardi, V., Raimondi, S., Lowenfel, A. B., & Maisonneuve, P. (2008). Smoking and colorectal cancer: A meta-analysis. *Journal of the American Medical Association, 300*(23), 2765–2778.

Boyle, P., & Langman, J. S. (2000). ABC of colorectal cancer. *British Medical Journal, 321*(7264), 805–808.

Bray, F., Ferlay, J., Soerjomataram, I., Siegel, R. L., Torre, L. A., & Jemal, A. (2018). Global cancer statistics 2018: GLOBOCAN estimates of incidence and mortality worldwide for 36 cancers in 185 countries. *CA: A Cancer Journal for Clinicians, 68*(6), 394–424.

Burkitt, D. P. (1971). Epidemiology of cancer of the colon and rectum. *Cancer, 28*, 3–13.

Burkitt, D. P. (1973). Epidemiology of large bowel disease: The role of fibre. *Proceedings of the Nutrition Society, 32*, 145–149.

Burkitt, D. P., Walker, A. R. P., & Painter, N. S. (1974). Dietary fiber and disease. *Journal of the American Medical Association, 229*, 1068–1072.

Caygill, C. P., & Hill, M. J. (1995). Fish, n-3 fatty acids and human colorectal and breast cancer mortality. *European Journal of Cancer Prevention, 4*, 329–332.

Center, M. M., & Jemal, A. E. (2009). International trends in colorectal cancer incidence rates. *Cancer Epidemiology, Biomarkers, and Prevention, 18*(6), 1688–1694.

Chlebowski, R. T., Wactawski-Wende, J. W., Ritenbaugh, C., Hubbell, F. A., Ascensao, J., Rebecca, J., … White, E. (2004). Estrogen plus progestin and colorectal cancer in postmenopausal women. *New England Journal of Medicine, 350*(10), 991–1004.

Cho, E., Smith-Warner, S. A., Ritz, J., van den Brandt, P. A., Colditz, G. A., Folsom, A. R., … Hunter, D. J. (2004). Alcohol intake and colorectal cancer: A pooled analysis of 8 cohort studies. *Annals of Internal Medicine, 140*(8), 603–613.

Duthie, S. (1999). Folic acid deficiency and cancer: Mechanisms of DNA instability. *British Medical Bulletin, 55*, 578–592.

Edwards, B. K., Ward, E., Kohler, B. A., Eheman, C., Zauber, A. G., Anderson, R. N., … Ries, L. A. (2009). Annual report to the nation on the status of cancer, 1975–2006, featuring colorectal cancer trends and impact of interventions (risk factors, screening, and treatment) to reduce future rates. *Cancer, 116*(3), 544–573.

Fearon, E. R. (2011). Molecular genetics of colorectal cancer. *Annual Review of Pathology: Mechanisms of Disease, 6*, 479–507.

Ferlay, J., Ervik, M., Lam, F., Colombet, M., Mery, L., Piñeros, M., … Bray, F. (2018). *Global cancer observatory: Cancer today*. Lyon, France: International Agency for Research on Cancer. Retrieved from https://gco.iarc.fr/today

Ferlay, J., Shin, H.-R., Bray, F., Forman, D., Mathers, C., & Parkin, D. M. (2010). Estimates of worldwide burden of cancer in 2008: GLOBOCAN 2008. *International Journal of Cancer, 127*(12), 2893–2917.

Ferlay, J., Soerjomataram, I., Ervik, M., Dikshit, R., Eser, S., Mathers, C., … Bray, F. (2013). *GLOBOCAN 2012 v1.0. Cancer incidence and mortality worldwide: IARC CancerBase No. 11 [Internet]*. Lyon, France: International Agency for Research on Cancer. Retrieved from http://globocan.iarc.fr

Frattini, M., Balestra, D., Suardi, S., Oggionni, M., Alberici, P., Radice, P., … Peirotti, M. A. (2004). Different genetic features associated with colon and rectal carcinogenesis. *Clinical Cancer Research, 10*, 4015–4021.

Freedman, D. M., Looker, A. C., Chang, S. C., & Graubard, B. L. (2007). Prospective study of serum vitamin D and cancer mortality in the United States. *Journal of the National Cancer Institute, 99*(21), 1594–1602.

Fuchs, C. S., Giovannucci, E. L., Colditz, G. A., Hunter, D. J., Stampfer, M. J., Rosner, B., … Willett, W. C. (1999). Dietary fiber and the risk of colorectal cancer and adenoma in women. *New England Journal of Medicine, 340*(3), 169–176.

Garcia, M., Jemal, A., Ward, E. M., Center, M. M., Hao, Y., Siegel, R. L., & Thun, M. J. (2007). *Global cancer facts & figures 2007*. Atlanta, GA: American Cancer Society. Retrieved from http://www.cancer.org/acs/groups/content/@nho/documents/document/globalfactsandfigures2007rev2p.pdf

Gardner, E. J. (1951). A genetic and clinical study of intestinal polyposis, a predisposing factor for carcinoma of the colon and rectum. *American Journal of Human Genetics, 3*, 167–176.

Garland, C. F., & Garland, F. C. (1980). Do sunlight and vitamin D reduce the likelihood of colon cancer? *International Journal of Epidemiology, 9*, 227–231.

Giovannucci, E. (2001). An updated review of the epidemiological evidence that cigarette smoking increases risk of colorectal cancer. *Cancer Epidemiology, Biomarkers, and Prevention, 10*, 725–731.

Giovannucci, E. (2007). Metabolic syndrome, hyperinsulinemia, and colon cancer: A review. *American Journal of Clinical Nutrition, 86*(3), 836–842.

Giovannucci, E., Colditz, G. A., Stampfer, M. J., & Willett, W. C. (1996). Physical activity, obesity and risk of colorectal cancer in women (United States). *Cancer Causes and Control, 7*, 253–263.

Gorham, E. D., Garland, C. F., Garland, F. C., Grant, W. B., Mohr, S. B., Lipkin, M., … Holick, M. F. (2005). Vitamin D and prevention of colorectal cancer. *Journal of Steroid Biochemistry and Molecular Biology, 97*, 179–194.

Greenwald, P., Lanza, E., & Eddy, G. A. (1987). Dietary fiber in the reduction of colon cancer risk. *Journal of the American Dietetic Association, 87*, 1178–1188.

Harris, R. E. (2007). COX-2 and the inflammogenesis of cancer. *Subcellular Biochemistry, 42*, 193–212.

Harris, R. E. (2009). Cyclooxygenase-2 (COX-2) blockade in the chemoprevention of cancers of the colon, breast, prostate, and lung. *Inflammopharmacology, 17*, 1–13.

Harris, R. E., Beebe-Donk, J., & Alshafie, G. A. (2008). Similar reductions in the risk of human colon cancer by selective and non-selective cyclooxygenase-2 (COX-2) inhibitors. *BMC Cancer, 8*(237). Retrieved from http://www.biomedcentral.com/1471-2407/8/237

Homann, N., Tillonen, J., & Salaspuro, M. (2000). Microbially produced acetaldehyde from ethanol may increase the risk of colon cancer via folate deficiency. *International Journal of Cancer, 86*, 169–173.

Howe, G. R., Benito, E., Castellato, R., Cornee, J., Esteve, J., Gallagher, R. P., … Shu, Z. (1992). Dietary intake of fiber and decreased risk of cancers of the colon and rectum: Evidence from the combined analysis of 13 case-control studies. *Journal of the National Cancer Institute, 84*, 1887–1896.

Kumar, V., Abbas, A. K., Fausto, N., & Astor, J. (2009). *Robbins and Cotran pathologic basis of disease* (8th ed.). Philadelphia, PA: W.B. Saunders.

Leppert, M., Dobbs, M., Scambler, P., O'Connell, P., Nakamura, Y., Stauffer, D., Woodward, S., … White, R. (1987). The gene for familial polyposis coli maps to the long arm of chromosome 5. *Science, 238*(4832), 1411–1413.

Levin, K. E., & Dozois, R. R. (1991). Epidemiology of large bowel cancer. *World Journal of Surgery, 15*(5), 562–567.

Lipkin, M., Reddy, B., Newmark, H., & Lamprecht, S. A. (1999). Dietary factors in human colorectal cancer. *Annual Review of Nutrition, 19*, 545–586.

Lynch, H. T., Guirgis, H. A., Lynch, P. M., & Harris, R. E. (1977). Familial cancer syndromes: A survey. *Cancer, 39*(4 Suppl.), 1867–1881.

Lynch, H. T., Lynch, P. M., & Harris, R. E. (1977). Proximal colon cancer in familial carcinoma of the colon exclusive of familial polyposis coli. *Lancet, 1*(8025), 1306–1307.

Lynch, H. T., Shaw, M. W., Magnuson, C. W., Larsen, A. L., & Krush, A. J. (1966). Hereditary factors in cancer: A study of two large midwestern kindreds. *Archives of Internal Medicine, 117*(2), 206–212.

MacLennan, S. C., MacLennan, A. H., & Ryan, P. (1991). Colorectal cancer and oestrogen replacement therapy: A meta-analysis of epidemiological studies. *Medical Journal of Australia, 162*, 491–493.

Matsumura, Y. (2001). Emerging trends of nutrition: Transition and trade-offs. Nutrition trends in Japan. *Asia Pacific Journal of Clinical Nutrition, 10*(Suppl.), S40–S47.

Mizoue, T., Inoue, M., Wakai, K., Nagata, C., Shimazu, T., Tsuji, I., … Tsugane, S. (2008). Alcohol drinking and colorectal cancer in Japanese: A pooled analysis of results from five cohort studies. *American Journal of Epidemiology, 167*(12), 1397–1406.

Nakaji, S., Shimoyama, T., Umeda, T., Sakamoto, J., Katsura, S., Sugawara, K., & Baxter, D. (2001). Dietary fiber showed no preventive effect against colon and rectal cancers in Japanese with low fat intake: An analysis from the results of nutrition surveys from 23 Japanese prefectures. *BMC Cancer, 1*, 1–14.

National Cancer Center, Japan. (2010). *Cancer statistics in Japan, 2010*. Tokyo, Japan: Author.

National Cancer Institute. (2007). *Colon cancer PDQ: Treatment options for colon cancer*. Bethesda, MD: Author.

Nelson, H. D., Humphrey, L. L., Nygren, P., Teutsch, S. M., & Allen, J. D. (2002). Postmenopausal hormone replacement therapy: Scientific review. *Journal of the American Medical Association, 288*(7), 872–881.

Noone, A. M., Howlader, N., Krapcho, M., Miller, D., Brest, A., Yu, M., … Cronin, K. A. (2018). *SEER cancer statistics review, 1975–2015*. Bethesda, MD: National Cancer Institute.

Park, Y., Hunter, D. J., Spiegelman, D., Bergkvist, L., Berrino, F., van den Brandt, P. A., … Smith-Warner, S. A. (2005). Dietary fiber intake and risk of colorectal cancer: A pooled analysis of prospective cohort studies. *Journal of the American Medical Association, 294*, 2849–2857.

Parkin, M. D., Bray, F., Ferlay, J., & Pisani, P. (2005). Global cancer statistics, 2002. *CA: A Cancer Journal for Clinicians, 55*, 74–108.

Reddy, B. S. (1995). Nutritional factors and colon cancer. *Critical Reviews in Food Science and Nutrition, 35*, 175–190.

Reddy, B. S., & Maeura, Y. (1984). Tumor promotion by dietary fat in azoxymethane induced colon carcinogenesis in female F344 rats: Influence of amount and source of dietary fat. *Journal of the National Cancer Institute, 72*, 746–750.

Street, M. E., de'Angelis, G., Camacho-Hübner, C., Giovannelli, G., Ziveri, M. A., Bacchini, P. L., … Savage, M. O. (2004). Relationships between serum IGF-1, IGFBP-2, interleukin-1beta and interleukin-6 in inflammatory bowel disease. *Hormone Research, 61*(4), 159–164.

Su, L. J., & Arab, L. (2004). Alcohol consumption and risk of colon cancer: Evidence from the national health and nutrition examination survey I epidemiologic follow-up study. *Nutrition and Cancer, 50*(2), 111–119.

Terry, P. D., Miller, A. B., & Rohan, T. E. (2002). Obesity and colorectal cancer risk in women. *Gut, 51*, 191–194.

Trock, B., Lanza, E., & Greenwald, P. (1990). Dietary fiber, vegetables, and colon cancer: Critical review and meta-analysis of epidemiological studies. *Journal of the National Cancer Institute, 82*, 650–661.

Wactawski-Wende, J., Morley Kotchen, J., & Anderson, G. L. (2006). Calcium plus vitamin D supplementation and the risk of colorectal cancer. *New England Journal of Medicine, 354*(7), 684–696.

Wei, E. S., Giovannucci, E., Wu, K., Rosner, B., Fuchs, C. S., Williett, W. C., & Colditz, G. A. (2004). Comparison of risk factors for colon and rectal cancer. *International Journal of Cancer, 108*(3), 433–442.

Willett, W. C., Stampfer, M. J., Colditz, G. A., Rosner, B. A., & Speizer, F. E. (1990). Relation of meat, fat, and fiber intake to the risk of colon cancer in a prospective study among women. *New England Journal of Medicine, 323*, 1664–1672.

Wong, J. M., de Souza, R., Kendall, C. W., Emam, A., & Jenkins, D. J. (2006). Colonic health: Fermentation and short chain fatty acids. *Journal of Clinical Gastroenterology, 40*(3), 235–243.

Wu, K., Giovannucci, E., Byrne, C., Platz, E. A., Fuchs, C., Willett, W. C., & Sinha, R. (2006). Meat mutagens and risk of distal colon Adenoma in a cohort of U.S. men. *Cancer Epidemiology, Biomarkers and Prevention, 15*(6), 1120–1125.

Wynder, E. L., Fujita, Y., Harris, R. E., Hirayama, T., & Hiyama, T. (1991). Comparative epidemiology of cancer between the United States and Japan: A second look. *Cancer, 67*(3), 746–763.

Wynder, E. L., Kajitani, T., Ishikawa, S., Dodo, H., & Takano, A. (1969). Environmental factors of cancer of the colon and rectum. II. Japanese epidemiological data. *Cancer, 23*, 1210–1220.

Yu, H., Harris, R. E., Gao, Y.-T., Gao, R., & Wynder, E. L. (1991). Comparative epidemiology of cancers of the colon, rectum, prostate and breast in Shanghai, China, versus the United States. *International Journal of Epidemiology, 20*(1), 76–81.

Zisman, A. L., Nickolov, A., Brand, R. E., Gorchow, A., & Roy, H. K. (2006). Associations between the age at diagnosis and location of colorectal cancer and the use of alcohol and tobacco. *Archives of Internal Medicine, 166*, 629–634.

© Andrew Brookes/Getty Images

CHAPTER 19

Epidemiology of Pancreatic Cancer

▶ Global Epidemiology of Pancreatic Cancer

Pancreatic cancer was diagnosed in 458,918 individuals and caused 432,242 deaths in the world population during 2018. In that year, pancreatic cancer caused 4.2% of all cancer deaths among men (226,910 deaths) and 4.9% among women (205,332 deaths). During the decade, 2008–2018, the annual number of cases of pancreatic cancer in the world population increased by 65% and the number of deaths from this malignancy increased by 62%. During the same period, the global age-adjusted annual mortality rate increased by 21% in men (from 4.2 to 5.1 per 100,000) and by 23% in women (from 3.1 to 3.8 per 100,000) (Bray et al., 2018; Ferlay et al., 2010). The global burden of pancreatic cancer is clearly rising due to not only population growth and aging, but also increasing exposure to certain risk factors such as tobacco, alcohol, and dietary fat in some populations.

The incidence rates of pancreatic cancer in 2018 were approximately fourfold higher in developed countries than in developing countries (7.3 versus 1.7 per 100,000 in men and 5.1 versus 1.4 per 100,000 in women). Likewise, the mortality rates were higher in developed versus developing countries (6.7 versus 1.8 per 100,000 in men and 4.7 versus 1.3 per 100,000 in women) (Bray et al., 2018; Ferlay et al., 2010). These rate differences are likely due to multiple factors including better diagnostic technology and greater exposure to dietary risk factors in the populations of developed nations.

The global age-adjusted incidence in 2018 was 38% higher in men than in women (5.5 versus 4.0 per 100,000), and the mortality from pancreatic cancer was 34% higher in men than in women (5.1 versus 3.8 per 100,000) (Bray et al., 2018). Gender differences in the rates of pancreatic cancer have been attributed to the greater prevalence of known risk factors, e.g., tobacco smoking and alcohol abuse, in men compared to women.

Regardless of gender, pancreatic cancer is usually fatal; survival rates 1 year after diagnosis are less than 20% even in developed nations such as the United States. As a consequence, the ratio of mortality to incidence is close to unity. Without treatment, survival after diagnosis is only 3–5 months (Hariharan, Saied, & Kocher, 2008; O'Sullivan & Kocher, 2007).

FIGURE 19.1 depicts the international variability in pancreatic cancer incidence and mortality rates in 2018. Regions with high incidence and mortality rates include affluent industrialized nations in North America, Europe, Northern Asia (Russia), Australia and New Zealand, and the southernmost nations of South America. Low rates were observed in Africa and Southern Asia. Notably, in China which has a population of 1.4 billion people, the incidence and mortality rates in 2018 were more than double the rates in 2008, thereby accounting for a significant fraction of the rising number of cases and deaths from pancreatic cancer during the last decade (Ferlay et al., 2010, 2013, 2018).

Estimated age-standardized incidence rates (World) in 2018, pancreas, both sexes, all ages

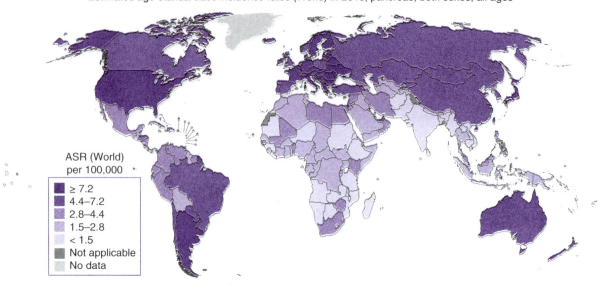

ASR (World)
per 100,000

- ≥ 7.2
- 4.4–7.2
- 2.8–4.4
- 1.5–2.8
- < 1.5
- Not applicable
- No data

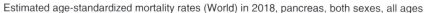

Estimated age-standardized mortality rates (World) in 2018, pancreas, both sexes, all ages

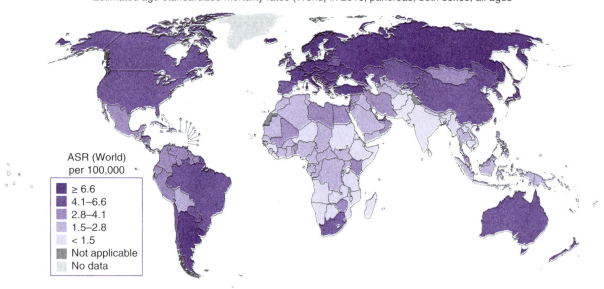

ASR (World)
per 100,000

- ≥ 6.6
- 4.1–6.6
- 2.8–4.1
- 1.5–2.8
- < 1.5
- Not applicable
- No data

FIGURE 19.1 Global Incidence and Mortality of Pancreatic Cancer, 2018.

Caption: ASR: Rates per 100,000 are age-standardized to the world population, 2000–2025.

Reproduced with permission from Ferlay, J., Ervik, M., Lam, F., Colombet, M., Mery, L., Piñeros, M., ... Bray, F. (2018). *Global cancer observatory: Cancer today*. Lyon, France: International Agency for Research on Cancer. Retrieved from https://gco.iarc.fr/today

▶ Pathogenesis of Pancreatic Cancer

The pancreas is a dual-functioning gland located deep in the abdomen just behind the stomach. Numerous pancreatic ducts communicate with the main (central) pancreatic duct that merges with the common bile duct to form the *ampulla of Vater* that empties into the duodenum (the upper small intestine). The anatomy of the pancreas is shown in **FIGURE 19.2**.

The pancreas functions as both an endocrine and an exocrine gland. Specialized endocrine cells of the *islets of Langerhans* are instrumental in the secretion of insulin and glucagon to maintain tight control of blood glucose. In contrast, specialized exocrine cells (called acinar cells) secrete powerful digestive enzymes as well as alkaline fluid into the pancreatic ducts that eventually drain into the main pancreatic duct and the duodenum (upper small intestine). The digestive enzymes include trypsin, lipase, and amylase, which break down protein, fats, and carbohydrates, respectively. Pancreatic fluids mix with bile from the liver in the ampulla of Vater prior to reaching the duodenum (the upper small intestine). A layer of specialized columnar epithelium circumferentially lines the pancreatic ducts as well as the main pancreatic duct.

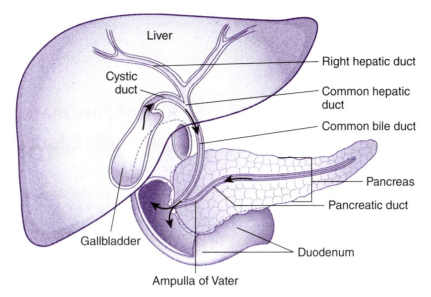

FIGURE 19.2 Anatomy of the Human Pancreas.

Most pancreatic cancers (approximately 99%) are adenocarcinomas that arise from the epithelial cells that line the ducts of the exocrine pancreas. The majority of this chapter is devoted to "carcinoma of the pancreas," which implies carcinoma arising from the epithelial lining of the exocrine portion of the pancreas. Only a small fraction (perhaps 1%–2%) of pancreatic tumors arise from the acinar cells of the pancreas or cells within the islets of Langerhans. These relatively rare tumors are discussed in a later section of this chapter.

Pancreatic cancer rates increase exponentially during the latter decades of the lifespan. Most cases are diagnosed after the age of 50 years with peak rates occurring in the age range 65–70 years. Furthermore, the majority of cases involve the head of the pancreas (60%–70%) rather than the body or tail of the gland (30%–40%). Because developing pancreatic tumors is difficult to palpate and there are no valid biomarkers of impending disease, it is believed that the genesis of these malignancies spans many years. Recent cellular and molecular studies suggest that pancreatic cancer develops over time by a progression of steps in the epithelial lining of the pancreatic ducts, from dysplasia to in situ carcinoma and, ultimately, invasive cancer (Ottenhof et al., 2009).

▶ **Tobacco Smoking and Pancreatic Cancer**

Tobacco smoking is a recognized risk factor for the development of pancreatic cancer. Wynder and colleagues first observed a significant dose response in the risk of pancreatic cancer with increasing number

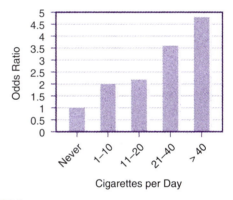

FIGURE 19.3 Risk of Pancreatic Cancer and Cigarette Smoking in Men.

Data from Wynder, E. L. (1975). An epidemiological evaluation of the causes of cancer of the pancreas. *Cancer Research, 35*(8), 2228–2233.

of cigarettes per day in chronic smokers (Wynder, 1975; Wynder, Mabuchi, & Maruchia, 1973). As shown in **FIGURE 19.3**, the risk increased nearly fivefold for smokers of two or more packs per day compared to never-smokers. Subsequently, many epidemiologic investigations have confirmed the etiologic impact of smoking tobacco in the development of this deadly malignancy. In a comprehensive meta-analysis of 82 studies conducted on four continents, chronic cigarette smoking increased the risk of developing pancreatic cancer by 74% compared to never smoking (summary relative risk [RR] = 1.74, 95% confidence interval [CI] = 1.61–1.87), and the risk elevation persisted 10 years after smoking cessation (Iodice, Gandini, Maisonneuve, & Lowenfels, 2008). Results were highly consistent for case–control studies (RR = 1.77) and cohort studies (RR = 1.70). The risk was also elevated for pipe or cigar smokers (RR = 1.47, 95% CI = 1.17–1.83). The public health implications of these results are enormous; for example, for populations with a smoking prevalence of 30%, the proportion of pancreatic cancer attributable to smoking is approximately 20%. Recent global estimates suggest that one in three adults smoke (World Health Organization [WHO], 2009), so it is evident that at least one-fifth of all pancreatic cancers are preventable by avoidance of the smoking habit.

Carcinogens from inhaled tobacco smoke can reach the pancreas through the circulatory system or through the bile. In particular, nitrosamines are activated in the liver and detoxified by liver enzymes of the cytochrome P-450 system (e.g., *CYP1A2*) or *n*-acetyl transferase enzymes. Recall that bile is secreted by the liver through the common cystic duct into the ampulla of Vater in the head of the pancreas. Notably, carcinogenic nitrosamines and their metabolites have been found in human bile (Hecht, 1998). Conceivably, some individuals may be genetically deficient in essential detoxification enzymes and as a consequence be at high risk for the development of pancreatic cancer due to sustained exposure to inhaled or ingested carcinogens (Lowenfels & Maisonneuve, 2006). Indeed, in a recent case–control investigation of genetic polymorphisms and pancreatic cancer, heavy smoking individuals genetically null for the glutathione-*S*-transferase enzyme (*GSTT1*) had markedly increased risk estimates compared to nonsmokers with normal *GSTT1* (Duell et al., 2002). Estimated odds ratios (OR) in the study were OR = 5.0, 95% CI = 1.8–14.5 for women, and OR = 3.2, 95% CI = 1.3–8.1 for men.

Alcohol and Pancreatic Cancer

The role of alcohol in the development of pancreatic cancer appears to be related to the dose and duration of alcohol consumption. The risk is increased by two- to threefold in heavy drinkers (i.e., consuming four or more drinks per day) (Olsen, Mandel, Gibson, Wattenberg, & Schuman, 1989; Ye et al., 2002) and the risk increase is higher per level of intake for certain ethnic groups; for example, risk estimates for African-American women are higher than for Caucasian women (Silverman et al., 1995). A recent pooled analysis of 14 prospective studies found that consumption of at least 30 g of alcohol daily (about two drinks) produced only a modest elevation in the risk (summary RR = 1.22, 95% CI = 1.03–1.45), whereas consumption of lesser amounts had no effect (Genkinger et al., 2009). Furthermore, some investigators caution that observed risk increases may be due to confounding with smoking (Ye et al., 2002; Zatonski et al., 1993). Nevertheless, there is no doubt that chronic alcohol abuse is a major cause of chronic pancreatitis, which in turn predisposes

to the development of pancreatic cancer. The association of chronic pancreatitis and pancreatic cancer is discussed in a later section of this chapter.

Risk of Pancreatic Cancer: Combined Effect of Tobacco and Alcohol

Talamini and colleagues recently published the results of a case–control study that examined both independent and combined effects of tobacco smoking and alcohol consumption in the development of pancreatic cancer. They compared 326 cases with incident pancreatic cancer to 652 hospital controls matched on age and gender without neoplastic disease. All subjects were ascertained and interviewed in hospitals in northern Italy during the period 1991–2008. Results revealed independent effects of tobacco smoking (OR = 2.04 for 20 or more pack years) and heavy alcohol consumption (OR = 2.03 for 21–34 drinks per week and OR = 3.42 for 35 or more drinks per week). The risk increased more than fourfold for chronic smokers and heavy drinkers (OR = 4.3) compared to never-smokers who consumed fewer than seven drinks per week. The authors suggest that the effects of tobacco and alcohol are additive, and together they account for approximately one-third of pancreatic cancer in Italy (Talamini et al., 2010).

Dietary Fat and Pancreatic Cancer

Fat and red meat consumption have been linked to the development of pancreatic cancer in a number of epidemiologic studies (Bueno de Mesquita, Moerman, Runia, & Maisonneuve, 1990; Chan, Wang, & Holly, 2007; Durbec, Chevillotte, Bidart, Berthezene, & Sarles, 1983; Farrow & Davis, 1990; Ghadirian, Simard, Baillargeon, Maisonneuve, & Boyle, 1991; Larsson, Hakanson, Permert, & Wolk, 2006; Mills, Beeson, Abbey, Fraser, & Phillips, 1988; Nöthlings et al., 2005; Raymond, Infante, Tuyns, Voirol, & Lowenfels, 1987; Stolzenberg-Solomon, Pietinen, Taylor, Virtamo, & Albanes, 2002; Wynder, 1975; Zhang, Zhao, & Berkel, 2005); however, results have not been consistent among all studies (Lin et al., 2006; Michaud, Giovannucci, Willett, Colditz, & Fuchs, 2003).

The U.S. National Institutes of Health–American Association of Retired Persons (AARP) Diet and Health Study was designed to provide definitive evidence on dietary factors and the development of a variety of chronic diseases including pancreatic cancer (Schatzkin et al., 2001). Using the NIH-AARP database, Thiébaut et al. (2009) examined the association between dietary fat and pancreatic cancer. Their investigation was based on the NIH-AARP cohort of 308,736 men and 216,737 women ages 51–70 years of age who completed a 124-item food frequency questionnaire in 1995–1996. Important findings of this study are summarized in the following paragraph.

Over an average follow-up of 6.3 years, 865 men and 472 women were diagnosed with exocrine pancreatic cancer (45.0 and 34.5 cases per 100,000 person-years, respectively). After multivariable adjustment and combination of data for men and women, pancreatic cancer risk was directly related to the intakes of total fat (highest versus lowest quintile, 46.8 versus 33.2 cases per 100,000 person-years, hazard ratio [HR] = 1.23, 95% CI = 1.03–1.46; P trend = 0.03), saturated fat (51.5 versus 33.1 cases per 100,000 person-years, HR = 1.36, 95% CI = 1.14–1.62; P trend < 0.001), and monounsaturated fat (46.2 versus 32.9 cases per 100,000 person-years, HR = 1.22, 95% CI = 1.02–1.46; P trend = 0.05) but not polyunsaturated fat. The associations were strongest for saturated fat from animal food sources (52.0 versus 32.2 cases per 100,000 person-years, HR = 1.43, 95% CI = 1.20–1.70; P trend < 0.001); specifically, intakes from red meat and dairy products were both statistically significantly associated with increased pancreatic cancer risk (HR = 1.27 and 1.19, respectively).

Of further note regarding findings of the NIH-AARP study of pancreatic cancer is that there were no consistent associations with polyunsaturated, saturated, or monounsaturated fats from plant food sources. Though there was no association with total intake of polyunsaturated fats (PUFAs) in this large comprehensive study, it is important to note that the high intake of dietary arachidonic acid (20:4), an omega-6 PUFA obtained primarily from animal foods, was significantly associated with the risk of developing pancreatic cancer (HR = 1.33, 95% CI = 1.12–1.59, P trend < 0.002). The investigators concluded that high intake of dietary fat of animal origin, particularly from red meat and dairy food sources, increases the risk of developing pancreatic cancer (Thiébaut et al., 2009).

Various hypotheses have been advanced to explain the link between high dietary fat and the development of pancreatic cancer. It is well known that diets with high fat content stimulate bile secretion by the liver, which in turn increases the gastrointestinal exposure to cholesterol, bile acids, and their metabolites. There is considerable experimental evidence that bile acids promote the development of gastrointestinal tumors both in vivo (Hill, 1991; Reddy, 1981; Reddy,

Weisburger, & Wynder, 1978) and in vitro (Kaibara, Yurugi, & Koga, 1984). Recent evidence also suggests that bile acids promote carcinogenesis by up-regulating cyclooxygenase-2 (COX-2) and prostaglandin production (Glinghammar & Rafter, 2001; Shirvani, Ouatu-Lascar, Kaur, Omary, & Triadafilopoulos, 2000; Zhang, Subbaramaiah, Altorki, & Dannenberg, 1998). Furthermore, bile acids have been found to induce COX-2 in pancreatic cancer cell lines (Tucker, Dannenberg, Yang, & Fahye, 2004). These findings, plus the significant effects of dietary fat and, specifically, arachidonic acid (the primary substrate of COX-2 in the inflammatory cascade) observed in the NIH-AARP Dietary Study (Thiébaut et al., 2009), suggest that up-regulation of COX-2 and excess production of prostaglandins may have an important role in the development of pancreatic cancer. This general process (called inflammogenesis) induces and promotes essential features of carcinogenesis (mutagenesis, mitogenesis, angiogenesis, reduced apoptosis, metastasis, and immunosuppression) (Harris, 2007).

▶ Chronic Pancreatitis and Pancreatic Cancer

Chronic pancreatitis refers to persistent inflammation of the pancreas, irrespective of the cause. This condition is clearly a risk factor for the development of pancreatic cancer. In an international multicenter historical cohort study of 2015 patients diagnosed with chronic pancreatitis, 56 new cases of pancreatic cancer developed over a mean follow-up period of 7.4 years, an incidence rate more than 16 times the expected rate (standardized incidence ratio = 16.5, 95% CI = 11.1–23.7) (Lowenfels et al., 1993). The cumulative risk after 20 years of follow-up was 4.0% (95% CI = 2.0–5.9) and the risk increase was independent of gender, country of origin, and type of pancreatitis.

The main cause of chronic pancreatitis among adults is chronic alcohol abuse. More than 70% of adult patients diagnosed with chronic pancreatitis have a long-term history of frequently drinking excessive amounts of alcoholic beverages. The majority of such patients report daily consumption of at least 150 g (more than 5 ounces) of alcohol for more than 5 years (Nair, Lawler, & Miller, 2007). The presence of gallstones (cholelithiasis) also predisposes affected individuals to the development of chronic pancreatitis. These two conditions, chronic alcohol abuse and cholelithiasis, account for about 90% of chronic pancreatitis in the United States. Autoimmune pancreatitis accounts for an additional 5%–6% of cases (Finkelberg, Sahani, Deshpande, & Brugge, 2006).

The pathophysiology of chronic pancreatitis has been characterized through detailed studies of alcoholic pancreatitis in both animals and humans (Witt, Apte, Keim, & Wilson, 2007). Alcohol is directly toxic to pancreatic tissue, and chronic exposure causes significant cell damage, necrosis, and inflammation (a process known as *necroinflammation*). In addition, the alcohol-induced destruction and destabilization of the epithelial lining of the pancreatic ducts permits the release of powerful digestive enzymes, thereby predisposing the gland to *autodigestion*. The progressive cascade of pathogenic events in chronic alcoholic pancreatitis involves chronic inflammation, cell necrosis, release of digestive enzymes, cell autodigestion, formation of reactive oxygen species, collagen deposition, fibrosis, and scarring of the pancreatic tissues. The inflammatory pathophysiology of chronic pancreatitis clearly provokes multiple mechanisms of carcinogenesis such as mitogenesis, mutagenesis, and angiogenesis (Harris, 2007).

Chronic pancreatitis induced by chronic cholelithiasis (gallstone formation) appears to follow a similar course (Yan & Li, 2006). Gallstones that travel down the common bile duct and become lodged in the ampulla of Vater can cause obstruction in the outflow of pancreatic digestive fluids. Backflow of these digestive fluids into the pancreas predisposes the ductal epithelium to autodigestion. The end result is persistent necroinflammation that progresses to chronic pancreatitis.

▶ Germline Mutations and Pancreatic Cancer

Various germline mutations have been identified that heighten the risk of developing pancreatic cancer. For example, hereditary pancreatitis is an autosomal dominant genetic condition caused by a mutation in the gene that encodes the powerful digestive enzyme trypsinogen. Carriers of the mutant gene produce abnormal trypsinogen that is resistant to autolysis, thereby causing autodigestion of the pancreas, necroinflammation, and chronic pancreatitis. Such individuals have a 40% lifetime risk of developing pancreatic cancer (Whitcomb, 1999).

Cystic fibrosis is an autosomal recessive genetic condition caused by a deleterious mutation in the transmembrane conductance regulator gene (*CFTR*) located on the long arm of chromosome 7. The protein encoded by *CFTR* is essential for normal function of the chloride ion channel of cell membranes and homeostatic regulation of concentrations of electrolytes in sweat, digestive enzymes, and mucus. The extremely viscid mucinous secretions characteristic of this condition result in cystic dilatation, necroinflammation, and fibrosis within the pancreas, lungs, and other organs, hence the name cystic fibrosis. Chronic pancreatitis develops early in patients with cystic fibrosis, with a consequent fivefold increase in the risk of early onset pancreatic cancer (Maisonneuve, Marshall, & Lowenfels, 2007). Cystic fibrosis is one of the more common genetic conditions among Caucasians, occurring in one of every 3200 newborns. The median life expectancy for individuals with cystic fibrosis is only 30–35 years.

Familial breast/ovarian cancer is often caused by a heritable mutation in either of two tumor suppressor genes, *BRCA-1* or *BRCA-2*. Females who inherit mutant alleles of *BRCA-1* or *BRCA-2* are not only at high risk for developing breast cancer and/or ovarian cancer, but also at increased risk for the development of other tumors, including pancreatic cancer. Both *BRCA-1* and *BRCA-2* are tumor suppressor genes that are essential for precise DNA replication in cell division. Mutant forms of a third gene (called *PAL-B2* because it interacts with *BRCA-2*) also increase pancreatic cancer risk as well as breast cancer risk (Chen et al., 2008).

The Familial Atypical Mole and Melanoma (FAMM) syndrome is a rare genetic disorder giving rise to multiple dysplastic pigmented moles of the skin that can progress to malignant melanoma. There is also an increase in the risk of developing pancreatic cancer. One form of the FAMM syndrome is caused by a mutation in the gene that encodes *p16*, an important cell cycle regulating protein (Hussussian et al., 1994).

Peutz–Jeghers syndrome is a rare autosomal dominant disorder characterized by the development of benign hamartomatous polyps in the gastrointestinal tract and hyperpigmented macules on the lips and oral mucosa (Boardman et al., 1998). This syndrome is caused by a mutant tumor suppressor gene known as STK11 located on chromosome 19. Mutations in this gene result in an altered serine/threonine protein kinase that markedly increases the risk of gastrointestinal tumors including pancreatic cancer (Jenne et al., 1998).

Lynch syndrome (hereditary nonpolyposis coli colon cancer, HNPCC) is characterized by a high lifetime risk for the development of colon cancer. The cause of HNPCC is an inherited (germline) mutation in at least one of a set of genes that normally repair DNA, the mismatch repair genes. This genetic disorder also carries an increase in the risk of developing pancreatic cancer.

Somatic Mutations in Pancreatic Cancer

Somatic mutations involving base pair changes in DNA occasionally occur in specific cells of specific tissues of the human body. The phenotypic effects of such mutations persist in the lineage of the cell of origin.

The *K-ras* gene product communicates signals from outside the cell to the nucleus, a process known as *signal transduction*. Somatic mutations of the *K-ras* gene can lead to its permanent activation, thereby causing inappropriate signaling inside the cell even in the absence of extracellular stimuli. Because *K-ras* signal transduction stimulates cell division, its deregulation may result in heightened cell proliferation and malignant transformation (Goodsell, 1999).

Somatic mutations of *K-ras* have been observed in up to 90% of certain malignancies such as colon cancer, lung cancer, and pancreatic cancer (Almoguera et al., 1988). Somatic mutations of *K-ras* have also been detected in premalignant lesions of these organs (Moskaluk, Hruban, & Kern, 1997). Molecular studies also suggest that mutational activation of *K-ras* coupled with disabling mutations in tumor suppressor genes such as *p53* and *p16* accentuate carcinogenesis (Ghaneh, Costello, & Neoptolemos, 2007; Moskaluk et al., 1997; Pellegata et al., 1994). Although specific mutagenic stimuli of persistent *K-ras* mutations have not yet been clearly identified (Crous-Bou et al., 2009), most factors that are associated with the development of pancreatic cancer (e.g., tobacco, alcohol, bile acids, reactive oxygen species, and inflammatory factors) do have significant mutagenic potential. Clearly, the oncogenic activation of *K-ras* is likely to play a key role in the initiation and promotion of pancreatic ductal adenocarcinoma.

Epigenetics of Pancreatic Cancer

Epigenetics refers to the study of changes in the expression of genes without any alteration in the base pair sequence of the DNA. Down-regulation of genetic expression has generally been linked to DNA methylation as opposed to up-regulation, which may be a result of DNA acetylation.

Because pancreatic cancer often develops subsequent to chronic pancreatitis and necroinflammation, it is notable that the inducible COX-2 gene that encodes the chief regulatory enzyme of the inflammatory cascade is markedly overexpressed in a high percentage of pancreatic adenocarcinomas; furthermore, positive immunostaining for COX-2 is localized to malignant epithelial cells whereas COX-2 staining is negative in noncancerous pancreatic tissues (Tucker et al., 1999). In addition, studies of pancreatic cancer cell lines show that bile acids effectively up-regulate the inducible COX-2 gene (Tucker et al., 2004). These findings suggest that bile acids could promote pancreatic cancer by up-regulation of the inducible COX-2 gene.

Obesity, Diabetes Mellitus Type 2, and Pancreatic Cancer

Twin epidemics of obesity and diabetes mellitus type 2 have emerged in many populations throughout the world. Both conditions are independently associated with the development of pancreatic cancer, and obesity is associated with the onset of diabetes.

An early meta-analysis of 20 epidemiologic studies determined a twofold elevation in the risk of pancreatic cancer among individuals with a 5-year history of diabetes mellitus type 2 (Everhart & Wright, 1995). In a more recent meta-analysis of 36 epidemiologic studies (17 case–control and 19 cohort studies involving 9220 cases), the adjusted summary OR was 1.83 (95% CI = 1.66–1.89) (Huxley, Ansary-Moghaddam, Berrington de González, Barzi, & Woodward, 2005). These results support a modest causal association of type 2 diabetes in the genesis of pancreatic cancer.

A major problem with studies of the association of pancreatic cancer and diabetes is that because both conditions evolve in the same organ over a period of many years, it is difficult to determine the causal pathway. The question becomes, does diabetes predispose to pancreatic cancer or the reverse? Drawing conclusions regarding the role of diabetes in causing pancreatic cancer is thus subject to a form of bias known as *reverse causality bias*. In fact, more than 70% of pancreatic cancer cases present with glucose intolerance (Gullo, Pezzilli, & Morselli-Labate, 1994; Schwarts, Zeidler, Moossa, Kuku, & Rubenstein, 1978).

The issue of reverse causality in regard to pancreatic cancer and diabetes has been discussed in some detail by various investigators. Currently, there is no general consensus as to a cause and effect relationship between these conditions. One argument *against* such a relationship is the fact that rates of pancreatic cancer have remained constant or declined in many nations even though prevalence rates of obesity and type 2 diabetes have increased dramatically. Nevertheless, in subjects with long-standing type 2 diabetes, the pancreas is exposed to hyperinsulinemia for years, and because cultures of pancreatic cancer cells have been found to express insulin receptors, it is conceivable that hyperinsulinemia could serve as a promoter of pancreatic cancer (Wang, Herrington, Larrson, & Permert, 2003).

Islet Cell Tumors

Islet cell tumors of the pancreas arise from endocrine cells in the *islets of Langerhans*. Although such tumors may involve any of the hormone-producing islet cells (alpha cells produce glucagon, beta cells produce insulin, delta cells produce somatostatin, PP cells produce pancreatic polypeptide, and epsilon cells produce ghrelin), most are beta cell tumors (also called insulinomas because the beta cells elaborate insulin). Insulinomas are clinically characterized by attacks of hyperinsulinism and hypoglycemia. Islet cell tumors are a component of Zollinger–Ellison syndrome, defined by the triad of recalcitrant peptic ulcer, hypersecretion of gastrin (gastrinoma), and pancreatic islet cell tumor. Islet cell tumors also occur in multiple endocrine neoplasia syndrome (MEN I),

which may include adenomas of the pituitary gland, the thyroid and parathyroid glands, and the adrenal cortex in combination with peptic ulcer. Most islet cell tumors are benign (less than 10% are malignant carcinomas). Malignant islet cell tumors constitute only about 1% of all cases of pancreatic cancer (Bellizzi & Frankel, 2004). Germline and somatic mutations and epigenetic suppression of multiple tumor suppressor genes that regulate nucleosome remodeling have been linked to the development of these rare pancreatic tumors (Elsässer, Allis, & Lewis, 2011).

Prevention of Pancreatic Cancer

There are currently no proven methods of preventing the development of pancreatic cancer, nor are there satisfactory tests or imaging procedures that can be used to screen the population for early lesions of the pancreas. Nevertheless, there are steps that can be taken to reduce the risk. These include complete avoidance of tobacco and alcohol; maintenance of a healthy weight through regular exercise; eating a diet rich in fruits, vegetables, and whole grains; and maintenance of blood glucose within normal limits.

References

Almoguera, C., Shibata, D., Forrester, K., Martin, J., Arnheim, N., & Perucho, M. (1988). Most human carcinomas of the exocrine pancreas contain mutant *c-K-ras* genes. *Cell, 53*, 549–554.

Bellizzi, A. M., & Frankel, W. L. (2004). Pancreatic pathology: A practical review. *LabMedicine, 40*, 417–426.

Boardman, L. A., Thibodeau, S. N., Schaid, D. J., Lindor, N. M., McDonnell, S. K., Burgart, L. J., … Hartmann, L. C. (1998). Increased risk for cancer in patients with the Peutz–Jeghers syndrome. *Annals of Internal Medicine, 128*(11), 896–899.

Bray, F., Ferlay, J., Soerjomataram, I., Siegel, R. L., Torre, L. A., & Jemal, A. (2018). Global cancer statistics 2018: GLOBOCAN estimates of incidence and mortality worldwide for 36 cancers in 185 countries. *CA: A Cancer Journal for Clinicians, 68*(6), 394–424.

Bueno de Mesquita, H. B., Moerman, C. J., Runia, S., & Maisonneuve, P. (1990). Are energy and energy-providing nutrients related to exocrine carcinoma of the pancreas? *International Journal of Cancer, 46*(3), 435–444.

Chan, J. M., Wang, F., & Holly, E. A. (2007). Pancreatic cancer, animal protein and dietary fat in a population-based study, San Francisco Bay Area, California. *Cancer Causes and Control, 18*(10), 1153–1167.

Chen, P., Liang, J., Wang, Z., Zhou, X., Chen, L., Li, M., … Wang, H. (2008). Association of common PALB2 polymorphisms with breast cancer risk: A case-control study. *Clinical Cancer Research, 14*(18), 5931–5937.

Crous-Bou, M., Porta, M., Morales, E., Lopez, T., Carrato, A., Puigdomènech, E., … PANKRAS II Study Group. (2009). Past

medical conditions and *K-ras* mutations in pancreatic ductal adenocarcinoma: A hypothesis-generating study. *Cancer Causes and Control, 20*, 591–599.

Duell, E. J., Holly, E. A., Bracci, P. M., Liu, M., Wiencke, J. K., & Kelsey, K. T. (2002). A population-based, case control study of polymorphisms in carcinogen-metabolizing genes, smoking, and pancreatic adenocarcinoma risk. *Journal of the National Cancer Institute, 94*(4), 297–306.

Durbec, J. P., Chevillotte, G., Bidart, J. M., Berthezene, P., & Sarles, H. (1983). Diet, alcohol, tobacco and risk of cancer of the pancreas: A case-control study. *British Journal of Cancer, 47*(4), 463–470.

Elsässer, S. J., Allis, C. D., & Lewis, P. W. (2011). New epigenetic drivers of cancers. *Science, 331*(6021), 1145–1146.

Everhart, J., & Wright, D. (1995). Diabetes mellitus as a risk factor for pancreatic cancer. A meta-analysis. *Journal of the American Medical Association, 273*(20), 1605–1609.

Farrow, D. C., & Davis, S. (1990). Diet and the risk of pancreatic cancer in men. *American Journal of Epidemiology, 132*(3), 423–431.

Ferlay, J., Ervik, M., Lam, F., Colombet, M., Mery, L., Piñeros, M., … Bray, F. (2018). *Global cancer observatory: Cancer today.* Lyon, France: International Agency for Research on Cancer. Retrieved from https://gco.iarc.fr/today

Ferlay, J., Shin, H.-R., Bray, F., Forman, D., Mathers, C., & Parkin, D. M. (2010). Estimates of worldwide burden of cancer in 2008: GLOBOCAN 2008. *International Journal of Cancer, 127*(12), 2893–2917.

Shirvani, V. N., Ouatu-Lascar, R., Kaur, B. S., Omary, M. B., & Triadafilopoulos, G. (2000). Cyclooxygenase 2 expression in Barrett's esophagus and adenocarcinoma: *Ex vivo* induction by bile salts and acid exposure. *Gastroenterology, 118*, 487–496.

Silverman, D. T., Brown, L. M., Hoover, R. N., Schiffman, M., Lilemoe, K. D., Schoenberg, J. B., & Pottern, L. M. (1995). Alcohol and pancreatic cancer in blacks and whites in the United States. *Cancer Research, 55*(21), 4899–905.

Stolzenberg-Solomon, R. Z., Pietinen, P., Taylor, P. R., Virtamo, J., & Albanes, D. (2002). Prospective study of diet and pancreatic cancer in male smokers. *American Journal of Epidemiology, 155*(9), 783–792.

Talamini, R., Polesil, J., Gallus, S., Dal Maso, L., Zucchetto, A., Negri, E., … La Vecchia, C. (2010). Tobacco smoking, alcohol consumption and pancreatic cancer risk: A case-control study in Italy. *European Journal of Cancer, 46*(2), 370–376.

Thiébaut, A. C. M., Jiao, L., Silverman, D. T., Cross, A. J., Thompson, F. E., Subar, A. F., … Stolzenberg-Solomon, R. Z. (2009). Dietary fatty acids and pancreatic cancer in the NIH-AARP Diet and Health Study. *Journal of the National Cancer Institute, 101*, 1001–1011.

Tucker, O. N., Dannenberg, A. J., Yang, E. K., & Fahye, T. J. (2004). Bile acids induce cyclooxygenase-2 expression in human pancreatic cancer cell lines. *Carcinogenesis, 25*(3), 419–423.

Tucker, O. N., Dannenberg, A. J., Yang, E. K., Zhang, F., Teng, L., Daly, J. M., … Fahey, T. J. (1999). Cyclooxygenase-2 expression is upregulated in human pancreatic cancer. *Cancer Research, 59*, 987–990.

Wang, F., Herrington, M., Larrson, J., & Permert, J. (2003). The relationship between diabetes and pancreatic cancer. *Molecular Cancer, 2*(4), 1476–4598.

Whitcomb, D. (1999). Hereditary pancreatitis: New insights into acute and chronic pancreatitis. *Gut, 45*(3), 317–322.

Witt, H., Apte, M. V., Keim, V., & Wilson, J. S. (2007). Chronic pancreatitis: Challenges and advances in pathogenesis, genetics, diagnosis, and therapy. *Gastroenterology, 132*, 1557–1573.

World Health Organization. (2009). *Report on the global tobacco epidemic, 2009*. Geneva, Switzerland: Author.

Wynder, E. L. (1975). An epidemiological evaluation of the causes of cancer of the pancreas. *Cancer Research, 35*(8), 2228–2233.

Wynder, E. L., Mabuchi, K., & Maruchia, N. (1973). Epidemiology of cancer of the pancreas. *Journal of the National Cancer Institute, 50*, 645–667.

Yan, M. X., & Li, Y. Q. (2006). Gallstones and chronic pancreatitis: The black box in between. *Postgraduate Medical Journal, 82*, 254–258.

Ye, W., Lagergren, J., Weiderpass, E., Nyrén, O., Adami, H. O., & Ekbom, A. (2002). Alcohol abuse and the risk of pancreatic cancer. *Gut, 51*(2), 236–239.

Zatonski, W. A., Boyle, P., Przewozniak, K., Maisonneuve, P., Drosik, K., & Walker, A. M. (1993). Cigarette smoking, alcohol, tea and coffee consumption and pancreas cancer risk: A case-control study from Opole, Poland. *International Journal of Cancer, 53*(4), 601–607.

Zhang, F., Subbaramaiah, K., Altorki, N., & Dannenberg, A. J. (1998). Dihydroxy bile acids activate the transcription of cyclooxygenase-2. *Journal of Biological Chemistry, 273*, 2424–2428.

Zhang, J., Zhao, Z., & Berkel, H. J. (2005). Animal fat consumption and pancreatic cancer incidence: Evidence of interaction with cigarette smoking. *Annals of Epidemiology, 15*(7), 500–508.

CHAPTER 20

Epidemiology of Primary Liver Cancer: Hepatocellular Carcinoma and Cholangiocarcinoma

▶ Liver Function and Anatomy

The human liver is a vital organ that regulates a number of life-sustaining functions, including the synthesis of important proteins (e.g., albumin, clotting factors, and complement); metabolism and regulation of lipids, carbohydrates, and certain steroidal hormones (e.g., estrogens and androgens); synthesis and regulation of cholesterol and cholesterol byproducts (e.g., bile acids and fat-soluble vitamins A, D, E, and K); production and secretion of bile acids for digestion; the formation, storage, and release of glycogen for the regulation of blood glucose; and detoxification of chemicals and harmful substances.

The liver is located in the upper right quadrant of the abdomen. Its normal weight in adults is between 1400 and 1600 g. The liver receives a dual blood supply from the hepatic portal vein and hepatic arteries. The hepatic portal vein carries venous blood drained from the spleen and gastrointestinal tract, and the hepatic arteries supply arterial blood. Oxygen is provided from both sources (approximately half from the hepatic portal vein and half from the hepatic arteries). The gallbladder, which is located just beneath the liver,

stores and concentrates bile produced by the liver and regulates bile secretion into the duodenum for the digestion of dietary fat (O'Brien & Gottlieb, 1979) (**FIGURE 20.1**).

The liver is organized into thousands of small lobules separated by bands of connective tissue. The parenchyma (tissue) within each lobule consists primarily of polygonal hepatocytes that carry out the multiple biosynthetic and metabolic functions of the liver. The hepatocytes are arranged in microscopic functional units called acini that are distributed within the lobules. Each acinus consists of hepatocytes arranged in concentric zones about hepatic arterioles and portal venules in order to facilitate selective secretion/excretion of cellular metabolites. The products of cellular synthesis and metabolism enter the blood in the sinusoids that are adjoined to the acini. Sinusoids are vascular channels that are lined by fenestrated endothelium and heavily populated by *Kupffer cells* (see the following description).

Hepatocytes are responsible for an amazing array of biochemical functions. Their cytoplasm is laden with mitochondria that are responsible for oxidative phosphorylation and energy production, and the oxidation

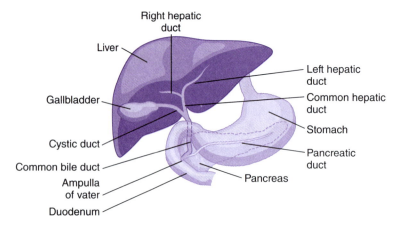

FIGURE 20.1 Anatomy of the Liver, Gallbladder, and Related Organs.

of fatty acids. Also within the cytoplasm, the smooth endoplasmic reticulum is the site of synthesis of cholesterol and bile acids; conjugation of bilirubin, drugs, and steroids; for excretion, metabolism of drugs and steroids; and breakdown of glycogen. The rough endoplasmic reticulum is the site of protein synthesis. The multiple synthetic and metabolic pathways of hepatocytes are dependent upon the presence and functional integrity of a variety of essential enzymes (e.g., the mixed function oxidase system [enzymes that oxidize toxic compounds for metabolism and excretion], cytochrome oxidase [a mitochondrial enzyme essential for respiration], and cytochrome P450 enzymes [oxidizing enzymes involved in metabolism and bioactivation of lipids, steroids, and drugs]).

The liver is the detoxification center of the human body. For example, the urea cycle metabolizes ammonia, the principle byproduct of protein breakdown. Ammonia is highly toxic to cells, whereas urea is nontoxic and readily condensed in urine by the kidneys for excretion. One of the enzymes present in hepatocytes is alcohol dehydrogenase, which catalyzes the conversion of alcohol to nontoxic metabolites for excretion. As discussed later in this chapter, genetic variability in the alcohol dehydrogenase enzyme system influences the risk of developing alcoholic cirrhosis of the liver.

Kupffer cells are large phagocytic cells of the innate immune system that circulate throughout the sinusoidal network of the liver parenchyma. They were first observed by the German scientist Karl Wilhelm von Kupffer in 1876 (Haubrich, 2004). Kupffer cells phagocytize senescent red blood cells and hepatocytes and break down hemoglobin and other cellular constituents (O'Brien & Gottlieb, 1979).

In 1951, novel fat-storage cells lining the hepatic sinusoids were discovered by Ito (1951). These *Ito cells* actively store lipids and retinoids and are apparently involved in liver fibrosis during the development and progression of cirrhosis (Geerts, 2001).

▶ Hepatocellular Carcinoma and Cholangiocarcinoma

There are two separate and distinctly different forms of primary liver cancer. Hepatocellular carcinoma arises from the cells of the liver per se (called hepatocytes) whereas cholangiocarcinoma (biliary cancer) arises from the epithelial lining of the gallbladder or the biliary ducts. Hepatocellular carcinoma is much more common than biliary cancer, accounting for approximately 93% of all primary liver cancers. Each type has its own set of epidemiologic parameters, so hepatocellular carcinoma and cholangiocarcinoma are discussed individually in the following sections of this chapter.

▶ Hepatocellular Carcinoma

Global Epidemiology of Hepatocellular Carcinoma

Hepatocellular carcinoma is the fifth most common malignancy in the world and the third most common cause of death due to cancer. During 2018, liver cancer was diagnosed in 841,080 individuals and caused 781,631 deaths in the world population. This malignancy has an extremely poor prognosis; nearly as many people die from the disease as are diagnosed. The ratio of deaths to incident cases in 2018 was 0.93. Most hepatocellular carcinomas are nonresectable at the time of diagnosis, and the disease is usually fatal within 3–6 months (American Cancer Society, 2007; Bray et al., 2018; Ferlay et al., 2010, 2013, 2018).

During the decade 2008–2018, the annual number of liver cancer cases and deaths each increased by 12.5%. In contrast, during the same period, the annual age-adjusted mortality decreased by 29% in women (from 6.5 to 4.6 per 100,000) and by 13% in men (from

14.6 to 12.7 per 100,000). The 2018 age-adjusted incidence and mortality rates in men were nearly three-fold higher than in women (Bray et al., 2018).

The 2018 age-adjusted incidence and mortality rates of liver cancer were highest in Egyptian men (49.0 and 48.2 per 100,000, respectively). The most likely cause is the high seroprevalence of hepatitis C virus (HCV) in the Egyptian population. It is widely accepted that HCV was inadvertently introduced and spread in the Egyptian population during 1950–1980 by a mass program of contaminated parenteral injections of tartrate compounds for the treatment of schistosomiasis. Liver cancer in the Egyptian population

can therefore be viewed as an iatrogenic effect of this program (Frank et al., 2000).

Rates of liver cancer reported in 2018 were also high in sub-Saharan Africa, Eastern and Southeastern Asia, and Melanesia (South Pacific islands north of Australia) (**FIGURE 20.2**). More than 84% of new cases occurred in developing countries in areas where oncogenic liver viruses (particularly hepatitis B virus (HBV) and HCV) are endemic. Chronic exposure to aflatoxins from moldy grains and chronic alcohol abuse are independent risk factors that can synergistically interact with oncogenic hepatitis viruses to markedly heighten the risk of developing hepatocellular

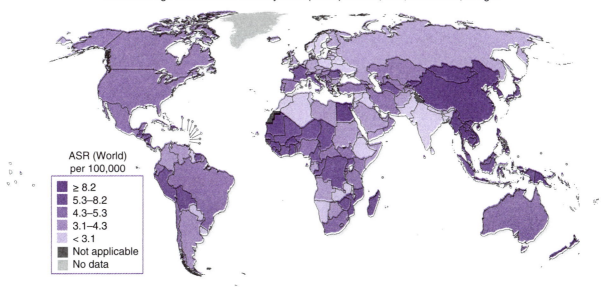

FIGURE 20.2 Global Incidence and Mortality of Liver Cancer, 2018.

Caption: ASR: Rates per 100,000 are age-standardized to the world population, 2000–2025.

Reproduced with permission from Ferlay, J., Ervik, M., Lam, F., Colombet, M., Mery, L., Piñeros, M., ... Bray, F. (2018). *Global cancer observatory: Cancer today.* Lyon, France: International Agency for Research on Cancer. Retrieved from https://gco.iarc.fr/today

carcinoma. The burden of hepatocellular carcinoma is particularly extreme in China, where more than half of new cases are diagnosed (Bray et al., 2018; Ferlay et al., 2010, 2013, 2018; Parkin, Bray, Ferlay, & Pisani, 2005).

Global Patterns of Hepatocellular Carcinoma

Hepatocellular carcinoma shows two main epidemiologic patterns, the predominant one being in China, sub-Saharan Africa, Southeast Asia, and the Amazon basin. In these regions, liver viruses are endemic, and the initial infection usually occurs during the perinatal period. In the populations of these regions, hepatocellular carcinomas are diagnosed early in life, sometimes during adolescence, and the peak incidence occurs before the age of 50.

A less common pattern of late onset is evident in North America and Western Europe. In the populations of these regions the onset of hepatocellular carcinoma occurs late in life, usually after the age of 60. This pattern is primarily a consequence of sustained damage to liver cells from chronic alcohol abuse or late onset viral hepatitis.

In the United States, the annual age-adjusted incidence rates of invasive liver cancer increased by more than twofold in women during 1975–2007 (from 1.6 to 3.6 cases per 100,000) and by nearly threefold in men (from 3.9 to 11.9 cases per 100,000). Consistent with their higher rates of chronic exposure to alcohol and liver viruses, incidence rates among African-American men and women exceed Caucasians' by about 75% (Alterkruse et al., 2010).

Pathogenesis of Hepatocellular Carcinoma

Hepatocellular carcinoma is initiated and promoted by sustained recursive damage to hepatocytes due to infection by oncogenic liver viruses, chronic exposure to aflatoxins, chronic alcohol abuse, or a combination of these factors. Though the exact sequence of events may differ from person to person, the cellular mechanisms involved include early fatty change (the appearance of lipid-containing vacuoles in hepatocytes), chronic inflammation and cell necrosis (termed *necroinflammation*), wound healing and regeneration of hepatocytes, and late stage fibrosis leading to the eventual formation of fibrotic nodules (cirrhosis of the liver).

The cellular processes of necroinflammation and wound healing incite several mechanisms of cancer development (mutagenesis, cell proliferation, angiogenesis, dysfunctional apoptosis, immunosuppression, and metastasis). Hepatocellular carcinoma may develop with or without liver cirrhosis; for example,

chronic viral hepatitis alone may produce cancer in a noncirrhotic liver. Cirrhosis (scarring) of the liver is invariably associated with chronic alcohol abuse, and severe cirrhosis of the liver markedly increases the risk of developing primary liver cancer, particularly in individuals suffering from chronic active hepatitis. The fibrotic nodules characteristic of alcoholic liver cirrhosis may occur in either a micronodular pattern or as large macronodules of coalesced foci of micronodules (O'Brien & Gottlieb, 1979).

Liver Viruses and Hepatocellular Carcinoma

Two liver viruses, HBV and HCV, account for 75% of the new cases of liver cancer worldwide and 85% of cases in developing countries (Parkin, Pisani, Muñoz, & Ferlay, 1999). In high-risk areas where HBV and HCV are endemic, 10%–20% of young individuals become chronic carriers of HBV or HCV. Among those who suffer from chronic viral hepatitis, the annual incidence rates per 100,000 range from 400 to 800 for men and from 120 to 180 for women (Nguyen, Law, & Dore, 2009). Among such individuals, the cumulative risk of developing hepatocellular carcinoma by age 65 years is nearly 33% in men and 10% in women.

The relative risk of developing liver cancer is increased by more than 20-fold for those chronically infected with either HBV or HCV compared to noninfected individuals and more than 100-fold for those infected by both viruses (Donato, Boffetta, & Puoti, 1998). Based on current estimates of the attributable fraction for each virus, approximately 50%–55% of hepatocellular carcinomas are caused by HBV and 20%–25% by HCV (Kirk, Bah, & Montesano, 2006). Because HBV causes far more infections than HCV, particularly in the younger generations, the global pattern of chronic HBV infections roughly simulates the global distribution of liver cancer (Hou, Liu, & Gu, 2005). It is important to note that HBV and HCV have both been classified as human carcinogens by the International Agency for Research on Cancer (IARC, 1994).

Hepatitis B Virus and Hepatocellular Carcinoma

Blumberg, Alter, and Visnich (1965) discovered the HBV by its novel "Australia antigen" in the serum of a patient with leukemia. Blumberg later developed the diagnostic test and vaccine for HBV and in 1976 was awarded the Nobel Prize in Medicine for these achievements (Blumberg, 2002). Dane first identified HBV in the serum of hepatitis patients using electron microscopy (Dane, 1970). A few years later, the genome of HBV was sequenced (Galibert, Mandart, Fitoussi, Tiollais, & Charnay, 1979) and antibody testing of viral antigens developed (Bonino, Chiaberge, Maran, & Piantino, 1987).

HBV is highly endemic in developing regions of the world that are heavily populated, such as Southeast Asia, China, sub-Saharan Africa, and the Amazon basin. In these high-risk regions, up to 95% of the population shows past or present serological evidence of HBV infection, and a significant fraction (15%–20%) become chronic carriers of the HBV surface antigen (HBsAg) (Kirk et al., 2004). The global distribution of hepatocellular carcinoma correlates with the geographic prevalence of chronic carriers of HBV, who number nearly 400 million worldwide (**FIGURE 20.3**).

Epidemiologic studies have demonstrated that there is a consistent and specific causal association between chronic HBV infection and hepatocellular carcinoma. In a landmark study, Beasley and colleagues followed 22,707 male Taiwanese health workers for more than a decade with nearly complete follow-up. Incidence rates of hepatocellular carcinoma among carriers of the HBsAg were approximately 100 times higher than among noncarriers (495 versus 5 per 100,000 per year) (Beasley, Huang, Lin, & Chien, 1981). In a meta-analysis of 32 studies, Donato et al. (1998) determined that the overall risk of developing hepatocellular carcinoma was increased by approximately 20-fold for individuals positive for the HBsAg and with no evidence of co-infection by HCV. Nevertheless, relative risk estimates from case–control and cohort studies show wide variability, ranging from 5 to 100, presumably due to genotypic differences in

HBV strains (Yu & Chen, 1994). Furthermore, the risk estimates vary depending on the presence/absence of other risk factors (e.g., HCV infection, chronic alcohol abuse, and aflatoxin exposure). These risk factors and combinations of risk factors involving HBV are discussed in the following sections of this chapter.

HBV is spread through contact with infected body fluids, and the only natural host is human. Blood is the most important vehicle for transmission, but other body fluids have also been implicated including semen, breast milk, and saliva. In regions of the world where HBV is endemic, most HBV infections occur during infancy or early childhood. Vertical transmission from mother to baby can occur during childbirth when the newborn passes through the birth canal, or later through contaminated saliva or breast milk. High rates of child-to-child transmission have also been documented in certain populations. Most acute HBV infections are asymptomatic and therefore left untreated. Because babies and young children may not have fully developed immune systems, once infected they are far more susceptible to persistence of the virus than adults. Therefore, acute HBV infections acquired during the perinatal period or early in childhood often progress to chronic infections that persist for many years (Shapiro, 1993).

Antibodies against the HBsAg develop in exposed individuals after an incubation period of a few weeks. Individuals who remain HBsAg positive for at least 6 months are considered to be hepatitis B carriers (Shapiro, 1993; Zuckerman, 1996). In young individuals who become chronic carriers of HBV, the rates of liver cancer begin to rise during adolescence and reach peak values by age 50 (Parkin et al., 2005).

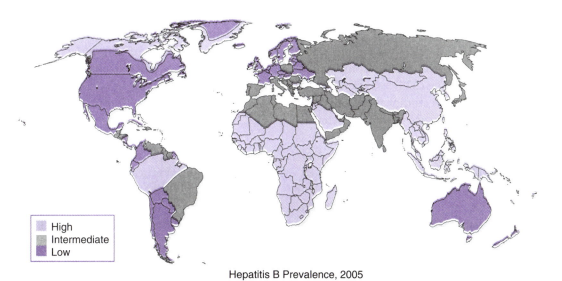

High
Intermediate
Low

Hepatitis B Prevalence, 2005

FIGURE 20.3 Global Seroprevalence of Hepatitis B Virus (HBV).

Data from Centers for Disease Control and Prevention. (2012). Infectious disease related to travel: Hepatitis B. In *CDC travelers' health yellow book*. Retrieved from http://wwwnc.cdc.gov/travel/yellowbook/2014/chapter-3-infectious-diseases-related-to-travel/hepatitis-b

Transmission of HBV in adults occurs through unprotected sexual contact with an infected individual or by using contaminated needles and syringes for the intravenous injection of illicit drugs. The virus can also be transmitted by transfusion with contaminated blood or blood products in countries without effective screening programs for donor blood. Nevertheless, immunocompetent adults who become infected by HBV usually clear the virus without treatment; less than 1% of individuals who become infected during adulthood will develop chronic hepatitis B.

The genome of HBV is made of circular DNA, but it is unusual because the DNA is not fully double-stranded. Furthermore, HBV replicates by reverse transcriptase, similar to the RNA viruses. At least four serotypes and eight genotypic strains of HBV have been identified. The process of carcinogenesis induced by chronic HBV infection involves interaction of the HBV genotype with the host immune system and infiltration of infected foci of hepatocytes by cytotoxic (killer) T lymphocytes (Zuckerman, 1996). Integration of the viral genome into the host DNA is a prominent feature of carcinogenesis that may induce overexpression of oncogenes and dysfunction of tumor suppressor genes (Kew, 1996).

Although all strains of HBV appear to be capable of sustaining long-term infections associated with liver damage, cirrhosis, and carcinogenesis, molecular epidemiologic studies suggest that there are genotypic differences in the pathogenesis of cirrhosis, carcinogenicity, and response to therapy. For example, individuals who carry genotype C are likely to have antibodies against the viral precore antigen, HBeAg, which is indicative of a high viral load and increased cirrhosis and carcinogenesis (Cao, 2009). In a prospective study of 11,893 men conducted in Taiwan (Yang et al., 2002), investigators observed a much higher incidence rate of hepatocellular carcinoma among men positive for both HBsAg and HBeAg (1169 cases per 100,000 person-years, relative risk [RR] = 60.2) compared to men positive for HBsAg alone (324 cases per 100,000 person-years, RR = 9.6). Other studies also suggest that viral load and viral replication are important determinants of liver cirrhosis and cancer risk in individuals suffering from chronic HBV infection (Chen et al., 2006; Iloeje et al., 2007). Furthermore, therapeutic trials show that individuals infected by genotypes A or B respond better to interferon therapy than individuals with other HBV genotypes (Cao, 2009). As will be discussed later in this chapter, effective vaccines that target the viral envelope (HBsAg) are now available that provide long-term immunity against HBV infection as well as protection against liver carcinogenesis (Vandamme & Van Herck, 2007).

Hepatitis C Virus and Hepatocellular Carcinoma

The studies of Harvey J. Alter and colleagues at the U.S. National Institutes of Health during the 1970s demonstrated that most patients who developed hepatitis following transfusion were not infected by either hepatitis A or B virus (Alter, 1995, 1997). Subsequently, in the laboratories of Michael Houghton, a novel virus named HCV was identified in patients with non-A non-B hepatitis (Choo et al., 1989; Kuo et al., 1989). Screening methods for detecting HCV in donor blood have markedly reduced the risk of post-transfusion hepatitis (Tanaka et al., 1994).

HCV is endemic in many parts of the world, particularly in those nations with impoverished populations, poor living conditions, and substandard sanitation. In these nations, seropositive rates range from 10% to 15% and high rates of transmission have no doubt persisted for centuries. Recent estimates suggest that HCV has infected nearly 200 million people worldwide and infects 3–4 million more people per year (World Health Organization, 2009). The seroprevalence of HCV is highest in certain countries of Africa, Asia, and South America (**FIGURE 20.4**). Egypt has the highest seroprevalence (approximately 20%), which likely resulted from the inadvertent spread of HCV by a now-discontinued mass campaign of parenteral treatment of schistosomiasis (infection by an endemic parasitic worm) (Frank et al., 2000).

HCV is transmitted by exposure to contaminated blood. In developed countries such as the United States, most infections were once caused by transfusions with contaminated blood or blood products. Fortunately, accurate methods of screening the blood supply have been developed and are in use; as a consequence, there has not been a documented posttransfusion-related case of hepatitis C in the United States for more than a decade. Currently, the primary route of HCV transmission in the United States is by intravenous injection of illicit drugs using contaminated needles (Campbell et al., 2006).

In less developed countries, the primary sources of HCV infection are unsterilized injection equipment and transfusion of inadequately screened blood and blood products. Vertical transmission from an infected mother to her child can occur during the birthing process, particularly when the mother is coinfected by the human immunodeficiency virus (HIV).

Sexual contact with an HCV-infected individual is believed to be an inefficient method of transmission; nevertheless, circumstances and any untoward events causing exposure to contaminated blood could facilitate transmission. Prison inmates are at high risk

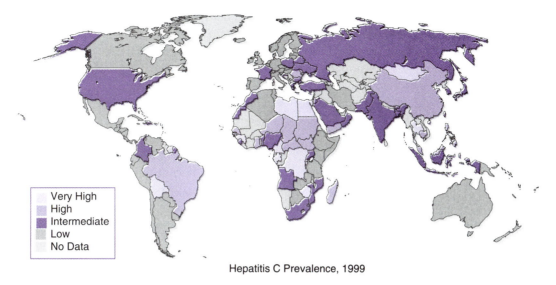

Hepatitis C Prevalence, 1999

FIGURE 20.4 Seroprevalence of Hepatitis C Virus.

Data from Centers for Disease Control and Prevention. (2012). Infectious diseases related to travel: Hepatitis C. In *CDC travelers' health yellow book*. Retrieved from http://wwwnc.cdc.gov/travel/yellowbook/2014/chapter-3-infectious-diseases-related-to-travel/hepatitis-c

of being infected either by injecting drugs using contaminated needles or by sexual transmission; a survey conducted in California found that 82% of subjects diagnosed with hepatitis C had previously been incarcerated (McGovern et al., 2006).

The HCV is a small, single-stranded RNA virus (50 nm in diameter). Like HBV and other liver viruses, HCV has a tropism for the liver, where it tends to persist in the cytoplasm of hepatocytes. Six major genotypes of HCV have been identified, and host responses to acute HCV infection vary. The virus can be detected in the blood by polymerase chain reaction (PCR) within 1–3 weeks after infection, and antibodies against HCV usually develop within 15 weeks. The acute phase of infection lasts up to 6 months and is treatable with antiviral drugs plus interferon. Chronic hepatitis C, defined as infection persisting for more than 6 months, is much more resistant to therapy (Caruntu & Benea, 2006).

The natural course of chronic hepatitis C varies considerably from one person to another. Nevertheless, HCV usually persists in the hepatocytic cell population of the liver, even in immunocompetent individuals who become infected. It is estimated that 60%–70% of infected adults will develop chronic hepatitis C. Furthermore, over a period of 10–30 years, 20%–30% of chronically infected individuals progress to liver cirrhosis and some develop hepatocellular carcinoma. Without treatment, it is estimated that more than 50% of patients with chronic hepatitis C will develop cirrhosis of the liver (National Institutes of Health, 2002). Concomitant alcohol abuse and/or co-infection with HIV are cofactors that hasten progression of liver cirrhosis. Males also tend to have more rapid disease progression than females.

FIGURE 20.5 Relative Risk of Hepatocellular Carcinoma: Effects of HBV and HCV Infection.

Data from Donato, F., Boffetta, P., & Puoti, M. A. (1998). Meta-analysis of epidemiological studies on the combined effect of hepatitis B and C virus infections in causing hepatocellular carcinoma. *International Journal of Cancer, 75*, 347–354.

Chronic hepatitis C and progressive liver cirrhosis may lead to loss of liver function and accumulation of ammonia and other toxic substances, jaundice, hepatic encephalopathy, ascites, portal hypertension, and bleeding varices. Chronic infection by HCV and subsequent cirrhosis of the liver resulting in liver failure is the leading reason for liver transplantation in the United States.

A meta-analysis of 32 studies that examined hepatocellular carcinoma and chronic hepatitis due to HBV and/or HCV provides convincing evidence that chronic infection by either virus alone markedly increases the risk of developing this malignancy and that chronic co-infection by both viruses further increases the risk (Donato et al., 1998). Two distinct patterns of risk are evident (**FIGURE 20.5**). In nations where HBV is highly endemic (sub-Saharan Africa,

China, Taiwan, South Korea, and Vietnam), HBV risk exceeds HCV risk and the markedly increased risk due to co-infection with both viruses is consistent with synergism. A different pattern is apparent in Japan and Mediterranean nations where HCV is more prominent. In these populations, HCV risk exceeds HBV risk, but the risk due to co-infection is more consistent with an additive model.

Coinfection with Human Immunodeficiency Virus and Hepatitis C Virus: Liver Cirrhosis and Hepatocellular Carcinoma

Approximately 30% of HIV-infected patients in the United States are also infected with HCV. The increasing rates of HIV and HCV co-infection have arisen due to blood-borne transmission of both viruses in association with high-risk behavior (e.g., IV drug use and unprotected sex with multiple partners). Even though overall survival has improved for HIV-infected individuals due to highly active antiretroviral therapy (HAART), it has been demonstrated in clinical studies that patients coinfected with HIV and HCV have more rapid progression of liver cirrhosis and are at increased risk of liver failure and hepatocellular carcinoma compared to those infected by only HCV (Ding, Gui, Zhang, Gao, & Yang, 2009; Giordano, Kramer, Souchek, Richardson, & El Serag, 2004). In a recent meta-analysis, Chen, Ding, Seage, and Kim (2009) observed that coinfected individuals have increased mortality primarily due to liver disease that is unrelated to HIV disease progression. Indeed, hepatocellular carcinoma has become the leading cause of non-AIDS-related death among coinfected individuals (Wilcox, 2009).

Aflatoxins and Hepatocellular Carcinoma

Aflatoxins are mycotoxins produced by certain species of the fungus *Aspergillus*, most notably *Aspergillus flavus* and *Aspergillus parasiticus*. When conditions of high humidity and heat prevail, these fungi readily colonize and contaminate grain before harvest and during storage. A wide variety of crops are frequently affected including cereals (maize, sorghum, pearl millet, rice, wheat), oilseeds (peanut, soybean, sunflower, cotton), spices (chili peppers, black pepper, coriander, turmeric, ginger), and tree nuts (almond, pistachio, walnut, coconut, brazil nut). Humans are exposed to aflatoxins by consumption of moldy grains (Williams et al., 2004). Exposure rates are highest in populations with high rates of hepatocellular carcinoma,

particularly in the nations of sub-Saharan Africa and in certain provinces of southern China (Montesano, Hainaut, & Wild, 1997).

Aflatoxins are toxic and potent carcinogens in the liver where they are metabolized to form reactive (highly mutagenic) epoxides. Among the many different forms of aflatoxins that have been identified, aflatoxin B_1, which is produced by both *Aspergillus flavus* and *Aspergillus parasiticus*, is considered the most toxic. Recent molecular studies have found that aflatoxin B_1 can specifically mutate and hence deactivate p53, a tumor suppressor gene that is critical for control of cell division (Montesano et al., 1997; Stern et al., 2001).

Chronic exposure to aflatoxins independently increases the risk of developing hepatocellular carcinoma. Early epidemiologic investigations using urinary metabolites of aflatoxins as biomarkers of exposure determined five- to sixfold increases in the risk with exposure to metabolites of aflatoxin B_1 (Ross et al., 1992; Wang et al., 1996). Furthermore, aflatoxin exposure in combination with chronic hepatitis B or C has been found to synergistically increase hepatocarcinogenesis. It is estimated that chronic exposure to aflatoxins plus concomitant liver infection by HBV increases the risk of developing hepatocellular carcinoma by up to 60-fold (Groopman, 1993; Sylla, Diallo, Castegnaro, & Wild, 1999; Yeh et al., 1989).

Alcohol Abuse, Cirrhosis of the Liver, and Hepatocellular Carcinoma

Cirrhosis of the liver is characterized by replacement of necrotic liver tissue by fibrosis, scar tissue, and regenerative nodules. The most common causes of this devastating condition are chronic alcohol abuse and chronic hepatitis due to HBV and/or HCV infection. Alcoholic cirrhosis of the liver develops in 10%–20% of individuals who drink heavily, usually for a decade or more. The process is accelerated when alcohol abuse is combined with chronic hepatitis.

Heavy chronic alcohol consumption (greater than 80 g [just under three ounces] daily for more than a decade) is estimated to increase the risk of developing hepatocellular carcinoma by more than fivefold, and if severe alcoholic liver cirrhosis develops, the risk approaches 1% per year (Morgan, Mandayam, & Jamal, 2004). Furthermore, chronic alcohol abuse in combination with chronic hepatitis C doubles the risk compared to hepatitis C alone, and even in the absence of liver cirrhosis and hepatitis, alcohol abuse increases the risk of hepatocellular carcinoma by more than fourfold (Chiesa et al., 2000). Alcohol is the primary risk factor for hepatocellular carcinoma in the populations of many developed nations, such as the United States and Italy.

Other Risk Factors for Hepatocellular Carcinoma

Acute and chronic hepatic porphyrias are inherited genetic disorders in heme biosynthesis that predispose to the development of hepatocellular carcinoma. Heme is the oxygen-binding component of hemoglobin in red blood cells and is also a key element of many enzymes of the P-450 system in the liver. This enzyme family is important in converting potentially harmful substances such as alcohol, drugs, and carcinogens to inactive metabolites destined for excretion. Thus, the pathogenesis of hepatocellular carcinoma in genetic carriers of this heme disorder may be due to inadequate detoxification and persistence of harmful substances in the liver.

In patients with acute hepatic porphyria, the calculated risk of hepatocellular carcinoma is increased 61-fold compared to normal individuals (Kauppinen & Mustajoki, 1988); furthermore, the risk increase appears to be several-fold higher in women who carry this genetic disorder compared to men (Andant, Puy, Faivre, & Deybach, 1998). Both active and latent genetic carriers of acute hepatic porphyrias are at risk, and patients with acute hepatic porphyria should be monitored for hepatocellular carcinoma.

Several other risk factors appear to modify the risk of developing hepatocellular carcinoma. These include cigarette smoking, obesity, and certain comorbid conditions such as hemochromatosis (excess deposition of iron in the liver and other organs) and Wilson's disease (excess deposition of copper in the liver). Also, vinyl chloride, a compound used in the plastics industry, can cause a rare form of liver cancer called *hepatic angiosarcoma* that appears many years after exposure (Baxter, 1976; Chuang, La Vecchia, & Boffetta, 2009).

Prevention of Hepatocellular Carcinoma

Primary prevention of the majority of liver cancer cases worldwide is now feasible, thanks to the development of a vaccine against HBV. This has been shown to be effective in preventing infection in childhood. A dramatic demonstration of the results of community vaccination is already available from Taiwan, where HBV immunization of newborns was introduced in 1984; for children ages 6–9 years in birth cohorts receiving vaccination, there was a dramatic decrease in the incidence of liver cancer (Chang et al., 1997; Thomas & Zhu, 2005).

▶ Cholangiocarcinoma

Epidemiology of Cholangiocarcinoma

Cholangiocarcinoma is an uncommon malignancy that arises from the epithelial lining of the gallbladder or bile ducts that drain bile from the liver into the small intestine. In 2018, 219,420 new cases of gallbladder cancer were diagnosed in the world population (97,396 in men and 122,024 in women), and 165,087 people died from this malignancy (70,168 men and 94,919 women). The age-standardized incidence and mortality rates per 100,000 were 2.2 and 1.6 in men, and 2.4 and 1.8 in women, respectively. Among afflicted individuals, approximately 56% were women, and the incidence and mortality rates for women were approximately 10% higher than for men. As discussed in a later section of this chapter, the higher rates in women may be partially attributable to their higher rates of cholelithiases (gallstones and biliary stones) compared to men.

During the decade 2008–2018, the annual number of new cases and deaths from cholangiocarcinoma each increased by 51%. Increases in the annual incidence and mortality rates also occurred during this period, e.g., both rates increased by 23% in men and approximately 10% in women (Bray et al., 2018; Ferlay et al., 2010). These global trends reflect the impact of multiple factors including population growth and aging, as well as potential increases in predisposing risk factors.

The annual incidence of cholangiocarcinoma is high in China and other regions of Southeast Asia, which is attributable to endemic liver parasites. The annual incidence in northern Thailand has been estimated at 135 per 100,000 in men and 43 per 100,000 in women compared to only 1–2 cases per 100,000 in the United States (Green et al., 1991). The incidence is also high in other regions in which liver flukes are endemic (e.g., the Caribbean, Andean nations of South America, North Africa, and the Middle East) (**FIGURE 20.6**). Without complete resection, cholangiocarcinoma has an extremely poor prognosis; as a consequence, the mortality/incidence ratio is high (~0.80), and mortality and incidence rates show similar patterns (Ferlay et al., 2010, 2013, 2018).

Global Trends in Cholangiocarcinoma

Cholangiocarcinoma is divisible into intrahepatic and extrahepatic disease. Intrahepatic disease refers to the gallbladder and ducts within the liver, whereas extrahepatic disease refers only to the biliary ducts outside the liver.

Estimated age-standardized incidence rates (World) in 2018, gallbladder, both sexes, all ages

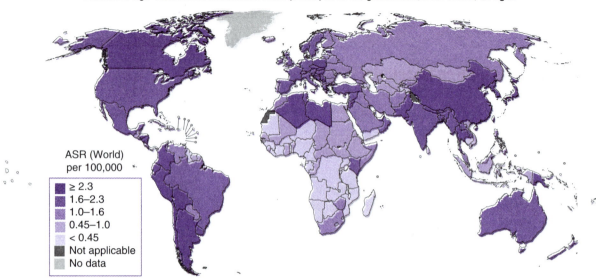

Estimated age-standardized mortality rates (World) in 2018, gallbladder, both sexes, all ages

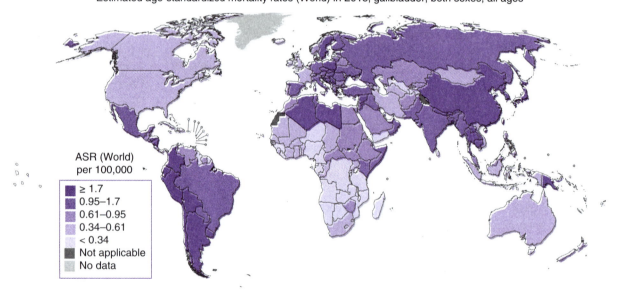

FIGURE 20.6 Global Incidence and Mortality Rates of Cholangiocarcinoma, 2018.

Caption: ASR: Rates per 100,000 are age-standardized to the world population, 2000–2025.

Reproduced with permission from Ferlay, J., Ervik, M., Lam, F., Colombet, M., Mery, L., Piñeros, M., ... Bray, F. (2018). *Global cancer observatory: Cancer today*. Lyon, France: International Agency for Research on Cancer. Retrieved from https://gco.iarc.fr/today

Patel examined chronological trends in the annual mortality rates of each subtype using data reported by the World Health Organization during 1980–1997. Mortality estimates were available for the men and women of 22 nations with population-based tumor registries. Regions represented included North America, Australia/New Zealand, Western Europe, Central Europe, Scandinavia, Asia, and the Middle East. Trend analysis revealed that the mortality rates of people with intrahepatic tumors increased on average by 6.9% per year in men and 5.1% in women, whereas the rates for those with extrahepatic tumors declined by 0.3% in men and 1.3% women. The reasons for the increasing occurrence of intrahepatic

cholangiocarcinoma are unclear; improved diagnostic methods may be partially responsible, but the prevalence of potential risk factors for cholangiocarcinoma such as HBV and HCV infections have also been increasing in some populations during this time frame. The diverging trends of these two subtypes of cholangiocarcinoma may be related to the high rate of cholecystectomies to remove symptomatic gallstones in some populations (Patel, 2001, 2002).

Risk Factors for Cholangiocarcinoma

Chronic biliary tract inflammation is a major risk factor for the development of cholangiocarcinoma.

The association between chronic parasitic infection of the biliary tract and cholangiocarcinoma is obvious in regions of high endemicity (e.g., in Far Eastern nations such as Taiwan). Additional risk factors in underserved nations include viral hepatitis and HIV disease. In Western nations there is a distinctly different profile of risk factors including alcoholic and nonalcoholic cirrhosis of the liver, congenital liver abnormalities (choledochal cysts), hepatolithiasis (liver stones), and cholelithiasis (gallstones).

Liver Flukes and Cholangiocarcinoma

In certain regions of Southeast Asia, North Africa, and South America, chronic colonization of the liver and biliary tract by liver flukes is a major public health problem. The technical term for this parasitic infection is *fasciolosis*. Two species of liver flukes, *Opisthorchis viverrini* (found in Thailand, Laos, and Malaysia) and *Clonorchis sinensis* (found in Japan, Korea, and Vietnam) markedly heighten the risk of developing cholangiocarcinoma (Watanapa, 1996; Watanapa & Watanapa, 2002). The highest annual incidence rates (334 and 104 per 100,000 for males and females, respectively) were observed in the northern Thailand province of Khon Kaen, where *O. viverrini* is endemic (Green et al., 1991). In an epidemiologic study in Pusan, Korea, infection by *Clonorchis sinensis* was associated with a threefold increase in the risk (Shin et al., 1996).

Fasciolosis is also a human health problem in Central America (Puerto Rico, Cuba, and Caribbean islands), the Andean countries of South America (Bolivia, Peru, Ecuador, and Bolivia), and coastal regions of North Africa and the Middle East. The life cycle of liver flukes involves a larval stage in snails and an encysted larval stage (metacercaria) in fish. Human infection results from the consumption of uncooked (raw) freshwater fish contaminated with the metacercarial form of the parasite (Markell & Voge, 1976).

In a recent meta-analysis of case–control studies of cholangiocarcinoma, the odds ratios (ORs) were highest for individuals chronically infected with liver flukes (summary OR = 4.8) but also consistently elevated for individuals with hepatitis B (summary OR = 2.6) or hepatitis C (summary OR = 1.8) (Shin et al., 2010).

Primary Sclerosing Cholangitis and Cholangiocarcinoma

In developed countries such as the United States, the most common risk factor for the development of cholangiocarcinoma is the presence of *primary sclerosing cholangitis*, a rare inflammatory disease of the bile ducts. Primary sclerosing cholangitis has a prevalence in the United States of 6 per 100,000 people. The mean age at diagnosis is 40 years of age, and 70% of cases are men. The development of primary sclerosing cholangitis is associated with other inflammatory conditions such as ulcerative colitis and Crohn's disease. Epidemiologic investigations suggest that up to 30% of individuals with primary sclerosing cholangitis may eventually develop cholangiocarcinoma (Rosen, Nagorney, Wiesner, Coffey, & LaRusso, 1991).

Cholelithiasis and Cholangiocarcinoma

Cholelithiasis refers to biliary stones in either the gallbladder or the biliary ducts. Biliary stones are formed by solidification of bile components, principally cholesterol. Cholesterol stones are predominantly found in women and obese individuals. If left untreated, these formations may cause obstruction of the biliary tree and chronic inflammation and malignant transformation of the biliary epithelium. Approximately one-third of patients who develop cholangiocarcinoma report a medical history of cholelithiasis. However, due to the high prevalence of cholelithiasis in many populations, some have argued that its association with cholangiocarcinoma is spurious rather than etiologic.

To clarify the risk factors for cholangiocarcinoma, investigators in Taiwan conducted a large case–control study of 5157 cases of cholangiocarcinoma and 20,628 disease-free controls matched to the cases by age, gender, and time of diagnosis. In the analysis, cases and their matched controls were subdivided into intrahepatic cholangiocarcinoma (within the gallbladder and liver) and extrahepatic cholangiocarcinoma (within the biliary ducts outside the liver). Results revealed that multiple inflammatory and cystic conditions are associated with substantial increases in the risk for the development of both intrahepatic and extrahepatic cholangiocarcinoma. Risk factors included medical history of choledochal cysts, cholangitis, cholecystitis, and cholelithiasis. After adjustment for other factors, cholelithiasis increased the risk of intrahepatic cholangiocarcinoma (OR = 4.3) and extrahepatic cholangiocarcinoma (OR = 3.3). Other major independent risk factors included cirrhosis of the liver and viral hepatitis (Chang, Tsai, & Chen, 2013).

Ionizing Radiation and Cholangiocarcinoma

Thorotrast, a radiologic contrast medium, was widely used throughout the world from 1920 to 1950. This ionizing compound has a half-life of 400 years and is retained in the liver, where it caused the eventual development of cholangiocarcinoma in some patients many years after their exposure. Thorotrast was banned from use in the United States in the 1950s due to its carcinogenicity (Zhu, Lauwers, & Tanabe, 2004).

Prevention and Control of Cholangiocarcinoma

Cholangiocarcinoma is difficult to diagnose and frequently presents at a later stage when no effective therapeutic intervention is possible. Primary prevention is therefore critical to reduce the risk of developing this malignancy. In areas endemic for liver flukes, effective prevention involves control of foodborne infection and/or mass anthelmintic therapy. Other strategies include avoidance of excessive alcohol intake, elimination of tobacco use, vaccination against HBV, prevention of HCV and HIV transmission, and excision of the gallbladder and common bile duct in patients with obstructive/inflammatory conditions of the biliary tree.

References

Alter, M. J. (1995). Epidemiology of hepatitis C in the West. *Seminars in Liver Disease, 15*, 5–14.

Alter, M. J. (1997). Epidemiology of hepatitis C. *Hepatology, 3*(Suppl. 1), 62S–65S.

Alterkruse, S. F., Kosary, C. L., Krapcho, M., Neyman, N., Aminou, R., Waldron, W., … Edwards, B. K. (2010). *SEER cancer statistics review, 1975–2007.* Bethesda, MD: Surveillance Epidemiology and End Results, National Cancer Institute, National Institutes of Health.

American Cancer Society. (2007). *Global cancer facts and figures, 2007.* Atlanta, GA: Author.

Andant, C., Puy, H., Faivre, J., & Deybach, J. C. (1998). Acute hepatic porphyrias and primary liver cancer. *New England Journal of Medicine, 338*, 1853–1854.

Baxter, P. J. (1976). Epidemiological studies of PVC manufacturers and fabricators, and primary angiosarcoma of the liver. *Proceedings of the Royal Society of Medicine, 69*(4), 297–299.

Beasley, R. P., Huang, L. Y., Lin, C., & Chien, C. (1981). Hepatocellular carcinoma and HBV: A prospective study of 22,707 men in Taiwan. *Lancet, 2*, 1129–1133.

Blumberg, B. S. (2002). Baruch Blumberg—Hepatitis B and beyond. Interviewed by Pam Das. *Lancet Infectious Diseases, 2*(12), 767–771.

Blumberg, B. S., Alter, H. J., & Visnich, S. (1965). A 'new' antigen in leukemia sera. *Journal of the American Medical Association, 252*(2), 252–257.

Bonino, F., Chiaberge, E., Maran, E., & Piantino, P. (1987). Serological markers of HBV infectivity. *Annali dell'Istituto Superiore di Sanità, 24*(2), 217–223.

Bray, F., Ferlay, J., Soerjomataram, I., Siegel, R. L., Torre, L. A., & Jemal, A. (2018). Global cancer statistics 2018: GLOBOCAN estimates of incidence and mortality worldwide for 36 cancers in 185 countries. *CA: A Cancer Journal for Clinicians, 68*(6), 394–424.

Campbell, J., Hagan, H., Latka, M., Garfein, R., Golub, E., Coady, M., … Strathdee, S. A. (2006). High prevalence of alcohol use among hepatitis C virus antibody positive injection drug users in three U.S. cities. *Drug and Alcohol Dependence, 81*(3), 259–265.

Cao, G. W. (2009). Clinical relevance and public health significance of hepatitis B virus genomic variations. *World Journal of Gastroenterology, 15*(46), 5761–5769.

Caruntu, F. A., & Benea, L. (2006). Acute hepatitis C virus infection: Diagnosis, pathogenesis, treatment. *Journal of Gastrointestinal and Liver Diseases, 15*(3), 249–256.

Chang, J. S., Tsai, C.-R., & Chen, L.-T. (2013). Medical risk factors associated with cholangiocarcinoma in Taiwan: A population-based case-control study. *PLoS ONE, 8*(7), e69981. doi:10.1371/journal.pone.0069981.

Chang, M. H., Chen, C. J., Lai, M. S., Hsu, H. M., Wu, T. C., Kong, M. S., … Chen, D. S. (1997). Universal hepatitis B vaccination in Taiwan and the incidence of hepatocellular carcinoma in children. *New England Journal of Medicine, 336*(26), 1855–1859.

Chen, C. J., Yang, H. I., Su, J., Jen, C.-L., You, S. L., Lu, S. N., … Iloeje, U. H. (2006). Risk of hepatocellular carcinoma across a biological gradient of serum hepatitis B virus DNA level. *Journal of the American Medical Association, 295*(1), 65–73.

Chen, T. Y., Ding, E. L., Seage, G. R., III., & Kim, A. Y. (2009). Meta-analysis: Increased mortality associated with hepatitis C in HIV-infected persons is unrelated to HIV disease progression. *Clinical Infectious Diseases, 49*(10), 1605–1615.

Chiesa, R., Donato, F., Tagger, A., Favret, M., Ribero, M. L., Nardi, G., … Callea, F. (2000). Etiology of hepatocellular carcinoma in Italian patients with and without cirrhosis. *Cancer Epidemiology, Biomarkers and Prevention, 9*, 213–216.

Choo, Q., Kuo, G., Weiner, A., Overby, L., Bradley, D., & Houghton, M. (1989). Isolation of a cDNA clone derived from a blood-borne non-A, non-B viral hepatitis genome. *Science, 244*(4902), 359–362.

Chuang, S.-C., La Vecchia, C., & Boffetta, P. (2009). Liver cancer: Descriptive epidemiology and risk factors other than HBV and HCV infection. *Cancer Letters, 286*, 9–14.

Dane, D. (1970). Virus-like particles in serum of patients with Australia-antigen-associated hepatitis. *Lancet, 295*, 695–698.

Ding, L. P., Gui, X. E., Zhang, Y. X., Gao, S. C., & Yang, R. R. (2009). Impact of human immunodeficiency virus infection on the course of hepatitis C virus infection. A meta-analysis. *World Journal of Gastroenterology, 28*(3), 996–1008.

Donato, F., Boffetta, P., & Puoti, M. A. (1998). Meta-analysis of epidemiological studies on the combined effect of hepatitis B and C virus infections in causing hepatocellular carcinoma. *International Journal of Cancer, 75*, 347–354.

Ferlay, J., Ervik, M., Lam, F., Colombet, M., Mery, L., Piñeros, M., … Bray, F. (2018). *Global cancer observatory: Cancer today.* Lyon, France: International Agency for Research on Cancer. Retrieved from https://gco.iarc.fr/today.

Ferlay, J., Shin, H.-R., Bray, F., Forman, D., Mathers, C., & Parkin, D. M. (2010). Estimates of worldwide burden of cancer in 2008: GLOBOCAN 2008. *International Journal of Cancer, 127*(12), 2893–2917.

Ferlay, J., Soerjomataram, I., Ervik, M., Dikshit, R., Eser, S., Mathers, C., ... Bray, F. (2013). *GLOBOCAN 2012 v1.0. Cancer incidence and mortality worldwide: IARC CancerBase No. 11* [Internet]. Lyon, France: International Agency for Research on Cancer. Retrieved from http://globocan.iarc.fr

Frank, C., Mohamed, M., Strickland, G., Lavanchy, D., Arthur, R., Magder, L., ... Sallam, I. (2000). The role of parenteral anti-schistosomal therapy in the spread of hepatitis C virus in Egypt. *Lancet, 355*(9207), 887–891.

Galibert, F., Mandart, E., Fitoussi, F., Tiollais, P., & Charnay, P. (1979). Nucleotide sequence of the hepatitis B virus genome (subtype ayw) cloned in *E. coli. Nature, 281*(5733), 646.

Geerts, A. (2001). History, heterogeneity, developmental biology and functions of quiescent hepatic stellate cells. *Seminars in Liver Disease, 21*, 311–335.

Giordano, T. P., Kramer, J. R., Souchek, J., Richardson, P., & El Serag, H. B. (2004). Cirrhosis and hepatocellular carcinoma in HCV-infected veterans with and without hepatitis C virus: A cohort study, 1992–2001. *Archives of Internal Medicine, 164*, 2249–2254.

Green, A., Uttaravichien, T., Bhudhisawasdi, V., Chartbanchachai, W., Elkins, D. B., Marieng, E. O., ... Haswell-Elkins, M. R. (1991). Cholangiocarcinoma in northeast Thailand. A hospital-based study. *Tropical and Geographical Medicine, 43*(1–2), 193–198.

Groopman, J. D. (1993). Molecular dosimetry methods for assessing human aflatoxin exposure. In D. L. Easton & J. D. Groopman (Eds.), *The toxicology of aflatoxins: Human health, veterinary and agricultural significance* (pp. 259–279). London: Academic Press.

Haubrich, W. S. (2004). Kupffer of Kupffer cells. *Gastroenterology, 127*(1), 16.

Hou, J., Liu, Z., & Gu, F. (2005). Epidemiology and prevention of hepatitis B virus infection. *International Journal of Medical Sciences, 2*, 50–57.

Iloeje, U. H., Yang, H. I., Jen, C. L., Su, J., Wang, L. Y., You, S. L., & Chen, C. J. (2007). Risk and predictors of mortality associated with chronic hepatitis B infection. *Clinical Gastroenterology and Hepatology, 5*(8), 921–931.

International Agency for Research on Cancer. (1994). IARC monographs on the evaluation of carcinogenic risks in humans. *International Agency for Research on Cancer, 59*, 1–253.

Ito, T. (1951). Cytological studies on stellate cells of Kupffer and fat storing cells in the capillary wall of human liver (abstract). *Acta Anatomica Japan, 26*, 42.

Kauppinen, R., & Mustajoki, P. (1988). Acute hepatic porphyria and hepatocellular carcinoma. *British Journal of Cancer, 57*(1), 117–120.

Kew, M. C. (1996). Hepatitis B and C viruses and hepatocellular carcinoma. *Clinics in Laboratory Medicine, 16*, 395–406.

Kirk, G. D., Bah, E., & Montesano, R. (2006). Molecular epidemiology of human liver cancer: Insights into etiology, pathogenesis and prevention from The Gambia, West Africa. *Carcinogenesis, 27*(10), 2070–2082.

Kirk, G. D., Lesi, O. A., Mendy, M., Akano, A. O., Sam, O., Goedert, J. J., ... Montesano, W. H. (2004). The Gambia Liver Cancer Study: Infection with hepatitis B and C and the risk of hepatocellular carcinoma in West Africa. *Hepatology, 39*(1), 211–219.

Kuo, G., Choo, Q., Alter, H., Gitnick, G., Redeker, A., Purcell, R., ... Houghton, M. (1989). An assay for circulating antibodies to a major etiologic virus of human non-A, non-B hepatitis. *Science, 244*(4902), 362–364.

Markell, E. K., & Voge, M. (1976). *Medical parasitology* (4th ed.). Philadelphia, PA: W. B. Saunders.

McGovern, B., Wurcel, A., Kim, A., Schulze zur Wiesch, J., Bica, I., Zaman, M., ... Lauer, G. (2006). Acute hepatitis C virus infection in incarcerated injection drug users. *Clinics in Infectious Diseases, 42*(12), 1663–1670.

Montesano, R., Hainaut, P., & Wild, C. P. (1997). Hepatocellular carcinoma: From gene to public health. *Journal of the National Cancer Institute, 898*, 1844–1851.

Morgan, T. R., Mandayam, S., & Jamal, M. M. (2004). Alcohol and hepatocellular carcinoma. *Gastroenterology, 127*(5 Suppl. 1), S87–S96.

National Institutes of Health. (2002). NIH consensus statement on management of hepatitis C. *Science Statements, 19*(3), 1–46.

Nguyen, V. T. T., Law, M. G., & Dore, G. J. (2009). Hepatitis B-related hepatocellular carcinoma: Epidemiological characteristics and disease burden. *Journal of Viral Hepatitis, 16*(7), 453–463.

O'Brien, M., Gottlieb, L. S. (1979). The liver and biliary tract. In S. L. Robbins & R. S. Cotran (Eds.), *Pathologic Basis of Disease* (pp. 1009–1091). Philadelphia: W.B. Saunders.

Parkin, D. M., Bray, F., Ferlay, J., & Pisani, P. (2005). Global cancer statistics, 2002. *CA: A Cancer Journal for Clinicians, 55*, 74–108.

Parkin, D. M., Pisani, P., Muñoz, N., & Ferlay, J. (1999). The global health burden of infection associated cancer. In R. A. Weiss, V. Beral, & R. Newton (Eds.), *Infections and human cancer: Cancer surveys* (Vol. 33, pp. 5–33). New York, NY: Cold Spring Harbor Laboratory Press.

Patel, T. (2001). Increasing incidence and mortality of primary intrahepatic cholangiocarcinoma in the United States. *Hepatology, 33*(6), 1353–1357.

Patel, T. (2002). Worldwide trends in mortality from biliary tract malignancies. *BMC Cancer, 2.* doi:10.1186/1471-2407-2-10.

Rosen, C., Nagorney, D., Wiesner, R., Coffey, R., & LaRusso, N. (1991). Cholangiocarcinoma complicating primary sclerosing cholangitis. *Annals of Surgery, 213*(1), 21–25.

Ross, R. K., Yuan, J. M., Yu, M. C., Wogan, G. N., Qian, G. S., Tu, J. T., ... Groopman, J. D. (1992). Urinary aflatoxin biomarkers and risk of hepatocellular carcinoma. *Lancet, 339*(8799), 943–946.

Shapiro, C. N. (1993). Epidemiology of hepatitis B. *Pediatric Infectious Disease Journal, 12*(5), 433–437.

Shin, H., Lee, C., Park, H., Seol, S., Chung, J., Choi, H., ... Shigemastu, T. (1996). Hepatitis B and C virus, *Clonorchis sinensis* for the risk of liver cancer: A case-control study in Pusan, Korea. *International Journal of Epidemiology, 25*(5), 933–940.

Shin, H. R., Oh, J. K., Masuyer, E., Curado, M. P., Bouvard, V., Fang, Y. Y., ... Hong, S. T. (2010). Epidemiology of cholangiocarcinoma: An update focusing on risk factors. *Cancer Science, 101*(3), 579–585.

Stern, M. C., Umbach, D. M., Yu, M. C., London, S. J., Zhang, Z. Q., & Taylor, J. A. (2001). Hepatitis B, aflatoxin B(1), and p53 codon 249 mutation in hepatocellular carcinomas from Guangxi, People's Republic of China, and a meta-analysis of existing studies. *Cancer Epidemiology, Biomarkers and Prevention, 10*(6), 617–625.

Sylla, A., Diallo, M. S., Castegnaro, J. J., & Wild, C. P. (1999). Interactions between hepatitis B virus infection and exposure to aflatoxins with the development of hepatocellular carcinoma: A molecular epidemiological approach. *Mutation Research, 428*, 187–196.

Tanaka, H., Hiyama, T., Tsukuma, H., Okubo, Y., Yamano, H., Kitada, A., & Fujimoto, I. (1994). Prevalence of second generation antibody to hepatitis C antibody among voluntary blood donors in Osaka, Japan. *Cancer Causes and Control, 5,* 409–413.

Thomas, M., & Zhu, A. (2005). Hepatocellular carcinoma: The need for progress. *Journal of Clinical Oncology, 23*(13), 2892–2899.

Vandamme, P., & Van Herck, K. (2007). A review of the long-term protection after hepatitis A and B vaccination. *Travel Medicine and Infectious Disease, 5*(2), 79–84.

Wang, L. Y., Hatch, M., Chen, C. J., Levin, B., You, S. L., Lu, S. N., … Santella, R. M. (1996). Aflatoxin exposure and risk of hepatocellular carcinoma in Taiwan. *International Journal of Cancer, 67*(5), 620–625.

Watanapa, P. (1996). Cholangiocarcinoma in patients with opisthorchiasis. *British Journal of Surgery, 83*(8), 1062–1064.

Watanapa, P., & Watanapa, W. (2002). Liver fluke-associated cholangiocarcinoma. *British Journal of Surgery, 89*(8), 962–970.

Wilcox, R. D. (2009). Hepatocellular carcinoma and HIV: Is there an association? *HIV Clinician, 21*(4), 11–12.

Williams, J. H., Phillips, T. D., Jolly, P. E., Stiles, J. K., Jolly, C. M., & Aggarwal, D. (2004). Human aflatoxicosis in developing countries: A review of toxicology, exposure, potential health consequences, and interventions. *American Journal of Clinical Nutrition, 80*(5), 1106–1122.

World Health Organization. (2009). *Death and DALY estimates for 2004 by cause for WHO member states (persons, all ages).* Geneva, Switzerland: Author.

Yang, H. I., Lu, S. N., Liaw, Y. F., You, S. L., Su, C. A., Wang, L. Y., … Chen, C. J. (2002). Hepatitis B e antigen and the risk of hepatocellular carcinoma. *New England Journal of Medicine, 347*(3), 168–174.

Yeh, F. S., Yu, M. C., Mo, C. C., Luo, S., Tong, M. J., & Henderson, B. E. (1989). Hepatitis B virus, aflatoxins, and hepatocellular carcinoma in southern Guangxi, China. *Cancer Research, 49,* 2506–2509.

Yu, M. W., & Chen, C. J. (1994). Hepatitis B and C viruses in the development of hepatocellular carcinoma. *Critical Reviews in Oncology/Hematology, 17,* 71–91.

Zhu, A., Lauwers, G., & Tanabe, K. (2004). Cholangiocarcinoma in association with Thorotrast exposure. *Journal of Hepato-Biliary-Pancreatic Surgery, 11*(6), 430–433.

Zuckerman, A. J. (1996). Hepatitis viruses. In S. Baron et al. (Eds.), *Baron's medical microbiology* (4th ed., pp. 849–863). Galveston, TX: University of Texas Medical Branch.

CHAPTER 21

Epidemiology of Breast Cancer

▶ Anatomy and Function of the Mammary Gland

The human female breast consists primarily of fat and glandular tissues. Each breast contains a complex network of sac-like lobules (milk glands) that produce breast milk and ducts that carry milk from the lobules to the nipple openings during breastfeeding. Adult women have 15–20 distinct clusters of lobules in each breast, which are called the breast lobes. Each breast lobe contains 20–40 lobules. Small ducts emanate from the lobules of the breast and join together and branch into increasingly larger ducts that carry breast milk to openings at the surface of the nipple. Adipose tissue (fat) furnishes the energy for lactation and is the most abundant tissue of the human female breast. Connective tissue and ligaments provide structural support and nerves provide sensation to the breast. The breast also contains blood vessels, lymph vessels, and lymph nodes (**FIGURE 21.1**).

In both males and females, immature breast tissues develop during embryogenesis and childhood; however, further development and maturation of the breast occurs exclusively in females in preparation for reproduction and lactation. Development and maturation of the human female breast begins at puberty concurrent with the onset of menarche, usually around 11–12 years of age. Under the primary influence of ovarian steroidal hormones (estrogen and progesterone) and the pituitary hormone prolactin, a complex network of breast lobes, milk glands (lobules), and milk ducts develops. These glandular structures are surrounded and interlaced by abundant adipose tissue.

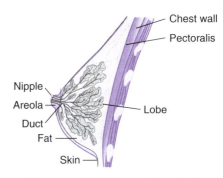

FIGURE 21.1 Anatomy of the Human Female Breast.

Mature breast development is typically complete by the age of 17–18 years. During the first pregnancy, the milk glands undergo further maturation in preparation for lactation. Lactation (the secretion and excretion of breast milk) following childbirth is stimulated by the pituitary hormones, oxytocin and prolactin. Concurrent with aging, the onset of menopause, and the depletion of ovarian hormones, the breast undergoes involution characterized by a decrease in glandular breast tissue and a relative increase in the surrounding adipose tissue (Hutson, Cowan, & Bird, 1985).

▶ Global Burden of Breast Cancer

Among women, breast cancer is the most commonly diagnosed cancer and the leading cause of cancer death. Invasive breast cancer was diagnosed in 2,088,849 women in 2018 and caused 626,679 deaths. Globally, breast cancer has now surpassed lung cancer as the leading cause of cancer death among women (Bray et al., 2018; Ferlay et al., 2010, 2013, 2018).

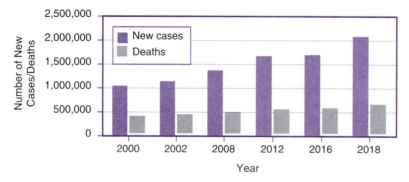

FIGURE 21.2 Global Increase in Breast Cancer, 2000–2018.

Data from Parkin, D. M., Bray, F., Ferlay, J., & Pisani, P. (2001). Estimating the world cancer burden: GLOBOCAN 2000. *International Journal of Cancer, 94,* 153–156; Ferlay, J., Bray, F., Pisani, P., & Parkin, D. M. (2004). *GLOBOCAN 2002. Cancer incidence, mortality, and prevalence worldwide.* IARC Cancer Base No. 5, version 2.0. Lyon, France: IARC Press. Retrieved from http://www-dep.iarc.fr; Ferlay, J., Shin, H.-R., Bray, F., Forman, D., Mathers, C., & Parkin, D. M. (2010). Estimates of worldwide burden of cancer in 2008: GLOBOCAN 2008. *International Journal of Cancer, 127*(12), 2893–2917; Ferlay, J., Soerjomataram, I., Ervik, M., Dikshit, R., Eser, S., Mathers, C., ... Bray, F. (2013). *GLOBOCAN 2012 v1.0. Cancer incidence and mortality worldwide: IARC CancerBase No. 11.* [Internet]. Lyon, France: International Agency for Research on Cancer. Retrieved from http://globocan.iarc.fr; Fitzmaurice, C., Allen, C., Barber, R. M., et al., Global Burden of Disease Cancer Collaboration. (2017). Global, regional, and national cancer incidence, mortality, years of life lost, years lived with disability, and disability-adjusted life-years for 32 cancer groups, 1990 to 2015: A systematic analysis for the Global Burden of Disease Study. *JAMA Oncology, 3*(4), 524–548; Fitzmaurice, C., Akinyemiju, T. F., Al Lami, F. H., et al., Global Burden of Disease Cancer Collaboration. (2018). Global, regional, and national cancer incidence, mortality, years of life lost, years lived with disability, and disability-adjusted life-years for 29 cancer groups, 1990 to 2016: A systematic analysis for the Global Burden of Disease Study. *JAMA Oncology.* Published online June 02, 2018. doi:10.1001/jamaoncol.2018.2706.

The global burden of breast cancer has increased sharply in the 21st century. During the time span 2000–2018, the reported annual numbers of new cases and deaths increased by 98% and 68%, respectively, and the age-adjusted annual incidence rate rose by approximately 19% (**FIGURE 21.2**). In 2018, the age-adjusted incidence rate of breast cancer in women was 46.3 per 100,000 and the mortality rate was 13.0 per 100,000. Breast cancer is rare in men, with annual incidence rates of less than 1 per 100,000 (Bray et al., 2018; Bray, McCarron, & Parkin, 2004; Ferlay et al., 2010, 2013, 2018; Fitzmaurice et al., 2017, 2018; Parkin, Bray, Ferlay, & Pisani, 2001).

As discussed in the following sections of this chapter, the rising worldwide burden of breast cancer undoubtedly reflects the impact of multiple factors, including population growth, increasing longevity, enhanced screening (mammography), therapy, and changes in risk factors including late childbearing, lack of breastfeeding, intake of exogenous hormones, intake of diets high in fat and calories, lack of exercise, and increasing obesity (Bray et al., 2004; Harris, Casto, & Harris, 2014).

As shown in **FIGURE 21.3**, the age-adjusted incidence rates of breast cancer in 2018 were highly variable among the 185 member nations of the World Health Organization (WHO) that reported data to the International Agency for Cancer Research (IARC), ranging from relatively low rates of 20–40 per 100,000 women in developing countries of Asian and Africa to markedly higher rates of 80–110 cases per 100,000 in developed countries of North America, Europe, and Australia/New Zealand. The lifetime risk of breast cancer was also higher among women living in developed versus developing countries, e.g., 1 in 8 for U.S. women compared to 1 in 66 for Chinese women. Despite the extreme variability in the incidence rates

among nations, breast cancer was the most commonly diagnosed malignancy in the women of 154 of the 185 member nations of WHO (Bray et al., 2018; Ferlay, Bray, Pisani, & Parkin, 2004; Ferlay et al., 2010, 2013, 2018; Garcia et al., 2007).

Breast cancer mortality rates in 2018 showed a much narrower range than the incidence rates. In general, incidence rates of breast cancer were higher in women living in developed countries compared to those in underdeveloped countries (54 versus 31 per 100,000), whereas mortality rates were higher in less developed nations where access to screening and therapy is limited (14.9 versus 11.6 per 100,000) (Figure 21.3). Nevertheless, breast cancer was the leading cause of cancer death in the women of 103 of the 185 member nations of WHO (Ferlay et al., 2018). Fiji, a small island in the Southwest Pacific, had the highest breast cancer mortality in 2018 (36.9 per 100,000), and it is notable that the prevalence of obesity among *iTaukei* women who are native to Fiji is currently about 60% (Lin et al., 2016).

▶ Breast Cancer Detection, Staging, and Survival

Mammography is a radiographic imaging process using low-dose X-rays to assist in the detection and diagnosis of breast cancer. The goal of mammography as a screening tool is to detect breast tumors early in their growth and development so they can be completely excised by qualified breast surgeons. Screening mammography together with effective biopsy, accurate pathologic evaluation, and surgical excision of breast tumors have been shown to reduce the mortality from breast cancer by approximately 30% in women over the age of 50 years. Because of the difficulty in discriminating normal active mammary glands from

Estimated age-standardized incidence rates (World) in 2018, breast, all ages

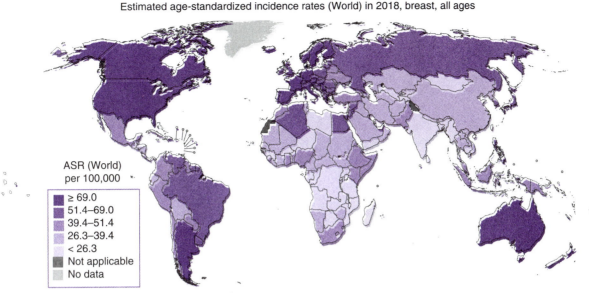

Estimated age-standardized mortality rates (World) in 2018, breast, all ages

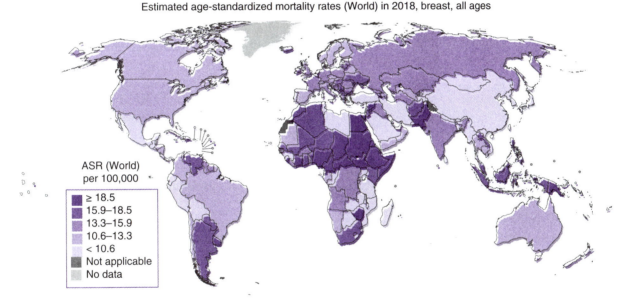

FIGURE 21.3 Global Incidence and Mortality Rates of Breast Cancer, 2018.

Caption: ASR: Rates per 100,000 are age-standardized to the world population, 2000–2025.

Reproduced with permission from Ferlay, J., Ervik, M., Lam, F., Colombet, M., Mery, L., Piñeros, M., … Bray, F. (2018). *Global cancer observatory: Cancer today.* Lyon, France: International Agency for Research on Cancer. Available from: https://gco.iarc.fr/today, accessed [09 October 2018].

abnormal neoplastic growths in women during their reproductive years, there is controversy about the value of screening for breast cancer by mammography in premenopausal women (before age 50). Currently, the American National Cancer Institute recommends that women initiate biannual screening for breast cancer by mammography at age 40–49, whereas after age 50, screening is recommended on an annual basis. Other imaging techniques such as ultrasound, magnetic resonance imaging (MRI), and positron emission tomography (PET) are now being widely used by physicians to assist in the evaluation and diagnosis of breast tumors. Breast self-examination (BSE) and

physician examination are also considered essential components of regular breast care.

▶ Pathology of Breast Cancer

Tumor staging refers to the microscopic evaluation of tissue by a pathologist to assess size, exact anatomic location, growth, and spread of a cancerous lesion. It is important to realize that although imaging procedures are important for the identification of suspicious lesions, the ultimate diagnosis of breast cancer (or any other malignant neoplasm) must be confirmed

TABLE 21.1 Breast Cancer Survival by Stage at Detection

Stage at Diagnosis	Description of Stage at Diagnosis	Five-Year Survival Rate (%)
0	Carcinoma in situ (no invasion)	100%
I	Tumor <2 cm with no lymphatic spread	100%
IIA	Tumor ≥2 cm with no lymphatic spread	93%
IIB	Spread to axillary lymph nodes	82%
IIIA	Spread to axillary and other lymph nodes	72%
IIIB	Spread to lymph nodes and opposite breast	59%
IV	Widespread metastatic cancer	22%

Data from American Joint Committee on Cancer (AJCC). (2010). Breast cancer staging. In S. B. Edge, D. R. Byrd, C. C. Compton, A. G. Fritz, F. L. Greene, & A. Trotti (Eds.)., *Cancer staging manual* (7th ed., pp. 347–376). New York, NY: Springer-Verlag.

by microscopic examination of cancerous tissue (obtained by biopsy) by a qualified pathologist.

Breast cancer survival is highest when tumors are detected prior to breaching the basement membrane upon which most solid tumors develop and invading contiguous tissues or lymph nodes (carcinoma in situ, stage I), whereas survival is lowest with late detection after tumors have spread (metastasized) to other sites (**TABLE 21.1**). Early stage breast cancer is effectively "cured" by complete surgical excision with clear margins (no evidence of spread beyond the surgical margins) whereas later stage disease is much more resistant to therapy and is conventionally treated by a combination of treatment modalities including chemotherapy, radiation therapy, and hormonal therapy and immunomodulation (AJCC, 2010).

Mechanisms of Breast Carcinogenesis

Breast cancer arises from the epithelial cells that line the ductal and glandular structures of the mammary

gland. Breast carcinogenesis is most probably due to excess stimulation of these cells by estrogen. Estrogen is a powerful mitogen that stimulates cell proliferation by activating estrogen receptors of the cell surface membrane. Sustained excessive estrogen stimulation may lead to heightened proliferation and atypia of the mammary epithelium, which are believed to be forerunners of breast cancer.

Breast cancer primarily occurs in women, although occasionally breast tumors do develop in men, particularly in association with Klinefelter's syndrome, where there is an extra X chromosome in the karyotype (XXY) or following ingestion of synthetic estrogens such as diethylstilbestrol, which has been used for the treatment of cancer of the prostate.

Several theories have been proposed to explain breast carcinogenesis. Perhaps the best known of these theories relates breast cancer risk to the sustained stimulus of estrogen over many years. The "estrogen stimulus" theory of breast cancer postulates that the risk is enhanced with a sustained continuum of estrogen cycles unbroken by pregnancy or other mechanisms of estrogen ablation such as ovariectomy. As discussed later in this chapter, both endogenous and exogenous factors may potentially increase estrogen stimulus of the mammary gland in association with breast cancer development.

A derivative of the estrogen stimulus hypothesis is the "estrogen window" hypothesis (Korenman, 1980). This postulate states that human breast cancer is induced by environmental carcinogens in a susceptible mammary gland, and that susceptibility is due to unopposed estrogen stimulation early in life during the onset of puberty (menses) and later in life with the onset of menopause. By this theory, susceptibility to induction of breast cancer declines with establishment of normal luteal phase progesterone secretion and becomes very low during pregnancy.

Risk Factors for Breast Cancer

Several risk factors have been identified that increase a woman's chance of developing breast cancer. Nevertheless, cause and effect cannot be established in most individual cases. The classical risk factors of breast cancer were first established in an early case–control study of breast cancer cases and matched controls conducted in 1923 by Dr. Janet Elizabeth Lane-Claypon in the United Kingdom. Dr. Lane-Claypon compared 500 women with breast cancer (cases) to 500 women of similar age with no history of cancer (controls) in the first documented epidemiologic case–control study (Winkelstein, 2006). Her groundbreaking study was the first to elucidate the well-known profile of classical breast cancer risk factors including familial and genetic predisposition, early menses, delayed reproductive history, nulliparity, absence of lactation, late menopause, and the natural process of aging (Lane-Claypon, 19–26).

Early Menarche and Late Menopause

Menarche and menopause mark the onset and cessation of ovarian activity and reproduction in women. During the reproductive years, estrogens are produced by the ovaries, whereas after menopause the source of circulating estrogens is biosynthesis in fat and muscle cells catalyzed by the enzyme aromatase.

An international team of investigators recently examined data on menarche and menopause from 117 epidemiologic studies including 118,964 women with invasive breast cancer and 306,091 controls. Compared to menarche at 13 years of age or menopause at 50 years of age, breast cancer risk was found to increase slightly for each year of earlier menarche (relative risk [RR] = 1.05) and each year of older menarche (RR = 1.03) (Collaborative Group on Hormonal Factors in Breast Cancer, 2012).

Nulliparity and Age at First Pregnancy

Pregnancy induces anatomic and physiologic changes in the female breast. During gestation, the ductal network of the breast expands, and the mammary epithelium differentiates into alveolar structures (glands) that secrete breast milk during lactation. In particular, the differentiation and maturation of the female breast at first pregnancy influences breast cancer risk.

MacMahon and colleagues conducted an international case–control study of pregnancy and breast cancer involving 4323 cases and 12,699 controls from seven areas of the world. Compared to nulliparous women, mothers who reported having their first full-term pregnancy before 20 years of age had a 50% reduced risk of developing breast cancer; furthermore, the risk reduction was about 60% compared to women who had their first child after 35 years of age (MacMahon et al., 1970). Recent studies provide evidence that early age at first birth is associated with reduced risk of developing only those tumors that are positive for estrogen and progesterone receptors (Ma, Bernstein, Pike, & Ursin, 2006; Ursin et al., 2005).

Genetic Predisposition to Breast Cancer

A strong family history (breast cancer in a first-degree or second-degree relative) increases the risk of breast cancer by three- to fivefold. Genetic or familial predisposition is identifiable for approximately 5%–10%

of women diagnosed with breast cancer. Hallmarks of familial predisposition to breast cancer include early age of onset, an excess of bilateral disease, and breast cancer in familial association with other malignancies such as ovarian cancer and endometrial cancer.

Two heritable genetic mutations have been identified that predispose to familial breast and ovarian cancer, *BRCA-1* and *BRCA-2*. The *BRCA-1* gene was discovered in 1990 by King and colleagues and is located on the long arm of chromosome 17 (Hall et al., 1990). Subsequently, a second breast cancer gene, *BRCA-2*, was identified on the long arm of chromosome 13 (Wooster et al., 1994). A mutation in either *BRCA* gene predisposes heterozygous female carriers to both breast cancer and, to a lesser extent, ovarian cancer. The lifetime risk of breast cancer among women who carry a single mutation in either *BRCA-1* or *BRCA-2* is approximately 85%, whereas the lifetime ovarian cancer risk for women with a *BRCA-1* mutation is 54%, compared to 24% for women with a *BRCA-2* mutation (King, Marks, Mandell, & New York Breast Cancer Study Group, 2003).

Both *BRCA-1* and *BRCA-2* are tumor suppressor genes that upon transcription form proteins essential for the repair of double-strand DNA breaks (Boulton, 2006). Mutated *BRCA* genes result in proteins that do not function properly in DNA repair, thereby promoting accumulation of genetic errors and carcinogenesis.

Breast cancer has also been observed in individuals with Cowden's disease and Sipple syndrome, two rare genetic conditions caused by germline autosomal dominant mutations (Eng, 1998). Cowden's disease is caused by a mutated tumor suppressor gene called *PTEN* located on chromosome 11 that normally helps regulate cell division and cell senescence (apoptosis). Mutations in the *PTEN* gene cause the development of small benign papules of the skin and mucous membranes (called hamartomas) and often result in thyroid lesions such as goiter, follicular adenomas, and thyroid cancer, as well as breast cancer, uterine cancer, and renal cancer. Sipple syndrome is caused by a variant of a proto-oncogene called *RET* located on chromosome 10 that regulates an important cellular growth factor (transforming growth factor beta or TGF-β). Carriers of the *RET* mutation develop malignancies of the endocrine system (specifically medullary thyroid cancer, pheochromocytoma, and occasionally breast cancer) (Lima & Smith, 1971).

Hormone Replacement Therapy and Postmenopausal Breast Cancer

Approximately 75% of breast cancers are diagnosed in women after they undergo menopause.

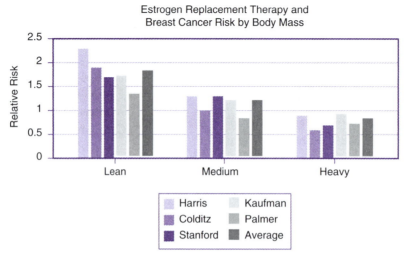

FIGURE 21.4 Body Mass and Breast Cancer Risk.

Data from Harris, R. E., Namboodiri, K. K., Farrar, W. B., Solano, S. M., & Wynder, E. L. (1996). Hormone replacement therapy and breast cancer risk. *Journal of the American Medical Association, 275*(15), 1158.

Several investigations have examined the association between hormone replacement therapy and postmenopausal breast cancer risk, and most have reported a modest increase in breast cancer risk with estrogen alone but a greater risk for estrogen plus progestin. For example, in the Million Women Study conducted in the United Kingdom, current use of estrogen alone increased the risk of invasive breast cancer by 30% compared to a twofold risk increase with current use of estrogen plus progestin (Beral & Million Woman Study Collaborators, 2003). Similar results were observed in the randomized clinical trial of estrogen plus progestin and the prospective observational cohort of postmenopausal women of the Women's Health Initiative (WHI) in the United States. The WHI results showed that breast cancer risk doubled after about 5 years of using estrogen plus progestin but declined soon after discontinuation of hormone therapy (Chlebowski et al., 2009).

Results of studies of hormone replacement therapy involving only estrogen are less clear, with some studies finding an increase in the risk of breast cancer whereas others report either no effect or a decrease in the risk. In the WHI clinical trial of conjugated equine estrogen (CEE) versus placebo for women who had undergone hysterectomy prior to enrollment, the risk of invasive breast cancer was *reduced* by 23% in women who received CEE (Anderson et al., 2004). However, 40% of the women in the trial also reported having bilateral oophorectomies prior to enrollment, and an alternative explanation of results is that discontinuation of estrogen replacement among oophorectomized women in the placebo arm may have heightened their risk by removing feedback inhibition of estrogen biosynthesis in breast tissues.

Several studies show consistency in observing an interaction between body mass and estrogen

replacement therapy (ERT) in elevating the risk of breast cancer in postmenopausal women (Colditz et al., 1992; Harris, Namboodiri, Farrar, Solano, & Wynder, 1996; Kaufman et al., 1991; Palmer, Rosenberg, Clarke, Miller, & Shapiro, 1991; Stanford et al., 1995). Specifically, lean women who receive ERT after menopause have been found to be at significantly higher risk than heavier women (**FIGURE 21.4**). One possible explanation for this is that lean women who receive ERT may have relatively higher concentrations of exogenous estrogens per unit of breast tissue, thereby increasing carcinogenesis.

▶ Body Mass and Postmenopausal Breast Cancer

Body mass index (BMI) shows differential effects on premenopausal versus postmenopausal breast cancer risk. Before menopause, BMI shows little association with risk, whereas after menopause, the risk of breast cancer increases two- to threefold among women with high BMI, presumably due to heightened estrogen biosynthesis through conversion of other steroids to estrogen by the enzyme aromatase in adipose tissue. The elevated risk of postmenopausal disease is most evident among women who gain excessive weight throughout the reproductive years and have no exposure to exogenous estrogens after menopause (Harris, Namboodiri, & Wynder, 1992).

Dietary Fat and Breast Cancer

From an etiologic perspective, it is of interest that rates of breast cancer are changing in populations that historically have been at low risk, whereas the rates have remained relatively constant in populations at higher risk. For example, breast cancer mortality rates among Japanese, Indian, and Chinese women have increased approximately threefold in the past two decades whereas rates for women in the United States, United Kingdom, and Sweden have declined (**FIGURE 21.5**). Concurrently, the Japanese, Indian, and Chinese diets have also changed dramatically with higher intakes of fat and calories; however, other risk factors may also be involved because birth rates are declining, age at first pregnancy is being delayed, the practice of breast-feeding is decreasing, and nulliparity is increasing in these populations.

A well-known but controversial hypothesis of breast cancer etiology is known as the *dietary fat hypothesis.* An extension of this hypothesis states that breast cancer development is due to intake of certain types of essential polyunsaturated fatty acids (PUFAs) that increase inflammation and estrogen biosynthesis

and thus promote breast cancer development (Harris, 2002). Karmali and colleagues first observed the divergent effects of omega-6 versus omega-3 PUFAs in animal models of breast carcinogenesis. Their studies clearly show that proinflammatory omega-6 fatty acids such as linoleic acid promote tumor development and metastasis whereas anti-inflammatory omega-3 fatty acids such as linolenic acid are inhibitory (Karmali, Adams, & Trout, 1993).

Important supportive evidence for the dietary fat hypothesis of breast cancer comes from chronological studies of Japanese women. Over the past half century, the age-adjusted breast cancer mortality rate among Japanese women has increased more than twofold, rising from less than 5 deaths per 100,000 in 1950 to nearly 12 deaths per 100,000 in 2006 (Kawamura & Sobue, 2005; Saika & Sobue, 2009). Notably, this gradual increase in breast cancer mortality among Japanese women closely parallels a threefold increase in per capita fat consumption over the same time period (**FIGURE 21.6**). In 1950, less than 10% of kilocalories were derived from fat, whereas in 2005 the level had risen to nearly 30% (Harris, 2002; Minami et al., 2004).

Although the correlated time trends of breast cancer rates and per capita dietary changes in certain populations support a role for dietary fat, analytic (case–control and cohort) studies of diet and breast cancer have yielded inconsistent results, perhaps due to the difficulty of accurately assessing dietary exposure on an individual basis. Consequently, there is controversy among epidemiologists regarding the role of dietary fat or other dietary factors in the genesis of breast cancer.

Oral Contraceptives and Premenopausal Breast Cancer

Oral contraceptive (OC) use has been found to influence the development of breast cancer in premenopausal women but not postmenopausal women

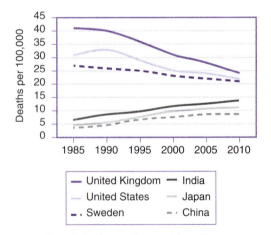

FIGURE 21.5 Trends in Breast Cancer Mortality.

Caption: Mortality rates are age-standardized to the world population, 2000.

Data from Ferlay, J., Bray, F., Pisani, P., & Parkin, D. M. (2004). *GLOBOCAN 2002. Cancer incidence, mortality, and prevalence worldwide.* IARC Cancer Base No. 5, version 2.0. Lyon, France: IARC Press. Retrieved from http://www-dep.iarc.fr; Ferlay, J., Shin, H.-R., Bray, F., Forman, D., Mathers, C., & Parkin, D. M. (2010). Estimates of worldwide burden of cancer in 2008: GLOBOCAN 2008. *International Journal of Cancer, 127*(12), 2893–2917; Ferlay, J., Soerjomataram, I., Ervik, M., Dikshit, R., Eser, S., Mathers, C., ... Bray, F. (2013). *GLOBOCAN 2012 v1.0. Cancer incidence and mortality worldwide: IARC CancerBase No. 11* [Internet]. Lyon, France: International Agency for Research on Cancer. Retrieved from http://globocan.iarc.fr

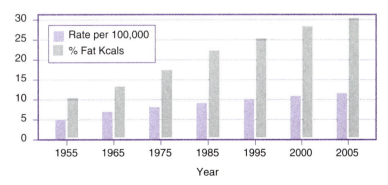

FIGURE 21.6 Breast Cancer and Dietary Fat, Japan, 1955–2005.

Data from Harris, R. E. (2002). Epidemiology of breast cancer and nonsteroidal anti-inflammatory drugs: Extension of the dietary fat hypothesis of breast cancer. In R. E. Harris (Ed.), *COX-2 blockade in cancer prevention and therapy* (pp. 57–68). Totowa, NJ: Humana Press; Minami, Y., Tsubono, Y., Nishino, Y., Ohuchi, N., Shibuya, D., & Hisamichi, S. (2004). The increase of female breast cancer incidence in Japan: Emergence of birth cohort effect. *International Journal of Cancer, 108*(6), 901–906; Kawamura, T., & Sobue, T. (2005). Comparison of breast cancer mortality in five countries: France, Italy, Japan, the UK, and the USA from the WHO Mortality Database (1960–2000). *Japan Journal of Clinical Oncology, 35*(12), 758–759; Saika, K., & Sobue, T. (2009). Epidemiology of breast cancer in Japan and the US. *Japanese Medical Association Journal, 52*(1), 39–44.

(Mills, Beeson, Phillips, & Fraser, 1989; Romieu, Berlin, & Colditz, 1990). In a meta-analysis of 34 studies, OC use was found to increase the risk of premenopausal breast cancer in parous women (odds ratio [OR] = 1.29) and nulliparous women (OR = 1.24), and the association was stronger when OCs were used before the first full-term pregnancy (OR = 1.44) (Kahlenborn, Modugno, Potter, & Severs, 2006). Conceivably, the OC content of estrogen and progestin heightens cancer risk by inducing hyperplasia of the breast epithelium in some premenopausal women.

Alcohol and Breast Cancer

Some investigations have noted a weak association between moderate alcohol consumption and breast cancer risk (Willett, Stampfer, & Colditz, 1989). However, the results of independent studies are mixed, and this too is a controversial issue in breast cancer epidemiology (Harris & Wynder, 1988; Wynder & Harris, 1989).

In a meta-analysis of the relationship of alcohol and breast cancer that included estimates of risk for drinkers versus nondrinkers from 89 separate studies, 29 studies reported odds ratios less than 1.0, 60 studies reported estimates greater than 1.0, and the combined estimate of risk was 1.11, suggesting there is a weak association. Nevertheless, the analysis also revealed the presence of significant heterogeneity among risk estimates (Key et al., 2006). Furthermore, studies of some populations reveal discordant results. For example, in a meta-analysis of studies of breast cancer and alcohol among Chinese women, alcohol consumption actually showed an *inverse* association with the risk of breast cancer (Li, Yang, & Cao, 2011).

Although alcohol per se is not carcinogenic, its primary metabolite, acetaldehyde, does have potent carcinogenic properties. Although alcohol metabolism occurs primarily in the liver, the responsible enzyme, alcohol dehydrogenase, can also be expressed in other tissues, including the mammary epithelium. Thus, it is conceivable that in women who are chronic drinkers, the local metabolism of alcohol may expose breast tissues to acetaldehyde (Crabb, Matsumoto, Chang, & You, 2004).

Other Breast Cancer Risk Factors

Certain endogenous conditions may also modulate the development of cancer of the breast. Fibrocystic disease with hyperplasia and/or atypia appears, in some instances, to antedate the development of cancer of the breast. In case–control studies, this condition elevates the risk of breast cancer by about two- to threefold.

Thyroid dysfunction has also been observed in association with breast cancer in some studies (Smyth, 1997). In particular, hypothyroidism may elevate breast cancer risk in certain individuals. The physiologic basis for this is, presumptively, the antiestrogenic effect of thyroxin; that is, when thyroxin levels are diminished, estrogen levels rise, thereby enhancing breast cancer risk.

It is noteworthy that the highest risk target organ for development of breast cancer is the contralateral (opposite) breast of a woman who has already manifested unilateral disease. In addition, the familial breast cancer patient has a markedly enhanced risk for development of malignancy in the contralateral breast (about 50% over 20 years, postmastectomy) (Harris, Lynch, & Guirgis, 1978).

Many studies in biochemical epidemiology have been performed with the objective of identifying a biochemical marker of breast cancer risk. The various subtypes of estrogens (estradiol, estrone, and estriol) and their ratios, androgens and other steroids, polypeptide hormones such as prolactin, and various indices of these parameters have been tried; however, no single parameter or index of parameters has been developed that accurately predicts an individual's risk for developing cancer of the breast.

▶ Mammographic Breast Density and Postmenopausal Breast Cancer Risk

Appearance of the breast on mammogram facilitates partition of tissues into radiolucent areas consisting of primarily adipose (fat) and radiodense areas consisting of primarily fibrous and glandular tissues. John Wolfe, a radiologist in Detroit, Michigan, was the first to describe differences in breast cancer risk associated with variations in the mammographic appearance of the breast (Wolfe, 1976). Many subsequent studies have consistently found that among postmenopausal women who undergo screening mammography, those with a high ratio of dense glandular tissue to adipose tissue have an elevated risk of developing breast cancer compared to those with low ratios (Boyd et al., 2005; McCormack & dos Santos Silva, 2006; Yaghjyan et al., 2011; Yaghjyan, Colditz, Rosner, & Taminmi, 2013).

In a meta-analysis of 42 studies involving more than 14,000 cases and 226,000 controls, the composite risk estimates increased in a dose-dependent fashion with increasing breast density, and women with breast densities of 75% or more had nearly five times higher

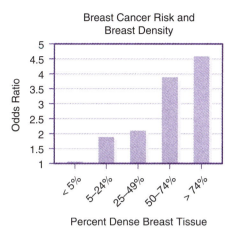

FIGURE 21.7 Mammographic Breast Density and Risk of Breast Cancer.

McCormack, V. A., & dos Santos Silva, I. (2006). Breast density and parenchymal patterns as markers of breast cancer risk: A meta-analysis. *Cancer Epidemiology, Biomarkers and Prevention, 15,* 1159–1169.

risk of developing breast cancer than those with breast densities less than 5% (**FIGURE 21.7**). The investigators concluded that "this marker has great potential to be used for research into the etiology and prevention of breast cancer" (McCormack & dos Santos Silva, 2006).

Conundrum of Mammographic Breast Density

The observed association of high mammographic breast density with the risk of breast cancer presents a conundrum. This association appears to be confounded by age and body mass, two factors that *increase* breast cancer risk but *decrease* the glandular component of mammary tissues. Furthermore, in a recent study of 9232 women with confirmed diagnoses of invasive breast cancer, high mammographic density was *not* associated with the risk of dying from breast cancer. Instead, there was a paradoxical *increase* in the risk of dying from breast cancer associated with *low* breast density, particularly in obese women (Gierach et al., 2012).

Legislation Requiring Disclosure of Mammographic Density

Despite uncertainties regarding the biological interpretation of mammographic density, the findings relating "dense breasts" to higher breast cancer risk have prompted legislation requiring full disclosure of mammography findings to patients. In the United States, laws requiring disclosure have been passed in Connecticut, Texas, Virginia, California, and New York, and a bill calling for a federal law has been introduced in the House of Representatives. Under these laws, women who have dense breast tissue by mammography must

be told not only that their risk of developing breast cancer is increased, but also that dense breast tissue can mask the detection of cancerous tumors.

Despite the association between mammographic density and the risk of breast cancer, it must be remembered that most women with radiodense breasts will *not* develop breast cancer. It is emphasized that the discrimination of small breast tumors from normal glandular tissues by mammography (or other imaging techniques) is extremely difficult because both tissues are radiodense. The only sure way of making this determination is by microscopic examination of a biopsy specimen by a trained pathologist.

▶ Male Breast Cancer

Male breast cancer is rare and accounts for only a small fraction of breast cancer cases (0.6% in 2016). Genetic factors heighten the risk of breast cancer development in men including Klinefelter's syndrome in which men inherit an extra X chromosome (47 XXY karyotype), mutations of BRCA1 and BRCA2 genes, Cowden's syndrome which is due to mutations in the PTEN tumor suppressor gene, and in general, a positive family history of breast cancer. Other risk factors include hormonal disorders that increase levels of circulating estrogens such as gravid obesity, chronic alcohol abuse, testicular anomalies (e.g., cryptorchidism [undescended testes]), and exposure to synthetic forms of estrogen (e.g. diethylstilbestrol therapy for advanced prostate cancer) (Weiss, Moysich, & Swede, 2005).

▶ Prevention of Breast Cancer

Breastfeeding and Breast Cancer

An early case–control study by Janet Lane-Claypon in Great Britain found that early pregnancy and breastfeeding protect against the development of breast cancer. Recent meta-analyses provided confirmation of these effects. An international collaborative team of investigators examined data from 47 epidemiologic studies conducted in 30 different countries that included information on breastfeeding patterns and other aspects of childbearing for 50,302 women with invasive breast cancer and 96,973 controls. Results showed that each birth reduced the risk of developing breast cancer by 7.0%, and among parous women, each year of breastfeeding reduced the risk by an additional 4.3% (Collaborative Group on Hormonal Factors in Breast Cancer, 2002).

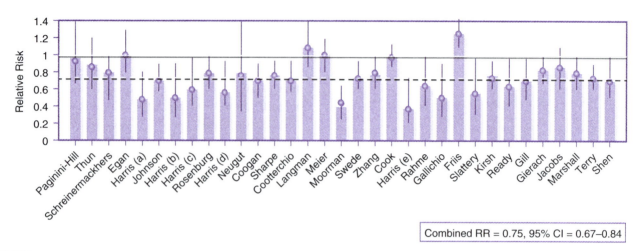

FIGURE 21.8 Breast Cancer and Nonsteroidal Anti-inflammatory Drugs (NSAIDs).

Data from Harris, R. E. (2009). Cyclooxygenase-2 (COX-2) blockade in the chemoprevention of cancers of the colon, breast, prostate, and lung. *Inflammopharmacology, 17,* 1–13; Harris, R. E., Casto, B. C., & Harris, Z. M. (2014). Cyclooxygenase-2 (COX-2) and the inflammogenesis of breast cancer. *World Journal of Clinical Oncology, 5*(4), 677–692.

Selective Estrogen Receptor Modulators and Breast Cancer

Breast cancer specimens ascertained by biopsy or surgical procedures (mastectomy) are routinely subjected to laboratory analysis of estrogen receptors (ERs) and progesterone receptors (PRs). Breast tumors that are positive for ERs/PRs may respond to hormone therapy by administration of antiestrogenic compounds such as tamoxifen. Such compounds are called *selective estrogen receptor modulators (SERMs)* because they inhibit the interaction of estrogen with the estrogen receptor. Tamoxifen is now being offered to women treated for early stage breast cancer for protection against the development of second primary cancer in the contralateral breast.

Large independent clinical trials have been performed to examine the preventive activity of tamoxifen. Although a U.S. trial showed beneficial effects (Fisher et al., 1998), the results of two European trials were negative (Powles et al., 1998; Veronesi et al., 1998). In a fourth randomized clinical trial conducted in European centers, tamoxifen administration reduced the incidence of breast cancer by 32% compared to the control group, but despite this benefit, there was a significant *excess* of deaths in the tamoxifen group (25 versus 11 deaths, *P* < 0.03) (Cuzick et al., 2002). Nevertheless, the U.S. FDA approved tamoxifen for use as a preventive agent in high-risk women. This action tends to disregard adverse side effects of the drug including increased risks of endometrial cancer, ER-negative breast cancer, colon cancer, pulmonary embolus, and other thrombotic events.

Nonsteroidal Anti-inflammatory Drugs and Breast Cancer

Many epidemiologic studies have noted a significant preventive effect of nonsteroidal anti-inflammatory drugs (NSAIDs) against breast cancer. A meta-analysis of these investigations suggests that the risk of breast cancer is reduced by approximately 25% with regular use of common over-the-counter NSAIDs such as aspirin and ibuprofen (**FIGURE 21.8**) (Harris, 2009; Harris et al., 2014). Studies in molecular epidemiology and in animals suggest that this effect is manifest primarily due to blockade of cyclooxygenase isoenzymes (COX) that catalyze biosynthesis of inflammatory prostaglandins, particularly the inducible isoform, cyclooxygenase-2 (COX-2) (Harris, 2007). Nevertheless, recent investigations provide evidence that lipoxygenase enzymes (LOX) that catalyze biosynthesis of inflammatory leukotrienes may also contribute to mammary carcinogenesis, suggesting that blockade of both COX and LOX enzymes may have greater potential for breast cancer chemoprevention (Kennedy & Harris, 2018; Schneider & Pozzi, 2011).

▶ Summary of Breast Cancer Epidemiology

Breast cancer is a multifactorial disease promoted by sustained heightened exposure to endogenous or exogenous estrogens. There is a rising worldwide trend in breast cancer incidence that undoubtedly reflects the impact of multiple factors, including screening (mammography) and increases in risk factors, including late childbearing, lack of breastfeeding, intake of exogenous hormones, intake of diets high in fat and calories, lack of exercise, and obesity. Incidence rates of breast cancer vary widely and are higher in developed countries such as the United States and United Kingdom and lower in developing countries such as India and China. Breast cancer risk appears to increase with high intake of essential polyunsaturated fats that promote inflammation and estrogen biosynthesis. Reproductive risk factors include early menses, nulliparity, late first pregnancy, absence of lactation, and late menopause, all of which increase exposure to endogenous estrogens. ERT and high body mass increase breast cancer risk in postmenopausal women. Identifiable genetic factors account for only a small fraction of breast cancer cases. Studies in cancer control show that annual screening with mammography after age 50 is effective in detecting early breast

lesions when they can be surgically excised with a high probability of long-term survival. Furthermore, the risk of developing breast cancer is increased among women with higher levels of dense breast tissue based on mammography. Breast cancer prevention may be aided by taking synthetic or natural compounds with anti-inflammatory or anti-estrogenic activity. Additional studies in molecular epidemiology are needed to more clearly delineate the way in which breast cancer risk factors interact to impact the natural history of this disease.

References

American Joint Committee on Cancer (AJCC). (2010). Breast cancer staging. In S. B. Edge, D. R. Byrd, C. C. Compton, A. G. Fritz, F. L. Greene, & A. Trotti (Eds.), *Cancer staging manual* (7th ed., pp. 347–376). New York, NY: Springer-Verlag.

Anderson, G. L., Limacher, M., Assaf, A. R., Bassford, T., Beresford, S. A., Black, H., … Wassertheil-Smoller, S. (2004). Effects of conjugated equine estrogen in postmenopausal women with hysterectomy: The Women's Health Initiative randomized controlled trial. *Journal of the American Medical Association, 291*(14), 1701–1712.

Beral, V., & Million Women Study Collaborators. (2003). Breast cancer and hormone-replacement therapy in the Million Women Study. *Lancet, 362*(9382), 419–427.

Boulton, S. J. (2006). Cellular functions of the BRCA tumour-suppressor proteins. *Biochemical Society Transactions, 34*(5), 633–645.

Boyd, N. F., Rommens, J. M., Vogt, K., Lee, V., Hopper, J. L., Yaffe, M. J., & Paterson, A. D. (2005). Mammographic breast density as an intermediate phenotype for breast cancer. *Lancet Oncology, 6*(10), 798–808.

Bray, F., Ferlay, J., Soerjomataram, I., Siegel, R. L., Torre, L. A., & Jemal, A. (2018). Global cancer statistics 2018: GLOBOCAN estimates of incidence and mortality worldwide for 36 cancers in 185 countries. *CA: A Cancer Journal for Clinicians, 68*(6), 394–424.

Bray, F., McCarron, P., & Parkin, D. M. (2004). The changing global patterns of female breast cancer incidence and mortality. *Breast Cancer Research, 6*(6), 229–239.

Chlebowski, R. T., Kuller, L. H., Prentice, R. L., Stefanick, M. L., Manson, J. E., Gass, M., … Anderson, G. (2009). Breast cancer after use of estrogen plus progestin in postmenopausal women. *New England Journal of Medicine, 360*(6), 573–587.

Colditz, G. A., Stampfer, M. J., Willett, W. C., Hunter, D. J., Manson, J. E., Hennekens, C. H., … Speizer, F. E. (1992). Type of postmenopausal hormone use and risk of breast cancer: 12-year follow-up from the Nurses' Health Study. *Cancer Causes and Control, 3*, 433–439.

Collaborative Group on Hormonal Factors in Breast Cancer. (2002). Breast cancer and breastfeeding: Collaborative reanalysis of individual data from 47 epidemiological studies in 30 countries, including 50,302 women with breast cancer and 96,973 women without the disease. *Lancet, 360*(9328), 187–195.

Collaborative Group on Hormonal Factors in Breast Cancer. (2012). Menarche, menopause, and breast cancer risk: Individual participant meta-analysis, including 118,964 women with breast cancer from 117 epidemiological studies. *Lancet Oncology, 13*(11), 1141–1151.

Crabb, D. W., Matsumoto, M., Chang, D., & You, M. (2004). Overview of the role of alcohol dehydrogenase and aldehyde dehydrogenase and their variants in the genesis of alcohol-related pathology. *Proceedings of the Nutrition Society, 63*, 49–63.

Cuzick, J., Forbes, J., Edwards, R., Baum, M., Cawthorn, S., Coates, A., … IBIS Investigators. (2002). First results from the International Breast Cancer Intervention Study (IBIS-I): A randomised prevention trial. *Lancet, 360*(9336), 817–824.

Eng, C. (1998). Genetics of Cowden syndrome: Through the looking glass of oncology. *International Journal of Oncology, 12*(3), 701–710.

Ferlay, J., Bray, F., Pisani, P., & Parkin, D. M. (2004). *GLOBOCAN 2002. Cancer incidence, mortality, and prevalence worldwide.* IARC Cancer Base No. 5, version 2.0. Lyon, France: IARC Press. Retrieved from www.dep.iarc.fr

Ferlay, J., Ervik, M., Lam, F., Colombet, M., Mery, L., Piñeros, M., … Bray, F. (2018). *Global cancer observatory: Cancer today.* Lyon, France: International Agency for Research on Cancer. Retrieved from https://gco.iarc.fr/today

Ferlay, J., Shin, H.-R., Bray, F., Forman, D., Mathers, C., & Parkin, D. M. (2010). Estimates of worldwide burden of cancer in 2008: GLOBOCAN 2008. *International Journal of Cancer, 127*(12), 2893–2917.

Ferlay, J., Soerjomataram, I., Ervik, M., Dikshit, R., Eser, S., Mathers, C., … Bray, F. (2013). *GLOBOCAN 2012 v1.0. Cancer incidence and mortality worldwide: IARC CancerBase No. 11* [Internet]. Lyon, France: International Agency for Research on Cancer. Retrieved from http://globocan.iarc.fr

Fisher, B., Costantino, J. P., Wickerham, D. L., Redmond, C. K., Kavanah, M., Cronin, W. M., … Wolmark, N. (1998). Tamoxifen for prevention of breast cancer: Report of the National Surgical Adjuvant Breast and Bowel Project P-1 Study. *Journal of the National Cancer Institute, 90*, 1371–1388.

Fitzmaurice, C., Akinyemiju, T. F., Al Lami, F. H., Alam, T., Alizadeh-Navaei, R., Allen, C., … Global Burden of Disease Cancer Collaboration. (2018). Global, regional, and national cancer incidence, mortality, years of life lost, years lived with disability, and disability-adjusted life-years for 29 cancer groups, 1990 to 2016: A systematic analysis for the Global Burden of Disease Study. *JAMA Oncology.* Online publication. doi:10.1001/jamaoncol.2018.2706.

Fitzmaurice, C., Allen, C., Barber, R. M., Barregard, L., Bhutta, Z. A., Brenner, H., … Global Burden of Disease Cancer Collaboration. (2017). Global, regional, and national cancer incidence, mortality, years of life lost, years lived with disability, and disability-adjusted life-years for 32 cancer groups, 1990 to 2015: A systematic analysis for the Global Burden of Disease Study. *JAMA Oncology, 3*(4), 524–548.

Garcia, M., Jemal, A., Ward, E. M., Center, M. M., Hao, Y., Siegel, R. L., & Thun, M. J. (2007). *Global cancer facts and figures 2007.* Atlanta, GA: American Cancer Society.

Gierach, G. L., Ichikawa, L., Kerlikowske, K., Brinton, L. A., Farhat, G. N., Vacek, P. M., & Sherman, M. E. (2012). Relationship between mammographic density and breast cancer death in the Breast Cancer Surveillance Consortium. *Journal of the National Cancer Institute, 104*, 1218–1227.

Hall, J. M., Lee, M. K., Newman, B., Morrow, J. E., Anderson, L. A., Huey, B., & King, M. C. (1990). Linkage of early-onset familial breast cancer to chromosome 17q21. *Science, 250*(4988), 1684–1689.

Harris, R. E. (2002). Epidemiology of breast cancer and nonsteroidal anti-inflammatory drugs: Extension of the dietary fat hypothesis of breast cancer. In R. E. Harris (Ed.), *COX-2 blockade in cancer prevention and therapy* (pp. 57–68). Totowa, NJ: Humana Press.

Harris, R. E. (2007). COX-2 and the inflammogenesis of cancer. *Subcellular Biochemistry, 42*, 193–212.

Harris, R. E. (2009). Cyclooxygenase-2 (COX-2) blockade in the chemoprevention of cancers of the colon, breast, prostate, and lung. *Inflammopharmacology, 17*, 1–13.

Harris, R. E., Casto, B. C., & Harris, Z. M. (2014). Cyclooxygenase-2 (COX-2) and the inflammogenesis of breast cancer. *World Journal of Clinical Oncology, 5*(4), 677–692.

Harris, R. E., Lynch, H. T., & Guirgis, H. A. (1978). Familial breast cancer: Risk to the contralateral breast. *Journal of the National Cancer Institute, 60*, 955–960.

Harris, R. E., Namboodiri, K. K., Farrar, W. B., Solano, S. M., & Wynder, E. L. (1996). Hormone replacement therapy and breast cancer risk. *Journal of the American Medical Association, 275*(15), 1158.

Harris, R. E., Namboodiri, K. K., & Wynder, E. L. (1992). Breast cancer risk: Effects of estrogen replacement therapy and body mass. *Journal of the National Cancer Institute, 84*, 1575–1582.

Harris, R. E., & Wynder, E. L. (1988). Breast cancer and alcohol consumption: A study in weak associations. *Journal of the American Medical Association, 259*(19), 2867–2871.

Hutson, S. W., Cowen, P. N., & Bird, C. C. (1985). Morphometric studies of age related changes in normal human breast and their significance for evolution of mammary cancer. *Journal of Clinical Pathology, 38*, 281–287.

Kahlenborn, C., Modugno, F., Potter, D. M., & Severs, W. B. (2006). Oral contraceptive use as a risk factor for premenopausal breast cancer: A meta-analysis. *Mayo Clinic Proceedings, 81*(10), 1290–1302.

Karmali, R. A., Adams, L., & Trout, J. R. (1993). Plant and marine n-3 fatty acids inhibit experimental metastasis of rat mammary adenocarcinoma cells. *Prostaglandins Leukotrienes and Essential Fatty Acids, 48*, 309–314.

Kaufman, D. W., Palmer, J. R., de Mouzon, J., Rosenberg, L., Stolley, P. D., Warshauer, E., … Shapiro, S. (1991). Estrogen replacement therapy and the risk of breast cancer: Results from the case-control surveillance study. *American Journal of Epidemiology, 134*, 1375–1385.

Kawamura, T., & Sobue, T. (2005). Comparison of breast cancer mortality in five countries: France, Italy, Japan, the UK, and the USA from the WHO Mortality Database (1960–2000). *Japan Journal of Clinical Oncology, 35*(12), 758–759.

Kennedy, B. M., & Harris, R. E. (2018). Cyclooxygenase and lipoxygenase gene expression in the inflammogenesis of breast cancer. *Inflammopharmacology, 26*(4), 909–923.

Key, J., Hodgson, S., Omar, R. Z., Jensen, T. K., Thompson, S. G., Boobis, A. R., … Elliott, P. (2006). Meta-analysis of studies of alcohol and breast cancer with consideration of the methodological issues. *Cancer Causes and Control, 17*(6), 759–770.

King, M. C., Marks, J. H., Mandell, J. B., & New York Breast Cancer Study Group. (2003). Breast and ovarian cancer risks due to inherited mutations in BRCA1 and BRCA2. *Science, 302*(5645), 643–646.

Korenman, S. G. (1980). Oestrogen window hypothesis of the aetiology of breast cancer. *Lancet, 315*, 700–701.

Lane-Claypon, J. E. (1926). *A further report on cancer of the breasts, with special reference to its associated antecedent conditions.* London, UK: HMSO. Report on Public Health and Medical Subjects No. 32.

Li, Y., Yang, H., & Cao, J. (2011). Association between alcohol consumption and cancers in the Chinese population—A systematic review and meta-analysis. *PLOS One, 6*(4), e18776. doi:10.1371/journal.pone.0018776.

Lima, J. B., & Smith, P. D. (1971). Sipple's syndrome (pheochromocytoma and thyroid carcinoma) with bilateral breast carcinoma. *American Journal of Surgery, 1*(6), 732–735.

Lin, S., Tukana, I., Linhart, C., Morrell, S., Taylor, R., Vatucawaqa, P., … Zimmet, P. (2016). Diabetes and obesity trends in Fiji over 30 years. *Journal of Diabetes, 8*, 533–543.

Ma, H., Bernstein, L., Pike, M. C., & Ursin, G. (2006). Reproductive factors and breast cancer risk according to joint estrogen and progesterone receptor status: A meta-analysis of epidemiological studies. *Breast Cancer Research, 8*(4), R43.

MacMahon, B., Cole, P., Lin, T. M., Lowe, C. R., Mirra, A. P., Ravnihar, B., … Yuasa, S. (1970). Age at first birth and breast cancer risk. *Bulletin of the World Health Organization, 43*(2), 209–221.

McCormack, V. A., & dos Santos Silva, I. (2006). Breast density and parenchymal patterns as markers of breast cancer risk: A meta-analysis. *Cancer Epidemiology, Biomarkers and Prevention, 15*, 1159–1169.

Mills, P. K., Beeson, L., Phillips, R. L., & Fraser, G. E. (1989). Prospective study of exogenous hormone use and breast cancer in Seventh-Day Adventists. *Cancer, 64*, 591–597.

Minami, Y., Tsubono, Y., Nishino, Y., Ohuchi, N., Shibuya, D., & Hisamichi, S. (2004). The increase of female breast cancer incidence in Japan: Emergence of birth cohort effect. *International Journal of Cancer, 108*(6), 901–906.

Palmer, J. R., Rosenberg, L., Clarke, E. A., Miller, D. R., & Shapiro, S. (1991). Breast cancer risk after estrogen replacement therapy: Results from the Toronto Breast Cancer Study. *American Journal of Epidemiology, 134*, 1386–1395.

Parkin, D. M., Bray, F., Ferlay, J., & Pisani, P. (2001). Estimating the world cancer burden: GLOBOCAN 2000. *International Journal of Cancer, 94*, 153–156.

Powles, T., Eeles, R., Ashley, S., Easton, D., Chang, J., Dowsett, M., … Davey, J. (1998). Interim analysis of the incidence of breast cancer in the Royal Marsden Hospital tamoxifen randomised chemoprevention trial. *Lancet, 352*, 98–101.

Romieu, I., Berlin, J. A., & Colditz, G. (1990). Oral contraceptives and breast cancer. Review and meta-analysis. *Cancer, 66*(11), 2253–2263.

Saika, K., & Sobue, T. (2009). Epidemiology of breast cancer in Japan and the US. *Japan Medical Association Journal, 52*(1), 39–44.

Schneider, C., & Pozzi, A. (2011). Cyclooxygenases and lipoxygenases in cancer. *Cancer Metastasis Reviews, 30*, 277–294.

Smyth, P. P. (1997). The thyroid and breast cancer: A significant association? *Annals of Medicine, 3*, 189–191.

Stanford, J. L., Weiss, N. S., Voight, L. F., Daling, J. R., Habel, L. A., & Rossing, M. A. (1995). Combined estrogen and progestin hormone replacement therapy in relation to risk of breast cancer in middle-aged women. *Journal of the American Medical Association, 274*, 137–142.

Ursin, G., Bernstein, L., Lord, S. J., Karim, R., Deapen, D., Press, M. F., … Spirtas, R. (2005). Reproductive factors and subtypes of breast cancer defined by hormone receptor and histology. *British Journal of Cancer, 93*(3), 364–371.

Veronesi, U., Maisonneuve, P., Costa, A., Sacchini, V., Maltoni, C., Robertson, C., … Boyle, P. (1998). Prevention of breast cancer with tamoxifen: Preliminary findings from the Italian randomised trial among hysterectomised women. Italian Tamoxifen Prevention Study. *Lancet, 352*, 93–97.

Weiss, J. R., Moysich, C. K., & Swede, H. (2005). Epidemiology of male breast cancer. *Cancer Epidemiology, Biomarkers and Prevention, 14*(1), 20–26.

Willett, W. C., Stampfer, M. J., & Colditz, G. A. (1989). Does alcohol consumption influence the risk of developing breast cancer? Two views (15a). In V. T. DeVita Jr., S. Hellman, & S. A. Rosenberg (Eds.), *Important advances in oncology, 1989* (pp. 267–281). Philadelphia, PA: J. B. Lippincott.

Winkelstein Jr., W. (2006). Janet Elizabeth Lane-Claypon: A forgotten epidemiologic pioneer. *Epidemiology, 17*(6), 705.

Wolfe, J. N. (1976). Risk for breast cancer development determined by mammographic parenchymal pattern. *Cancer, 37*, 2486–2492.

Wooster, R., Neuhausen, S. L., Mangion, J., Quirk, Y., Ford, D., Collins, N., … Stratton, M. R. (1994). Localization of a breast cancer susceptibility gene, BRCA2, to chromosome 13q12–13. *Science, 265*(5181), 2088–2090.

Wynder, E. L., & Harris, R. E. (1989). Does alcohol consumption influence the risk of developing breast cancer? Two views (15b). In V. T. DeVita Jr., S. Hellman, & S. A. Rosenberg (Eds.), *Important advances in oncology, 1989* (pp. 267–281). Philadelphia, PA: JB Lippincott.

Yaghjyan, L., Colditz, G. A., Collins, L. C., Schnitt, S. J., Rosner, B., Vachon, C., & Tamimi, R. M. (2011). Mammographic breast density and subsequent risk of breast cancer in postmenopausal women according to tumor characteristics. *Journal of the National Cancer Institute, 103*, 1–11.

Yaghjyan, L., Colditz, G. A., Rosner, B., & Taninmi, R. M. (2013). Mammographic breast density and subsequent risk of breast cancer in postmenopausal women according to the time since the mammogram. *Cancer Epidemiology, Biomarkers and Prevention, 22*(6), 1110–1117.

CHAPTER 22

Epidemiology of Ovarian Cancer

Global Epidemiology of Ovarian Cancer

During 2018, ovarian cancer was diagnosed in 295,414 women and caused 184,799 deaths in the world population. During the 21st century (2000–2018), the annual number of cases increased by 54% and the number of deaths from ovarian cancer increased by 62%. Ovarian cancer currently accounts for approximately 3.4% of all female cancers and about 4.4% of cancer deaths in women (Bray et al., 2018; Ferlay et al., 2010, 2013, 2018; Fitzmaurice et al., 2017, 2018). Most new cases (80%–90%) are diagnosed either during or after menopause, and the peak incidence occurs during the fifth decade of life (American Cancer Society, 2009; National Cancer Institute, 2009).

The 2018 global patterns of ovarian cancer incidence and mortality shown in **FIGURE 22.1** are somewhat like those of breast cancer. High incidence rates were observed among women living in industrialized areas such as the United States, Canada, Europe, Australia, New Zealand, Japan, and the Russian Federation. Nevertheless, some less developed countries (e.g., Central African countries such as Niger, Ghana, and Ethiopia and South American counties such as Columbia, Argentina, and Guyana) also had high incidence rates of ovarian cancer. In contrast, mortality rates of ovarian cancer were highest in countries of Eastern Europe, Central Africa, and the island nations of Southeastern Asia. On average, incidence rates were about 19% higher in developed nations than in developing nations (7.0 versus 5.9 per 100,000), whereas mortality rates were about 5% higher in developing

nations than in developed nations (4.0 versus 3.8 per 100,000) (Bray et al., 2018; Ferlay et al., 2018).

Ovarian Cancer: The "Silent Killer"

Ovarian cancer develops silently over a period of many years without clinically detectable signs or symptoms. At the time of diagnosis, more than 70% of ovarian cancers have spread to lymph nodes, surrounding tissues of the peritoneum, or beyond (**FIGURE 22.2**). Because of the failure to detect ovarian cancers at an early stage when treatment is more likely to be of benefit to the patient, ovarian cancer generally has an extremely poor prognosis. Worldwide, the 5-year survival rate for ovarian cancer is only about 30% (Parkin, Bray, Ferlay, & Pisani, 2005).

Pathophysiology of the Human Ovary

Ovarian pathophysiology is complex. The gland is covered by surface epithelium and the inner core (the cortex) consists of multiple cell types. Follicles within the cortex contain the oocytes (eggs), granulosa cells, and theca cells. Granulosa cells surround and nourish the oocytes in response to follicular stimulating hormone (FSH) secreted by the pituitary gland. Theca cells respond to luteinizing hormone (LH) and synthesize androgens that are subsequently aromatized to estrogens by the granulosa cells. On ovulation, the remnant

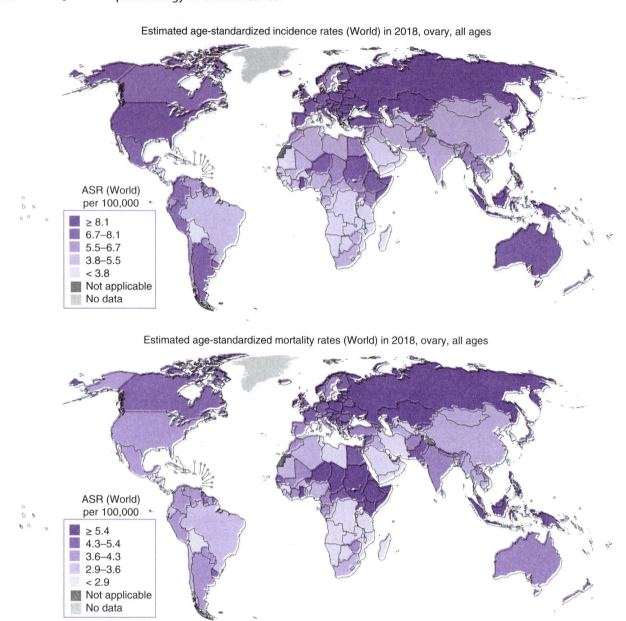

FIGURE 22.1 Global Incidence and Mortality of Ovarian Cancer, 2018.

Caption: ASR: Rates per 100,000 are standardized to the world population, 2000–2025.

Reproduced with permission from Ferlay, J., Ervik, M., Lam, F., Colombet, M., Mery, L., Piñeros, M., … Bray, F. (2018). *Global cancer observatory: Cancer today*. Lyon, France: International Agency for Research on Cancer. Retrieved from https://gco.iarc.fr/today, accessed [09 October 2018].

of the follicle (the corpus luteum) secretes progesterone as well as estrogen. Various structures and cell types of the human ovary are shown in **FIGURE 22.3** (Kumar, Abbas, & Aster, 2014).

▶ Pathogenesis of Ovarian Cancer

Ovarian cancer usually arises from the epithelial cells at the surface of the ovary. Dr. Mahmoud Fathalla originally proposed that the genesis of this malignancy is likely related to incessant ovulation and repetitive

disruption and wound healing of the surface epithelium coincident with the menstrual cycle during the reproductive years (Fathalla, 1971). Incessant ovulation could cause sustained exposure of the ovarian epithelium to hormones and growth factors secreted by the ovarian cortex (Scully, 1995) as well as increase the inflammatory microenvironment of cytokines and prostaglandins, leading to cell damage and oxidative stress (Ness & Cottreau, 1999). In support of the incessant ovulation model, several epidemiologic studies have determined that the number of successive ovulatory cycles uninterrupted by pregnancy, lactation, and/ or contraception increases the risk of ovarian cancer

(Risch, Marrett, & Howe, 1994). The natural repetitive cyclic process of ovulation may thus increase the chance of spontaneous somatic mutations and/or epigenetic changes that alter the expression of tumor suppressor genes and oncogenes in favor of carcinogenesis.

However, the incessant ovulation model does not explain the increased risk of ovarian cancer in women who are infertile due to anovulation (absence of ovulation). Such women may be at risk due to excessive stimulation of the ovary by gonadotropic hormones secreted by the pituitary gland, namely FSH and LH. Ovulation and ovarian secretion of estrogen and progesterone during the menstrual cycle depend upon normal functioning of the hypothalamic–pituitary–ovarian axis; reciprocally, abnormalities in this system may result in anovulation, loss of hormonal feedback control, and hypersecretion of gonadotropins (**FIGURE 22.4**). Indeed, as a woman undergoes menopause, the diminished ovarian secretion of estrogen and progesterone results in loss of feedback inhibition, thereby resulting in marked elevations in FSH and LH secreted by the pituitary gland (Chakravarti et al., 1976). These perimenopausal events (diminished ovarian hormones and excess pituitary gonadotropins) are temporally related to the onset of ovarian cancer in the postmenopausal years (Choi, Wong, Huang, & Leung, 2007; Helzlsouer, Alberg, & Gordon, 1995). Furthermore, gonadotropin levels in ovarian cyst and peritoneal fluid appear to be associated with ovarian cancer incidence (Kramer, Leeker, & Jager, 1998), and cell membrane receptors for FSH are overexpressed in a high percentage of ovarian carcinomas as well as preneoplastic lesions of the ovarian surface epithelium (Choi, Choi, Auersperg, & Leung, 2004; Zheng et al., 2000). Up-regulation of FSH, in particular, appears to be related to the growth, survival, and metastasis of ovarian cancer cells and may involve other growth factors mediated by a complex array of intracellular signaling pathways (Choi et al., 2007). Finally, it has been hypothesized that ovarian cancer is etiologically linked to the excessive production of androgens and diminished levels of progesterone, which upset the balance of the ovarian hormonal milieu resulting in carcinogenesis (Risch, 1998).

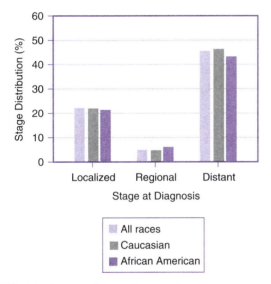

FIGURE 22.2 Ovarian Cancer Stage at Detection.

Data from Horner, M. J., Ries, L. A. G., Krapcho, M., Neyman, N., Aminou, R., Howlader, N., . . . Edwards, B. K. (Eds). *SEER Cancer Statistics Review, 1975–2006*. Bethesda, MD: National Cancer Institute.

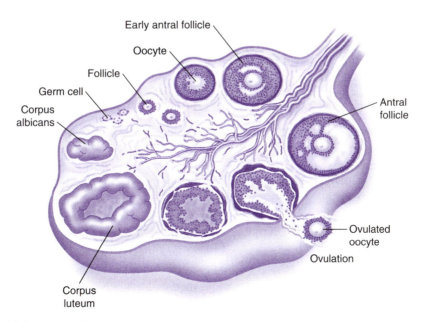

FIGURE 22.3 Anatomy of the Human Ovary.

FIGURE 22.4 The Hypothalamus–Pituitary–Ovarian Axis.

▶ Risk Factors for Ovarian Cancer

Several risk factors have been identified that increase a woman's chance of developing ovarian cancer. Because the ovarian epithelium contains many of the same cell membrane receptors as the ductal epithelium of the mammary gland, the reproductive risk factor profile for ovarian cancer is like that of breast cancer. These risk factors include familial and genetic predisposition plus reproductive events that increase the cumulative months of ovulation, rupture of the ovarian surface epithelium, and exposure to hormones of the menstrual cycle (early menses, delayed reproductive history, nulliparity, absence of lactation, late menopause, and the natural process of aging).

Reciprocally, reproductive factors such as pregnancy, lactation, and oral contraceptive use that interrupt the menstrual cycle have consistently been observed to be protective. These factors are discussed in greater detail in a following section of this chapter.

Genetic Predisposition to Ovarian Cancer

A strong family history (ovarian cancer in a first-degree or second-degree relative) increases the risk of ovarian cancer by three- to fivefold. Genetic or familial predisposition is identifiable for approximately 5%–10% of women diagnosed with ovarian cancer. Hallmarks of familial predisposition to ovarian cancer include early age of onset, an excess of bilateral disease, and ovarian cancer in familial association with other malignancies such as breast cancer, endometrial cancer, and colorectal cancer.

Two heritable genetic mutations have been identified that predispose to familial breast and ovarian cancer, *BRCA-1* and *BRCA-2*. The *BRCA-1* gene was discovered in 1990 by King and colleagues and is located on the long arm of chromosome 17 (Hall et al., 1990). Subsequently, a second breast cancer gene, *BRCA-2*, was identified on the long arm of

chromosome 13 (Wooster et al., 1994). A mutation in either *BRCA* gene predisposes heterozygous female carriers to both breast cancer and, to a lesser extent, ovarian cancer. The lifetime risk of breast cancer among women who carry a single mutation in either *BRCA-1* or *BRCA-2* is approximately 85%, whereas the lifetime ovarian cancer risk for women with a *BRCA-1* mutation is 54% compared to 24% for women with a *BRCA-2* mutation (King, Marks, Mandell, & New York Breast Cancer Study Group, 2003).

Both *BRCA-1* and *BRCA-2* are tumor suppressor genes that upon transcription form proteins essential for the repair of double-strand DNA breaks (Boulton, 2006). Mutated *BRCA* genes result in proteins that do not function properly in DNA repair, thereby promoting accumulation of genetic errors and carcinogenesis. Population studies have identified high gene frequencies of *BRCA-1* and *BRCA-2* among women of Ashkenazi Jewish descent and high frequencies of *BRCA-1* among women of Greenlander origin (Harboe et al., 2009).

Another genetic condition that predisposes to ovarian cancer is hereditary nonpolyposis colorectal cancer (HNPCC), also called Lynch syndrome (named after Henry T. Lynch, who characterized the genetic and clinical features of HNPCC). The cause of HNPCC is an inherited (germline) mutation in at least one of a set of genes that normally repair DNA, the mismatch-repair genes. In 1993, the first of the HNPCC genes (*MSH2*) was discovered on chromosome 2 by a team of international investigators (Aaltonen et al., 1993). Soon after, *MLH1* was discovered on chromosome 3 (Aaltonen et al., 1994). Mutations in these two genes account for approximately 90% of the known HNPCC families. Lynch syndrome accounts for a small percentage of all colorectal cancer cases, perhaps 1%–3%. Women in HNPCC families are also at increased risk of developing cancers of the uterine lining (endometrium), colon, ovary, and stomach (Offit & Kauff, 2006).

Fertility Agents and Ovarian Cancer

Results of several case–control studies suggest a link between the use of fertility drugs and the development of ovarian cancer. In general, fertility drugs (e.g., clomiphene citrate) stimulate the secretion of FSH and LH by the pituitary gland to help stimulate ovulation. In a meta-analysis of 12 studies, Whittemore et al. (1992) found that infertile women who had taken any form of fertility drugs were 2.7 times more likely to develop ovarian cancer than women who had never taken these medications. It is important to point out that there was no increase in cancer risk among the women who used fertility drugs and subsequently became pregnant. Nevertheless, a subsequent study by Rossing, Daling, Weiss,

Moore, and Self (1994) also found more than a twofold increase in the risk of ovarian cancer among women who had used clomiphene citrate for at least 1 year. Controversy remains regarding the exact nature of the increased risk, and it is difficult to reconcile whether it is due to use of the fertility agent or the underlying pathologies of infertility (Holschneider & Berek, 2000).

Polycystic ovary syndrome (also called Stein–Leventhal syndrome) is a relatively common female endocrine disorder affecting approximately 5%–10% of women of reproductive age. This syndrome is a leading cause of female infertility that develops when the ovaries are stimulated to produce excessive amounts of male hormones (androgens), particularly testosterone, either through the release of excessive LH by the anterior pituitary gland or through high levels of insulin in the blood (hyperinsulinemia) (Carmina, 2004). One small case–control study observed a 2.5-fold increase in the risk of ovarian cancer in women with polycystic ovary syndrome (Schildkraut, Schwingl, Bastos, Evanoff, & Hughes, 1996); however, this finding has not been confirmed in prospective studies (Coulam, Annegers, & Kranz, 1983; Pierpoint, McKeigue, Isaacs, Wild, & Jacobs, 1998).

Other Risk Factors for Ovarian Cancer

Many other potential risk factors have been examined in epidemiologic investigations of ovarian cancer. One factor that has received considerable attention in the media is perineal dusting with talcum powder, a practice that has been observed to increase the risk of ovarian cancer by some investigators (Cramer et al., 1999). Meta-analyses of 16 case–control studies determined a modest increase in the risk (the summary relative risk was 1.3), but also reflected heterogeneity among studies (Huncharek, Geschwind, & Kupelnick, 2003). Furthermore, the biological basis of talc carcinogenicity remains controversial because inhaled talc in mining and milling operations has not been found to be associated with the development of pulmonary tumors (Muscat & Huncharek, 2008).

Ecological studies of ovarian cancer and dietary factors have noted positive correlations between milk consumption, lactase persistence (a measure of lactose digestion), and the incidence of ovarian cancer (Cramer, 1989; Rose, Boyar, & Wynder, 1986). However, analytic studies have yielded conflicting results, some finding a positive association of lactose intake with ovarian cancer development and others finding no association (Larsson, Bergkvist, & Wolk, 2004; Risch, Jain, Marrett, & Howe, 1994). It has been hypothesized that galactose, a component sugar of the disaccharide lactose, might increase the risk of

ovarian cancer either by direct toxicity to the oocytes or by inducing high concentrations of gonadotropins, thereby stimulating the proliferation of the ovarian surface epithelium (Harlow et al., 1991).

Findings from both case–control and cohort epidemiologic studies suggest there is a dose–response relationship between body mass index and the risk of developing ovarian cancer, particularly among postmenopausal women. In a large prospective study of 94,525 women aged 50–71 years, Leitzmann et al. (2009) observed that obesity increased the risk of ovarian cancer by 80% in postmenopausal women with no history of hormone replacement therapy. In a meta-analysis of 28 epidemiologic studies, Olsen et al. (2007) found significant increases in the risk of developing ovarian cancer with obesity (summary relative risk = 1.3) or being overweight (summary relative risk = 1.2); however, there is lack of agreement regarding the timing of the development of ovarian cancer in relation to adiposity (Schouten et al., 2008). In general, the epidemiologic findings support the hypothesis that long-term adiposity enhances aromatase-catalyzed estrogen biosynthesis that in turn increases the genesis of ovarian cancer.

The use of exogenous hormones (estrogen replacement therapy [ERT]) has been studied extensively in relation to various forms of cancer, including ovarian cancer. In a meta-analysis of 19 case–control studies and eight cohort studies, the risk increase was approximately 20% in ever-users versus never-users, and the risk increased with the duration of use (Zhou et al., 2008). A prospective study of nearly 1 million women in the United Kingdom found that current ERT users were about 20% more likely to develop and die from ovarian cancer than never-users (Beral, Million Women Study Collaborators, Bull, Green, & Reeves, 2007). Biologically, the ovarian surface epithelium has cell membrane receptors that are responsive to estrogen, and it is conceivable that ERT may stimulate cell proliferation and other cellular events related to carcinogenesis through modulation of estrogen receptors.

It has been hypothesized that circulating androgens may be involved in the development of ovarian cancer (Risch, 1998). Furthermore, in one study, the synthetic male hormone danazol was linked to the development of ovarian cancer (Cottreau, Ness, Modugno, Allen, & Goodman, 2003). Danazol is sometimes prescribed to women who suffer from endometriosis, a condition associated with dysplasia and bleeding of the endometrium. However, there is consistent evidence that endometriosis is a risk factor for the development of ovarian cancer; for example, a pooled analysis of eight case–control studies found a summary relative risk of 1.7 (Ness, Cramer, Goodman, Kruger Kjaer, & Mallin, 2002), and a large cohort study of Swedish women found a 1.3-fold increase in the risk of ovarian cancer among women with endometriosis (Melin, Sparén, & Bergqvist, 2007). Because the use of danazol is confounded by the presence of endometriosis, additional studies will be required to determine whether this drug truly increases the risk of ovarian cancer.

▶ Protective Reproductive Factors and Ovarian Cancer

Interruption of the menstrual cycle by a first pregnancy early in the reproductive years or by sustained use of oral contraceptives has been found to be protective against the development of ovarian cancer in several studies. For example, in a multicenter population-based case–control study of 436 cases and 3833 controls, the estimated relative risks of epithelial ovarian cancer were 0.6 for women who had ever been pregnant, 0.6 for women who had ever breast fed, and 0.5 for women who had ever used oral contraceptives, and there was a strong trend in decreasing risk with increasing cumulative months of pregnancy (Gwinn, Lee, Rhodes, Layde, & Rubin, 1990). Overall, women with multiple children have risk reductions in the range of 40%–60% compared to nulliparous women (Adami et al., 1994; Hankinson et al., 1995; Risch, Marrett & Howe, 1994). Lactation also confers a slight additional reduction in the risk of ovarian cancer (Rosenblatt & Thomas, 1993).

During the reproductive years, estrogens are produced by the ovaries; in contrast, after menopause, estrogen biosynthesis is catalyzed by the enzyme aromatase in fat and muscle cells. Some investigations have therefore focused on the differential impact of reproductive factors on the risk of developing ovarian cancer in the premenopausal years versus the postmenopausal years. In a large study of 896 cases and 967 controls, Moorman et al. (2008) observed that interruption of the menstrual cycle by either pregnancy or oral contraception conferred protection, but the effect tended to diminish with age during the postmenopausal years.

▶ Oral Contraceptives and Ovarian Cancer

Several epidemiologic investigations have observed significant reductions in the risk of ovarian cancer in women who used oral contraceptives (Franceschi et al., 1991; Gross & Schlesselman, 1994; Narod et al., 1998; Schlesselman, 1995). Recently, a comprehensive meta-analysis of 45 epidemiologic studies comparing

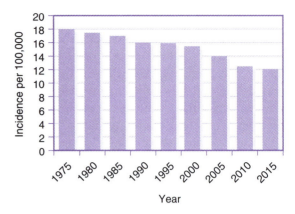

FIGURE 22.5 Ovarian Cancer Incidence in Caucasian Women, 1975–2015, United States.

Data from American Cancer Society. (2009). *Cancer facts and figures. Statistics for 2009.* Atlanta, GA: Author; Horner, M. J., Ries. L. A. G., Krapcho, M., Neyman, N., Aminou, R., Howlader, N., . . . Edwards, B. K. (Eds.). *SEER cancer statistics review, 1975–2006.* Bethesda, MD: National Cancer Institute; Torre, L. A., Trabert, B., DeSantis, C. E., Miller, K. D., Samimi, G., & Runowicz, C. D. (2018). Ovarian cancer statistics, 2018. *CA: A Cancer Journal for Clinicians, 68,* 284–296; Noone, A. M., Howlader, N., Krapcho, M., Miller, D., Brest, A., Yu, M., . . . Cronin, K. A. (Eds.). (2018). *SEER cancer statistics review, 1975–2015.* Bethesda, MD: National Cancer Institute.

23,257 cases with 87,303 controls determined that the use of oral contraceptives reduced the risk by as much as 29% per 5 years of use (Collaborative Group on Epidemiological Studies of Ovarian Cancer, 2008). Furthermore, the rates of ovarian cancer appear to be declining in some countries as a consequence of widespread oral contraceptive use. For example, the incidence and mortality rates of ovarian cancer in the United States have declined by 33% since 1975 when oral contraceptive pills were approved for use by premenopausal women (Noone et al., 2018; Torre et al., 2018) (**FIGURE 22.5**). Oral contraceptives interfere with the pituitary hormones, FSH, and LH, thereby reducing proliferation of epithelial cells at the surface of the ovary and diminishing their potential for carcinogenesis.

▶ Screening for Ovarian Cancer

No screening tools have proven successful in detecting ovarian cancer at an early stage (in situ or localized, stage I) when it can be effectively treated by complete surgical excision. Consequently, more than 70% of these tumors are diagnosed after they have metastasized to contiguous tissue and/or nearby lymph nodes. The overall survival rate is poor, with a 5-year survival rate below 50%, even in developed countries such as the United States. Elevated levels of a small antigenic protein called CA-125 secreted by ovarian cancer cells are usually present and measurable at the time of diagnosis; however, this biomarker has only shown value in monitoring cancer regression or progression, and thus far has not proven useful for screening and early detection (Bast et al., 1981, 1998).

References

Aaltonen, L. A., Peltomiki, P., Leach, F. S., Sistonen, P., Pylkkanen, L., Mecklin, J. P., … de la Chapelle, A. (1993). Clues to the pathogenesis of familial colorectal cancer. *Science, 260,* 812–816.

Aaltonen, L. A., Peltomiki, P., Mecklin, J. P., Jirvinen, H., Jass, J. R., Green, J. S., … de la Chapelle, A. (1994). Replication errors in benign and malignant tumors from hereditary nonpolyposis colorectal cancer patients. *Cancer Research, 54,* 1645–1648.

Adami, H. O., Hsieh, C. C., Lambe, M., Persson, I., Ekbom, A., Adami, H. O., … Janson, P. O. (1994). Parity, age at first childbirth, and risk of ovarian cancer. *Lancet, 344*(8932), 1250–1254.

American Cancer Society. (2009). *Cancer facts and figures.* Atlanta, GA.

Bast, R. C., Feeney, M., Lazarus, H., Nadler, L. M., Colvin, R. B., & Knapp, R. C. (1981). Reactivity of a monoclonal antibody with human ovarian carcinoma. *Journal of Clinical Investigations, 68*(5), 1331–1337.

Bast, R. C., Xu, F. J., Yu, Y. H., Barnhill, S., Zhang, Z., & Mills, G. B. (1998). CA 125: The past and the future. *International Journal of Biological Markers, 13*(4), 179–187.

Beral, V., Million Women Study Collaborators, Bull, D., Green, J., & Reeves, G. (2007). Ovarian cancer and hormone replacement therapy in the Million Women Study. *Lancet, 369*(9574), 1703–1710.

Boulton, S. J. (2006). Cellular functions of the BRCA tumour-suppressor proteins. *Biochemical Society Transactions, 34*(5), 633–645.

Bray, F., Ferlay, J., Soerjomataram, I., Siegel, R. L., Torre, L. A., & Jemal, A. (2018). Global cancer statistics 2018: GLOBOCAN estimates of incidence and mortality worldwide for 36 cancers in 185 countries. *CA: A Cancer Journal for Clinicians, 68*(6), 394–424.

Carmina, E. (2004). Diagnosis of polycystic ovary syndrome: From NIH criteria to ESHRE-ASRM guidelines. *Minerva Ginecologica, 56*(1), 1–6.

Chakravarti, S., Collins, W. P., Forecast, J. D., Newton, J. R., Oram, D. H., & Studd, J. W. (1976). Hormonal profiles after the menopause. *British Medical Journal, 2,* 784–787.

Choi, J. H., Choi, K. C., Auersperg, N., & Leung, P. C. (2004). Overexpression of follicle-stimulating hormone receptor activates oncogenic pathways in preneoplastic ovarian surface epithelial cells. *Journal of Clinical Endocrinology and Metabolism, 89,* 5508–5516.

Choi, J. H., Wong, A. S. T., Huang, H. F., & Leung, P. C. K. (2007). Gonadotropins and ovarian cancer. *Endocrine Reviews, 28*(4), 440–461.

Collaborative Group on Epidemiological Studies of Ovarian Cancer. (2008). Ovarian cancer and oral contraceptives: Collaborative reanalysis of data from 45 epidemiological studies including 23,257 women with ovarian cancer and 87,303 controls. *Lancet, 371,* 303–314.

Cottreau, C. M., Ness, R. B., Modugno, F., Allen, G. O., & Goodman, M. T. (2003). Endometriosis and its treatment with danazol or Lupron in relation to ovarian cancer. *Clinical Cancer Research, 9,* 5142–5144.

Coulam, C. B., Annegers, J. F., & Kranz, J. S. (1983). Chronic anovulation syndrome and associated neoplasia. *Obstetrics and Gynecology, 61,* 403–407.

Cramer, D. W. (1989). Lactase persistence and milk consumption as determinants of ovarian cancer risk. *American Journal of Epidemiology, 130*(5), 904–910.

Cramer, D. W., Liberman, R. F., Titus-Ernstoff, L., Welch, W. R., Greenberg, E. R., Baron, J. A., & Harlow, B. L. (1999). Genital talc exposure and risk of ovarian cancer. *International Journal of Cancer, 81,* 351–356.

Fathalla, M. F. (1971). Incessant ovulation—A factor in ovarian neoplasia? *Lancet, 2*(7716), 163.

Ferlay, J., Ervik, M., Lam, F., Colombet, M., Mery, L., Piñeros, M., … Bray, F. (2018). *Global cancer observatory: Cancer today.* Lyon, France: International Agency for Research on Cancer. Retrieved from https://gco.iarc.fr/today

Ferlay, J., Shin, H.-R., Bray, F., Forman, D., Mathers, C., & Parkin, D. M. (2010). Estimates of worldwide burden of cancer in 2008: GLOBOCAN 2008. *International Journal of Cancer, 127*(12), 2893–2917.

Ferlay, J., Soerjomataram, I., Ervik, M., Dikshit, R., Eser, S., Mathers, C., … Bray, F. (2013). *GLOBOCAN 2012 v1.0. Cancer incidence and mortality worldwide: IARC CancerBase No. 11* [Internet]. Lyon, France: International Agency for Research on Cancer. Retrieved from http://globocan.iarc.fr

Fitzmaurice, C., Akinyemiju, T. F., Al Lami, F. H., Alam, T., Alizadeh-Navaei, R., Allen, C., … Global Burden of Disease Cancer Collaboration. (2018). Global, regional, and national cancer incidence, mortality, years of life lost, years lived with disability, and disability-adjusted life-years for 29 cancer groups, 1990 to 2016: A systematic analysis for the Global Burden of Disease Study. *JAMA Oncology.* Online publication. doi:10.1001/jamaoncol.2018.2706.

Fitzmaurice, C., Allen, C., Barber, R. M., Barregard, L., Bhutta, Z. A., Brenner, H., … Global Burden of Disease Cancer Collaboration. (2017). Global, regional, and national cancer incidence, mortality, years of life lost, years lived with disability, and disability-adjusted life-years for 32 cancer groups, 1990 to 2015: A systematic analysis for the Global Burden of Disease Study. *JAMA Oncology, 3*(4), 524–548.

Franceschi, S., Parazzini, F., Negri, E., Booth, M., La Vecchia, C., Beral, V., … Trichopoulos, D. (1991). Pooled analysis of three European case-control studies of epithelial ovarian cancer: III. Oral contraceptive use. *International Journal of Cancer, 49,* 61–65.

Gross, T. P., & Schlesselman, J. J. (1994). The estimated effect of oral contraceptive use on the cumulative risk of epithelial ovarian cancer. *Obstetrics and Gynecology, 83,* 419–424.

Gwinn, M. L., Lee, N. C., Rhodes, P. H., Layde, P. M., & Rubin, G. L. (1990). Pregnancy, breast feeding, and oral contraceptives and the risk of epithelial ovarian cancer. *Journal of Clinical Epidemiology, 43*(6), 559–568.

Hall, J. M., Lee, M. K., Newman, B., Morrow, J. E., Anderson, L. A., Huey, B., & King, M. C. (1990). Linkage of early-onset familial breast cancer to chromosome 17q21. *Science, 250*(4988), 1684–1689.

Hankinson, S. E., Colditz, G. A., Hunter, D. J., Willett, W. C., Stampfer, M. J., Rosner, B., … Speizer, F. E. (1995). A prospective study of reproductive factors and risk of epithelial ovarian cancer. *Cancer, 76,* 284–290.

Harboe, T. L., Eiberg, E. H., Kern, E. P., Ejlertsen, B., Nedergaard, E. L., Timmermans-Wielenga, V., … Bisgaard, M. L. (2009). A high frequent BRCA1 founder mutation identified in the Greenlandic population. *Familial Cancer, 8,* 413–419.

Harlow, B. L., Cramer, D. W., Geller, J., Willett, W. C., Bell, D. A., & Welch, W. R. (1991). The influence of lactose consumption on the association of oral contraceptive use and ovarian cancer risk. *American Journal of Epidemiology, 134,* 445–453.

Helzlsouer, K. J., Alberg, A. J., & Gordon, G. B. (1995). Serum gonadotropins and steroid hormones in the development of ovarian cancer. *Journal of the American Medical Association, 274*, 1926–1930.

Holschneider, C. H., & Berek, J. S. (2000). Ovarian cancer: Epidemiology, biology and prognostic factors. *Seminars in Surgical Oncology, 19*, 3–10.

Huncharek, M., Geschwind, J. F., & Kupelnick, B. (2003). Perineal application of cosmetic talc and risk of invasive epithelial ovarian cancer: A meta-analysis of 11,933 subjects from sixteen observational studies. *Anticancer Research, 23*, 1955–1960.

King, M. C., Marks, J. H., Mandell, J. B., & New York Breast Cancer Study Group. (2003). Breast and ovarian cancer risks due to inherited mutations in BRCA1 and BRCA2. *Science, 302*(5645), 643–646.

Kramer, S., Leeker, M., & Jager, W. (1998). Gonadotropin levels in ovarian cyst fluids: A predictor of malignancy? *International Journal of Biological Markers, 13*, 165–168.

Kumar, V., Abbas, A. K., & Aster, J. C. (2014). *Robbins and Cotran pathologic basis of disease* (9th ed.). Philadelphia, PA: Mosby & Saunders.

Larsson, S. C., Bergkvist, L., & Wolk, A. (2004). Milk and lactose intakes and ovarian cancer risk in the Swedish Mammography Cohort. *American Journal of Clinical Nutrition, 80*(5), 1353–1357.

Leitzmann, M. F., Koebnick, C., Danforth, K. N., Brinton, L. A., Moore, S. C., Hollenbeck, A. R., … Lacey, J. V. (2009). Body mass index and risk of ovarian cancer. *Cancer, 155*(4), 812–822.

Melin, A., Sparén, P., & Bergqvist, A. (2007). The risk of cancer and the role of parity among women with endometriosis. *Human Reproduction, 22*(11), 3021–3026.

Moorman, P. G., Calingaert, B., Palmieri, R. T., Iversen, E. S., Bentley, R. C., Halabi, S., … Schildkraut, J. M. (2008). Hormonal risk factors for ovarian cancer in premenopausal and postmenopausal women. *American Journal of Epidemiology, 167*(9), 1059–1069.

Muscat, J. E., & Huncharek, M. S. (2008). Perineal talc use and ovarian cancer: A critical review. *European Journal of Cancer Prevention, 17*, 139–146.

Narod, S. A., Risch, H., Moslehi, R., Dorum, A., Neuhausen, S., Olsson, H., … Klijn, J. G. M. (1998). Oral contraceptives and the risk of hereditary ovarian cancer. *New England Journal of Medicine, 339*, 424–428.

National Cancer Institute. (2009). *Cancer statistics, 2009.* Bethesda, MD.

Ness, R. B., & Cottreau, C. (1999). Possible role of ovarian epithelial inflammation in ovarian cancer. *Journal of the National Cancer Institute, 91*, 1459–1467.

Ness, R. B., Cramer, D. W., Goodman, M. T., Kruger Kjaer, S., & Mallin, K. (2002). Infertility, fertility drugs, and ovarian cancer: A pooled analysis of case–control studies. *American Journal of Epidemiology, 155*, 217–224.

Noone, A. M., Howlader, N., Krapcho, M., Miller, D., Brest, A., Yu, M., … Cronin, K. A. (Eds.). (2018). *SEER cancer statistics review, 1975–2015.* Bethesda, MD: National Cancer Institute.

Offit, K., & Kauff, N. D. (2006). Reducing the risk of gynecologic cancer in the Lynch syndrome. *New England Journal of Medicine, 354*(3), 293–295.

Olsen, C. M., Green, A. C., Whiteman, D. C., Sadeghi, S., Kolahdooz, F., & Webb, P. M. (2007). Obesity and the risk of epithelial ovarian cancer: A systematic review and meta-analysis. *European Journal of Cancer, 43*, 690–709.

Parkin, M. D., Bray, F., Ferlay, J., & Pisani, P. (2005). Global cancer statistics, 2002. *CA: A Cancer Journal for Clinicians, 55*, 74–108.

Pierpoint, T., McKeigue, P. M., Isaacs, A. J., Wild, S. H., & Jacobs, H. S. (1998). Mortality of women with polycystic ovary syndrome at long-term follow-up. *Journal of Clinical Epidemiology, 51*, 581–586.

Risch, H. A. (1998). Hormonal etiology of epithelial ovarian cancer, with a hypothesis concerning the role of androgens and progesterone. *Journal of the National Cancer Institute, 90*, 1774–1786.

Risch, H. A., Jain, M., Marrett, L. D., & Howe, G. R. (1994). Dietary lactose intake, lactose intolerance, and the risk of epithelial ovarian cancer in southern Ontario (Canada). *Cancer Causes and Control, 5*, 540–548.

Risch, H. A., Marrett, L. D., & Howe, G. R. (1994). Parity, contraception, infertility, and the risk of epithelial ovarian cancer. *American Journal of Epidemiology, 140*, 585–597.

Rose, D. P., Boyar, A. P., & Wynder, E. L. (1986). International comparisons of mortality rates for cancer of the breast, ovary, prostate, and colon, and per capita food consumption. *Cancer, 58*, 2363–2371.

Rosenblatt, K. A., & Thomas, D. B. (1993). Lactation and the risk of epithelial ovarian cancer. The WHO Collaborative Study of Neoplasia and Steroid Contraceptives. *International Journal of Epidemiology, 22*, 192–197.

Rossing, M. A., Daling, J. R., Weiss, N. S., Moore, D. E., & Self, S. G. (1994). Ovarian tumors in a cohort of infertile women. *New England Journal of Medicine, 331*, 771–776.

Schildkraut, J. M., Schwingl, P. J., Bastos, E., Evanoff, A., & Hughes, C. (1996). Epithelial ovarian cancer risk among women with polycystic ovary syndrome. *Obstetrics and Gynecology, 88*(4 Pt 1), 554–559.

Schlesselman, J. J. (1995). Net effect of oral contraceptive use on the risk of cancer in women in the United States. *Obstetrics and Gynecology, 85*(5 Pt 1), 793–801.

Schouten, L. J., Rivera, C., Hunter, D. J., Spiegelman, D., Adami, H. O., Arslan, A., … Smith-Warner, S. A. (2008). Height, body mass index, and ovarian cancer: A pooled analysis of 12 cohort studies. *Cancer Epidemiology, Biomarkers and Prevention, 17*, 902–912.

Scully, R. E. (1995). Pathology of ovarian cancer precursors. *Journal of Cellular Biochemistry, 23*(Suppl.), 208–218.

Torre, L. A., Trabert, B., DeSantis, C. E., Miller, K. D., Samimi, G., & Runowicz, C. D. (2018). Ovarian cancer statistics, 2018. *CA: A Cancer Journal for Clinicians, 68*, 284–296.

Whittemore, A. S., Harris, R., & Itnyre, J. (1992). Characteristics relating to ovarian cancer risk: Collaborative analysis of 12 U.S. case-control studies. II. Invasive epithelial ovarian cancers in white women. *American Journal of Epidemiology, 136*, 1184–1203.

Wooster, R., Neuhausen, S. L., Mangion, J., Quirk, Y., Ford, D., Collins, N., … Stratton, M. R. (1994). Localization of a breast cancer susceptibility gene, BRCA2, to chromosome 13q12–13. *Science, 265*(5181), 2088–2090.

Zheng, W., Lu, J. J., Luo, F., Zheng, Y., Feng, Y., Felix, J. C., … Pike, M. (2000). Ovarian epithelial tumor growth promotion by follicle-stimulating hormone and inhibition of the effect by luteinizing hormone. *Gynecologic Oncology, 76*, 80–88.

Zhou, B., Sun, Q., Cong, R., Gu, H., Tang, N., Yang, L., & Wang, B. (2008). Hormone replacement therapy and ovarian cancer risk: A meta-analysis. *Gynecologic Oncology, 108*(3), 641–651.

CHAPTER 23

Epidemiology of Cancer of the Corpus Uteri: Endometrial Cancer, Uterine Sarcoma, and Choriocarcinoma

▶ Global Impact of Cancer of the Corpus Uteri

Worldwide, cancer of the *corpus uteri* (body of the uterus) was diagnosed in 382,069 women and caused 89,929 deaths during 2018. Cancer of the corpus uteri currently accounts for 4.4% of cancer cases and 2.4% of cancer deaths among women. The global age-adjusted incidence rate in 2018 was 8.4 per 100,000 and the mortality rate was 1.8 per 100,000 (Bray et al., 2018; Parkin, Bray, Ferlay, & Pisani, 2001).

The 2018 incidence rates of corpus uteri cancer were highest in developed countries of North America, the Russian Federation, Western Europe, and Scandinavia (>15 cases per 100,000) and lowest in underdeveloped countries of Southeast Asia and Africa (<3 cases per 100,000) (**FIGURE 23.1**). In general, developed countries also had higher mortality rates than developing countries. On average, the incidence of corpus uteri cancer was threefold higher in developed versus developing countries (11.1 versus 3.3 per 100,000), and the mortality was approximately 67% higher in developed versus developing countries

(2.0 versus 1.2 per 100,000) (Bray et al., 2018; Ferlay et al., 2018). Due to shared risk factors that heighten exposure to both endogenous and exogenous estrogens, the global pattern of corpus uteri cancer shows similarities to those of breast cancer and ovarian cancer.

The global burden of cancer of the corpus uteri has increased sharply in the 21st century. During 2000–2018, reported numbers of new cases and deaths have doubled (**FIGURE 23.2**) (Bray et al., 2018; Bray, Dos Santos Silva, Moller, & Weiderpass, 2005; Ferlay, Bray, Pisani, & Parkin, 2004, 2010, 2013; Fitzmaurice et al., 2018; Parkin et al., 2001; Parkin, Bray, Ferlay, & Pisani, 2005). These increases are predominantly due to increasing rates of endometrial cancer, which accounts for over 90% of malignancies of the corpus uteri. As discussed in the following sections of this chapter, the rising worldwide burden of endometrial cancer undoubtedly reflects the impact of multiple factors, including better detection and therapy plus heightened exposure to certain risk factors, including late childbearing, lack of breastfeeding, intake of exogenous hormones, intake of diets high in fat and calories, lack of exercise, and in particular, increasing rates of obesity and diabetes mellitus (Bray, Dos Santos Silva, Moller, & Weiderpass, 2005).

Estimated age-standardized incidence rates (World) in 2018, corpus uteri, all ages

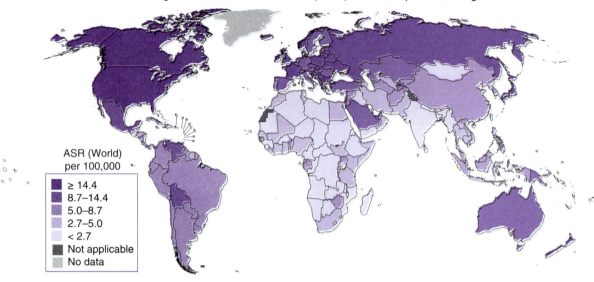

ASR (World)
per 100,000

- ≥ 14.4
- 8.7–14.4
- 5.0–8.7
- 2.7–5.0
- < 2.7
- Not applicable
- No data

Estimated age-standardized mortality rates (World) in 2018, corpus uteri, all ages

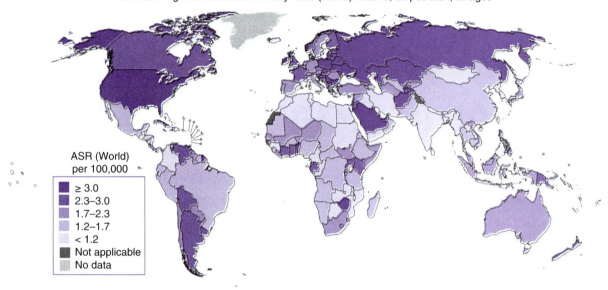

ASR (World)
per 100,000

- ≥ 3.0
- 2.3–3.0
- 1.7–2.3
- 1.2–1.7
- < 1.2
- Not applicable
- No data

FIGURE 23.1 Global Rates of Cancer of the Corpus Uteri.

Caption: ASR: Rate per 100,000 Standardized to the World Population, 2000–2025.

Reproduced with permission from Ferlay, J., Ervik, M., Lam, F., Colombet, M., Mery, L., Piñeros, M., … Bray, F. (2018). *Global cancer observatory: Cancer today.* Lyon, France: International Agency for Research on Cancer. Retrieved from https://gco.iarc.fr/today

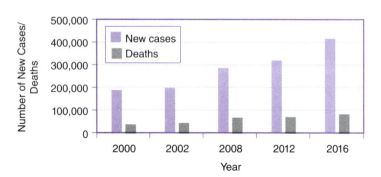

FIGURE 23.2 Global Increase in Cancer of the Corpus Uteri, 2000–2016.

Data from Ferlay, J., Bray, F., Pisani, P., & Parkin, D. M. (2004). *GLOBOCAN 2002. Cancer incidence, mortality, and prevalence worldwide.* IARC Cancer Base No. 5, version 2.0. Lyon, France: IARC Press. Retrieved from http://www-dep.iarc.fr; Ferlay, J., Shin, H.-R., Bray, F., Forman, D., Mathers, C., & Parkin, D. M. (2010). Estimates of worldwide burden of cancer in 2008: GLOBOCAN 2008. *International Journal of Cancer, 127*(12), 2893–2917; Ferlay, J., Soerjomataram, I., Ervik, M., Dikshit, R., Eser, S., Mathers, C., … Bray, F. (2013). *GLOBOCAN 2012 v1.0. Cancer incidence and mortality worldwide: IARC CancerBase No. 11* [Internet]. Lyon, France: International Agency for Research on Cancer. Retrieved from http://globocan.iarc.fr; Parkin, D. M., Bray, F., Ferlay, J., & Pisani, P. (2001). Estimating the world cancer burden: GLOBOCAN 2000. *International Journal of Cancer, 94*, 153–156.

▶ Malignant Tumors of the Corpus Uteri

Approximately 92% of malignant tumors of the corpus uteri are *endometrial carcinomas* that arise from the epithelial lining of the endometrium. Histologically, more than 90% of endometrial carcinomas are adenocarcinomas that show glandular characteristics under the microscope (Kosary, 2007).

Sarcomas derived from connective tissues of the uterus do occur, but infrequently; for example, leiomyosarcoma of smooth muscle cells and stromal sarcoma of other connective tissues account for about 3% of all uterine cancers (Kosary, 2007). Sarcomas can arise not only in the uterus, but also in many other anatomic sites such as subcutaneous tissue, the peritoneal cavity, the stomach, and omental tissues surrounding the gastrointestinal tract (Kumar, Abbas, & Aster, 2014). Uterine sarcomas are briefly discussed in a later section of this chapter.

Two additional subtypes of corpus uterine cancer, carcinosarcomas and mixed malignant Müllerian tumors, consist of a mixture of glandular and connective tissues. Consequently, the exact histological classification of such tumors as endometrial carcinomas or sarcomas is controversial and has been debated by pathologists for many years (Kanthan & Senger, 2011). Mixed malignant Müllerian tumors and carcinosarcomas account for about 5% of corpus uteri tumors (Kosary, 2007).

Choriocarcinoma is a very rare type of uterine malignancy that occasionally develops during pregnancy. The epidemiology of choriocarcinoma is included in a later section of this chapter.

▶ Endometrial Cancer Versus Cervical Cancer: Cellular Origins

When combined with cervical cancer, malignant neoplasms of the corpus uteri and the endometrium account for more than two-thirds of all invasive malignancies that develop in the female genital tract (Platz & Benda, 1995). Though they border one another, the cellular populations that give rise to endometrial cancer and cervical cancer are distinctly different.

Endometrial cancer arises from the cuboidal epithelial cells that line the body of the uterus above the cervix, whereas cervical cancer arises from the squamous epithelial cells that line the cervix. The corpus uterus is the hollow pear-shaped organ in which the placenta is implanted, and where the fetus develops during pregnancy. The endometrium per se refers to the innermost glandular layer of the corpus uterus. The anatomic distinction between the endometrium and the cervix can be seen in **FIGURE 23.3** (Kumar et al., 2014).

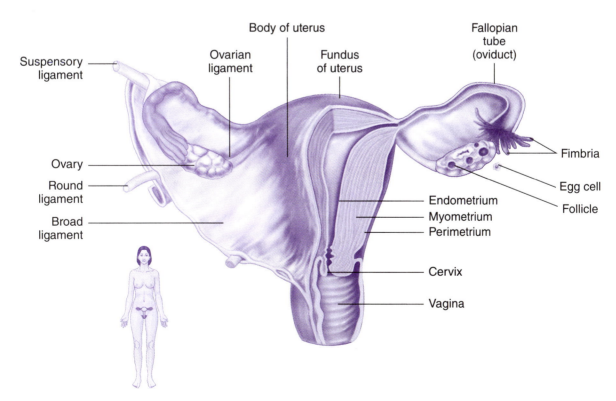

FIGURE 23.3 Female Reproductive Anatomy.

In world population studies by the International Association of Cancer Research (IARC), cases that are pathologically confirmed as endometrial cancer or cancer of the body of the uterus (*corpus uteri*) are all coded under the *International Code of Disease* as ICD 54. In contrast, cervical cancer is coded separately as ICD 53. It should be noted that cases of *unspecified uterine cancer* are coded as ICD 55, which are allocated to endometrial cancer or cervical cancer according to the differential age distributions of these tumors (Loos et al., 2004).

▶ Trends in Endometrial Cancer

In developed regions of the world, endometrial cancer has surpassed cervical cancer as the leading gynecological malignancy in women (Sankaranarayanan & Ferlay, 2006). As shown in **FIGURES 23.4** and **23.5**, the annual incidence rates of endometrial cancer among U.S. women have trended upward since 2000 and are now 3–4 times higher than cervical cancer rates, which continue to decline (Duong, Wilson, Ajani, Singh, &

Eheman, 2011; Hayat, Howlader, Reichman, & Edwards, 2007; Howlader et al., 2012). Recent increases in the incidence of endometrial cancer and declining rates of cervical cancer are also evident in Great Britain, Western Europe, Scandinavia, and Australia (Bray et al., 2005; Evans et al., 2011; Purdie & Green, 2001; Saso et al., 2011). These trends undoubtedly reflect greater exposure to major risk factors for endometrial cancer (e.g., obesity, insulin resistance, estrogen replacement therapy, tamoxifen) plus the significant impact of successful screening for precancerous cervical lesions by Papanicolaou cytological testing (the Pap test).

In contrast to the pattern in developed nations, women living in underdeveloped nations have markedly higher rates of cervical cancer than endometrial cancer. This is due to the high rates of genital infections by oncogenic strains of human papillomavirus (HPV) in women living in underdeveloped nations. Although HPV infections account for virtually all cases of cervical cancer, their role in the genesis of endometrial cancer is negligible.

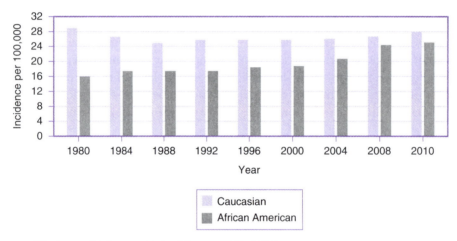

FIGURE 23.4 Incidence of Endometrial Cancer, United States, 1980–2010.

Data from Howlader, N., Noone, A. M., Krapcho, M., Garshell, J., Neyman, N., Altekruse, S. F., ... Cronin, K. A. (Eds.). (2012, November). *SEER cancer statistics review, 1975–2010*. Bethesda, MD: National Cancer Institute. Retrieved from http://seer.cancer.gov/csr/1975_2010

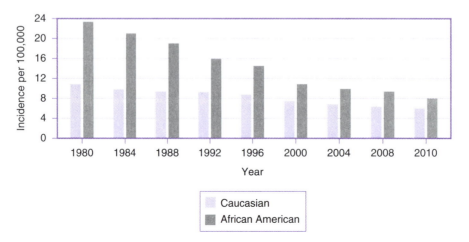

FIGURE 23.5 Incidence of Cervical Cancer, United States, 1980–2010.

Data from Howlader, N., Noone, A. M., Krapcho, M., Garshell, J., Neyman, N., Altekruse, S. F., ... Cronin, K. A. (Eds.). (2012, November). *SEER cancer statistics review, 1975–2010*. Bethesda, MD: National Cancer Institute. Retrieved from http://seer.cancer.gov/csr/1975_2010/

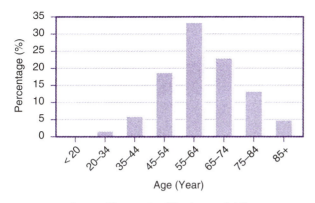

FIGURE 23.6 Age at Diagnosis of Endometrial Cancer.

Data from National Cancer Institute. *Fast stats*. Retrieved from http://seer.cancer.gov/faststats

▶ Endometrial Cancer: Postmenopausal Age of Onset

The vast majority of cases of endometrial cancer (nearly 95%) are detected in postmenopausal women after the age of 45 years (**FIGURE 23.6**). Based on data from the United States collected during 2006–2010, the median age at diagnosis is 62 years (National Cancer Institute, n.d.).

▶ Subtypes of Endometrial Cancer

Endometrial cancers can be classified according to their dependence (or lack of dependence) on estrogen for growth and development. Type 1 cancers are estrogen-dependent and positive for estrogen receptors (ER-positive) (Bender, Buekers, & Leslie, 2011). They develop in women in association with obesity, hyperlipidemia, hyperestrogenism, anovulatory uterine bleeding, infertility, late onset of menopause, and hyperplasia of the epithelial lining of the endometrium (Bokhman, 1983). Type 1 endometrial cancers are typically low-grade, well-differentiated adenocarcinomas that have a favorable prognosis. Type 1 tumors are also called *endometrioid endometrial carcinomas*. They account for about 90% of all endometrial cancers (Felix et al., 2010).

Type 2 endometrial cancers are non-estrogen-dependent and are ER-negative. Type 2 endometrial cancers are typically high-grade serous carcinomas associated with poor survival. They account for about 10% of all endometrial cancers (Amant et al., 2005).

▶ Models of Endometrial Carcinogenesis

Similar molecular mechanisms may be at work in the genesis of endometrial cancer and breast cancer. Both tumors arise from epithelial cell populations that are rich in estrogen and progesterone receptors (PRs) and thus responsive to ovarian fluctuations in estrogen and progesterone during the menstrual cycle in premenopausal women and to other sources of estrogen in postmenopausal women. Consequently, sustained exposure to estrogen, particularly in the absence of progesterone (unopposed estrogen), may lead to an increasing mitotic rate and atypical hyperplasia of the mammary epithelium or endometrial epithelium, which increases the chance of cancer development (Key & Pike, 1988a, 1988b). Sources of excessive estrogen exposure may be endogenous, exogenous, or both, as discussed later in this section.

Barry Sherman and Stanley Korenman originally proposed that heightened *endogenous* exposure to unopposed estrogen is most likely to occur during two windows of time: early in life at menarche when menstruation begins and later in life at menopause when menstrual cycles cease. They postulated that exposure to unopposed estrogen occurs in association with abnormal maturation of follicles (containing unfertilized eggs) as well as irregular or deficient progesterone production by the corpus luteum (the remnant follicle after ovulation). Their theory of corpus luteum dysfunction as the cause of unopposed estrogen and heightened breast cancer risk is called the *estrogen window hypothesis* (Korenman, 1980; Sherman & Korenman, 1974).

In considering the estrogen window hypothesis of either breast cancer or endometrial cancer, it is essential to review key features of the human female menstrual cycle, as shown in **FIGURE 23.7**. During the *follicular proliferative phase*, which lasts about 10 days in an ordinary 28-day cycle, follicular stimulating hormone (FSH) is secreted by the pituitary gland, which stimulates maturation of ovarian follicles containing unfertilized eggs. The maturing ovarian follicles secrete increasing amounts of estrogen, causing accelerated cell proliferation and thickening of the endometrial epithelium. Both FSH and estrogen peak at the time of ovulation, which involves the rupture of one follicle and release of its unfertilized egg into the fallopian tube. After ovulation, luteinizing hormone (LH) from the pituitary gland stimulates the *luteal secretory phase* of the cycle, which lasts for about 14 days. During this phase, the corpus luteum secretes progesterone, which induces the development of spiral arteries and stromal edema of the endometrium. In the absence of fertilization, the *menstrual phase* of the cycle occurs, which lasts about 4 days. During menses, the endometrial lining is shed, and blood and tissue are discharged from the uterus.

According to the *estrogen window hypothesis*, unopposed estrogen due to corpus luteum dysfunction

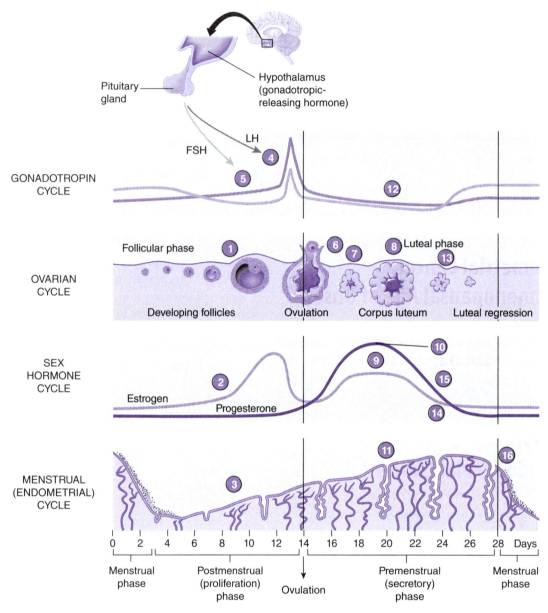

FIGURE 23.7 Pituitary and Ovarian Hormones in the Menstrual Cycle.

Caption: Endometrial cancer risk is increased by exposure to unopposed estrogen and inflammatory factors. Inflammation and wound healing are present with the shedding and repair of the endometrium during menstruation. Unopposed estrogen is present in anovulatory cycles because no corpus luteum forms and progesterone is absent.

during anovulatory cycles of the perimenopausal time window elevates the risk of cancer development in the epithelial tissues of the mammary gland and the endometrium (Korenman, 1980; Sherman & Korenman, 1974). With cessation of menstruation at menopause, the ovaries abruptly discontinue secretion of both estrogen and progesterone. However, in some women this biological phenomenon opens a window of time during which irregular or anovulatory cycles occur, resulting in heightened exposure to unopposed estrogen from either continuing production of estrogen in the absence of progesterone or amplified enzymatic conversion of other steroids to estrogen by aromatase in fat and muscle. An earlier time window of unopposed estrogen may also occur

in young women around the time of menarche when anovulatory menstrual cycles are more likely to occur (Korenman, 1980).

Several factors must be considered in assessing a woman's level of exposure to excessive levels of unopposed estrogen. These include reproductive history (pregnancy and lactation), long-term use of oral contraceptives, surgical history (e.g., hysterectomy and oophorectomy), postmenopausal estrogen replacement therapy (with or without progesterone), obesity, and chronic cigarette smoking (Key & Pike, 1988a, 1988b; Sherman, Wallace, & Korenman, 1981).

An alternative model postulates that the chronic repetitive inflammatory process of menstruation may also play an important role in the genesis of endometrial cancer. The shedding and repair of the endometrium during menstruation obviously includes inflammation and wound healing as physiologic components. Thus, in the absence of a pregnancy, the endometrium is cyclically exposed to chronic repetitive inflammation involving the release of multiple inflammatory factors (prostaglandins, cytokines, and growth factors) that could influence the initiation and progression of endometrial malignancies (Modugno, Ness, Chen, & Weiss, 2005).

▸ Risk Factors for Endometrial Cancer

Estrogenic risk factors for endometrial cancer are broadly divisible into (1) reproductive hallmarks and medical conditions that heighten exposure to *endogenous estrogens* and (2) lifestyle choices that result in exposure to *exogenous estrogens*. Conversely, avoidance of excessive exposure to estrogen reduces the risk. Genetic factors play a minor role. The profile of endometrial cancer risk factors is like those for breast cancer and ovarian cancer.

Factors that increase the risk include early menarche, nulliparity, late menopause, obesity, type 2 diabetes mellitus, estrogen replacement therapy, and use of medications that modulate ERs. Factors that decrease the risk include high parity, late age at last pregnancy, the use of oral contraceptives, and tobacco smoking (Purdie & Green, 2001; Schottenfeld, 1995). Removal of the endometrium and/or the ovaries by hysterectomy and/or oophorectomy for conditions other than cancer must be considered in the assessment of risk.

Reproductive Hallmarks and Endometrial Cancer

Early menarche, nulliparity, and late menopause have all been consistently found to increase the risk of developing endometrial cancer. Conversely, late menarche, high parity, and early menopause are associated with decreases in risk. Unlike breast cancer, early age at first full-term pregnancy has no effect on the risk of endometrial cancer. Rather, *late age at a last pregnancy* appears to reduce the risk (MacMahon, 1974; McPherson, Sellers, Potter, Bostick, & Folsom, 1996; Purdie & Green, 2001).

Recently, a team of investigators analyzed data from the European Prospective Investigation into Cancer and Nutrition (EPIC) to re-examine the association of menstrual and reproductive factors and the risk of developing endometrial cancer. In the EPIC database, 1017 incident cases of endometrial cancer were identified among 302,618 women enrolled for study from 10 European countries (Denmark, France, Germany, Greece, Italy, the Netherlands, Norway, Spain, Sweden, and the United Kingdom). Results revealed significant risk reductions associated with late menarche, early menopause, past use of oral contraceptives (OC), high parity, and shorter time since last full-term pregnancy. Compared to nulliparous women, parous women had a 35% reduction in the risk of developing endometrial cancer. Among parous women, the number of full-term pregnancies and the age at last pregnancy were inversely related to risk. After multivariate adjustment, late age at menarche, early age at menopause, and duration of OC use showed similar risk reductions of 7%–8% per year of menstrual life, whereas the decreased risk associated with cumulative duration of full-term pregnancies was stronger (22% per year). The investigators concluded that:

> … our findings confirmed a reduction in risk of endometrial cancer with factors associated with a lower cumulative exposure to estrogen and/or higher exposure to progesterone, such as increasing number of full-term pregnancies and shorter menstrual lifespan and, therefore, support an important role of hormonal mechanisms in endometrial carcinogenesis (Dossus et al., 2010).

Polycystic Ovary Syndrome and Premenopausal Endometrial Cancer

Certain menstrual cycle irregularities increase the risk of developing endometrial cancer in premenopausal women. One such condition is *polycystic ovary syndrome* (also known as Stein–Leventhal syndrome) wherein women of reproductive age develop bilateral ovarian cysts in association with prolonged anovulation, infertility, excess ovarian secretion of androgens, masculinizing symptoms (e.g., hirsutism), and endometriosis (Radosh, 2009). A recent prevalence study suggests that about 7% of U.S. women are afflicted with polycystic ovary syndrome (Azziz et al., 2004).

The link between polycystic ovary syndrome and endometrial cancer was first observed more than half a century ago (Dockerty, Loveday, & Foust, 1951; Jackson & Dockerty, 1957; Speert, 1949). In a recent study of Australian women, the medical history of polycystic ovary syndrome was assessed among 156 cases and 398 controls under the age of 50 years. Results showed that women with polycystic ovaries had a fourfold increase in risk compared to healthy women (Fearnley et al., 2010). One mechanism underlying this association is that during anovulatory menstrual cycles the endometrium receives increased exposure to estrogens unopposed by progesterone (Jafari, Javaheri, & Ruiz, 1978; Navaratnarajah, Pillay, & Hardiman, 2008).

Granulosa Cell Ovarian Tumors and Endometrial Cancer

Granulosa cell tumors of the ovary occasionally occur in association with heterogeneous symptoms of the female genital tract, including menstrual cycle irregularities, infertility, vaginal bleeding, pelvic pain, and uterine pathologies. These tumors are uncommon and account for only 2%–5% of all ovarian malignancies. Because human ovarian granulosa cells secrete estrogen, women who develop granulosa cell ovarian tumors manifest marked increases in circulating estrogens, which in turn stimulate ERs in other tissues such as the endometrium. Consequently, women who develop ovarian granulosa cell tumors are prone to the development of endometrial hyperplasia and endometrial carcinoma. Granulosa cell tumors also typically secrete inhibin, a polypeptide hormone that regulates FSH secretion by the anterior pituitary gland. Due to hyperestrogenism and hormonal imbalance, endometrial cancer develops in about 10% of women with ovarian granulosa cell tumors (Malmström, Högberg, Risberg, & Simonsen, 1994; Schumer & Cannistra, 2003).

In a molecular study of tissue samples of granulosa cell ovarian tumors, 90 of 93 cases (97%) manifested a somatic mutation that mapped to the same location in the *FOXL2* gene on chromosome 3. Because *FOXL2* is required for the normal development and function of granulosa cells in ovarian tissue, further studies of its mutant form may aid in diagnosis and provide new modalities and molecular targets for prevention and therapeutic intervention (Shah et al., 2009).

Endometriosis and Endometrial Cancer

Endometriosis is the abnormal presence of endometrial glands in the myometrium (muscle) of the female genital tract (e.g., ovaries, uterine ligaments, vagina). This is a common gynecologic condition with a prevalence of about 10% among women of reproductive age (Viganò, Parazzini, Somigliana, & Vercellini, 2004). The pathogenesis of endometriosis is most often attributed to retrograde implantation of endometrial glands external to the uterus during menstruation. Although endometriosis has been linked to the development of ovarian cancer, current evidence *does not*

support an association between endometriosis and the development of endometrial cancer (Brinton, Gridley, Persson, Baron, & Bergqvist, 1997).

Obesity and Endometrial Cancer

The role of obesity as a significant risk factor for endometrial cancer has been firmly established. In a meta-analysis of 16 epidemiologic studies, the pooled relative risk (RR) for obese women compared to women of normal weight was elevated nearly twofold (RR = 1.85, 95% confidence interval 1.30–2.65, $P < 0.0001$). In the study, women with a body mass index (BMI) of 30 or more were compared to those with a BMI less than 25. The largest of the studies included in the meta-analysis was a prospective examination of 103,882 women who participated in the American Association of Retired Persons Diet and Health Study, which was designed to address the effects of dietary and lifestyle factors on cancer risk. In this investigation, similar increases in risk were observed for obese women (RR = 3.03) and women who had gained more than 20 kg (44 pounds) since age 18 (RR = 2.75) (Chang et al., 2007). The association among obesity, excess adiposity, and the development of endometrial cancer is biologically plausible because obese women tend to have higher endogenous estrogen levels than lean women due to aromatization of androstenedione in adipose tissue. Obese women have also been found to have reduced levels of sex hormone–binding globulin compared to lean women, which increases the bioavailability of estrogens (Simpson & Brown, 2011).

Diabetes Mellitus and Endometrial Cancer

Many epidemiologic investigations have observed that women with a medical history of diabetes mellitus are at increased risk of developing endometrial cancer. The role of both type 1 and type 2 diabetes was examined in a meta-analysis of 16 studies (3 cohort and 13 case–control studies) including data on 96,003 subjects and 7596 cases of endometrial cancer. Summary relative risk estimates revealed a twofold risk increase for type 2 diabetics (RR = 2.10) and a threefold increase for type 1 diabetics (RR = 3.15) (Friberg, Orsini, Mantzoros, & Wolk, 2007).

The biological basis of this association may be related to hyperinsulinemia due to the insulin resistance of type 2 diabetes or insulin therapy for type 1 diabetes; that is, chronically elevated levels of circulating insulin may stimulate the proliferation of endometrial epithelium by binding to insulin receptors in endometrial tissues (Nagamani & Stuart, 1998). Hyperinsulinemia may also increase exposure to bioactive estrogens by decreasing the activity of sex hormone–binding globulin (Nestler et al., 1991). Furthermore, obesity is a major risk factor for type 2 diabetes, and the presence of both conditions has been found to synergistically increase the risk of developing endometrial cancer (Lucenteforte et al., 2007).

Hormone Replacement and Endometrial Cancer

In the early 1970s, the incidence of endometrial cancer abruptly doubled among Caucasian women in the United States (**FIGURE 23.8**). This phenomenon was observed shortly after a marked increase in estrogen replacement therapy (equine estrogens) for the treatment of hot flashes at the time of menopause in some U.S. women (Purdie & Green, 2001).

Subsequent epidemiologic studies consistently revealed significant increases in the risk of developing endometrial cancer among women who received estrogen replacement therapy. In an international study of 425 cases and 792 controls, the use of estrogen replacement therapy was found to increase the risk of developing early stage endometrial cancer by more than fivefold and late stage cancer by more than threefold. Furthermore, the risk persisted for more than 10 years after discontinuation of use (Shapiro et al., 1985).

Another striking example of the link between endometrial cancer and estrogen replacement therapy comes from a longitudinal study of postmenopausal women in a California retirement community. In this investigation, women who reported any exposure to estrogen replacement therapy had a relative risk of 10 compared to women with no exposure and women with 15 years of exposure, who had a relative risk

of 20 (Paganini-Hill, Ross, & Henderson, 1989). A meta-analysis of 30 studies found a summary relative risk of 2.3 among women who had ever received estrogen replacement therapy and a 10-fold risk increase after 10 or more years of use (Grady, Gebretsadik, Kerlikowske, Ernster, & Petitti, 1995).

Fortunately, the administration of progesterone in each treatment cycle has been found to mitigate the deleterious mitogenic effects of unopposed estrogen therapy. The decline in the incidence of endometrial cancer to pre-1970 levels during the 1980s (shown in Figure 23.8) is ascribed to the introduction of progesterones as part of the hormonal replacement regimen (Ziel, Finkle, & Greenland, 1998).

Despite some evidence suggesting that the estrogen plus progesterone regimens do not increase the risk of developing endometrial cancer, recent studies have provided mixed results on this controversial issue. In a study of 541 incident cases of endometrial cancer detected among 30,379 postmenopausal women enrolled in the Breast Cancer Detection Demonstration Project (BCDDP), endometrial cancer risk increased by 0.38 per year of estrogen plus progesterone use, and the risk remained elevated for more than 10 years after the cessation of use (Lacey et al., 2005).

In sharp contrast, a study of 433 incident cases of endometrial cancer among 73,211 women enrolled in the National Institutes of Health–AARP Diet and Health Study during 1995–2000 found that estrogen plus progesterone regimens neither increased nor decreased the risk of developing endometrial cancer (Lacey et al., 2007).

Further complicating this issue is the impact of hormone replacement therapy on the risk of developing other medical conditions. In the Women's Health

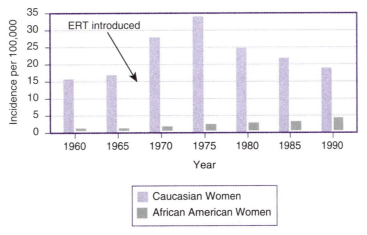

FIGURE 23.8 Incidence of Endometrial Cancer Among Women in San Francisco, California, United States, 1960–1990.
Data from Purdie, D. M., & Green, A. C. (2001). Epidemiology of endometrial cancer. *Best Practice and Research Clinical Obstetrics and Gynaecology, 16*(3), 341–354.

Initiative (WHI), a placebo-controlled randomized clinical trial in which 8506 postmenopausal women received estrogen plus progesterone and 8102 women received a placebo, significant risk increases were noted in the treated group for coronary heart disease, stroke, pulmonary embolism, and breast cancer whereas risk reductions were observed for colorectal cancer and hip fracture. Notably, the overall health risks exceeded the health benefits. The authors stated that "despite decades of accumulated observational evidence, the balance of risks and benefits for hormone use in healthy postmenopausal women remains uncertain" (Rossouw et al., 2002).

Selective Estrogen Receptor Modulators (SERMs) and Endometrial Cancer

Randomized clinical trials of breast cancer patients conducted in the 1970s found that tamoxifen, a drug that selectively modulates ERs, reduces the risk of cancer of the contralateral breast as well as the recurrence of breast cancer. These results soon led to the approval of tamoxifen for routine use as adjuvant therapy for women with breast cancer (Jordan, 1997). However, follow-up studies of women who received tamoxifen determined that they had an increased incidence of endometrial cancer (Fisher et al., 1994). In a case–control study of 324 cases of endometrial cancer and 671 controls, the use of tamoxifen for 2–4 years was found to double the risk of endometrial cancer; longer duration of use quadrupled the risk. Notably, results of this study also showed that combined exposure to tamoxifen and estrogen replacement therapy in obese women increased the risk of developing endometrial cancer by almost ninefold (Bernstein et al., 1999). Molecular studies indicate that tamoxifen has estrogenic effects on the endometrial epithelium and may also have genotoxic properties, which may account for its association with endometrial cancer (Brown, 2009).

Radiation Therapy and Endometrial Cancer

Women who develop primary cancers of the pelvic organs (kidneys, urinary bladder, colon, rectum, cervix, vulva, or vagina) may receive therapeutic radiation. Such patients have an increased risk of developing second primary malignancies in tissues that are inadvertently exposed to high dosages of ionizing radiation (Boice et al., 1985). In a study of 205 cases with radiation-associated endometrial cancer, the mean latency period between diagnosis of the primary pelvic tumor and the onset of endometrial cancer was 110 months.

Radiation-associated endometrial cancers are typically poorly differentiated advanced-stage malignancies that carry a grave prognosis (Kumar et al., 2009).

Oral Contraceptives and Endometrial Cancer

Standard regimens of oral contraceptives currently in use involve the administration of estrogen and progesterone during the menstrual cycle to prevent pregnancy by suppressing ovulation. In most oral contraceptive regimens, the progesterone component prevents the surge of LH from the pituitary gland that is required for the release of the ovum from the ovary.

A significant body of scientific evidence suggests that use of oral contraceptives decreases the risk of some gynecologic malignancies, including ovarian cancer and endometrial cancer. In a highly instructive meta-analysis of 11 studies of oral contraceptive use and endometrial cancer, the duration of use was found to be inversely related to the risk. Compared to women with no exposure, 12 years of using oral contraceptives was estimated to reduce the risk of developing endometrial cancer by 72% (**FIGURE 23.9**). Furthermore, the data suggested that the protective effect of oral contraceptive use persisted after discontinuation; for example, 20 years after stopping use, the risk in former users was 50% below that of women who never used oral contraceptives (Schlesselman, 1997).

Smoking and Endometrial Cancer

Several epidemiologic studies have consistently found that women who smoke cigarettes are at *reduced risk* of developing endometrial cancer. In a meta-analysis of 34 epidemiologic studies (20 prospective and 24 case–control studies), the combined relative risk for ever-smokers compared to never-smokers was reduced by 19% (RR = 0.81), and heavier smoking was

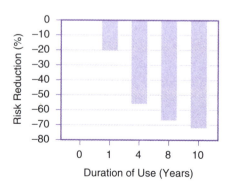

FIGURE 23.9 Endometrial Cancer Risk and Oral Contraceptive Use.

Data from Schlesselman, J. J. (1997). Risk of endometrial cancer in relation to use of combined oral contraceptives. A practitioner's guide to meta-analysis. *Human Reproduction, 12*, 1851–1863.

found to be inversely related to the risk. Estimated risk reductions were stronger in postmenopausal women (RR = 0.71) and women who received estrogen replacement therapy (RR = 0.45) (Zhou et al., 2008). The biological basis of the inverse association of smoking and the risk of endometrial cancer remains to be clarified. Some studies suggest that circulating estrogens is decreased, and androgens are increased in smokers (Michnovicz, Hershcopf, Naganuma, Bradlow, & Fishman, 1986); however, interactions of chronic smoking with weight, diet, and exercise make the issue highly complex.

Exercise and Endometrial Cancer

Sedentary behavior may contribute to the development of endometrial cancer, and reciprocally, physical activity may be protective. In a meta-analysis of nine prospective studies, women who reported high levels of physical activity reduced their risk of developing endometrial cancer by about 25% compared to inactive women (Moore, Gierach, Schatzkin, & Matthews, 2010). Biologically, physical activity reduces obesity and central adiposity and can lead to favorable changes in the balance of endogenous estrogens and androgens.

Diet and Endometrial Cancer

Among the dietary factors that have been studied, coffee consumption has shown the most consistent inverse association with the risk of endometrial cancer. In a meta-analysis of two cohort studies (201 cases) and seven case–control studies (2409 cases), regular coffee drinkers versus nondrinkers had an overall 20% reduction in risk, and heavy coffee consumers (four or more cups per day) reduced their risk by 36% (Bravi et al., 2009).

More recently, investigators in the Nurse's Health Study (NHS) examined coffee consumption and endometrial cancer risk among 27,470 female participants over a period of 26 years during 1980–2006. A total of 672 incident cases of endometrial cancer were diagnosed in the study. Results revealed that women consuming four or more cups of coffee daily had a 25% lower risk than women consuming less than one cup daily (Je, Hankinson, Tworoger, DeVivo, & Giovannucci, 2011). Biologically, high concentrations of caffeine are present in most blends of coffee (60–100 mg per cup), and caffeine has antioxidant properties that may inhibit carcinogenesis. High levels of coffee and caffeine intake have also been found to improve insulin sensitivity and reduce levels of endogenous estrogens, factors thought to reduce the risk (Kotsopoulos, Eliassen,

Missmer, Hankinson, & Tworoger, 2009; Wu, Willett, Hankinson, & Giovannucci, 2005).

Aspirin and Endometrial Cancer

Regular intake of aspirin and other nonsteroidal anti-inflammatory drugs (NSAIDs) appears to protect against the development of many forms of cancer. To examine the effects of NSAIDs on the development of endometrial cancer, a team of investigators examined data from the Australian National Endometrial Cancer Study (ANECS), a population-based study of 1398 cases and 740 controls. Results revealed that women who reported taking two or more regular aspirin tablets per week reduced their risk of developing endometrial cancer by nearly 50% compared to those reporting no intake. Ever use of non-aspirin NSAIDs (e.g., ibuprofen) was also associated with a significant decrease in the risk, and the observed risk reductions with aspirin/NSAID use were similar for both type 1 and type 2 endometrial cancer. Systematic review of the published literature identified nine studies of NSAIDs and endometrial cancer. A pooled meta-analysis of these data revealed a significant risk reduction with regular aspirin use, particularly in obese women (Neill et al., 2013). These results demonstrate chemopreventive effects of aspirin and other NSAIDs against the development of endometrial cancer. Biologically, aspirin and other NSAIDs block the cyclooxygenase-2 (COX-2) enzyme that triggers the prostaglandin inflammatory cascade (Harris, 2002, 2007).

Hysterectomy and Endometrial Cancer

Hysterectomy, the surgical removal of the uterus, is a frequent major surgical procedure among women of reproductive age in developed nations such as the United States. Women who have had a hysterectomy for conditions other than cancer obviously eliminate their risk of developing endometrial cancer; failure to remove these women from the population at risk leads to an underestimate of endometrial cancer incidence (Jamison, Noone, Ries, Lee, & Edwards, 2013). Correction of incidence rates of endometrial cancer becomes very important in populations with high prevalence rates of hysterectomy.

In a study of endometrial cancer and hysterectomy utilizing data from the Surveillance, Epidemiology, and End Results (SEER) cancer registries and the Behavioral Risk Factor Surveillance System (BRFSS) of the United States during 1992–2008, the observed prevalence of hysterectomy among women of reproductive age was 41% for Caucasians and 47% for African Americans.

Correction for hysterectomy increased the annual incidence rates by 73% and 90%, respectively, 136 per 100,000 for Caucasians and 115 per 100,000 for African-American women 50 years and older. The authors concluded that "comparisons of rates of endometrial cancer among racial groups may be misleading in the absence of denominator correction for hysterectomy prevalence" (Jamison et al., 2013).

Molecular Genetics of Endometrial Cancer
Tumor Suppressor Genes and Endometrial Cancer

Loss of function of the *PTEN* tumor suppressor gene located on the long arm of human chromosome 10 is a frequent event in the genesis of type 1 (estrogen-dependent) endometrial cancer. In a recent molecular study of endometrial cancer tissues, somatic *PTEN* mutations were identified by immunohistochemistry in 64% of cases (Djordjevic et al., 2012). Somatic mutations in *PTEN* have been found to elevate the risk of not only endometrial cancer, but also prostate cancer and glioblastoma (Sansal & Sellers, 2004; Steck et al., 1997).

Endometrial cancer also occurs in Cowden's disease, a rare genetic condition caused by a germline mutation in *PTEN*. Cowden's disease is characterized by a spectrum of neoplasms, including cancers of the breast, thyroid, and endometrium, plus the presence of multiple hamartomas (small benign papules of the skin and mucous membranes) (Eng, 1998).

The *PTEN* gene encodes the enzymatic protein *phosphatase and tensin homolog*, which functions as a tumor suppressor by dephosphorylating protein kinase B (*PKB*, also known as *Akt*). Normal *PTEN* function is important in regulating the intracellular *PKB/Akt* signaling pathway to maintain tight control of the rates of cell division and programmed cell-death (apoptosis) (Lee et al., 1999).

Normal *PTEN* function may be compromised by germline mutations, somatic mutations, or epigenetic mechanisms such as DNA methylation (Djordjevic et al., 2012). The silencing of *PTEN* in estrogen-responsive tissues (e.g., the endometrial epithelium) leads to constitutive activation of the *PKB/Akt* signaling cascade, which results in uncontrolled cell proliferation and enhanced cell survival, thereby increasing the risk of dysplasia and cancer development. Interestingly, progesterone counteracts the loss of *PTEN* function, and the administration of progesterone-containing agents has proven effective in the treatment of endometrial dysplasia and localized endometrial cancer (Luo, Manning, & Cantley, 2003; Zheng, Baker, & Mutter, 2004).

In contrast to type 1 (estrogen-dependent) endometrial cancer, type 2 (non-estrogen-dependent) is commonly associated with *p53* mutations that result in abnormal accumulation of abnormal *p53* protein and deregulation of the cell cycle. Mutations in *p53* lead to excessive cell proliferation, hyperplasia, and malignant transformation of the endometrial epithelium (Okuda et al., 2010).

Oncogenes and Endometrial Cancer

Mutational events that enhance rather than suppress the function of certain genes have been detected in tissue studies of endometrial cancer, particularly type 1 endometrial cancer (endometrioid endometrial cancer). Genes that increase carcinogenesis by somatic mutations or epigenetic mechanisms leading to their activation or overexpression are called *proto-oncogenes*. Mutated forms of two such proto-oncogenes, *K-ras* and β-*catenin*, have been observed in excess in studies of endometrial cancer tissues. Molecular studies suggest that mutated forms of these proto-oncogenes stimulate cell proliferation and inhibit apoptosis (Okuda et al., 2010; Peifer, 1997; Sasaki et al., 1993).

Lynch Syndrome and Endometrial Cancer

Endometrial cancer is a significant component of Lynch syndrome (hereditary nonpolyposis colorectal cancer), named after Henry T. Lynch who documented two large kindreds with this autosomal dominant syndrome (Lynch, Shaw, Magnuson, Larsen, & Krush, 1966). The cause of Lynch syndrome is an inherited (germline) mutation in at least one of a set of genes that normally repair DNA, the mismatch repair genes. Mutant forms of two mismatch repair genes, *MSH2* and *MLH1*, account for over 90% of cases with Lynch syndrome (Aaltonen et al., 1993, 1994). Women who inherit either of these genes have a markedly increased lifetime risk (40%–60%) of developing not only colorectal cancer, but also endometrial cancer. Germline mutations in mismatch repair genes account for about 2% of all prevalent cases of endometrial cancer and about 9% of cases that are diagnosed before the age of 50 years (Meyer, Broaddus, & Lu, 2009).

▶ Summary: Epidemiology of Endometrial Cancer

In developed regions of the world, endometrial cancer has surpassed cervical cancer as the leading gynecological malignancy in women, and incidence rates appear to be rising in these populations. Most cases

(90%) are diagnosed in postmenopausal women. Factors that increase exposure to estrogen in the absence of progesterone (unopposed estrogen) increase the risk (e.g., early menarche, anovulatory menstrual cycles, nulliparity, late menopause, estrogen replacement therapy, and in particular, obesity). Reciprocally, factors that decrease estrogen exposure reduce the risk (e.g., oral contraceptives and tobacco smoking). Current evidence also suggests that women who drink coffee or take aspirin regularly are at lower risk. Therapy of breast cancer patients with tamoxifen, a selective estrogen receptor modulator (SERM), has consistently been found to increase their risk of developing endometrial cancer.

Somatic mutations causing loss of function of the *PTEN* tumor suppressor gene, which regulates cell division and apoptosis, are found in more than 60% of type 1 (estrogen-dependent) endometrial tumors whereas *p53* mutations are more common in type 2 (non-estrogen-dependent) tumors. Germline mutations in mismatch repair genes that also predispose to colorectal cancer have been observed in familial endometrial cancer.

Certain medical conditions also increase the risk (e.g., polycystic ovaries, estrogen-secreting granulosa cell ovarian tumors, and diabetes mellitus). Excision of the uterus by hysterectomy for an unrelated medical condition (e.g., fibroids) removes the target tissue and eliminates the risk.

Most women manifest symptoms of endometrial cancer (postmenopausal bleeding, pain, discomfort, pelvic mass) prior to the metastatic spread of cancer cells. The size and location of endometrial tumors can be precisely determined by transvaginal ultrasound; however, the presence of cancer must be confirmed by endometrial biopsy and pathologic examination of cancerous tissues under the microscope. Surgical excision by total hysterectomy and bilateral salpingo-oophorectomy is the treatment of choice for endometrial cancer. For all stages taken together, the overall 5-year survival rate is 80% among women who receive timely and appropriate treatment (Amant et al., 2005).

Epidemiology of Uterine Sarcoma

Uterine sarcomas are relatively rare forms of uterine cancer that arise from smooth muscle (myometrium) or connective tissues of the uterus. Among U.S. women, these tumors account for less than 5% of all uterine malignancies. Due to their low incidence, very few epidemiologic investigations have been conducted to identify risk factors for these tumors. Furthermore, recent pathologic studies of uterine sarcomas have led to an important change in the classification of one type of uterine sarcoma called *uterine carcinosarcoma.* Although this malignant tumor is very aggressive with poor survival, it is now classified as a high-grade endometrial adenocarcinoma and has been renamed *malignant mixed Müllerian tumor* (McCluggage, 2002).

Due to the low incidence of uterine sarcomas plus the recent change in pathologic classification and nomenclature, members of the Epidemiology of Endometrial Cancer Consortium designed an international study to combine all data from published cohort and case–control studies to re-examine the risk factors for uterine sarcoma in comparison to malignant mixed Müllerian tumor and endometrioid endometrial carcinoma. Data from 15 studies (10 case–control studies and 5 cohort studies) were combined and analyzed for this purpose. Pooled data for 229 uterine sarcomas, 244 malignant mixed Müllerian tumors, 7623 endometrioid endometrial carcinomas, and 28,829 controls without cancer were available for analysis (Felix et al., 2013).

Results from the analysis of this large pooled database were in general agreement with the findings from previous smaller studies. In general, the findings reflect a pattern of shared risk factors for uterine sarcoma and type 1 (endometrioid) endometrial carcinoma. Obesity and postmenopausal hormone replacement therapy were associated with increases in the risk whereas cigarette smoking, parity, and oral contraceptive use were associated with risk reductions. Notably, a history of diabetes mellitus increased the risk of developing uterine sarcoma more than twofold. Analysis by subtype of uterine sarcoma (endometrial stromal sarcoma and leiomyosarcoma) revealed associations like those for all uterine sarcomas combined. The risk pattern for malignant mixed Müllerian tumors was not strikingly different from that of uterine sarcoma or endometrioid endometrial carcinoma. The investigators concluded that "associations between menstrual, hormonal, and anthropometric risk factors and uterine sarcoma were similar to those identified for endometrioid endometrial carcinoma" (Felix et al., 2013).

Uterine Leiomyoma (Uterine Fibroids)

Leiomyomas (colloquially known as fibroids) are benign tumors that frequently develop in the smooth muscle (myometrium) of the uterus. Uterine fibroids are, in fact, the most common of all tumors that afflict the female population. Prevalence estimates for women living in developed nations suggest that up to 25% of women develop these benign tumors, typically during their reproductive years. Uterine fibroids are the most frequent indication for hysterectomy in premenopausal women and therefore present a major public health issue (Flake, Andersen, & Dixon, 2003; Kumar, Abbas, & Aster, 2014; Stewart, 2001).

Leiomyomas usually arise during the premenopausal years in association with excessive secretion of estrogen and progesterone by the ovaries. Several lines of evidence support their dependence on stimulation of ERs and PRs in smooth muscle. During pregnancy, when estrogen and progesterone levels increase dramatically, existing leiomyomas experience rapid growth and development, which subsides after delivery. Conversely, oophorectomy induces atrophy of existing leiomyomas, and primary tumors rarely arise after menopause when estrogen and progesterone levels are low.

Risk factors for leiomyoma are like the risk factors for endometrial cancer and breast cancer. They include early menarche (before age 12 years), late first pregnancy (after age 30 years), nulliparity, late menopause, obesity, and exposure to exogenous estrogens (hormone replacement therapy) in the postmenopausal years or exposure to SERMs (e.g., tamoxifen) as adjuvant therapy for ER-positive breast cancer. Reciprocally, factors that decrease the risk appear to lower exposure to estrogen or have anti-estrogenic effects. For example, the inverse association of chronic tobacco smoking and leiomyoma risk has been attributed to the anti-estrogenic effect of nicotine exposure (Flake et al., 2003). It is important to emphasize that nearly all known risk factors for leiomyoma involve sustained excess exposure to estrogens and/or activation of cell membrane ERs.

Several epidemiologic investigations have noted that African-American women have earlier average onset and two- to threefold higher rates of uterine fibroids than Caucasian women (Stewart, 2001). In a recent study, leiomyoma tissues from African-American women were found to have significantly higher concentrations of aromatase than tissues from women of other ethnic groups. Because aromatase is the enzyme responsible for the conversion of androgens to estrogens in fat and muscle, this finding may help account for the higher prevalence and earlier incidence of leiomyoma in the female African-American population (Ishikawa et al., 2009).

Uterine Leiomyosarcoma

Uterine leiomyosarcomas arise from the smooth muscle (myometrium) of the uterus. These tumors are extremely rare, and whether or not they are derived from preexisting benign leiomyomas (fibroids) remains a highly controversial issue (Hodge & Morton, 2007; Kumar, Abbas, & Aster, 2014). The peak incidence of leiomyosarcomas occurs during the perimenopausal years between ages 45 and 60 years. In a recent population-based study of uterine sarcomas in Scandinavian women, the annual incidence of leiomyosarcoma was estimated at about 4–5 cases per million for the period 2003–2007 (Koivisto-Korander, Martinsen, Weiderpass, Leminen, & Pukkala, 2012). In the U.S. population, the estimated annual rates of leiomyosarcoma for women over 35 years of age during 1989–1999 were higher for African-American women than women of all other ethnic groups (15 cases per million versus 9 cases per million) (Brooks, Zhan, Cote, & Baquet, 2004). Leiomyosarcomas have the capability to metastasize to distant organs (e.g., lungs, liver, bones, and brain); consequently, 5-year survival rates are less than 50%.

Like its benign counterpart leiomyoma, the etiology of leiomyosarcoma appears to be linked to excessive exposure to exogenous sources of estrogen, such as hormone replacement therapy (Schwartz et al., 1996) or sustained exposure to SERMs (e.g., tamoxifen) as adjunct therapy for breast cancer (Arenas et al., 2006). Other risk factors include a history of pelvic radiation, history of diabetes, and obesity (Felix et al., 2013).

Endometrial Stromal Sarcoma

Endometrial stromal sarcomas arise from connective tissues of the uterus. These tumors are less common than leiomyomas with annual incidence rates of about 2–3 per million in European women and 5–6 per million in U.S. women (Brooks et al., 2004; Koivisto-Korander et al., 2012). Similar patterns of risk have been observed for all uterine sarcomas, regardless of subtype. In general, risk increases are associated with chronic excessive exposure to endogenous estrogens due to reproductive factors (early menarche, late first pregnancy, nulliparity, or late menopause) or exposure to exogenous estrogens or ER modulators (postmenopausal hormone replacement or adjunct breast cancer therapy with tamoxifen). Reciprocally, risk decreases are associated with anti-estrogenic factors such as chronic cigarette smoking and long-term use of oral contraceptives (Arenas et al., 2006; Schwartz et al., 1996). A novel finding from the analysis of a large pooled database extracted from epidemiologic studies of uterine sarcomas is a significant link with diabetes mellitus (Felix et al., 2013).

▶ Epidemiology of Choriocarcinoma

Choriocarcinomas are rare tumors that develop from trophoblastic cells called *syncytiotrophoblasts* and *cytotrophoblasts* that ordinarily form the chorionic membranes of the placenta. Although the majority of choriocarcinomas develop in the uterus, they can also arise in extrauterine sites such as the ovaries or the fallopian tubes in association with an ectopic pregnancy, and even in the male testes. Approximately 50% of choriocarcinomas develop from *hydatidiform moles*, 20% in association with spontaneous abortions and miscarriages, 20%–30% in normal pregnancies, and 2%–3% in ectopic pregnancies (Kumar et al., 2014).

During the early stages of a normal pregnancy, projections of the chorionic membranes called *chorionic villi* invade the endometrium and absorb nutrients essential for fetal growth and development. However, the trophoblastic cells that form the chorionic membranes occasionally manifest abnormal proliferation and differentiation and form a neoplastic lesion.

The most common form of gestational choriocarcinoma arises from a precursor lesion known as a *hydatidiform mole*. Hydatidiform moles are vesicular (grapelike) tumors that arise due to the implantation of nonviable eggs in the uterus. These cells are void of maternal DNA and may contain various combinations of paternal DNA. Implantation of a nonviable egg in the uterine wall induces aberrant development of placental chorionic tissues that are swollen (hydropic) and void of circulation. About 1 in 40 hydatidiform moles eventually progress to gestational choriocarcinomas. Gestational choriocarcinomas are typically diagnosed during the fourth or fifth month of pregnancy. A key diagnostic feature is excessive secretion of β human chorionic gonadotropin by the syncytiotrophoblasts.

In a study of women of reproductive age in the United States during 1973–1982, choriocarcinomas were detected in about 1 in 24,000 pregnancies, and significant effects of race and age were observed. African-American women had a twofold increase in the incidence compared to Caucasians, and women ages 40–44 years had an 8.6-fold increase compared to those ages 20–24 years. Incidence rates were also increased in teen pregnancies (Brinton, Bracken, & Connelly, 1986). Subsequent studies of diverse populations have noted increases in the incidence of gestational trophoblastic disease for women in underdeveloped areas (e.g., southeast Asia, India, and Africa) and have confirmed that women in the extreme classes of gestational age (under 20 and over 40 years) are at increased risk (Di Cintio, Parazzini, Rosa, Chatenoud, & Benzi, 1997).

Because syncytiotrophoblasts within choriocarcinomas secrete human chorionic gonadotropin (hCG), a marked elevation in the blood level of this hormone can serve as an early biomarker of tumor development. Nevertheless, choriocarcinomas are often detected after metastatic spread to other anatomic sites (e.g., lungs, liver, and bones). Fortunately, most of these tumors are extremely sensitive to treatment with methotrexate and other chemotherapeutic agents. With appropriate therapy, the cure rate for gestational choriocarcinoma exceeds 90% (Lurain & Nejad, 2005).

References

Aaltonen, L. A., Peltomiki, P., Leach, F. S., Sistonen, P., Pylkkanen, L., Mecklin, J.-P., … de la Chappelle, A. (1993). Clues to the pathogenesis of familial colorectal cancer. *Science, 260,* 812–816.

Aaltonen, L. A., Peltomiki, P., Mecklin, J.-P., Jirvinen, H., Jass, J. R., Green, J. S., … de la Chappelle, A. (1994). Replication errors in benign and malignant tumors from hereditary nonpolyposis colorectal cancer patients. *Cancer Research, 54,* 1645–1648.

Amant, F., Moerman, P., Neven, P., Timmerman, D., Van Limbergen, E., & Vergote, I. (2005). Endometrial cancer. *Lancet, 366,* 491–505.

Arenas, M., Rovirosa, A., Henandez, V., Ordi, J., Jorcano, S., Mellado, B., & Biete, A. (2006). Uterine sarcomas in breast cancer patients treated with tamoxifen. *International Journal of Gynecologic Cancer, 16,* 861–865.

Azziz, R., Woods, K. S., Reyna, R., Key, T. J., Knochenhauer, E. S., & Yildiz, B. O. (2004). The prevalence and features of the polycystic ovary syndrome in an unselected population. *Journal of Clinical Endocrinology and Metabolism, 89*(6), 2745–2749.

Bender, D., Buekers, T., & Leslie, K. K. (2011). Hormone receptors and endometrial cancer. *Proceedings in Obstetrics and Gynecology, 2*(1), 1–25.

Bernstein, L., Deapen, D., Cerhan, J. R., Schwartz, S. M., Liff, J., McGann-Maloney, E., … Ford, L. (1999). Tamoxifen therapy for breast cancer and endometrial cancer risk. *Journal of the National Cancer Institute, 91,* 1654–1662.

Boice, J. D., Jr., Day, N. E., Andersen, A., Brinton, L. A., Brown, R., Choi, N. W., … Flannery, J. T. (1985). Second cancers following radiation treatment for cervical cancer. An international collaboration among cancer registries. *Journal of the National Cancer Institute, 74*(5), 955–975.

Bokhman, J. V. (1983). Two pathogenetic types of endometrial carcinoma. *Gynecologic Oncology, 15*(1), 10–17.

Bravi, F., Scotti, L., Bosetti, C., Gallus, S., Negri, E., La Vecchia, C., & Tavani, A. (2009). Coffee drinking and endometrial cancer risk: A metaanalysis of observational studies. *American Journal of Obstetrics and Gynecology, 200*(2), 130–135.

Bray, F., Dos Santos Silva, I., Moller, H., & Weiderpass, E. (2005). Endometrial cancer incidence trends in Europe: Underlying determinants and prospects for prevention. *Cancer Epidemiology, Biomarkers and Prevention, 14*(5), 1132–1142.

Bray, F., Ferlay, J., Soerjomataram, I., Siegel, R. L., Torre, L. A., & Jemal, A. (2018). Global cancer statistics 2018: GLOBOCAN estimates of incidence and mortality worldwide for 36 cancers in 185 countries. *CA: A Cancer Journal for Clinicians, 68*(6), 394–424.

Brinton, L. A., Bracken, M. B., & Connelly, R. R. (1986). Choriocarcinoma incidence in the United States. *American Journal of Epidemiology, 123*(6), 1094–1100.

Brinton, L. A., Gridley, G., Persson, I., Baron, J., & Bergqvist, A. (1997). Cancer risk after a hospital discharge diagnosis of endometriosis. *American Journal of Obstetrics and Gynecology, 176*(3), 572–579.

Brooks, S. E., Zhan, M., Cote, T., & Baquet, C. R. (2004). Surveillance, epidemiology, and end results analysis of 2677 cases of uterine sarcoma 1989–1999. *Gynecologic Oncology, 93*, 204–208.

Brown, K. (2009). Is tamoxifen a genotoxic carcinogen in women? *Mutagenesis, 24*(5), 391–404.

Chang, S.-C., Lacey, J. V., Brinton, L. A., Harge, P., Adams, K., Mouw, T., … Leitzmann, M. F. (2007). Lifetime weight history and endometrial cancer risk by type of menopausal hormone use in the NIH-AARP Diet and Health Study. *Cancer Epidemiology, Biomarkers and Prevention, 16*(4), 723–730.

Di Cintio, E., Parazzini, F., Rosa, C., Chatenoud, L., & Benzi, G. (1997). The epidemiology of gestational trophoblastic disease. *General and Diagnostic Pathology, 143*(2–3), 103–108.

Djordjevic, B., Hennessy, B. T., Li, J., Barkoh, B. A., Luthra, R., Mills, G. B., & Broaddus, R. R. (2012). Clinical assessment of PTEN loss in endometrial carcinoma: Immunohistochemistry outperforms gene sequencing. *Modern Pathology, 25*, 699–708.

Dockerty, M. B., Loveday, S. B., & Foust, G. T. (1951). Carcinoma of the corpus uteri in young women. *American Journal of Obstetrics and Gynecology, 61*, 966–981.

Dossus, L., Allen, N., Kaaks, R., Bakken, K., Lund, E., Tjonneland, A., … Riboli, E. (2010). Reproductive risk factors and endometrial cancer: The European Prospective Investigation into Cancer and Nutrition. *International Journal of Cancer, 127*, 442–451.

Duong, L. M., Wilson, R. J., Ajani, U. A., Singh, S. D., & Eheman, C. R. (2011). Trends in endometrial cancer incidence rates in the United States, 1999–2006. *Journal of Women's Health, 20*(8), 1157–1163.

Eng, C. (1998). Genetics of Cowden syndrome: Through the looking glass of oncology. *International Journal of Oncology, 12*(3), 701–710.

Evans, T., Sany, O., Pearman, P., Ganesan, R., Blann, A., & Sundar, S. (2011). Differential trends in the rising incidence of endometrial cancer by type: Data from a U.K. population-based registry from 1994 to 2006. *British Journal of Cancer, 104*(9), 1505–1510.

Fearnley, E. J., Marquart, L., Spurdle, A. B., Weinstein, P., Webb, P. M., & Australian Ovarian Cancer Study Group and Australian National Endometrial Cancer Study Group. (2010). Polycystic ovary syndrome increases the risk of endometrial cancer in women aged less than 50 years: An Australian case-control study. *Cancer Causes and Control, 21*(12), 2303–2308.

Felix, A. S., Cook, L. S., Gaudet, M. M., Rohan, T. E., Schouten, L. J., Setiawan, V. W., … Brinton, L. A. (2013). The etiology of uterine sarcomas: A pooled analysis of the Epidemiology of Endometrial Cancer Consortium. *British Journal of Cancer, 108*(3), 727–734.

Felix, A. S., Weissfeld, J. L., Stone, R. A., Bowser, R., Chivukula, M., Edwards, R. P., & Linkov, F. (2010). Factors associated with type I and type II endometrial cancer. *Cancer Causes and Control, 21*(11), 1851–1856.

Ferlay, J., Bray, F., Pisani, P., & Parkin, D. M. (2004). *GLOBOCAN 2002. Cancer incidence, mortality, and prevalence worldwide. IARC Cancer Base No. 5, version 2.0.* Lyon, France: IARC Press. Retrieved from http://www-dep.iarc.fr

Ferlay, J., Ervik, M., Lam, F., Colombet, M., Mery, L., Piñeros, M., … Bray, F. (2018). *Global cancer observatory: Cancer today.* Lyon, France: International Agency for Research on Cancer. Retrieved from https://gco.iarc.fr/today

Ferlay, J., Shin, H.-R., Bray, F., Forman, D., Mathers, C., & Parkin, D. M. (2010). Estimates of worldwide burden of cancer in 2008: GLOBOCAN 2008. *International Journal of Cancer, 127*(12), 2893–2917.

Ferlay, J., Soerjomataram, I., Ervik, M., Dikshit, R., Eser, S., Mathers, C., … Bray, F. (2013). *GLOBOCAN 2012 v1.0. Cancer incidence and mortality worldwide: IARC CancerBase No. 11* [Internet]. Lyon, France: International Agency for Research on Cancer. Retrieved from http://globocan.iarc.fr

Fisher, B., Costantino, J. P., Redmond, C. K., Fisher, E. R., Wickerham, D. L., & Cronin, W. M. (1994). Endometrial cancer in tamoxifen-treated breast cancer patients: Findings from the National Surgical Adjuvant Breast and Bowel Project (NSABP) B-14. *Journal of the National Cancer Institute, 86*, 527–537.

Fitzmaurice, C., Allen, C., Barber, R. M., Barber, R. M., Barregard, L., Bhutta, Z. A., … Global Burden of Disease Cancer Collaboration. (2017). Global, regional, and national cancer incidence, mortality, years of life lost, years lived with disability, and disability-adjusted life-years for 32 cancer groups, 1990–2015: A systematic analysis for the Global Burden of Disease Study. *JAMA Oncology, 3*(4), 524–548.

Fitzmaurice, C., Akinyemiju, T. F., Al Lami, F. H., Alam, T., Alizadeh-Navaei, R., Allen, C., … Global Burden of Disease Cancer Collaboration. (2018). Global, regional, and national cancer incidence, mortality, years of life lost, years lived with disability, and disability-adjusted life-years for 29 cancer groups, 1990–2016: A systematic analysis for the Global Burden of Disease Study. *JAMA Oncology.* Online publication. doi:10.1001/jamaoncol.2018.2706.

Flake, G. P., Andersen, J., & Dixon, D. (2003). Etiology and pathogenesis of uterine leiomyomas: A review. *Environmental Health Perspectives, 111*(8), 1037–1054.

Friberg, E., Orsini, N., Mantzoros, C. S., & Wolk, A. (2007). Diabetes mellitus and risk of endometrial cancer: A meta-analysis. *Diabetologia, 50*(7), 1365–1374.

Grady, D., Gebretsadik, T., Kerlikowske, K., Ernster, V., & Petitti, D. (1995). Hormone replacement therapy and endometrial cancer risk: A meta-analysis. *Obstetrics and Gynecology, 85*, 304–313.

Harris, R. E. (2002). Cyclooxygenase-2 blockade in cancer prevention and therapy: Widening the scope of impact. In R. E. Harris (Ed.), *Cyclooxygenase-2 blockade in cancer prevention and therapy* (pp. 341–365). Totowa, NJ: Human Press.

Harris, R. E. (2007). Cyclooxygenase-2 (COX-2) and the inflammogenesis of cancer. *Subcellular Biochemistry, 42*, 93–126.

Hayat, M. J., Howlader, N., Reichman, M. E., & Edwards, B. K. (2007). Cancer statistics, trends, and multiple primary cancer analyses from the Surveillance, Epidemiology, and End Results (SEER) program. *Oncologist, 12*(1), 20–37.

Hodge, J. C., & Morton, C. C. (2007). Genetic heterogeneity among uterine leiomyomata: Insights into malignant progression. *Human Molecular Genetics, 16*(1), 7–13.

Howlader, N., Noone, A. M., Krapcho, M., Garshell, J., Neyman, N., Altekruse, S. F., … Cronin, K. A. (Eds.). (2012, November). *SEER cancer statistics review, 1975–2010.* Bethesda, MD: National Cancer Institute. Retrieved from http://seer.cancer.gov/csr/1975_2010/

Ishikawa, H., Reierstad, S., Demura, M., Rademaker, A. W., Kasai, T., Inoue, M., … Bulun, S. E. (2009). High aromatase expression in uterine leiomyoma tissues of African-American women. *Journal of Clinical Endocrinology and Metabolism, 94*(5), 1752.

Jackson, R., & Dockerty, M. B. (1957). The Stein–Leventhal syndrome: Analysis of 43 cases with special reference to association with endometrial carcinoma. *American Journal of Obstetrics and Gynecology, 73*, 161–173.

Jafari, K., Javaheri, G., & Ruiz, G. (1978). Endometrial adenocarcinoma and the Stein-Leventhal syndrome. *Obstetrics and Gynecology, 51*, 97–100.

Jamison, P. M., Noone, A. M., Ries, L. A., Lee, N. C., & Edwards, B. K. (2013). Trends in endometrial cancer incidence by race and histology with a correction for the prevalence of hysterectomy, SEER 1992–2008. *Cancer Epidemiology, Biomarkers and Prevention, 22*(2), 233–241.

Je, Y., Hankinson, S. E., Tworoger, S. S., DeVivo, I., & Giovannucci, E. (2011). A prospective cohort study of coffee consumption and risk of endometrial cancer over a 26-year follow-up. *Cancer Epidemiology, Biomarkers and Prevention, 20*(12), 2487–2495.

Jordan, V. C. (1997). Tamoxifen: The herald of a new era of preventive therapeutics [editorial]. *Journal of the National Cancer Institute, 89*, 747–749.

Kanthan, R., & Senger, J. L. (2011). Uterine carcinosarcomas (malignant mixed Müllerian tumours): A review with special emphasis on the controversies in management. *Obstetrics and Gynecology International, 2011*, d470795.

Key, T. J., & Pike, M. C. (1988a). The dose-effect relationship between 'unopposed' oestrogens and endometrial mitotic rate: Its central role in explaining and predicting endometrial cancer risk. *British Journal of Cancer, 57*(2), 205–212.

Key, T. J., & Pike, M. C. (1988b). The role of oestrogens and progestogens in the epidemiology and prevention of breast cancer. *European Journal of Cancer and Clinical Oncology, 24*(1), 29–43.

Koivisto-Korander, R., Martinsen, J. I., Weiderpass, E., Leminen, A., & Pukkala, E. (2012). Incidence of uterine leiomyosarcoma and endometrial stromal sarcoma in Nordic countries: Results from NORDCAN and NOCCA databases. *Maturitas, 72*(1), 56–60.

Korenman, S. G. (1980). Oestrogen window hypothesis of the aetiology of breast cancer. *Lancet, 315*(8170), 700–701.

Kosary, C. L. (2007). Cancer of the corpus uteri. In L. A. G. Ries, J. L. Young, G. E. Keel, M. P. Eisner, Y. D. Lin, & M.-J. Horner (Eds.), *SEER survival monograph: Cancer survival among adults: U.S. SEER program, 1988–2001, patient and tumor characteristics* (NIH Pub. No. 07-6215). Bethesda, MD: National Cancer Institute.

Kotsopoulos, J., Eliassen, A. H., Missmer, S. A., Hankinson, S. E., & Tworoger, S. S. (2009). Relationship between caffeine intake and plasma sex hormone concentrations in premenopausal and postmenopausal women. *Cancer, 115*(12), 2765–2774.

Kumar, S., Shah, J. P., Bryant, C. S., Seward, S., Ali-Fehmi, R., Morris, R. T., & Malone, J. M., Jr. (2009). Radiation-associated endometrial cancer. *Obstetrics and Gynecology, 113*(2 Pt 1), 319–325.

Kumar, V., Abbas, A. K., & Aster, J. C. (2014). *Robbins and Cotran pathologic basis of disease* (9th ed.). Philadelphia, PA: Mosby & Saunders.

Lacey, J. V., Jr., Brinton, L. A., Lubin, J. H., Sherman, M. E., Schatzkin, A., & Schairer, C. (2005). Endometrial carcinoma risks among menopausal estrogen plus progestin and unopposed estrogen users in a cohort of postmenopausal women. *Cancer Epidemiology, Biomarkers and Prevention, 14*(7), 1724–1731.

Lacey, J. V., Jr., Leitzmann, M. F., Chang, S. C., Mouw, T., Hollenbeck, A. R., Schatzkin, A., & Brinton, L. A. (2007). Endometrial cancer and menopausal hormone therapy in the National Institutes of Health-AARP Diet and Health Study cohort. *Cancer, 109*(7), 1303–1311.

Lee, J. O., Yang, H., Georgescu, M. M., Di Cristofano, A., Maehama, T., Shi, Y., … Pavletich, N. P. (1999). Crystal structure of the PTEN tumor suppressor: Implications for its phosphoinositide phosphatase activity and membrane association. *Cell, 99*(3), 323–334.

Loos, A. H., Bray, F., McCarron, P., Weiderpass, E., Hakama, M., & Parkin, D. M. (2004). Sheep and goats: Separating cervix and corpus uteri from imprecisely coded uterine cancer deaths, for studies of geographical and temporal variations in mortality. *European Journal of Cancer, 40*, 2794–2803.

Lucenteforte, E., Bosetti, C., Talamini, R., Montella, M., Zucchetto, A., Pelucchi, C., … La Vecchia, C. (2007). Diabetes and endometrial cancer: Effect modification by body weight, physical activity and hypertension. *British Journal of Cancer, 97*(7), 995–998.

Luo, J., Manning, B. D., & Cantley, L. C. (2003). Targeting the PI3K-Akt pathway in human cancer: Rationale and promise. *Cancer Cell, 4*, 257–262.

Lurain, J. R., & Nejad, B. (2005). Secondary chemotherapy for high-risk gestational trophoblastic neoplasia. *Gynecologic Oncology, 97*(2), 618–623.

Lynch, H. T., Shaw, M. W., Magnuson, C. W., Larsen, A. L., & Krush, A. J. (1966). Hereditary factors in cancer: A study of two large Midwestern kindreds. *Archives of Internal Medicine, 117*(2), 206–212.

MacMahon, B. (1974). Risk factors for endometrial cancer. *Gynecologic Oncology, 2*(2–3), 122–129.

Malmström, H., Högberg, H., Risberg, B., & Simonsen, E. (1994). Granulosa cell tumors of the ovary: Prognostic factors and outcome. *Gynecologic Oncology, 52*(1), 50–55.

McCluggage, W. G. (2002). Uterine carcinosarcomas (malignant mixed Mullerian tumors) are metaplastic carcinomas. *International Journal of Gynecologic Cancer, 12*(6), 687–690.

McPherson, C. P., Sellers, T. A., Potter, J. D., Bostick, R. M., & Folsom, A. R. (1996). Reproductive factors and risk of endometrial cancer. The Iowa Women's Health Study. *American Journal of Epidemiology, 143*(12), 1195–1202.

Meyer, L. A., Broaddus, R. R., & Lu, K. H. (2009). Endometrial cancer and Lynch syndrome: Clinical and pathologic considerations. *Cancer Control, 16*(1), 14–22.

Michnovicz, J. J., Hershcopf, R. J., Naganuma, H., Bradlow, H. L., & Fishman, J. (1986). Increased 2-hydroxylation of estradiol as a possible mechanism for the anti-estrogenic effect of cigarette smoking. *New England Journal of Medicine, 315*(21), 1305–1319.

Modugno, F., Ness, R. B., Chen, C., & Weiss, N. S. (2005). Inflammation and endometrial cancer: A hypothesis. *Cancer Epidemiology, Biomarkers and Prevention, 14*, 2480.

Moore, S. C., Gierach, G. L., Schatzkin, A., & Matthews, C. E. (2010). Physical activity, sedentary behaviours, and the prevention of endometrial cancer. *British Journal of Cancer, 103*(7), 933–938.

Nagamani, M., & Stuart, C. A. (1998). Specific binding and growth promoting activity of insulin in endometrial cancer cells in culture. *American Journal of Obstetrics and Gynecology, 179*, 6–12.

National Cancer Institute. (n.d.). *Fast Stats: An interactive tool for access to SEER cancer statistics. Surveillance Research Program.* Retrieved from http://seer.cancer.gov/faststats

Navaratnarajah, R., Pillay, O. C., & Hardiman, P. (2008). Polycystic ovary syndrome and endometrial cancer. *Seminars in Reproductive Medicine, 26*(1), 62–71.

Neill, A. S., Nagle, C. M., Protani, M. M., Obermair, A., Spurdle, A. B., Webb, P. M., & Australian National Endometrial Cancer Study Group. (2013). Aspirin, nonsteroidal anti-inflammatory drugs, paracetamol and risk of endometrial cancer: A case-control study, systematic review and meta-analysis. *International Journal of Cancer, 132*(5), 1146–1155.

Nestler, J. E., Powers, L. P., Matt, D. W., Steingold, K. A., Plymate, S. R., Rittmaster, R. S., ... Blackard, W. G. (1991). A direct effect of hyperinsulinemia on serum sex hormone-binding globulin levels in obese women with the polycystic ovary syndrome. *Journal of Clinical Endocrinology and Metabolism, 72*, 83–89.

Okuda, T., Sekizawa, A., Purwosunu, Y., Nagatsuka, M., Morioka, M., Hayashi, M., & Okai, T. (2010). Genetics of endometrial cancers. *Obstetrics and Gynecology International, 2010.* doi:10.1155/2010/984013.

Paganini-Hill, A., Ross, R. K., & Henderson, B. E. (1989). Endometrial cancer and patterns of use of oestrogen replacement therapy: A cohort study. *British Journal of Cancer, 59*(3), 445–447.

Parkin, D. M., Bray, F., Ferlay, J., & Pisani, P. (2001). Estimating the world cancer burden: GLOBOCAN 2000. *International Journal of Cancer, 94*, 153–156.

Parkin, D. M., Bray, F., Ferlay, J., & Pisani, P. (2005). Global cancer statistics, 2002. *CA: A Cancer Journal for Clinicians, 55*, 74–108.

Peifer, M. (1997). β-Catenin as oncogene—The smoking gun. *Science, 275*(5307), 1752.

Platz, C. E., & Benda, J. A. (1995). Female genital tract cancer. *Cancer, 75*, 270–294.

Purdie, D. M., & Green, A. C. (2001). Epidemiology of endometrial cancer. *Best Practice and Research Clinical Obstetrics and Gynaecology, 16*(3), 341–354.

Radosh, L. (2009). Drug treatments for polycystic ovary syndrome. *American Family Physician, 79*(8), 671–676.

Rossouw, J. E., Anderson, G. L., Prentice, R. L., LaCroix, A. Z., Kooperberg, C., Stefanick, M. L., ... Ockene, J., Writing Group for the Women's Health Initiative Investigators. (2002). Risks and benefits of estrogen plus progestin in healthy postmenopausal women: Principal results from the Women's Health Initiative randomized controlled trial. *Journal of the American Medical Association, 288*(3), 321–333.

Sankaranarayanan, R., & Ferlay, J. (2006). Worldwide burden of gynaecological cancer: The size of the problem. *Best Practice and Research Clinical Obstetrics and Gynaecology, 20*(2), 207–225.

Sansal, I., & Sellers, W. R. (2004). The biology and clinical relevance of the PTEN tumor suppressor pathway. *Journal of Clinical Oncology, 22*(14), 2954–2963.

Sasaki, H., Nishii, H., Takahashi, H., Tada, A., Furusato, M., Terashima, Y., ... Boyd, J. (1993). Mutation of the Ki-ras protooncogene in human endometrial hyperplasia and carcinoma. *Cancer Research, 53*(8), 1906–1910.

Saso, S., Chatterjee, J., Georgiou, E., Ditri, A. M., Smith, J. R., & Ghaem-Maghami, S. (2011). Endometrial cancer. *BMJ, 343*, d3954.

Schlesselman, J. J. (1997). Risk of endometrial cancer in relation to use of combined oral contraceptives. A practitioner's guide to meta-analysis. *Human Reproduction, 12*, 1851–1863.

Schottenfeld, D. (1995). Epidemiology of endometrial neoplasia. *Journal of Cellular Biochemistry, 59*(Suppl. 23), 151–159.

Schumer, S. T., & Cannistra, S. A. (2003). Granulosa cell tumor of the ovary. *Journal of Clinical Oncology, 21*(6), 1180–1189.

Schwartz, S. M., Weiss, N. S., Daling, J. R., Gammon, M. D., Liff, J. M., Watt, Z. J., ... Thompson, W. D. (1996). Exogenous sex hormone use, correlates of endogenous hormone levels, and the incidence of histologic types of sarcoma of the uterus. *Cancer, 77*(4), 717–724.

Shah, S. P., Köbel, M., Senz, J., Morin, R. D., Clarke, B. A., Wiegand, K. C., & Huntsman, D. G. (2009). Mutation of *FOXL2* in granulosa-cell tumors of the ovary. *New England Journal of Medicine, 360*, 2719–2720.

Shapiro, S., Kelly, J. P., Rosenberg, L., Kaufman, D. W., Helmrich, S. P., Rosenshein, N. B., ... Schottenfeld, D. (1985). Risk of localized and widespread endometrial cancer in relation to recent and discontinued use of conjugated estrogens. *New England Journal of Medicine, 313*, 969–972.

Sherman, B. M., & Korenman, S. G. (1974). Inadequate corpus luteum function: A pathophysiological interpretation of human breast cancer epidemiology. *Cancer, 33*, 1306–1312.

Sherman, B. M., Wallace, R. B., & Korenman, S. G. (1981). Corpus luteum dysfunction and the epidemiology of breast cancer: A reconsideration. *Breast Cancer Research and Treatment, 1*(4), 287–296.

Simpson, E. R., & Brown, K. A. (2011). Obesity, aromatase and breast cancer. *Expert Review of Endocrinology and Metabolism, 6*(3), 383–395.

Speert, H. (1949). Carcinoma of the endometrium in young women. *Journal of Surgery, Gynaecology and Obstetrics, 88*, 332–336.

Steck, P. A., Pershouse, M. A., Jasser, S. A., Yung, W. K., Lin, H., Ligon, A. H., ... Tavtigian, S. V. (1997). Identification of a candidate tumour suppressor gene, MMAC1, at chromosome 10q23.3 that is mutated in multiple advanced cancers. *Nature Genetics, 15*(4), 356–362.

Stewart, E. A. (2001). Uterine fibroids. *Lancet, 357*(9252), 293–298.

Viganò, P., Parazzini, F., Somigliana, E., & Vercellini, P. (2004). Endometriosis: Epidemiology and etiological factors. *Best Practice and Research Clinical Obstetrics and Gynecology, 18*(2), 177–200.

Wu, T., Willett, W. C., Hankinson, S. E., & Giovannucci, E. (2005). Caffeinated coffee, decaffeinated coffee, and caffeine in relation to plasma C-peptide levels, a marker of insulin secretion, in U.S. women. *Diabetes Care, 28*, 1390–1396.

Zheng, W., Baker, H. E., & Mutter, G. L. (2004). Involution of PTEN-null endometrial glands with progestin therapy. *Gynecologic Oncology, 92*(3), 1008–1013.

Zhou, B., Yang, L., Sun, Q., Cong, R., Gu, H., Tang, N., ... Wang, B. (2008). Cigarette smoking and the risk of endometrial cancer: A meta-analysis. *American Journal of Medicine, 121*(6), 501–508.

Ziel, H. K., Finkle, W. D., & Greenland, S. (1998). Decline in incidence of endometrial cancer following increase in prescriptions for opposed conjugated estrogens in a prepaid health plan. *Gynecologic Oncology, 68*, 253–255.

CHAPTER 24

Epidemiology of Cervical Cancer

▶ Global Burden of Cervical Cancer

Cancer of the uterine cervix is the third most common cancer diagnosed among women worldwide (behind only breast cancer and colorectal cancer). During 2018, 569,847 new cases were diagnosed, and 311,365 women died from cervical cancer. During 2000–2018, the annual number of cases of cervical cancer increased by 21% and the annual number of deaths increased by 33%. Nearly 85% of the new cases were diagnosed in women living in less-developed regions where cervical cancer was the second leading cause of cancer death among women ranking behind only breast cancer. Despite the increasing annual number of cases and deaths, the incidence and mortality rates of cervical cancer have declined in many populations worldwide. The global age-adjusted incidence rate of cervical cancer in 2018 was 13.1 per 100,000, a reduction of approximately 19% since 2002, and the mortality rate from cervical cancer was 6.9 per 100,000, a reduction of 23% since 2002. The increasing global burden of cervical cancer is primarily due to high incidence and mortality rates in populous nations of sub-Saharan Africa and Southeast Asia (Bray et al., 2018; Parkin, Bray, Ferlay, & Pisani, 2005).

The highest incidence and mortality rates of cervical cancer are persisting in sub-Saharan African, Melanesia, Latin America, and the Caribbean, and certain nations of South America (Bolivia and Guyana), and Asia (Mongolia, India, and Indonesia) (**FIGURE 24.1**). The public health burden due to cervical cancer in these nations reflects the virtual absence of screening programs for the detection and treatment of precancerous lesions of the uterine cervix. On average in 2018, the age-adjusted incidence in less developed nations was 75% higher than in developed nations (18.2 per 100,000 versus 10.4 per 100,000), and the mortality was threefold high in less developed nations compared to developed nations (12.2 versus 4.1 per 100,000) (Bray et al., 2018; Ferlay et al., 2010, 2013, 2018).

The women of most developed nations and certain other nations such as China have relatively low rates. The incidence and mortality rates of cervical cancer have declined dramatically among women of developed countries since the introduction and widespread use of screening for cervical dysplasia in the mid-20th century (Ferlay, Bray, Pisani, Parkin, 2004; Ferlay et al., 2010, 2013, 2018; Fitzmaurice et al., 2017, 2018).

▶ Early Detection of Cervical Dysplasia

The early detection and appropriate treatment of premalignant conditions of the cervical mucosa (e.g., cervical dysplasia) reflects a major triumph of modern medicine over a life-threatening disease process. In the early decades of the 20th century, cancer of the cervix was the leading cause of cancer mortality among U.S. women. Since 1955, mortality due to cervical cancer has declined by 74%; today, cancer of the cervix ranks 14th in female cancer mortality, accounting for approximately 4000 deaths per year in the United States (Jemal et al., 2009).

Estimated age-standardized incidence rates (World) in 2018, cervix uteri, all ages

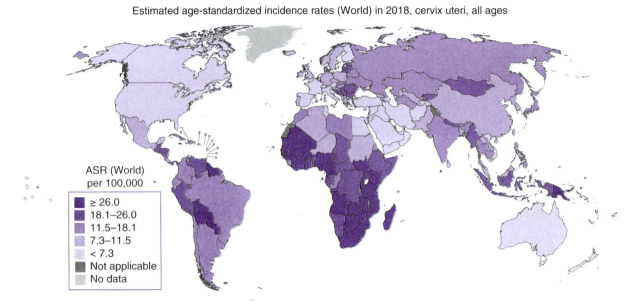

Estimated age-standardized mortality rates (World) in 2018, cervix uteri, all ages

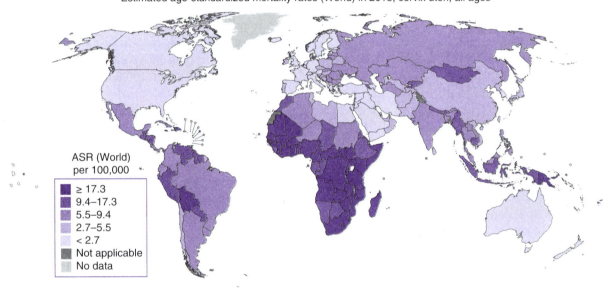

FIGURE 24.1 Global Incidence and Mortality Rates of Cervical Cancer, 2018.

Caption: ASR: Rates per 100,000 are age-standardized to the world population, 2000–2025.

Reproduced with permission from Ferlay, J., Ervik, M., Lam, F., Colombet, M., Mery, L., Piñeros, M., ... Bray, F. (2018). *Global cancer observatory: Cancer today*. Lyon, France: International Agency for Research on Cancer. Retrieved from https://gco.iarc.fr/today

The dramatic reduction in cervical cancer among women of developed nations is due largely to the effectiveness of the Papanicolaou–Traut cytological test (Papanicolaou & Traut, 1943). The *Pap test*, which was introduced in the United States around 1950, provides a quick, safe, affordable, and accurate means of detecting precancerous dysplastic lesions of the cervix that can be cured by simple surgery or other ablative techniques. It is important to note that in situ cervical cancer is 100% curable by appropriate surgical excision. Furthermore, advanced-stage cervical cancer that has not spread beyond the cervix is 80%–90% curable by appropriate surgery. The importance of cervical screening coupled with appropriate therapy

is underscored by differences in cervical cancer mortality in populations with high versus low screening rates. Public health programs to inform and educate the population as to the efficacy of cervical screening by appropriate implementation of Papanicolaou cytological testing at an early age are therefore imperative. Evaluation of the Pap smear has also resulted in critical information regarding carcinogenesis, and in fact, more is known about the natural history of cervical cancer than about any other malignancy.

Although the Pap test has produced substantial declines in cervical cancer incidence and mortality, it is noteworthy that marked disparities persist among the subpopulations within certain nations,

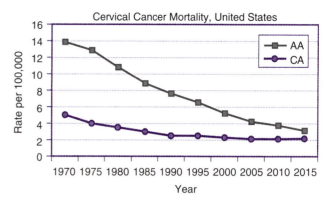

FIGURE 24.2 Trends in Incidence and Mortality Rates of Cervical Cancer in U.S. Women, 1970–2015.

Caption: AA: African Americans; CA: Caucasian Americans.

Data from Noone, A. M., Howlader, N., Krapcho, M., Miller, D., Brest, A., Yu, M., Ruhl, J., ... Cronin, K. A. (2018). *SEER Cancer Statistics Review, 1975–2015.* Bethesda, MD: National Cancer Institute.

perhaps due to excess risk, lack of screening, and limited healthcare access (Sherman, Wang, Carreon, & Devesa, 2005). For example, among U.S. women, the incidence and mortality rates for African Americans are still nearly twice those of Caucasians (Howlader et al., 2011) (**FIGURE 24.2**).

▶ Pathogenesis of Cervical Cancer

Cancer of the uterine cervix almost always originates at the squamocolumnar junction at the cervical os in the transitional area between the cervix and the vagina. It is at this border that the columnar epithelium of the cervix transforms into the squamous cell epithelium of the vagina. The vast majority (95%) of cervical cancers are of the squamous cell variety; however, a few adenocarcinomas evolve from the cervical glands, and in fact some of the cervical malignancies are of the mixed variety (i.e., adenosquamous carcinomas) (Kumar, Abbas, Nelson, & Mitchell, 2007).

Carcinoma of the cervix arises in a series of stepwise epithelial changes ranging from progressively more severe dysplasia to carcinoma in situ and, ultimately, invasive carcinoma (**FIGURE 24.3**). Although carcinoma of the cervix may occur at any age following puberty, the peak incidence is at about 30–40 years of age for in situ lesions and 40–50 years of age for invasive cancer.

Several questions remain regarding the risk factors associated with cervical carcinoma and cervical dysplasia. One feature of mild cervical dysplasia is the tendency for a large percentage of cases to spontaneously remiss; that is, individuals with mild dysplasia when followed over time may spontaneously undergo resolution. Although the reason for this is unknown, it is certainly a subject worthy of study by prospective epidemiologic methods.

▶ Risk Factors for Cervical Cancer

Results of early epidemiologic studies of cervical cancer strongly suggested that the disease was related to the sexual transmission of an oncogenic agent, most probably a virus, from male to female at an early age. Factors that were consistently observed to increase the risk included early age at first intercourse, high parity, multiple sexual partners, contact with "high-risk" (promiscuous) male sexual partners, and cigarette smoking. Observed differences in risk for certain subpopulations of women were also related to sexual behavior, including the higher incidence of cervical cancer in lower socioeconomic groups; the higher incidence in married women, which increases with the number of marriages and children; the rarity of cervical cancer in virgins and nuns; and the high incidence in prostitutes. Although herpes simplex virus type 2 (HSV2) was once suspected as the etiologic agent, it is now believed that infection by certain strains of human papillomavirus (HPV) is the most important risk factor in the genesis of cervical malignancies.

HPV and Cervical Cancer

It is now quite clear that oncogenic subtypes of human papillomavirus (HPV-16 and HPV-18) are necessary agents in the pathogenesis of cervical cancer (Walboomers et al., 1999). The link between cervical cancer and HPV infection was first suggested by Harald zur Hausen in Germany (zur Hausen, 1976). Professor zur Hausen and colleagues demonstrated the presence of HPV strains 16 and 18 in cancerous tissues from cervical cancer patients (Boshart et al., 1984; Dürst, Gissmann, Ikenberg, & zur Hausen, 1983). Strong etiologic evidence came from an epidemiologic case–control study in which HPV DNA was

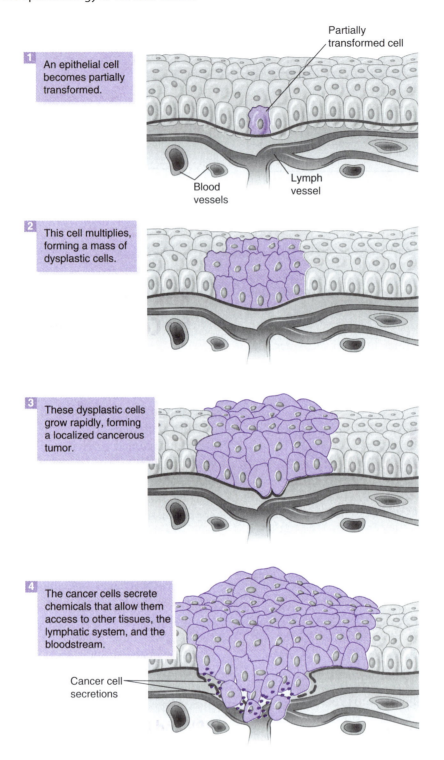

1 An epithelial cell becomes partially transformed.

Partially transformed cell

Blood vessels

Lymph vessel

2 This cell multiplies, forming a mass of dysplastic cells.

3 These dysplastic cells grow rapidly, forming a localized cancerous tumor.

4 The cancer cells secrete chemicals that allow them access to other tissues, the lymphatic system, and the bloodstream.

Cancer cell secretions

FIGURE 24.3 Progression of Cervical Cancer.

detected by hybridization techniques in 75%–100% of patients with cervical condylomas, precancerous cervical dysplasia, and invasive cervical carcinoma (Muñoz et al., 1992). Although there is an overlap in HPV strains, strains 6 and 11 are found most frequently in benign condylomas (vulvar condyloma acuminatum) whereas oncogenic HPV strains such as 16, 18, and 31 are more often present in carcinoma of the cervix (**FIGURE 24.4**). Cancer develops when the

DNA from the oncogenic strains becomes integrated with the DNA of infected cervical cells, leading to overexpression of certain viral genes (E6 and E7) that in turn inactivate tumor suppressor genes such as *p53* and *Rb* (Münger & Howley, 2002).

Molecular epidemiologic studies also indicate that HPV infection coupled with low-dose nitrosamines in the cervical mucosa of cigarette smokers may accentuate carcinogenesis (Gunnell et al., 2006).

Hypothetical Scheme for the Role of Human
Papillomavirus in Cervical Neoplasia

FIGURE 24.4 Human Papillomavirus (HPV) Infection and Cervical Cancer.

It has also been shown that HPV strains 16 and 18 (but not 6 and 11) interact with the *ras* oncogene in causing transformed tumorigenic foci in cultured cervical cells (Prokopakis, Sourvinos, Koumantaki, Koumantakis, & Spandidos, 2002). Furthermore, male partners of women with cervical cancer have been found to exhibit lesions of the genitalia harboring high-risk strains HPV-16 and HPV-18. Certain strains of HPV are also suspected as oncogenic agents in a variety of other squamous cell tumors or proliferative lesions of the skin and mucous membranes.

Immunosuppression and Cervical Cancer

Immunosuppression places women at high risk for infection by oncogenic strains of HPV, thereby increasing the risk of cervical cancer (Stentella et al., 1998). Indeed, women who are seropositive for the human immunodeficiency virus (HIV) are at extremely high risk for development of cervical cancer. Apparently, this is due to a synergistic interaction between HIV and oncogenic HPV strains. Antecedent infection by HIV compromises the immune system and predisposes sexually active women to co-infection by strains of HPV that cause cervical cancer.

Tobacco Use and Cervical Cancer

Although infection by high-risk strains of HPV (e.g., HPV-16 and HPV-18) is the strongest risk factor for cervical cancer, the risk appears to be modified by cigarette smoking and other forms of tobacco use. Winkelstein initially postulated that tobacco smoking may play a role in the development of cervical cancer, and several epidemiologic investigations have since found that smoking is associated with an increase in cervical cancer risk (Winkelstein, 1977, 1990). A meta-analysis of nine studies conducted between 1977 and 1990 revealed a significant effect of ever versus never smoking (odds ratio [OR] = 1.46) (Sood, 1991); a subsequent meta-analysis of 21 studies found a significant effect of current smoking (OR = 1.83) (Gandini et al., 2008). Nevertheless, with the elucidation of oncogenic HPV infection as the dominant cause of cervical cancer, these early epidemiologic results stimulated controversy as to whether the observed association with smoking was causal or simply due to confounding of smoking with sexual behavioral factors related to HPV infection.

In order to rule out confounding variables, several investigators designed epidemiologic studies to estimate the effects of tobacco use in the presence of HPV infection. Castle and colleagues conducted a 10-year prospective investigation of smoking and other factors among 1812 women who tested positive for oncogenic HPV DNA at baseline. They found that among the HPV-positive women, smoking one or more packs of cigarettes daily increased the risk more than fourfold (OR = 4.3) compared to nonsmokers (Castle et al., 2002). In a subsequent investigation, Plummer and colleagues pooled international data from 10 case–control studies of invasive and in situ cervical carcinoma utilizing only those women who tested positive for HPV DNA. Their study included data on tobacco use among 1463 cases with invasive cervical cancer, 211 cases with cervical carcinoma in situ, and 254 female controls without cancer. Compared to HPV-positive controls who were nonsmokers, the risk of developing squamous cell cervical cancer among the HPV-positive cases was significantly increased for current smokers (OR = 2.30) and ex-smokers (OR = 1.80) (Plummer et al., 2003). A team of Swedish investigators conducted a nested population-based case–control study to examine interactions between cigarette smoking and HPV-16 in the development of in situ cervical cancer. Archival cervical smears were tested for HPV-16 by polymerase chain reaction

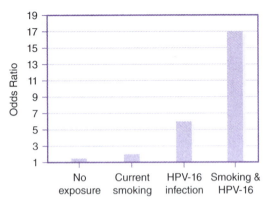

FIGURE 24.5 Synergism of Cigarette Smoking and HPV-16 Infection in the Pathogenesis of Cervical Cancer.

Data from Gunnell, A. S., Tran, T. N., Torrång, A., Dickman, P. W., Sparén, P., Palmgren, J., & Ylitalo, N. (2006). Synergy between cigarette smoking and human papillomavirus type 16 in cervical cancer in situ development. *Cancer Epidemiology, Biomarkers and Prevention, 15*(11), 2141–2147.

(PCR) analysis in 375 cases and 363 age-matched disease-free controls. On average, cases were diagnosed 9 years after collection of cervical smears. At the time of diagnosis, data on smoking and other risk factors were collected for each participant by a telephone interview. Results revealed independent effects of smoking and HPV-16 infection and effect modification of combined exposure. Current smoking versus nonsmoking adjusted for HPV-16 status increased the risk nearly twofold (OR = 1.7), whereas HPV-16 positive versus negative status adjusted for smoking increased the risk more than eightfold (OR = 8.4). Among nonsmokers, women who were positive for HPV-16 had more than a fivefold increase in risk (OR = 5.6) compared to women who were HPV-16 negative, whereas among smokers, HPV-16 positive women had more than a 14-fold increase in risk (OR = 14.4) compared to women who were HPV-16 negative. Nonsmoking women with a high viral load of HPV-16 had a sixfold increase in risk (OR = 5.9) compared to women who were HPV-16 negative, whereas among smokers, women with a high viral load of HPV-16 had a 27-fold increase in risk (OR = 27.0) compared to those who were negative for HPV-16 (**FIGURE 24.5**). These results clearly suggest that smoking synergistically increases the risk of developing cervical cancer among women with HPV-16 infection (Gunnell et al., 2006).

Inflammogenesis of Cervical Cancer

Cyclooxygenase-1 and cyclooxygenase-2 (COX-1 and COX-2) are the chief rate-limiting enzymes of inflammation and the prostaglandin cascade. Low levels of the COX-1 isoform are produced constitutively in certain tissues such as the gastric mucosa, whereas much higher levels of the COX-2 isoform can be induced by a variety of pro-inflammatory stimuli, including

tobacco smoke. Sustained COX-2 expression in a tissue is generally accepted as a biomarker of chronic inflammation.

In recent years, many molecular biologists have consistently and independently demonstrated that COX-2 is expressed in most epithelial neoplasms, including those of the uterine cervix. Although not detectable in normal cervical epithelium, COX-2 expression is a prominent feature of early stage premalignant lesions of the cervix as well as in situ cervical cancer and invasive cervical cancer (Harris, 2007).

Molecular studies have also shown that chronic inflammation of the cervical mucosa enhances HPV-induced carcinogenesis. According to one model, because HPV infection of the cervix by itself is not highly inflammatory, infection by other viruses (e.g., herpes simplex virus 2) and/or bacteria (e.g., *Chlamydia trachomatis*) and/or exposure to other inflammatory factors (e.g., tobacco metabolites) may be necessary to promote carcinogenesis. An important finding is that in HPV-infected women, carcinogenesis is tightly linked to *integration* of oncogenic HPV DNA into the host DNA. Notably, reactive oxygen and nitrogen species (ROS and RNS) generated by inflammation readily induce double-strand breaks in both host and viral DNA, thereby facilitating integration of HPV DNA into the DNA of infected cervical epithelium. Following integration of oncogenic HPV DNA, there is overexpression of viral oncogenes *E6* and *E7*, which accelerates carcinogenesis by interfering with key tumor suppressor genes such as *p53* and *Rb* (Williams, Filippova, Soto, & Duerksen-Hughes, 2011).

▶ Prevention of Cervical Cancer

Prevention of cervical cancer relies on avoidance of HPV infection and other risk factors (HIV infection and smoking) coupled with early detection and effective ablation of premalignant lesions of the uterine cervix. Strains of HPV are spread by sexual intercourse, oral sex, anal sex, or any other contact involving the genitalia. Preventive strategies include abstinence from sexual contact, monogamy, condom use, avoidance of tobacco, regular screening by Papanicolaou cytological testing (yearly Pap tests for sexually active women), and vaccination against high-risk HPV strains.

HPV Vaccination

Two effective vaccines have now been developed and are approved for use against high-risk HPV strains in the United States and Europe (McNeil, 2006).

In randomized clinical trials, Gardasil (Merck) prevented infection by HPV types 6, 11, 16, and 18 in up to 98% of those vaccinated; Cervarix (GlaxoSmith-Kline) prevented infections by HPV strains 16 and 18 in 92% of recipients over a 4-year follow-up period. These vaccines are effective only if administered to young females prior to HPV exposure. Unfortunately, their relatively high cost may prohibit widespread HPV vaccination programs in impoverished nations (Singh, 2005). Furthermore, vaccination should not be considered a replacement for screening because the known oncogenic HPV strains account for only about 70% of cervical cancer overall.

Visual Inspection for Detection of Cervical Neoplasia

In populations with limited access to healthcare facilities, direct visual inspection of the uterine cervix after staining with acetic acid or Lugol's iodine has proven very effective in the detection of precancerous lesions (Sherris et al., 2009). Direct visual inspection procedures eliminate the need for transport of specimens and laboratory testing, require very little equipment, and provide women with immediate test results. A range of medical professionals, including doctors, nurses, and professional midwives, can effectively perform the procedure, provided they receive adequate training and supervision. Furthermore, such screening tests have been shown to perform equal to or better than cervical cytology in accurately identifying precancerous lesions. A major advantage of direct visual inspection is that women can be screened and treated in a single visit. One efficacious treatment option is cryotherapy (freezing), a relatively simple and inexpensive method by which cervical lesions can be immediately removed by the primary care physician (Denny et al., 2005).

References

Boshart, M., Gissmann, L., Hans Ikenberg, H., Kleinheinz, A., Wolfram Scheurlen, W., & zur Hausen, H. (1984). A new type of papilloma virus DNA, its presence in genital cancer biopsies and in cell lines derived from cervical cancer. *EMBO Journal, 3*(5), 1151–1157.

Bray, F., Ferlay, J., Soerjomataram, I., Siegel, R. L., Torre, L. A., & Jemal, A. (2018). Global cancer statistics 2018: GLOBOCAN estimates of incidence and mortality worldwide for 36 cancers in 185 countries. *CA: A Cancer Journal for Clinicians, 68*(6), 394–424.

Castle, P. E., Wacholder, S., Lorincz, A. T., Scott, D. R., Sherman, M. E., Glass, A. G., … Schiffman, M. (2002). A prospective study of high-grade cervical neoplasia risk among human papillomavirus-infected women. *Journal of the National Cancer Institute, 94*(18), 1406–1404.

Denny, L., Kuhn, L., De Souza, M., Pollack, A. E., Dupree, W., & Wright, T. C., Jr. (2005). Screen-and-treat approaches for cervical cancer prevention in low-resource settings: A randomized controlled trial. *Journal of the American Medical Association, 294*(17), 2173–2181.

Dürst, M., Gissmann, L., Ikenberg, H., & zur Hausen, H. (1983). A papillomavirus DNA from a cervical carcinoma and its prevalence in cancer biopsy samples from different geographic regions. *Proceedings of the National Academy of Sciences, 80*(12), 3812–3815.

Ferlay, J., Bray, F., Pisani, P., & Parkin, D. M. (2004). *GLOBOCAN 2002. Cancer incidence, mortality, and prevalence worldwide. IARC CancerBase No. 5*, version 2.0. Lyon, France: IARC Press. Retrieved from http://www-dep.iarc.fr

Ferlay, J., Ervik, M., Lam, F., Colombet, M., Mery, L., Piñeros, M., … Bray, F. (2018). *Global cancer observatory: Cancer today*. Lyon, France: International Agency for Research on Cancer. Retrieved from https://gco.iarc.fr/today

Ferlay, J., Shin, H.-R., Bray, F., Forman, D., Mathers, C., & Parkin, D. M. (2010). Estimates of worldwide burden of cancer in 2008: GLOBOCAN 2008. *International Journal of Cancer, 127*(12), 2893–2917.

Ferlay, J., Soerjomataram, I., Ervik, M., Dikshit, R., Eser, S., Mathers, C., … Bray, F. (2013). *GLOBOCAN 2012 v1.0. Cancer incidence and mortality worldwide: IARC CancerBase No. 11* [Internet]. Lyon, France: International Agency for Research on Cancer. Retrieved from http://globocan.iarc.fr

Fitzmaurice, C., Akinyemiju, T. F., Al Lami, F. H., Alam, T., Alizadeh-Navaei, R., Allen, C., … Global Burden of Disease Cancer Collaboration. (2018). Global, regional, and national cancer incidence, mortality, years of life lost, years lived with disability, and disability-adjusted life-years for 29 cancer groups, 1990 to 2016: A systematic analysis for the Global Burden of Disease Study. *JAMA Oncology*. Online publication. doi:10.1001/jamaoncol.2018.2706.

Fitzmaurice, C., Allen, C., Barber, R. M., Barregard, L., Bhutta, Z. A., Brenner, H., … Global Burden of Disease Cancer Collaboration. (2017). Global, regional, and national cancer incidence, mortality, years of life lost, years lived with disability, and disability-adjusted life-years for 32 cancer groups, 1990 to 2015: A systematic analysis for the Global Burden of Disease Study. *JAMA Oncology, 3*(4), 524–548.

Gandini, S., Botteri, E., Iodice, S., Boniol, M., Lowenfels, A. B., Maisonneuve, P., & Boyle, P. (2008). Tobacco smoking and cancer: A meta-analysis. *International Journal of Cancer, 12*(1), 155–164.

Gunnell, A. S., Tran, T. N., Torrång, A., Dickman, P. W., Sparén, P., Palmgren, J., & Ylitalo, N. (2006). Synergy between cigarette smoking and human papillomavirus type 16 in cervical cancer in situ development. *Cancer Epidemiology, Biomarkers and Prevention, 15*(11), 2141–2147.

Harris, R. E. (2007). Cyclooxygenase-2 (COX-2) and the inflammogenesis of cancer. *Subcellular Biochemistry, 42*, 93–126.

Howlader, N., Noone, A. M., Krapcho, M., Neyman, N., Aminou, R., Waldron, W., … Edwards, B. K. (Eds.). (2011). *SEER Cancer Statistics Review, 1975–2008*. Bethesda, MD: National Cancer Institute.

Jemal, A., Siegel, R., Ward, E., Hao, Y., Xu, J., & Thun, M. J. (2009). Cancer statistics, 2009. *CA: A Cancer Journal for Clinicians, 59*, 225–249.

Kumar, V., Abbas, A. K., Nelson, F., & Mitchell, R. N. (2007). *Robbins basic pathology* (8th ed., pp. 718–721). Philadelphia, PA: Elsevier Saunders.

McNeil, C. (2006). Who invented the VLP cervical cancer vaccines? *Journal of the National Cancer Institute, 98*(7), 433.

Münger, K., & Howley, P. M. (2002). Human papillomavirus immortalization and transformation functions. *Virus Research, 89*(2), 213–228.

Muñoz, N., Bosch, F. X., de Sanjose, S., Tafur, L., Izarzugaza, I., Gili, M., … Shah, K. (1992). The causal link between human papillomavirus and invasive cervical cancer: A population-based case-control study in Colombia and Spain. *International Journal of Cancer, 52*, 743–749.

Noone, A. M., Howlader, N., Krapcho, M., Miller, D., Brest, A., Yu, M., Ruhl, J., … Cronin, K. A. (2018). *SEER Cancer Statistics Review, 1975–2015*. Bethesda, MD: National Cancer Institute.

Papanicolaou, G. N., & Traut, H. F. (1943). *Diagnosis of uterine cancer by the vaginal smear*. New York, NY: Commonwealth Fund.

Parkin, M., Bray, F., Ferlay, J., & Pisani, P. (2005). Global cancer statistics, 2002. *CA: A Cancer Journal for Clinicians, 55*(2), 74–108.

Plummer, M., Herrero, R., Franceschi, S., Meijer, C. J., Snijders, P., Bosch, F. X., … IARC Multi-centre Cervical Cancer Study Group. (2003). Smoking and cervical cancer: Pooled analysis of the IARC multi-centric case-control study. *Cancer Causes and Control, 14*(9), 805–814.

Prokopakis, P., Sourvinos, G., Koumantaki, Y., Koumantakis, E., & Spandidos, D. A. (2002). *K-ras* mutations and HPV infection in cervicitis and intraepithelial neoplasias of the cervix. *Oncology Reports, 9*, 129–133.

Sherman, M. E., Wang, S. S., Carreon, J., & Devesa, S. S. (2005). Mortality trends for cervical squamous and adenocarcinoma in the United States. Relation to incidence and survival. *Cancer, 103*, 1258–1264.

Sherris, J., Wittet, S., Kleine, A., Sellors, J., Luciani, S., Sankaranarayanan, R., & Barone, M. A. (2009). Evidence-based alternative cervical cancer screening approaches in low-resource settings. *International Perspectives on Sexual and Reproductive Health, 35*(3), 147–152.

Singh, N. (2005). HPV and cervical cancer: Prospects for prevention through vaccination. *Indian Journal of Medical and Pediatric Oncology, 26*(1), 20–23.

Sood, A. K. (1991). Cigarette smoking and cervical cancer: Meta-analysis and critical review of recent studies. *American Journal of Preventive Medicine, 7*(4), 208–213.

Stentella, P., Frega, A., Ciccarone, M., Cipriano, L., Tinari, A., Tzantzoglou, S., & Pachì, A. (1998). HPV and intraepithelial neoplasia recurrent lesions of the lower genital tract: Assessment of the immune system. *European Journal of Gynaecological Oncology, 19*(5), 466–469.

Walboomers, J. M., Jacobs, M. V., Manos, M. M., Bosch, F. X., Kummer, J. A., Shah, K. V., … Muñoz, N. (1999). Human papillomavirus is a necessary cause of invasive cervical cancer worldwide. *Journal of Pathology, 189*, 12–19.

Winkelstein, W., Jr. (1977). Smoking and cancer of the uterine cervix: Hypothesis. *American Journal of Epidemiology, 106*(4), 257–259.

Winkelstein, W., Jr. (1990). Smoking and cervical cancer—Current status: A review. *American Journal of Epidemiology, 131*, 945–957.

Williams, V. M., Filippova, M., Soto, U., & Duerksen-Hughes, P. J. (2011). HPV-DNA integration and carcinogenesis: Putative roles for inflammation and oxidative stress. *Future Virology, 6*(1), 45–57.

zur Hausen, H. (1976). Condylomata acuminata and human genital cancer. *Cancer Research, 36*, 530.

CHAPTER 25

Epidemiology of Vaginal, Vulvar, and Anal Cancer

▶ Global Burden of Vaginal, Vulvar, and Anal Cancer

Epidemiologic features of vaginal, vulvar, and anal cancer are in many respects quite similar to those of cervical cancer because all are etiologically linked to infection of the respective tissues by oncogenic strains of human papillomavirus (HPV). However, cervical cancer is by far the most common of all HPV-related malignancies, with a global mortality burden among women that is nearly 10-fold higher than the combined mortality of malignancies of the vagina, vulva, and anus. Worldwide in 2018, invasive cervical cancer was diagnosed in 569,847 women and caused 311,365 deaths whereas cancers of the vagina, vulva, and anus were diagnosed in 90,180 women and caused 32,795 deaths. Anal cancer also afflicted 20,196 men in 2018, causing an additional 9618 deaths in the male population. The annual number of deaths from these malignancies has increased by about 15% in women and 20% in men over the past two decades (Bray et al., 2018; de Martel et al., 2012; Ferlay et al., 2010; Forman et al., 2012; Parkin & Bray, 2006).

In contrast to cervical cancer, malignancies of the vagina and vulva are relatively rare and account for less than 0.5% of all female cancers and less than 5% of malignancies of the female genital tract. Likewise, anal cancer is an uncommon lesion of the lower gastrointestinal tract accounting for about 0.3% of all cancers and 2%–3% of malignancies of the gastrointestinal tract in both men and women. Most vaginal, vulvar, and anal malignancies (90%–95%) are squamous cell carcinomas (SCCs) that arise from the stratified epithelium that covers these anatomic sites. Adenocarcinomas are the most common of the other malignancies that arise in tissues of the vagina, vulva, or anus (Hamilton & Aaltonen, 2000; Tavassoli & Devilee, 2003a, 2003b).

▶ Human Papillomavirus in Vaginal, Vulvar, and Anal Carcinoma

Human papillomaviruses are DNA viruses capable of infecting the skin and mucous membranes of humans. Although most of the more than 150 HPV subtypes do not cause disease, a few strains may cause condyloma acuminata (warts) or carcinomas of the anogenital and/or oropharyngeal mucosa. Genital infections by HPV are common, and most (~90%) resolve spontaneously over time without treatment. However, persisting infections by low-risk strains (HPV-6 and HPV-11) predispose to condyloma development, and chronic infections by high-risk strains (HPV-16 and HPV-18) predispose to carcinoma development of the anogenital tissues (cervix, vagina, vulva, and anus).

TABLE 25.1 PAF and HPV-Attributable Cases of Vaginal, Vulvar, and Anal Cancer, 2008

Cancer Site	PAF (%)	Incident Cases	Attributable Cases
Vagina	70	13,000	9100
Vulva	43	27,000	11,610
Anus	88	27,000	23,760
Total	66	67,000	44,470

Data from de Martel, C., Ferlay, J., Franceschi, S., Vignat, J., Bray, F., Forman, D., & Plummer, M. (2012). The global burden of cancers attributable to infections in the year 2008: A review and synthetic analysis. *Lancet Oncology*, 13, 607–615.

Nobel laureate Harald zur Hausen and colleagues first suggested that certain HPV strains are carcinogenic in human tissues of the cervix and elsewhere (zur Hausen, 1976, 1977). Using polymerase chain reaction (PCR) assays, they demonstrated the presence of HPV DNA in virtually all cancerous tissues from cervical cancer patients and premalignant (precursor) lesions of the uterine cervix (Boshartb et al., 1984; zur Hausen, 2002). Subsequent molecular studies have documented the presence of HPV DNA in a high proportion of other anogenital carcinomas as well as their precursor lesions. The current consensus is that virtually all cervical cancers are caused by HPV infections and that two types (HPV-16 and HPV-18) are responsible for about 70% of cases. Furthermore, chronic anogenital infections due to oncogenic HPV strains are estimated to cause approximately 88% of anal cancers, 70% of vaginal cancers, and 43% of vulvar cancers (de Martel et al., 2012; De Vuyst, Clifford, Nascimento, Madeleine, & Franceschi, 2009; Parkin, 2006; Parkin & Bray, 2006).

Population Attributable Fraction and Human Papillomavirus Infection

To gauge the overall population impact of HPV infection in the genesis of carcinomas of the vagina, vulva, and anus, investigators at the International Agency for Research on Cancer (IARC) estimated a parameter known as the population attributable fraction (PAF) for each of these malignancies. The PAF is an estimate of the proportion of cases of a specific disease (in this case, cancer) that could theoretically be avoided if exposure to a specific risk factor (in this case, HPV infection) was eliminated.

METHODOLOGY

Population Attributable Fraction (PAF)

The standard formula for estimating the population attributable fraction is $PAF = f_e (I_e - I_o)/I$, where f_e = frequency of exposure in the general population, I_e = incidence with exposure, I_o = incidence without exposure, and I = overall incidence. Note that since the Relative Risk $(RR) = I_e / I_o$ and overall incidence $I = f_e I_e + (1 - f_e) I_o$, an alternative formula is

$$PAF = f_e (RR - 1) / [f_e (RR - 1) + 1].$$

The PAF can also be approximated by the following formula: $PAF = f_c (RR - 1)/RR$, where f_c = the prevalence of *exposed cases* in the population. As the RR increases, the latter formula approaches $PAF = f_c$, which can be viewed as the upper limit of the PAF. The number of cases attributable to the risk factor can be obtained by the following formula:

Attributable Cases = PAF × (Incident Cases).

Estimates of the PAF and the number of cases of vaginal cancer, vulvar cancer, and anal cancer caused by HPV infection are given in **TABLE 25.1**. Using PAF estimates of 70%, 43%, and 88% for vaginal, vulvar, and anal cancer, respectively, the IARC investigators estimated that HPV infection accounted for nearly 45,000 new cases (66%) of these malignancies in 2008 (de Martel et al., 2012; De Vuyst et al., 2009).

Molecular Mechanisms of Carcinogenesis by Human Papillomavirus

Cancer develops when the DNA from oncogenic HPV strains, particularly HPV-16, HPV-18, HPV-31, and HPV-33, integrate with the DNA of host cells in

Model of HPV and Carcinogenesis

Cofactors: Tobacco, HIV, HSV2

FIGURE 25.1 Molecular Mechanisms of HPV and Carcinogenesis. Steps in the Model: (1) HPV Infection; (2) Integration of HPV DNA into Epithelial Cell DNA (Lysogeny); (3) Expression of Viral Proteins (*E6*, *E7*); (4) Disruption of *p53*, *Rb*, *ras*, and Telomerase Gene Function; and (5) Loss of Cell Cycle Control, Accelerated Cell Proliferation, Failure of Apoptosis, and Immortalization of Cell Lineage.

the cervix, vagina, vulva, anus, and/or other tissues. The integration of viral genes into the genome of the invaded epithelial cell (called lysogeny) leads to the overexpression of certain viral genes (*E6* and *E7*) that in turn inactivate tumor suppressor genes such as *P53* and *Rb* (Münger, Scheffner, Huibregtse, & Howley, 1992) or up-regulate proto-oncogenes such as *ras* and *telomerase* (Kiyono et al., 1998; Matlashewskil et al., 1987; zur Hausen, 2002). Potential cofactors include chronic exposure to tobacco carcinogens, systemic HIV-related immunosuppression and coinfection by other genital viruses (such as herpes simplex virus 2 [HSV2]), and bacteria. Key steps in the carcinogenic process are illustrated in **FIGURE 25.1**.

▶ Global Pattern of Vaginal, Vulvar, and Anal Squamous Cell Cancers

Because HPV is the predominant risk factor in the genesis of SCCs of the cervix, vagina, vulva, and anus, the global distributions of these malignancies should closely follow the global distribution of HPV genital infections. Nevertheless, marked differences in the timely diagnosis and reporting of anogenital cancers in different populations have confounded efforts to discern their true global pattern. Currently, the worldwide patterns of anogenital cancer incidence rates reflect not only the underlying risk due to factors such as HPV infection, but also the impact of screening, early detection, and curative removal of premalignant lesions in women living in more developed nations (Parkin & Bray, 2006).

Recently, data from 194 published studies were pooled to assess the global burden and pattern of HPV cervical infections in asymptomatic women. In all studies, HPV DNA was detected in cytological cervical specimens using PCR assays or hybrid capture (detection of denatured HPV DNA with complementary RNA probes). The global distribution of HPV infections is shown in **FIGURE 25.2**. The prevalence of HPV infection in cervical tissues is high (over 20%) among asymptomatic women living in sub-Saharan Africa, Central America, South America, and Southeast Asia and low (less than 10%) in those living in North America, Western Europe, Scandinavia, and Oceania (Bruni et al., 2010). This pattern is a virtual image of the distribution of cervical cancer incidence and presumably approximates the global pattern of vaginal, vulvar, and anal carcinoma (Forman et al., 2012).

▶ Human Immunodeficiency Virus in Vaginal, Vulvar, and Anal Carcinoma

Patients with acquired immune deficiency syndrome (AIDS) due to infection by human immunodeficiency virus (HIV) are at markedly increased risk of developing certain malignancies, most notably Kaposi's sarcoma and non-Hodgkin's lymphoma. Chronic HIV infection also has been found to accelerate the risk of developing multiple other cancers, including those related to HPV infection.

Using data collected in the multicenter AIDS–Cancer Match Registry Study in the United States, investigators at the National Cancer Institute (NCI) examined the incidence of HPV-associated malignancies among 309,365 patients with HIV/AIDS (257,605 men and 51,760 women) during the period 1978–1996. Their study revealed that among patients with HIV/AIDS, all HPV-associated cancers occurred in significant excess of the expected rates in the general population. Invasive malignancies of the cervix, vagina, vulva, and anus were increased more than fivefold among HIV-infected women, and malignancies of the anus and penis were increased by 38-fold and fourfold, respectively, among HIV-infected men (**FIGURE 25.3**). Furthermore, invasive tumors were diagnosed earlier (~10 years on average) in HIV/AIDS patients than cases from the general population, suggesting that HIV-related immunosuppression hastens the progression of HPV-related cancer (Frisch, Biggar, & Goedert, 2000).

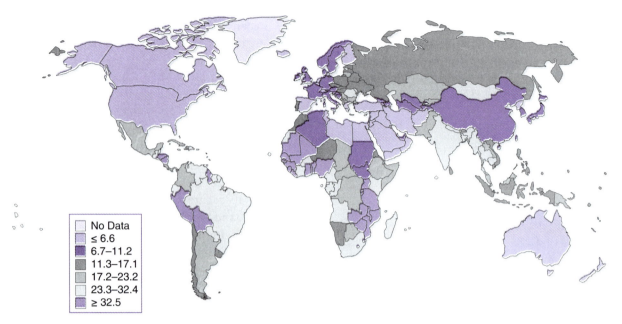

FIGURE 25.2 Prevalence of Human Papillomavirus (HPV) Cervical Infection in Asymptomatic Women, 2008.

Data from Bruni, L., Diaz, M., Castellsagué, X., Ferrer, E., Bosch, F. X., & de Sanjosé, S. (2010). Cervical human papillomavirus prevalence in 5 continents: Meta-analysis of 1 million women with normal cytological findings. *Journal of Infectious Disease, 202,* 1789–1799; Forman, D., de Martel, C., Lacey, C. J., Soerjomataram, I., Lortet-Tieulent, J., Bruni, L., … Franceschi, S. (2012). Global burden of human papillomavirus and related diseases. *Vaccine, 30*(Suppl. 5), F12–F23.

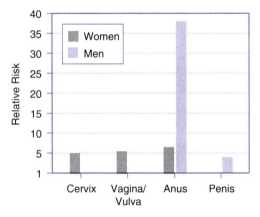

FIGURE 25.3 Relative Risk of HPV-Related Cancer in Women and Men With HIV/AIDS.

Data from Frisch, M., Biggar, R. J., & Goedert, J. J. (2000). Human papillomavirus-associated cancers in patients with human immunodeficiency virus infection and acquired immunodeficiency syndrome. *Journal of the National Cancer Institute, 92*(18), 1500–1510.

▶ Epidemiology of Vaginal Cancer

Vaginal cancer is an uncommon malignancy accounting for less than 0.3% of all female cancers and about 1%–2% of malignancies of the female genital tract. Estimates of the annual incidence ranged from 0.3 to 0.7 per 100,000 among populations sampled in 2002 (Parkin & Bray, 2006). During 2008, approximately 13,000 new cases of vaginal cancer were diagnosed in the world population; of these, 8000 occurred in women living in underdeveloped countries (de Martel et al., 2012). Five-year survival rate depends on the stage at detection and is far better for women with localized tumors (70%) than those with advanced

disease (15%). Based on available survival data, more than 7000 women die annually from metastatic vaginal cancer (Ferlay et al., 2010).

Most vaginal malignancies (90%–95%) are SCCs that arise from the vaginal epithelium distal to the opening of the cervix. The other prominent cell type of vaginal cancer is clear cell adenocarcinoma, which is caused by in utero exposure to diethylstilbestrol (DES).

Age at Diagnosis of Vaginal Cancer

The onset of vaginal cancer differs markedly according to the histologic cell type. SCCs of the vagina are predominantly diagnosed late in life, whereas clear cell adenocarcinomas develop much earlier (**FIGURE 25.4**). This difference relates to the timing of exposure to etiologic agents. SCCs are linked to exposure to oncogenic HPV strains through sexual activity with multiple partners, coinfection by HIV, and chronic cigarette smoking, whereas clear cell adenocarcinomas arise due to in utero exposure to a carcinogenic agent (DES).

Vaginal Cancer in the United States

The incidence of vaginal cancer varies by age and race. In a study of women based on 39 population-based cancer registries in the United States, 1370 cases of in situ vaginal cancer and 5430 cases of invasive cancer were detected during 1998–2003. The annual age-adjusted incidence estimated for all women was 0.18 per 100,000 for in situ cancer and 0.69 for invasive

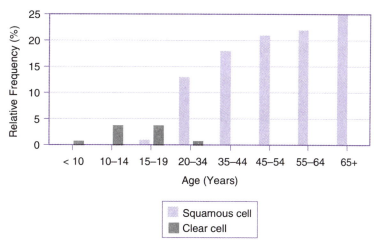

FIGURE 25.4 Age at Diagnosis of Vaginal Cancer by Histology.

Caption: The relative frequency of clear cell adenocarcinoma among all cases of vaginal carcinoma is approximately 10% of the level shown in the chart.

Data from Howlader, N., Noone, A. M., Krapcho, M., Garshell, J., Neyman, N., Altekruse, S. F., . . . Cronin, K. A. (Eds.). (2013). *SEER cancer statistics review, 1975–2010.* Bethesda, MD: National Cancer Institute. Retrieved from http://seer.cancer.gov/csr/1975_2010/; National Cancer Institute. (2011). *Diethylstilbestrol (DES) and cancer.* Bethesda, MD: National Cancer Institute.

cancer. Cases of in situ cancer were diagnosed an average of 10 years earlier (58 years) than cases of invasive cancer (68 years). The annual incidence of invasive vaginal cancer was highest among African-American women (1.06 per 100,000) and lowest among women of Asian and Pacific Island origin (0.50 per 100,000). Rates were intermediate for Caucasian and Hispanic women (0.65 and 0.87 per 100,000, respectively) (Wu et al., 2008).

Risk Factors for Squamous Cell Carcinoma of the Vagina

Squamous cell carcinoma of the vagina has a similar profile of risk factors as cervical cancer. Current evidence suggests that malignant transformation of the vaginal epithelium is most often a consequence of chronic genital infection by oncogenic strains of HPV, particularly HPV-16 and HPV-18. In fact, this type of malignancy is often diagnosed as a second primary tumor among women who were formerly treated for cervical dysplasia or cervical cancer (Brinton, Nasca, Mallin, Schairer, et al., 1990; Choo & Anderson, 1982; Gallup, Talledo, Shah, & Hayes, 1987). Other cofactors also increase the risk, including cigarette smoking and infection by the genital herpes simplex virus (HSV2) and/or HIV.

Human Papillomavirus and Vaginal Carcinoma

Investigators at the IARC examined the prevalence of HPV in vulvar, vaginal, and anal carcinoma and premalignant lesions called intraepithelial neoplasia using

the data from 93 studies conducted in 26 countries of Asia, Europe, North America, Latin America, and Oceania. In all studies included for meta-analysis, the presence of HPV DNA in tissue samples was detected by PCR assays. Prevalence estimates for vaginal lesions were obtained by pooling the data from 14 of these studies. The prevalence of HPV was 70% among 136 vaginal carcinomas and 94% among 298 vaginal intraepithelial neoplasms (VAINs). Among HPV-positive cases of vaginal carcinoma, 80% were positive for HPV-16, 10% were positive for HPV-18, and the remaining cases were positive for either HPV-6 or HPV-11. These results clearly indicate that oncogenic strains of HPV (particularly HPV-16 and HPV-18) play a significant role in the genesis of vaginal carcinoma (De Vuyst et al., 2009).

Vaginal Intraepithelial Neoplasia

Microscopic studies of cytological specimens of suspicious lesions of the vaginal epithelium clearly reveal the presence of premalignant foci of abnormally proliferating cells called *vaginal intraepithelial neoplasia (VAIN)*. Similar to cervical intraepithelial neoplasia (CIN), these lesions are graded as VAIN1, VAIN2, or VAIN3, reflecting the likelihood of transition to invasive carcinoma. Of these, VAIN3 is synonymous with carcinoma in situ, which may progress to invasive squamous cell carcinoma if cancer cells breach the basement membrane (National Cancer Institute, 2011).

Women who develop VAIN are most often premenopausal with coexisting CIN. In a series of 121 VAIN cases, the mean age at diagnosis was 35 years and the lesions were typically multifocal and located in the upper third of the vagina in association with CIN (Dodge, Eltabbakh, Mount, Walker, & Morgan, 2001). In a meta-analysis of tissue specimens from women with vaginal neoplasia, HPV DNA was detected in 100% of 107 cases with VAIN1, 90% of 191 cases with VAIN2 or VAIN3, and 70% of 136 cases with invasive vaginal carcinoma (De Vuyst et al., 2009). These results suggest that in some women, persisting HPV infection of the vaginal epithelium is sufficient to cause progression of VAIN to invasive vaginal carcinoma, whereas in others, additional risk factors likely contribute to malignant transformation.

Web of Causation in Vaginal Carcinoma

Factors other than HPV may be involved in the causal pathway leading to vaginal cancer. This is illustrated by the results of a population-based case–control study conducted in the state of Washington in the United States. In the study, 156 women with squamous cell vaginal carcinoma were compared to 2041 age-matched controls without cancer. Effects were quantified by estimating odds ratios (ORs). Notably, tumors of the cervix or the anus preceded the diagnosis of vaginal cancer in 30% of the cases. Women with vaginal cancer were more likely to have five or more sexual partners (OR = 3.1), first intercourse before age 17 years (OR = 2.0), and be current smokers at diagnosis (OR = 2.1) than controls. The presence of antibodies to HPV-16 was the strongest risk factor (OR = 4.3); furthermore, HPV-16 DNA was detected in 80% of cases with in situ vaginal cancer and 60% of cases with invasive vaginal cancer. Nevertheless, independent risk increases were also noted among women with antibodies to HPV-18 (OR = 2.0) and genital HSV2 (OR = 2.1). Finally, there was an increasing dose response in risk with the duration of cigarette smoking, peaking at more than 30 years of tobacco addiction (OR = 2.8). These findings suggest a web of causation that includes multiple risk factors (e.g., early sexual activity with several partners) leading to chronic infection of the cervical, anal, and vaginal epithelium by HPV-16, HPV-18, and/or HSV2 coupled with chronic tobacco smoking (Daling et al., 2002). Though not assessed in this study, immunosuppression due to HIV/AIDS also increases the risk.

Cigarette Smoking and Squamous Cell Vaginal Carcinoma

Only a small percentage (~10%) of women infected with oncogenic strains of HPV develop squamous cell carcinoma of the vagina. One cofactor that significantly heightens malignant transformation is chronic cigarette smoking.

An international team of investigators recently examined associations of HPV infection and smoking with the development of SCCs of the vulva and vagina in a case–control study of Danish women. A total of 182 cases with SCCs of the vulva or vagina were compared to 164 women with adenocarcinomas of the corpus uteri and 518 population controls without cancer. Women with uterine adenocarcinomas and women without cancer manifested similar characteristics, and the two control groups were pooled in the final analysis of data. Tumor specimens were examined for the presence of HPV DNA by PCR assays. Univariate analyses revealed that current smoking significantly increased the risk of vulvar SCC (OR = 2.69) and vaginal SCC (OR = 1.68). However, stratification by the presence/absence of HPV DNA revealed that tobacco smoking increased the risk among HPV-positive women (OR = 2.78) *but not among HPV-negative women* (OR = 1.03). These results suggest that tobacco carcinogens interact with oncogenic strains of HPV to synergistically heighten the risk (Madsen, Jensen, van den Brule, Wohlfahrt, & Frisch, 2008).

Human Immunodeficiency Virus in Vaginal Carcinoma

Based on data from the AIDS–Cancer Match Registry Study in the United States, women with AIDS have a 5.8-fold increased incidence of developing invasive vulvar/vaginal cancer compared to women from the general population (**FIGURE 25.3**). On average, invasive tumors emerged at an earlier age in AIDS patients, suggesting that HIV-related immunosuppression markedly accelerates the progression of HPV-related in situ lesions of the vulva or vagina to invasive carcinoma (Frisch et al., 2000).

Clear Cell Adenocarcinoma of the Vagina

Clear cell adenocarcinomas of the vagina are caused by in utero exposure to diethylstilbestrol (DES). From 1940 to 1971, a routine practice in the United States and throughout Europe was to administer DES to pregnant women with first trimester bleeding in order to prevent miscarriage and premature labor and delivery. It is estimated that DES was prescribed to 5–10 million women in the United States and millions more in Europe. It was eventually discovered that daughters of these DES-treated women developed clear cell adenocarcinoma of the vagina at an exceptionally high rate. This tumor is extraordinarily rare and, unlike other forms of vaginal cancer that are usually diagnosed late in life, clear cell vaginal adenocarcinomas stimulated by in utero DES exposure are most often diagnosed during adolescence (Herbst & Anderson, 1991; National Cancer Institute, 2011).

In 1970, Arthur Herbst and Robert Scully reported characteristics of a series of seven rare vaginal adenocarcinomas diagnosed in young women, 15–22 years of age, during a 2-year window of time at Massachusetts General Hospital and one other hospital in Boston. Six of the tumors were pathologically classified as clear cell adenocarcinomas of the vagina. Prior to this time, there were only a few case reports of this rare type of malignancy occurring in young women (Herbst & Scully, 1970).

Shortly after the initial cluster of cases was identified, a retrospective case–control investigation was conducted comparing exposures in eight young women with clear cell vaginal adenocarcinomas to four matched controls per case. Seven of the eight mothers of these patients had been treated with DES during the first trimester of pregnancy ($P < 0.00001$). The investigators concluded that "maternal ingestion of stilbestrol during early pregnancy appears to have enhanced the risk of vaginal adenocarcinoma developing years later in the offspring exposed" (Herbst, Ulfelder, & Poskanzer, 1971).

Following these early reports, the carcinogenic impact of in utero DES exposure was confirmed by several independent studies, and a registry of DES-exposed daughters was established. The risk of developing clear cell vaginal adenocarcinoma by age 24 years among women who were exposed to DES in utero was estimated at approximately 1 per 1000, more than 40 times higher than among unexposed

women (Herbst, 1981; Herbst & Anderson, 1991; Herbst, Cole, Colton, Robboy, & Scully, 1977). Clear cell adenocarcinoma is often preceded by a condition known as vaginal adenosis (the presence of abnormal glandular foci in the vaginal epithelium). In 1972, DES administration to pregnant women was discontinued in the United States; however, its use continued in Europe until 1978 (National Cancer Institute, 2011).

By 1981, 400 cases of clear cell adenocarcinoma of the vagina had been diagnosed among young women born after 1940. The number of cases peaked in the United States in 1975 and has since declined (**FIGURE 25.5**). The age-specific incidence rates of this tumor are highest among young women aged 15–22 years, with a peak incidence at age 19. Furthermore, DES-exposed women are at high risk for a multitude of other adverse reproductive events, including stillbirth, neonatal death, ectopic pregnancy, miscarriage, pre-eclampsia, and infertility (Herbst, 1981; Herbst & Anderson, 1991).

Some studies suggest that the risk of breast cancer may be elevated in DES-exposed daughters. Investigators in the United States compared the incidence of breast cancer in a cohort of 4817 women with prenatal DES exposure to that in a matched cohort of 2073 women with no exposure. During follow-up, 102 cases of clear cell vaginal adenocarcinoma were diagnosed among DES-exposed women compared to 26 cases in unexposed women. Exposure to DES increased the incidence of breast cancer approximately twofold by age 40 (RR = 2.05) and by nearly fourfold by age 50 (RR = 3.85) (Palmer et al., 2006). The NCI has therefore recommended that DES-exposed daughters have regular mammograms and yearly medical checkups that include careful pelvic examination to identify premalignant lesions (National Cancer Institute, 2011).

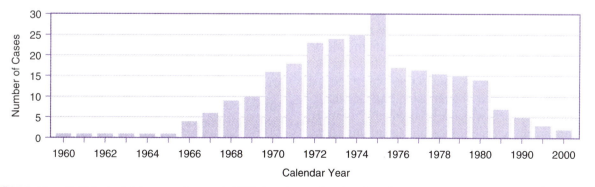

FIGURE 25.5 Clear Cell Vaginal Adenocarcinoma in DES-daughters. *Caption:* Data Points are Moving Averages of Published Numbers of Cases.

Data from Herbst, A. L. (1981). Clear cell adenocarcinoma and the current status of DES-exposed females. *Cancer, 48*, 484–488.

▶ Epidemiology of Vulvar Cancer

Carcinoma of the vulva accounts for about 1%–2% of all malignancies of the female genitalia. Estimates of the incidence of vulvar cancer ranged from 0.5 to 1.5 per 100,000 among populations sampled in 2002 (Parkin & Bray, 2006). Worldwide, vulvar cancer was diagnosed in 27,000 women during 2008 and caused nearly 15,000 deaths (de Martel et al., 2012; Ferlay et al., 2010; Parkin, 2006). This tumor rarely manifests in women under the age of 60 years and is often preceded by premalignant dysplastic lesions called *vulvar intraepithelial neoplasia (VIN)*. As is true for CIN and VAIN, higher grades of VIN increase the likelihood of progression to invasive cancer of the vulva. Carcinoma in situ of the vulva (also called *Bowen's disease*) has been found to progress to invasive cancer over a period of 5–10 years. Like vaginal cancer and cervical cancer, most malignant tumors (90%–95%) of the vulva are SCCs that arise from the stratified epithelium covering the vulva. Other histologies include malignant melanomas, Bartholin gland adenocarcinomas that arise in the sweat glands, Paget tumors, sarcomas, and basal cell carcinomas.

Squamous Cell Carcinoma of the Vulva

More than 90% of vulvar malignancies are SCCs; however, two independent pathways of vulvar carcinogenesis have been postulated corresponding to two distinct subtypes of SCCs of the vulva (Andersen, Franquemont, Williams, Taylor, & Crum, 1991; Bloss et al., 1991).

The classic, warty, or Bowenoid type is predominantly associated with chronic infection by HPV-16, HPV-18, or HPV-33 and is found in younger women (often prior to menopause). Factors associated with malignant transformation of the vulvar mucosa in HPV-infected women include early age at first intercourse, multiple sexual partners, HIV infection, genital HSV2 infection, and cigarette smoking.

The keratinizing, differentiated, or simplex type occurs in older postmenopausal women, is *not* related to HPV infection, and is associated with inflammatory vulvar dystrophies such as lichen sclerosis and chronic venereal granulomatous disease. In this type, the cancer cells are usually well differentiated and classically manifest *keratin pearls*, which are foci of keratinization within concentric layers of cancerous squamous cells.

Ethnic Differences and Time Trends in Vulvar Cancer

A team of investigators examined data from 39 population-based tumor registries in the United States covering 83% of the population during 1983–2003 and assessed patterns of vulvar cancer by age, race, ethnicity, and histology. During this time period, 12,554 in situ vulvar tumors and 18,066 invasive tumors were diagnosed. SCCs accounted for 77% of in situ vulvar malignancies and 75% of invasive tumors. On average, in situ tumors were diagnosed about 20 years earlier (49 years) than invasive tumors (69 years). For all women, the annual incidence was 1.2 per 100,000 for in situ cancer and 1.7 per 100,000 for invasive cancer. The annual rate of invasive cancer was highest in Caucasians (1.8 per 100,000), intermediate in African-American and Hispanic women (1.3 per 100,000), and lowest in Asian and Pacific Islanders (0.4 per 100,000). In contrast to many other forms of cancer, vulvar cancer rates are higher among Caucasian women than African-American women, suggesting the presence of different risk factor profiles (Saraiya et al., 2008).

In a separate study, a rising trend was observed in the age-adjusted incidence of both invasive vulvar cancer and in situ tumors among U.S. women during 1973–2004. Based on data from nine registries of the Surveillance, Epidemiology, and End Results (SEER) program, the rate of in situ vulvar cancer increased 74% (3.5% annually), and the rate of invasive vulvar cancer increased 21% (1.0% annually) during the 21-year time period of study. The age-adjusted incidence rate of invasive vulvar cancer during 1997–2004 was 2.5 cases per 100,000 among all women, 2.8 per 100,000 among Caucasians, and 2.0 per 100,000 in African Americans. Speculative reasons for the increase in vulvar cancer rates include rising rates of infection by oncogenic strains of HPV and greater numbers of immunocompromised patients due to HIV infections (Bodelon, Madeleine, Voigt, & Weiss, 2009).

Human Papillomavirus and Vulvar Carcinoma

The prevalence of HPV in vulvar carcinoma was examined in a meta-analysis of data from 93 studies conducted on four continents using PCR assays for detection of HPV seropositivity. Prevalence estimates for vulvar lesions were obtained by pooling the data from 63 of these studies. The prevalence of HPV was 68% in 90 cases of VIN1, 85% in 1061 cases of VIN2 or VIN3, but only 40% in 1873 cases of invasive vulvar carcinoma. The prevalence of HPV strains differed by grade of neoplasia: HPV-6 (22%), HPV-16 (10%), and HPV-11 (9%) in VIN1; HPV-16 (72%), HPV-18 (5%), and HPV-33 (8%) in VIN2/3; and HPV-16 (32%), HPV-18 (4%), and HPV-33 (5%) in invasive carcinoma. Notably, the prevalence of HPV was markedly higher in basaloid (warty) vulvar carcinomas (70%) compared to keratinized tumors (13%). These results support the existence of different etiologies of carcinoma of the vulva, one process related to infection by HPV-16, HPV-18, or HPV-33 and another that is independent of HPV and related to different inflammatory and/or infectious agents (De Vuyst et al., 2009).

Cigarette Smoking and Vulvar Carcinoma

Cigarette smoking has been consistently implicated as a risk factor for SCCs of the female genital tract including the vulva (Daling et al., 1992). Effects of smoking on vulvar cancer were examined in a population-based case–control study of 400 women with in situ vulvar carcinoma, 110 women with invasive carcinoma, and 1403 age-matched controls in the Seattle, Washington, area. Serum samples were analyzed for antibodies against oncogenic HPV strains and HSV2. Current smokers were at increased risk (OR = 3.6 for in situ carcinoma and OR = 2.8 for invasive carcinoma). Independent effects were also observed for HPV infection or HSV2 infection. Notably, vulvar carcinoma risk was increased 18.8-fold among women who were current smokers and seropositive for HPV-16 compared to nonsmokers who were seronegative for HPV-16. The investigators concluded that current smoking and infection by either HPV or HSV2 are risk factors for vulvar carcinoma and that HPV-16 infection and smoking synergistically increase the risk (Madeleine, Daling, & Schwartz, 1997).

Condyloma Acuminata of the Vulva

Condyloma acuminata (genital warts) are associated with sexually transmitted viruses, particularly certain strains of HPV (e.g., HPV-6 and HPV-11) and genital HSV2. These lesions consist of proliferating squamous epithelium with atypical morphology. Though controversial, some studies suggest that their presence may heighten the risk of developing vulvar carcinoma. In a case–control study of 209 vulvar cancer patients and 348 age-matched controls from the same communities, several risk factors were examined, including history of genital warts. The findings revealed a marked increase in risk (OR = 15.2) among those women who reported a medical history of condyloma acuminata. Furthermore, women with a history of this condition who were smokers had a 35-fold increase in the risk of developing vulvar cancer compared to women with neither exposure (Brinton, Nasca, Mallin, Baptiste, et al., 1990).

Human Immunodeficiency Virus and Vulvar Carcinoma

Immunosuppression due to HIV/AIDS appears to be a strong risk factor for vulvar carcinoma. In a case–control study, investigators at the University of Witwatersrand in Johannesburg, South Africa, compared 53 women with vulvar carcinoma to 556 women without cancer ascertained from three tertiary care hospitals in Johannesburg and Soweto. Seropositivity for HIV was found to significantly increase the vulvar cancer risk (adjusted OR = 4.8) (Sitas et al., 2000). This estimate for South African women is like findings from the AIDS–Cancer Match Registry Study in the United States in which women with HIV/AIDS had a 5.8-fold increased incidence of developing invasive vulvar/vaginal cancer compared to women from the general population (Figure 25.3) (Frisch et al., 2000). These results, together with several published case reports, indicate that HIV-associated immunosuppression increases the likelihood of chronic infection by high-risk HPV types that predispose to intraepithelial neoplasia and carcinoma of the vulva (Elit, Voruganti, & Simunovic, 2005).

Vulvar Lichen Sclerosis and Vulvar Carcinoma

Vulvar lichen sclerosis is an insidious inflammatory condition that is most commonly found in older postmenopausal women, but can also develop in girls prior to menarche. Characteristic signs of lichen sclerosis are leukoplakia (white glistening plaques of the vulvar mucous membranes) and unrelenting pruritus (itching). Etiologically, this condition has been linked to preexisting dermatologic autoimmune conditions, estrogen deficiency in prepubertal girls and postmenopausal women, and certain bacterial and viral infections. However, the exact cause remains enigmatic (van de Nieuwenhof, van der Avoort, & de Hullu, 2008).

Patients with vulvar lichen sclerosis are at high risk for the development of squamous cell carcinoma of the vulva. Pathologic studies of cases with vulvar carcinoma reveal that 50%–60% of malignant specimens manifest lichen sclerosis (Kagie, Kenter, Herman, Trimbos, & Fleuren, 1997; Rouzier et al., 2001). In an Italian study of 211 patients with lichen sclerosis, three had developed vulvar carcinoma after 20 months, a 247-fold increase compared to age-matched women in the general population (Carli et al., 1995). Nevertheless, the absolute cancer risk in women with lichen sclerosis is small and can be attenuated with appropriate therapy (Canavan & Cohen, 2002).

Granulomatous Disease and Vulvar Carcinoma

An early report of young women with invasive vulvar carcinoma in the West Indies noted that the majority of cases (66%) had a prior history of sexually transmitted granulomatous diseases of the vulva (Hay & Cole, 1969). Similar findings were reported in a later review of 119 patients with primary invasive cancer of the vulva diagnosed during 1958–1973 at University Hospital of the West Indies, Kingston, Jamaica. Of these cases, 77 (65%) were premenopausal and in 51% of cases, vulvar carcinoma coexisted or followed previous chronic vulvar granulomatous disease and showed rapid tumor progression (Sengupta, 1980). Granuloma inguinale and lymphogranuloma venereum are granulomatous conditions caused by sexually transmitted organisms (*Donovania granulomatis* and *Chlamydia trachomatis*, respectively).

Recent studies suggest that *C. trachomatis* infection may be a component of a complex web of causation of lichen sclerosis and vulvar cancer. In a study of Polish women, 80 women with vulvar disease (30 with vulvar cancer and 50 with lichen sclerosis) were tested for the presence of *C. trachomatis* antibodies. Serum antibodies to *C. trachomatis* were detected in 50% of women with vulvar cancer and 16% of women with lichen sclerosis (Olejek et al., 2009).

▶ Epidemiology of Anal Carcinoma

Anal cancer is relatively uncommon, comprising only 2%–3% of all gastrointestinal malignancies. Estimates of the annual incidence of anal cancer vary widely (0.1–3.0 per 100,000), and in most populations the rates in women are approximately double the rates in men. Exceptions are populations with higher levels of male HPV transmission (e.g., San Francisco) wherein men have higher rates (Parkin & Bray, 2006). During 2008, approximately 27,000 cases were diagnosed worldwide, 15,000 in women and 12,000 in men, and in that year, 15,000 people died from anal cancer (de Martel et al., 2012; Ferlay et al., 2010; Parkin, 2006).

Most anal malignancies (~90%) are SCCs, with the remainder consisting predominantly of adenocarcinomas. Sarcomas and malignant melanomas very rarely develop from tissues of the anal canal (Salmo & Haboubi, 2011).

The incidence of anal cancer has more than doubled in some populations in recent years in association with increasing rates of sexually transmitted infections such as HPV, HSV2, and HIV. Other significant risk factors include receptive anal intercourse, history of condyloma acuminata (genital warts), and chronic cigarette smoking. From an etiologic perspective, anal cancer has more similarities to genital malignancies than to gastrointestinal tract cancer.

Trends in Anal Cancer

Although anal cancer is rare, the rates of squamous cell anal carcinoma have increased significantly in some populations in recent years. In the United States, population-based tumor registries of the SEER program of the NCI reported 11,231 squamous cell anal carcinomas and 1791 anal adenocarcinomas during the period 1973–2009. During this 26-year period, the annual rates of squamous cell anal carcinomas increased threefold in men (from 1.0 to 3.0 per 100,000) and nearly twofold in women (1.3–2.4 per 100,000), whereas the rates of adenocarcinomas remained stable at approximately 0.25 per 100,000 (Johnson, Madeleine, Newcomer, Schwartz, & Daling, 2004; Nelson, Levine, Bernstein, Smith, & Lai, 2013).

Rising trends in the incidence of anal cancer and high-grade anal intraepithelial neoplasia (AIN2/3) have also been observed in the Danish population. Using data from the Danish Cancer Registry and the Danish Registry of Pathology, investigators at the Danish Cancer Society examined trends in the incidence of invasive anal carcinoma (2198 cases) and AIN2/3 (608 cases) among Danish men and women during 1978–2008. Approximately 65% of these tumors developed in women. During the 30-year period of study, the age-standardized incidence rate of anal cancer increased from 0.68 to 1.48 per 100,000 person-years in women and from 0.45 to 0.80 per 100,000 person-years in men, and there was a corresponding 5% annual increase in AIN2/3 cases. Increases of 4% per year were noted for HPV-related squamous cell and transitional cell carcinomas in men and women, but there were no increases in the incidence of adenocarcinomas. The investigators suggest the need for intensified screening and HPV vaccination to reduce the burden of anal cancer (Nielsen, Munk, & Kjaer, 2012).

Human Papillomavirus and Anal Carcinoma

The prevalence of HPV in anal carcinoma and anal intraepithelial neoplasia (AIN) was examined in a meta-analysis of data from 93 studies conducted on four continents using PCR assays for detection of

HPV DNA. Prevalence estimates for anal lesions were obtained by pooling the data from 29 of these studies. The prevalence of HPV was 84% among 955 invasive anal carcinomas and 93% among 1280 cases of AIN. Among cases of anal carcinoma, the most frequent strains detected were HPV-16 (73%), HPV-18 (5%), and HPV-6 (5%). Notably, among cases of AIN2 or AIN3 that were co-infected with HIV, 66% were positive for multiple strains of HPV. Although the most common strains were HPV-16 (55%), HPV-18 (26%), and HPV-58 (21%), several other strains (e.g., HPV-31, HPV-33, HPV-45, HPV-58) were also detected in 10%–20% of the HIV-positive AIN2/AIN3 cases. In contrast, among AIN2/3 cases that were *negative* for HIV, coinfection by multiple HPV strains was relatively infrequent (13%) and the prevalence of HPV-16 increased with increasing grade of neoplasia (e.g., 30% in AIN1, 75% in AIN2/3, and 85% in invasive carcinoma). These results support the view that immunosuppression due to HIV coinfection allows a broader range of HPV types to persist and contribute to malignant transformation of the anal mucosa, whereas in the absence of HIV, the process appears to be primarily driven by chronic infection with HPV-16 (De Vuyst et al., 2009).

Human Immunodeficiency Virus and Anal Carcinoma

The association between AIDS and anal carcinoma was examined in 309,365 men and women with AIDS (257,605 men and 51,760 women) using data collected in the multicenter AIDS–Cancer Match Registry Study during the period 1978–1996. Compared to the general population, the incidence rates of invasive and in situ anal cancers increased more than 100-fold in AIDS-afflicted men and women less than 30 years of age. Across all age groups, the incidence of invasive carcinoma of the anus increased 7-fold among HIV-infected women and 38-fold among HIV-infected men (Figure 25.3). The relative risk (RR) among Caucasians with AIDS was more than double that of other ethnic groups (RR = 55 versus RR = 22) (Frisch et al., 2000).

To examine the impact of HIV-related immunosuppression on the genesis of anal neoplasia, investigators in San Francisco, California, compared the progression of squamous intraepithelial neoplasia of the anal mucosa in 346 HIV-positive and 262 HIV-negative homosexual men. Subjects were examined at defined intervals using anal cytology, anoscopy with biopsy of visible lesions, HPV and HIV testing, level of CD4 lymphocytes, and data on medical history and lifestyle. After 2 years of follow-up, the incidence of anal squamous intraepithelial neoplasia among men who were free of disease at baseline was 20% in HIV-positive men and 8% in HIV-negative men. Low-grade lesions progressed to higher grade lesions in 62% of HIV-positive men and 36% of HIV-negative men. The relative risk of disease progression in HIV-positive compared to HIV-negative men was 2.4, and the risk increased to 3.1 in HIV-positive men with CD4 counts less than 200 per cubic millimeter. Infection with multiple HPV strains increased the risk of disease progression in HIV-positive men (RR = 2.0) and HIV-negative men (RR = 5.1). The findings suggest that HPV infection per se stimulates the progression of AIN to invasive carcinoma and that co-infection with HIV synergistically heightens the risk of malignant transformation by reducing the immune response (Palefsky et al., 1998).

Australian investigators conducted a review and meta-analysis of published data on the prevalence of HPV-16 and the incidence of anal cancer in men who have sex with men (MSM). Data were pooled from 53 studies that included 31 estimates of HPV prevalence and 9 estimates of anal cancer incidence. The prevalence of HPV-16 was threefold higher in HIV-positive MSM than HIV-negative MSM (35.4% versus 12.5%), and the incidence of anal cancer was ninefold higher among HIV-positive MSM than HIV-negative MSM (46 versus 5 per 100,000) (Machalek et al., 2012).

Investigators of the North American AIDS Cohort Collaboration on Research and Design (NA-ACCORD) compared anal cancer incidence rates among 34,189 HIV-positive and 113,260 HIV-negative individuals from 13 cohorts followed during 1996–2007. Among HIV-positive subjects, 55% were MSM, 19% were other men, and 26% were women. Among HIV-negative subjects, 90% were men and 10% were women. Anal cancer incidence rates per 100,000 person-years were considerably higher among HIV-positive risk groups (131 for HIV-positive MSM, 46 for other HIV-positive men, 30 for HIV-positive women, 2 for HIV-negative men, and 0 for HIV-negative women). A striking finding was the increasing incidence of anal cancer with increasing prevalence of MSM among the 13 cohorts (**FIGURE 25.6**). Based on linear regression analysis, the projected incidence of anal cancer was 28 per 100,000 for a population with 0% MSM and 146 per 100,000 for a population with 100% MSM, a 5.2-fold increase in anal cancer risk. Though their study lacked data on HPV infection as well as other risk factors, the investigators suggest that HPV vaccination and enhanced cytological screening for AIN should be considered for all HIV-positive individuals (Silverberg et al., 2012).

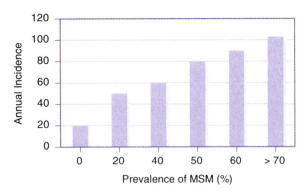

FIGURE 25.6 Incidence of Anal Cancer in MSM.

Caption: Annual incidence rates per 100,000 person-years are mean values estimated from 13 separate cohorts according to their prevalence of MSM. One outlier representing less than 0.5% of exposure time was omitted from the calculations.

Data from Silverberg, M. J., Lau, B., Justice, A. C., Engels, E., Gill, M. J., Goedert, J. J., . . . North American AIDS Cohort Collaboration on Research and Design (NA-ACCORD) of IeDEA. (2012). Risk of anal cancer in HIV-infected and HIV-uninfected individuals in North America. *Clinical Infectious Disease, 54*(7), 1026–1034.

▶ Primary Prevention of HPV-Related Vaginal, Vulvar, and Anal Cancer

Effective quadrivalent vaccines (e.g., Gardasil) have been developed against oncogenic strains of HPV (HPV-16 and HPV-18) and strains that cause genital warts (HPV-6 and HPV-11). Preliminary results of randomized clinical trials show up to 100% efficacy in preventing infection by these viruses and reducing the risk of precancerous lesions of the cervical, vaginal, and vulvar epithelium among young women who received the vaccine prior to infection. Results suggest that protection against infection by these HPV strains persists for up to 5 years after vaccination (Cutts et al., 2007; Markowitz et al., 2007).

Clinical trials have recently been conducted to assess the value of quadrivalent vaccination against HPV-16, HPV-18, HPV-6, and HPV-11 to prevent the development of AIN and anal cancer in MSM. In a double-blinded international trial, 602 healthy MSM, ages 16–26, were randomized to receive either the quadrivalent vaccine or placebo. After 3 years of follow-up, the rates of AIN and anal carcinoma related to infection by HPV-6, HPV-11, HPV-16, or HPV-18 were reduced by 75% and 95%, respectively, in those who received the three-shot vaccine regimen compared to those receiving placebo, and no serious adverse events or reactions were reported. These findings support the use of quadrivalent HPV vaccine in high-risk groups (e.g., MSM) to reduce the anal cancer risk (Palefsky et al., 2011).

Recently, a new 9-valent HPV vaccine has been developed (Gardasil) and was licensed in Europe for the prevention of cancers and precancerous lesions of the cervix, vulva, vagina, and anus plus genital warts caused by HPV6, 11, 16, 18, 31, 33, 45, 52, and 58. The 9-valent vaccine protects against strains not covered by the quadrivalent vaccine has important preventive potential for approximately 90% of HPV-related malignancies (Hartwig, St Guily, Dominiak-Felden, Alemany, & de Sanjosé, 2017).

Given that a substantial proportion of cervical cancers as well as noncervical cancers are caused by HPV-16 and HPV-18, current HPV vaccines may hold great promise in reducing the burden of HPV-associated malignancies in the human population. Nevertheless, because HPV vaccines do not totally eliminate the risk of developing HPV-related malignancies, cytological screening is still recommended in order to detect premalignant lesions and minimize cancer incidence and mortality. Furthermore, it seems advisable to target certain high-risk groups such as MSM and HIV-seropositive individuals for intensified screening, even those who are well controlled on antiretroviral therapy (Cutts et al., 2007; Gillison, Chaturvedi, & Lowy, 2008; Lowy & Schiller, 2006; Palefsky, 2000).

▶ Screening for Squamous Cell Vaginal, Vulvar, and Anal Cancer

Dramatic reductions in cervical cancer incidence and mortality among women of developed nations are due largely to the effectiveness of the Papanicolaou-Traut cytological test (Papanicolaou & Traut, 1943). The *Pap test*, which was introduced in the United States around 1950, provides a quick, safe, affordable, and accurate means of detecting precancerous dysplastic lesions of the cervix that can be cured by simple surgery or other ablative techniques.

In the absence of symptoms or major risk factors, the Pap test is *not* routinely used for screening the vagina of the female genital tract. However, if symptoms are present (e.g., bleeding unrelated to the menstrual period, pelvic pain, palpable mass), the Pap test is an effective diagnostic tool for the detection of dysplastic lesions of the squamous cell epithelium of the vagina (VAIN), vulva (VIN), and anus (AIN). These are like cervical dysplasia and are graded according to the depth of abnormal cells in the vaginal epithelium (**TABLE 25.2**).

It is important to note that all VAIN, VIN, and AIN lesions including in situ carcinomas of the vagina, vulva, or anus are up to 100% curable by

TABLE 25.2 Classification of Premalignant Lesions of the Urogenital Tract

Classification	Description
VAIN1, VIN1, AIN1	Dysplastic cells in the outermost one-third of the epithelium
VAIN2, VIN2, AIN2	Dysplastic cells in the outermost two-thirds of the epithelium
VAIN3, VIN3, AIN3	Dysplastic cells in more than two-thirds of the epithelium without breaching the basement membrane (also called *carcinoma in situ*)

Data from Holschneider, C. H. (2013). *Vulvar intraepithelial neoplasia*. Retrieved from http://www.uptodate.com/contents/vulvar-intraepithelial-neoplasia; Holschneider, C. H., & Berek, J. S. (2013). *Vaginal intraepithelial neoplasia*. Retrieved from http://www.uptodate.com/contents/vaginal-intraepithelial-neoplasia; Palefsky, J. M., & Cranston, R. D. (2013). *Anal intraepithelial neoplasia, diagnosis, screening, prevention and treatment*. Retrieved from http://www.uptodate.com/contents/anal-intraepithelial-neoplasia

surgical excision or other forms of ablative therapy. Furthermore, localized tumors that have not spread to the inguinal lymph nodes are curable in 90% of cases by appropriate therapy (Batista & Martins, 2012; Holschneider, 2013; Holschneider & Berek, 2013; Palefsky & Cranston, 2013).

References

Andersen, W. A., Franquemont, D. W., Williams, H., Taylor, P. T., & Crum, C. P. (1991). Vulvar squamous cell carcinoma and papillomaviruses: Two separate entities. *American Journal of Obstetrics and Gynecology, 165*, 335–336.

Batista, T. P., & Martins, M. R. (2012). Vaginal cancer. *International Journal of Cancer Research and Prevention, 5*(3–4), 235–246.

Bloss, J. D., Liao, S. Y., Wilczynski, S. P., Macri, C., Walker, J., Peake, M., & Berman, M. L. (1991). Clinical and histologic features of vulvar carcinomas analyzed for human papillomavirus status: Evidence that squamous cell carcinoma of the vulva has more than one etiology. *Human Pathology, 22*(7), 711–718.

Bodelon, C., Madeleine, M. M., Voigt, L. F., & Weiss, N. S. (2009). Is the incidence of invasive vulvar cancer increasing in the United States? *Cancer Causes and Control, 20*(9), 1779–1782.

Boshartb, M., Gissmann, L., Ikenberg, H., Kleinheinz, A., Scheurlen, W., & zur Hausen, H. (1984). A new type of papillomavirus DNA, its presence in genital cancer biopsies and in cell lines derived from cervical cancer. *EMBO Journal, 3*(5), 1151–1157.

Bray, F., Ferlay, J., Soerjomataram, I., Siegel, R. L., Torre, L. A., & Jemal, A. (2018). Global cancer statistics 2018: GLOBOCAN estimates of incidence and mortality worldwide for 36 cancers in 185 countries. *CA: A Cancer Journal for Clinicians, 68*(6), 394–424.

Brinton, L. A., Nasca, P. C., Mallin, K., Baptiste, M. S., Wilbanks, G. D., & Richart, R. M. (1990). Case-control study of cancer of the vulva. *Obstetrics and Gynecology, 75*(5), 859–866.

Brinton, L. A., Nasca, P. C., Mallin, K., Schairer, C., Rosenthal, J., Rothenberg, R., … Richart, R. M. (1990). Case-control study of *in situ* and invasive carcinoma of the vagina. *Gynecological Oncology, 38*, 49–54.

Bruni, L., Diaz, M., Castellsagué, X., Ferrer, E., Bosch, F. X., & de Sanjosé, S. (2010). Cervical human papillomavirus prevalence in 5 continents: Meta-analysis of 1 million women with normal cytological findings. *Journal of Infectious Diseases, 202*, 1789–1799.

Canavan, T. P., & Cohen, D. (2002). Vulvar cancer. *American Family Physician, 66*(7), 1269–1275.

Carli, P., Cattaneo, A., De, M. A., Biggeri, A., Taddei, G., & Giannotti, B. (1995). Squamous cell carcinoma arising in vulval lichen sclerosus: A longitudinal cohort study. *European Journal of Cancer Prevention, 4*(6), 491–495.

Choo, Y. C., & Anderson, D. G. (1982). Neoplasms of the vagina following cervical carcinoma. *Gynecological Oncology, 14*, 125–132.

Cutts, F. T., Franceschi, S., Goldie, S., Castellsague, X., de Sanjose, S., Garnett, G., … Markowitz, L. (2007). Human papillomavirus and HPV vaccines: A review. *Bulletin of the World Health Organization, 85*(9), 719–726.

Daling, J. R., Madeleine, M. M., Schwartz, S. M., Shera, K. A., Carter, J. J., McKnight, B., … Tamimi, H. (2002). A population-based study of squamous cell vaginal cancer: HPV and cofactors. *Gynecological Oncology, 84*(2), 263–270.

Daling, J. R., Sherman, K. J., Hislop, T. G., Mandelson, M., Beckmann, A. M., & Weiss, N. S. (1992). Cigarette smoking and the risk of anogenital cancer. *American Journal of Epidemiology, 135*, 180–189.

de Martel, C., Ferlay, J., Franceschi, S., Vignat, J., Bray, F., Forman, D., & Plummer, M. (2012). The global burden of cancers attributable to infections in the year 2008: A review and synthetic analysis. *Lancet Oncology, 13*, 607–615.

De Vuyst, H., Clifford, G. M., Nascimento, M. C., Madeleine, M. M., & Franceschi, S. (2009). Prevalence and type distribution of human papillomavirus in carcinoma and intraepithelial neoplasia of the vulva, vagina and anus: A meta-analysis. *International Journal of Cancer, 124*(7), 1626–1636.

Dodge, J. A., Eltabbakh, G. H., Mount, S. L., Walker, R. P., & Morgan, A. (2001). Clinical features and risk of recurrence among patients with vaginal intraepithelial neoplasia. *Gynecological Oncology, 83*(2), 363–369.

Elit, L., Voruganti, S., & Simunovic, M. (2005). Invasive vulvar cancer in a woman with human immunodeficiency virus: Case report and review of the literature. *Gynecological Oncology, 98*(1), 151–154.

Ferlay, J., Shin, H.-R., Bray, F., Forman, D., Mathers, C., & Parkin, D. M. (2010). Estimates of worldwide burden of cancer in 2008: GLOBOCAN 2008. *International Journal of Cancer, 127*(12), 2893–2917.

Forman, D., de Martel, C., Lacey, C. J., Soerjomataram, I., Lortet-Tieulent, J., Bruni, L., … Franceschi, S. (2012). Global burden of human papillomavirus and related diseases. *Vaccine, 30*(Suppl. 5), F12–F23.

Frisch, M., Biggar, R. J., & Goedert, J. J. (2000). Human papilloma virus-associated cancers in patients with human immunodeficiency virus infection and acquired immunodeficiency syndrome. *Journal of the National Cancer Institute, 92*(18), 1500–1510.

Gallup, D. G., Talledo, E., Shah, K. J., & Hayes, C. (1987). Invasive squamous cell carcinoma of the vagina: A 14 year study. *Obstetrics and Gynecology, 69*, 782–785.

Gillison, M. L., Chaturvedi, A. K., & Lowy, D. R. (2008). HPV prophylactic vaccines and the potential prevention of noncervical cancers in both men and women. *Cancer, 113*(10 Suppl.), 3036–3046.

Hamilton, S. R., & Aaltonen, L. A. (2000). Tumours of the anal canal. In S. R. Hamilton & L. A. Aaltonen (Eds.), *Pathology and genetics of tumours of the digestive system* (pp. 145–156). World Health Organization Classification of Tumours. Lyon, France: IARC Press.

Hartwig, S., St Guily, J. L., Dominiak-Felden, G., Alemany, L., & de Sanjosé, S. (2017). Estimation of the overall burden of cancers, precancerous lesions, and genital warts attributable to 9-valent HPV vaccine types in women and men in Europe. *Infectious Agents and Cancer, 12*, 19.

Hay, D. M., & Cole, F. M. (1969). Primary invasive carcinoma of the vulva in Jamaica. *Journal of Obstetrics and Gynaecology of the British Commonwealth, 76*(9), 821–830.

Herbst, A. L. (1981). Clear cell adenocarcinoma and the current status of DES-exposed females. *Cancer, 48*, 484–488.

Herbst, A. L., & Anderson, D. (1991). Clear cell adenocarcinoma of the vagina and cervix secondary to intrauterine exposure to diethylstilbestrol. *Cancer, 67*(7), 1971–1978.

Herbst, A. L., Cole, P., Colton, T., Robboy, S. J., & Scully, R. E. (1977). Age-incidence and risk of diethylstilbestrol-related clear cell adenocarcinoma of the vagina and cervix. *American Journal of Obstetrics and Gynecology, 128*, 43–50.

Herbst, A. L., & Scully, R. E. (1970). Adenocarcinoma of the vagina in adolescence. A report of 7 cases including 6 clear-cell carcinomas (so-called mesonephromas). *Cancer, 25*(4), 745–757.

Herbst, A. L., Ulfelder, H., & Poskanzer, D. C. (1971). Adenocarcinoma of the vagina—Association of maternal stilbestrol therapy with tumor appearance in young women. *New England Journal of Medicine, 284*, 878–881.

Holschneider, C. H. (2013). *Vulvar intraepithelial neoplasia.* Retrieved from www.uptodate.com/contents/vulvar-intraepithelial-neoplasia

Holschneider, C. H., & Berek, J. S. (2013). *Vaginal intraepithelial neoplasia.* Retrieved from www.uptodate.com/contents/vaginal-intraepithelial-neoplasia

Howlader, N., Noone, A. M., Krapcho, M., Garshell, J., Neyman, N., Altekruse, S. F., … Cronin, K. A. (Eds.). (2013). *SEER cancer statistics review, 1975–2010.* Bethesda, MD: National Cancer Institute. Retrieved from http://seer.cancer.gov/csr/1975_2010/

Johnson, L. G., Madeleine, M. M., Newcomer, L. M., Schwartz, S. M., & Daling, J. R. (2004). Anal cancer incidence and survival: The surveillance, epidemiology, and end results experience, 1973–2000. *Cancer, 101*(2), 281.

Kagie, M. J., Kenter, G. G., Herman, J., Trimbos, J. B., & Fleuren, G. J. (1997). The relevance of various vulvar epithelial changes in the early detection of squamous cell carcinoma of the vulva. *International Journal of Gynecological Cancer, 7*(1), 50–57.

Kiyono, T., Foster, S. A., Koop, J. I., McDougall, J. K., Galloway, D. A., & Klingelhutz, A. J. (1998). Both Rb/p16INK4a inactivation and telomerase activity are required to immortalize human epithelial cells. *Nature, 396*(6706), 84–88.

Lowy, D. R., & Schiller, J. T. (2006). Prophylactic human papillomavirus vaccines. *Journal of Clinical Investigation, 116*(5), 1167–1173.

Machalek, D. A., Poynten, M., Jin, F., Fairley, C. K., Farnsworth, A., Garland, S. M., … Grulich, A. E. (2012). Anal human papillomavirus infection and associated neoplastic lesions in men who have sex with men: A systematic review and meta-analysis. *Lancet Oncology, 13*(5), 487–500.

Madeleine, M. M., Daling, J. R., & Schwartz, S. M. (1997). Cofactors with human papillomavirus in a population-based study of vulvar cancer. *Journal of the National Cancer Institute, 89*(20), 1516–1523.

Madsen, B. S., Jensen, H. L., van den Brule, A. J., Wohlfahrt, J., & Frisch, M. (2008). Risk factors for invasive squamous cell carcinoma of the vulva and vagina—Population-based case-control study in Denmark. *International Journal of Cancer, 122*(12), 2827–2834.

Markowitz, L. E., Dunne, E. F., Saraiya, M., Lawson, H. W., Chesson, H., Unger, E. R., & Centers for Disease Control and Prevention Advisory Committee on Immunization Practices. (2007). Quadrivalent human papillomavirus vaccine: Recommendations of the Advisory Committee on Immunization Practices (ACIP). *Morbidity and Mortality Weekly Report Recommendation Report, 56*(RR-2), 1–24.

Matlashewskil, G., Schneider, J., Banks, L., Jones, N., Murray, A., & Crawford, L. (1987). Human papillomavirus type 16 DNA cooperates with activated *ras* in transforming primary cells. *EMBO Journal, 6*(6), 1741–1746.

Münger, K., Scheffner, M., Huibregtse, J. M., & Howley, P. M. (1992). Interactions of HPV E6 and E7 oncoproteins with tumour suppressor gene products. *Journal of Cancer Survivorship, 12*, 197–217.

National Cancer Institute. (2011). *Diethylstilbestrol (DES) and cancer.* Bethesda, MD: National Cancer Institute.

Nelson, R. A., Levine, A. M., Bernstein, L., Smith, D. D., & Lai, L. L. (2013). Changing patterns of anal canal carcinoma in the United States. *Journal of Clinical Oncology, 31*(12), 1569–1575.

Nielsen, A., Munk, C., & Kjaer, S. K. (2012). Trends in incidence of anal cancer and high-grade anal intraepithelial neoplasia in Denmark, 1978–2008. *International Journal of Cancer, 130*(5), 1168–1173.

Olejek, A., Kozak-Darmas, I., Kellas-Sleczka, S., Jarek, A., Wiczkowski, A., Krol, W., & Stencel-Gabriel, K. (2009). Chlamydia trachomatis infection in women with lichen sclerosis vulvae and vulvar cancer. *Neuro Endocrinology Letters, 30*(5), 671–674.

Palefsky, J. M. (2000). Anal squamous intraepithelial lesions in human immunodeficiency virus-positive men and women. *Seminars in Oncology, 27*(4), 471–479.

Palefsky, J. M., & Cranston, R. D. (2013). *Anal intraepithelial neoplasia, diagnosis, screening, prevention and treatment.*

Retrieved from www.uptodate.com/contents/anal-intraepithelial -neoplasia

Palefsky, J. M., Giuliano, A. R., Goldstone, S., Moreira, E. D., Jr, Aranda, C., Jessen, H., … Garner, E. I. (2011). HPV vaccine against anal HPV infection and anal intraepithelial neoplasia. *New England Journal of Medicine, 365*(17), 1576–1585.

Palefsky, J. M., Holly, E. A., Hogeboom, C. J., Ralston, M. L., DaCosta, M. M., Botts, R., … Darragh, T. M. (1998). Virologic, immunologic, and clinical parameters in the incidence and progression of anal squamous intraepithelial lesions in HIV-positive and HIV-negative homosexual men. *Journal of Acquired Immune Deficiency Syndromes and Human Retrovirology, 17*(4), 314–319.

Palmer, J. R., Wise, L. A., Hatch, E. E., Troisi, R., Titus-Ernstoff, L., Stohsnitter, W., … Hoover, R. N. (2006). Prenatal diethylstilbestrol exposure and risk of breast cancer. *Cancer Epidemiology, Biomarkers and Prevention, 15*(8), 1509–1514.

Papanicolaou, G. N., & Traut, H. F. (1943). *Diagnosis of uterine cancer by the vaginal smear.* New York, NY: Commonwealth Fund.

Parkin, D. M. (2006). The global health burden of infection-associated cancers in the year 2002. *International Journal of Cancer, 118*(12), 3030–3044.

Parkin, D. M., & Bray, F. (2006). Chapter 2: The burden of HPV-related cancers. *Vaccine, 24*(Suppl. 3), S3/11–S3/25.

Rouzier, R., Morice, P., Haie-Meder, C., Lhomme, C., Avril, M. F., Duvillard, P., & Castaigne, D. (2001). Prognostic significance of epithelial disorders adjacent to invasive vulvar carcinomas. *Gynecological Oncology, 81*, 414–419.

Salmo, E., & Haboubi, N. (2011). Anal cancer: Pathology, staging, and evidence-based minimum data set. *Colorectal Disease, 13*, 11–20.

Saraiya, M., Watson, M., Wu, X., King, J. B., Chen, V. W., Smith, J. S., & Giuliano, A. R. (2008). Incidence of in situ and invasive vulvar cancer in the US, 1998–2003. *Cancer, 113*(10 Suppl.), 2865–2872.

Sengupta, B. S. (1980). Vulvar carcinoma in premenopausal Jamaican women. *International Journal of Gynaecology and Obstetrics, 17*(6), 526–530.

Silverberg, M. J., Lau, B., Justice, A. C., Engels, E., Gill, M. J., Goedert, J. J., … North American AIDS Cohort Collaboration on Research and Design (NA-ACCORD) of IeDEA. (2012). Risk of anal cancer in HIV-infected and HIV-uninfected individuals in North America. *Clinical Infectious Diseases, 54*(7), 1026–1034.

Sitas, F., Pacella-Norman, R., Carrara, H., Patel, M., Ruff, P., Sur, R., … Beral, V. (2000). The spectrum of HIV-1 related cancers in South Africa. *International Journal of Cancer, 88*, 489–492.

Tavassoli, F. A., & Devilee, P. (2003a). Tumours of the vagina. In F. A. Tavassoli & P. Devilee (Eds.), *Pathology and genetics of tumours of the breast and female genital organs* (pp. 291–311). World Health Organization Classification of Tumours. Lyon, France: IARC Press.

Tavassoli, F. A., & Devilee, P. (2003b). Tumours of the vulva. In F. A. Tavassoli & P. Devilee (Eds.), *Pathology and genetics of tumours of the breast and female genital organs* (pp. 313–334). World Health Organization Classification of Tumours. Lyon, France: IARC Press.

van de Nieuwenhof, H. P., van der Avoort, I. A., & de Hullu, J. A. (2008). Review of squamous premalignant vulvar lesions. *Critical Reviews in Oncology/Hematology, 68*(2), 131–156.

Wu, X., Matanoski, G., Chen, V. W., Saraiya, M., Coughlin, S. S., King, J. B., & Tao, X. G. (2008). Descriptive epidemiology of vaginal cancer incidence and survival by race, ethnicity, and age in the United States. *Cancer, 113*(10 Suppl.), 2873–2882.

zur Hausen, H. (1976). Condyloma acuminata and human genital cancer. *Cancer Research, 36*, 794.

zur Hausen, H. (1977). Human papilloma viruses and their possible role in squamous cell carcinoma. *Current Topics in Microbiology and Immunology, 78*, 1–30.

zur Hausen, H. (2002). Papillomaviruses and cancer: From basic studies to clinical application. *Nature Reviews: Cancer, 2*(5), 342–350.

CHAPTER 26

Epidemiology of Prostate Cancer

▶ Global Burden of Prostate Cancer

Carcinoma of the prostate is the second most common form of cancer in men (behind only lung cancer) and is now the fifth leading cause of cancer deaths worldwide. In 2018, 1,276,106 new cases were diagnosed, and 358,989 men died of prostate cancer. These data reflect a marked increase in the global burden of prostate cancer. During 2000–2018, the number of new cases of prostate cancer more than doubled and the number of deaths increased by 76%. Despite these dramatic increases in the annual numbers of prostate cancer cases and deaths, the annual age-adjusted incidence increased only 16% (from 25.3 to 29.3 per 100,000) and the annual mortality rate decreased by 7% (from 8.2 to 7.6 per 100,000) during the same period (Bray et al., 2018; Ferlay, Bray, Pisani, & Parkin, 2004; Ferlay et al., 2010, 2013, 2018; Fitzmaurice et al., 2017, 2018; Parkin, Bray, Ferlay, & Pisani, 2001, 2005) (**FIGURE 26.1**).

Among men living in developed countries, prostate cancer is diagnosed more often than any other form of male cancer and is the third leading cause of death from cancer. Disease survival in developed countries is high, and the ratio of mortality to incidence is relatively low (0.30 in 2018), which is primarily due to screening of asymptomatic men by prostate-specific antigen (PSA) and the early detection of small latent carcinomas of the prostate. Among men living in developing countries, prostate cancer is diagnosed less often but tumors are usually detected late in development, resulting in higher mortality and a much higher mortality-to-incidence ratio (0.79) (Bray et al., 2018).

There is marked variability in the international incidence and mortality rates of prostate cancer. Incidence rates tend to be high in developed nations such as the United States, Canada, Australia, New Zealand, and the nations of Western Europe and Scandinavia (~80 cases per 100,000 in 2018), whereas the rates are relatively low in populations of Asia and Africa (~20 cases per 100,000) (Bray et al., 2018; Ferlay et al., 2010, 2013, 2018) (**FIGURE 26.2**).

In sharp contrast to the global pattern of incidence rates, mortality rates of prostate cancer tend to be higher in developing areas such as Southern and Central Africa, Central America, the Caribbean, and South America. Men of West African descent living on the small Caribbean island of Barbados had the highest age-adjusted mortality in 2018 (48 deaths per 100,000) (Figure 26.2). Furthermore, certain ethnic groups within countries have exceedingly high mortality rates; for example, African Americans living in the United States have one of the highest age-adjusted death rates from prostate cancer in the world (annual rate ~37 deaths per 100,000). Their rate is more than double that of Caucasian or Hispanic Americans (less than 18 deaths per 100,000) (**FIGURE 26.3**). By comparison, native Asian men have annual mortality rates less than five deaths per 100,000 (American Cancer Society [ACS], 2009; Ferlay et al., 2010, 2013, 2018; Ito, 2014; Noone et al., 2018; Parkin et al., 2005). As discussed in the following sections of this chapter, the wide variation in the incidence and mortality of prostate cancer is influenced by many factors, including diet, lifestyle, genetics, screening, and therapy.

▶ Age-Specific Risk of Prostate Cancer

The incidence of invasive cancer of the prostate increases dramatically in men over the age of 50 years. The disease is rare until age 50, after which the risk increases exponentially (**TABLE 26.1**). The lifetime risk of developing invasive disease is approximately 1 in 6 among U.S. Caucasian men (ACS, 2009).

In addition to the clinically overt forms of prostate cancer, there is an even more frequent biologic form

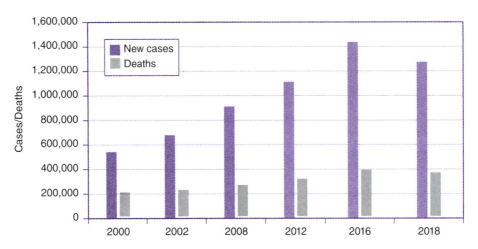

FIGURE 26.1 Increasing Global Burden of Prostate Cancer, 2000–2018.

Data from Ferlay, J., Bray, F., Pisani, P., & Parkin, D. M. (2004). *GLOBOCAN 2002. Cancer incidence, mortality, and prevalence worldwide.* IARC Cancer Base No. 5, version 2.0. Lyon, France: IARC Press; Ferlay, J., Shin, H.-R., Bray, F., Forman, D., Mathers, C., & Parkin, D. M. (2010). Estimates of worldwide burden of cancer in 2008: GLOBOCAN 2008. *International Journal of Cancer, 127*(12), 2893–2917; Ferlay, J., Soerjomataram, I., Ervik, M., Dikshit, R., Eser, S., Mathers, C., . . . Bray, F. (2013). *GLOBOCAN 2012 v1.0. Cancer incidence and mortality worldwide: IARC CancerBase No. 11* [Internet]. Lyon, France: International Agency for Research on Cancer. Retrieved from http://globocan.iarc.fr; Parkin, D. M., Bray, F., Ferlay, J., & Pisani, P. (2001). Estimating the world cancer burden: GLOBOCAN 2000. *International Journal of Cancer, 94,* 153–156; Parkin, D. M., Bray, F., Ferlay, J., & Pisani, P. (2005). Global cancer statistics, 2002. CA: *A Cancer Journal for Clinicians, 55,* 74–108; Fitzmaurice, C., Allen, C., Barber, R. M., Barregard, L., Bhutta, Z. A., Brenner, H., . . . Global Burden of Disease Cancer Collaboration. (2017). Global, regional, and national cancer incidence, mortality, years of life lost, years lived with disability, and disability-adjusted life-years for 32 cancer groups, 1990 to 2015: A systematic analysis for the Global Burden of Disease Study. *JAMA Oncology, 3*(4), 524–548; Fitzmaurice, C., Akinyemiju, T. F., Al Lami, F. H., Alam, T., Alizadeh-Navaei, R., Allen, C., . . . Global Burden of Disease Cancer Collaboration. (2018, June). Global, regional, and national cancer incidence, mortality, years of life lost, years lived with disability, and disability-adjusted life-years for 29 cancer groups, 1990 to 2016: A systematic analysis for the Global Burden of Disease Study. *JAMA Oncology.* Published online June 02, 2018. doi:10.1001/jamaoncol.2018.2706.

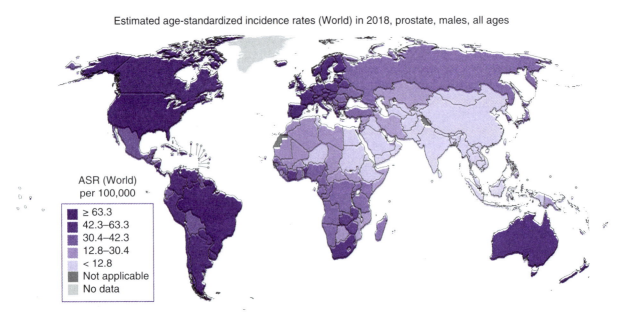

FIGURE 26.2 Global Incidence and Mortality Rates of Prostate Cancer, 2018.

Estimated age-standardized mortality rates (World) in 2018, prostate, males, all ages

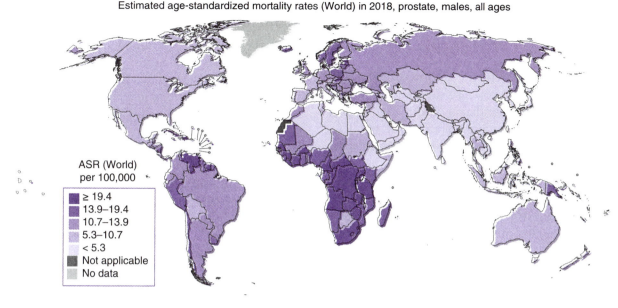

ASR (World)
per 100,000

- ≥ 19.4
- 13.9–19.4
- 10.7–13.9
- 5.3–10.7
- < 5.3
- Not applicable
- No data

FIGURE 26.2 CONTINUED

Caption: ASR: Rates per 100,000 are age-standardized to the world population, 2000–2025.

Reproduced with permission from Ferlay, J., Ervik, M., Lam, F., Colombet, M., Mery, L., Piñeros, M., . . . Bray, F. (2018). *Global cancer observatory: Cancer today*. Lyon, France: International Agency for Research on Cancer. Available from: https://gco.iarc.fr/today, accessed [09 October 2018].

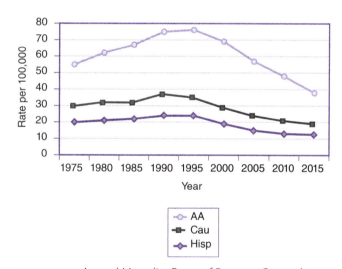

FIGURE 26.3 Annual Mortality Rates of Prostate Cancer by Ethnicity, United States, 1990–2015.

AA: African Americans; Cau: Caucasian Americans; Hisp: Hispanic Americans.

Caption: Rates per 100,000 are age-adjusted to the U.S. male population, 2000.

Data from American Cancer Society. (2009). *Cancer facts and figures*. Atlanta, GA: National Cancer Institute (2018).

TABLE 26.1 Age-Specific Incidence of Prostate Cancer in U.S. Men	
Age (Years)	**Cumulative Risk of Invasive Prostate Cancer**
45	1 in 2500
50	1 in 476
55	1 in 120
60	1 in 43
65	1 in 21
70	1 in 9
75	1 in 7
Lifetime	1 in 6

Data from American Cancer Society. (2009). *Cancer facts and figures*. Atlanta, GA: Author.

of prostate cancer that is discovered as an incidental finding either at postmortem examination or in a surgical specimen removed for other reasons (e.g., in the treatment of benign prostatic hypertrophy [BPH]). In almost all these incidental findings, the lesions are small and composed only of microscopic foci of malignant cells. This form of prostatic cancer is called *occult* or *latent* prostate cancer.

In postmortem studies of unselected men, occult prostate cancer can be identified in about 10% of subjects between 50 and 59 years of age, rising to a prevalence of 40%–50% in those over the age of 70. It is noteworthy that in most of these subjects (95%) these occult lesions were absolutely unsuspected and clinically asymptomatic (Robbins & Cotran, 1979).

Anatomy and Function of the Prostate Gland

The prostate gland encircles the urethra at the base of the urinary bladder. The normal adult gland is 3–4 cm in diameter, slightly larger than a walnut, and weighs 7–16 g. The organ is composed of a network of ductules lined by epithelial cells admixed with muscular and fibrous cells. Its main function is to produce the fluid portion of semen. Prostatic fluid is continually produced and secreted by epithelial cells lining the extensive network of prostate ductules. Prostatic fluid is rich in the proteins, minerals, and other compounds necessary for maintenance and nourishment of the sperm. The anterior portion of the prostate gland also aids in the control of urine flow from the bladder.

The prostate gland is roughly divisible into four zones: the transition zone, the central zone, the peripheral zone, and the anterior fibromuscular zone. These zones are shown with other nearby structures (bladder, vas deferens, seminal vesicles, ejaculatory ducts, and verumontanum) in **FIGURE 26.4**. The *vas deferens* carries sperm from each testicle to the ejaculatory duct. The *seminal vesicles* are paired tubular glands that secrete seminal fluid into the ejaculatory ducts. Seminal fluid is a mixture of proteins, enzymes, fructose, and other compounds that are essential in maintaining viable sperm. The *verumontanum* refers to the union of the vas deferens with the ejaculatory duct at the point of entry of seminal fluid into the urethra.

The *transition zone* encircles the urethra as it passes through the gland just below the bladder. The transition zone contains about 5%–10% of the glandular tissue of the prostate. Epithelial cells of the transition zone carry estrogen receptors and are thus predominantly responsive to estrogen stimulation. It

is this zone that enlarges in the condition known as *BPH*. Approximately 20% of prostate adenocarcinomas arise from the epithelium of the transition zone.

The *central zone* is a cone-shaped region that surrounds the ejaculatory ducts that carry seminal fluid from the seminal vesicles into the urethra. This zone constitutes about 25% of glandular tissue of the prostate. Epithelial cells in the central zone carry primarily estrogen receptors. Less than 5% of prostate adenocarcinomas arise from the epithelium of the central zone.

The *peripheral zone* comprises the outer 70% of the prostate. This zone is situated in the posterolateral portion of the gland and is palpable through the rectum. The epithelial cells lining the ductules of the peripheral zone are responsible for the synthesis and secretion of most of the prostatic fluid. These cells are laden with androgen receptors (ARs) and are therefore responsive to stimulation by androgens (testosterone and dihydrotestosterone [DHT]). Approximately 70%–75% of prostate adenocarcinomas arise from the epithelium of the peripheral zone.

The *anterolateral zone* lies in the anterior portion of the prostate and is devoid of glandular tissue. This zone consists of fibromuscular tissue, and its primary function is to propel urine and semen through the urethra during urination and ejaculation, respectively.

BPH is an extremely common disorder that affects men over the age of 50. The hyperplastic nodules of BPH typically arise from the transitional zone of the prostate gland, perhaps due to the balance between androgens and estrogens. There is long-standing controversy regarding the development of cancer from BPH (Robbins & Cotran, 1979).

DHT, the active form of testosterone, mediates prostatic epithelial cell division through interactions with ARs on the cell membrane. Whereas nodular hyperplasia tends to develop centrally in the prostate, prostate cancer usually arises in the posterior lobe and peripheral zone of the prostate gland (McNeal, 1981). For this reason, most experts do not believe that nodular hyperplasia is a precursor lesion of prostate cancer; rather, microscopic carcinomas appear to arise from focal areas of dysplasia in the peripheral zone of the prostate gland (McNeal, 1993). Subsequently, over a period of many years, these very small lesions increase in size and acquire invasive potential.

Pathogenesis of Prostate Cancer

Prostate cancer arises from the epithelial lining of the prostatic ducts that channel prostatic fluids into the ejaculatory ducts of the prostate gland. Histologically,

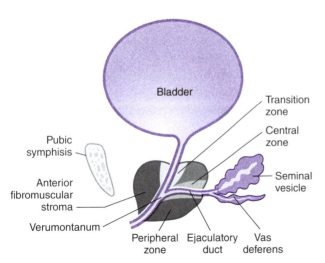

FIGURE 26.4 Zones of the Prostate Gland.

nearly all cancerous tumors are adenocarcinomas that display prominent glandular features.

The pathogenesis of prostate cancer and BPH are both related to the endocrine system. Androgens acting through ARs on the cell membranes of prostatic epithelium play critical roles in prostate development and growth as well as the pathogenesis of BPH and prostate cancer (Zhu, 2005). Studies over the years have demonstrated that there are two natural potent androgens acting at the same ARs in mammals, including humans (Zhu, Katz, & Imperato-McGinley, 1998). Although testosterone is the primary androgen synthesized and secreted by the testes, DHT converted from testosterone by the enzyme 5α-reductase (5αRD) is the main androgen in the prostate. Two forms of 5α-reductase have been identified: 5αRD-1 and 5αRD-2 (Russell & Wilson, 1994). Cellular effects of both enzymes are mediated by their activation of AR in prostatic tissues.

Early studies by Rose and colleagues demonstrated higher levels of the active metabolite of testosterone, DHT, in prostatic fluid of cases with prostate cancer compared to controls with other urologic conditions (Rose, Laaksa, Satarouta, & Wynder, 1984). International metabolic epidemiologic studies by Ross and colleagues revealed that African Americans have higher average serum levels of testosterone than Caucasian Americans (Ross et al., 1986) and that native Japanese and Chinese men have significantly lower average 5α-reductase activity than either African Americans or Caucasian Americans (Ross et al., 1992). These differences suggested a hormonal basis for the high prostate cancer rates observed in African-American men compared to the relatively low rates in Asian men.

More recently, molecular studies have shown that prostate cancer tissues overexpress both the 5αRD-1 and 5αRD-2 isozymes whereas BPH tissues overexpress only the 5αRD-2 isozyme. It has also been demonstrated in animal studies that both forms of 5α-reductase can be markedly up-regulated by high intake of dietary fat (Cai, Imperato-McGinley, & Zhu, 2006). This observation provides an important mechanistic link between dietary fat intake and the genesis of prostate cancer (see the following section on "Dietary Fat and Prostate Cancer"). Furthermore, the molecular link between 5α-reductase activity and prostate carcinogenesis has motivated the development and investigation of drugs such as finasteride that inhibit 5α-reductase.

▶ Finasteride and Prostate Cancer

In 1993, a large placebo-controlled randomized clinical trial, the Prostate Cancer Prevention Trial

(PCPT), was initiated to determine if the 5α-reductase inhibitor, finasteride, could prevent prostate cancer. The study enrolled 18,882 men aged 55 years or older randomized to receive either finasteride (5 mg daily) or placebo. About 4% of participants were African-American men. After 7 years of follow-up, 18% of men receiving finasteride developed prostate cancer compared to 24% in the placebo group, a risk reduction of 25%. However, the men who did develop prostate cancer while receiving finasteride were more likely to have high-grade tumors with high metastatic potential. Furthermore, the men taking finasteride reported significantly more sexual side effects (impotence) than men on placebo. Final results were based on analysis of 9060 participants, only about half the men who initially enrolled in the study (Thompson et al., 2003).

▶ Dietary Fat and Prostate Cancer

Ecological correlation studies show a strong positive correlation between diets high in fat and calories with prostate cancer incidence and mortality (CCCIS, 2010; Matsumura, 2001; WHO, 2009; Wynder et al., 1991). Within countries, chronological trends in prostate cancer rates tend to follow in close parallel with per capita trends in dietary fat intake. For example, prostate cancer rates in Japanese men have increased nearly fivefold over a 50-year period since 1955, seemingly in response to the rising level of fat in the Japanese diet (**FIGURE 26.5**).

West and colleagues examined associations of prostate cancer with dietary intakes of fat, protein, carbohydrate, and certain vitamins and minerals in a population-based case–control study in Utah. Dietary data were ascertained from 358 cases and 679 controls group-matched by age and county of residence. For older cases with aggressive tumors, significant associations were observed for the highest versus lowest quartiles of intake of total fat (odds ratio [OR] = 2.9), saturated fat (OR = 2.2), monounsaturated fat (OR = 3.6), polyunsaturated fat (OR = 2.7), and total energy (OR = 2.5). Results suggest that dietary fat increases the risk of aggressive prostate cancer in elderly men (West, Slattery, Robison, Fench, & Mahoney, 1991).

Giovannucci and colleagues examined the association of dietary fat and prostate cancer in a prospective cohort of 51,529 U.S. men aged 40–75 years in the Health Professionals Follow-Up Study. After 5 years, men reporting fat intake in the highest quintile experienced a 79% increase in the risk of invasive prostate

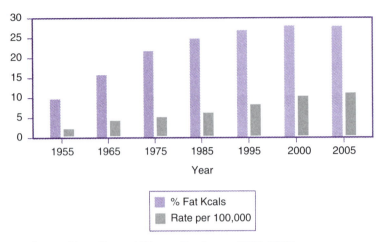

FIGURE 26.5 Trends in Prostate Cancer Mortality and Dietary Fat, Japan, 1955–2005.

Data from Center for Cancer Control and Information Services. (2010). *Cancer statistics in Japan, 2010*. Tokyo, Japan: Author; Wynder, E. L., Fujita, Y., Harris, R. E., Hirayama, T., & Hiyama, T. (1991). Comparative epidemiology of cancer between the United States and Japan: A second look. *Cancer, 67*(3), 746–763; Matsumura, Y. (2001). Emerging trends of nutrition: Transition and trade-offs. Nutrition trends in Japan. *Asia Pacific Journal of Clinical Nutrition, 10*(Suppl.), S40–S47.

cancer compared to men in the lowest quintile. Notably, fat derived from consumption of red meat produced a 2.6-fold increase in the risk (Giovannucci et al., 1993).

Neuhouser and colleagues examined the association of prostate cancer and various dietary factors in a prospective cohort of 12,025 U.S. men followed over an 11-year period. In men with a family history of prostate cancer, high intake of essential omega-6 polyunsaturated fatty acids produced a 2.6-fold increase in the risk of invasive disease (Neuhouser et al., 2007).

Animal studies support an important etiologic link between prostate cancer development and intake of specific types of dietary fat. Zhu and colleagues found that feeding young rats a diet high in a-linoleic acid from corn oil induced high levels of plasma DHT and 5αRD-2 expression in the prostate gland, thus suggesting a potential molecular mechanism for dietary fat stimulation of prostate growth and pathogenesis (Cai et al., 2006). Their studies also suggest that insulin-like growth factor (IGF-1) increases with intake of dietary fat and may be involved in mediating the effects of androgens in the prostate gland.

Using a transgenic model of prostate cancer, Aaronson and colleagues identified strong tumor promotion by essential omega-6 polyunsaturated fats from corn oil (α-linoleic acid) that are common in the U.S. diet (Kobayashi et al., 2008). Mechanistically, omega-6 polyunsaturated fatty acids are readily converted by the cyclooxygenase and lipoxygenase pathways to eicosanoids, such as prostaglandin E2, leukotrienes, and hydroxyl derivatives of fatty acids. These inflammatory eicosanoids have long been implicated in the pathogenesis of cancer and are believed to play important roles in tumor promotion, progression, and metastasis. Reciprocally, essential omega-3 polyunsaturated fatty acids such as gamma-linolenic acid that inhibit the inflammatory cascade have been found to inhibit conversion of testosterone to its active metabolite, DHT (Pham & Ziboh, 2002; Rose & Connolly, 1991).

The differential effects of omega-6 versus omega-3 fatty acids on androgen metabolism suggest an important etiological link between the balance of essential fatty acids in the diet and prostate carcinogenesis. As discussed previously, international studies reflect marked differences in the rates of prostate cancer. African Americans have the highest rates and Asian men the lowest, but Asian men who migrate to the United States transition to higher rates after a single generation (Parkin et al., 2005). This pattern correlates with the 5α-reductase activity among ethnic groups. There is high 5α-reductase activity in African Americans and low activity in Asian men; furthermore, Asian males who live in North America have higher 5α-reductase activity when compared to males in their home countries (Ross et al., 1992). As pointed out by Yuan-Shan Zhu and Julianne Imperato-McGinley (2009), "These data indicate that differences in 5a-reductase activity may be ethnically and environmentally determined and may be related to differences in prostate cancer development." Indeed, the totality of evidence indicates that the "Westernized lifestyle," which incorporates high fat/high calorie diets and, in particular, high levels of inflammatory omega-6 fatty acids, enhances the risk for malignant transformation of the prostate gland.

▶ Genetics of Prostate Cancer

Prostatic cancer also shows a strong familial component. In studies by Meikle and Stanish (1982), brothers of cases had four times higher cumulative rates of prostate cancer than brothers-in-law or males of the general population, thereby reflecting the existence of genetic factors that increase the risk of neoplastic development in the prostate gland. Logically, discovery of mutations and genetic polymorphisms that influence prostate carcinogenesis might be expected in components of the androgen axis that regulate testosterone, DHT, 5α-reductase, and the ARs. One such mutation has already been discovered in African-American men with a family history of prostate cancer, a genetic defect in the receptor for the male hormone androgen (testosterone) that may contribute to the development of prostate cancer and its progression (Hu et al., 2010).

▶ Prostate Cancer and Sexual Activity

Another factor that may impact on prostate cancer risk is sexual activity. Declining activity with age may relate to changing ratios of testosterone and estrogen, which in turn may stimulate enhanced proliferation of prostatic glandular epithelium.

▶ Supplemental Antioxidants and Prostate Cancer

The findings of several observational studies plus two randomized clinical trials indicated that supplemental intake of selenium and vitamin E might be effective in preventing the development of prostate cancer. Both agents scavenge reactive oxygen species (ROS) and are thus classifiable as *antioxidants*. In 2001, a large randomized placebo-controlled clinical trial, the Selenium and Vitamin E Cancer Prevention Trial (SELECT), was initiated to determine whether selenium, vitamin E, or both could prevent prostate cancer. A total of 35,533 men aged 55 years or older were recruited for study from 427 participating sites in the United States, Canada, and Puerto Rico. After more than 5 years of follow-up, supplemental selenium or vitamin E, alone or in combination, produced no effect on the risk of developing invasive prostate cancer. In fact, the data showed two concerning trends: a slight increase in the incidence of prostate cancer in men taking supplemental vitamin E and a slight increase in the incidence of type 2 diabetes in men taking supplemental selenium (Lippman et al., 2008). Notably, with continued follow-up of men in the SELECT trial, these adverse effects of supplemental vitamin E

and selenium became statistically significant (Klein et al., 2011). The results of SELECT and several other studies have shown that taking antioxidants such as vitamin E may actually accelerate the progression of cancer. Nobel laureate James Watson recently suggested that antioxidants enhance cancer progression by scavenging ROS that effectively induce apoptosis of cancer cells. In particular, the enhanced destruction of ROS by the introduction of supplemental antioxidants may spur cancer growth by disabling apoptotic cancer cell death, particularly in late stage malignancies (Watson, 2013).

▶ Nonsteroidal Anti-inflammatory Drugs and Prostate Cancer

In the past two decades, traditional nonsteroidal anti-inflammatory drugs (NSAIDs) with cyclooxygenase-2 (COX-2) blocking activity have consistently shown potential in the chemoprevention of several forms of malignant neoplasms, including prostate cancer. In a meta-analysis of 17 epidemiologic studies, regular intake of aspirin, ibuprofen, or other over-the-counter NSAIDs was found to reduce the risk of prostate cancer by 27% (Harris, 2009).

Such effects are manifest primarily through COX-2–dependent molecular mechanisms. For example, NSAIDs reduce COX-2–catalyzed formation of specific inflammatory prostaglandins (particularly PGE-2) that promote key cellular processes in cancer development, including mutagenesis, mitogenesis, angiogenesis, deregulation of apoptosis, immunosuppression, and metastasis (Harris, 2007).

▶ Screening for Prostate Cancer

Screening for prostate cancer using serum PSA gained favor in the United States and other developed countries during the 1990s. It is estimated that 20 million PSA tests are performed annually in North America and possibly 20 million more outside North America (De Angelis, Rittenhouse, Mikolajczyk, Blair Shamel, & Semjonow, 2007). A high level of serum PSA (>4 ng/mL) when coupled with digital rectal examination (DRE), ultrasonography, and directed biopsy of suspicious prostatic tissue can be effective in identifying men with invasive disease confined to the prostate gland that can be completely surgically excised without recurrence. Nevertheless, PSA screening is controversial because prostate cancer often develops so slowly that it will never lead to symptoms during a man's lifetime. Furthermore, prostatectomy for removal of a cancerous prostate gland often produces major debilitating side effects such as urinary incontinence, erectile dysfunction, and impotence. The major consideration for any screening protocol is to weigh the benefits of early detection and lifesaving treatment against the risk of harm from unnecessary intervention.

Results of two large randomized clinical trials of PSA screening have now been published. The European Randomized Study of Screening for Prostate Cancer evaluated PSA testing versus no screening among 182,000 men aged 50–74 years. After 9 years of follow-up, the results did show 20% fewer deaths in the treated group; however, the study also found that many men were treated unnecessarily, resulting in a high rate of major side effects (Schröder et al., 2009). Another randomized study of 76,693 men in the United States compared PSA plus DRE to "usual care" in the detection and treatment of prostate cancer. After 7 years of follow-up, there were actually 13% fewer deaths in the "usual care" group (Andriole et al., 2009).

After careful review of the scientific evidence, the U.S. Preventive Services Task Force concluded that the data were insufficient to recommend screening for men under 75 and that men 75 and older should not be screened (U.S. Preventive Services Task Force, 2008). Rather, clinicians are now advised to use a process of shared decision-making with each patient that includes candid discussion about the potential risks and benefits of screening. A telling statement from the investigator who initially discovered PSA, Dr. Richard J. Ablin, underscores the controversial nature of routinely screening asymptomatic men for prostate cancer using the PSA test. Dr. Ablin states, "I never dreamed that my discovery four decades ago would lead to such a profit-driven public health disaster. The medical community must confront reality and stop the inappropriate use of PSA screening. Doing so would save billions of dollars and rescue millions of men from unnecessary, debilitating treatments" (Ablin, 2010).

▶ Zinc and Survival of Prostate Cancer

Zinc is an essential mineral with known antioxidant and anti-inflammatory effects. Zinc is an important cofactor in DNA repair, apoptosis, and cellular immunity. Notably, the concentration of zinc is higher in prostate tissue than any other tissue in the human body. Recently, Epstein and colleagues examined the level of dietary zinc as a potential predictor of survival among 525 Swedish men diagnosed with invasive prostate cancer during 1989–1995. Swedish men have one of the highest annual mortality rates from prostate cancer in the world (22 deaths per 100,000). After a median follow-up time of 6.4 years, 218 cases (42%) had died of prostate cancer. Zinc intake was estimated based on its average content in grains, meat, dairy products, fruits, and vegetables consumed by the individual patients. Results revealed that high dietary zinc intake (>15.6 mg per day) was associated with a reduced risk of death due to prostate cancer (hazard ratio = 0.64), whereas zinc intake was not associated with mortality from other causes. The protective effect of high dietary zinc was stronger among men diagnosed with localized tumors (hazard ratio = 0.24). These results suggest that high intake of dietary zinc may have therapeutic benefit in men diagnosed with prostate cancer, particularly among those with localized tumors at the time of diagnosis (Epstein et al., 2011).

References

Ablin, R. J. (2010). The great prostate mistake. *New York Times*, p. A27.

American Cancer Society. (2009). *Cancer facts and figures*. Atlanta, GA.

Andriole, G. L., Crawford, E. D., Grubb, R. L., Buys, S. S., Chia, D., Church, T. R., … Berg, C. D. (2009). Mortality results from a randomized prostate-cancer screening trial. *New England Journal of Medicine, 360*(13), 1310–1319.

Bray, F., Ferlay, J., Soerjomataram, I., Siegel, R. L., Torre, L. A., & Jemal, A. (2018). Global cancer statistics 2018: GLOBOCAN estimates of incidence and mortality worldwide for 36 cancers in 185 countries. *CA: A Cancer Journal for Clinicians, 68*(6), 394–424.

Cai, L. Q., Imperato-McGinley, J., & Zhu, Y. S. (2006). Regulation of prostate 5α-reductase-2 gene expression and prostate weight by dietary fat and caloric intake in the rat. *Prostate, 66*, 738–748.

Center for Cancer Control and Information Services. (2010). *Cancer statistics in Japan, 2010*. Tokyo, Japan: Author.

De Angelis, G., Rittenhouse, H. G., Mikolajczyk, S. D., Blair Shamel, L., & Semjonow, A. (2007). Twenty years of PSA: From prostate antigen to tumor marker. *Reviews in Urology, 9*(3), 113–123.

Epstein, M. M., Kasperzyk, J. L., Andrén, O., Giovannucci, E. L., Wolk, A., Håkansson, N., … Mucci, L. A. (2011). Dietary zinc and prostate cancer survival in a Swedish cohort. *American Journal of Clinical Nutrition, 93*(3), 586–593.

Ferlay, J., Bray, F., Pisani, P., & Parkin, D. M. (2004). *GLOBOCAN 2002. Cancer incidence, mortality, and prevalence worldwide*. IARC Cancer Base No. 5, version 2.0. Lyon, France: IARC Press.

Ferlay, J., Ervik, M., Lam, F., Colombet, M., Mery, L., Piñeros, M., … Bray, F. (2018). *Global cancer observatory: Cancer today.* Lyon, France: International Agency for Research on Cancer. Retrieved from https://gco.iarc.fr/today.

Ferlay, J., Shin, H.-R., Bray, F., Forman, D., Mathers, C., & Parkin, D. M. (2010). Estimates of worldwide burden of cancer in 2008: GLOBOCAN 2008. *International Journal of Cancer, 127*(12), 2893–2917.

Ferlay, J., Soerjomataram, I., Ervik, M., Dikshit, R., Eser, S., Mathers, C., … Bray, F. (2013). *GLOBOCAN 2012 v1.0. Cancer incidence and mortality worldwide: IARC Cancer Base No. 11* [Internet]. Lyon, France: International Agency for Research on Cancer. Retrieved from http://globocan.iarc.fr

Fitzmaurice, C., Akinyemiju, T. F., Al Lami, F. H., Alam, T., Alizadeh-Navaei, R., Allen, C., … Global Burden of Disease Cancer Collaboration. (2018, June). Global, regional, and national cancer incidence, mortality, years of life lost, years lived with disability, and disability-adjusted life-years for 29 cancer groups, 1990 to 2016: A systematic analysis for the Global Burden of Disease Study. *JAMA Oncology.* Online publication. doi:10.1001/jamaoncol.2018.2706.

Fitzmaurice, C., Allen, C., Barber, R. M., Barregard, L., Bhutta, Z. A., Brenner, H., … Global Burden of Disease Cancer Collaboration. (2017). Global, regional, and national cancer incidence, mortality, years of life lost, years lived with disability, and disability-adjusted life-years for 32 cancer groups, 1990 to 2015: A systematic analysis for the Global Burden of Disease Study. *JAMA Oncology, 3*(4), 524–548.

Giovannucci, E., Eric, B., Rimm, E. B., Colditz, G. A., Stampfer, M. J., Ascherio, A., & Willett, W. A. (1993). A prospective study of dietary fat and risk of prostate cancer. *Journal of the National Cancer Institute, 85*(19), 1571–1579.

Harris, R. E. (2007). COX-2 and the inflammogenesis of cancer. *Subcellular Biochemistry, 42*, 193–212.

Harris, R. E. (2009). Cyclooxygenase-2 (COX-2) blockade in the chemoprevention of cancers of the colon, breast, prostate and lung. *Inflammopharmacology, 17*, 1–13.

Hu, S. Y., Liu, T., Liu, Z., Ledet, E., Velasco-Gonzalez, C., Mandal, D. M., & Koochekpour, S. (2010). Identification of a novel germline missense mutation of the androgen receptor in African American men with familial prostate cancer. *Asian Journal of Andrology, 12*(3), 336–343.

Ito, K. (2014). Prostate cancer in Asian men. *Nature Reviews Urology, 11*, 197–212.

Klein, E. A., Thompson, I. M., Tangen, C. M., Crowley, J. J., Lucia, M. S., Goodman, P. J., & Baker, L. H. (2011). Vitamin E and the risk of prostate cancer. The Selenium and Vitamin E Cancer Prevention Trial (SELECT). *Journal of the American Medical Association, 306*(14), 1549–1556.

Kobayashi, N., Barnard, R. J., Said, J., Hong-Gonzalez, J., Corman, D. M., Ku, M., … Aronson, W. J. (2008). Effect of low-fat diet on development of prostate cancer and Akt phosphorylation in the *Hi-Myc* transgenic mouse model. *Cancer Research, 68*(8), 3066–3073.

Lippman, S. M., Klein, E. A., Goodman, P. J., Lucia, M. S., Thompson, I. M., Ford, L. G., … Coltman, C. A. (2008). Effect of selenium and vitamin E on risk of prostate cancer and other cancers: The Selenium and Vitamin E Cancer Prevention Trial (SELECT). *Journal of the American Medical Association, 301*(1), 39–51.

Matsumura, Y. (2001). Emerging trends of nutrition: Transition and trade-offs. Nutrition trends in Japan. *Asia Pacific Journal of Clinical Nutrition, 10*(Suppl.), S40–S47.

McNeal, J. (1981). Normal and pathologic anatomy of prostate. *Urology, 17*(Suppl. 3), 11–16.

McNeal, J. (1993). Prostatic microcarcinomas in relation to cancer origin and the evolution to clinical cancer. *Cancer, 71*, 984–991.

Meikle, A. W., & Stanish, W. M. (1982). Familial prostatic cancer risk and low testosterone. *Journal of Clinical Endocrinology and Metabolism, 54*, 1104–1108.

Neuhouser, M. L., Barnett, M. J., Kristal, A. R., Ambrosone, C. B., King, I., Thornquist, M., & Goodman, G. (2007). Omega-6 PUFA increase and dairy foods decrease prostate cancer risk in heavy smokers. *Journal of Nutrition, 137*, 1821–1827.

Noone, A. M., Howlader, N., Krapcho, M., Miller, D., Brest, A., Yu, M., … Cronin, K. A. (Eds.). (2018). *SEER cancer statistics review, 1975–2015.* Bethesda, MD: National Cancer Institute.

Parkin, D. M., Bray, F., Ferlay, J., & Pisani, P. (2001). Estimating the world cancer burden: GLOBOCAN 2000. *International Journal of Cancer, 94*, 153–156.

Parkin, D. M., Bray, F., Ferlay, J., & Pisani, P. (2005). Global cancer statistics, 2002. *CA: A Cancer Journal for Clinicians, 55*, 74–108.

Pham, H., & Ziboh, V. A. (2002). 5 alpha-reductase-catalyzed conversion of testosterone to dihydrotestosterone is increased in prostatic adenocarcinoma cells: Suppression by 15-lipoxygenase metabolites of gamma-linolenic and eicosapentaenoic acids. *Journal of Steroid Biochemistry and Molecular Biology, 82*(4–5), 393–400.

Robbins, S. L., & Cotran, R. S. (1979). *Pathologic basis of disease* (2nd ed.). Philadelphia, PA: W. B. Saunders.

Rose, D. P., & Connolly, J. M. (1991). Effects of fatty acids and eicosanoid synthesis inhibitors on the growth of two human prostate cancer cell lines. *Prostate, 18*(3), 243–254.

Rose, D. P., Laaksa, K., Satarouta, M., & Wynder, E. L. (1984). Hormone levels in prostatic fluid in healthy Finns and prostate cancer patients. *European Journal of Cancer and Clinical Oncology, 20*, 1317–1324.

Ross, R., Bernstein, L., Judd, H., Hanisch, R., Pike, M., & Henderson, B. (1986). Serum testosterone levels in healthy young black and white men. *Journal of the National Cancer Institute, 76*(1), 45–48.

Ross, R. K., Bernstein, L., Lobo, R. A., Shimizu, H., Stanczyk, F. Z., Pike, M. C., & Henderson, B. E. (1992). 5-Alpha-reductase activity and risk of prostate cancer among Japanese and US white and black males. *Lancet, 339*(8798), 887–889.

Russell, D. W., & Wilson, J. D. (1994). Steroid 5 alpha-reductase: Two genes/two enzymes. *Annual Review of Biochemistry, 63*, 25–61.

Schröder, F. H., Hugosson, J., Roobol, M. J., Tammela, T. L. J., Ciatto, S. Nelen, V., … Auvinen, A. (2009). Screening and prostate cancer mortality in a randomized European study. *New England Journal of Medicine, 360*(13), 1320.

Thompson, I. M., Goodman, P. J., Tangen, C. M., Lucia, M. S., Miller, G. J., Ford, L. G., … Coltman, C. A. (2003). The influence of finasteride on the development of prostate cancer. *New England Journal of Medicine, 349*, 215–224.

U.S. Preventive Services Task Force. (2008). Screening for prostate cancer: US Preventive Services Task Force recommendation statement. *Annals of Internal Medicine, 149*(3), 185–191.

Watson, J. (2013). Oxidants, antioxidants and the current incurability of metastatic cancers. *Open Biology,* 3. doi:10.1098/rsob.120144.

West, D. W., Slattery, M. L., Robison, L. M., Fench, T. K., & Mahoney, A. W. (1991). Adult dietary intake and prostate cancer risk in Utah: A case-control study with special emphasis on aggressive tumors. *Cancer Causes and Control, 2*, 85–94.

World Health Organization. (2009). *Death and DALY estimates for 2004 by cause for WHO member states (persons, all ages).* Geneva, Switzerland: Author. Retrieved from www.who.int /healthinfo/global_burden_disease/estimates_country/en/

Wynder, E. L., Fujita, Y., Harris, R. E., Hirayama, T., & Hiyama, T. (1991). Comparative epidemiology of cancer between the United States and Japan: A second look. *Cancer, 67*(3), 746–763.

Zhu, Y. S. (2005). Molecular basis of steroid action in the prostate. *Cellscience, 1*, 27–55.

Zhu, Y. S., & Imperato-McGinley, J. (2009). 5α-Reductase isozymes and androgen actions in the prostate. *Annals of the New York Academy of Sciences, 1155*, 43–56.

Zhu, Y. S., Katz, M. D., & Imperato-McGinley, J. (1998). Natural potent androgens: Lessons from human genetic models. *Bailliere's Clinical Endocrinology and Metabolism, 12*, 83–113.

CHAPTER 27

Epidemiology of Testicular Cancer

▶ Anatomy of the Testis and Spermatogenesis

Each testis consists of approximately 250 lobules separated by fibrous strands. Each lobule consists of loose connective tissue and a network of tubules called *seminiferous tubules.* Each seminiferous tubule is lined by a basement membrane that supports the germinal epithelium. The germinal epithelium is made up of primordial germ cells or spermatogonia, from which sperm arise. Spermatogonia are stem cells that proliferate by mitosis. As spermatogonia move away from the basement membrane, they undergo meiosis to form immature sperm called *spermatids.*

Two important cell types, Sertoli cells and Leydig cells, stimulate and regulate the process of spermatogenesis. Sertoli cells are nurse cells that secrete estrogen and other hormones in response to the pituitary hormone, follicular stimulating hormone (FSH). Leydig cells secrete testosterone in response to the pituitary hormone, luteinizing hormone (LH). The process of spermatogenesis involves both mitotic and meiotic divisions of germinal epithelial cells under the influence of testosterone and estrogen.

Each day in the adult male, millions of immature spermatids travel through the seminiferous tubules into a network of efferent ductules in the central portion of the testis called the *rete testis.* Cilia within ductules of the rete testis assist the transport of spermatozoa

into an extratesticular structure called the *epididymis.* The epididymis is a rich source of glucose and energy, and it is within this organ that the spermatozoa complete the maturation process to form sperm. Mature sperm cells are transported from the epididymis into a muscular tube called the *vas deferens* that transports sperm into bilateral saccular structures called *seminal vesicles* near the prostate gland. Within the seminal vesicles, sperm cells are mixed with prostatic fluids to form semen for ejaculation through the urethra (**FIGURE 27.1**) (Kumar, Abbas, & Aster, 2014).

▶ Pathology of Testicular Cancer

Ninety-five percent of all tumors of the testis are germ cell neoplasms. The International Agency for Research on Cancer (IARC) recognizes four specific types of germ cell tumors: seminomas, embryonal carcinomas, malignant teratomas, and choriocarcinomas. These lesions can be combined into two histologic groups: seminomas and nonseminomas. Further classification beyond the two main histologic categories (seminoma and nonseminoma) appears to have limited relevance in etiologic or clinical settings (Bray et al., 2006).

Based on pathological review, about 50% of testicular germ cell tumors are seminomas, 40% are nonseminomas, and 5%–10% consist of components of both cell types. These malignancies are believed to arise from precursor carcinomas in situ (Dieckmann

FIGURE 27.1 Spermatogenesis and Anatomy of the Testis.

& Skakkebaek, 1999; Leendert, Loooijenga, & Oosterhuis, 2013; Sandberg, Meloni, & Suijkerbuijk, 1996; Skakkebaek, 1972).

Seminomas primarily occur in adult men, but rarely in infants. These tumors *do not* express fetal proteins such as alpha fetoprotein, but some *do* express human chorionic gonadotropin. Seminomas consist of sheets of round tumor cells growing in a monotonous morphologic pattern. Lymphocytic infiltration is a common feature of these tumors. They tend to be radiosensitive and are therefore usually curable by a combination of surgical excision and radiotherapy.

Nonseminomas include embryonal carcinomas, immature (malignant) teratomas, and choriocarcinomas. These tumors *do* express alpha fetoprotein, and the majority are diagnosed before age 30. The morphology of nonseminomas is highly variable, and in some cases their appearance is bizarre. For example, teratomas often show characteristics of early fetal development and contain immature remnants of various body parts.

Teratomas and yolk sac tumors constitute a distinct group of rare nonseminomas of the testes that develop in prepubertal boys and are typically found during the first 4 years of life. Such tumors have been reported among male infants, usually in association with congenital anomalies and chromosomal anomalies.

Germ cell tumors are slightly more common in men than women. In women, they occasionally arise from the ovarian, placental, or uterine tissues. Choriocarcinomas are distinct from other nonseminomas in that they secrete human chorionic gonadotropin (hCG). These rare tumors can arise in the placenta or other uterine tissues during pregnancy and are composed of two specific cell types of the chorionic membranes, cytotrophoblasts and syncytiotrophoblasts. Testicular choriocarcinomas are quite rare.

▶ Global Epidemiology of Testicular Cancer

Incidence and Mortality

Testicular cancer accounts for less than 1% of all malignant neoplasms in males. Nevertheless, testicular cancer is the most common malignancy in young men under 40 years of age. During 2018, 71,105 incident cases were diagnosed, and 9507 deaths were attributed to testicular cancer in the world population. During 2000–2018, the annual number of new cases increased by 44% whereas the number of deaths from testicular cancer increased by only 9%. The age-adjusted incidence of testicular cancer in 2018 was 1.7 per 100,000 and the age-adjusted mortality rate was 0.2 per 100,000 (Bray et al., 2018).

The annual age-adjusted incidence of testicular cancer worldwide has remained stable during the last decade (1.5–1.7 cases per 100,000 men). However, the incidence rates vary more than 20-fold among nations, ranging from less than 1.0 per 100,000 in Asian and African/African-American populations to over 12 per 100,000 in Norway and Croatia (Bray et al., 2018; Ferlay et al., 2010, 2013, 2018) (**FIGURE 27.2**).

The annual mortality rate of testicular cancer worldwide has also remained stable during the last decade (0.2–0.3 deaths per 100,000 men). Mortality rates are highest in nations with high incidence rates and where access to therapy is limited; for example, during 2018, men living in Mexico, Argentina, and Niger had mortality rates exceeding 0.8 deaths per 100,000 (Bray et al., 2018; Ferlay et al., 2010, 2013, 2018) (Figure 27.2).

Within nations, the incidence of testicular cancer varies markedly by race, with blacks and other non-white races exhibiting extremely low rates in comparison to white populations. In the United States, the incidence of testicular cancer in 2012 was about five times higher among Caucasians than African Americans. Furthermore, the annual incidence has steadily increased over time in some populations, particularly in developed nations (Bray et al., 2006; Rosen, Jayram, Drazer, & Eggener, 2011; Zheng et al., 1996). For example, the incidence more than doubled in Great Britain during 1975–2010 (Cancer Research UK, 2011) (**FIGURE 27.3**).

Several investigators have examined the rising incidence of testicular cancer that has occurred primarily in populations of the developed world, and various hypotheses have been advanced to explain the trend. One possible explanation is the widespread use of scanning and imaging equipment in developed nations,

which has led to earlier and more accurate detection of testicular tumors. There is also heightened awareness among urologists about the development of such tumors in adolescents and young men, particularly those with conditions of low fertility. Another hypothesis suggests that exposure to estrogenic hormones during fetal development may compromise mitosis and meiosis of the testicular germ cells (Huyghe, Matsuda, & Thonneau, 2003). One recent finding of importance is the higher rate of testicular cancer in men who are HIV-positive compared to those who are HIV-negative (Lyter, Bryant, Thackeray, Rinaldo, & Kingsley, 1995). The high rate of HIV-positive men living in underserved populations may therefore herald emerging epidemics of testicular cancer in these populations.

In the face of rising incidence rates of testicular cancer, mortality rates are steadily declining in many populations. For example, in Great Britain, testicular cancer incidence increased from 3 to 7.5 per 100,000 during 1970–2010, an increase of nearly 4% per year; in contrast, mortality for the same period fell from 1.2 to 0.2 per 100,000, a *decrease* of about 2% per year (Figure 27.3). Similar patterns are evident for the United States, Australia, New Zealand, China, and most Western European and Scandinavian nations (Shanmugalingam, Soultati, Chowdhury, Rudman, & Van Hemelrijck, 2013). The declining mortality rates of testicular cancer are a consequence of the high cure rates for this malignancy due to multidisciplinary therapy involving surgery, chemotherapy, and radiation.

Age Distribution of Testicular Cancer

Most cases of testicular cancer (more than 70%) are diagnosed in young men between the ages of 20 and 40 years. Nonseminomas tend to occur prior to age 30 whereas seminomas show a slightly later age of onset pattern (**FIGURE 27.4**).

▶ Cytogenetics and Genetics of Testicular Germ Cell Tumors

Testicular germ cell tumor karyotypes are characterized by *aneuploidy*, which means that the chromosome number is not an exact multiple of the usual haploid number (23 in humans). The usual diploid number of chromosomes in human cells is 46 (22 autosomes plus XX in women or XY in men). In contrast, the karyotypes of germ cell tumors often approach triploidy, with chromosome numbers ranging from 50 to 70 (median ~60). According to one model, nondisjunction produces abnormal tetraploid cells that develop into carcinoma

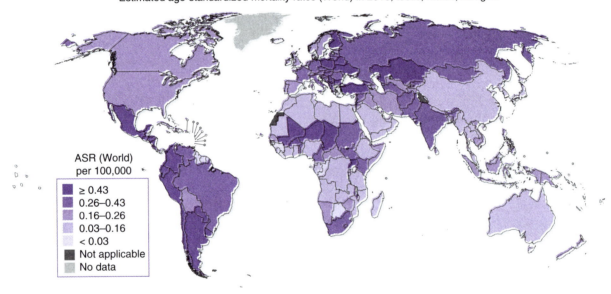

FIGURE 27.2 Global Incidence and Mortality Rates of Testicular Cancer, 2012.

Reproduced with permission from Ferlay, J., Ervik, M., Lam, F., Colombet, M., Mery, L., Piñeros, M., . . . Bray, F. (2018). *Global cancer observatory: Cancer today*. Lyon, France: International Agency for Research on Cancer. Available from: https://gco.iarc.fr/today, accessed [09 October 2018].

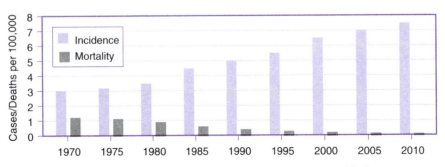

FIGURE 27.3 Trends in Testicular Cancer Incidence and Mortality in Great Britain, 1970–2010.

Data from Cancer Research UK. (2011). *UK cancer information service*. Retrieved from http://www.cancerresearchuk.org; Shanmugalingam, T., Soultati, A., Chowdhury, S., Rudman, S., & Van Hemelrijck, M. (2013). Global incidence and outcome of testicular cancer. *Journal of Clinical Epidemiology, 5*, 417–427.

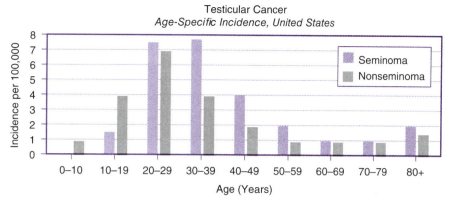

FIGURE 27.4 Age Distribution of Testicular Cancer, United States.

Data from Zheng, T., Holford, T. R., Ma, Z., Ward, B. A., Flannery, J., & Boyle, P. (1996). Continuing increase in incidence of germ-cell testis cancer in young adults: Experience from Connecticut, USA, 1935–1992. *International Journal of Cancer, 65*, 723–729.

in situ. Subsequently, tetraploid cells of carcinoma in situ lose chromosomes or develop other chromosomal aberrations that result in invasive germ cell cancer (Dieckmann & Skakkebaek, 1999; Frigyesi et al., 2004).

There is a frequent appearance (~80%) of an iso-chromosome of the short arm of chromosome 12 called *i(12p)* in testicular germ cell tumors of all cell types. This hybrid chromosome typically consists of two combined short arms of chromosome 12. The exact role of *i(12p)* in the development of testicular cancer is unknown. Notably, in tumors without *i(12p)*, other structural changes of chromosome 12 have been identified. These findings suggest that amplification of certain genes on the short arm of chromosome 12 may play a role in the genesis of germ cell tumors (Sandberg et al., 1996).

▶ Risk Factors for Testicular Cancer

Risk factors for testicular cancer include prior history of unilateral disease, familial history, cryptorchidism (maldescended testes), infertility, infection, and certain congenital anomalies and germline mutations.

Cryptorchidism (Maldescended Testes)

A major risk factor for the development of testicular cancer is *cryptorchidism* or *maldescended testicle*. In a review of nine case–control studies, cryptorchidism was found to increase the risk of developing testicular cancer by nearly sixfold (summary relative risk = 5.8) (Chilvers & Pike, 1992). In a large case–control study conducted in Great Britain, 794 men with testicular cancer were compared to age-matched controls without disease. Results revealed that an undescended testis increased the risk nearly fourfold (odds ratio [OR] = 3.8), and inguinal hernia nearly doubled the

risk (OR = 1.9). The risk was also elevated among men who reported infertility (OR = 2.7). Notably, the investigators found that the excess risk associated with an undescended testis was eliminated in men who underwent orchiopexy (surgical repositioning of the testis) before the age of 10 years (Forman et al., 1994).

Orchiopexy before puberty decreases the risk of testicular cancer but may not completely attenuate excess risk. In a Swedish cohort of 16,983 men who underwent orchiopexy between 1964 and 1999 and were followed for a total of 209,984 person-years, 56 cases of testicular cancer were identified. Among those who were treated before 13 years of age, the relative risk of testicular cancer compared with the general population was 2.2. Among those who were treated at age 13 or later, the relative risk was 5.4. These findings clearly show that orchiopexy should be performed prior to puberty to minimize the risk of developing testicular cancer (Pettersson, Richiardi, Nordenskjold, Kaijser, & Akre, 2007). Furthermore, pathologic studies of biopsy specimens from patients with cryptorchidism reveal that deviations from normal spermatogenesis become more evident and the absence of germ cells more pronounced with delay of orchiopexy beyond only a few months of age (Abou-Zeid, Mousa, Soliman, Hamza, & Hay, 2011; Huff et al., 2001).

Familial History of Testicular Cancer

In genetic studies of index cases (probands) with testicular cancer, approximately 1.3% report having at least one blood relative (father, brother, or son) also afflicted with the disease (Dieckmann & Pichlmeier, 1997; Dong, Lönnstedt, & Hemminki, 2001). In a study of 4659 cases among Swedish men, fathers, sons, and brothers of afflicted subjects had risk increases of 3.8, 3.9, and 8.3, respectively. An international consortium that identified 461 families with 985 cases found that the clinical and pathologic features of familial testicular germ cell tumors were like those of nonfamilial cases (Mai et al., 2010).

At least 25 rare hereditary disorders have been identified in isolated cases of testicular cancer. These include certain congenital and genetic anomalies such as Klinefelter's syndrome (XXY genotype), Down's syndrome (trisomy 21), the Li–Fraumeni syndrome (*p53* germline mutation), and many others; however, there is no apparent unifying role of these diverse genetic defects in malignant transformation of germ cells of the testes. One X-linked gene, *Xq27*, may heighten the risk of testicular cancer by predisposing to undescended testes (Lutke Holzik et al., 2003).

Infection and Testicular Cancer

The incidence of testicular germ cell tumors, particularly seminomas, is markedly higher among HIV-infected men compared to HIV-negative men. In the Pittsburgh component of the Multicenter AIDS Cohort Study (MACS), the rate of seminoma was 20-fold higher than expected among 430 HIV-positive patients compared to the general male population of Pennsylvania. The investigators suggest that immunosuppression due to HIV infection may heighten the risk of seminoma development (Lyter et al., 1995).

Other infectious agents have been examined in studies of testicular cancer. In a hospital-based case–control study conducted in Washington, D.C., infection histories and other risk factors were examined among 271 cases with testicular cancer and 259 controls matched by age, race, and other factors. One infectious condition, mumps orchitis, occurred in six cases and only one control subject (OR = 5.8), suggesting an etiologic association (Brown, Pottern, & Hoover, 1987).

Many subsequent studies have examined the potential role of mumps orchitis and other childhood infections in the development of testicular germ cell cancer. Using existing data from the U.S. Servicemen's Testicular Tumor Environmental and Endocrine Determinants (STEED) study, a team of investigators evaluated the association between common childhood infections and testicular germ cell tumors by comparing 767 cases and 928 age-matched controls. They also conducted a meta-analysis of mumps, mumps orchitis, and testicular cancer. Results of the case–control study revealed that a history of orchitis was associated with an increase in the risk (OR = 2.4); however, this association was limited to orchitis diagnosed within

1 calendar year of the date of diagnosis (OR = 23.1) and not before that date (OR = 1.2). In the meta-analysis, estimates of testicular cancer risk due to orchitis were elevated in studies conducted prior to 1990 (pooled OR = 9.1), but the addition of more recent studies dramatically attenuated the estimate (pooled OR = 1.8). The authors of the study concluded that their data *do not* support an association between testicular cancer and mumps orchitis (Trabert, Graubard, Erickson, & McGlynn, 2012). Nevertheless, in view of recent outbreaks of mumps in the United States and other developed countries, it seems prudent to continue assessment of mumps orchitis and development of testicular cancer.

Personal History of Testicular Cancer

Patients with a history of unilateral testicular germ cell cancer carry an approximate 25–50-fold increased risk of developing a contralateral tumor. Follow-up studies of patients with unilateral disease consistently reveal that approximately 5% eventually develop contralateral germ cell tumors (Dieckmann & Loy, 1996; Holstein & Lauke, 1996).

Teratomas and Yolk Sac Tumors

Testicular teratomas and yolk sac tumors of prepubertal boys are rare, with an annual rate of about 1.2 per million. Most testicular teratomas are diploid without apparent chromosomal aberrations. Infantile testicular teratomas are usually benign and are curable by orchidectomy. In contrast, yolk sac tumors typically show aneuploidy (often near tetraploidy) and have invasive malignant potential, thus requiring combination therapy (Holstein & Lauke, 1996).

▶ Prevention and Therapy of Testicular Cancer

Rapid detection of cryptorchidism (undescended testis) and timely surgical correction (orchiopexy) are essential in lowering the risk of developing testicular cancer. The optimal time of surgery is at about 6 months of age, after which spontaneous descent is rare. Males who undergo orchiopexy remain at elevated risk, particularly those who undergo surgical correction after puberty.

Regular self-examination is advised in order to detect tumors as early as possible. Suspicious testicular masses on palpation should be imaged by ultrasound and/or magnetic resonance imaging (MRI) to identify size, location, and morphological features. Biopsy and microscopic examination of tissue are necessary to confirm the presence of cancer.

Testicular cancer is treatable by surgery, radiation therapy, and chemotherapy. Data from the Surveillance, Epidemiology, and End Results (SEER) Program of the U.S. National Cancer Institute suggest that up to 95% of cases are curable with early detection and appropriate chemotherapy (Brenner, 2002); however, survival is low for patients with advanced malignancies living in regions with no access to therapy.

References

AbouZeid, A. A., Mousa, M. H., Soliman, H. A., Hamza, A. F., & Hay, S. A. (2011). Intra-abdominal testis: Histological alterations and significance of biopsy. *Journal of Urology, 85*(1), 269–274.

Bray, F., Ferlay, J., Soerjomataram, I., Siegel, R. L., Torre, L. A., & Jemal, A. (2018). Global cancer statistics 2018: GLOBOCAN estimates of incidence and mortality worldwide for 36 cancers in 185 countries. *CA: A Cancer Journal for Clinicians, 68*(6), 394–424.

Bray, F., Lorenzo, R., Ekbom, A., Forman, D., Pukkala, E., Cuninkova, M., & Moller, H. (2006). Testicular seminoma and nonseminoma share the same etiology? Evidence from an age-period-cohort analysis of incidence trends in eight European countries. *Cancer Epidemiology, Biomarkers and Prevention, 15*, 652–658.

Brenner, H. (2002). Long-term survival rates of cancer patients achieved by the end of the 20th century: A period analysis. *Lancet, 360*, 1131–1135.

Brown, L. M., Pottern, L. M., & Hoover, R. N. (1987). Testicular cancer in young men: The search for causes of the epidemic increase in the United States. *Journal of Epidemiology and Community Health, 41*, 349–354.

Cancer Research UK. (2011). *UK cancer information service.* Retrieved from www.cancerresearchuk.org

Chilvers, C., & Pike, M. C. (1992). Cancer risk in the undescended testicle. *European Urology Update Series, 1*, 74–79.

Dieckmann, K.-P., & Loy, V. (1996). Prevalence of contralateral testicular intraepithelial neoplasia in patients with testicular germ cell neoplasms. *Journal of Clinical Oncology, 14*, 3126–3132.

Dieckmann, K.-P., & Pichlmeier, U. (1997). The prevalence of familial testicular cancer: An analysis of two patient populations and a review of the literature. *Cancer, 80*(10), 1954–1960.

Dieckmann, K.-P., & Skakkebaek, N. E. (1999). Carcinoma in situ of the testis: Review of biological and clinical features. *International Journal of Cancer, 83*, 815–822.

Dong, C., Lönnstedt, I., & Hemminki, K. (2001). Familial testicular cancer and second primary cancers in testicular cancer patients by histological type. *European Journal of Cancer, 37*(15), 1878–1885.

Ferlay, J., Ervik, M., Lam, F., Colombet, M., Mery, L., Piñeros, M., … Bray, F. (2018). *Global cancer observatory: Cancer today.* Lyon, France: International Agency for Research on Cancer. Retrieved from https://gco.iarc.fr/today.

Ferlay, J., Soerjomataram, I., Ervik, M., Dikshit, R., Eser, S., Mathers, C., … Bray, F. (2013). *GLOBOCAN 2012 v1.0. Cancer incidence and mortality worldwide: IARC CancerBase No. 11* [Internet]. Lyon, France: International Agency for Research on Cancer. Retrieved from http://globocan.iarc.fr

Forman, D., Pike, M. C., Davey, G., Dawson, S., Baker, K., Chilvers, C. E. D., … Coupland, C. A. C. (1994). Aetiology of testicular cancer: Association with congenital abnormalities, age at puberty, infertility and exercise. *BMJ, 308*, 1393–1399.

Frigyesi, A., Gisselsson, D., Hansen, G. B., Soller, M., Mitelman, F., & Höglund, M. (2004). A model for karyotypic evolution in testicular germ cell tumors. *Genes, Chromosomes and Cancer, 40*(3), 172–178.

Holstein, A. F., & Lauke, H. (1996). Histologic diagnostics of early testicular germ cell tumor. *International Journal of Urology, 3*, 165–172.

Huff, D. S., Fenig, D. M., Canning, D. A., Carr, M. G., Zderic, S. A., & Snyder, H. M. (2001). Abnormal germ cell development in cryptorchidism. *Hormone Research, 55*(1), 11–17.

Huyghe, E., Matsuda, T., & Thonneau, P. (2003). Increasing incidence of testicular cancer worldwide: A review. *Journal of Urology, 170*, 5–11.

Kumar, V., Abbas, A. K., & Aster J. C. (2014). *Robbins and Cotran pathologic basis of disease* (9th ed.). Philadelphia, PA: Mosby & Saunders.

Looijenga, L. H., & Oosterhuis, J. W. (2013). Pathobiology of germ cell tumors-applying the gossip test. *The International of Journal Developmental Biology, 57*(2–4), 289–296.

Lutke Holzik, M. F., Sijmons, R. H., Sleijfer, D. T., Sonneveld, D. J., Hoekstra-Weebers, J. E., van Echten-Arends, J., & Hoekstra, H. J. (2003). Syndromic aspects of testicular carcinoma. *Cancer, 97*(4), 984–992.

Lyter, D. W., Bryant, J., Thackeray, R., Rinaldo, C. R., & Kingsley, L. A. (1995). Incidence of human immunodeficiency virus-related and nonrelated malignancies in a large cohort of homosexual men. *Journal of Clinical Oncology, 13*(10), 2540–2546.

Mai, P. L., Friedlander, M., Tucker, K., Phillips, K. A., Hogg, D., Jewett, M. A., … Greene, M. H. (2010). The International Testicular Cancer Linkage Consortium: A clinicopathologic descriptive analysis of 461 familial malignant testicular germ cell tumor kindred. *Urologic Oncology, 28*(5), 492–499.

Pettersson, A., Richiardi, L., Nordenskjold, A., Kaijser, M., & Akre, O. (2007). Age at surgery for undescended testis and risk of testicular cancer. *New England Journal of Medicine, 356*(18), 1835–1841.

Rosen, A., Jayram, G., Drazer, M., & Eggener, S. E. (2011). Global trends in testicular cancer incidence and mortality. *European Urology, 60*(2), 374–379.

Sandberg, A. A., Meloni, A. M., & Suijkerbuijk, R. F. (1996). Reviews of chromosome studies in urological tumors. III. Cytogenetics and genes in testicular tumors. *Journal of Urology, 144*, 1531–1556.

Shanmugalingam, T., Soultati, A., Chowdhury, S., Rudman, S., & Van Hemelrijck, M. (2013). Global incidence and outcome of testicular cancer. *Journal of Clinical Epidemiology, 5*, 417–427.

Skakkebaek, N. E. (1972). Possible carcinoma in situ of the testis. *Lancet, 2*(7776), 516–517.

Trabert, B., Graubard, B. I., Erickson, R. L., & McGlynn, K. A. (2012). Childhood infections, orchitis and testicular germ cell tumours: A report from the STEED study and a meta-analysis of existing data. *British Journal of Cancer, 106*, 1331–1334.

Zheng, T., Holford, T. R., Ma, Z., Ward, B. A., Flannery, J., & Boyle, P. (1996). Continuing increase in incidence of germ-cell testis cancer in young adults: Experience from Connecticut, USA, 1935–1992. *International Journal of Cancer, 65*, 723–729.

© Andrew Brookes/Getty Images

CHAPTER 28

Epidemiology of Carcinoma of the External Male Genitalia: Penis and Scrotum

▶ Global Epidemiology of Penile Cancer

Carcinoma of the penis is an uncommon and potentially mutilating disease with a heterogeneous etiology. This malignancy is predominantly found in men who were not circumcised shortly after birth and is rarely found in populations where neonatal circumcision is routine (Maden et al., 1993; Schoen, Oehrli, Colby, & Machin, 2000). Nevertheless, sexually transmitted infectious agents such as oncogenic human papillomaviruses (HPVs) may cause disease even in circumcised men.

In 2018, 34,475 men were diagnosed with cancer of the penis and 15,138 deaths were attributed to this malignancy. The estimated number of new cases in 2018 was 33% higher than the annual number reported in 2002. The age-adjusted incidence and mortality rates of penile cancer in 2018 were 0.80 per 100,000 and 0.35 per 100,000, respectively (Bray et al., 2018; IARC, 2007; Parkin & Bray, 2006).

Carcinomas of the penis are rare among men living in developed countries but are relatively common among the male populations of some underdeveloped nations. In 2018, age-adjusted incidence rates less than 1.0 per 100,000 were observed in developed nations such as the United States, Canada, Australia, New Zealand, and Western European and Scandinavian nations, whereas the rates greater than 1 per 100,000 were observed in India and most nations of South America and Southern Africa. The global mortality rates in 2018 had a similar pattern as the incidence rates; for example, mortality rates in North America and Europe were low (0.10–0.20 per 100,000) compared to the higher rates in India and nations of South America and Southern Africa (0.5–1.1 per 100,000) (Ferlay et al., 2018) (**FIGURE 28.1**).

Incidence rates of penile cancer are very low among Israeli Jewish men (0.1 per 100,000) who are circumcised shortly after birth and among Muslim men (0.2 per 100,000) who are circumcised during childhood. In contrast, rates are much higher (3–10 per 100,000) among men living in certain parts of the world where circumcision is rare. Several high-risk populations have been identified in regions of Uganda, India, Thailand, Puerto Rico, Paraguay, Brazil, and elsewhere in which penile cancer accounts for 10%–22% of all malignancies in men (Barnholtz-Sloan et al., 2007; Bleeker et al., 2008; Morris et al., 2011; Shabbir, Barod, Hegart, & Minhasa, 2013).

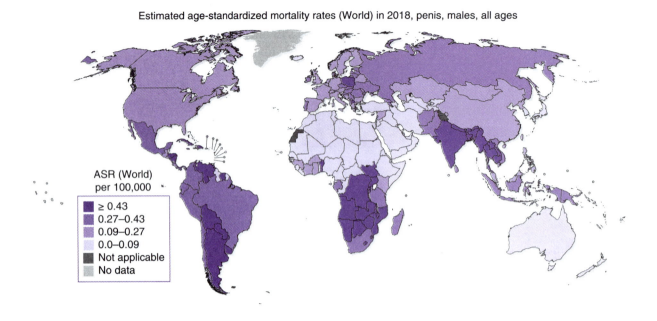

Estimated age-standardized mortality rates (World) in 2018, penis, males, all ages

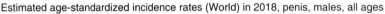

Estimated age-standardized incidence rates (World) in 2018, penis, males, all ages

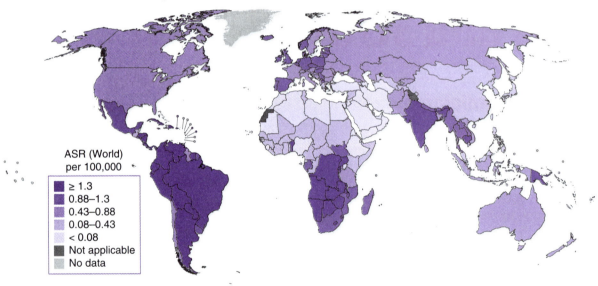

FIGURE 28.1 Global Incidence and Mortality Rates of Penile Cancer, 2018.

Caption: ASR: Rates per 100,000 are age-standardized to the world population, 2000–2025.

Reproduced with permission from Ferlay, J., Ervik, M., Lam, F., Colombet, M., Mery, L., Piñeros, M., ... Bray, F. (2018). *Global cancer observatory: Cancer today*. Lyon, France: International Agency for Research on Cancer. Retrieved from https://gco.iarc.fr/today

▶ Penile Cancer in the United States

In 2013, cancer of the penis was diagnosed in 1570 men and caused 310 deaths in the United States. A team of investigators from the University of Hawaii examined incidence and mortality rates of penile cancer among U.S. men using population-based data from the Surveillance, Epidemiology, and End Results (SEER) program of the National Cancer Institute and the National Program for Cancer Registries of the

Centers for Disease Control and Prevention. During 1998–2003, 4967 men were diagnosed with histologically confirmed squamous cell carcinoma of the penis—less than 1% of all malignant neoplasms in males. Overall, the annual age-adjusted rate was 0.81 cases per 100,000 men. Incidence rates among Caucasians and African Americans were similar to the overall rate. Pacific Islanders had the lowest rate (0.37 per 100,000) and Hispanics the highest (1.32 per 100,000). The age-adjusted annual mortality rate for all men was low (0.18 per 100,000); however, mortality rates were about 50% higher among African-American and

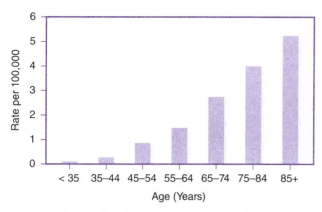

FIGURE 28.2 Age-Specific Annual Incidence of Penile Cancer, United States, 1973–2002.

Data from Barnholtz-Sloan, J. S., Maldonado, J. L., Pow-san, J., & Guiliano, A. R. (2007). Incidence trends in primary malignant penile cancer. *Urologic Oncology: Seminars and Original Investigations, 25*(5), 361–367.

Hispanic men and those living in regions of low socio-economic status (Hernandez et al., 2008).

▶ Age-Specific Incidence of Penile Cancer

Penile cancer is diagnosed predominantly in elderly men, although onset in young adult males does occur. The median age at diagnosis of penile cancer is about 68 years of age. The incidence increases steadily throughout life, and the rates are highest for elderly men, age 70 years or older (**FIGURE 28.2**).

▶ Pathology and Histology

The vast majority (>95%) of penile malignancies are squamous cell carcinomas that arise from the epithelium covering the organ. Other rare forms include basal cell carcinoma, melanoma, lymphoma, and sarcoma. Approximately 75% of squamous cell carcinomas are either flat ulcerative lesions or papillary tumors that typically show keratinization. Most remaining squamous cell carcinomas exhibit wart-like features characteristic of infection by certain strains of HPV.

Pathogenesis of Squamous Cell Penile Carcinoma

Like other malignancies derived from epithelium, squamous cell carcinomas of the penis appear to evolve through a stepwise process. Over a period of several years, early dysplastic lesions develop and progress to carcinomas in situ. A variety of names have been given to penile carcinoma in situ, including Bowen's disease, Bowenoid papulosis, and erythroplasia of Queyrat.

Subsequently, cancer cells breach the basement membrane leading to invasive carcinoma, which has the capability of disseminating to lymph nodes and other tissues.

Premalignant Lesions of Penile Carcinoma

Lichen sclerosis is characterized by white atrophic plaques on the glans and prepuce (foreskin) of the penis. These plaques may enlarge and coalesce to form sclerotic masses. In a study of 86 cases of uncircumcised Italian men with lichen sclerosis, five lesions (5.8%) exhibited malignant features and four of these were found to be positive for HPV (Nasca, Innocenzi, & Micali, 1999). In a second study, the clinical and pathology records of 130 Italian men with confirmed lichen sclerosis were reviewed to quantify the presence of premalignant and malignant lesions. Eleven of these cases (8.4%) had lesions with malignant histopathological features (Barbagli et al., 2006).

Leukoplakia refers to solitary or multiple white scaly plaques, often involving the glans and/or meatus. Such lesions arise due to chronic irritation and inflammation and are often found very near squamous cell carcinomas. Furthermore, areas of dysplasia that can progress to cancer are present in up to 20% of cases with penile leukoplakia (Mikhail, 1980; Schellhammer, Jordan, Robey, & Spaulding, 1992).

A penile *cutaneous horn* is a keratotic lesion that develops from epithelial cells on the surface of pre-existing lesions such as pigmented nevi, warts, or abrasions in response to chronic inflammation. Such lesions have been observed in association with invasive carcinoma.

Condyloma acuminata (genital warts) can arise on the penis as well as other anogenital sites of both men and women. Although usually benign, malignant transformation has been observed in association with oncogenic subtypes of HPV infection, particularly HPV-16 and HPV-18. The association of HPV infection with the development of penile carcinoma is discussed in greater detail in the section of this chapter on risk factors.

▶ Risk Factors for Carcinoma of the Penis

Several early studies identified poor genital hygiene, smegma retention, and phimosis (unretractable foreskin) as risk factors for penile cancer. More recently, infection of the genitalia by oncogenic strains of HPV, particularly HPV-16, has been confirmed to play an etiologic role in a subset of cases. Conditions such as penile rash, abrasion, urethral stricture, and inflammation have also been found to increase the risk. Inflammation may be a key component of tumor development or progression because most penile cancers arise at sites of infection, chronic irritation, or injury (Bleeker et al., 2008).

Circumcision and Penile Cancer

Multiple studies have found that neonatal circumcision reduces the risk of carcinoma of the penis by 60%–70%. The first evidence that circumcision prevented the development of penile cancer was reported in 1932 by Anthony Wolbarst from New York. In the study, 1103 cases of penile cancer from more than 200 U.S. hospitals were reviewed and none were Jewish, despite 3% of the hospital population being Jewish and hence circumcised (Wolbarst, 1932). Based on these data, Wolbarst suggested that circumcision in early life protects against the development of penile cancer and advocated the practice of universal circumcision, which stimulated considerable controversy and debate regarding the risk versus benefit ratio of the procedure. This controversy still rages, although a recent report from the American Academy of Pediatrics (AAP) has concluded that the health benefits of infant circumcision outweigh the risks (AAP, 2012).

FIGURE 28.3 shows the global prevalence of circumcision by country. Overall, about one-third of all men have been circumcised. Prevalence rates of circumcision are highest among Jewish and Muslim men and men living in industrialized nations. The incidence and mortality rates of penile cancer tend to be lower in those countries with a higher prevalence of circumcision (Morris et al., 2011).

Despite the controversial nature of the practice of childhood circumcision, numerous studies provide strong evidence that early circumcision markedly reduces the risk of developing penile cancer later in life. In 1947, a hospital-based case–control study was conducted among U.S. military personnel in which 139 cases with penile cancer were compared to 356 controls of similar age and ethnicity. Circumcision during childhood was infrequent among cases compared to controls (1.4% vs. 17.7%, odds ratio [OR] = 0.07), suggesting a 93% reduction in risk associated with early circumcision (Schrek & Lenowitz, 1947).

A 1991 review noted that 592 cases of invasive penile cancer reported by five major cancer centers in the United States included *no* men circumcised in infancy, even though more than 80% of men surveyed during the 1960s had neonatal circumcision (Schoen, 1991).

In a systematic review of the literature on circumcision and penile carcinoma, eight studies were identified that reported estimates of ORs or other data suitable for meta-analysis. Study populations included men from the United States, Europe, and China. Circumcision in childhood/adolescence was found to be protective against the development of invasive cancer of the penis (summary OR = 0.33), but there was little evidence of an association with either intraepithelial neoplasia or carcinoma in situ (Larke, Thomas, dos Santos Silva, & Weiss, 2011).

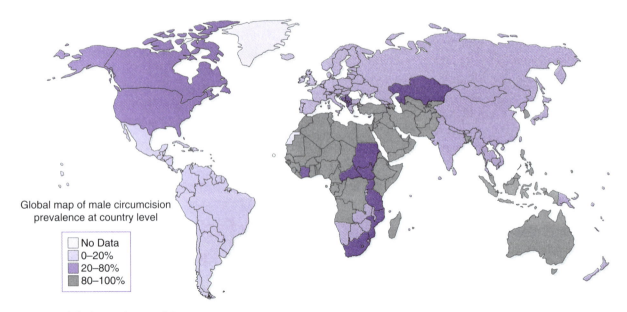

Global map of male circumcision prevalence at country level

☐ No Data
☐ 0–20%
☐ 20–80%
☐ 80–100%

FIGURE 28.3 Global Prevalence of Circumcision, 2006.

Reproduced with permission of The World Health Organization report of 14 December 2007. Male circumcision: Global trends and determinants of prevalence, safety, and acceptability. This report is the result of collaborative work between the London School of Hygiene and Tropical Medicine, the World Health Organization, and the Joint United Nations Programme on HIV/AIDS (UNAIDS).

Phimosis and Penile Cancer

Phimosis refers to circumferential fibrosis of preputial tissue (foreskin) in uncircumcised men that leads to narrowing and inability to retract the penile foreskin over the glans penis. This condition leads to the accumulation of smegma beneath the foreskin and predisposes to chronic inflammation and infection. Phimosis is found in about 1% of uncircumcised men, but rarely in circumcised men. In a study of uncircumcised schoolboys conducted in Denmark, the incidence of phimosis among 3355 adolescent boys aged 14–17 years was 1.1% (Oster, 1968).

Several studies have found that phimosis among uncircumcised men is associated with an approximate 10-fold higher risk of penile cancer, whereas uncircumcised men with no history of phimosis are not at elevated risk (Brinton et al., 1991; Daling et al., 2005; Madsen, Brule, Jensen, Wohlfahrt, & Frisch, 2008; Schoen et al., 2000; Tseng, Morgenstern, Mack, & Peters, 2001). The true predisposing factor for penile cancer associated with lack of circumcision therefore appears to be phimosis. Obviously, removal of the foreskin by circumcision virtually negates the development of phimosis, thereby reducing the risk of developing penile cancer.

Human Papillomavirus (HPV)

Investigators at the Fred Hutchinson Cancer Center in Seattle, Washington conducted a population-based case–control study of penile cancer among men living in the region. They compared 110 men with carcinoma of the penis to 355 male disease-free control subjects frequency-matched to the cases on age and date of diagnosis. Tumor tissues from 67 of the cases were tested for HPV DNA by polymerase chain reaction (PCR). Increased ORs were noted for uncircumcised men compared to men circumcised at birth (OR = 3.2), smokers compared to nonsmokers (OR = 2.8), and men with a history of genital warts compared to men with no history (OR = 5.9). Among 67 tumor specimens, 49% were positive for HPV DNA, and 70% of these were positive for HPV-16 DNA. Risk increases were also noted for those men who reported persistent smegma and/or rashes and ulcerations of the penis. Notably, cases reported a greater number of sexual partners than controls (28% of cases reported 30 or more sexual partners compared to 10% of controls). These results implicate absence of early circumcision, high sexual activity, infection with HPV, and smoking as risk factors for the development of carcinoma of the penis (Maden et al., 1993).

In a subsequent case–control study, investigators in Seattle compared men with carcinoma in situ (*n* = 75) or invasive cancer (*n* = 62) of the penis to 671 disease-free controls from the general population. Blood samples were tested for HPV-16 and genital herpes simplex virus (HSV2), and tumor specimens from the cases were tested for HPV DNA. Risk factors for invasive penile cancer included smoking versus nonsmoking (OR = 4.5) and absence versus presence of circumcision in childhood (OR = 2.3). Among uncircumcised men, medical history of phimosis increased the risk of invasive penile cancer more than 11-fold (OR = 11.4), whereas those with no history of phimosis were not at increased risk. The proportion of HPV positivity was similar for carcinoma in situ and invasive cancer and did not vary with subgrouping for any of the other risk factors. Among tumor specimens from all cases, 80% were positive for HPV DNA and 69% of these were positive for HPV-16 DNA. The investigators concluded that HPV-16 infection is a strong risk factor for penile cancer and that elimination of phimosis by early circumcision is protective (Daling et al., 2005).

Investigators in Denmark conducted a case–control study of penile carcinoma among Danish men, a population in which childhood circumcision is rare. They compared cases with invasive (*n* = 53) or in situ (*n* = 18) squamous cell carcinomas of the penis to 86 controls with prostate cancer and 103 disease-free population controls. Tissue samples were examined by PCR to detect HPV DNA. Overall, 24 tumors (65%) were positive for HPV, and 92% of these were positive for HPV-16. Penile cancer risk increased with lifetime number of female sex partners, number of female sex partners before age 20, early age at first intercourse, penile–oral sex, history of anogenital warts, and never having used condoms. Medical histories of phimosis or priapism (persisting painful erection) at least 5 years before diagnosis were also significant risk factors. The investigators concluded that sexually transmitted HPV-16 infection and phimosis are major risk factors for the development of squamous cell carcinoma of the penis (Madsen et al., 2008).

In a systematic review of 31 studies that included 1466 men with penile carcinomas, 47% of cases were positive for HPV, and the majority of these were positive for either HPV-16 (60%) or HPV-18 (13%) (Miralles-Guri et al., 2009). In contrast, HPV infection in the foreskins of otherwise healthy men without penile cancer ranges from 0% to 6% (Grussendorf-Conen, Meinhof, de Villiers, & Gissmann, 1987; Varma et al., 1991).

Human Immunodeficiency Virus Infection

Recent case reports have documented that combined infection by HPV and human immunodeficiency virus (HIV) may accelerate the progression of squamous cell carcinoma of the penis (Aboulafia & Gibbons, 2001; Théodore et al., 2002). These reports raise the specter of synergism between HPV and HIV due to the immunosuppressive effects of HIV.

Tobacco and Penile Cancer

Cigarette smoking has been identified as a risk factor for penile carcinoma in several epidemiologic studies. ORs from these studies suggest there is an approximate two- to fourfold increase in the risk among chronic smokers compared to nonsmokers (Daling et al., 2005; Hellberg, Valentin, Eklund, & Nilsson, 1987; Maden et al., 1993). Other forms of chronic tobacco use (chewing tobacco and snuff) have also been noted to increase the risk (Harish & Ravi, 1995).

Psoralen and Ultraviolet A Radiation

Certain treatments have been linked to the genesis of cancer of the external male genitalia (penis and scrotum). Psoralen and ultraviolet A radiation (PUVA) is a form of photochemotherapy that is administered in several treatment sessions to patients with severe psoriasis. Long-term PUVA therapy has been found to increase the risk of developing squamous cell carcinoma of the skin and malignant melanoma (Stern, Nichols, & Väkevä, 1997). When whole-body PUVA is administered, patients are in a standing position, and the external male genitalia may therefore be exposed to excess ultraviolet (UV) radiation. In a cohort of 892 U.S. men treated with PUVA and followed on average for 12 years after therapy, 14 patients (1.6%) subsequently developed penile and scrotal tumors, and the incidence of invasive squamous cell carcinoma was 286 times higher than in the general male population. Furthermore, the estimates of risk increased significantly with increasing exposure to PUVA (as well as ultraviolet B radiation), suggesting that chronic exposure to ultraviolet radiation may incite malignant transformation of the external male genitalia (Stern, 1990).

▶ Cancer of the Scrotum

Cancer of the scrotum was the first documented malignancy arising from an occupational exposure. In 1775, Percival Pott described the development of cancer of the scrotum among chimney sweeps in England. He called this tumor the "chimney-sweeper's cancer" and attributed the condition to "a lodgment of soot in the rugae of the scrotum" (Pott, 1775).

Scrotal cancer has also been reported in men with other occupational exposures (e.g., coal tar, arsenic, and mineral oil). Carcinoma of the scrotum is exceedingly rare in most populations. In the United States, the annual incidence is approximately 5–10 cases per 10 million men (Wright, Morgan, & Lin, 2008). Most cases are thought to arise because of poor genital hygiene coupled with chronic exposure to irritating and inflammatory agents. Unfortunately, patients with scrotal lesions often delay seeking medical attention for several months and even years, thereby diminishing successful therapy and survival (Azike, 2009).

▶ Molecular Carcinogenesis

The molecular carcinogenesis of penile cancer may involve both HPV-related and HPV-independent mechanisms. The primary mechanism of HPV-related carcinogenesis has been elucidated in studies of cervical carcinogenesis. Oncogenic strains of HPV (e.g., HPV-16) express oncoproteins E6 and E7 that bind to and inactivate *p53* and *Rb* tumor suppressor gene products, respectively, resulting in loss of control of cell division and apoptosis (Scheffner et al., 1994; zur Hausen, 2002).

Other HPV-independent mechanisms may also contribute to penile carcinogenesis. For example, immunohistochemistry has demonstrated that the inducible inflammatory enzymecyclooxygenase-2 (COX-2) is overexpressed in human samples of penile intraepithelial neoplasia and carcinoma, suggesting that chronic inflammation may play a key role in the development of some penile malignancies (Golijanin et al., 2004).

▶ Preventive Strategies

Preventive strategies should target the major risk factors for penile carcinoma, including phimosis in uncircumcised men, promiscuous sexual activity, infection with HPV-16 or other oncogenic HPV strains, and cigarette smoking.

Circumcision during infancy largely negates phimosis as a risk factor for penile cancer. Furthermore, a recent meta-analysis of randomized trials of sexually active heterosexual men in Africa found that circumcision reduced the incidence of HIV by 50%–60% over a period of 24 months (Doyle, Kahn, Hosang, & Carroll, 2010; Siegfried, Muller, Deeks, & Volmink, 2009; Uthman, Popoola, Uthman, & Aremu, 2010). Because of these studies, the World Health

Organization (WHO) has included circumcision as a key component of a comprehensive program for HIV control in sub-Saharan Africa and other areas with high endemic rates of HIV (WHO, 2012). Other options for prevention of penile cancer include vaccination against oncogenic HPV strains, condom use

to prevent virus transmission, protective clothing to prevent excess exposure to UV radiation during phototherapy for dermatologic conditions, and health education to prevent smoking, promote smoking cessation, and improve genital hygiene (Bleeker et al., 2008; Shabbir et al., 2013).

References

Aboulafia, D. M., & Gibbons, R. (2001). Penile cancer and human papilloma virus (HPV) in a human immunodeficiency virus (HIV)-infected patient. *Cancer Investigation, 19*(3), 266–272.

American Academy of Pediatrics. (2012). Circumcision policy statement. *Pediatrics, 130*(3), 585–586.

Azike, J. E. (2009). A review of the history, epidemiology and treatment of squamous cell carcinoma of the scrotum. *Rare Tumors, 1*(1), e17.

Barbagli, G., Palminteri, E., Mirri, F., Guazzoni, G., Turini, D., & Lazzeri, M. (2006). Penile carcinoma in patients with genital lichen sclerosus: A multicenter survey. *Journal of Urology, 175*(4), 1359–1363.

Barnholtz-Sloan, J. S., Maldonado, J. L., Pow-sang, J., & Guiliano, A. R. (2007). Incidence trends in primary malignant penile cancer. *Urologic Oncology: Seminars and Original Investigations, 25*(5), 361–367.

Bleeker, M. C. G., Heideman, D. A. M., Snijders, P. J. F., Horenblas, S., Dillner, J., & Meijer, C. J. L. (2008). Penile cancer: Epidemiology, pathogenesis and prevention. *World Journal of Urology, 27*(2), 141–150.

Bray, F., Ferlay, J., Soerjomataram, I., Siegel, R. L., Torre, L. A., & Jemal, A. (2018). Global cancer statistics 2018: GLOBOCAN estimates of incidence and mortality worldwide for 36 cancers in 185 countries. *CA: A Cancer Journal for Clinicians, 68*(6), 394–424.

Brinton, L. A., Li, J. Y., Rong, S. D., Huang, S., Xiao, B. S., Shi, B. G., … Dawsey, S. (1991). Risk factors for penile cancer: Results from a case-control study in China. *International Journal of Cancer, 47*(4), 504–509.

Daling, J. R., Madeleine, M. M., Johnson, L. G., Schwartz, S. M., Shera, K. A., Wurscher, M. A., … Krieger, J. N. (2005). Penile cancer: Importance of circumcision, human papillomavirus and smoking in in situ and invasive disease. *International Journal of Cancer, 116*(4), 606–616.

Doyle, S., Kahn, J., Hosang, N., & Carroll, P. (2010). The impact of male circumcision on HIV transmission. *Journal of Urology, 183*(1), 21–26.

Ferlay, J., Ervik, M., Lam, F., Colombet, M., Mery, L., Piñeros, M., … Bray, F. (2018). *Global cancer observatory: Cancer today.* Lyon, France: International Agency for Research on Cancer. Retrieved from https://gco.iarc.fr/today

Golijanin, D., Tan, J. Y., Kazior, A., Cohen, E. G., Russo, P., Dalbagni, G., … Dannenberg, A. J. (2004) Cyclooxygenase-2 and microsomal prostaglandin E synthase-1 are overexpressed in squamous cell carcinoma of the penis. *Clinical Cancer Research, 10*(3), 1024–1031.

Grussendorf-Conen, E. I., Meinhof, W., de Villiers, E. M., & Gissmann, L. (1987). Occurrence of HPV genomes in penile smears of healthy men. *Archives of Dermatological Research, 279*(Suppl.), S73–S75.

Harish, K., & Ravi, R. (1995). The role of tobacco in penile carcinoma. *British Journal of Urology, 75*(3), 375–377.

Hellberg, D., Valentin, J., Eklund, T., & Nilsson, S. (1987). Penile cancer: Is there an epidemiological role of smoking and sexual behavior? *British Medical Journal, 295*(6609), 1306–1308.

Hernandez, B. Y., Barnholtz-Sloan, J., German, R. R., Giuliano, A., Goodman, M. T., King, J. B., … Villalon-Gomez, J. M. (2008). Burden of invasive squamous cell carcinoma of the penis in the United States, 1998–2003. *Cancer, 113*(10 Suppl.), 2883–2891.

International Agency for Research on Cancer. (2007). *Cancer incidence in five continents* (Vol. 9, IARC Scientific Publication No. 160). Lyon, France: Author.

Larke, N. L., Thomas, S. L., dos Santos Silva, I., & Weiss, H. A. (2011). Male circumcision and penile cancer: A systematic review and meta-analysis. *Cancer Causes and Control, 22*(8), 1097–1110.

Maden, C., Sherman, K. J., Beckmann, A. M., Hislop, T. G., Teh, C. Z., Ashley, R. L., & Daling, J. R. (1993). History of circumcision, medical conditions, and sexual activity and risk of penile cancer. *Journal of the National Cancer Institute, 85*(1), 19–24.

Madsen, B. S., Brule, A. J., Jensen, H. L., Wohlfahrt, J., & Frisch, M. (2008). Risk factors for squamous cell carcinoma of the penis—population-based case–control study in Denmark. *Cancer Epidemiology, Biomarkers and Prevention, 17*(10), 2683–2691.

Mikhail, G. R. (1980). Cancers, precancers, and pseudocancers on the male genitalia. A review of clinical appearances, histopathology, and management. *Journal of Dermatological Surgery and Oncology, 6*(12), 1027–1035.

Miralles-Guri, C., Bruni, L., Cubilla, A. L., Castellsagué, X., Bosch, F. X., & de Sanjosé, S. (2009). Human papillomavirus prevalence and type distribution in penile carcinoma. *Journal of Clinical Pathology, 62*(10), 870–878.

Morris, B. J., Gray, R. H., Castellsague, X., Bosch, F. X., Halperin, D. T., Waskett, J. H., & Hankins, C. A. (2011). The strong protective effect of circumcision against cancer of the penis. *Advances in Urology, 2011*. doi.org/10.1155/2011/812368.

Nasca, M. R., Innocenzi, D., & Micali, G. (1999). Penile cancer among patients with genital *lichen sclerosus. Journal of the American Academy of Dermatology, 41*(6), 911–914.

Oster, J. (1968). Further fate of the foreskin: Incidence of preputial adhesions, phimosis and smegma among Danish schoolboys. *Archive of Diseases in Childhood, 43*, 200–203.

Parkin, D. M., & Bray, F. (2006). The burden of HPV-related cancer. *Vaccine, 24*(Suppl. 3), 11–25.

Pott, P. (1775). Cancer scroti. In S. J. Earle (Ed.), *The chirurgical works of Percivall Pott* (Vol. 3, pp. 177–183). London, England: James Webster.

Scheffner, M., Romanczuk, H., Munger, K., Huibregtse, J. M., Mietz, J. A., & Howley, P. M. (1994). Functions of human papillomavirus proteins. *Current Topics in Microbiology and Immunology, 186*, 83–99.

Schellhammer, P. F., Jordan, G. H., Robey, E. L., & Spaulding, J. T. (1992). Premalignant lesions and nonsquamous malignancy of the penis and carcinoma of the scrotum. *Urologic Clinics of North America, 19*(1), 131–142.

Schoen, E. J. (1991). The relationship between circumcision and cancer of the penis. *CA: A Cancer Journal for Clinicians, 41*(5), 306–309.

Schoen, E. J., Oehrli, M., Colby, C., & Machin, G. (2000). The highly protective effect of newborn circumcision against invasive penile cancer. *Pediatrics, 105*(3), E36.

Schrek, R., & Lenowitz, H. (1947). Etiologic factors in carcinoma of the penis. *Cancer Research, 7*, 180–187.

Shabbir, M., Barod, R., Hegart, P. K., & Minhasa, S. (2013). Primary prevention and vaccination for penile cancer. *Therapeutic Advances in Urology, 5*(3), 161–169.

Siegfried, N., Muller, M., Deeks, J. J., & Volmink, J. (2009). Male circumcision for prevention of heterosexual acquisition of HIV in men. *Cochrane Database of Systematic Reviews, 2*, CD003362. doi:10.1002/14651858.

Stern, R. S. (1990). Genital tumors among men with psoriasis exposed to psoralens and ultraviolet A radiation (PUVA) and ultraviolet B radiation. The Photochemotherapy Follow-up Study. *New England Journal of Medicine, 322*(16), 1093–1097.

Stern, R. S., Nichols, K. T., & Väkevä, L. H. (1997). Malignant melanoma in patients treated for psoriasis with methoxsalen (psoralen) and ultraviolet A radiation (PUVA). *New England Journal of Medicine, 336*, 1041–1045.

Théodore, C., Androulakis, N., Spatz, A., Goujard, C., Blanchet, C. P., & Wibault, P. (2002). An explosive course of squamous cell penile cancer in an AIDS patient. *Annals of Oncology, 13*(3), 475–479.

Tseng, H. F., Morgenstern, H., Mack, T., & Peters, R. K. (2001). Risk factors for penile cancer: Results of a population-based case–control study in Los Angeles County (United States). *Cancer Causes and Control, 12*(3), 267–277.

Uthman, O. A., Popoola, T. A., Uthman, M. M., & Aremu, O. (2010). Economic evaluations of adult male circumcision for prevention of heterosexual acquisition of HIV in men in sub-Saharan Africa: A systematic review. *PLoS ONE, 5*(3), e9628.

Varma, V. A., Sanchez-Lanier, M., Unger, E. R., Clark, C., Tickman, R., Hewan-Lowe, K., … Swan, D. C. (1991). Association of human papillomavirus with penile carcinoma: A study using polymerase chain reaction and *in situ* hybridization. *Human Pathology, 22*(9), 908–913.

Wolbarst, A. (1932). Circumcision and penile cancer. *Lancet, 219*(5655), 150–153.

World Health Organization. (2012). *Use of devices for adult male circumcision in public health HIV prevention programmes: Conclusion and executive summary of the WHO Technical Advisory Group on Innovation in Male Circumcision.* Geneva, Switzerland: Author.

Wright, J. L., Morgan, T. M., & Lin, D. W. (2008). Primary scrotal cancer: Disease characteristics and increasing incidence. *Urology, 72*(5), 1139–1143.

zur Hausen, H. (2002). Papillomaviruses and cancer: From basic studies to clinical application. *Nature Reviews Cancer, 2*(5), 342–350.

CHAPTER 29

Epidemiology of Urinary Bladder Cancer

▶ Anatomy and Function of the Urinary Bladder

The urinary bladder is a muscular sac located in the lower pelvis. Basic structures and cell types are shown in **FIGURE 29.1**. Urine manufactured by the kidneys travels to the bladder through the ureters for storage prior to excretion. In normal adults, the urinary bladder holds 300–600 mL of urine. The bladder wall consists of smooth muscle that contracts during urination. Urine passes out of the body through the urethra, which is longer in men than women (approximately 20 cm versus 4 cm). In men, the prostate gland encircles the urethra just below the bladder. The urinary bladder is lined by multiple layers of transitional epithelium (called *urothelium*), which expands or contracts depending on the volume of urine contained. When the bladder is empty, transitional epithelial cells are cuboidal in shape; when the bladder is full, they are flat (Kumar, Abbas, & Aster, 2014).

▶ Global Epidemiology of Bladder Cancer

Cancer of the urinary bladder afflicts 3–4 times more men than women. During 2018, 549,393 new cases were diagnosed in the world population and 199,922 people died from bladder cancer. Of these, 424,082 cases (77%) and 148,270 deaths (74%) occurred in men. During 2008–2018, the annual number of cases of bladder cancer increased 42% and the annual number of deaths increased 33%. The 2018 age-adjusted incidence rate in men was 9.6 cases per 100,000 compared to 2.4 per 100,000 in women, and the mortality rate was 3.2 deaths per 100,000 in men compared to 0.9 per 100,000 in women. Annual incidence and mortality rates in men have declined by 5% and 20%, respectively, since 2002, indicating that the increasing global burden of bladder cancer is primarily a consequence of increasing population growth and aging (Bray et al., 2018; Ferlay et al., 2010, 2013, 2018; Parkin, Bray, Ferlay, & Pisani, 2001, 2005).

FIGURE 29.2 shows the global distributions of incidence and mortality rates of bladder cancer among men in 2018. Age-adjusted incidence rates exceeding 20 per 100,000 were observed in the United States, Canada, and most western European nations, whereas India, China, and most nations of sub-Saharan Africa had incidence rates less than 5 per 100,000. Mortality rates were less variable and tended to be higher in less developed countries with limited access to therapy. On average, developed nations had higher incidence and mortality (12.1 and 3.2 per 100,000, respectively) than developing nations (3.6 and 2.0 per 100,000), but the mortality-to-incidence ratio in developed nations (0.26) was only about half that of developing nations (0.56) (Bray et al., 2018; Ferlay et al., 2018).

Incidence rates of transitional cell carcinoma of the bladder urothelium exceed 15 per 100,000 among

FIGURE 29.1   Anatomy of the Urinary Bladder in Men and Women.

men of North America, Western Europe, Scandinavia, and other regions where the prevalence of smoking is high. Incidence rates are also high among men of Eastern Mediterranean and North African countries, particularly in Egypt (20 per 100,000), where squamous cell bladder cancer arises due to chronic infection by the parasitic worm *Schistosoma haematobium*. Mortality is exceedingly high (over 10 deaths per 100,000) for the male populations of Latvia, Lebanon, Syria, and Egypt (Ferlay et al., 2010, 2013, 2018; Parkin, Bray, Ferlay, & Pisani, 2001, 2005).

▶ Pathogenesis of Urinary Bladder Cancer

In developed countries of North America, Europe, and Australia, most bladder cancers (approximately 95%) are transitional cell carcinomas that arise from the epithelial cell lining of the bladder (called

the urothelium). The progression of carcinogenesis appears similar to other forms of cancer with epithelial cell origin. The urothelium undergoes a stepwise progression of changes from mild to severe dysplasia that results in the formation of noninvasive papillary carcinoma in situ and ultimately invasive cancer that penetrates the basement membrane. The evolutionary progression of carcinogenesis in the urinary bladder is believed to occur over many years, usually 2–3 decades. Often, transitional cell carcinomas of the urinary bladder show multiple cancerous foci at the time of diagnosis, a phenomenon known as *field cancerization*.

In developing nations of Africa and Southern Asia, the predominant histological type of bladder cancer is squamous cell carcinoma, which arises due to chronic infection by the parasitic worm *Schistosoma haematobium*. Chronic infection of the bladder by these parasites (called *bilharziasis*) causes sustained local inflammation, irritation, and subsequent reparative hyperplasia and squamous metaplasia in which

Estimated age-standardized incidence rates (World) in 2018, bladder, males, all ages

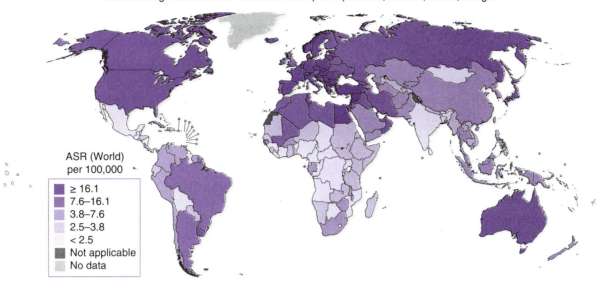

Estimated age-standardized mortality rates (World) in 2018, bladder, males, all ages

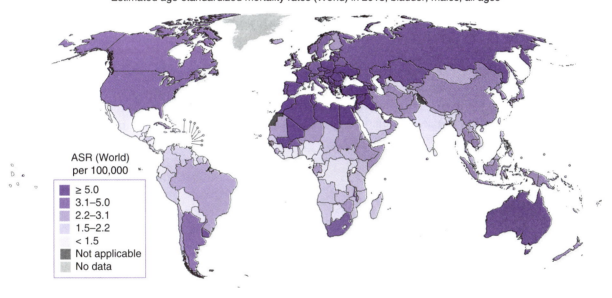

FIGURE 29.2 Global Incidence and Mortality Rates of Bladder Cancer in Men, 2018.

Caption: ASR: Rates per 100,000 are age-standardized to the world population, 2000–2025.

Reproduced with permission from Ferlay, J., Ervik, M., Lam, F., Colombet, M., Mery, L., Piñeros, M., . . . Bray, F. (2018). *Global cancer observatory: Cancer today.* Lyon, France: International Agency for Research on Cancer. Available from: https://gco.iarc.fr/today, accessed [09 October 2018].

the normal urothelial cells are replaced by squamous cells. These changes in the bladder mucosa eventually progress to squamous cell carcinoma.

▶ Risk Factors for Urinary Bladder Cancer

Tobacco Use and Urinary Bladder Cancer

The dominant risk factor for transitional cell urinary bladder cancer is cigarette smoking, which accounts

for about two-thirds of new cases in men and one-third of new cases in women. Epidemiologic cohort and case–control studies have consistently observed two- to threefold increases in the relative risk of developing transitional cell bladder cancer among chronic smokers compared to nonsmokers, as well as dose–response relationships with the number of cigarettes smoked and duration of smoking. Cigarette smoking shows similar effects for men and women as well as for individuals with different ethnic backgrounds (Boffetta, 2008).

Urinary bladder carcinogenesis associated with smoking is primarily the result of aromatic amines and arylamines present in cigarette smoke that reach the bladder mucosa (e.g., benzidine, 4-aminobiphenyl, 2-naphthylamine, and 4-chloro-ortho-toluidine) (Patrianakos & Hoffman, 1979). Molecular investigations show that these compounds are ultimately biotransformed (activated) in the acidic environment of the bladder to form potent DNA-reactive carcinogens (Vineis et al., 1990). Detoxification enzymes compete with activating enzymes for these procarcinogens to facilitate their excretion in the urine. Genetic differences in these enzymes are discussed in the following section on "Genetic Factors and Urinary Bladder Cancer."

Interestingly, individuals who smoke black (air-cured) tobacco are at a two- to threefold higher risk than smokers of blonde (flue-cured) tobacco, a difference attributable to the higher levels of highly carcinogenic arylamines in black tobacco (Vineis, 1994). The common practice of smoking black tobacco may thus explain the high rates of bladder cancer observed among men in Spain, Italy, the Netherlands, and Uruguay.

Notably, cigarette smoking also independently increases the risk of developing squamous cell carcinoma of the bladder and may, in fact, interact synergistically with other risk factors (Fortuny et al., 1999). As discussed in the following section, chronic schistosomiasis infection is the key risk factor for development of squamous cell carcinoma of the urinary bladder.

Schistosomiasis and Urinary Bladder Cancer

Squamous cell carcinomas of the bladder occur frequently in conjunction with infection by the trematode *Schistosoma haematobium*. The parasite is endemic in the Nile River, but is also found throughout Africa, in certain parts of Southeast Asia, on the islands of Cyprus, and in southern Portugal. It has been estimated that 85% of Egyptians become infected with this parasite in their lifetimes, which accounts for the astounding fact that bladder cancer accounts for 30% of all malignant neoplasms in Egypt (el-Mawla, el-Bolkainy, & Khaled, 2001).

Schistosome worms mature in the liver and migrate to the plexus of blood vessels that nourish the bladder and pelvic organs. The female worms may deposit their eggs in the walls of the bladder, uterus, prostate, or other pelvic organs. This parasitic infection can result in chronic inflammation of the bladder urothelium, which may ultimately produce squamous metaplasia and carcinoma.

The schistosomes are diecious, and the two sexes mature and reproduce in the vascular system. The eggs are laid in small blood vessels that are then liberated into the lumen of the intestines or the urinary bladder. Schistosome eggs subsequently hatch when they reach fresh water, and the newborn form of the worm (the miracidium) swims in search of an appropriate snail host. After infestation of the snail, the miracidium develops into another form called the cercariae, which is liberated into the fresh water again and capable of penetrating the skin of swimmers and bathers. Upon penetration of human skin, the parasite reaches the circulation and the liver, and the cycle repeats itself (**FIGURE 29.3**).

Molecular studies also suggest that bladder carcinogenesis associated with chronic schistosomiasis may be promoted by co-infection with certain viruses and bacteria, particularly in immunocompromised patients. For example, oncogenic strains of human papillomavirus (HPV-16, HPV-18, and HPV-52) have been found in cancerous urothelial tissues of such patients (Boucher & Anderson, 1997).

Environmental Risk Factors for Urinary Bladder Cancer

Several environmental and occupational factors increase the risk of bladder cancer. These include occupational exposure to arylamines such as 2-naphthylamine, 4-aminobiphenyl, benzidine, and other compounds and intermediates in the synthesis of azo dyes and pigments used in the textile, printing, plastic, rubber, and cable industries. Long-term exposure to these compounds among workers in these industries increases the risk of bladder cancer by about 50% (Scélo & Brennan, 2007).

Workers in aluminum production, auramine O (yellow) and magenta dye manufacturing, and coal gasification may also be at increased risk because of sustained exposure to a variety of chemicals that reach the bladder mucosa, including polycyclic aromatic hydrocarbons, polychlorinated biphenyls, formaldehyde, and solvents. The uncertainty surrounding the hazards posed by these occupations is partly attributable to the difficulty of measuring past exposure to specific chemical agents (Kogevinas et al., 2003; Mannetje et al., 1999).

Pharmacologic Agents and Urinary Bladder Cancer

The analgesic medication phenacetin was once widely used in European nations until the drug was linked to cancers of the renal pelvis and urinary bladder (Hoover & Fraumeni, 1981; Johansson & Wahlqvist, 1977). A case–control investigation found more than

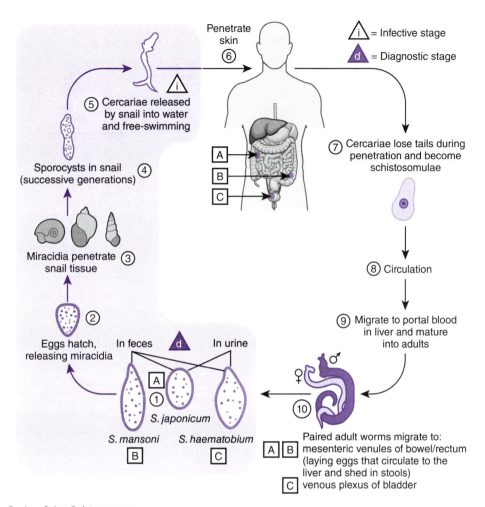

FIGURE 29.3 Life Cycle of the Schistosomes.

Courtesy of Centers for Disease Control and Prevention, *DPDx - Laboratory Identification of Parasitic Diseases of Public Health Concern-HH,* http://www.cdc.gov/dpdx/schistosomiasis/

a sixfold increase in the risk of bladder cancer development due to heavy phenacetin ingestion among women (Piper, Tonascia, & Matanoski, 1985). Phenacetin compounds were removed from the U.S. market in 1983 and have now been discontinued worldwide.

Certain chemotherapeutic agents used in cancer therapy also increase the risk of developing bladder cancer. For example, cyclophosphamide, an alkylating agent used to treat advanced malignancies, has been linked to bladder cancer development. This agent has strong immunosuppressive side effects and sometimes causes a disease known as hemorrhagic cystitis. This condition is associated with cellular atypia and a 10-fold increase in the risk of developing transitional cell carcinoma of the urinary bladder (Hoover & Fraumeni, 1981).

Fluid Intake, Arsenic, and Urinary Bladder Cancer

It is important to ingest plenty of water and fluids (drinking 8–10 eight-ounce glasses of water per day

is recommended) to continually flush the renal system and protect against diseases of the urinary tract, including bladder cancer. In a 10-year prospective cohort study of 47,909 men, the risk of bladder cancer was reduced by about 50% among men who consumed, on average, 84 ounces of fluids daily compared to those consuming 43 ounces (Michaud et al., 1999). Nevertheless, certain contaminants of drinking water, including chlorination disinfection by-products, nitrates, and arsenic, have been linked to bladder carcinogenesis (Cantor, 1997).

A 50-year longitudinal study documented marked increases in bladder and lung cancer mortality related to ingestion of arsenic-contaminated drinking water by the population residing in northern Chile. Observed cancer rates were highest 10–20 years after peak concentrations of arsenic were detected in the drinking water, suggesting a long latency period. Peak rates of bladder cancer were elevated 6-fold in men and nearly 14-fold in women. Cancer rates declined dramatically following installation of water treatment plants to eliminate arsenic from the drinking water (Marshall et al., 2007; Smith, Goycolea, Haque, & Biggs, 1998).

Genetic Factors and Urinary Bladder Cancer

The relative risk of bladder cancer is influenced by the smoking habit as well as genetically determined enzymes that either activate or detoxify arylamines that enter the human system via tobacco smoke or contaminated environments. For example, first-degree relatives of patients with bladder cancer have a two-fold increased risk of developing the disease compared to the general population, whereas there is a fivefold increase in the risk for individuals with a positive family history who are also chronic smokers.

Exposure to arylamines (e.g., from tobacco smoke or the environments of certain occupations) is known to increase the risk of bladder cancer. The metabolism of arylamines occurs in the liver and the urinary bladder through specific enzymatic reactions. The first step takes place in the liver, where nitrogen oxidation of arylamines is catalyzed by enzymes of the P450 system. Subsequently in the bladder, the *N*-hydroxylamines can be either detoxified and excreted or activated to form potent DNA-reactive carcinogens.

The enzyme arylamine *N*-acetyltransferase 2 (NAT2) is involved in the detoxification of various bladder carcinogens, including carcinogenic arylamines (Vineis et al., 1990). A specific dominant mutation in the *NAT2* gene results in slow metabolism of arylamines. Consequently, individuals with the *NAT2* slow acetylation mutation are at higher risk of developing bladder cancer than those without the mutation (Risch, Wallace, Bathers, & Sim, 1995; Vineis et al., 1990). Furthermore, a synergistic interaction is present involving the *NAT2* slow acetylation mutation and heavy smoking, which translates to a greatly increased risk of developing bladder cancer in individuals with both these risk factors compared to nonsmokers who do not carry the *NAT2* mutation (Marcus, Vineis, & Rothman, 2000).

Other enzymatic reactions also modulate the potential carcinogenicity of arylamines in the urinary bladder. Notably, levels of the ubiquitous enzyme beta-glucuronidase are present in the bladder. At urine pH 5.6, this enzyme is capable of splitting various urinary conjugates into carcinogenic elements. The glutathione-S-transferase M1 (*GSTM1*) null genotype also increases the risk of bladder cancer, although it apparently has no interaction with smoking status (Yu et al., 1995).

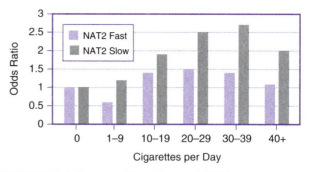

FIGURE 29.4 Influence of Smoking and NAT2 Genotypes on the Risk of Bladder Cancer.

Data from Garcia-Closas, M., Malats, N., Silverman, D., Dosemeci, M., Kogevinas, M., Hein, D. W., . . . Rothman, N. (2005). NAT2 slow acetylation and GSTM2 null genotypes increase bladder cancer risk: Results from the Spanish Bladder Cancer Study and meta-analyses. *Lancet, 36*(9486), 649–659.

A team of international investigators examined *NAT2*, *GSTM1*, and smoking in a large case–control study of bladder cancer in Spain involving 1150 cases and 1149 controls matched to the cases by age, gender, and location. The investigators also conducted a meta-analysis of data on these factors from 31 studies involving 5096 cases of bladder cancer and 6519 disease-free controls. Results from the case–control study revealed significant increases in risk associated with the slow acetylation *NAT2* genotype and the null *GSTM1* genotype. Notably, influence of the slow acetylation *NAT2* genotype became stronger with increasing intensity of smoking (**FIGURE 29.4**). Summary estimates of risk from the meta-analysis suggest that among smokers, the *NAT2* slow acetylation genotype increases bladder cancer risk by 40% compared to other genotypes, and the null *GSTM1* genotype increases the risk by 50% (Garcia-Closas et al., 2005).

Ethnic Variation in Urinary Bladder Cancer

In the United States, the annual incidence of bladder cancer is twice as high in Caucasian-American men than African-American men (41 versus 20 per 100,000 in 2007) and 24% higher in Caucasian-American women compared to African-American women (9.4 versus 7.6 per 100,000 in 2007) (Altekruse et al., 2007). These ethnic differences have persisted for decades (**FIGURE 29.5**) and they pertain primarily to transitional cell bladder cancer that is related to cigarette smoking and other sources of exposure to arylamines (Risch et al., 1995).

The persistently higher incidence rates of bladder cancer in Caucasians versus African Americans in the United States prompted investigations of genetic polymorphisms of smoking and *NAT2* in these populations. In a study restricted to smokers, Richie and colleagues demonstrated that the frequency of slow

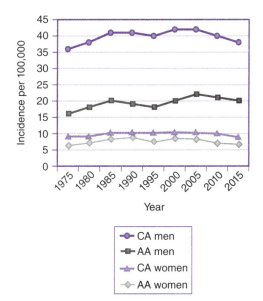

FIGURE 29.5 Trends in the Incidence of Bladder Cancer, United States, 1975–2015.

Data from Altekruse, S. F., Kosary, C. L., Krapcho, M., Neyman, N., Aminou, R., Waldron, W., & Edwards, B. K. (Eds.). (2007). *SEER cancer statistics review, 1975–2007.* Bethesda, MD: National Cancer Institute. Retrieved from http://seer.cancer.gov /csr/1975_2007; Noone, A. M., Howlader, N., Krapcho, M., Miller, D., Brest, A., Yu, M., ... Cronin, K. A. (Eds.). *SEER cancer statistics review, 1975–2015.* Bethesda, MD: National Cancer Institute.

NAT2 acetylators was twofold higher in Caucasians than African Americans (64% versus 36%). Furthermore, Caucasians smoked an average of eight cigarettes per day more than African-American smokers. These observations (high smoking-related arylamine exposure coupled with slow genetically regulated *NAT2* acetylation and delayed detoxification in Caucasians) provide a genetic by environmental basis for the ethnic divergence in the incidence rates of bladder cancer (Muscat et al., 2008).

Despite their relatively low incidence rates of bladder cancer, African Americans typically have more advanced disease at the time of diagnosis and poor survival compared to Caucasians (Underwood, Dunn, Williams, & Lee, 2009). Thus, racial disparity continues to exist in bladder cancer presentation and survival in the United States (Underwood et al., 2009).

▶ Prevention of Bladder Cancer

For the primary prevention of urinary bladder cancer, avoid chronic exposure to tobacco or tobacco smoke, arsenic, benzene, arylamines, azo dyes, and any other chemicals known to irritate the urothelium. In regions where the schistosome parasite is endemic, protect against contracting schistosomiasis by avoiding swimming or wading in contaminated water. Infected individuals should immediately be treated with antiparasitic agents (e.g., praziquantel). It is also important to continually flush the renal system and bladder by daily intake of 8–10 glasses of clean water.

References

Altekruse, S. F., Kosary, C. L., Krapcho, M., Neyman, N., Aminou, R., Waldron, W., & Edwards, B. K. (Eds.). (2007). *SEER cancer statistics review, 1975–2007.* Bethesda, MD: National Cancer Institute. Retrieved from http://seer.cancer.gov /csr/1975_2007/

Boffetta, P. (2008). Tobacco smoking and risk of bladder cancer. *Scandinavian Journal of Urology and Nephrology, 42*(S218), 45–54.

Boucher, N. R., & Anderson, J. B. (1997). Human papillomavirus and bladder cancer. *International Urogynecology Journal, 8,* 354–357.

Bray, F., Ferlay, J., Soerjomataram, I., Siegel, R. L., Torre, L. A., & Jemal, A. (2018). Global cancer statistics 2018: GLOBOCAN estimates of incidence and mortality worldwide for 36 cancers in 185 countries. *CA: A Cancer Journal for Clinicians, 68*(6), 394–424.

Cantor, K. P. (1997). Drinking water and cancer. *Cancer Causes and Control, 8*(3), 292–308.

el-Mawla, N. G., el-Bolkainy, M. N., & Khaled, H. M. (2001). Bladder cancer in Africa: Update. *Seminars in Oncology, 28*(2), 174–178.

Ferlay, J., Bray, F., Pisani, P., & Parkin, D. M. (2004). *GLOBOCAN 2002. Cancer incidence, mortality, and prevalence worldwide. IARC Cancer Base No. 5, version 2.0.* Lyon, France: IARC Press.

Ferlay, J., Ervik, M., Lam, F., Colombet, M., Mery, L., Piñeros, M., ... Bray, F. (2018). *Global cancer observatory: Cancer today.* Lyon, France: International Agency for Research on Cancer. Retrieved from https://gco.iarc.fr/today

Ferlay, J., Shin, H.-R., Bray, F., Forman, D., Mathers, C., & Parkin, D. M. (2010). Estimates of worldwide burden of cancer in 2008: GLOBOCAN 2008. *International Journal of Cancer, 127*(12), 2893–2917.

Ferlay, J., Soerjomataram, I., Ervik, M., Dikshit, R., Eser, S., Mathers, C., ... Bray, F. (2013). *GLOBOCAN 2012 v1.0, cancer incidence and mortality worldwide: IARC CancerBase No. 11* [Internet]. Lyon, France: International Agency for Research on Cancer. Retrieved from http://globocan.iarc.fr

Fortuny, J., Kogevinas, M., Chang-Claude, J., González, C. A., Hours, M., Jöckel, K. H., ... Bofetta, P. (1999). Tobacco, occupation and non-transitional-cell carcinoma of the bladder: An international case-control study. *International Journal of Cancer, 80*(1), 44–46.

Garcia-Closas, M., Malats, N., Silverman, D., Dosemeci, M., Kogevinas, M., Hein, D. W., ... Rothman, N. (2005). NAT2 slow acetylation and GSTM2 null genotypes increase bladder cancer risk: Results from the Spanish Bladder Cancer Study and meta-analyses. *Lancet, 36*(9486), 649–659.

Hoover, R., & Fraumeni, J. F., Jr. (1981). Drug-induced cancer. *Cancer, 47,* 1071.

Johansson, S., & Wahlqvist, L. (1977). Tumours of urinary bladder and ureter associated with abuse of phenacetin-containing analgesics. *Acta Pathologica Microbiologica Scandinavica [A], 85,* 768–774.

Kogevinas, M., 't Mannetje, A., Cordier, S., Ranft, U., González, C. A., Vineis, P., ... Boffetta, P. (2003). Occupation and bladder cancer among men in Western Europe. *Cancer Causes and Control, 14*(10), 907–914.

Kumar, V., Abbas, A. K., & Aster, J. C. (2014). *Robbins and Cotran pathologic basis of disease* (9th ed.). Philadelphia, PA: Mosby & Saunders.

Mannetje, A., Kogevinas, M., Chang-Claude, J., Cordier, S., González, C. A., Hours, M., ... Boffetta, P. (1999). Occupation and bladder cancer in European women. *Cancer Causes and Control, 10*(3), 209–217.

Marcus, P. M., Vineis, P., & Rothman, N. (2000). NAT2 slow acetylation and bladder cancer risk: A meta-analysis of 22 case–control studies conducted in the general population. *Pharmacogenetics, 10*, 115–122.

Marshall, G., Ferreccio, C., Yuan, Y., Bates, M. N., Steinmaus, C., Selvin, S., ... Smith, A. H. (2007). Fifty-year study of lung and bladder cancer mortality in Chile related to arsenic in drinking water. *Journal of the National Cancer Institute, 99*, 920–928.

Michaud, D. S., Spiegelman, D., Clinton, S. K., Rimm, E. B., Curhan, G. C., Willett, W. C., & Giovannucci, E. L. (1999). Fluid intake and the risk of bladder cancer in men. *New England Journal of Medicine, 340*, 1390–1397.

Muscat, J. E., Pittman, B., Kleinman, W., Lazarus, P., Steven, D., Stellman, S. D., & Richie, J. P., Jr. (2008). Comparison of CYP1A2 and NAT2 phenotypes between black and white smokers. *Biochemical Pharmacology, 76*(7), 929–937.

Noone, A. M., Howlader, N., Krapcho, M., Miller, D., Brest, A., Yu, M., ... Cronin, K. A. (Eds.). *SEER cancer statistics review, 1975–2015.* Bethesda, MD: National Cancer Institute.

Parkin, D. M., Bray, F., Ferlay, J., & Pisani, P. (2001). Estimating the world cancer burden: GLOBOCAN 2000. *International Journal of Cancer, 94*, 153–156.

Parkin, D. M., Bray, F., Ferlay, J., & Pisani, P. (2005). Global cancer statistics, 2002. *CA: A Cancer Journal for Clinicians, 55*, 74–108.

Patrianakos, C., & Hoffman, D. (1979). Chemical studies of tobacco smoke. LXIV. On the analysis of aromatic amines in cigarette smoke. *Journal of Analytical Chemistry, 3*, 150–154.

Piper, J. M., Tonascia, J., & Matanoski, G. M. (1985). Heavy phenacetin use and bladder cancer in women aged 20–49 years. *New England Journal of Medicine, 313*(5), 292–295.

Risch, A., Wallace, D. M. A., Bathers, S., & Sim, E. (1995). Slow *N*-acetylation genotype is a susceptibility factor in occupational and smoking related bladder cancer. *Human Molecular Genetics, 4*, 231–236.

Scélo, G., & Brennan, P. (2007). The epidemiology of bladder and kidney cancer. *Nature Clinical Practice Urology, 4*, 205–217.

Smith, A. H., Goycolea, M., Haque, R., & Biggs, M. L. (1998). Marked increase in bladder and lung cancer mortality in a region of Northern Chile due to arsenic in drinking water. *American Journal of Epidemiology, 147*, 660–669.

Underwood, W., III, Dunn, R., Williams, C., & Lee, C. (2009). Gender and geographic influence on the racial disparity in bladder cancer mortality in the US. *Journal of the American College of Surgeons, 202*(2), 284–290.

Vineis, P. (1994). Epidemiology of cancer from exposure to arylamines. *Environmental Health Perspectives, 102*(Suppl. 6), 7–10.

Vineis, P., Caporaso, N., Tannenbaum, S. R., Skipper, P. L., Glogowski, J., Bartsch, H., ... Kadlubar, F. (1990). Acetylation phenotype, carcinogen-hemoglobin adducts, and cigarette smoking. *Cancer Research, 50*, 3002–3004.

Yu, M. C., Ross, R. K., Chan, K. K., Henderson, B. E., Skipper, P. L., Tannenbaum, S. R., & Coetzee, G. A. (1995). Glutathione *S*-transferase M1 genotype affects aminobiphenyl–hemoglobin adduct levels in white, black, and Asian smokers and nonsmokers. *Cancer Epidemiology, Biomarkers and Prevention, 4*, 861–864.

CHAPTER 30

Epidemiology of Kidney Cancer

▶ Anatomy and Function of the Kidneys

The human kidneys are paired organs that perform multiple functions that are essential for life. They excrete waste products of metabolism, regulate the body's concentration of water and salt, maintain the acid–base balance of the blood, regulate blood pressure, and secrete important hormones, including erythropoietin, renin, and prostaglandins. These physiological functions necessarily require a high degree of structural complexity (Robbins & Cotran, 1979).

Kidneys are bean-shaped organs weighing about 150 g that are in the retroperitoneal cavity. Individual renal arteries branching from the abdominal aorta supply blood to the kidneys. The kidneys filter about 17 L of blood per day, producing a derived specialized filtrate of about 1 L of urine.

Urea is the most abundant of the nitrogen-containing waste products excreted by the kidneys. Urea is formed from ammonia or amino acids by a series of reactions known as the urea cycle, which occurs primarily in the liver. Ammonia arising from the metabolism of amino acids and nitrogen-containing compounds is rapidly transported by red bloods cells to the liver, where it enters the urea cycle.

Ammonia itself is highly toxic and cannot be filtered by the kidneys. In contrast, its breakdown product, urea, is colorless, odorless, highly soluble in water, and nontoxic in humans. Urea formed in the liver is transported in the blood to the kidneys, where it is freely filtered by the glomeruli and becomes a major constituent of urine.

The basic functional unit of the kidney is the nephron (**FIGURE 30.1**). Each kidney contains up to 1 million nephrons that carry out the essential functions of the kidney. Each nephron receives unfiltered blood from an afferent arteriole, which divides into capillaries of the glomerulus. The glomerulus is contained in a structure known as *Bowman's capsule*. The glomerulus filters urea and other waste products from the blood. The glomerular filtrate enters Bowman's space, diffuses into the renal tubule, and then travels along the renal tubule, which is lined by a single layer of specialized endothelial cells and surrounded by capillaries. As the glomerular filtrate traverses the renal tubule, salt, water, glucose, and other small molecules are reabsorbed from the filtrate into the blood, and additional waste products (e.g., ammonia, hydrogen, and potassium ions) are secreted from the blood into the urine. Urine exits the nephron via collecting ducts at the end of the renal tubule. Filtered arteriole blood exits the nephron through the efferent arteriole.

▶ Global Epidemiology of Kidney Cancer

Kidney cancer causes significant morbidity and mortality worldwide. In 2018, 403,262 new cases were diagnosed (254,507 in men and 148,755 in women) and 175,098 individuals died from kidney cancer (113,822 men and 61,276 women). The global age-adjusted incidence and mortality rates in men (6.0 per 100,000 and 2.6 per 100,000) were more than twofold

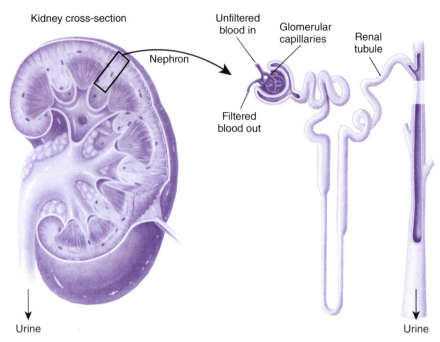

Kidney cross-section

Unfiltered blood in

Glomerular capillaries

Renal tubule

Nephron

Filtered blood out

Urine

Urine

FIGURE 30.1 The Nephron of the Kidney.

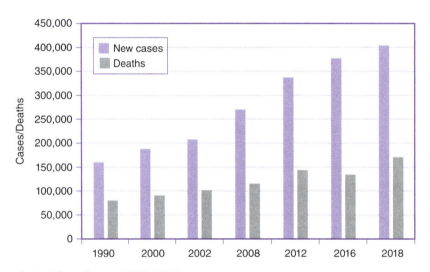

FIGURE 30.2 Global Trends in Kidney Cancer, 1990–2018.

Caption: Values for 2016 are Means of 2015 and 2016 Data.

Data from Ferlay, J., Shin, H. R., Forman, D., Mathers, C., & Parkin, D. M. (2010). Estimates of worldwide burden of cancer in 2008. *International Journal of Cancer, 127*(12), 2893–2917; Ferlay, J., Soerjomataram, I., Ervik, M., Dikshit, R., Eser, S., Mathers, C., . . . Bray, F. (2013). *GLOBOCAN 2012 v1.0, cancer incidence and mortality worldwide: IARC CancerBase No. 11* [Internet]. Lyon, France: International Agency for Research on Cancer. Retrieved from http://globocan.iarc.fr; Parkin, D. M., Bray, F., Ferlay, J., & Pisani, P. (2005). Global cancer statistics, 2002. *CA: A Cancer Journal for Clinicians, 55*, 74–108; Parkin, D. M., Pisani, P., & Ferlay, J. (1999a). Global cancer statistics. *CA: A Cancer Journal for Clinicians, 49*(1), 33–64; Parkin, D. M., Pisani, P., & Ferlay, J. (1999b). Estimates of the worldwide incidence of 25 major cancers in 1990. *International Journal of Cancer, 80*(6), 827–841; Fitzmaurice, C., Allen, C., Barber, R. M., Barregard, L., Bhutta, Z. A., Brenner, H., . . . Global Burden of Disease Cancer Collaboration. (2017). Global, regional, and national cancer incidence, mortality, years of life lost, years lived with disability, and disability-adjusted life-years for 32 cancer groups, 1990 to 2015: A systematic analysis for the Global Burden of Disease Study. *JAMA Oncology, 3*(4), 524–548; Fitzmaurice, C., Akinyemiju, T. F., Al Lami, F. H., Alam, T., Alizadeh-Navaei, R., Allen, C., . . . Global Burden of Disease Cancer Collaboration. (2018). Global, regional, and national cancer incidence, mortality, years of life lost, years lived with disability, and disability-adjusted life-years for 29 cancer groups, 1990 to 2016: A systematic analysis for the Global Burden of Disease Study. *JAMA Oncology*. Online publication. doi:10.1001/jamaoncol.2018.2706.

higher than women (3.1 per 100,000 and 1.1 per 100,000) (Bray et al., 2018).

The annual number of new cases of kidney cancer and deaths due to this malignancy more than doubled in the world population during 1990–2018 (**FIGURE 30.2**). In contrast to these huge increases in new cases and deaths, the annual age-adjusted incidence and mortality rates of kidney cancer changed relatively little during the same period, suggesting

that the increasing global burden of this malignancy has largely been driven by the growth and aging of the world population (Bray et al., 2018; Ferlay, Shin, Forman, Mathers, & Parkin, 2010; Ferlay et al., 2010, 2013, 2018; Fitzmaurice et al., 2017, 2018; Parkin, Bray, Ferlay, & Pisani, 2005; Parkin, Pisani, & Ferlay, 1999a, 1999b).

It is notable that recent studies provide evidence that the annual incidence and mortality rates of kidney cancer are increasing in some populations. For example, based on data collected by tumor registries of the *Surveillance, Epidemiology and End Results* (SEER) program in the United States, there was a persistent upward trend in the incidence and mortality of renal cell carcinomas (the major histological cell type of kidney cancer) during 1975–2009 (Gandaglia et al., 2014). Recent increases in the incidence and mortality rates of kidney cancer have also been observed in other countries, particularly Eastern European nations (Wong et al., 2017). Furthermore, during the past decade, 2008–2018, the annual incidence and mortality rates of kidney cancer increased slightly in the world population (by 18% and 16%, respectively) (Bray et al., 2018; Parkin & Bray, 2010). Although the rising incidence rates noted in some developing countries may be partially attributable to improvements in imaging techniques, better detection does *not* explain the increases in mortality (Hollingsworth, Miller, Daignault, & Hollenbeck, 2006). Rather, global increases in the three major risk factors for kidney cancer—cigarette smoking, obesity, and hypertension—may at least be partially responsible for the accelerating global burden of kidney cancer. The epidemiologic evidence linking these factors to the development of the most common form of kidney cancer, renal cell carcinoma, is discussed later in this chapter.

▶ Global Pattern of Kidney Cancer

FIGURE 30.3 shows the global distributions of incidence and mortality rates of kidney cancer among men in 2018. As shown, there is considerable geographic variability in both the incidence and mortality. Nations of North America, Europe, and Australia/New Zealand, as well as Argentina in South America had the highest reported incidence rates, and Asian and African populations had the lowest. The 2018 annual incidence rates in populations of more developed nations, approximately 10–20 per 100,000 for men and 5–10 per 100,000 for women, were fivefold higher than corresponding rates in less developed nations, 2 per 100,000 for men and 1 per 100,000 for women. Mortality rates showed a similar pattern; e.g., the 2018 average rates were 2–3 times higher in developed nations (3.2 in men and 1.3 in women) than in developing nations (1.1 in men and 0.6 in women) (Bray et al., 2018; Ferlay, Bray, Pisani, & Parkin, 2004; Ferlay et al., 2013, 2018; Weikert & Ljungberg, 2010). Although such differences may partially reflect specific effects of

lifestyle and environmental exposures, it is likely that they are largely attributable to underreporting due to lack of diagnostic imaging and detection in underdeveloped nations.

▶ Kidney Cancer Mortality

Historically, the classic triad of clinical signs (flank pain, hematuria, and palpable mass) in a patient usually led to the detection of a large tumor of the kidney at a later stage of development. Such tumors had often metastasized to other anatomic sites by the time they were diagnosed, making treatment difficult and prognosis poor.

In the current practice of medicine, kidney tumors are often detected incidentally at a relatively early stage of development during imaging studies of the abdomen for other conditions. As with all forms of cancer, early detection of kidney cancer is essential for successful therapy and prolonged patient survival. Kidney tumors detected at an early stage often respond well to treatment and, therefore, survival rates have improved, and mortality rates have stabilized or declined in many developed nations of the world (Pantuck, Zisman, & Belldegrun, 2001). Nevertheless, in less developed nations without sophisticated methods of early detection, the upward trend in mortality is continuing.

▶ Types of Kidney Cancer

Renal cell carcinoma, arising from epithelial cells that line the renal tubules, is the most common type of kidney cancer, accounting for approximately 85%–90% of all malignant kidney tumors. Because these cells normally secrete a variety of vasoactive and regulatory hormones (e.g., renin, erythropoietin, antidiuretic hormone), such tumors often manifest symptoms of hypertension, polycythemia, and other metabolic disturbances.

Transitional cell carcinomas, arising from epithelial cells at the junction of the renal pelvis and the ureter, constitute 5%–10% of malignant kidney tumors. Microscopically, transitional cell carcinomas of the renal pelvis are like urothelial carcinomas of the urinary bladder. Transitional epithelial cells are intermediate between flat squamous cells and tall columnar cells. This type of epithelium lines the collecting ducts in the renal pelvis, the ureters, and the urinary bladder (Kumar, Abbas, & Aster, 2014).

Wilms' tumor (named after the German surgeon, Max Wilms, who first described it) accounts for

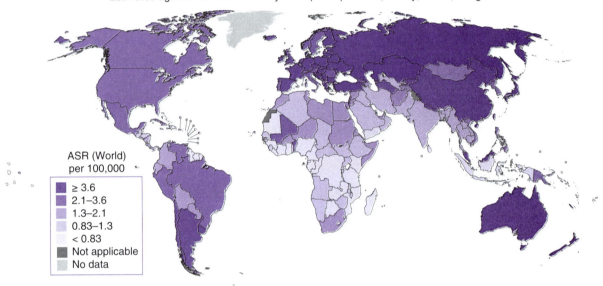

FIGURE 30.3 Global Incidence and Mortality Rates of Kidney Cancer in Men, 2018.

Caption: ASR: Rates per 100,000 are age-standardized to the world population, 2000–2025.

Reproduced with permission from Ferlay, J., Ervik, M., Lam, F., Colombet, M., Mery, L., Piñeros, M., . . . Bray, F. (2018). *Global cancer observatory: Cancer today*. Lyon, France: International Agency for Research on Cancer. Available from: https://gco.iarc.fr/today, accessed [09 October 2018].

about 5% of malignant kidney tumors. This tumor occurs almost exclusively in children under the age of 10 years, usually before the age of 5 years. Wilms' tumors are composed of mixed stromal and epithelial cells with abortive configurations of renal glomeruli and tubules. As discussed in the following sections of this chapter, Wilms' tumor most often arises in children with heritable genetic susceptibility, in contrast to the adult forms of kidney cancer that are predominantly associated with exposure to certain environmental risk factors (Kim & Chung, 2006; Robbins & Cotran, 1979).

▶ **Pathologic Subtypes of Renal Cell Carcinoma**

Histological examination of renal cell carcinomas reveals four distinct subtypes: clear cell, papillary, chromophobe, and collecting duct tumors. Clear cell tumors make up about 85% of all renal cell carcinomas. They arise from the proximal tubules of the kidney and are genetically characterized by deletions and other abnormalities of the short arm of chromosome 3. An important finding in the field of cancer genetics is that the genetic abnormalities of clear cell tumors of the kidney invariably involve the von Hippel–Lindau gene. The remaining subtypes consist of papillary carcinomas (~10%), chromophobe tumors (~5%), and collecting duct (Bellini) tumors (<1%), all of which have been found in association with a variety of chromosomal abnormalities.

▶ Risk Factors for Renal Cell Carcinoma

The web of causation of renal cell carcinoma includes three major risk factors that are modifiable: cigarette smoking, obesity, and hypertension. Although epidemiologic studies have clearly established that each of these factors has an etiologic link with renal cell carcinoma, the underlying physiologic mechanisms and interactions remain to be elucidated. Specific dietary factors and certain other environmental factors have also shown effects in some studies, although the evidence supporting their role has been inconsistent. A notable finding from molecular analyses of renal cell tumors (clear cell subtype) is the presence of abnormalities in the von Hippel–Lindau gene, a tumor–suppressor gene with pleiotropic (multiple) effects on tumor growth and development (Chow, Dong, & Devesa, 2010; Pascual & Borque, 2008).

Gender Differences in Kidney Cancer

Renal cell carcinoma occurs in a male-to-female ratio of approximately 1.6:1 in most populations studied. A recent analysis by the U.S. SEER database also shows that men present with significantly larger and higher-grade tumors than women, and women have a slightly higher 5-year survival rate than men (69% for women versus 65% for men) (Aron, Nguyen, Stein, & Gill, 2008). Although the exact reasons for these differences have not been clarified, it is probable that men have higher levels of exposure to tobacco and other toxic compounds than women, and women are traditionally more health conscious than men.

Smoking and Renal Cell Carcinoma

There is compelling evidence to support a causal link between cigarette smoking and the development of renal cell carcinomas. Hunt and colleagues examined this association in a meta-analysis of 24 epidemiologic investigations: 19 case–control studies of 8032 cases and 13,800 controls, and 5 cohort studies of

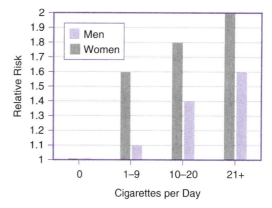

FIGURE 30.4 Relative Risk of Renal Cell Carcinoma by Intensity of Cigarette Smoking.

Data from Hunt, J. D., van der Hel, O. L., McMillan, G. P., Boffetta, P., & Brennan, P. (2005). Renal cell carcinoma in relation to cigarette smoking: Meta-analysis of 24 studies. *International Journal of Cancer, 114*, 101–108.

1326 cases among 1,457,754 participants. Combined estimates of relative risk (RR) for ever smokers compared to never smokers were RR = 1.38 for all subjects, RR = 1.54 for men, and RR = 1.22 for women. Furthermore, there were significant dose responses in the risk with increasing intensity of smoking in both men and women (**FIGURE 30.4**), and significant risk reductions were evident in former smokers. The investigators concluded that cigarette smoking is clearly implicated in the etiology of renal cell carcinoma (Hunt, van der Hel, McMillan, Boffetta, & Brennan, 2005). It is also noteworthy that two case–control studies suggest there may be an association between exposure to environmental smoke and the risk of developing renal cell carcinoma, although further studies will be needed to confirm this (Hu & Ugnat, 2005; Theis, Dolwick Grieb, Burr, Siddiqui, & Asal, 2008).

Obesity and Renal Cell Carcinoma

Numerous epidemiologic investigations suggest there is an association between obesity and the risk of developing renal cell carcinoma. In a recent meta-analysis of 21 cohort studies involving 15,144 cases, the combined estimates of RR were elevated for overweight (body mass index [BMI]: 25–29.9, RR = 1.3) and obese subjects (BMI: 30–39.9, RR = 1.8) compared to those of normal weight (BMI: 20–24.9). Risk elevations were similar for obese men (RR = 1.6) and obese women (RR = 2.0), and each unit of BMI increase above 25 produced a risk increase of approximately 7% (Wang & Xu, 2014). These results are in agreement with earlier meta-analyses and suggest that obese people have a nearly twofold increase in the risk of developing renal cell carcinomas compared to those of normal weight (Bergström et al.,

2001; Ildaphonse, George, & Mathew, 2009; Mathew, George, & Ildaphonse, 2009).

Hypertension and Renal Cell Carcinoma

Regulation of blood pressure is an important kidney function, and as such, hypertension has been extensively examined as a risk factor for the development of renal cell carcinoma. As discussed in the following paragraphs, several epidemiologic studies of hypertension and renal cell carcinoma in different populations show reasonable consistency in revealing an association; nevertheless, whether hypertension is a cause or an effect of this malignancy remains a topic of high controversy.

Chow and colleagues examined the health records of 363,992 Swedish men who underwent at least one physical examination during 1971–1992 and were followed until death or the end of the study in 1995. Cases of kidney cancer (759 with renal cell carcinoma and 136 with transitional cell carcinoma of the renal pelvis) were identified through cross-linkage of data with the nationwide Swedish Cancer Registry. Results revealed that obesity and hypertension independently increased the risk of developing renal cell carcinoma but not transitional cell carcinoma, whereas smoking was a risk factor for both forms of kidney cancer (Chow, Gridley, Fraumeni, & Järvholm, 2000).

Choi and colleagues examined the association between death from kidney cancer and baseline hypertension in a large cohort of 576,562 Korean men who were studied during 1992–2001. Hypertension was found to significantly increase the risk (RR = 2.43), and the risk was particularly high among cigarette smokers (RR = 8.18) (Choi, Jee, Sull, & Nam, 2005).

Flaherty and colleagues examined hypertension, thiazide use, BMI, weight change, and smoking as risk factors for renal cell carcinoma in prospective cohorts being followed in the United States. The study population included 118,191 women enrolled in the U.S. Nurses' Health Study and 48,953 men enrolled in the Health Professionals Follow-Up Study. Analysis was based on 155 incident cases reported during 24 years of follow-up for women, and 110 incident cases reported during 12 years of follow-up for men. With adjustment for other variables, hypertension significantly increased the risk of cancer development in both women (RR = 1.9) and men (RR = 1.8). Risk increases were also noted for obesity and chronic smoking, but there was no increase with thiazide use (Flaherty et al., 2005).

Vatten and colleagues conducted a prospective cohort study of blood pressure and renal cell carcinoma in 36,728 women and 35,688 men in Norway. Compared to normotensive individuals, women with elevated blood pressure (systolic blood pressure exceeding 150 mm Hg) had twice the risk of developing renal cell carcinoma (RR = 2.0); however, results were inconsistent for men (Vatten, Trichopoulos, Holmen, & Nilsen, 2007).

Weikert and colleagues examined blood pressure and renal cell carcinoma in the European Prospective Investigation into Cancer and Nutrition (EPIC). Blood pressure was measured in 296,638 men and women recruited in eight European countries during 1992–1998. Information on the use of antihypertensive medications was available for 254,935 of these individuals. During an average follow-up of more than 6 years, 250 cases of renal cell carcinoma were detected. Elevated blood pressure (systolic blood pressure exceeding 160 mm Hg) was found to be an independent risk factor (RR = 2.48). Risk estimates did not differ by gender or type of antihypertensive medication, and individuals taking antihypertensive medications were not found to be at increased risk unless blood pressure was poorly controlled (Weikert et al., 2008).

Corrao and colleagues conducted a meta-analysis of 18 studies that examined the association of renal cell carcinoma with hypertension and use of antihypertensive medications. The pooled estimate of risk for hypertension was significantly increased (odds ratio [OR] = 1.62). Risk increases were also noted for use of antihypertensive medications, although effects were attenuated with adjustment for other factors (Corrao, Scotti, Bagnardi, & Sega, 2007).

What is clear from these studies is that hypertension is independently associated with a significant increase in the risk of developing renal cell carcinoma in both men and women. What is as yet unclear is the sequence of pathogenesis. Does malignant transformation induce changes in renin and other vasoactive substances in the kidney that increase blood pressure, or does an increase in the blood pressure cause malignant transformation?

Diabetes Mellitus and Kidney Cancer

Because type 2 diabetes is etiologically linked to chronic diseases of the kidney (nephrosis and nephritis), it is logical to examine the association between diabetes and kidney cancer. Investigators at the Karolinska Institute in Sweden recently examined this association by meta-analysis of nine prospective cohort studies involving patients from Europe, Asia, and North America. Across all studies, individuals with diabetes were at increased risk for the development of kidney cancer compared to those without diabetes (combined RR = 1.42). However, there was statistically significant heterogeneity among studies, and the association with diabetes was stronger in women (RR = 1.70) than in men (RR = 1.26). Additional studies designed to assess the time interval between the onset of diabetes and development of kidney cancer are needed to provide definitive evidence of a causal link (Larsson & Wolk, 2010).

Genetic Abnormalities in Renal Cell Carcinoma

Renal cell carcinomas occasionally occur in a familial setting in association with certain genetic abnormalities; however, only a small fraction of cases (about 4%) report a positive family history of kidney cancer (Lipworth, Tarone, Lund, & McLaughlin, 2009). Familial cases often develop multifocal and/or bilateral tumors at a relatively early age. Among the heritable cancer syndromes, the most important are the von Hippel–Lindau (VHL) syndrome and Birt–Hogg–Dubé syndrome.

von Hippel–Lindau Syndrome and Renal Cell Carcinoma

The von Hippel–Lindau syndrome is a rare autosomal dominant cancer syndrome with a prevalence rate of about 1 in 36,000 individuals. This syndrome is caused by a mutant tumor–suppressor gene called the von Hippel–Lindau (*VHL*) gene. Approximately one-third of patients who carry a mutant form of the *VHL* gene develop renal cell carcinoma (clear cell type). Other clinical characteristics include retinal angiomas, hemangioblastomas of the central nervous system, islet cell pancreatic tumors, and pheochromocytomas of the adrenal glands. The syndrome is named after the physicians who first described its clinical signs in afflicted patients. The German ophthalmologist Eugen von Hippel first described the angiomas of the eye (von Hippel, 1904), and the Swedish pathologist Arvid Lindau first described the angiomas of the cerebellum and spine (Lindau, 1927).

The *VHL* gene, which is located on the short arm of chromosome 3, regulates the transcription of other genes that encode proteins critical for cell division and function such as hypoxia-inducible factor (HIF), vascular endothelial growth factor (VEGF), platelet-derived growth factor (PDGF), and transforming growth factors (TGF-a and TGF-b). Mutations in the *VHL* gene accelerate tumor initiation, growth, and development.

von Hippel–Lindau Gene and Sporadic Renal Cell Carcinoma

It has recently been discovered that mutations of the *VHL* gene are common not only in von Hippel–Lindau syndrome, but also in sporadic (nonfamilial) cases of clear cell renal carcinoma. In a study of 187 Japanese patients with malignancy, 108 tumor samples were found to have *VHL* abnormalities (98 with *VHL* mutations and 10 with *VHL* hypermethylation) (Yao et al., 2002). In a more recent study of 205 clear cell tumors ascertained from patients in Central Europe, investigators found *VHL* abnormalities in 91% of cases (82.4% with *VHL* mutations and 8.3% with *VHL* hypermethylation). These studies suggest that most clear cell tumors of the kidney arise in association with genetic or epigenetic modifications of a single gene, the *VHL* gene (Nickerson et al., 2008). Indeed, the *VHL* gene has potential as a biomarker, a prognostic indicator, and/or a target for molecular therapy.

Birt–Hogg–Dubé Syndrome

Birt–Hogg–Dubé syndrome is a rare autosomal dominant syndrome that has been identified in about 50 families worldwide. This syndrome is characterized by renal cancer, renal and pulmonary cysts, and benign tumors of the hair follicles (Birt, Hogg, & Dubé, 1977). It is caused by mutations in the folliculin gene (*FLCN*), a tumor–suppressor gene located on the short arm of chromosome 17 (Toro et al., 2008).

Occupational Exposures and Renal Cell Carcinoma

A few epidemiologic investigations have examined exposure to toxic compounds and the risk of developing renal cell carcinomas. Mandel and colleagues conducted an international case–control study involving 1732 incident cases of renal cell carcinoma and 2309 controls from centers in Australia, Denmark, Germany, Sweden, and the United States. Significant associations were found for occupational exposures to asbestos (RR = 1.4), cadmium (RR = 2.0), petroleum products (RR = 1.6), and dry-cleaning solvents (RR = 1.4) (Mandel et al., 1995). Synergism involving environmental exposures have also been noted in some studies. For example, in an early case–control study of cadmium exposure and renal cancer, the combination of cadmium exposure and cigarette smoking was found to increase the risk more than fourfold (Kolonel, 1976).

Development of renal cell carcinoma has been found in association with somatic genetic mutations in the von Hippel–Lindau (*VHL*) tumor–suppressor gene. As already discussed, the *VHL* gene functions by controlling steps in the cell cycle and, if mutated, cell proliferation continues unabated. Brauch and colleagues studied 151 cases of renal cell carcinoma (clear cell type), 44 of whom had long-term occupational exposure to trichloroethylene, an industrial solvent, and 107 cases without exposure. Somatic mutations were detected in tumor specimens from 33 of the 44 (75%) cases exposed to trichloroethylene, whereas such mutations were totally absent in tumors from the 107 nonexposed cases. Results suggest that exposure to trichloroethylene may trigger mutational events in the *VHL* gene that are associated with the development of renal cell carcinoma (Brauch et al., 1999).

Acquired Cystic Kidney Disease and Renal Cell Carcinoma

Acquired cystic kidney disease develops in approximately 50% of patients who are maintained on chronic hemodialysis and peritoneal dialysis for kidney failure. A major complication of this condition is the development of renal cell carcinoma. Follow-up studies of patients with acquired cystic kidney disease suggest that their risk of developing renal cell carcinoma is 50-fold higher than in the general population. Careful surveillance of dialysis patients by periodic ultrasonography and computerized tomography is recommended for the early detection of such tumors (Brennan, Stilmant, Babayan, & Siroky, 1991; Truong, Krishnan, Cao, Barrios, & Suki, 1995).

Analgesics and Renal Cell Carcinoma

Although some studies have found an association between renal cell carcinoma and heavy or long-term use of analgesics, others have not. Chow studied associations in 440 cases of renal cell carcinoma, spouses of 151 cases, and 691 control subjects. No significant excess risk was observed with regular use of aspirin, acetaminophen, or combinations of these agents. The investigators concluded that the use of analgesics is not likely to pose a significant risk for the development of renal cell carcinoma (Chow et al., 2000).

Risk Factors for Transitional Cell Carcinoma of the Renal Pelvis

The profile of risk factors associated with the development of transitional cell carcinomas of the renal pelvis is essentially the same as for transitional cell carcinomas of the urinary bladder. The dominant risk factor is chronic exposure to tobacco smoke, which has been found to elevate the risk two- to threefold compared to nonsmokers (Boffetta, 2008). Carcinogenesis associated with smoking is primarily the result of aromatic amines and arylamines present in cigarette smoke that reach the mucosal lining of the renal pelvis, ureters, and urinary bladder.

Several environmental and occupational factors increase the risk including occupational exposure to arylamines such as 2-naphthylamine, 4-aminobiphenyl, benzidine, and other compounds and intermediates in the synthesis of azo-dyes and pigments used in the textile, printing, plastic, rubber, and cable industries. Long-term exposure to these compounds among workers in these industries increases the risk by about 50% (Vineis, 1994).

The analgesic medication phenacetin was once widely used in European nations until the drug was linked to cancers of the renal pelvis and urinary bladder (Hoover & Fraumeni, 1981; Johansson & Wahlqvist, 1977). A case–control investigation found more than a sixfold increase in the risk of bladder cancer development due to heavy phenacetin ingestion among women (Piper, Tonascia, & Matanoski, 1985). Phenactin compounds were removed from the U.S. market in 1983 and have now been discontinued worldwide (Chow, McLaughlin, Linet, Niwa, & Mandel, 1994).

Prevention of Kidney Cancer

The rising global trajectory in the incidence and mortality rates of renal cancer during the past 25 years can be partially explained by greater use of imaging technologies such as ultrasound, computed tomography, and magnetic resonance imaging. Nevertheless, despite increased early detection and surgical excision of small renal tumors, mortality rates of kidney cancer are continuing to rise throughout the world.

Three major risk factors—smoking, hypertension, and obesity—significantly increase the risk of developing kidney cancer. These factors constitute a web of causation that has contributed to the rising global burden of kidney cancer. (The prevalence of obesity has reached pandemic proportions, and the rates of smoking and hypertension are also increasing in many populations.) Effective preventive strategies must therefore reverse the trajectory of these factors through control of weight and blood pressure and prevention of tobacco use.

References

Aron, M., Nguyen, M. M., Stein, R. J., & Gill, I. S. (2008). Impact of gender in renal cell carcinoma: An analysis of the SEER database. *European Urology, 54*(1), 133–142.

Bergström, A., Hsieh, C. C., Lindblad, P., Lu, C. M., Cook, N. R., & Wolk, A. (2001). Obesity and renal cell cancer—A quantitative review. *British Journal of Cancer, 85*(7), 984–990.

Birt, A. R., Hogg, G. R., & Dubé, W. J. (1977). Hereditary multiple fibrofolliculomas with trichodiscomas and acrochordons. *Archives of Dermatology, 113*(12), 1674–1677.

Boffetta, P. (2008). Tobacco smoking and risk of bladder cancer. *Scandinavian Journal of Urology and Nephrology, 42*(S218), 45–54.

Brauch, H., Weirich, G., Hornauer, M. A., Störkel, S., Wöhl, T., & Brüning, T. (1999). Trichloroethylene exposure and specific somatic mutations in patients with renal cell carcinoma. *Journal of the National Cancer Institute, 91*(10), 854–861.

Bray, F., Ferlay, J., Soerjomataram, I., Siegel, R. L., Torre, L. A., & Jemal, A. (2018). Global cancer statistics 2018: GLOBOCAN estimates of incidence and mortality worldwide for 36 cancers in 185 countries. *CA: A Cancer Journal for Clinicians, 68*(6), 394–424.

Brennan, J. F., Stilmant, M. M., Babayan, R. K., & Siroky, M. B. (1991). Acquired renal cystic disease: Implications for the urologist. *British Journal of Urology, 67*(4), 342–348.

Choi, M. Y., Jee, S. H., Sull, J. W., & Nam, C. M. (2005). The effect of hypertension on the risk for kidney cancer in Korean men. *Kidney International, 67*(2), 647–652.

Chow, W. H., Dong, L. M., & Devesa, S. S. (2010). Epidemiology and risk factors for kidney cancer. *Nature Reviews Urology, 7*, 245–257.

Chow, W. H., Gridley, G., Fraumeni, J. F., Jr., & Järvholm, B. N. (2000). Obesity, hypertension, and the risk of kidney cancer in men. *New England Journal of Medicine, 343*(18), 1305–1311.

Chow, W. H., McLaughlin, J. K., Linet, M. S., Niwa, S., & Mandel, J. S. (1994). Use of analgesics and risk of renal cell cancer. *International Journal of Cancer, 59*(4), 467–470.

Corrao, G., Scotti, L., Bagnardi, V., & Sega, R. (2007). Hypertension, antihypertensive therapy and renal-cell cancer: A meta-analysis. *Current Drug Safety, 2*(2), 125–133.

Ferlay, J., Bray, F., Pisani, P., & Parkin, D. M. (2004). *GLOBOCAN 2002. Cancer incidence, mortality, and prevalence worldwide. IARC Cancer Base No. 5, version 2.0.* Lyon, France: IARC Press.

Ferlay, J., Ervik, M., Lam, F., Colombet, M., Mery, L., Piñeros, M., … Bray, F. (2018). *Global cancer observatory: Cancer today.* Lyon, France: International Agency for Research on Cancer. Retrieved from https://gco.iarc.fr/today

Ferlay, J., Shin, H. R., Forman, D., Mathers, C., & Parkin, D. M. (2010). Estimates of worldwide burden of cancer in 2008. *International Journal of Cancer, 127*(12), 2893–2917.

Ferlay, J., Soerjomataram, I., Ervik, M., Dikshit, R., Eser, S., Mathers, C., … Bray, F. (2013). *GLOBOCAN 2012 v1.0, cancer incidence and mortality worldwide: IARC CancerBase No. 11* [Internet]. Lyon, France: International Agency for Research on Cancer. Retrieved from http://globocan.iarc.fr

Fitzmaurice, C., Akinyemiju, T. F., Al Lami, F. H., Alam, T., Alizadeh-Navaei, R., Allen, C., … Global Burden of Disease Cancer Collaboration. (2018). Global, regional, and national cancer incidence, mortality, years of life lost, years lived with disability, and disability-adjusted life-years for 29 cancer groups, 1990 to 2016: A systematic analysis for the Global Burden of Disease Study. *JAMA Oncology.* Online publication. doi:10.1001/jamaoncol.2018.2706.

Fitzmaurice, C., Allen, C., Barber, R. M., Barregard, L., Bhutta, Z. A., Brenner, H., … Global Burden of Disease Cancer Collaboration. (2017). Global, regional, and national cancer incidence, mortality, years of life lost, years lived with disability, and disability-adjusted life-years for 32 cancer groups, 1990 to 2015: A systematic analysis for the Global Burden of Disease Study. *JAMA Oncology, 3*(4), 524–548.

Flaherty, K. T., Fuchs, C. S., Colditz, G. A., Stampfer, M. J., Speizer, F. E., Willett, W. C., & Curhan, G. C. (2005). A prospective study of body mass index, hypertension, and smoking and the risk of renal cell carcinoma (United States). *Cancer Causes and Control, 16*(9), 1099–1106.

Gandaglia, G., Ravi, P., Abdollah, F., Abd-El-Barr, A., Becker, A., Popa, I., … Sun, M. (2014). Contemporary incidence and mortality rates of kidney cancer in the United States. *Canadian Urological Association Journal, 8*(7–8), 247–252.

Hollingsworth, J. M., Miller, D. C., Daignault, S., & Hollenbeck, B. K. (2006). Rising incidence of small renal masses: A need to reassess treatment effect. *Journal of the National Cancer Institute, 98*, 1331–1334.

Hoover, R., & Fraumeni, J. F., Jr. (1981). Drug-induced cancer. *Cancer, 47*(5 Suppl.), 1071–1080.

Hu, J., & Ugnat, A. M. (2005). Active and passive smoking and risk of renal cell carcinoma in Canada. *European Journal of Cancer, 41*, 770–778.

Hunt, J. D., van der Hel, O. L., McMillan, G. P., Boffetta, P., & Brennan, P. (2005). Renal cell carcinoma in relation to cigarette smoking: Meta-analysis of 24 studies. *International Journal of Cancer, 114*, 101–108.

Ildaphonse, G., George, P. S., & Mathew, A. (2009). Obesity and kidney cancer risk in men: A meta-analysis (1992–2008). *Asian Pacific Journal of Cancer Prevention, 10*, 279–286.

Johansson, S., & Wahlqvist, L. (1977). Tumours of urinary bladder and ureter associated with abuse of phenacetin-containing analgesics. *Acta Pathologica Microbiologica Scandinavica [A], 85*, 768–774.

Kim, S., & Chung, D. H. (2006). Pediatric solid malignancies: Neuroblastoma and Wilms' tumor. *Surgical Clinics of North America, 86*(2), 469–487.

Kolonel, L. N. (1976). Association of cadmium with renal cancer. *Cancer, 37*, 1782–1787.

Kumar, V., Abbas, A. K., & Aster, J. C. (2014). *Robbins and Cotran pathologic basis of disease* (9th ed.). Philadelphia, PA: Mosby & Saunders.

Larsson, S. C., & Wolk, A. (2010). Diabetes mellitus and incidence of kidney cancer: A meta-analysis of cohort studies. *Diabetologia, 54*(5), 1013–1018.

Lindau, A. (1927). Zur Frage der Angiomatosis Retinae und Ihrer Hirncomplikation. *Acta Ophthalmologica, 4,* 193–226.

Lipworth, L., Tarone, R. E., Lund, L., & McLaughlin, J. K. (2009). Epidemiologic characteristics and risk factors for renal cell cancer. *Clinical Epidemiology, 2009*(1), 33–43.

Mandel, J. S., McLaughlin, J. K., Schlehofer, B., Mellemgaard, A., Helmert, U., Lindblad, P., ... Adami, H.-O. (1995). International renal-cell cancer study. IV. Occupation. *International Journal of Cancer, 61*(5), 601–605.

Mathew, A., George, P. S., & Ildaphonse, G. (2009). Obesity and kidney cancer risk in women: A meta-analysis (1992–2008). *Asian Pacific Journal of Cancer Prevention, 10,* 471–478.

Nickerson, M. L., Jaeger, E., Shi, Y., Durocher, J. A., Mahurkar, S., Zaridze, D., ... Moore, L. E. (2008). Improved identification of von Hippel-Lindau gene alterations in clear cell renal tumors. *Clinical Cancer Research, 14*(15), 4726–4734.

Pantuck, A. J., Zisman, A., & Belldegrun, A. S. (2001). The changing natural history of renal cell carcinoma. *Journal of Urology, 166*(5), 1611–1623.

Parkin, D. M., Bray, F., Ferlay, J., & Pisani, P. (2005). Global cancer statistics, 2002. *CA: A Cancer Journal for Clinicians, 55,* 74–108.

Parkin, D. M., Pisani, P., & Ferlay, J. (1999a). Global cancer statistics. *CA: A Cancer Journal for Clinicians, 49*(1), 33–64.

Parkin, D. M., Pisani, P., & Ferlay, J. (1999b). Estimates of the worldwide incidence of 25 major cancers in 1990. *International Journal of Cancer, 80*(6), 827–841.

Pascual, D., & Borque, A. (2008). Epidemiology of kidney cancer. *Advances in Urology, 2008,* 782381.

Piper, J. M., Tonascia, J., & Matanoski, G. M. (1985). Heavy phenacetin use and bladder cancer in women aged 20–49 years. *New England Journal of Medicine, 313*(5), 292–295.

Robbins, S. L., & Cotran, R. S. (1979). *Pathologic basis of disease* (2nd ed.). Philadelphia, PA: W. B. Saunders.

Theis, R. P., Dolwick Grieb, S. M., Burr, D., Siddiqui, T., & Asal, N. R. (2008). Smoking, environmental tobacco smoke and risk of renal cell cancer: A population-based case-control study. *BMC Cancer, 8,* 387.

Toro, J. R., Wei, M. H., Glenn, G. M., Weinreich, M., Toure, O., Vocke, C., ... Linehan, W. M. (2008). *BHD* mutations, clinical and molecular genetic investigations of Birt–Hogg–Dubé syndrome: A new series of 50 families and a review of published reports. *Journal of Medical Genetics, 45*(6), 321–331.

Truong, L. D., Krishnan, B., Cao, J. T., Barrios, R., & Suki, W. N. (1995). Renal neoplasm in acquired cystic kidney disease. *American Journal of Kidney Diseases, 26*(1), 1–12.

Vatten, L. J., Trichopoulos, D., Holmen, J., & Nilsen, T. I. (2007). Blood pressure and renal cancer risk: The HUNT Study in Norway. *British Journal of Cancer, 97*(1), 112–114.

Vineis, P. (1994). Epidemiology of cancer from exposure to arylamines. *Environmental Health Perspectives, 102*(Suppl. 6), 7–10.

von Hippel, E. (1904). Ueber eine sehr seltene Erkrankung der Netzhaut. *Albrecht von Graefes Archiv für Ophthalmologie, 59,* 83–106.

Wang, F., & Xu, Y. (2014). Body mass index and risk of renal cell cancer: A dose-response meta-analysis of published cohort studies. *International Journal of Cancer, 135*(7), 1673–1686.

Weikert, S., Boeing, H., Pischon, T., Weikert, C., Olsen, A., Tjonneland, A., ... Riboli, E. (2008). Blood pressure and risk of renal cell carcinoma in the European prospective investigation into cancer and nutrition. *American Journal of Epidemiology, 167*(4), 438–446.

Weikert, S., & Ljungberg, B. (2010). Contemporary epidemiology of renal cell carcinoma: Perspectives of primary prevention. *World Journal of Urology, 28*(3), 247–252.

Wong, M. C. S., Goggins, W. B., Yip, B. H. K., Fung, F. D. H., Leung, C., Fang, Y., ... Ng, C. F. (2017). Incidence and mortality of kidney cancer: Temporal patterns and global trends in 39 countries. *Scientific Reports, 7,* 15698.

Yao, M., Yoshida, M., Kishida, T., Nakaigawa, N., Baba, M., Kobayashi, K., ... Kondo, K. (2002). VHL tumor suppressor gene alterations associated with good prognosis in sporadic clear-cell renal carcinoma. *Journal of the National Cancer Institute, 94*(20), 1569–1575.

© Andrew Brookes/Getty Images

CHAPTER 31

Epidemiology of Cancers of the Thyroid and Parathyroid

▶ Thyroid Gland: Anatomy and Function

The human thyroid is a butterfly-shaped gland located in the anterior neck inferior to the thyroid cartilage (also known as the Adam's apple). The word *thyroid* means "shield," which describes the basic shape of the thyroid cartilage.

The thyroid produces iodine-containing thyroid hormones, the principal ones being triiodothyronine (T_3) and thyroxine (T_4). Triiodothyronine is 2–3 times more potent than thyroxine, and considerably more T_4 is produced than T_3 (20:1 ratio). These circulating hormones are essential in regulating the rate of metabolism in the body. Inside the cell, T_3 and T_4 stimulate energy production by the mitochondria and promote glucose catabolism, protein synthesis, lipolysis, and excretion of cholesterol. Thyroid hormones also influence growth and development in early life and participate in several essential physiologic functions throughout life, such as maintenance of normal cardiac rhythm, muscle tone, and neuronal function in the sympathetic nervous system (Kumar, Abbas, & Aster, 2014).

The functional unit of the thyroid is the thyroid follicle. The thyroid is composed of thousands of spherical thyroid follicles, each of which contains a material called *colloid* that contains iodide (the storage form of iodine) and thyroglobulin (the glycoprotein bound to thyroid hormones). Thyroid hormones are synthesized by cuboidal epithelial cells that line the thyroid follicles. The essential substrates for biosynthesis are the amino acid tyrosine and the mineral iodine. The biosynthesis of thyroid hormones (T_3 and T_4) is regulated by peptide hormones secreted by the hypothalamus and the anterior pituitary gland. In response to low blood levels of thyroid hormones or neurological signals, the hypothalamus secretes a protein called *thyroid-releasing hormone (TRH)* into special blood vessels connected to the pituitary gland, which in turn triggers the anterior pituitary to secrete a second protein called *thyroid-stimulating hormone (TSH)* or thyrotropin into the blood. In response to TSH, receptors on the cell membranes of thyroid epithelial cells (thyrotropin receptors) activate the biosynthetic pathway for the production of thyroid hormones (T_3 and T_4). Thyroid hormones are stored in a glycoprotein called thyroglobulin, which also is synthesized in the thyroid epithelium. Thyroid hormones are secreted into the blood from the thyroglobulin (colloid) stored within thyroid follicles. Thyroid hormones (T_3 and T_4) are transported in the blood bound to a carrier protein known as *thyroxine-binding globulin*. The secretion and release of T_3 and T_4 are regulated by blood levels of thyroid hormones (i.e., low levels stimulate the release of active T_3 and T_4) (**FIGURE 31.1**).

Special cells of the thyroid gland called *C cells* produce a polypeptide hormone called *calcitonin* that helps regulate calcium homeostasis throughout the body. Relatively small parathyroid glands (usually four) are located at the periphery of the thyroid gland.

FIGURE 31.1 The Hypothalamus–Pituitary Axis: Feedback Control of the Thyroid Gland.

The parathyroid glands synthesize parathyroid hormone (PTH), which together with calcitonin and the active form of vitamin D, regulate levels of calcium and phosphorous in the blood, the bones, and most other tissues (Kumar et al., 2014).

▶ Benign Adenomas of the Thyroid Gland

Thyroid nodules arising from thyroid follicles are relatively common and are detected approximately three times more often in women than in men. Approximately 90%–95% of solitary thyroid nodules are benign, and treatment by simple excision is curative; however, careful histological examination of tissue is always necessary to rule out malignant transformation. Like thyroid cancer (discussed in the next section), the major risk factors for thyroid adenoma include radiation exposure, iodine deficiency or excess, and personal and/or familial history of thyroid disorders.

The thyroid gland is extremely sensitive to radiation exposure. Elaine Ron and Alina Brenner at the Radiation Epidemiology Branch of the U.S. National Cancer Institute recently reviewed major studies of cohorts of individuals exposed to radiation from various sources to evaluate dosage effects on the development of thyroid adenomas and other nonmalignant thyroid disorders. They found that a wide range of doses of ionizing radiation increased the risk of developing benign thyroid adenomas and nodules in a variety of populations and settings. Their findings suggest that the elevation in risk continues for decades following exposure (Ron & Brenner, 2010). Investigators in New York monitored the incidence of thyroid adenomas in a cohort of 2657 infants given X-ray treatment for thymus enlargement and a comparison cohort of 4833 untreated siblings. Individuals in these cohorts were followed for up to 50 years. The observed rates of thyroid adenoma increased in a linear dose response with the level of radiation, and risk increases persisted throughout the entire follow-up period. Exposure levels of 6 Gy increased the relative risk more than sixfold. (1 Gy is approximately equivalent to 100 rads of ionizing radiation.) Other significant risk factors included a personal medical history and/or a family history of thyroid disorders (Shore, Hildreth, Dvoretsky, Pasternack, & Andresen, 1993). The question of whether thyroid adenomas can undergo malignant transformation has been debated for decades. To address this question, Franceschi et al. conducted a pooled analysis of 12 case–control studies including 2094 women and 425 men with cancer of the thyroid and age-matched control groups of 3248 women and 928 men who were disease-free. Significant risk increases were noted for history of goiter (odds ratio [OR] = 5.9) and history of benign thyroid adenomas (OR = 29.9 in women and 18 cases versus 0 controls in men). The investigators concluded that goiter and benign nodules/adenomas were strong risk factors for malignant transformation in the thyroid gland (Franceschi et al., 1999).

Recent pathological studies suggest that a subset of thyroid adenomas display atypical morphology, a pathologic entity known as *atypia*, and that such neoplasms may represent an intermediate step in the progression of adenoma to invasive carcinoma. More studies are needed to clarify the molecular features of premalignant lesions of the thyroid to determine their potential for malignant transformation and establish definitive guidelines for diagnosis and treatment (McHenry & Phitayakorn, 2011; Vasko et al., 2004).

▶ Malignant Tumors of the Thyroid and Parathyroid

Malignant tumors of the thyroid gland are rare. Nevertheless, all thyroid nodules must be carefully examined under the microscope to distinguish benign from malignant tumors. Approximately 90%–95% of thyroid malignancies are carcinomas that arise from the cuboidal epithelium that lines the thyroid follicles. These cells normally synthesize thyroid hormones (T_3 and T_4) and thyroglobulin.

Pathologists routinely classify thyroid carcinomas into various subtypes. The most common subtype is *papillary carcinoma*, which constitutes about 70% of all thyroid malignancies. Papillary thyroid carcinoma is an encapsulated, well-differentiated tumor that shows a papillary growth pattern (finger-like projections) under the microscope. The second most common subtype is *follicular carcinoma*, which constitutes about 30% of thyroid cancers. Follicular thyroid carcinoma also consists of well-differentiated cells, but the growth pattern lacks papillary formations. A small subset of thyroid malignancies consists of *medullary thyroid carcinomas*, which arise from the parafollicular C cells that secrete calcitonin (a polypeptide hormone that helps regulate calcium and phosphorous in bone remodeling). Medullary thyroid carcinomas constitute only 5%–10% of all thyroid malignancies.

Malignancies of the *parathyroid glands* are distinct from thyroid cancer and are discussed in a separate section of this chapter. Parathyroid tumors arise from cells that secrete PTH (a polypeptide hormone that increases calcium levels in the blood).

▶ Global Burden of Thyroid Cancer

Cancer of the thyroid afflicts 3–4 times more women than men. During 2018, 567,233 new cases were diagnosed in the world population, and 41,071 people died from thyroid cancer. Of these, 436,344 cases (77%) and 25,514 deaths (62%) occurred in women. The age-adjusted incidence rate in women was triple the rate in men (10.2 per 100,000 versus 3.1 per 100,000) whereas the mortality rates were similar (0.5 per 100,000 in women and 0.4 per 100,000 in men) (Bray et al., 2018).

During 2000–2018, the annual number of incident cases of thyroid cancer detected in the world population increased more than fourfold, whereas the number of deaths changed relatively little (**FIGURE 31.2**). Age-adjusted incidence and mortality rates actually show inverse trends. During 2002–2018, the incidence more than tripled among women (3.3 versus 10.2 per 100,000), whereas the mortality declined by 38% (0.8 versus 0.5 per 100,000). As discussed in a later section of this chapter, the inverse trends of incidence and mortality may largely reflect the increased early detection of small papillary thyroid tumors that were treated by complete surgical resection (Bray et al., 2018; Ferlay et al., 2004, 2010, 2013, 2018; Fitzmaurice et al., 2017, 2018; Parkin, Bray,

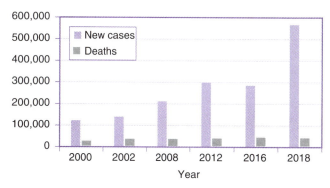

FIGURE 31.2 Global Trends of Thyroid Cancer, 2000–2018.

Caption: Values for 2016 are means for the years 2015 and 2016.

Data from Bray, F., Ferlay, J., Soerjomataram, I., Siegel, R. L., Torre, L. A., & Jemal, A. (2018). Global cancer statistics 2018: GLOBOCAN estimates of incidence and mortality worldwide for 36 cancers in 185 countries. *CA: A Cancer Journal for Clinicians, 68*(6), 394–424; Ferlay, J., Shin, H. R., Forman, D., Mathers, C., & Parkin, D. M. (2010). Estimates of worldwide burden of cancer in 2008. *International Journal of Cancer, 127*(12), 2893–2917; Ferlay, J., Soerjomataram, I., Ervik, M., Dikshit, R., Eser, S., Mathers, C., ... Bray, F. (2013). *GLOBOCAN 2012 v1.0. Cancer incidence and mortality worldwide: IARC CancerBase No. 11* [Internet]. Lyon, France: International Agency for Research on Cancer. Retrieved from http://globocan.iarc.fr; Parkin, D. M., Bray, F., Ferlay, J., & Pisani, P. (2001). Estimating the world cancer burden: GLOBOCAN 2000. *International Journal of Cancer, 94*, 153–156; Parkin, D. M., Bray, F., Ferlay, J., & Pisani, P. (2005). Global cancer statistics, 2002. *CA: A Cancer Journal for Clinicians, 55*, 74–108; Fitzmaurice, C., Allen, C., Barber, R. M., Barregard, L., Bhutta, Z. A., Brenner, H., ... Global Burden of Disease Cancer Collaboration. (2017). Global, regional, and national cancer incidence, mortality, years of life lost, years lived with disability, and disability-adjusted life-years for 32 cancer groups, 1990 to 2015: a systematic analysis for the Global Burden of Disease Study. *JAMA Oncology. 3*(4), 524–548; Fitzmaurice, C., Akinyemiju, T. F., Al Lami, F. H., Alam, T., Alizadeh-Navaei, R., Allen, C., ... Global Burden of Disease Cancer Collaboration. (2018). Global, regional, and national cancer incidence, mortality, years of life lost, years lived with disability, and disability-adjusted life-years for 29 cancer groups, 1990 to 2016: A systematic analysis for the Global Burden of Disease Study. *JAMA Oncology.* Published online June 02, 2018. doi:10.1001/jamaoncol.2018.2706.

Ferlay, & Pisani, 2005; Parkin, Pisani, & Ferlay, 1999a, 1999b; Parkin et al., 1992).

FIGURE 31.3 shows the global distributions of incidence and mortality rates of thyroid cancer among women in 2018. Incidence rates are markedly higher in developed countries than developing countries; for example, the average age-adjusted incidence in U.S. and Canadian women (~26 per 100,000) is 10–20 times higher than the incidence among women living in India and sub-Saharan Africa (1–2 per 100,000). In contrast, mortality rates of thyroid cancer show a much narrower range, e.g., approximately 0.4 deaths per 100,000 in Africa and Asia compared to 0.3 deaths per 100,000 in Australia, Canada, and the United States. The highest mortality rate in 2018 was observed among women living in the South Pacific island nation of Samoa (~5 deaths per 100,000) and rates were also exceptionally high among women in Indonesia, the Philippines, and other Melanesian island nations (Ferlay et al., 2018). Factors contributing to the high thyroid cancer mortality rates in female populations of the Pacific Islands include the lack of access to medical services (Alto, 1997) plus the clustering of likely risk factors such as iodine deficiency, multiparity, and obesity. Interactions of risk factors for thyroid cancer are complex as discussed in following sections of this chapter.

Estimated age-standardized incidence rates (World) in 2018, thyroid, females, all ages

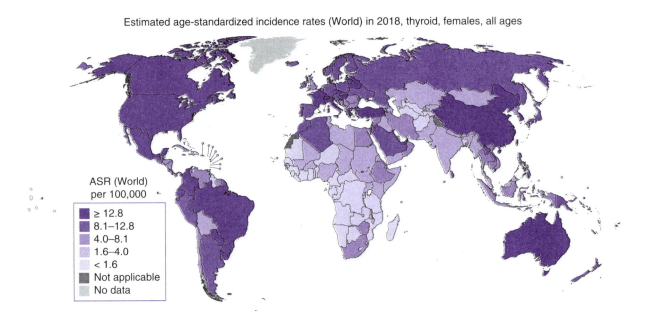

Estimated age-standardized mortality rates (World) in 2018, thyroid, females, all ages

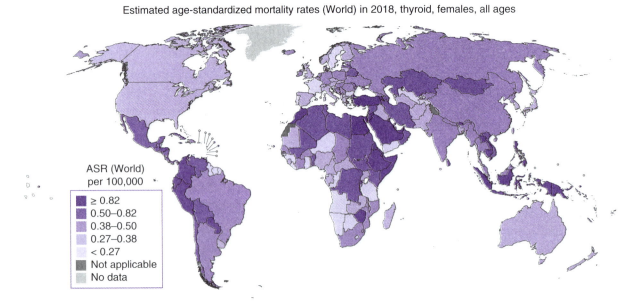

FIGURE 31.3 Global Incidence and Mortality Rates of Thyroid Cancer in Women, 2018.

Caption: ASR: Rates per 100,000 are age-standardized to the world population, 2000–2025.

Reproduced with permission from Ferlay, J., Ervik, M., Lam, F., Colombet, M., Mery, L., Piñeros, M., . . . Bray, F. (2018). *Global cancer observatory: Cancer today.* Lyon, France: International Agency for Research on Cancer. Available from: https://gco.iarc.fr/today, accessed [09 October 2018].

▶ Trends in Papillary and Follicular Thyroid Carcinoma

The incidence of thyroid cancer has increased dramatically in most developed countries during the past few decades; for example, in the United States the incidence rates have more than tripled since the 1970s increasing from less than 5 cases per 100,000 in 1970 to more than 15 cases per 100,000 in 2015. However, mortality has remained relatively constant over the same period at around 5 deaths per million (**FIGURE 31.4**).

To explore reasons for the increasing incidence of thyroid cancer in the U.S. population, Davies and Welch examined the annual incidence of pathologic subtypes of thyroid cancer for the period 1973–2002 using registry data from the Surveillance, Epidemiology, and End Results (SEER) system of the U.S. National Cancer Institute. As shown in **FIGURE 31.5**, the annual incidence of thyroid cancer increased 142% during the study period, from 3.6 per 100,000 to 8.7 per 100,000. This increase was almost entirely attributed to the corresponding 185% increase in the incidence of papillary thyroid carcinoma, from 2.7 per 100,000 to 7.7 per 100,000. In contrast, the incidence

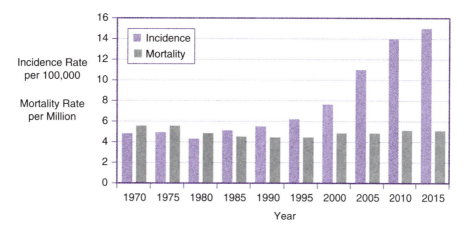

FIGURE 31.4 Incidence and Mortality of Thyroid Cancer, 1970–2015, United States.

Data from Noone, A. M., Howlader, N., Krapcho, M., Miller, D., Brest, A., Yu, M., … Cronin, K. A. (2018). *SEER cancer statistics review, 1975–2015.* Bethesda, MD: National Cancer Institute.

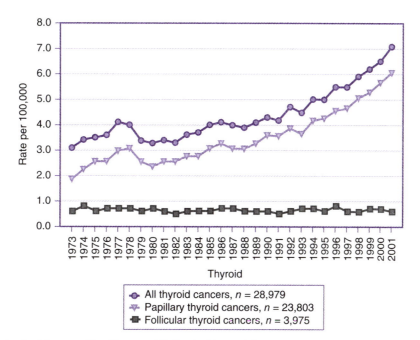

FIGURE 31.5 Trends in the Incidence of Papillary and Follicular Thyroid Carcinoma, 1973–2003, United States.

Data from Davies, L., & Welch, H. G. (2006). Increasing incidence of thyroid cancer in the United States, 1973–2002. *Journal of the American Medical Association, 295*(18), 2164–2167.

of follicular thyroid carcinoma did not change during the study period, and the mortality rates of thyroid cancer actually *declined* from 0.57 per 100,000 in 1973 to 0.47 per 100,000 in 2003. The investigators suggest that enhanced diagnostic scrutiny is the most likely explanation for these trends. They point out that ultrasound is routinely used to identify thyroid nodules that are only a few millimeters in diameter, and fine-needle aspiration and pathologic examination of specimens from small papillary tumors have been adopted as standard practice. The observed trends are therefore largely explainable by the increased early detection of small papillary thyroid tumors that were treated by complete surgical resection (Davies & Welch, 2006).

Risk Factors for Thyroid Cancer

Gender and Thyroid Cancer

Thyroid cancer as well as other thyroid disorders predominate in women. For example, iodine deficiency that causes nontoxic (simple) goiter, and autoimmune forms of thyroid disease (e.g., Graves' disease and Hashimoto's thyroiditis) are 2–3 times more common in women than in men.

Behavioral differences between men and women may partially explain the excess of thyroid disease in women. It is well known that women seek medical attention more often than men and may thus be more likely than men to undergo screening and diagnostic procedures that detect thyroid disorders.

Alternatively, biological gender differences may preferentially predispose women to thyroid disorders including thyroid neoplasms. For example, serum levels of TSH, a known promoter of thyroid hyperplasia, are elevated by menarche, pregnancy, surgical menopause (oophorectomy), use of oral contraceptives, and estrogen replacement therapy (Yao, Chiu, Strugnell, Gill, & Wiseman, 2011). However, the results of epidemiologic studies of these factors are mixed and do not provide clear evidence of causality (Negri et al., 1999; Sakoda & Horn-Ross, 2002; Yao et al., 2011). The genesis of thyroid autoimmunity and its predominance in females remains enigmatic. One hypothesis postulates incompatibility of X chromosomes. Because either the paternal or the maternal X chromosome is inactivated in cell lineages early during embryogenesis, the genotype of the human female is actually a mosaic of active and inactivated paternal and maternal X chromosomes. This phenomenon was described by Mary Lyon in 1961 and is called the *Lyon hypothesis* (Lyon, 1961). Inactivated X chromosomes are called *Barr*

bodies, named after Murray Barr, who first described them (Barr & Bertram, 1949). Conceivably, incompatibility of the paternal and maternal X chromosomes might lead to immunoreactivity, particularly if thyroid tissues contain the active X chromosome from one parent and immune cells contain the active X chromosome from the other parent.

Other mechanisms might also heighten the predisposition of women to autoimmune thyroiditis as well as other forms of autoimmunity. During pregnancy, fetal cells can cross the placenta and enter the maternal circulation, and these cells may survive in maternal tissues such as the thyroid gland, a condition known as *microchimerism*. Interestingly, microchimerism in thyroid specimens and circulating fetal cells in blood samples have been found to be more common in patients with autoimmune thyroiditis than normal controls. Further research is needed to characterize the autoimmune effects of fetal cells in maternal blood and tissues (Lepez, Vandewoestyne, & Deforce, 2013).

Radiation Exposure and Thyroid Cancer

In 1950, Duffy and Fitzgerald reported that 9 out of 28 children with thyroid cancer had a history of external head and neck irradiation (Duffy & Fitzgerald, 1950). Soon after that, case reports of thyroid cancer in young atomic bomb survivors appeared in the literature (Fujimoto, Yamamoto, Numata, & Mori, 1959). There is now convincing evidence that the incidence of thyroid malignancies increased markedly in populations exposed to excessive radioactive fallout in Japan following the atomic bombing in World War II and in Russia after the Chernobyl nuclear reactor accident (Boice, 1998, 2006). Furthermore, a recent study suggests the presence of synergism between radiation exposure and iodine deficiency in elevating the risk of developing thyroid cancer (Cardis et al., 2005).

Cardis and colleagues conducted a case–control study of thyroid cancer and exposure to radioactive fallout from the Chernobyl nuclear reactor accident in combination with dietary intake of iodine and iodine supplements. Cases and controls were ascertained from Belarus and the Russian Federation population living near the reactor at the time of the accident. Questionnaire data on diet were obtained from 276 patients with pathologically confirmed thyroid cancer and 1300 healthy control subjects matched by age and gender. Radiation exposure was estimated by a comprehensive dose-reconstruction program considering both inhaled and ingested radioactive particles. The major contribution to dose was from drinking milk contaminated with radioactive iodine isotopes, particularly I^{131}. Dietary iodine and dietary supplements containing potassium iodide were also examined as cofactors in the study. Like many other investigations, the overall risk of thyroid cancer increased with increasing dose of radioactivity. Notably, subjects with low iodine intake and 1 Gy of total radiation exposure had high odds ratios ranging from 4.85 to 8.44, whereas those with similar radiation exposure who took potassium iodide supplements were *not* at increased risk (OR = 1.08). These results indicate that diets deficient in iodine potentiate the risk of radiation-induced thyroid cancer and suggest that iodine supplementation has a protective effect against carcinogenesis (Cardis et al., 2005).

Dietary Factors and Thyroid Cancer

Goodman and colleagues conducted a population-based case–control study of thyroid cancer, diet, and other factors in Hawaii, which has one of the highest incidence rates of thyroid cancer in the world. Cases with pathologically confirmed thyroid cancer (51 men and 140 women) were compared to 113 male and 328 female controls matched on age and gender. The risk of thyroid cancer increased with increasing body weight in both men and women. Men and women in the highest quartiles of weight had fivefold and twofold increases in thyroid cancer risk, respectively, compared to those in the lowest quartiles. Risk increases were also observed among heavier women who used fertility drugs or experienced miscarriages or stillbirths at first pregnancy. Results suggest a dose response relationship between body weight and thyroid carcinogenesis with potential effect modification due to fertility drugs and/or reproductive failure (Goodman, Kolonel, & Wilkens, 1992; Goodman, Yoshizawa, & Kolonel, 1988). Interestingly, certain inflammatory adipokines secreted by adipocytes (fat cells) in obese individuals have been linked to carcinogenesis (Barb, Pazaitou-Panayiotou, & Mantzoros, 2006; Vona-Davis & Rose, 2007). It is therefore conceivable that the increased storage of fat associated with weight gain could induce adipocytes to secrete inflammatory adipokines that target the thyroid gland.

In another case–control study conducted in the Hawaiian population, women with high iodine intake who took fertility drugs or suffered miscarriage or stillbirth at first pregnancy were found to be at exceptionally high risk for the development of thyroid cancer. Women with high iodine intake who suffered a first pregnancy miscarriage had an odds ratio of 4.8, and women with high iodine intake who used fertility drugs had an odds ratio of 7.3 (Kolonel, Hankin, Wilkens, Fukunaga, &

Hinds, 1990). These results tend to contradict the more recent findings of Cardis et al. (2005), who observed protective effects of supplemental potassium iodide. Clearly, additional investigations are needed in order to clarify the impact of radiation, iodine, body mass, female reproduction, and other risk factors on thyroid carcinogenesis in different populations.

Nonmalignant Thyroid Disorders and Thyroid Cancer

Several nonmalignant thyroid disorders have been found to be associated with thyroid cancer. The most prominent of these associations involve autoimmune conditions and autoantibodies against thyroglobulin and other thyroid-specific factors.

The most commonly encountered diseases of the thyroid gland involve either an overactive gland (hyperthyroidism) or an underactive gland (hypothyroidism). Early screening surveys conducted among adults in the United States and Great Britain reflect prevalence rates of thyroid abnormalities of approximately 6% (Baldwin & Rowitt, 1978; Tunbridge et al., 1977; Wang & Crapo, 1997). The most prevalent thyroid condition is enlargement of the thyroid gland, which is commonly called a *goiter*. Goiters fall into two broad categories: inflammatory (toxic) goiters that cause hyperthyroidism (e.g., Graves' disease) and noninflammatory (nontoxic) goiters that cause hypothyroidism (e.g., iodine deficiency).

Thyroiditis refers to any inflammatory condition of the thyroid gland. Thyroiditis can lead to hyperthyroidism (as in Graves' disease) or hypothyroidism (as in Hashimoto's thyroiditis). These inflammatory conditions are believed to have an autoimmune basis, and both have been linked to the development of thyroid adenomas and thyroid cancer.

Hyperthyroidism

Hyperthyroidism refers to an overactive thyroid. Symptoms of hyperthyroidism are due to the overproduction of thyroid hormones (T_3 and T_4) by the thyroid gland. The most common cause of hyperthyroidism is an autoimmune form of thyroiditis known as *Graves' disease*, named after the Irish physician Robert J. Graves, who first described the condition in 1835 (Weetman, 2000).

Hypothyroidism

Hypothyroidism refers to an underactive thyroid gland, which results in a deficiency of thyroid hormones (T_3 and T_4). Hypothyroid disorders occur when the thyroid gland is inactive or underactive because of improper formation from birth, lack of iodine, removal or iatrogenic inactivation (ablation) of the thyroid gland, or autoimmune conditions such as Hashimoto's thyroiditis. Symptoms of hypothyroidism include abnormal weight gain, fatigue, baldness, temperature intolerance (typically cold), and in some cases thyroid enlargement (nontoxic goiter).

Human Leukocyte Antigen (HLA) Locus and Autoimmune Thyroiditis

The *HLA* locus on chromosome 6 encodes a variety of molecules that are related to autoimmune conditions. The two classical forms of thyroiditis, Graves' disease (a common cause of hyperthyroidism) and Hashimoto's thyroiditis (which causes hypothyroidism), are both known to have an autoimmune basis related to specific genes of the HLA locus.

Genes of the HLA locus play a major role in the immune response to foreign antigens as well as the recognition of self versus non-self in immune reactions. The six major genes of the HLA locus are all located on the short arm of chromosome 6 (Levinson, 2006). Specific HLA genes encode cell-surface antigen-presenting proteins that regulate the processing of bacterial antigens by T lymphocytes and the formation of antibodies by B lymphocytes. The profile of cell membrane HLA proteins differentiates self from non-self in the immune response; perturbations in the system occasionally result in the formation of antibodies that are directed against self. Such autoantibodies are capable of selectively stimulating and/or destroying certain tissues of the body, thereby causing autoimmune disease.

Genetic variants at the HLA locus have been found to increase susceptibility to Graves' disease and Hashimoto's thyroiditis. For example, results of HLA genotyping studies of cases and controls suggest that individuals who carry the HLA-DR3 allele have 3–4 times higher risk of developing Graves' disease than noncarriers (Farid, Stone, & Johnson, 1980; Jacobson & Tomer, 2007b; Zamani et al., 2000) and that HLA-DR3 carriers have approximately twice the higher risk of developing Hashimoto's thyroiditis than noncarriers (Jacobson, Huber, & Tomer, 2008; Tandon, Zhang, & Weetman, 1991). It is hypothesized that the HLA-DR3 protein may heighten susceptibility through its special affinity for thyroid antigens, thereby creating an autoimmune response directed against the thyroid gland. Furthermore, there is increasing evidence suggesting that interactions between thyroglobulin and genetic variants of the HLA-DR3 allele enhance susceptibility

to the development of Graves' disease (Jacobson & Tomer, 2007a).

Another candidate gene for conferring susceptibility to the development of autoimmune thyroid disorders is the cytotoxic T lymphocyte associated antigen-4 (*CTLA-4*). The normal *CTLA-4* gene product helps to regulate the response of T lymphocytes to antigenic stimuli. It apparently provides a negative signal to the T cell, thus limiting autoimmune responses and maintaining self-tolerance (Chambers & Allison, 1997). Significant associations have consistently been observed between Graves' disease and certain allelic forms of *CTLA-4*, whereas associations with Hashimoto's thyroiditis are less clear (Chistiakov & Turakulov, 2003).

Other susceptibility-genes have also been identified. For example, variants of the gene that encodes vitamin D-binding protein have been linked to the development of Graves' disease. Vitamin D-binding protein facilitates the transport and release of vitamin D in blood and tissues, and the active form of vitamin D works in concert with calcitonin, parathyroid, and thyroid hormones to regulate calcium and phosphorous homeostasis. Graves' disease combined with low serum vitamin D leads to poor absorption of calcium and related symptoms of muscle wasting, bone resorption, and nervous system dysfunction (Herman-Bonert & Friedman, 2004).

German investigators studied genetic polymorphisms of vitamin D-binding protein among 561 individuals in families with an offspring affected by either Graves' disease (95 pedigrees) or Hashimoto's thyroiditis (92 pedigrees). They found that allelic variants of vitamin D-binding protein confer susceptibility to the development of Graves' disease but not Hashimoto's thyroiditis (Pani et al., 2002). In a subsequent genetic case–control study of Graves' disease and vitamin D-binding protein, Polish investigators compared single nucleotide polymorphisms of 332 cases to 185 healthy control subjects. They found a specific polymorphism at codon 420 involving substitution of lysine for threonine that significantly increased the risk of disease and decreased the level of serum vitamin D (Kurylowicz, Ramos-Lopez, Bednarczuk, & Badenhoop, 2006). These results suggest that genetic regulation of vitamin D activity plays a role in thyroid autoimmunity and the development of Graves' disease.

Graves' Disease

Graves' disease, also called diffuse toxic goiter, is believed to arise because of autoimmune reactions.

Graves' disease affects approximately 0.5% of the U.S. population and is the underlying cause of up to 80% of all cases of hyperthyroidism. The clinical signs and symptoms of this condition result from excess stimulation of the thyroid gland by autoantibodies, resulting in inflammation of the thyroid gland (thyroiditis) and overproduction of T_3 and T_4 hormones. Molecular studies suggest that circulating IgG antibodies bind to and activate thyrotropin receptors of the thyroid epithelium, causing hypertrophy and hyperplasia of thyroid follicles. This process results in increased production of thyroid hormones, thyroid enlargement, and goiter formation. The peak incidence of Graves' disease is between 20 and 40 years of age. Symptoms include enlargement of the thyroid gland (goiter), protruding eyes (exophthalmos), palpitations, excess sweating, diarrhea, weight loss, muscle weakness, and unusual sensitivity to heat. Notably, Graves' disease is diagnosed 5–10 times more often in women than men (Brent, 2008; Weetman, 2000). As shown by the age-specific rates for Swedish women and men in **FIGURE 31.6**, the marked female excess of this condition is evident throughout life (Hemminki, Li, Sundquist, & Sundquist, 2010).

Genetic studies suggest that Graves' disease has a significant hereditary component. A nationwide population-based study of twins ascertained from the Danish Twin Registry during 1953–1976 revealed a concordance rate of 35% among monozygous twins compared to 3% for dizygous twins. In regression models, genetic factors accounted for 79% of the liability to development of Graves' disease compared to 21% for environmental factors. Based on these findings, the investigators suggested that "genetic factors play a major role in the etiology of Graves' disease" (Brix, Kyvik, Christensen, & Hegedus, 2001).

A national genetic study of Graves' disease was conducted in Sweden using data from the Swedish Multigeneration Register linked to the Swedish Hospital Discharge Register for the years 1987–2007. Standard incidence ratios were calculated based on familial relationships of 15,743 patients hospitalized for Graves' disease during this period. Standard incidence ratios were increased 5-fold in families with an affected sibling and more than 300-fold in families with two affected siblings. The standard incidence ratio in twins was 16.5. The incidence of Graves' disease was also increased in families with other auto-immune conditions such as Addison's disease, type 1 diabetes mellitus, Hashimoto's thyroiditis, pernicious anemia, myasthenia gravis, lupus erythematosus, and scleroderma. Surprisingly, the standard incidence ratio was also increased among spouses of affected individuals, suggesting that environmental factors may also be involved in the genesis of Graves' disease (Hemminki et al., 2010). Interestingly, cigarette smoking has been linked to the development of multiple autoimmune diseases, including rheumatoid arthritis, systemic lupus erythematosus, multiple sclerosis, and Graves' disease (Costenbader & Karlson, 2006; Manji et al., 2006). Notwithstanding, the genetic factors that influence the thyroid autoimmunity involved in Graves' disease clearly outweigh the environmental factors (Jacobson & Tomer, 2007a, 2007b).

Graves' Disease, Autoimmune Thyroiditis, and Thyroid Cancer

An association between Graves' disease and the development of thyroid cancer was reported more than 60 years ago (Pemberton & Black, 1948). Several lines of evidence suggest that patients with Graves' disease may be at increased risk for the development of benign thyroid adenomas and thyroid carcinoma. A review of 450 surgically treated patients during 1982–1994 revealed that 36 of 450 (8%)

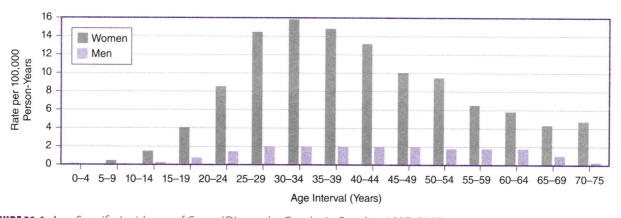

FIGURE 31.6 Age-Specific Incidence of Graves' Disease by Gender in Sweden, 1987–2007.

Data from Hemminki, K., Li, X., Sundquist, J., & Sundquist, K. (2010). The epidemiology of Graves' disease: Evidence of a genetic and an environmental contribution. *Journal of Autoimmunity, 34*(3), J307–J313.

had thyroid carcinomas, 33 of which were papillary tumors (Pellegriti, Belfiore, Giuffrida, Lupo, & Vigneri, 1998). In a European multicenter study of 557 patients who were surgically treated for Graves' disease, thyroid cancer was detected among 3.9% of all patients and 15% of those patients with nodules (Kraimps et al., 2000). A review of the malignancy rate in multiple studies of surgically resected thyroid nodules suggests that approximately 1.7%–2.5% of nodules from Graves' patients manifest thyroid cancer compared to only 0.25% of nodules from other patients, reflecting a 7- to 10-fold risk increase of thyroid cancer among patients with Graves' disease (Belfiore, Russo, Vigneri, & Filetti, 2001).

Specific antithyroid antibodies have been linked to the development of thyroid cancer in several investigations. In a U.S. study of 253 patients with thyroid cancer and 2247 patients with benign thyroid nodules, fine-needle aspiration biopsy was performed on all subjects and specimens were tested for the presence/absence of antibodies against thyroglobulin. Results revealed that thyroid cancer was significantly associated with elevated antibodies against thyroglobulin (OR = 1.57) (Azizi & Malchoff, 2011).

In an Italian study of 2053 patients with thyroid nodules, fine-needle aspirates were evaluated for the presence of a profile of antithyroid antibodies. Patients with thyroid nodules positive for antithyroid antibodies had more than double the risk of having thyroid cancer (OR = 2.2) (Boi et al., 2013).

In a retrospective study of 1638 Korean patients with thyroid nodules, ultrasound-guided aspirates were tested for antibodies against thyroglobulin. A higher frequency of malignant nodules tested positive for autoantibodies than did benign nodules (31% versus 21%), and patients who tested positive for thyroglobulin autoantibodies were at increased risk (OR = 1.6) compared to those who tested negative (Kim et al., 2010).

Autoantibodies against the receptor for TSH are a diagnostic characteristic of Graves' disease. Notably, these antibodies have been linked to the development and progression of thyroid cancer. In a study of serum samples from 27 patients with localized or metastatic thyroid cancer, 25 of 27 samples (93%) tested positive for TSH receptor antibodies compared to 0 of 51 samples from normal controls (Chinnappa et al., 2004).

In summary, evidence from both epidemiologic and immunological studies suggests that patients with Graves' disease or other forms of autoimmune thyroiditis develop antibodies against TSH receptors, thyroglobulin, and other thyroid-specific antigens that may elevate their risk of developing thyroid cancer.

Hashimoto's Thyroiditis

Hashimoto's thyroiditis is a chronic autoimmune disease in which the thyroid gland is gradually destroyed by the body's own immune system. The disorder was first described by the Japanese physician Dr. Hakaru Hashimoto (1912). It is diagnosed by clinical symptoms plus the presence of autoantibodies against thyroglobulin or other cellular components of the thyroid gland. Pathologic review of thyroidal tissue from patients reveals inflammation and striking infiltration by lymphocytes admixed with plasma cells, necrosis, and derangement of thyroid follicles plus goitrous enlargement of the gland. Without treatment, there is progressive depletion of thyroid follicles accompanied by hypothyroidism and loss of thyroid function (Rapoport, 1991).

Patients with Hashimoto's thyroiditis often have a family history of thyroid disorders, including Graves' disease and/or other autoimmune conditions such as type 1 diabetes, celiac disease, pernicious anemia, Addison's disease, and Sjogren's syndrome. Hashimoto's thyroiditis is typically diagnosed between the ages of 45 and 65 years and occurs 10–20 times more often in women than men (Vanderpump & Tunbridge, 2002). Certain genes of the HLA locus confer susceptibility to the development of this disorder (e.g., presence of the *HLA-DR5* gene increases the relative risk more than threefold). Furthermore, polymorphisms of the *CTLA-4* gene have also been implicated in the genesis of Hashimoto's thyroiditis (Chistiakov, 2005; Tomer, Barbesino, Greenberg, Concepcion, & Davies, 1999; Yesilkaya et al., 2008).

Hashimoto's Thyroiditis and Thyroid Cancer

The relationship between Hashimoto's thyroiditis and papillary thyroid carcinoma was first proposed by Dailey, Lindsay, and Skahen (1955). Since this initial description, the association between the two diseases has been highly debated in the literature and the relationship remains controversial. However, recent studies of patients from different populations provide evidence of a positive association.

In a study of 474 consecutive Taiwanese patients who underwent thyroidectomy and had a final pathological diagnosis of Hashimoto's thyroiditis, 133 patients (28%) had a preoperative diagnosis of thyroid cancer (based on pathologic examination of fine-needle aspirates), and an additional 114 patients (24%) had a postoperative diagnosis of thyroid cancer based on pathologic examination of the surgical specimens.

Most of the thyroid tumors (95%) were papillary carcinomas (Shih et al., 2007).

In a U.S. study of 217 cases with Hashimoto's thyroiditis and 1198 controls without thyroiditis who underwent thyroid surgery, 29% of the cases had papillary thyroid carcinoma versus 23% of controls (OR = 1.3). Among patients with Hashimoto's thyroiditis, 94% of the thyroid tumors were papillary carcinomas (Repplinger et al., 2008). In a meta-analysis of 38 studies, pathologic evidence of Hashimoto's thyroiditis was present in 938 (40.5%) of 2317 cases with thyroid cancer compared to 634 (21%) of 3019 controls with benign thyroid nodules or other thyroid disorders. Cases with thyroid cancer were nearly three times more likely to manifest Hashimoto's thyroiditis compared to controls with benign nodules (summary OR = 2.8) (Lee, Younghye, Choi, & Kim, 2013).

A variety of autoantibodies have been identified in patients with Hashimoto's thyroiditis. These include antibodies against thyroglobulin, thyroid peroxidase, and to a lesser extent, antibodies against TSH receptors. Chronic influx of auto-reactive T cells in thyroid tissues and polymorphisms in the *CTLA-4* gene in response to antigenic stimuli may also be involved in thyroid carcinogenesis.

▶ Iodine and Thyroid Function

Adequate intake of iodine is essential for the biosynthesis of thyroid hormones and maintenance of normal thyroid function. The normal range of serum iodine is approximately 40–80 ng/mL. Values consistently outside this range indicate the presence of thyroid disease: Low levels indicate hypothyroidism and high levels indicate hyperthyroidism.

Iodine Deficiency and Thyroid Disease

Nontoxic goiter, or simply "goiter," refers to enlargement of the thyroid gland in conjunction with hypothyroidism. As discussed later in this section, the dominant global cause of goiter is iodine deficiency. Enlargement of the thyroid gland in iodine-deficient children is progressive, initially involving diffuse hyperplasia and later the development of multiple nodules wherein the thyroid follicles are markedly distended by the presence of excess colloid. Goiter arising from iodine deficiency is very uncommon in developed countries because iodine is routinely added to salt and other foods for consumption. Indeed, iodized salt has been a prominent feature of the U.S. diet since 1924 (Marine, 1924; McClure, 1935).

The discovery of iodine as an essential mineral for normal function of the thyroid glands and the production of thyroid hormones provides a convincing example of the power of epidemiologic investigation. In 1905, a young physician trained at Johns Hopkins University, David Marine, began his residency training in pathology at Lakeside Hospital on the shores of Lake Erie in Cleveland, Ohio. His interest in thyroid disease was spiked by the high prevalence of goiters in dogs in the area, and he began a series of studies to elucidate the cause. Marine observed that dietary supplements of iodine in the form of iodized salt reduced the incidence of goiter in sheep and produced regression of goiters and reversal of hypothyroid symptoms in dogs (Marine, 1907). In pathologic studies, Marine found that large goitrous thyroids from dogs had lower levels of iodine than normal thyroids from healthy dogs (Marine & Williams, 1908). Marine was also called upon to investigate the high rate of "alleged thyroid carcinomas" in trout in a fish hatchery in northern Ohio. Pathologic studies revealed that the fish had goiters due to iodine deficiency, rather than thyroid carcinomas, and Marine demonstrated that goiter development was effectively prevented by the addition of iodine or foods high in iodine content to the trout hatchery water (Marine, 1914).

Marine soon translated these findings to the human population, showing in his clinic that children suffering from simple goiter responded to therapy with sodium iodide. Realizing the devastating problem of goiter in the Great Lakes region, Marine and his colleague, O. P. Kimball, organized and conducted a field intervention study using sodium iodide supplements in the diets of young girls in the Akron, Ohio, region. Girls in the fifth through eighth grades received 200 mg of sodium iodide for 10 consecutive days, and older girls received twice this amount. The dosing regimen was repeated every 6 months. A total of 2305 girls received the supplemental iodine compared to 2190 girls from a nearby region who did not. The results of this field experiment after 30 months of follow-up are summarized in **TABLE 31.1**.

After 30 months of observation, the chemopreventive value of the treatment with sodium iodide was remarkable. Among participants with normal thyroid glands at the beginning of the study, 347 of 1257 girls (27.6%) who did not receive iodine developed goiters compared to only 2 of 908 girls (0.2%) who did receive iodine. Substantial therapeutic effects were also evident. Among participants with enlarged thyroid glands at baseline, progression of disease was observed in only 0.2% of treated girls compared to 14.1% of controls, whereas regression of disease

TABLE 31.1 Effects of Sodium Iodide Supplementation in School Girls of Northern Ohio		
Size of Thyroid	**Treatment Group**	**Control Group**
Initially normal	$n = 908$	$n = 1257$
Unchanged	906 (99.8%)	910 (72.4%)
Enlarged	2 (0.2%)	347 (27.6%)
Initially enlarged	$n = 1282$	$n = 1048$
Unchanged	506 (39.5%)	755 (72.0%)
Increased	3 (0.2%)	148 (14.1%)
Decreased	773 (60.3%)	145 (13.8%)

Data from Marine, D., & Kimball, O. P. (1920). The prevention of simple goiter in man: Fourth paper. *Archives of Internal Medicine, 25,* 661–672.

was observed in 60.3% of treated girls compared to 13.8% of controls. Importantly, no toxic effects of the sodium iodide supplement were detected in the study (Marine, 1924; Marine & Kimball, 1917, 1920). The definitive evidence from this study was the crowning achievement of Marine's work on iodine deficiency as the causative factor in the development of hypothyroidism and simple goiter.

Cretinism and Iodine Deficiency

The health consequences of iodine deficiency often manifest early in life. These include abnormal neuronal development, mental retardation, congenital malformations, and hypothyroidism. Deleterious effects on reproduction such as spontaneous abortion, miscarriage, and infertility are also notable. Later in life, lack of iodine is also associated with intellectual impairment.

Cretinism is an anomaly that is caused by iodine deficiency in the developing fetus. Clinical manifestations of this condition depend on the gestational timing and severity of iodine and hormonal insufficiency in both the mother and fetus. In the absence of iodine, there is abnormal development and function of the fetal thyroid gland. This devastating condition typically manifests at birth or during infancy and is characterized by hypothyroidism, goiter, mental retardation, deaf-mutism, stunted growth, and other anomalies. Though extremely rare, there are case reports of thyroid cancer in young patients with cretinism (Fellman, Wojtowicz, & Pawlaczyk, 1968).

Endemic cretinism was once common in the Alpine populations of Southern Europe due to lack of iodine in their diets. As an example, in Switzerland, where the soil contains little iodine, cases of cretinism were once commonplace. In fact, the soils of many inland areas on all continents are iodine-deficient, and plants and animals grown there are correspondingly deficient. Populations living in such areas without outside food sources are therefore at high risk for the development of iodine deficiency diseases (Gaitan & Dunn, 1992).

Fortunately, the addition of iodine to table salt has virtually eliminated cretinism in developed countries. Furthermore, early detection of thyroid insufficiency in newborns and administration of thyroxine (T_4) can often be effective in reinstating thyroid function and normal growth and development. Nevertheless, in developing nations without such programs, the lack of dietary iodine remains the leading cause of preventable mental retardation in babies and small children.

Global Impact of Iodine Deficiency

Following the pioneering research of David Marine in the early 20th century, confirming evidence of the chemopreventive value of supplemental iodine soon became available from studies in Sweden, Switzerland, and many other nations. In the United States, iodized table salt containing 100 mg per kg of potassium iodide has been available since 1924. The U.S. Food and Drug Administration recommends 150 µg of iodine per day for both men and women.

Supplementing the diet with iodized salt is a simple, cost-effective method of ensuring adequate iodine intake, and successful population-based programs have increased around the world with the active encouragement and support of the World Health Organization (Holman & McCartney, 1960). According to recent survey data from the World Health Organization, 164 countries now have iodized-salt programs, and the percentage of households in the developing world that use iodized salt rose from about 20% in 1970 to 70% in 2000. Nevertheless, these estimates also suggest that iodine deficiency impacts approximately 2 billion people worldwide and causes a high burden of disease in many developing nations. For example, in India, it is estimated that 100 million suffer from iodine deficiency, 4 million from goiter, and 500,000 from cretinism. Other pockets of iodine deficiency are evident in the Western Pacific, Southeast Asia, Africa, and the Russian Federation (Andersson, Takkouche, Egli, Allen, & de Benoist, 2005). Continuing international efforts should therefore focus on implementing and sustaining iodine–supplementation programs in all nations (*Lancet*, 2008).

Iodine Deficiency and Thyroid Cancer

In 1928, the German pathologist Carl Wegelin published a report suggesting that the prevalence of occult thyroid carcinoma was 10-fold higher at autopsy among decedents from areas endemic for goiter versus those from nonendemic areas (Wegelin, 1928). Early epidemiologic data from the canton of Zurich in Switzerland provided supportive evidence of a link between iodine deficiency and thyroid cancer. Prior to the introduction of iodized salt, prevalence estimates of goiter in this region approached 100%, and up to 30% of young men were unfit for military service owing to the presence of large goiters (Bürgi, Supersaxo, & Selz, 1990; Wespi-Eggenberger, 1948). Following the introduction of iodized salt in 1923, goiters virtually disappeared in newborns and schoolchildren, and the mortality from thyroid cancer in the canton of Zurich gradually declined (the mortality rate for men was 2.1 per 100,000 before 1925, 1.4 during 1926–1935, and 0.6 after 1935), suggesting that iodized salt may have prevented not only goiter, but also thyroid cancer in this population (Wynder, 1952). Thyroid cancer mortality has continued to decline in the Swiss population concurrent with augmentation of national iodized salt programs and advances in early detection and therapy (Levi et al., 1990; Zimmerman, 2008).

Recent ecologic studies of the two predominant histological types of thyroid cancer, papillary and follicular carcinoma, suggest there may be an inverse association with iodine levels; that is, follicular thyroid carcinoma is associated with iodine deficiency, whereas papillary thyroid carcinoma is associated with iodine overload. In Poland, suspension of iodine prophylaxis (removal of iodized salt) in 1980 resulted in a rise in the incidence of follicular thyroid cancer whereas restoration of iodine prophylaxis produced a fall in the incidence of follicular tumors but a corresponding rise in the incidence of papillary tumors (Huszno et al., 2003).

Investigators in Northern California studied iodine intake and thyroid cancer in a retrospective study of 608 women with thyroid cancer and 558 age-matched controls from the same area. There were too few follicular cancers for evaluation (28 cases), so the analysis was limited to cases with papillary thyroid carcinoma. As expected, risk increases were noted for radiation exposure to the head and neck (OR = 2.3), history of goiter or thyroid nodules (OR = 3.7), and family history of thyroid disorders (OR = 2.5). After adjustment for these established risk factors, total dietary iodine intake was found to be *inversely* related to the risk of developing papillary thyroid cancer (e.g., OR = 0.49 for the highest versus the lowest quintile of intake). This protective effect of dietary iodine was primarily due to higher daily consumption of multivitamin pills containing 150 µg of iodine by women in the control group. Based on these findings, the investigators suggest that *moderately* high levels of dietary iodine may help *reduce* the risk of papillary thyroid cancer, possibly by maintaining normal thyroid levels of thyroxine and TSH. They also note that extraordinarily high levels of iodine consumption, which have resulted in substantially increased rates of papillary thyroid cancer in specific populations (e.g., Japanese consuming over 200 mg/day of iodine from seaweed), are more than 20 times higher than the average consumption among women in the highest quintile of iodine intake among the women in their study (Horn-Ross et al., 2001).

Iodine Overload and Thyroid Disease

In 1963, iodine prophylaxis was introduced into the severe goiter-endemic area in Salta, Argentina. Incident cases of thyroid cancer ascertained during the 15-year period before prophylaxis (59 cases) were compared to incident cases in the 16-year period after prophylaxis (85 cases). The relative frequency of papillary thyroid carcinomas rose by 80% after intervention, and thyroiditis was more frequent in patients with papillary carcinoma compared to those with nonpapillary tumors (35% versus 6%). Furthermore, three non-Hodgkin's B cell lymphomas were detected in the postintervention period, all in women over the age of 50 years. Numbers of incident cases of follicular and medullary carcinomas detected in the two periods were similar. These results indicate that high dietary intake of iodine may be associated with the development of thyroiditis, papillary thyroid carcinoma, and thyroid lymphoma (Harach, Escalante, & Day, 2002; Harach & Williams, 1995).

It is well established that excessive iodine intake is associated with thyroid autoimmunity. Several large population-based studies have demonstrated higher prevalence rates of individuals with thyroid autoantibodies in populations in which iodine intake was supplemented. In an epidemiologic study conducted in Slovenia, 676 13-year-old schoolchildren were followed over a period of 10 years after a mandatory governmental increase in the level of iodized salt from 10 to 25 mg of potassium iodide per kilogram. At baseline, thyroid volume was measured by ultrasound, and the iodine concentration was measured in urine samples. During the follow-up period, all incident cases of thyroid disease among Slovenian adults were examined by ultrasonography combined with measurement of serum levels of TSH, thyroid hormones, and antibodies to thyroglobulin and thyroid peroxidase. After the increase in iodine supplementation, the prevalence of goiter among children was reduced from 11% to 1%, corresponding to average increases in urinary iodine and decreases in thyroid volume. Among adults, the incidence of diffuse goiter gradually decreased by about 80%, from 35 per 100,000 in 1999 to 7 per 100,000 in 2009, and the incidence of Graves' disease was stable throughout the follow-up period. Conversely, the incidence of solitary and multinodular goiter increased by about 60%, from 30 per 100,000 to 48 per 100,000, and the incidence of Hashimoto's thyroiditis more than doubled (from 73 per 100,000 in 1999 to 166 per 100,000 in 2009) (Zaletel et al., 2011).

These results, and those of several other studies, suggest that iodine prophylaxis effectively changes the pattern of thyroid cancer. In iodine-deficient populations, iodine prophylaxis appears to shift the incidence of papillary thyroid carcinoma upward while decreasing the incidence of follicular carcinomas. Most studies have found increases in the incidence of Hashimoto's thyroiditis, hypothyroidism, and corresponding thyroid autoantibodies following increased salt iodization. Nevertheless, additional studies are needed to clarify the role of iodine intake and dosage in the prevention versus pathogenesis of thyroid cancer in different populations (Knobel & Medeiros-Neto, 2007).

Goitrogenic Dietary Factors and Thyroid Disorders

Goitrogens are dietary agents that suppress thyroid function and induce the formation of goiters, particularly in children. The principal goitrogens are isothiocyanate and the isoflavones (a class of phytoestrogens). These compounds inhibit the activity of thyroxine peroxidase, a key enzyme in the formation of thyroid hormones from iodine and tyrosine. Cruciferous vegetables such as broccoli, cauliflower, and cabbage contain high levels of isothiocyanate. Other sources include peanuts, spinach, peaches, and strawberries (Vanderpas, 2006). Soybeans and soy-based products contain high concentrations of isoflavones (Doerge & Sheehan, 2002).

Thiocyanate overload from consumption of cassava root has been found to be goitrogenic in Central Africa, particularly in association with selenium deficiency. The cassava root has low concentrations of iodine and selenium and high concentrations of isothiocyanate. Thilly and colleagues investigated dietary factors and thyroid disorders in children ages 5–7 years from goiter-endemic areas of Central Africa. Low serum levels of thyroxine (T_4) were associated with low selenium and high thiocyanate levels in children residing in regions where cassava is the principal source of carbohydrates in the diet. Furthermore, high rates of cretinism were observed among children with severe iodine and selenium deficiencies in combination with thiocyanate overload (Thilly et al., 1993).

High consumption of soy has also been linked to thyroid disorders in children. Early case reports document goiter development in infants on a soy diet (Hydovitz, 1960). Fort and colleagues studied 59 children with autoimmune thyroid disease, their 76 healthy siblings, and 54 healthy unrelated children. They found that the frequency of feedings with soy-based milk formulas in early life (31%) was significantly higher in children with autoimmune thyroid disease compared to healthy siblings and unrelated children (12%) (Fort, Moses, & Fasano, 1990). Thus, despite some beneficial health effects of soy, the issue of goitrogenic impact remains problematic.

Medullary Thyroid Cancer

Medullary thyroid cancer arises from the parafollicular calcitonin-secreting cells of the thyroid gland. Although most cases are sporadic (nonfamilial), approximately 25% involve heritable mutations of the

RET gene, a proto-oncogene located on chromosome 10 (Donis-Keller et al., 1993; Eng, 1999). The *RET* gene encodes a cell membrane receptor called *receptor tyrosine kinase* that activates signal transduction and complex cascades of biochemical reactions involving tyrosine phosphorylation within cells. The exact nature of these reactions depends upon the cell type (e.g., in parafollicular C cells, *RET* signaling induces excess biosynthesis of calcitonin).

Mutations of the *RET* gene or the *MENIN* gene (a tumor suppressor gene located on chromosome 11) cause distinct heritable syndromes known as *multiple endocrine neoplasia (MEN)* (Donis-Keller et al., 1993; Guru et al., 1998). Endocrine tumors of the MEN syndromes elaborate a variety of amines and peptides, depending on the tissue of origin. Individuals who manifest MEN syndromes are classified into two major groups: *MEN I* (adenomas of the pituitary gland, islet cell tumors of the pancreas, hyperplasia of the parathyroid glands, and peptic ulcers) and *MEN II* (medullary thyroid carcinoma, pheochromocytoma, and occasionally mucocutaneous neuroma). These syndromes show an autosomal dominant inheritance pattern (Carney, 1998; Werner, 1963).

Carriers of certain mutated forms of the *RET* gene have a high lifetime risk of developing medullary thyroid carcinoma and pheochromocytoma (a malignant tumor of the adrenal glands). The familial association of medullary thyroid cancer and pheochromocytoma is called the *Sipple syndrome* after the physician who first described it (Sipple, 1961). Early onset, typically between 15 and 20 years of age, is a prominent characteristic of hereditary medullary thyroid cancer.

▶ Prevention and Therapy of Thyroid Cancer

Strategies for the primary prevention of thyroid cancer include total avoidance of radiation exposure to the head and neck, maintenance of normal thyroid function by sufficient intake of iodine, and avoidance of goitrogens in the diet (e.g., soy products). For high-risk individuals, particularly those with a family or medical history of thyroid disorders, regular checkups by ultrasonography to detect nodules and other abnormalities of the thyroid gland may be advisable.

Fortunately, early detection of thyroid malignancies coupled with complete excision is usually curative. The 5-year survival rates for patients with stage I disease exceed 95%. Total thyroidectomy is the definitive surgery, followed by replacement of thyroid hormones with thyroxine (T_4). Graves' disease and Hashimoto's thyroiditis are often treated with oral doses of radioactive iodine, resulting in permanent destruction of cells in the thyroid and rendering them permanently inactive. Another treatment option for these conditions is surgery in which the thyroid gland is partially or fully removed. Patients who undergo thyroid ablation or thyroidectomy receive daily replacement thyroid hormone therapy.

▶ Epidemiology of Parathyroid Cancer

Parathyroid cancer is extremely rare, accounting for about 1% of all cases of parathyroidism and only 0.005% of all cancers. Virtually all parathyroid tumors secrete PTH and thus cause hypercalcemia.

During 1988–2003, 224 cases of parathyroid cancer were identified from the SEER system of tumor registries in the United States. Cases were equally distributed among men and women, and most (75%) were diagnosed between 45 and 80 years of age. The crude incidence rates appeared to increase slightly over time, from 3.6 cases per 10 million in 1988–1991 to 5.7 cases per 10 million in 2000–2003 (Lee, Jarosek, Virnig, Evasovich, & Tuttle, 2007).

In a long-term study of incident cases diagnosed during 1958–2010 in Australia, 18 of the 21 cases identified were diagnosed during the last 5 years of the study. Possible reasons for the dramatic increase in new cases of parathyroid cancer include increased detection due to ultrasonography and fine-needle aspiration, improved techniques of head and neck surgery, and immunohistochemistry for a protein called *parafibromin* (Brown et al., 2011).

Most parathyroid tumors are sporadic, but approximately 5% are associated with autosomal dominant hereditary cancer syndromes, including MEN I and MEN II, familial hyperparathyroidism, and a rare syndrome called *hyperparathyroidism jaw tumor syndrome (HPT-JT)*.

Carpten and colleagues at the U.S. National Institutes of Health discovered that HPT-JT is caused by germline mutations of a gene called *HRPT2* located on chromosome 1. The *HRPT2* gene encodes a protein called *parafibromin* that may help regulate cell division. In this syndrome, individuals develop hypercalcemia, jaw tumors, and renal lesions in childhood or early adulthood. Individuals with mutant forms of *HRPT2* have an increased risk of parathyroid cancer. Mutations of *HRPT2* were found in 14 affected families, all of which were thought to cause deficient or impaired function of parafibromin (Carpten et al., 2002).

Additional studies have confirmed the role of *HRPT2* mutations in the development of parathyroid cancer. Shattuck and colleagues identified *HRPT2* mutations in 10 of 15 sporadic parathyroid carcinomas thought to inactivate parafibromin protein (Shattuck et al., 2003), and Howell and colleagues found *HRPT2* mutations in 11 of 60 parathyroid tumors, 4 of 4 sporadic tumors, 5 of 5 tumors from patients with HPT-JT, and 2 tumors from patients with familial hyperparathyroidism (Howell et al., 2003). Mutations in the *MEN I* and *MEN II* genes have also been identified in both familial and

sporadic parathyroid tumors. These genes are found primarily in medullary tumors of the thyroid gland (Carney, 1998).

Other than genetic susceptibility linked to mutant forms of *HRPT2*, *MEN I*, and *MEN II*, risk factors associated with the development of parathyroid cancer have not been identified. Hyperparathyroidism has been observed in patients irradiated for acne or other disorders, and radiation exposure may also be a risk factor for parathyroid neoplasia (Brown et al., 2011). Nevertheless, there are currently no case reports of irradiation-induced parathyroid cancer.

References

Alto, W. (1997). Primary health care in Melanesia: Problems and potentials. *Papua and New Guinea Medical Journal, 39*(4), 315–320.

Andersson, M., Takkouche, B., Egli, I., Allen, H. E., & de Benoist, B. (2005). Current global iodine status and progress over the last decade towards the elimination of iodine deficiency. *Bulletin of the World Health Organization, 83*(7), 518–525.

Azizi, G., & Malchoff, C. D. (2011). Three-dimensional ultrasound images and fine-needle aspiration biopsy of a thyroid nodule. *Endocrine Practice, 17*(4), 659–661.

Baldwin, D. B., & Rowett, D. (1978). Incidence of thyroid disorders in Connecticut. *Journal of the American Medical Association, 239*, 742–744.

Barb, D., Pazaitou-Panayiotou, K., & Mantzoros, C. S. (2006). Adiponectin: A link between obesity and cancer. *Expert Opinions in Investigative Drugs, 15*, 917–931.

Barr, M. L., & Bertram, E. G. (1949). A morphological distinction between neurones of the male and female, and the behaviour of the nucleolar satellite during accelerated nucleoprotein synthesis. *Nature, 63*(4148), 676–677.

Belfiore, A., Russo, D., Vigneri, R., & Filetti, S. (2001). Graves' disease, thyroid nodules and thyroid cancer. *Clinical Endocrinology, 55*(86), 711–718.

Boi, F., Minerba, L., Lai, M. L., Marziani, B., Figus, B., Spanu, F., … Mariotti, S. (2013). Both thyroid autoimmunity and increased serum TSH are independent risk factors for malignancy in patients with thyroid nodules. *Journal of Endocrinological Investigation, 36*(5), 313–320.

Boice, J. D., Jr. (1998). Radiation and thyroid cancer: What more can be learned? *Acta Oncologica, 37*, 321–324.

Boice, J. D., Jr. (2006). Thyroid disease 60 years after Hiroshima and 20 years after Chernobyl. *Journal of the American Medical Association, 295*, 1060–1062.

Bray, F., Ferlay, J., Soerjomataram, I., Siegel, R. L., Torre, L. A., & Jemal, A. (2018). Global cancer statistics 2018: GLOBOCAN estimates of incidence and mortality worldwide for 36 cancers in 185 countries. *CA: A Cancer Journal for Clinicians, 68*(6), 394–424.

Brent, G. (2008). Graves' disease. *New England Journal of Medicine, 358*, 2594–2605.

Brix, T. H., Kyvik, K. O., Christensen, K., & Hegedus, L. (2001). Evidence for a major role of heredity in Graves' disease: A population-based study of two Danish twin cohorts. *Journal of Clinical Endocrinology and Metabolism, 86*, 930–934.

Brown, S., O'Neill, C., Suliburk, J., Sidhu, S., Sywak, M., Gill, A., … Delbridge, L. (2011). Parathyroid carcinoma: Increasing incidence and changing presentation. *ANZ Journal of Surgery, 81*(7–8), 528–532.

Bürgi, H., Supersaxo, Z., & Selz, B. (1990). Iodine deficiency diseases in Switzerland one hundred years after Theodor Kocher's survey: A historical review with some new goiter prevalence data. *Acta Endocrinologica (Copenhagen), 123*(6), 577–590.

Cardis, E., Kesminiene, A., Ivanov, V., Malakhova, I., Shibata, Y., Khrouch, V., … Williams, D. (2005). Risk of thyroid cancer after exposure to ^{131}I in childhood. *Journal of the National Cancer Institute, 97*, 724–732.

Carney, J. A. (1998). Familial multiple endocrine neoplasia syndromes: Components, classification, and nomenclature. *Journal of Internal Medicine, 243*(6), 425–432.

Carpten, J. D., Robbins, C. M., Villablanca, A., Forsberg, L., Presciuttini, S., Bailey-Wilson, J., … Hobbs, M. R. (2002). *HRPT2*, encoding parafibromin, is mutated in hyperparathyroidism-jaw tumor syndrome. *Nature Genetics, 32*(4), 676–680.

Chambers, C. A., & Allison, J. P. (1997). Co-stimulation in T cell responses. *Current Opinion in Immunology, 9*, 396–404.

Chinnappa, P., Taguba, L., Arciaga, R., Faiman, C., Siperstein, A., Mehta, A. E., … Gupta, M. K. (2004). Detection of thyrotropin-receptor messenger ribonucleic acid (mRNA) and thyroglobulin mRNA transcripts in peripheral blood of patients with thyroid disease: Sensitive and specific markers for thyroid cancer. *Journal of Clinical Endocrinology and Metabolism, 89*(8), 3705–3709.

Chistiakov, D. A. (2005). Immunogenetics of Hashimoto's thyroiditis. *Journal of Autoimmune Diseases, 2*, 1–10.

Chistiakov, D. A., & Turakulov, R. I. (2003). *CTLA-4* and its role in autoimmune thyroid disease. *Journal of Molecular Endocrinology, 31*, 21–36.

Costenbader, K. H., & Karlson, E. W. (2006). Cigarette smoking and autoimmune disease: What can we learn from epidemiology? *Lupus, 15*, 737–745.

Dailey, M. E., Lindsay, S., & Skahen, R. (1955). Relation of thyroid neoplasms to Hashimoto disease of the thyroid gland. *Archives of Surgery, 70*, 291–297.

Davies, L., & Welch, H. G. (2006). Increasing incidence of thyroid cancer in the United States, 1973–2002. *Journal of the American Medical Association, 295*(18), 2164–2167.

Doerge, D. R., & Sheehan, D. M. (2002). Goitrogenic and estrogenic activity of soy isoflavones. *Environmental Health Perspectives, 110*(Suppl. 3), 349–353.

Donis-Keller, H., Dou, S., Chi, D., Carlson, K. M., Toshima, K., Lairmore, T. C., … Wells, S. A., Jr. (1993). Mutations in the

RET proto-oncogene are associated with MEN 2A and FMTC. *Human Molecular Genetics, 2*(7), 851–856.

Duffy, B. J., Jr., & Fitzgerald, P. J. (1950). Cancer of the thyroid in children: A report of 28 cases. *Journal of Clinical Endocrinology and Metabolism, 10*, 1296–1308.

Eng, C. (1999). RET proto-oncogene in the development of human cancer. *Journal of Clinical Oncology, 17*(1), 380–393.

Farid, N. R., Stone, E., & Johnson, G. (1980). Graves' disease and HLA: Clinical and epidemiologic associations. *Clinical Endocrinology (Oxford), 13*, 535–544.

Fellman, K., Wojtowicz, M., & Pawlaczyk, B. (1968). [Thyroid cancer with thyroidal cretinism in an 13-year-old girl.] *Endokrynologia Polska, 19*(6), 605–609.

Ferlay, J., Bray, F., Pisani, P., & Parkin, D. M. (2004). *GLOBOCAN 2002. Cancer incidence, mortality, and prevalence worldwide. IARC Cancer Base No. 5, version 2.0.* Lyon: IARC Press.

Ferlay, J., Ervik, M., Lam, F., Colombet, M., Mery, L., Piñeros, M., … Bray, F. (2018). *Global cancer observatory: Cancer today.* Lyon, France: International Agency for Research on Cancer. Retrieved from https://gco.iarc.fr/today

Ferlay, J., Shin, H. R., Forman, D., Mathers, C., & Parkin, D. M. (2010). Estimates of worldwide burden of cancer in 2008. *International Journal of Cancer, 127*(12), 2893–2917.

Ferlay, J., Soerjomataram, I., Ervik, M., Dikshit, R., Eser, S., Mathers, C., … Bray, F. (2013). *GLOBOCAN 2012 v1.0. Cancer incidence and mortality worldwide: IARC CancerBase No. 11* [Internet]. Lyon: International Agency for Research on Cancer. Retrieved from http://globocan.iarc.fr

Fitzmaurice, C., Akinyemiju, T. F., Al Lami, F. H., Alam, T., Alizadeh-Navaei, R., Allen, C., … Global Burden of Disease Cancer Collaboration. (2018, June 2). Global, regional, and national cancer incidence, mortality, years of life lost, years lived with disability, and disability-adjusted life-years for 29 cancer groups, 1990 to 2016: A systematic analysis for the Global Burden of Disease Study. *JAMA Oncology.* doi:10.1001/jamaoncol.2018.2706.

Fitzmaurice, C., Allen, C., Barber, R. M., Barregard, L., Bhutta, Z. A., Brenner, H., … Global Burden of Disease Cancer Collaboration. (2017). Global, regional, and national cancer incidence, mortality, years of life lost, years lived with disability, and disability-adjusted life-years for 32 cancer groups, 1990 to 2015: A systematic analysis for the Global Burden of Disease Study. *JAMA Oncology, 3*(4), 524–548.

Fort, P., Moses, N., & Fasano, M. (1990). Breast and soy-formula feedings in early infancy and the prevalence of autoimmune thyroid disease in children. *Journal of the American College of Nutrition, 9*, 164–167.

Franceschi, S., Preston-Martin, S., Dal Maso, L., Negri, E., La Vecchia, C., Mack, W. J., … Ron, E. (1999). A pooled analysis of case-control studies of thyroid cancer. IV. Benign thyroid diseases. *Cancer Causes and Control, 10*(6), 583–595.

Fujimoto, Y., Yamamoto, T., Numata, J., & Mori, K. (1959). Two autopsy cases of thyroid cancer in young atomic bomb survivors. *Journal of the Hiroshima Medical Association, 12*, 519–524.

Gaitan, E., & Dunn, J. T. (1992). Epidemiology of iodine deficiency. *Trends in Endocrinology and Metabolism, 3*(5), 170–175.

Goodman, M. T., Kolonel, L. N., & Wilkens, L. R. (1992). The association of body size, reproductive factors and thyroid cancer. *British Journal of Cancer, 66*(6), 1180–1184.

Goodman, M. T., Yoshizawa, C. N., & Kolonel, L. N. (1988). Descriptive epidemiology of thyroid cancer. *Cancer (Phila.), 61*, 1272–1281.

Guru, S. C., Manickam, P., Crabtree, J. S., Olufemi, S. E., Agarwal, S. K., & Debelenko, L. V. (1998). Identification and characterization of the multiple endocrine neoplasia type 1 (*MEN1*) gene. *Journal of Internal Medicine, 243*(6), 433–439.

Harach, H. R., Escalante, D. A., & Day, E. S. (2002). Thyroid cancer and thyroiditis in Salta, Argentina: A 40-yr study in relation to iodine prophylaxis. *Endocrine Pathology, 13*(3), 175–181.

Harach, H. R., & Williams, E. D. (1995). Thyroid cancer and thyroiditis in the goitrous region of Salta, Argentina, before and after iodine prophylaxis. *Clinical Endocrinology, 43*(6), 701–706.

Hashimoto, H. (1912). Report on lymphomatous goiter. *Archiv für klinische Chirurgie, Berlin, 97*, 219–248.

Hemminki, K., Li, X., Sundquist, J., & Sundquist, K. (2010). The epidemiology of Graves' disease: Evidence of a genetic and an environmental contribution. *Journal of Autoimmunity, 34*(3), J307–J313.

Herman-Bonert, V., & Friedman, T. C. (2004). The thyroid gland. In C. C. J. Carpenter, R. C. Griggs, & J. Loscalzo (Eds.), *Cecil essentials of medicine* (6th ed., pp. 593–602). Philadelphia, PA: W. B. Saunders.

Holman, J. C. M., & McCartney, W. (1960). Iodized salt. In *Endemic goitre* (pp. 411–441). Geneva, Switzerland: World Health Organization.

Horn-Ross, P. L., Morris, S., Lee, M., West, D. W., Whittemore, A. S., McDougall, I. R., … Krone, M. R. (2001). Iodine and thyroid cancer risk among women in a multiethnic population, The Bay Area Thyroid Cancer Study. *Cancer Epidemiology, Biomarkers and Prevention, 20*, 979–985.

Howell, V. M., Haven, C. J., Kahnoski, K., Khoo, S. K., Petillo, D., Chen, J., … Teh, B. T. (2003). *HRPT2* mutations are associated with malignancy in sporadic parathyroid tumours. *Journal of Medical Genetics, 40*(9), 657–663.

Huszno, B., Szybiński, Z., Przybylik-Mazurek, E., Stachura, J., Trofimiuk, M., Buziak-Bereza, M., … Pantoflinski, J. (2003). Influence of iodine deficiency and iodine prophylaxis on thyroid cancer histotypes and incidence in endemic goiter area. *Journal of Endocrinological Investigation, 26*(2 Suppl.), 71–76.

Hydovitz, J. D. (1960). Occurrence of goiter in an infant on a soy diet. *New England Journal of Medicine, 262*, 351–353.

Jacobson, E. M., Huber, A., & Tomer, Y. (2008). The HLA gene complex in thyroid autoimmunity: From epidemiology to etiology. *Journal of Autoimmunity, 30*(1–2), 58–62.

Jacobson, E. M., & Tomer, Y. (2007a). The *CD40, CTLA-4,* thyroglobulin, TSH receptor, and *PTPN22* gene quintet and its contribution to thyroid autoimmunity: Back to the future. *Journal of Autoimmunity, 28*(2–3), 85–98.

Jacobson, E. M., & Tomer, Y. (2007b). The genetic basis of thyroid autoimmunity. *Thyroid, 17*, 949–961.

Kim, E. S., Baek, L. D. J., Lee, J. M., Kim, M. K., Kwon, H. S., Song, K. H., … Son, H. Y. (2010). Thyroglobulin antibody is associated with increased cancer risk in thyroid nodules. *Thyroid, 30*(9), 885–891.

Knobel, M., & Medeiros-Neto, G. (2007). Relevance of iodine intake as a reputed predisposing factor for thyroid cancer. *Archives of Endocrinology and Metabolism, 51*(5), 701–712.

Kolonel, L. N., Hankin, J. H., Wilkens, L. R., Fukunaga, F. H., & Hinds, M. W. (1990). An epidemiologic study of thyroid cancer in Hawaii. *Cancer Causes and Control, 1*(3), 223–234.

Kraimps, J. L., Bouin-Pineau, M. H., Mathonnet, M., De Calan, L., Roncery, J., Visset, J., … Barbier, J. (2000). Multicentre study of thyroid nodules in patients with Graves' disease. *British Journal of Surgery, 87*, 1111–1113.

Kumar, V., Abbas, A. K., & Aster, J. C. (2014). *Robbins and Cotran pathologic basis of disease* (9th ed.). Philadelphia, PA: Mosby & Saunders.

Kurylowicz, A., Ramos-Lopez, E., Bednarczuk, T., & Badenhoop, K. (2006). Vitamin D-binding protein (DBP) gene polymorphism is associated with Graves' disease and the vitamin D status in a Polish population study. *Experimental and Clinical Endocrinology and Diabetes, 114*(6), 329–335.

Lancet. (2008). Iodine deficiency—Way to go yet. *372*(9633), 88.

Lee, J.-H., Younghye, K., Choi, J.-W., & Kim, Y.-S. (2013). The association between papillary thyroid carcinoma and histologically proven Hashimoto's thyroiditis: A meta-analysis. *European Journal of Endocrinology, 168*, 343–349.

Lee, P. K., Jarosek, S. L., Virnig, B. A., Evasovich, M., & Tuttle, T. M. (2007). Trends in the incidence and treatment of parathyroid cancer in the United States. *Cancer, 109*(9), 1736–1741.

Lepez, T., Vandewoestyne, M., & Deforce, D. (2013). Fetal microchimeric cells in autoimmune thyroid diseases. *Chimerism, 4*(4), 111–118.

Levi, F., Franceschi, S., Te, V.-C., Negri, E., & La Vecchia, C. (1990). Descriptive epidemiology of thyroid cancer in the Swiss canton of Vaud. *Journal of Cancer Research and Clinical Oncology, 116*, 639–647.

Levinson, W. (2006). Major histocompatibility complex and transplantation. In W. Levinson (Ed.), *Review of medical microbiology and immunology* (9th ed., pp. 434–439). New York, NY: McGraw-Hill.

Lyon, M. F. (1961). Gene action in the X-chromosome of the mouse (*Mus musculus L.*). *Nature, 190*(4773), 372–373.

Manji, N., Carr-Smith, J. D., Boelaert, K., Allahabadia, A., Armitage, M., Chatterjee, V. K., … Franklyn, J. A. (2006). Influences of age, gender, smoking, and family history on autoimmune thyroid disease phenotype. *Journal of Clinical Endocrinology and Metabolism, 91*, 4873–4880.

Marine, D. (1907). On the occurrence and physiological nature of glandular hyperplasia of the thyroid (dog and sheep), together with remarks on important clinical (human) problems. *Johns Hopkins Bulletin, 18*, 359–365.

Marine, D. (1914). Further observations and experiments on goitre (so called thyroid carcinoma) in brook trout (*Salvelinus fontinalis*). *Journal of Experimental Medicine, 19*, 70–88.

Marine, D. (1924). Etiology and prevention of simple goiter. In *Harvey Lectures Series* (Vol. 19, pp. 96–122). Philadelphia, PA: Lippincott.

Marine, D., & Kimball, O. P. (1917). The prevention of simple goiter in man. *Journal of Laboratory and Clinical Medicine, 3*, 40–48.

Marine, D., & Kimball, O. P. (1920). The prevention of simple goiter in man: Fourth paper. *Archives of Internal Medicine, 25*, 661–672.

Marine, D., & Williams, W. W. (1908). The relation of iodine to the structure of the thyroid gland. *Archives of Internal Medicine, 1*, 349–384.

McClure, R. D. (1935). Goiter prophylaxis with iodized salt. *Science, 82*(2129), 370–371.

McHenry, C. R., & Phitayakorn, R. (2011). Follicular adenoma and carcinoma of the thyroid gland. *Oncologist, 16*(5), 585–593.

Negri, E., Dal Maso, L., Ron, E., La Vecchia, C., Mark, S. D., Preston-Martin, S., … Franceschi, S. (1999). A pooled analysis of case-control studies of thyroid cancer: II. Menstrual and reproductive factors. *Cancer Causes and Control, 10*, 143–155.

Noone, A. M., Howlader, N., Krapcho, M., Miller, D., Brest, A., Yu, M., … Cronin, K. A. (2018). *SEER cancer statistics review, 1975–2015.* Bethesda, MD: National Cancer Institute.

Pani, M. A., Regulla, K., Segni, M., Hofmann, S., Hüfner, M., Pasquino, A. M., … Badenhoop, K. (2002). A polymorphism within the vitamin D-binding protein gene is associated with Graves' disease but not with Hashimoto's thyroiditis. *Journal of Clinical Endocrinology and Metabolism, 87*, 2564–2567.

Parkin, D. M., Bray, F., Ferlay, J., & Pisani, P. (2001). Estimating the world cancer burden: GLOBOCAN 2000. *International Journal of Cancer, 94*, 153–156.

Parkin, D. M., Bray, F., Ferlay, J., & Pisani, P. (2005). Global cancer statistics, 2002. *CA: A Cancer Journal for Clinicians, 55*, 74–108.

Parkin, D. M., Muir, C. S., Whelan, S. L., Gao, Y. T., Ferlay, J., & Powell, J. (1992). *Cancer incidence in five continents. VI.* IARC Scientific Publ. No. 120. Lyon, France: International Agency for Research on Cancer.

Parkin, D. M., Pisani, P., & Ferlay, J. (1999a). Estimates of the worldwide incidence of 25 major cancers in 1990. *International Journal of Cancer, 80*(6), 827–841.

Parkin, D. M., Pisani, P., & Ferlay, J. (1999b). Global cancer statistics. *CA: A Cancer Journal for Clinicians, 49*(1), 33–64.

Pellegriti, G., Belfiore, A., Giuffrida, D., Lupo, L., & Vigneri, R. (1998). Outcome of differentiated thyroid cancer in Graves' patients. *Journal of Clinical Endocrinology and Metabolism, 83*, 2805–2809.

Pemberton, J. D., & Black, B. M. (1948). The association of carcinoma of the thyroid gland and exophthalmic goiter. *Surgery Clinics of North America, 28*, 935–952.

Rapoport, B. (1991). Pathophysiology of Hashimoto's thyroiditis and hypothyroidism. *Annual Review of Medicine, 42*, 91–96.

Repplinger, D., Bargren, A., Zhang, Y.-W., Adler, J., Haymart, M., & Chen, H. (2008). Is Hashimoto's thyroiditis a risk factor for papillary thyroid cancer? *Journal of Surgical Research, 150*(1), 49–52.

Ron, E., & Brenner, A. (2010). Non-malignant thyroid disease following a wide range of radiation exposures. *Radiation Research, 174*(6), 877–888.

Sakoda, L. C., & Horn-Ross, P. L. (2002). Reproductive and menstrual history and papillary thyroid cancer risk: The San Francisco Bay Area Thyroid Cancer Study. *Cancer Epidemiology, Biomarkers and Prevention, 11*(1), 1–57.

Shattuck, T. M., Välimäki, S., Obara, T., Gaz, R. D., Clark, O. H., Shoback, D., … Arnold, A. (2003). Somatic and germ-line mutations of the *HRPT2* gene in sporadic parathyroid carcinoma. *New England Journal of Medicine, 349*(18), 1722–1729.

Shih, M.-L., Lee, J. A., Hsieh, C.-B., Yu, J.-C., Liu, H. D., Kebebew, E., … Duh, Q.-Y. (2007). Thyroidectomy for Hashimoto's thyroiditis: Complications and associated cancers. *Thyroid, 18*(7), 729–734.

Shore, R. E., Hildreth, N., Dvoretsky, P., Pasternack, B., & Andresen, E. (1993). Benign thyroid adenomas among persons X-irradiated in infancy for enlarged thymus glands. *Radiation Research, 134*(2), 217–223.

Sipple, J. H. (1961). The association of pheochromocytoma with carcinoma of the thyroid gland. *American Journal of Medicine, 31*, 163–166.

Surveillance, Epidemiology, and End Results. *SEER data, 1973–2007.* Bethesda, MD: U.S. National Institutes of Health, National Cancer Institute.

Tandon, N., Zhang, L., & Weetman, A. P. (1991). HLA associations with Hashimoto's thyroiditis. *Clinical Endocrinology (Oxford), 34*, 383–386.

Thilly, C. H., Swennen, B., Bourdoux, P., Ntambue, K., Moreno-Reyes, R., Gillies, J., & Vanderpas, J. B. (1993). The epidemiology of iodine-deficiency disorders in relation to goitrogenic factors and thyroid-stimulating-hormone regulation. *American Journal of Clinical Nutrition, 57,* 267S–270S.

Tomer, Y., Barbesino, G., Greenberg, D. A., Concepcion, E., & Davies, T. F. (1999). Mapping the major susceptibility loci for familial Graves' and Hashimoto's diseases: Evidence for genetic heterogeneity and gene interactions. *Journal of Clinical Endocrinology and Metabolism, 84,* 4656–4664.

Tunbridge, W. M. G., Evered, D. C., Hall, R., Appleton, P. A., Brewis, M., Clark, F., … Smith, P. A. (1977). The spectrum of thyroid disease in a community: The Whickham survey. *Clinical Endocrinology, 7,* 481–493.

Vanderpas, J. (2006). Nutritional epidemiology and thyroid hormone metabolism. *Annual Review of Nutrition, 26,* 293–322.

Vanderpump, M. P., & Tunbridge, W. M. (2002). Epidemiology and prevention of clinical and subclinical hypothyroidism. *Thyroid, 12,* 839–847.

Vasko, V. V., Gaudart, J., Allasia, C., Savcehnko, V., Di Cristofaro, J., Saji, M., … De Micco, C. (2004). Thyroid follicular adenomas may display features of follicular carcinoma and follicular variant of papillary carcinoma. *European Journal of Endocrinology, 151,* 779–786.

Vona-Davis, L., & Rose, D. P. (2007). Adipokines as endocrine, paracrine, and autocrine factors in breast cancer risk and progression. *Endocrine-Related Cancer, 14,* 189–206.

Wang, C., & Crapo, L. M. (1997). The epidemiology of thyroid disease and the implications for screening. *Endocrinology and Metabolism Clinics of North America, 26*(1), 189–218.

Weetman, A. P. (2000). Graves' disease. *New England Journal of Medicine, 343,* 1236–1248.

Wegelin, C. (1928). Malignant disease of the thyroid gland and its relation to goiter in man and animal. *Cancer Review, 3,* 197–213.

Werner, P. (1963). Endocrine adenomatosis and peptic ulcer in a large kindred. Inherited multiple tumors and mosaic pleiotropism in man. *American Journal of Medicine, 35,* 205–212.

Wespi-Eggenberger, H. J. (1948). Untersuchungen über das Vorkommen und die Verhütung des Neugeborenenkropfes im Einzugsgebiet des Krankenhauses Frauenfeld. *Schweizerische medizinische Wochenschrift, 78,* 130–132.

Wynder, E. L. (1952). Some practical aspects of cancer prevention. *New England Journal of Medicine, 246,* 573–582.

Yao, R., Chiu, C. G., Strugnell, S. S., Gill, S., & Wiseman, S. M. (2011). Gender differences in thyroid cancer. *Expert Reviews in Endocrinology and Metabolism, 6*(2), 215–243.

Yesilkaya, E., Koc, A., Bideci, A., Camurdan, O., Boyraz, M., Erkal, O., … Cinaz, P. (2008). *CTLA4* gene polymorphisms in children and adolescents with autoimmune thyroid diseases. *Genetic Testing, 12*(3), 461–464.

Zaletel, K., Gaberšček, S., Pirnat, E., Krhin, B., & Hojker, S. (2011). Ten-year follow-up of thyroid epidemiology in Slovenia after increase in salt iodization. *Croatian Medical Journal, 52*(5), 615–621.

Zamani, M., Spaepen, M., Bex, M., Bouillon, R., & Cassiman, J. J. (2000). Primary role of the HLA class II DRB1*0301 allele in Graves' disease. *American Journal of Medical Genetics, 95*(5), 432–437.

Zimmerman, M. B. (2008). Research on iodine and goiter in the 19th and early 20th centuries. *The Journal of Nutrition, 138*(11), 2060–2063.

CHAPTER 32

Epidemiology of Adrenal Cancer

▶ Anatomy and Function of the Adrenal Glands

The adrenal glands are bilateral triangular structures positioned above and slightly behind the kidneys. Each gland consists of the adrenal cortex and the adrenal medulla (**FIGURE 32.1**).

The *adrenal cortex* consists of zones of cuboidal epithelial cells that actively synthesize and secrete steroid hormones. All steroid hormones are synthesized from cholesterol. Adrenal steroids include corticosteroids (cortisol), which regulate the metabolism of protein, fat, and carbohydrates, and mineralocorticoids (aldosterone), which regulate salt and water balance. The adrenal cortex also synthesizes low levels of androgens and estrogens that help modulate masculine and feminine characteristics.

The *adrenal medulla* consists of neuroendocrine cells called *chromaffin cells*. Chromaffin cells communicate with the sympathetic nervous system by virtue of synapses with splanchnic nerves in the adrenal medulla. These cells can be visualized by staining with chromium salts. They synthesize and secrete *catecholamines, epinephrine (adrenaline)*, and *norepinephrine (noradrenaline)*, which regulate blood pressure and modulate response to stress. When the human host is endangered, the adrenal medulla releases a burst of epinephrine (adrenaline) that spurs the body's "fight or flight" response (Kumar, Abbas, & Aster, 2014).

▶ Detection of Adrenal Tumors

Adrenal masses are often found incidentally during imaging studies for other conditions, such as diseases of the genitourinary and/or digestive tract. Such serendipitously discovered adrenal masses are called *incidentalomas*. Most adrenal masses are benign adenomas; only a small fraction (~10%) prove to be malignant on biopsy. Definitive differentiation of benign from malignant adrenal tumors is often problematic and requires careful evaluation of structural, clinical, hormonal, cytologic, and molecular features (Grumbach et al., 2003).

Diagnostic symptoms of adrenal tumors are often related to hormonal imbalance due to hypersecretion of specific hormones by dysplastic and malignant cells. Clinical signs and symptoms of adrenal cortical tumors include Cushing's syndrome, in which excessive production of cortisol influences the body's response to stress, metabolism of fat and protein, and immune function; Conn's disease, in which excessive production of aldosterone leads to increased salt retention, potassium depletion, and elevated blood pressure; and virilism due to excessive production of androgens. The dominant clinical manifestation of tumors of the adrenal medulla (neuroblastoma in children and pheochromocytoma in adults) is hypertension due to excessive production of catecholamines (epinephrine and norepinephrine). Measurement of the levels of these hormones in blood and urine aid in the differential diagnosis of adrenal tumors.

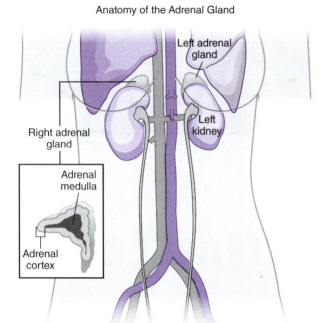

Anatomy of the Adrenal Gland

FIGURE 32.1 Anatomy of the Adrenal Gland.

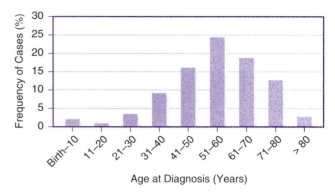

FIGURE 32.2 Age Distribution of Adrenal Cortical Carcinoma.

Data from Kerkhofs, T. M., Verhoeven, R. H., Van der Zwan, J. M., Dieleman, J., Kerstens, M. N., Links, T. P., ... Haak, H. R. (2013). Adrenocortical carcinoma: A population-based study on incidence and survival in the Netherlands since 1993. *European Journal of Cancer, 19*(11), 2579–2586.

Adrenal Cortical Carcinoma

Malignant tumors that arise from the adrenal cortex are called *adrenal cortical carcinomas*. Adrenal tumors that secrete adrenal steroids are classified as functional, whereas nonsecreting tumors are classified as nonfunctional. Most adrenal cortical carcinomas (90%) secrete steroids and are therefore functional.

Global Incidence and Mortality of Adrenal Cortical Carcinoma

Adrenal cortical carcinomas are rare, and accurate data on their incidence and mortality are lacking. A review of 1891 cases identified in published reports between 1952 and 1992 found that 58.6% of cases were female, with a first peak of onset in childhood and a second peak during the fifth decade of life (Wooten & King, 1993).

In the United States, the annual incidence estimated from Surveillance, Epidemiology, and End Results (SEER) data is less than one case per million. Adrenal cortical carcinoma accounts for only about 0.1% of all U.S. cancer deaths (Goodman, Gurney, Smith, & Olshan, 1999). Among children younger than 15 years of age, high annual rates have been reported in southern Brazil (3–4 cases per million) compared to only 0.3 per million worldwide (Ribeiro et al., 2000; Sandrini, Ribeiro, & DeLacerda, 1997). As discussed later in this chapter, a specific germline

mutation in the *p53* tumor–suppressor gene is responsible for more than 90% of Brazilian childhood cases (Ribeiro et al., 2001).

In a recent population-based study conducted in the Netherlands during 1993–2010, the age-adjusted annual incidence was estimated at about 1.2 per million, and 55% of 359 cases were female. The age at diagnosis ranged from 1 to 91 years of age, with a small early peak during childhood and a much higher peak in the fifth decade of life (**FIGURE 32.2**). The investigators noted a slight downward trend in the incidence (from 1.3 to 1.0 per million during the period of study), but no change in survival (Kerkhofs et al., 2013).

Risk Factors for Adrenal Cortical Carcinomas

In an exploratory study in which 176 decedent cases of adrenal cancer were compared to 352 age- and gender-matched controls, long-term use of oral contraceptives and heavy tobacco smoking were found to increase the risk of developing adrenal cortical carcinoma by approximately twofold (Hsing, Nam, Co Chien, McLaughlin, & Fraumeni, 1996).

In a subsequent study, the association between tobacco use and mortality due to adrenal cortical carcinoma was examined in a cohort of 248,046 male U.S. veterans. A total of 27 adrenal cancer deaths were observed during the period of study, 1954–1980. Relative to nonusers of any tobacco, the risk of dying from adrenal cancer was elevated more than fivefold among current cigarette smokers (relative risk [RR] = 5.1) and more than eightfold among those who smoked more than 20 cigarettes per day (RR = 8.4) (Chow, Hsing, McLaughlin, & Fraumeni, 1996).

Genetic Predisposition to Adrenal Cortical Carcinoma

Specific genetic syndromes have been identified that increase the risk of developing adrenal cortical carcinoma and several other malignant neoplasms. These include Li–Fraumeni syndrome, Beckwith–Wiedemann syndrome, Carney complex, and familial adenomatous polyposis.

Li–Fraumeni Syndrome

Li–Fraumeni syndrome is a rare hereditary condition caused by mutant forms of the *p53* tumor–suppressor gene located on the short arm of chromosome 17. The protein encoded by *p53* plays a critical role in a variety of cellular processes, including cell division, DNA repair, apoptosis, response to cellular stress, and regulation of embryo implantation and fertility (Mai et al., 2012).

Multiple germline mutations of *p53* have been identified that predispose to a wide range of malignant neoplasms, including adrenal cortical carcinoma, glioma, sarcoma, and leukemia in children and cancers of the lung, breast, and lymphatic system in adults. This bizarre profile of cancers characterizes the classic Li–Fraumeni syndrome. Indeed, multigenerational pedigrees have been reported in which the risk of cancer development among carriers of such mutations approaches 100% (Schneider, Zelley, Nichols, & Garber, 1999).

In contrast to the classic Li–Fraumeni syndrome, a few *p53* mutations have been identified that show diminished penetrance and tumor development limited to specific tissues. Notably, one such *p53* mutation has been identified as the primary cause of pediatric adrenal cortical carcinomas in southern Brazil.

In the contiguous Brazilian states of São Paulo and Paraná, the incidence of adrenal cortical carcinoma in children under age 15 years is estimated at 3–4 cases per million, which is 10–15 times higher than the global incidence of this malignancy. To explore the potential role of *p53* mutations, a team of international investigators conducted a genetic study of 36 cases of childhood adrenal cortical carcinoma and members of their families ascertained from this high incidence region. Samples of DNA from cases and family members were specifically probed for *p53* mutations by polymerase chain reaction analysis. Remarkably, 35 of the 36 cases had an identical germline point mutation of the p53 gene encoding a single base pair change (*p53* mutant *R337H*). However, unlike the Li–Fraumeni syndrome, there was no excess of other cancers among family members. The investigators concluded that a single *p53* mutation is responsible for the extraordinarily high incidence of childhood adrenal cortical carcinoma in this region; nevertheless, its effect appears to be limited to the adrenal glands, in sharp contrast to the profile of malignancies observed in the classic Li–Fraumeni syndrome. They speculate that exposure to an environmental mutagen might have caused the specific germ cell mutation in this population (Ribeiro et al., 2000).

Due to the extraordinarily high incidence of pediatric adrenocortical tumors in southern Brazil, where more than 90% of patients carry the germline *p53* mutation *R337H*, free newborn screening was offered at all hospitals in the state of Paraná. Parents of positive newborns were tested, and relatives in the carrier line were offered screening. Positive newborns and their relatives under the age of 15 years were offered surveillance (periodic clinical, laboratory, and ultrasound evaluations), and adrenal cortical tumors detected by imaging were surgically resected. Of 180,000 newborns offered screening, 171,649 (95.3%) were screened and 461 were identified as carriers. Screening of relatives identified an additional 228 carriers. Surveillance resulted in early detection and successful resection of 17 adrenal cortical tumors among carriers. Cancer histories and pedigrees were also obtained for 353 families in which 48 cases of adrenal cortical carcinoma were identified among 1704 carriers of the mutant gene. These findings provide an important example of a successful program of genetic screening and therapy for a life-threatening form of cancer in children (Custódio et al., 2013).

Beckwith–Wiedemann Syndrome

Beckwith–Wiedemann syndrome is characterized by overgrowth of certain cell populations during early human development resulting in asymmetry of legs, arms, and other bilateral structures of the body; macroglossia (large tongue); visceromegaly (enlarged abdominal organs); enlarged adrenal glands; abdominal and renal abnormalities; and hypoglycemia (low blood sugar). Children with Beckwith–Wiedemann syndrome have an approximate 20% risk of developing certain childhood cancers during the first few years of life (e.g., adrenal cortical carcinoma, neuroblastoma, retinoblastoma, Wilms tumor [nephroblastoma], and rhabdomyosarcoma). The incidence is approximately 1 per 13,700 live births (Shuman, Beckwith, Smith, & Weksberg, 2000; Weksberg, Shuman, & Smith, 2005).

Beckwith–Wiedemann syndrome has been linked to epigenetic events during childhood resulting in methylation of several genes on the short arm of chromosome 11. The affected genes encode specific growth factors, such as insulin growth factor (IGF-II), that regulate early growth and development. Overexpression of IGF-II is characteristic of adrenal cortical carcinoma in children with Beckwith–Wiedemann syndrome and is also found in 60%–90% of tumor specimens from sporadic cases (Barlaskar & Hammer, 2007).

Carney Complex

The *Carney complex* is a constellation of anomalies including cardiac and cutaneous myxomas (benign tumors of connective tissue), testicular and pituitary tumors, pigmented cutaneous nodular hyperplasia, and adrenal cortical adenomas. This autosomal dominant genetic condition is caused by germline mutations in the *PRKAR1A* gene located on the long arm of chromosome 17 (Barlaskar & Hammer, 2007). The *PRKAR1A* gene encodes a subunit of the enzyme protein kinase A, which is critical for the regulation of cell division. The normal catalytic function of protein kinase A is dependent upon cyclic adenosine monophosphate (AMP) and the integrity of the *PRKAR1A* subunit. When the *PRKAR1A* gene is mutated, protein kinase A is overexpressed, which leads to uncontrolled cell proliferation and tumor formation in certain tissues (Kirschner et al., 2000).

Familial Adenomatous Polyposis

A few reports have described an association between adrenal cortical adenomas and *familial adenomatous polyposis*, a hereditary syndrome caused by a germline inactivating mutation of the *adenomatous polyposis coli (APC)* tumor–suppressor gene (Gaujoux et al., 2010). The *APC* gene, which is located on the long arm of chromosome 5, regulates cadherin proteins that are involved in cell adhesion and contact inhibition of cell proliferation. Individuals who carry mutant forms of the *APC* gene develop florid adenomatous polyps of the colon and are at nearly 100% risk of developing colorectal cancer by the age of 40 years (Markowitz & Bertagnolli, 2009).

Telomerase Reverse Transcriptase Mutations

A team of investigators in the Netherlands recently examined tumors of the adrenal and extra-adrenal paraganglia to assess the frequency of mutations in the promoter region of the *telomerase reverse transcriptase (TERT)* gene. They found *TERT* promoter mutations

in 4 of 38 adrenal cortical carcinomas and 2 of 18 paragangliomas, whereas no mutations were found among 127 pheochromocytomas. Results suggest that activation of telomerase may be involved in the genesis of some adrenal cortical carcinomas and extra-adrenal paragangliomas (Papathomas et al., 2014).

▶ Tumors of the Adrenal Medulla: Neuroblastoma and Pheochromocytoma

The two principal tumors of the adrenal medulla are neuroblastoma and pheochromocytoma. Both tumors arise from neuroendocrine tissues of the adrenal medulla and thus may secrete catecholamines that influence the sympathetic nervous system. Nevertheless, there are distinct differences in the clinical and pathologic features of these tumors. For example, neuroblastomas are diagnosed primarily in children whereas their counterpart, pheochromocytomas, are diagnosed in adults.

Neuroblastoma

Neuroblastomas are tumors that arise from immature neuroendocrine cells in the adrenal medulla or other neuronal tissues of the thorax or abdomen. The famous German pathologist Rudolf Virchow was the first to describe an abdominal tumor of neural tissue that developed in a child. Most neuroblastomas (~80%) are found in children before the age of 5 years, and nearly half of all cases occur before the age of 2 years. These tumors constitute about 6%–10% of all childhood malignancies (Cheung & Dyer, 2013).

Neuroblastomas display unusual developmental characteristics in that they typically regress and disappear spontaneously if they appear in infants under the age of 1 year; alternatively, if they appear later in life, their prognosis is grim because they readily metastasize to other anatomic sites (e.g., bone marrow, bone, liver, brain, and lungs). Neuroblastomas secrete catecholamines, principally norepinephrine, and are thus associated with elevations in blood pressure. Unlike pheochromocytomas (discussed in the next section), neuroblastomas are *not* composed of more mature chromaffin cells that are stained brown by chromium salts.

Maternal Factors and Neuroblastoma

Because neuroblastomas are found almost exclusively in infants and children, gestational and maternal factors may be involved in their development. Preliminary studies suggest that certain gestational exposures influence the risk. These include opiates, folate deficiency, and gestational diabetes.

Investigators at the University of North Carolina evaluated associations of maternal use of specific medications during pregnancy and nursing with the risk of neuroblastoma development in offspring. The study included 504 incident–cases of neuroblastoma identified from hospital records in the United States and Canada during 1992–1994 and 504 disease-free controls from the same communities. Exposure data were collected from mothers of the cases and controls by structured telephone interviews. No associations were found with maternal exposure to diuretic agents, antibiotics, estrogens, progestins, sedatives, or anticonvulsant drugs; however, there was a significant association of neuroblastoma development with maternal use of opioid agonists, particularly codeine, during pregnancy or lactation (odds ratio [OR] = 3.4) (Cook et al., 2004).

In early 1997, a program was initiated by the Canadian government to fortify cereal grains with folic acid. This intervention was aimed at reducing the rate of fetal neural tube defects and possibly other childhood conditions. Investigators at the University of Toronto examined rates of neuroblastoma before and after folate fortification in the province of Ontario, Canada. Data on incident neuroblastoma cases during 1985–2000 were retrieved from the Pediatric Oncology Group of Ontario, which captures 95% of all pediatric cancers. Time series analysis revealed a significant 61% decline in the rate of neuroblastoma from 1.57 to 0.62 cases per 10,000 live births after folic acid fortification (French et al., 2003).

Investigators at the University of Washington in Seattle conducted a population-based case–control study of 240 cases of neuroblastoma and 2400 controls ascertained from cancer registry records collected during 1980–2004. They found significant associations of neuroblastoma with major congenital abnormalities of the heart and other organs (OR = 6.9) and maternal gestational diabetes (OR = 1.8) (Chow, Friedman, & Mueller, 2007).

Genetics of Neuroblastoma

Most neuroblastomas occur sporadically in the absence of specific germline mutations or chromosomal aberrations. Exceptions include Turner syndrome (45, X genotype and gonadal dysgenesis), Hirschsprung's disease (mutant RET proto-oncogene and failure of migration of neuroblasts from the neural crest during embryogenesis), and neurofibromatosis type 1 (mutant *NF1* gene and defective neurofibromin, a protein essential for nerve development).

Alfred Knudson and Louise Strong reviewed data on the age at diagnosis and occurrence of multiple tumors in sporadic cases and familial cases of neuroblastoma and pheochromocytoma ascertained by a review of the literature. Their review included 504 sporadic and 25 familial cases of neuroblastoma and 366 sporadic and 46 familial cases of pheochromocytoma. They concluded that for both tumors, predisposed individuals do not develop a tumor until a second genetic event occurs in a somatic cell. They suggest that the data on familial incidence, age at diagnosis, and multiplicity of tumors are compatible with a two-hit mutational model of tumor development. In sporadic cases, both events occur in somatic cells whereas in familial (hereditary) cases, one mutation occurs in germinal cells and is inherited and the second occurs in somatic cells (Knudson, 1971; Knudson & Strong, 1972).

Survival of Neuroblastoma

Neuroblastomas are responsible for about 15% of deaths from cancer in children. The genetic aberration most consistently associated with poor outcome is amplification of the *N-myc* proto-oncogene, which occurs in approximately 20% of primary tumors (Slavc et al., 1990). Long-term survival in this high-risk group, even with aggressive therapy, remains very low (~15%). Specific chromosomal aberrations (e.g., deletion of chromosomes 1p and 11q and gain of 17q) are also associated with poor prognosis. Stage 4S is a special category of neuroblastoma reserved for infants diagnosed before 1 year of age and who have resectable tumors and metastasis limited to the liver. Spontaneous regression of tumors in this group is high, and overall survival exceeds 85% (Brodeur, Hogarty, Mosse, & Maris, 2011).

In a recent investigation conducted by investigators of the U.S. Pediatric Cancer Genome Project, tissues from 104 patients with metastatic neuroblastoma were analyzed by polymerase chain reaction (PCR) analysis and other molecular methods to identify associated gene mutations. Notably, mutations in the α-*thalassemia/mental retardation syndrome X-linked* (*ATRX*) gene were identified in 14 of 32 tumor specimens (44%) from adolescents and young adults compared to 9 of 54 (17%) from children and 0 of 18 (0%) from infants. The *ATRX* gene encodes a protein that is intricately involved in chromatin remodeling, nucleosome assembly, and telomere maintenance. The observed *ATRX* mutations in neuroblastoma tissues were associated with the absence of the *ATRX* protein and the presence of long telomeres at the chromosomal tips. The authors suggest that the presence of *ATRX* mutations may help identify patients with progressive disease that can be targeted for new molecular therapies (Cheung et al., 2012).

Pheochromocytoma

Pheochromocytomas arise from chromaffin cells of the medulla of the adrenal gland or other anatomic sites where such cells exist in the sympathetic nervous system. Extra-adrenal pheochromocytomas (called *paragangliomas*) constitute about 10% of such tumors. These tumors are usually benign and are most often detected in adults in the age range of 20–50 years.

Pheochromocytomas hypersecrete catecholamines and thus cause marked elevations in blood pressure. Most pheochromocytomas (more than 90%) have no metastatic potential and are thus curable by excision.

Genetic Predisposition to Pheochromocytoma

A significant fraction of cases, perhaps 30%, occur in familial settings with multigenerational inheritance patterns. The most common of these hereditary conditions are von Hippel–Lindau disease (VHL) and the multiple endocrine neoplasia (MEN) syndromes.

Von Hippel–Lindau Disease

Von Hippel–Lindau disease (VHL) is a rare, autosomal dominant genetic condition that predisposes individuals to a spectrum of benign and malignant tumors of the central nervous system and certain other tissues. The condition is caused by a germline mutation in the von Hippel–Lindau tumor–suppressor gene on the short arm of chromosome 3. Carriers of the mutant gene typically develop multiple tumors, including hemangioblastomas of the retina and central nervous system, clear cell renal carcinomas, pheochromocytomas, pancreatic neuroendocrine tumors, pancreatic cysts, endolymphatic sac tumors, and epididymal papillary cystadenomas. The incidence of VHL is about 1 per 36,000 live births, and the penetrance of the mutated gene is over 90% by age 65 years (Richard, Gardie, Couvé, & Gad, 2012).

▶ Multiple Endocrine Neoplasia and Sipple Syndrome

Pheochromocytomas in combination with tumors of the thyroid and parathyroid glands make up a hereditary syndrome known as *MEN*. The MEN syndromes

are caused by heritable mutations of the *MENIN* gene, a tumor–suppressor gene located on chromosome 11, or the *RET* gene, a proto-oncogene located on chromosome 10 (Donis-Keller et al., 1993; Eng, 1999; Guru et al., 1998).

Endocrine tumors of the MEN syndromes elaborate a variety of amines and peptides depending upon the tissue of origin. Individuals who manifest MEN syndromes are classified into two major groups: MEN I (adenomas of the pituitary gland, islet cell tumors of the pancreas, hyperplasia of the parathyroid glands, and peptic ulcers) and MEN II (medullary thyroid carcinoma, pheochromocytoma, and occasionally mucocutaneous neuroma). These syndromes show an autosomal dominant inheritance pattern (Carney, 1998; Werner, 1963).

Mutant forms of the *MENIN* gene cause MEN I. The *MENIN* gene encodes a protein (menin) that has multiple functions within the cell nucleus. Specifically, menin regulates the transcription of certain genes involved in cell division such as TERT (Hashimoto et al., 2008).

Mutant forms of the *RET* gene cause MEN II. The *RET* gene encodes a cell membrane receptor called receptor tyrosine kinase that activates signal transduction and complex cascades of biochemical reactions involving tyrosine phosphorylation within cells. The exact nature of these reactions depends upon the cell type; for example, in parafollicular C cells, *RET* signaling induces excess biosynthesis of calcitonin (Eng, 1999).

Carriers of certain mutated forms of the *RET* gene have a high lifetime risk of developing medullary thyroid carcinoma and pheochromocytoma. The familial association of medullary thyroid cancer (a form of thyroid carcinoma that originates from the parafollicular C cells that secrete the hormone calcitonin) and pheochromocytoma is called the *Sipple syndrome* after the physician who first described it (Sipple, 1961). Early onset, typically 15–20 years of age, is a prominent characteristic of Sipple syndrome.

▶ Summary of Adrenal Cancer Epidemiology

Adrenal cancers are rare, with annual incidence rates of 1–2 per million in most populations. Adrenal tumors arise from either the cortex or the medulla of the adrenal glands. Adrenal tumors typically hypersecrete adrenal hormones specific for their cell of origin; for example, adenomas and carcinomas of the cortex secrete cortisol, aldosterone, or androgens whereas tumors of the medulla secrete catecholamines. Clinical signs and symptoms of these tumors are therefore associated with elevated levels of specific adrenal hormones.

Certain genetic syndromes caused by germline mutations are associated with the development of adrenal cortical tumors. The syndromes and mutated genes include Li–Fraumeni syndrome (*p53*), Beckwith–Wiedemann syndrome (IGF-II), Carney complex (*PRKAR1A*), and familial adenomatous polyposis (*APC*). Mutations in the promoter region of the TERT gene have also been identified in about 10% of adrenal cortical carcinomas. Chronic tobacco smoking and long-term use of oral contraceptives may also increase the risk. Notably, genetic screening for a specific germline *p53* mutation (*R337H*) conducted in southern Brazil has proven effective for the early detection and successful therapy of adrenal cortical tumors in children.

Neuroblastomas arise from immature neuroendocrine cells of the adrenal medulla. These tumors characteristically hypersecrete catecholamines that cause hypertension. They are responsible for about 15% of deaths from cancer in children. Because neuroblastomas are almost exclusively found in infants and children, gestational and maternal factors may be involved in their development. Maternal risk factors include use of opiates, folate deficiency, and gestational diabetes. Amplification of the *N-myc* proto-oncogene and disabling mutations of the X-linked *ATRX* tumor–suppressor gene are associated with poor outcome in patients with neuroblastoma.

Pheochromocytomas are tumors of the adrenal medulla that arise in adults. Most pheochromocytomas (more than 90%) are benign and have no metastatic potential. Nevertheless, these tumors also hypersecrete catecholamines and thus cause marked elevations in blood pressure. A significant fraction of cases, perhaps 30%, occur in familial settings with multigenerational inheritance patterns. The most common of these hereditary conditions are von Hippel–Lindau (VHL) disease and the MEN syndromes.

References

Barlaskar, F. M., & Hammer, G. D. (2007). The molecular genetics of adrenal cortical carcinoma. *Reviews in Endocrine and Metabolic Disorders, 8*(4), 343–348.

Brodeur, G. M., Hogarty, M. D., Mosse, Y. P., & Maris, J. M. (2011). Neuroblastoma. In P. A. Pizzo & D. G. Poplack (Eds.), *Principles and practice of pediatric oncology* (pp. 886–922). Philadelphia, PA: Lippincott Williams & Wilkins.

Carney, J. A. (1998). Familial multiple endocrine neoplasia syndromes: Components, classification, and nomenclature. *Journal of Internal Medicine, 243*(6), 425–432.

Cheung, N. K., & Dyer, M. A. (2013). Neuroblastoma: Developmental biology, cancer genomics and immunotherapy. *Nature Reviews Cancer, 13*, 397–411.

Cheung, N. K., Zhang, J., Lu, C., Parker, M., Bahrami, A., Tickoo, S. K., … Dyer, M. A. (2012). Association of age at diagnosis and genetic mutations in patients with neuroblastoma. *Journal of the American Medical Association, 307*(10), 1062–1071.

Chow, E. J., Friedman, D. L., & Mueller, B. A. (2007). Maternal and perinatal characteristics in relation to neuroblastoma. *Cancer, 109*(5), 983–992.

Chow, W. H., Hsing, A. W., McLaughlin, J. K., & Fraumeni, J. F. (1996). Smoking and adrenal cancer mortality among United States veterans. *Cancer Epidemiology, Biomarkers and Prevention, 5*(2), 79–80.

Cook, M. N., Olshan, A. F., Guess, H. A., Savitz, D. A., Poole, C., Blatt, J., … Pollock, B. H. (2004). Maternal medication use and neuroblastoma in offspring. *American Journal of Epidemiology, 159*(8), 721–731.

Custódio, G., Parise, G. A., Kiesel Filho, N., Komechen, H., Sabbaga, C. C., Rosati, R., … Figueiredo, B. C. (2013). Impact of neonatal screening and surveillance for the *TP53 R337H* mutation on early detection of childhood adrenocortical tumors. *Journal of Clinical Oncology, 31*(20), 2619–2626.

Donis-Keller, H., Dou, S., Chi, D., Carlson, K. M., Toshima, K., Lairmore, T. C., … Wells, S. A. Jr. (1993). Mutations in the RET proto-oncogene are associated with MEN 2A and FMTC. *Human Molecular Genetics, 2*(7), 851–856.

Eng, C. (1999). RET proto-oncogene in the development of human cancer. *Journal of Clinical Oncology, 17*(1), 380–393.

French, A. E., Grant, R., Weitzman, S., Ray, J. G., Vermeulen, M. J., Sung, L., … Koren, G. (2003). Folic acid food fortification is associated with a decline in neuroblastoma. *Clinical Pharmacological Therapy, 74*(3), 288–294.

Gaujoux, S., Pinson, S., Gimenez-Roqueplo, A. P., Amar, L., Ragazzon, B., Launay, P., … Bertherat, J. (2010). Inactivation of the APC gene is constant in adrenocortical tumors from patients with familial adenomatous polyposis but not frequent in sporadic adrenocortical cancers. *Clinical Cancer Research, 16*(21), 5133–5141.

Goodman, M. T., Gurney, J. G., Smith, M. A., & Olshan, A. F. (1999). Sympathetic nervous system tumors. In L. A. Ries, M. A. Smith, J. G. Gurney, Linet, M, Young, T. T., Bunin, J. L. (Eds.), *Cancer incidence and survival among children and adolescents: United States SEER program, 1975–1995.* Bethesda, MD: National Cancer Institute.

Grumbach, M. M., Biller, B. M., Braunstein, G. D., Campbell, K. K., Carney, J. A., Godley, P. A., … Wieand, H. S. (2003). Management of the clinically inapparent adrenal mass ("incidentaloma"). *Annals of Internal Medicine, 138*(5), 424–429.

Guru, S. C., Manickam, P., Crabtree, J. S., Olufemi, S. E., Agarwal, S. K., & Debelenko, L. V. (1998). Identification and characterization of the multiple endocrine neoplasia type 1 (MEN1) gene. *Journal of Internal Medicine, 243*(6), 433–439.

Hashimoto, M., Kyo, S., Hua, X., Tahara, H., Nakajima, M., Takakura, M., … Inoue, M. (2008). Role of menin in the regulation of telomerase activity in normal and cancer cells. *International Journal of Oncology, 33*(2), 333–340.

Hsing, A. W., Nam, J. M., Co Chien, H. T., McLaughlin, J. K., & Fraumeni, J. F. Jr. (1996). Risk factors for adrenal cancer: An exploratory study. *International Journal of Cancer, 65*(4), 432–436.

Kerkhofs, T. M., Verhoeven, R. H., Van der Zwan, J. M., Dieleman, J., Kerstens, M. N., Links, T. P., … Haak, H. R. (2013). Adrenocortical carcinoma: A population-based study on incidence and survival in the Netherlands since 1993. *European Journal of Cancer, 19*(11), 2579–2586.

Kirschner, L. S., Carney, J. A., Pack, S. D., Taymans, S. E., Giatzakis, C., Cho, Y. S., ... Stratakis, C. A. (2000). Mutations of the gene encoding the protein kinase A type I-alpha regulatory subunit in patients with the Carney complex. *Nature Genetics, 26*(1), 89–92.

Knudson, A. G. (1971). Mutation and cancer: Statistical study of retinoblastoma. *Proceedings of the National Academy of Sciences of the United States of America, 68*, 820–823.

Knudson, A. G., Jr., & Strong, L. C. (1972). Mutation and cancer: Neuroblastoma and pheochromocytoma. *American Journal of Human Genetics, 24*(5), 514–532.

Kumar, V., Abbas, A.K., & Aster, J. C. (2014). *Robbins and Cotran pathologic basis of disease* (9th ed.). Philadelphia, PA: Mosby & Saunders.

Mai, P. L., Malkin, D., Garber, J., Schiffman, J. D., Weitzel, J. N., Strong, L. C., ... Savage, S. A. (2012). Li-Fraumeni syndrome: Report of a clinical research workshop and creation of a research consortium. *Cancer Genetics, 205*(10), 479–487.

Markowitz, S. D., & Bertagnolli, M. M. (2009). Molecular basis of colorectal cancer. *New England Journal of Medicine, 361*, 2449–2460.

Papathomas, T., Oudijk, L., Zwarthoff, E. C., Post, E., Duijkers, F. A., van Noesel, M., ... Korpershoek, E. (2014). *TERT* promoter mutations in tumors originating from the adrenal gland and extra-adrenal paraganglia. *Endocrine Related Cancer.* ERC-13-0429 [Epub ahead of print].

Ribeiro, R. C., Michalkiewicz, E. L., Figueiredo, B. C., DeLacerda, L., Sandrini, F., Pianovsky, M. D., ... Sandrini, R. (2000). Adrenocortical tumors in children. *Brazilian Journal of Medical and Biological Research, 33*(10), 1225–1234.

Ribeiro, R. C., Sandrini, F., Figueiredo, B., Zambetti, G. P., Michalkiewicz, E., Lafferty, A. R., ... Sandrini, R. (2001). An inherited *p53* mutation that contributes in a tissue-specific manner to pediatric adrenal cortical carcinoma. *Proceedings of the National Academy of Sciences of the United States of America, 98*(16), 9330–9335.

Richard, S., Gardie, B., Couvé, S., & Gad, S. (2012). Von Hippel-Lindau: How a rare disease illuminates cancer biology. *Seminars in Cancer Biology, 23*(1), 26–37.

Sandrini, R., Ribeiro, R. C., & DeLacerda, L. (1997). Childhood adrenocortical tumors. *Journal of Clinical Endocrinology and Metabolism, 82*(7), 2027–2031.

Schneider, K., Zelley, K., Nichols, K. E., & Garber, J. (1999). Li-Fraumeni syndrome. In R. A. Pagon, M. P. Adam, H. H. Ardinger, D. Bird, C. R. Dolan, C. T. Fong, ... K. Stephens (Eds.), *GeneReviews.* Seattle, WA: University of Washington.

Shuman, C., Beckwith, J. B., Smith, A. C., & Weksberg, R. (2000). Beckwith-Wiedemann syndrome. In R. A. Pagon, M. P. Adam, H. H. Ardinger, D. Bird, C. R. Dolan, C. T. Fong, ... K. Stephens (Eds.), *GeneReviews.* Seattle, WA: University of Washington.

Sipple, J. H. (1961). The association of pheochromocytoma with carcinoma of the thyroid gland. *American Journal of Medicine, 31*, 163–166.

Slavc, I., Ellenbogen, R., Jung, W. H., Vawter, G. F., Kretschmar, C., Grier, H., & Korf, B. R. (1990). *myc* gene amplification and expression in primary human neuroblastoma. *Cancer Research, 50*, 1459–1463.

Weksberg, R., Shuman, C., & Smith, A. C. (2005). Beckwith-Wiedemann syndrome. *American Journal of Medical Genetics Part C: Seminars in Medical Genetics, 1137C*(1), 12–23.

Werner, P. (1963). Endocrine adenomatosis and peptic ulcer in a large kindred. Inherited multiple tumors and mosaic pleiotropism in man. *American Journal of Medicine, 35*, 205–212.

Wooten, M. D., & King, D. K. (1993). Adrenal cortical carcinoma. Epidemiology and treatment with mitotane and a review of the literature. *Cancer, 72*(11), 3145–3155.

CHAPTER 33

Epidemiology of Malignant Melanoma

▶ Global Epidemiology of Malignant Melanoma

During 2018, malignant melanoma of the skin was diagnosed in 287,723 individuals worldwide and caused 60,712 deaths. This potentially fatal form of skin cancer was detected slightly more frequently in men than women (150,698 new cases in men versus 137,025 in women, a male-to-female ratio of 1.10); nevertheless, the deaths from melanoma in men exceeded deaths in women by more than 34% (34,831 men and 25,881 women died from melanoma). Incidence and mortality rates of melanoma reflect a similar pattern; the incidence was 21% higher in men than women (3.5 per 100,000 in men and 2.9 per 100,000 in women), whereas the mortality was 60% higher in men (0.8 per 100,000 versus 0.5 per 100,000) (Bray et al., 2018).

The global burden of melanoma has increased dramatically in the 21st century (**FIGURE 33.1**). During 2000–2018, the annual number of cases more than doubled (from 133,000 to nearly 288,000 cases) and the annual deaths from melanoma increased by 65% (from 37,000 to 61,000 deaths) (Bray et al., 2018; Ferlay et al., 2010, 2013, 2018; Fitzmaurice et al., 2017, 2018; Parkin et al., 2001, 2005).

Malignant melanoma is most common in Caucasian populations living in sunny climates. High incidence rates are observed in Caucasian populations

of Australia, New Zealand, North America, Western Europe, Scandinavia, the Republic of South Africa, Northern Chile, and Papua New Guinea (**FIGURE 33.2**). Melanoma incidence is particularly high in Australia and New Zealand (~34 per 100,000 in 2018) and males in these nations have the highest mortality rates in the world (4.3 and 7.2 deaths per 100,000, respectively) (Ferlay et al., 2018).

The global pattern of malignant melanoma reflects the interactions of susceptible genotypes and phenotypes with cumulative exposure to ionizing radiation from the sun. Due to heavy diffuse melanin skin pigmentation that forms a protective barrier against cumulative radiation damage, populations living nearest the equator are *not* at the highest risk for development of melanoma. Rather, individuals without substantial melanin pigment in the epidermis are most susceptible to cumulative damage due to ultraviolet (UV) rays and the development of this potentially fatal malignancy of the skin. The highest mortality rates are observed among the fair-skinned populations of Australia, South Africa, and certain regions of South America, and progressively lesser rates are found depending on the degree of skin pigmentation coupled with the level of sun exposure. Furthermore, several investigators have suggested that the depletion of the ozone layer and the absence of cloud cover increase exposure to the sun and therefore heighten the risk – the Caucasian populations of Australia and New Zealand have the highest mortality,

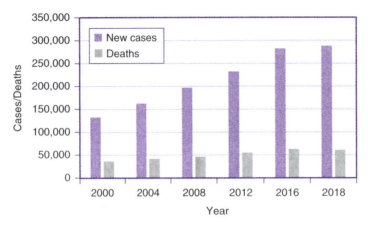

FIGURE 33.1 Global Trends of Malignant Melanoma, 2000–2018.

Data from Bray, F., Ferlay, J., Soerjomataram, I., Siegel, R. L., Torre, L. A., & Jemal, A. (2018). Global cancer statistics 2018: GLOBOCAN estimates of incidence and mortality worldwide for 36 cancers in 185 countries. *CA: A Cancer Journal for Clinicians, 68*(6), 394–424; Ferlay, J., Shin, H. R., Forman, D., Mathers, C., & Parkin, D. M. (2010). Estimates of worldwide burden of cancer in 2008. *International Journal of Cancer, 127*(12), 2893–2917; Ferlay, J., Soerjomataram, I., Ervik, M., Dikshit, R., Eser, S., Mathers, C., . . . Bray, F. (2013). *GLOBOCAN 2012 v1.0. cancer incidence and mortality worldwide: IARC CancerBase No. 11*; [Internet]. Lyon, France: International Agency for Research on Cancer. Retrieved from http://globocan.iarc.fr; Parkin, M., Bray, F., Ferlay, J., & Pisani, P. (2001). Estimating the world cancer burden: GLOBOCAN 2000. *International Journal of Cancer, 94*, 153–156; Parkin, M., Bray, F., Ferlay, J., & Pisani, P. (2005). Global cancer statistics, 2002. *CA: A Cancer Journal for Clinicians, 55*, 74–108; Fitzmaurice, C., Allen, C., Barber, R. M., Barregard, L., Bhutta, Z. A., Brenner, H., . . . Naghavi, M. (2017). Global, regional, and national cancer incidence, mortality, years of life lost, years lived with disability, and disability-adjusted life-years for 32 cancer groups, 1990 to 2015: A systematic analysis for the Global Burden of Disease Study. *JAMA Oncology, 3*(4), 524–548; Fitzmaurice, C., Akinyemiju, T. F., Al Lami, F. H., Alam, T., Alizadeh-Navaei, R., Allen. C., . . . Naghavi, M. (2018, June 02). Global, regional, and national cancer incidence, mortality, years of life lost, years lived with disability, and disability-adjusted life-years for 29 cancer groups, 1990 to 2016: A systematic analysis for the Global Burden of Disease Study. *JAMA Oncology*. Published online June 02, 2018. doi:10.1001/jamaoncol.2018.2706.

presumably because of the thinning ozone layer in the southern hemisphere over the past several decades (Carver, 1998). In recent decades, sharp increases in incidence and mortality have been observed in both sexes in many countries, even where rates were formerly low, such as Japan. In the Nordic countries, for example, the rate of increase since 1980 has averaged approximately 30% every 5 years (Parkin et al., 2005). Similar increases are evident in the U.S. population, where the incidence of malignant melanoma has more than tripled in men and women during the last three decades (Altekruse et al., 2009; Noone et al., 2018) (**FIGURE 33.3**).

▶ Pathogenesis of Malignant Melanoma

The cell of origin of malignant melanoma is the melanocyte, which resides in the basal layer of the epidermis. In this location, melanocytes are in contact with keratinocytes of the epidermis. Melanocytes synthesize melanin, a brownish-black pigment that is distributed to surrounding keratinocytes through dendritic projections (Gilchrest, Eller, Geller, & Yaar, 1999). The melanocyte population rests on a fibrous basement membrane that separates the epidermis from the dermis. When malignant melanoma first develops, the basement membrane forms a protective barrier that keeps the tumor cells confined (in situ). However, malignant melanocytes are unusual in their ability to breach the basement membrane and invade the underlying dermis (**FIGURE 33.4**). The high metastatic

potential of malignant melanoma is responsible for its significant impact on cancer mortality.

Damage to melanocytes caused by UV radiation is central to the pathogenesis of malignant melanoma (Gilchrest et al., 1999). For example, patients with *xeroderma pigmentosum* have a genetically inherited defect in the repair of DNA photoproducts induced by UV radiation (Cleaver, 1968); individuals with this condition are at greatly increased risk of developing malignant melanoma as well as squamous cell and basal cell carcinomas of the skin (Lambert, Kuo, & Lambert, 1995).

Both ultraviolet A (UVA) (wavelength: 320–400 nm) and ultraviolet B (UVB) (wavelength: 270–320 nm) radiations have deleterious effects on the DNA of melanocytes and other cells of the skin. UVB radiation induces the formation of pyrimidine dimers that, if incorrectly repaired, cause DNA mutations (Freeman et al., 1989). UVA radiation causes oxidative damage to DNA that is also potentially mutagenic (Meyskens, Farmer, & Anton-Culver, 2004; Pathak, 1991).

Melanin serves *photoprotective* functions in the skin: It absorbs UV photons and reactive oxygen species generated by the interaction of photons with cell membrane lipids and other cellular components (Pathak, 1995). Within cells, melanin forms a *supranuclear protective cap* about the nucleus, thereby shielding the nuclear DNA from damaging UV radiation (Kobayashi et al., 1998). The photoprotective property of melanin is illustrated by the phenomenon of tanning in response to UV radiation. Tanning is due to enhanced proliferation of melanocytes accompanied by increased synthesis and transfer of melanin

Estimated age-standardized incidence rates (World) in 2018, melanoma of skin, both sexes, all ages

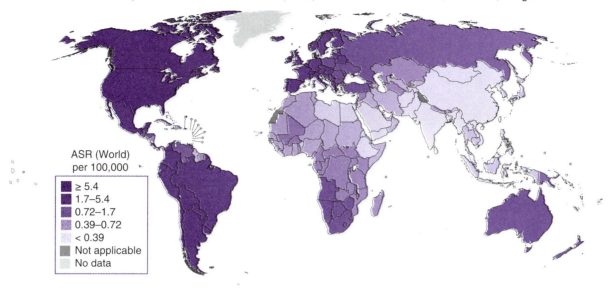

ASR (World)
per 100,000

- ≥ 5.4
- 1.7–5.4
- 0.72–1.7
- 0.39–0.72
- < 0.39
- Not applicable
- No data

Estimated age-standardized mortality rates (World) in 2018, melanoma of skin, both sexes, all ages

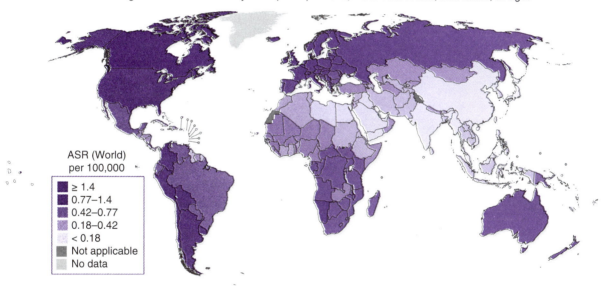

ASR (World)
per 100,000

- ≥ 1.4
- 0.77–1.4
- 0.42–0.77
- 0.18–0.42
- < 0.18
- Not applicable
- No data

FIGURE 33.2 Global Incidence and Mortality Rates of Malignant Melanoma, 2018.

Caption: ASR: Rates per 100,000 are age-standardized to the world population, 2000–2025.

Reproduced with permission from Ferlay, J., Ervik, M., Lam, F., Colombet, M., Mery, L., Piñeros, M., ... Bray, F. (2018). *Global cancer observatory: Cancer today.* Lyon, France: International Agency for Research on Cancer. Available from: https://gco.iarc.fr/today, accessed [09 October 2018].

to surrounding keratinocytes (Gilchrest, Park, Eller, & Yaar, 1998).

Numerous studies suggest that repeated intense exposure to UV radiation leads to the accumulation of cancer-causing mutations in melanocytes. As discussed later in this chapter, several genetic mutations have already been identified that cause dysfunction in melanin biosynthesis and dissemination, cell adhesion and communication, mechanisms of DNA repair, and regulation of the cell cycle.

In addition to the potential for inducing mutagenic changes in the DNA of melanocytes, UV radiation also causes inflammation and immunosuppression in the skin, both of which may play a role in carcinogenesis as well as the metastatic spread of cancer (Gilchrest et al., 1999). Several molecular studies have noted overexpression of cyclooxygenase-2 (COX-2), the chief regulatory enzyme of the inflammatory cascade, in the progression of malignant melanoma from dysplasia to invasive cancer (Denkert et al.,

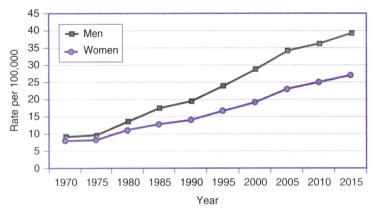

FIGURE 33.3 Annual Incidence of Malignant Melanoma in the United States, 1970–2015.

Caption: Incidence Rates per 100,000 are age-standardized to the U.S. population in 2000.

Data from Altekruse, S. F., Kosary, C. L., Krapcho, M., Neyman, N., Aminou, R., Waldron, W., ... Edwards, B. K. (Eds.). (2009). *SEER cancer statistics review, 1975–2007.* Bethesda, MD: National Cancer Institute; Noone, A. M., Howlader, N., Krapcho, M., Miller, D., Brest, A., Yu, M., ... Cronin, K. A. (2018). *SEER cancer statistics review, 1975–2015.* Bethesda, MD: National Cancer Institute.

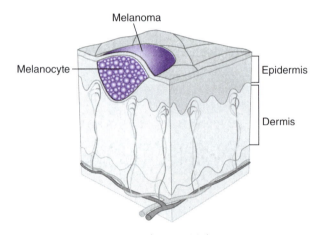

FIGURE 33.4 Cutaneous Malignant Melanoma.

2001; Goulet et al., 2003). In fact, some investigators have observed chemopreventive effects of nonsteroidal anti-inflammatory drugs against melanoma development (Gamba et al., 2013; Harris, Namboodiri, & Beebe-Donk, 2001), and selective anti-inflammatory COX-2 inhibiting agents such as celecoxib have shown significant therapeutic value in clinical trials of patients with metastatic malignant melanoma (Hakim et al., 2006).

Even low-dose UVB exposure can damage the Langerhans cells (circulating immune cells found in the epidermis) and produce significant immunosuppression (Tang & Udey, 1991). Thus, failure of the immune system to recognize and destroy malignant cells may also play a significant role in the expansion and promotion of clones of malignant melanocytes (Cruz, Paul, & Bergstresser, 1989).

A key feature in the progression of malignant melanoma is the unusual capacity of cancerous melanocytes to metastasize throughout the body. Homeostasis of the melanocytic population depends on many

features of the cellular milieu in the dermis and epidermis of the skin. In particular, keratinocytes in the epidermis keep melanocytic proliferation in check, and the basement membrane prevents melanocytes from migrating into the dermis. Melanocytes that become cancerous often lose important molecules called *cadherins* that modulate cell-to-cell adhesion and communication. Although signature mutations of malignant melanoma have not yet been identified, the metastatic potential of this form of cancer appears to be the result of complex epigenetic and genetic phenomena that result in the silencing of tumor suppression genes (e.g., p16, *K-ras*, E-cadherin, p53, etc.) and the activation of oncogenes that stimulate cell division (*BRAF, EGFR*), angiogenesis (*VEGF*), deregulation of apoptosis (telomerase), and metastasis (*C-MET*) (Rákosy et al., 2007; Rudolph et al., 2000; Satyamoorthy & Herlyn, 2002; Soubrane et al., 2006). Recent molecular investigations have identified mutations of the *BRAF* gene in up to 80% of malignant melanomas (Davies et al., 2002). Mutant *BRAF* protein stimulates deregulation of important mechanisms of carcinogenesis in melanocytes (e.g., cell division and apoptosis) and has been proposed as a molecular target for the therapy of malignant melanoma (Garber, 2009).

▶ Risk Factors for Malignant Melanoma

The primary risk factor for the development of malignant melanoma is excessive exposure to UV rays from the sun. Many epidemiologic investigations have also demonstrated that the risk increases with lighter pigmentation of the skin by melanin. Individuals with lightly pigmented skin are at the highest risk and individuals with darkly pigmented skin are at the lowest risk. Other phenotypic factors also increase the risk, including inability to tan, light eye color, red hair, and extensive freckling. Furthermore, the risk increases with the number of pigmented (melanocytic) nevi (see the following discussion). Although the risk of malignant melanoma development is clearly linked to cumulative exposure to the sun, the risk is heightened further by intense, intermittent exposure causing multiple sunburns, particularly during childhood and adolescence.

In contrast to other types of skin cancer, malignant melanoma frequently occurs in areas of the body that are intermittently exposed to the sun, such as the back in men and the lower legs in women, with relative sparing of more frequently exposed sites such as the face, hands, and forearms (Gilchrest et al., 1999). Furthermore, malignant melanoma is more likely to develop in persons with predominantly indoor occupations whose exposure to the sun is limited to weekends and vacations (Holman, Armstrong, & Heenan, 1986). Indeed, the marked increase in the incidence of malignant melanoma in recent decades may reflect the effects of intense intermittent exposures in individuals who vacation in sunny climates during the winter months (Westerdahl et al., 1992). The risk of malignant melanoma is specifically increased with exposures that induce sunburn; for example, a history of five or more severe sunburns during adolescence more than doubles the risk (Weinstock, 1996).

Pigmented Nevi and Malignant Melanoma

As pointed out in a review of melanoma epidemiology by Margaret Tucker, there are two broad categories of pigmented nevi, common and dysplastic, which carry different risks of melanoma development (Tucker, 2009). Dysplastic nevi, which carry a far greater risk, are characterized by size greater than 5 mm at largest diameter, a flat surface, irregular asymmetric shape, indiscriminate borders, and variability in the degree of pigmentation. In a meta-analysis of 46 epidemiologic studies, Gandini and colleagues examined dose responses in melanoma risk associated with the number of common or dysplastic nevi. Individuals with more than 100 common nevi had a relative risk of 6.4 compared to individuals with fewer than 15 common nevi, whereas even the presence of one solitary dysplastic nevus doubled the risk, and having 10 or more dysplastic nevi produced a 12-fold increase in the risk (Gandini et al., 2005).

Genetic Predisposition to Malignant Melanoma

Approximately 10% of melanoma cases diagnosed in the United States report that one or more relatives are also affected (Greene, 1998; Tucker, 2009). In case–control studies, individuals with a positive family history have roughly a twofold increased risk compared to individuals with no family history.

The familial atypical mole and melanoma (FAMM) syndrome is a rare genetic disorder giving rise to multiple dysplastic pigmented moles of the skin that invariably progress to malignant melanoma. Genetic linkage studies of members of families with the FAMM syndrome have identified two major susceptibility genes, *CDKN2A* and *CDK4*, both of which are inherited in an autosomal dominant pattern. Carriers of either mutant gene are at 100% risk of developing malignant melanoma during their lifetimes (Greene, 1998).

One form of the FAMM syndrome is caused by a mutation in *CDKN2A*, the gene that encodes p16, an important cell cycle regulating protein (Hussussian et al., 1994). The *CDKN2A* gene is located on the short arm of chromosome 9 (9p21). This gene normally codes for the tumor–suppressor protein p16, which is essential for the regulation of cell division (Monzon et al., 1998). Mutant forms of *CDKN2A* encode dysfunctional p16 protein that leads to loss of control of cell division and enhanced proliferation of melanocytes.

A second form of the FAMM syndrome is caused by a mutation in the *CDK4* gene, which maps to the long arm of chromosome 12 (12q13). This gene also codes for an oncogenic protein that is important for the regulation of cell division of melanocytes. Mutations in *CDK4* are very rare and have been detected in only a few families (Greene, 1998).

Individuals who carry certain polymorphisms or mutant alleles of a gene called *MC1R* (melanocortin receptor) are also at increased risk for the development of malignant melanoma. The *MC1R* gene plays an important role in melanin biosynthesis and pigmentation of the skin and hair. Mutant forms of *MC1R* are extremely common and may result in a highly susceptible phenotype: red hair, fair skin, numerous freckles, and inability to tan.

Ultraviolet Radiation from Tanning Beds

Many epidemiologic investigations have focused on the association between malignant melanoma and exposure to UV rays in tanning beds. In 2009, the

International Agency for Research on Cancer (IARC) released a report that categorized tanning beds as "carcinogenic to humans." This classification is based on a meta-analysis of 19 epidemiologic studies indicating that people who begin using tanning devices before age 30 are 75% more likely to develop melanoma (IARC, 2007; World Health Organization, 2009).

In a more recent meta-analysis, a team of European investigators examined data from 27 studies, including 18 conducted in Europe, 7 in the United States and Canada, and 2 in Australia. Their results are based on 11,428 cases of melanoma studied during 1981–2012. The combined results revealed that ever versus never use of tanning beds increased the risk of developing melanoma by 20% (summary relative risk [RR] = 1.20); furthermore, initiation of exposure before age 35 years nearly doubled the risk (summary RR = 1.87). Examination of data from studies that included data on frequency of using tanning beds revealed a 1.8% increase in melanoma risk for each additional annual tanning bed session. There was no evidence of heterogeneity among studies. These findings clearly link exposure to UV radiation in tanning beds to an increased risk of developing melanoma and suggest there is an urgent need to implement strict regulations regarding use of indoor tanning equipment (Boniol, Autier, Boyle, & Gandini, 2012).

A particularly disturbing finding is the increased risk of melanoma among young adults who begin using tanning beds at an early age. Investigators in Australia investigated the association between tanning bed use and the risk of early onset melanoma in a study of 604 cases diagnosed between ages 18 and 39 years and 479 controls matched by age, gender, and residence to the cases. The results revealed that ever versus never use of tanning beds significantly increased the risk of melanoma development by 41%, and more than 10 lifetime sessions doubled the risk (odds ratio [OR] = 2.01). The investigators concluded that exposure of adolescents and young adults to artificial UV radiation in tanning beds increases their risk of developing malignant melanoma at an early age (Cust et al., 2011). Indoor tanning equipment emits primarily UVA rays and, to a lesser extent, UVB rays. Powerful units may produce exposures 10–15 times stronger than midday sunlight, and repeated exposures delivered to the skin in 10- to 20-minute periods could enhance mutagenesis and other mechanisms of carcinogenesis.

Ozone Holes and Malignant Melanoma

The stratospheric ozone layer resides approximately 10–50 km above the earth and acts as a protective

FIGURE 33.5 Ozone Depletion in the Southern Hemisphere, September 2006.
Reproduced from National Aeronautics and Space Administration (NASA). (2006). *National ozone watch.* Goddard Space Flight Center. Retrieved from http://www.theozonehole.com/ozonehole2006.htm

shield against the sun's harmful UV rays, particularly UVB rays (wavelengths of 270–315 nm). The natural ozone shield has been gradually depleted by the atmospheric release of man-made chemicals such as chlorofluorocarbons (freons) and bromofluorocarbons (halons) that spark the catalytic destruction of ozone. Ozone destruction is most prominent around the polar regions of the earth, leading to "ozone holes" and penetration of the earth's atmosphere by UVB rays. Excessive exposure to UVB rays is linked to the development of malignant melanoma as well as other conditions such as cataracts (Norval et al., 2007). Such windows of UVB exposure appear to coincide roughly with the high mortality rates of malignant melanoma in the southern hemisphere of the world, particularly in the populations of Australia, New Zealand, and the southernmost tips of South America and Africa (NASA, 2006) (**FIGURE 33.5**).

▶ Malignant Melanoma and Parkinson's Disease

Early case reports noted that patients with Parkinson's disease treated with levodopa (a synthetic form of dopamine) developed malignant melanoma. More recently, epidemiologic evidence has accumulated suggesting there may be a link between Parkinson's disease and malignant melanoma. In a systematic review and meta-analysis of available data from 12 epidemiological studies, investigators at the *National Institutes of Environment Health Science* found significant increases in the odds ratios for both men (OR = 2.04) and women (OR = 1.52). When temporal data were examined, the development of melanoma was markedly increased after the diagnosis of Parkinson's disease (OR = 3.6) but the reciprocal association was not as strong (OR = 1.44) (Liu, Gao, Lu, & Chen, 2011).

Investigators at the *Shanghai Jiao Tong University School of Medicine* in China conducted an updated meta-analysis of the association that included 25 eligible studies involving 292,275 patients with Parkinson's disease. The pooled odds ratio from their study was significantly increased (OR = 1.83) and subgroup analysis revealed that patients with Parkinson's disease were at increased risk for melanoma (OR = 2.4) whereas the reciprocal association was not significant (Huang, Yang, Chen, & Xiao, 2015). The link between Parkinson's disease and malignant melanoma may somehow be related to the shared biosynthetic pathway of dopamine and melanin from tyrosine, but further research is needed to clarify the biological mechanisms involved.

▶ Prevention of Malignant Melanoma

The primary prevention of malignant melanoma is dependent upon minimizing exposure to intensive UV radiation from the sun, tanning beds, and other sources of radiation. Avoidance of intense sun exposure during peak times of the day, wearing protective clothing, and using sunscreen lotions can offer protection (Autier, 2005).

National and community programs of secondary prevention have also proven to be highly effective. The American Academy of Dermatology recommends annual inspection of the skin by a certified dermatologist for the detection and surgical removal of dysplastic pigmented nevi and other suspicious lesions prior to their progression to malignancy (American Academy of Dermatology, 2010). A special surgical technique called *Mohs surgery*, wherein repeated circumferential sections of tumor are removed and microscopically examined until cancer-free margins are evident, has been shown to be effective in treating in situ cutaneous malignant melanoma (Bene, Healy, & Coldiron, 2008).

References

Altekruse, S. F., Kosary, C. L., Krapcho, M., Neyman, N., Aminou, R., Waldron, W., … Edwards, B. K. (Eds.). (2009). *SEER cancer statistics review, 1975–2007*. Bethesda, MD: National Cancer Institute.

American Academy of Dermatology. (2010). *National skin cancer screening program, USA*. American Academy of Dermatology. Retrieved from https://www.aad.org

Autier, P. (2005). Cutaneous malignant melanoma: Facts about sunbeds and sunscreen. *Expert Review of Anticancer Therapy, 5*(5), 821–833.

Balch, C., Buzaid, A., Soong, S., Atkins, M., Cascinelli, N., Coit, D., … Thompson, J. (2001). Final version of the American Joint Committee on Cancer staging system for cutaneous melanoma. *Journal of Clinical Oncology, 19*(16), 3635–3648.

Bene, N. I., Healy, C., & Coldiron, B. M. (2008). Mohs micrographic surgery is accurate 95.1% of the time for melanoma in situ: A prospective study of 167 cases. *Dermatologic Surgery, 34*(5), 660–664.

Boniol, M., Autier, P., Boyle, P., & Gandini, S. (2012). Cutaneous melanoma attributable to sunbed use: Systematic review and meta-analysis. *BMJ, 345*, e4757. doi:10.1136/bmj.e4757.

Bray, F., Ferlay, J., Soerjomataram, I., Siegel, R. L., Torre, L. A., & Jemal, A. (2018). Global cancer statistics 2018: GLOBOCAN estimates of incidence and mortality worldwide for 36 cancers in 185 countries. *CA: A Cancer Journal for Clinicians, 68*(6), 394–424.

Buzaid, A. (2004). Management of metastatic cutaneous melanoma. *Oncology (Williston Park), 18*(11), 1443–1450.

Carver, G. (1998). *Part III. The science of the ozone hole*. Cambridge, UK: University of Cambridge, Center for Atmospheric Science.

Cleaver, J. E. (1968). Defective repair replication of DNA in xeroderma pigmentosum. *Nature, 218*, 652–656.

Cruz, P. D., Jr., Paul, R., & Bergstresser, P. R. (1989). Ultraviolet radiation, Langerhans' cells and skin cancer: Conspiracy and failure. *Archives of Dermatology, 125*(7), 975–979.

Cust, A. E., Armstrong, B. K., Goumas, C., Jenkins, M. A., Schmid, H., Hopper, J. L., … Mann, G. J. (2011). Sunbed use during adolescence and early adulthood is associated with increased risk of early-onset melanoma. *International Journal of Cancer, 128*(10), 2425–2435.

Davies, H., Bignell, G. R., Cox, C., Stephens, P., Edkins, S., Clegg, S., … Futreal, P. A. (2002). Mutations of the *BRAF* gene in human cancer. *Nature, 417*, 949–954.

Denkert, C., Köbel, M., Berger, S., Siegert, A., Leclere, A., Trefzer, U., & Hauptmann, S. (2001). Expression of cyclooxygenase 2 in human malignant melanoma. *Cancer Research, 61*(1), 303–308.

Ferlay, J., Ervik, M., Lam, F., Colombet, M., Mery, L., Piñeros, M., … Bray, F. (2018). *Global cancer observatory: Cancer today*. Lyon, France: International Agency for Research on Cancer. Retrieved from https://gco.iarc.fr/today

Ferlay, J., Shin, H. R., Forman, D., Mathers, C., & Parkin, D. M. (2010). Estimates of worldwide burden of cancer in 2008. *International Journal of Cancer, 127*(12), 2893–2917.

Ferlay, J., Soerjomataram, I., Ervik, M., Dikshit, R., Eser, S., Mathers, C., … Bray, F. (2013). *GLOBOCAN 2012 v1.0. cancer incidence and mortality worldwide: IARC CancerBase No. 11* [Internet]. Lyon, France: International Agency for Research on Cancer. Retrieved from http://globocan.iarc.fr

Fitzmaurice, C., Akinyemiju, T. F., Al Lami, F. H., Alam, T., Alizadeh-Navaei, R., Allen. C., … Naghavi, M. (2018, June 02). Global, regional, and national cancer incidence, mortality, years of life lost, years lived with disability, and disability-adjusted life-years for 29 cancer groups, 1990 to 2016: A systematic analysis for the Global Burden of Disease Study. *JAMA Oncology*. Online publication June 02, 2018. doi:10.1001/jamaoncol.2018.2706.

Fitzmaurice, C., Allen, C., Barber, R. M., Barregard, L., Bhutta, Z. A., Brenner, H., … Naghavi, M. (2017). Global, regional, and national cancer incidence, mortality, years of life lost, years lived with disability, and disability-adjusted life-years for 32 cancer groups, 1990 to 2015: A systematic analysis for the Global Burden of Disease Study. *JAMA Oncology, 3*(4), 524–548.

Freeman, S. E., Hacham, H., Gange, R. W., Maytum, D. J., Sutherland, J. C., & Sutherland, B. M. (1989). Wavelength dependence of pyrimidine dimer formation in DNA of human skin irradiated *in situ* with ultraviolet light. *Proceedings of the National Academy of the Sciences of the United States of America, 86*, 5605–5609.

Gamba, C. A., Swetter, S. M., Stefanick, M. L., Kubo, J., Desai, M., Spaunhurst, K. M., … Tang, J. Y. (2013). Aspirin is associated with lower melanoma risk among postmenopausal women. *Cancer, 119*(8), 1562–1569.

Gandini, S., Sera, F., Cattaruzza, M. S., Pasquini, P., Abeni, D., Boyle, P., & Melchi, C. F. (2005). Meta-analysis of risk factors for cutaneous melanoma: I. Common and atypical naevi. *European Journal of Cancer, 41*(1), 28–44.

Garber, K. (2009). Cancer research. Melanoma drug vindicates targeted approach. *Science, 326*(5960), 1619.

Gilchrest, B. A., Eller, M. S., Geller, A. C., & Yaar, M. (1999). The pathogenesis of melanoma induced by ultraviolet radiation. *New England Journal of Medicine, 340*(17), 1341–1348.

Gilchrest, B. A., Park, H. Y., Eller, M. S., & Yaar, M. (1998). The photobiology of the tanning response. In J. J. Nordlund, R. E. Boissy, V. J. Hearing, R. A. King, & J. P. Ortonne (Eds.), *The pigmentary system: Physiology and pathophysiology* (pp. 359–372). New York, NY: Oxford University Press.

Goulet, A. C., Einsphar, J. G., Alberts, D. S., Beas, A., Burk, C., Bhattacharyya, A., … Nelson, M. A. (2003). Analysis of cyclooxygenase 2 (COX-2) expression during malignant melanoma progression. *Cancer Biology Therapy, 2*(6), 713–718.

Greene, M. H. (1998). The genetics of hereditary melanoma and nevi. *Cancer, 86*(11), 2464–2477.

Hakim, R., Poggi, R., Pantaleo, M., Benedetti, G., Brandi, G., Zannetti, G., … Biasco, G. (2006). Phase II study of temozolomide and celecoxib in the treatment of metastatic melanoma. *Journal of Clinical Oncology, 24*(18S), 18015.

Harris, R. E., Namboodiri, K. A., & Beebe-Donk, J. (2001). Inverse association of malignant melanoma and non-steroidal anti-inflammatory drugs (NSAIDs) in women. *Oncology Reports, 8*, 655–657.

Holman, C. D. J., Armstrong, B. K., & Heenan, P. J. (1986). Relationship of cutaneous malignant melanoma to individual sunlight-exposure habits. *Journal of the National Cancer Institute, 76*, 403–414.

Huang, P., Yang, X. D., Chen, S. D., & Xiao, Q. (2015). The association between Parkinson's disease and melanoma: A systematic review and meta-analysis. *Translational Neurodegeneration, 4*, 21. doi:10.1186/s40035-015-0044-y.

Hussussian, C. J., Struewing, J. P., Goldstein, A. M., Higgins, P. A., Ally, D. S., Sheahan, M. D., … Dracopoli, N. C. (1994). Germline p16 mutations in familial melanoma. *Nature Genetics, 8*(1), 15–21.

International Agency for Research on Cancer, Working Group on Artificial Ultraviolet (UV) Light and Skin Cancer. (2007).

The association of use of sunbeds with cutaneous malignant melanoma and other skin cancers: A systematic review. *International Journal of Cancer, 120*(5), 1116–1122.

Kobayashi, N., Nakagawa, A., Muramatsu, T., Yamashin, Y., Shiral, T., Hashimoto, M. W., …. Mori, T. (1998). Supranuclear melanin caps reduce ultraviolet induced DNA photoproducts in human epidermis. *Journal of Investigative Dermatology, 110*, 806–810.

Lambert, W. C., Kuo, H. R., & Lambert, M. W. (1995). Xeroderma pigmentosum. *Dermatology Clinics, 13*, 169–209.

Liu, R., Gao, X., Lu, Y., & Chen, H. (2011). Meta-analysis of the relationship between Parkinson disease and melanoma. *Neurology, 76*(23), 2002–2009.

Meyskens, F. L., Jr., Farmer, P. J., & Anton-Culver, H. (2004). Etiologic pathogenesis of melanoma: A unifying hypothesis for the missing attributable risk. *Clinical Cancer Research, 10*(8), 2581–2583.

Monzon, J., Liu, L., Brill, H., Goldstein, A. M., Tucker, M. A., From, L., … Lassam, N. J. (1998). *CDKN2A* mutations in multiple primary melanomas. *New England Journal of Medicine, 338*(13), 879–887.

National Aeronautics and Space Administration (NASA). (2006). *National ozone watch*. Goddard Space Flight Center. Retrieved from http://www.theozonehole.com/ozonehole2006.htm

Noone, A. M., Howlader, N., Krapcho, M., Miller, D., Brest, A., Yu, M., … Cronin, K. A. (2018). *SEER cancer statistics review, 1975–2015*. Bethesda, MD: National Cancer Institute.

Norval, M., Cullen, A. P., de Gruijl, F. R., Longstreth, J., Takizawa, Y., Lucas, R. M., … van der Leun, J. C. (2007). The effects on human health from stratospheric ozone depletion and its interactions with climate change. *Photochemical and Photobiological Sciences, 6*(3), 232–251.

Parkin, M., Bray, F., Ferlay, J., & Pisani, P. (2001). Estimating the world cancer burden: GLOBOCAN 2000. *International Journal of Cancer, 94*, 153–156.

Parkin, M., Bray, F., Ferlay, J., & Pisani, P. (2005). Global cancer statistics, 2002. *CA: A Cancer Journal for Clinicians, 55*, 74–108.

Pathak, M. A. (1991). Ultraviolet radiation and the development of non-melanoma and melanoma skin cancer: Clinical and experimental evidence. *Skin Pharmacology, 4*(Suppl. 1), 85–94.

Pathak, M. A. (1995). Functions of melanin and protection by melanin. In L. Zeise, M. R. Chedekel, & T. B. Fitzpatrick (Eds.), *Melanin: Its role in human photoprotection* (pp. 125–134). Overland Park, KS: Valdenmar.

Rákosy, Z., Vízkeleti, L., Ecsedi, S., Vokó, Z., Bégány, A., Barok, M., … Balázs, M. (2007). EGFR gene copy number alterations in primary cutaneous malignant melanomas are associated with poor prognosis. *International Journal of Cancer, 121*(8), 1729–1737.

Rudolph, P., Schubert, C., Tamm, S., Heidorn, K., Hauschild, A., Michalska, I., … Parwaresch, R. (2000). Telomerase activity in melanocytic lesions: A potential marker of tumor biology. *American Journal of Pathology, 156*, 1425–1432.

Satyamoorthy, K., & Herlyn, M. (2002). Cellular and molecular biology of human melanoma. *Cancer Biology and Therapy, 1*(1), 12–15.

Soubrane, C., Mouawad, R., Sultan, V., Spano, J., Khayat, D., & Rixe, O. (2006). Soluble *VEGF-A* and lymphangiogenesis in metastatic malignant melanoma patients. *Journal of Clinical Oncology, 24*(18S), 8049.

Tang, A., & Udey, M. C. (1991). Inhibition of epidermal Langerhans cell function by low dose ultraviolet B radiation. Ultraviolet B radiation selectively modulates ICAM-1 (CD54) expression by murine Langerhans cells. *Journal of Immunology, 146*(10), 3347–3355.

Tucker, M. (2009). Melanoma epidemiology. *Hematology/Oncology Clinics of North America, 23*, 383–395.

Weinstock, M. A. (1996). Controversies in the role of sunlight in the pathogenesis of cutaneous melanoma. *Photochemistry and Photobiology, 63*, 406–410.

Westerdahl, J., Olsson, H., Ingvar, C., Brandt, L., Jonsson, P. E., & Moller, T. (1992). Southern travelling habits with special reference to tumour site in Swedish melanoma patients. *Anticancer Research, 12*, 1539–1542.

World Health Organization, International Agency for Research on Cancer Monograph Working Group. (2009). A review of human carcinogens—Part D: Radiation. *Lancet Oncology, 10*(8), 751–752.

CHAPTER 34

Epidemiology of Nonmelanoma Skin Cancer: Basal Cell, Squamous Cell, and Merkel Cell Skin Cancers

▶ Anatomy and Function of the Skin

The skin is the largest organ of the body, covering a surface area of approximately 2 square meters (21 square feet) and weighing about 4.5 kg (10 pounds) in the average adult. It serves as a protective barrier that protects internal tissues from exposure to trauma, ultraviolet (UV) radiation, temperature extremes, toxins, and bacteria. Other important functions include sensory perception, immunologic surveillance, thermoregulation, and control of fluid loss. The skin is also actively involved in the biosynthesis of vitamin D. Basic anatomy of the skin is depicted in **FIGURE 34.1**.

The skin consists of three layers: the epidermis, the dermis, and the subcutis. The outer layer of skin is called the epidermis, and it consists of layers of cells called *keratinocytes* that produce the protein keratin. Keratin is a durable but flexible protein that provides strength and elasticity to the skin. Basal cells and squamous cells of the epidermis are collectively called *keratinocytes* because both cell types produce keratin. The epidermis also contains *melanocytes*, which produce melanin, a pigment that absorbs radiant energy from the sun and protects the skin from the harmful effects of UV radiation. Immune cells called *Langerhans cells* (so named after the German pathologist Paul Langerhans, who discovered them in 1868) circulate in the epidermis and play an important role in immunosurveillance and defense against infection. The epidermis also contains neurosensory cells called *Merkel cells* that connect with nerve endings to transmit electrical impulses in response to touch.

The epidermis is separated from the dermis by the *basement membrane*, a thin fibrous membrane composed of glycoproteins and proteoglycans. This membrane anchors the epithelial cells to the underlying dermis and provides a mechanical barrier that prevents malignant cells from invading into deeper tissues.

The *dermis* is connective tissue made of collagen, elastic fibers, and reticular fibers. Its primary function is to sustain and support the epidermis. The major

433

FIGURE 34.1 Anatomic Features of Human Skin.

cell type in the dermis is the fibroblast, which secretes collagen and elastic fibers. The dermis also contains sweat glands, hair roots, nerves, blood vessels, and lymphatic vessels.

The subcutis (or subcutaneous tissue) that underlies the dermis consists primarily of lobules of adipose (fat) separated by connective tissues. The subcutis cushions the body and provides insulation for thermoregulation of internal organs. The adipose of the subcutis also serves as an energy reserve in times of food shortage.

Nonmelanoma Skin Cancer

This chapter focuses on nonmelanoma skin cancers, which make up about 95% of all skin cancers. Melanomas arising from melanocytes of the epidermis make up the remaining 5% of skin cancers. The two principal forms of nonmelanoma skin cancer are basal cell carcinoma and squamous cell carcinoma. These two cell types make up over 99% of all nonmelanoma skin cancers. In a German survey of 12,956 cases, 82% of nonmelanoma skin cancers were basal cell carcinomas, 17% were squamous cell carcinomas, and fewer than 1% were classified as other histological forms (Katalinic, Kunze, & Schäfer, 2003).

Basal cell carcinoma is the most common form of human cancer. These tumors arise from the keratinized basal cells of the epidermis, which are in contact with the basement membrane. Basal cell carcinomas most often develop from the skin of the face, neck, or upper trunk that has been damaged by intermittent blistering sunburns during childhood or adolescence. Although basal cell carcinomas rarely metastasize to

distant organs, they can invade and damage contiguous tissues (de Gruijl, 1999; Miller, 1995).

Squamous cell carcinoma is the second most common human cancer. These tumors arise from keratinized squamous cells in the uppermost cell layers of the epidermis. Squamous cell carcinomas of the skin occasionally develop because of continuous sun exposure throughout life. These tumors nearly always develop due to malignant transformation of sun-induced precancerous skin lesions known as *actinic keratoses*. Exposed skin of the face, neck, and backs of the hands are the most common sites of cumulative sun damage leading to tumor development. In contrast to basal cell carcinomas, squamous cell carcinomas *do* have the potential to metastasize to other organs through the lymph and blood (Armstrong & Kricker, 2001).

Merkel cell carcinoma is a rare malignancy that is briefly discussed in this chapter. This form of cancer arises from the neurosensory Merkel cells of the epidermis. Merkel cell carcinoma tends to be highly aggressive with the potential for rapid and widespread metastasis.

Global Burden of Nonmelanoma Skin Cancer

Investigators at the Institute for Health Metrics and Evaluation (IHME) reported that during 2016, 1.52 million individuals (848,000 men and 673,000 women) were diagnosed with nonmelanoma skin cancer in the world population. Basal cell carcinomas accounted for 886,000 cases (451,000 in men and 436,000 in women) and squamous cell carcinomas accounted for 635,000 cases (397,000 in men and 238,000 in women). All of the 53,000 deaths from nonmelanoma skin cancer (35,000 men and 18,000 women) were attributed to squamous cell carcinomas. The age-adjusted mortality rate for squamous cell carcinoma in men was more than double the rate in women (1.3 per 100,000 versus 0.5 per 100,000) (Fitzmaurice et al., 2018).

▶ Age-Specific Incidence of Nonmelanoma Skin Cancer

Byfield and colleagues examined claims data filed during 2009–2010 in a large national managed healthcare system in the United States in order to characterize the age-specific incidence of nonmelanoma skin cancers. Estimates were based on 47,451 incident cases identified during 2010 from a population of 6.61 million individuals enrolled in the system. **FIGURE 34.2** shows the age-specific incidence of nonmelanoma skin cancer. The incidence rises sharply with age, ranging from approximately 1 case per 100,000 among individuals under the age of 25 years to 209 cases per 100,000 among individuals 75 years of age or older. The data revealed an excess of male cases compared to female cases (54.5% versus 45.5%), and only 16 cases (0.03%) showed evidence of metastatic spread at the time of diagnosis (Byfield, Chen, Yim, & Reyes, 2013).

Staples and colleagues estimated age-specific incidence rates of the two major forms of nonmelanoma skin cancer, basal cell and squamous cell carcinomas, based on national survey data collected in Australia during 2002 (**FIGURE 34.3**). The Australian population has the highest rates of nonmelanoma skin cancer in the world, and it is indeed striking that the 2002

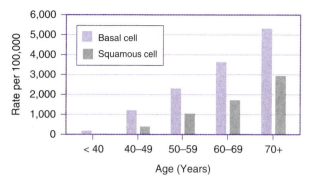

FIGURE 34.3 Age-Specific Incidence of Basal Cell and Squamous Cell Carcinoma in Australia.

Data from Staples, M. P., Elwood, M., Burton, R. C., William, J. L., Marks, R., & Giles, G. G. (2006). Non-melanoma skin cancer in Australia: The 2002 national survey and trends since 1985. *Medical Journal of Australia, 184*, 6–10.

Australian rates were 10–20 times higher than the corresponding age-specific rates for the U.S. population shown in Figure 34.2 (Staples et al., 2006).

The age-specific incidence rates shown in Figure 34.3 reflect a clear difference in the pathogenesis of basal cell versus squamous cell carcinoma. Note that the rate ratio of basal cell to squamous cell carcinoma for individuals under 40 years of age is 29.0 (203 versus 7 per 100,000), whereas after age 40 the rate ratios progressively decline from 2.9 for individuals ages 40–49 years to 1.8 for individuals over 70 years of age. The sharper increase in the risk of squamous cell carcinoma compared to basal cell carcinoma with aging is a possible consequence of the effects of cumulative sun damage (Staples et al., 2006).

▶ Global Incidence and Mortality of Nonmelanoma Skin Cancer

The incidence of nonmelanoma skin cancer is highly correlated with the level of solar radiation and varies inversely with the degree of skin pigmentation among populations. For example, among Caucasians in the United States, nonmelanoma skin cancer constitutes 20%–30% of all neoplasms, whereas among African Americans such lesions are infrequent and make up less than 1% of all neoplasms (Gloster & Neal, 2005; Ridky, 2007).

Australia has the highest reported incidence of nonmelanoma skin cancer in the world. A national survey of the Australian population conducted in 2002 found an age-adjusted rate of 1409 cases per 100,000 (977 per 100,000 for basal cell carcinoma and 432 per 100,000 for squamous cell carcinoma). The incidence of nonmelanoma skin cancer in men was 49% higher than in women (1712 versus 1148 per 100,000).

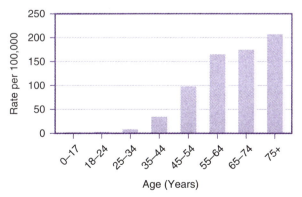

FIGURE 34.2 Age-Specific Incidence of Nonmelanoma Skin Cancer in Members of a U.S. Healthcare Plan, 2010.

Data from Byfield, S. D., Chen, D., Yim, Y. M., & Reyes, C. (2013). Age distribution of patients with advanced non-melanoma skin cancer in the United States. *Archives of Dermatologic Research, 305*(9), 845–850.

Based on these data, approximately 70% of Australian men and 60% of Australian women develop nonmelanoma skin cancer by 75 years of age (Australian Institute of Health and Welfare & Cancer Australia, 2008).

The major predisposing factors in the Australian population are light skin pigmentation, high ambient levels of UV light due to the South Polar ozone hole, and cultural emphasis on outdoor activities and sun exposure throughout life (Arthey & Clarke, 1995; Staples, Marks, & Giles, 1998; Staples et al., 2006).

Incidence rates of nonmelanoma skin cancer reported for Caucasians living in the United States and other developed countries are considerably less than the Australian rates. For example, during 1994-1995, the age-adjusted incidence of squamous cell carcinoma in Australian men was more than fivefold higher than U.S. men (419 versus 81 per 100,000), and eightfold higher in Australian women than in U.S. women (228 versus 26 per 100,000). Nevertheless, within certain ethnic groups living in regions that have high UV exposure, the incidence rates of nonmelanoma skin cancer are more similar to the Australian rates; e.g., in 1996, the incidence rate of squamous cell skin cancer among non-Hispanic Caucasian males living in Southern Arizona (364 per 100,000) was only about 13% less than the Australian rate (Harris, Griffith, & Moon, 2001; Miller & Weinstock, 1994).

In other developed nations, reported incidence rates of nonmelanoma skin cancer for Caucasians vary between 100 and 200 cases per 100,000. For example, in Ireland, the incidence of nonmelanoma skin cancer during 1994–2011 was 156 per 100,000, 110 for basal cell carcinoma and 46 for squamous cell carcinoma (Ireland National Cancer Registry, 2013).

In Asian populations, the incidence rates of nonmelanoma skin cancer are considerably less than in Caucasian populations. Published estimates of the incidence of basal cell carcinoma are 6.4 and 5.8 per 100,000 for Chinese men and women, respectively, and 16.5 per 100,000 for Japanese men and women. Notably, the rates of skin cancer in populations with predominantly dark skin pigmentation are comparatively very low; for example, rates for African populations are in the range of 1–2 per 100,000 (Gloster & Neal, 2005).

FIGURE 34.4 shows the global pattern of incidence and mortality of nonmelanoma skin cancer among men in 2018. Estimated incidence rates varied widely from high values exceeding 200 per 100,000 among men in Australia and New Zealand to much lower values of approximately 1 per 100,000 in India and China. Though Australian men continue to have the highest age-adjusted incidence rates of nonmelanoma skin cancer in the world (234 per 100,000 in 2018),

the annual rate has fallen 80% since 2002. Similarly, the annual incidence rate among men in the United States (85 per 100,000 in 2018) has declined more than 80% over the past two decades. Mortality rates in 2018 were less than 2 deaths per 100,000 for most nations, although men in several nations of Southern Africa had higher mortality rates from nonmelanoma skin cancer (Ferlay et al., 2018). The higher death rates among dark-skinned males of these populations are related to the high rate of aggressive squamous cell carcinomas that arise from *Marjolin ulcers* (e.g., chronic nonhealing wounds, ulcerations, burns, scars, and inflammatory conditions such as discoid lupus, lichen sclerosis, and lichen planus) of the lower extremities rather than malignancies of the upper extremities that are due to sun exposure (Gohara, 2015).

▶ Longitudinal Trends in Basal Cell and Squamous Cell Carcinomas of the Skin

Longitudinal investigations of multiple cohorts provide evidence that the incidence of nonmelanoma skin cancer (basal cell and squamous cell carcinomas) has increased among Caucasian populations of several different regions. As discussed in this section, increases have been noted for males and females of all age groups and particularly in younger individuals.

Four national surveys were conducted in the Australian population during 1985–2002 to determine trends in the incidence of nonmelanoma skin cancer. Results reflect an overall increase of 35% for basal cell carcinoma (from 657 to 884 per 100,000) and 233% for squamous cell carcinoma (from 166 to 387 per 100,000) (**FIGURE 34.5**). The increases were similar for men and women and tended to occur primarily among older individuals (Staples, Marks, & Giles, 1998; Staples et al., 2006).

Investigators in the United States examined trends in the annual incidence of basal cell carcinoma in two large prospective cohorts of older adults: 95,743 women from the Nurses' Health Study (1986–2006) and 44,428 men from the Health Professionals' Follow-up Study (1988–2006). All participants in these cohorts were between 40 and 50 years of age at baseline. During the follow-up periods, age-adjusted incidence rates increased markedly in women (from 519 to 1019 per 100,000) and men (from 606 to 1488 per 100,000) (**FIGURE 34.6**). The investigators suggested that several factors may have contributed to these trends, including increasing susceptibility with greater longevity and heightened exposure to solar radiation

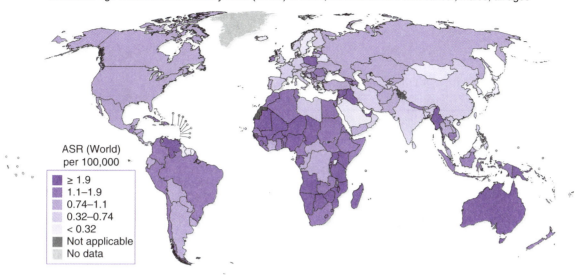

Estimated age-standardized mortality rates (World) in 2018, non-melanoma skin cancer, males, all ages

ASR (World)
per 100,000
- ≥ 1.9
- 1.1–1.9
- 0.74–1.1
- 0.32–0.74
- < 0.32
- Not applicable
- No data

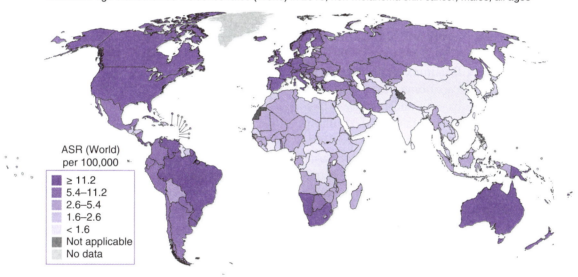

Estimated age-standardized incidence rates (World) in 2018, non-melanoma skin cancer, males, all ages

ASR (World)
per 100,000
- ≥ 11.2
- 5.4–11.2
- 2.6–5.4
- 1.6–2.6
- < 1.6
- Not applicable
- No data

FIGURE 34.4 Global Incidence and Mortality of Nonmelanoma Skin Cancer in Men, 2018.

Reproduced with Permission from Ferlay, J., Ervik, M., Lam, F., Colombet, M., Mery, L., Piñeros, M., . . . Bray, F. (2018). *Global cancer observatory: Cancer today*. Lyon, France: International Agency for Research on Cancer. Retrieved from https://gco.iarc.fr/today

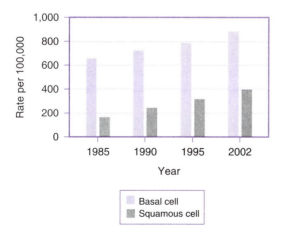

FIGURE 34.5 Trends in the Incidence of Basal Cell and Squamous Cell Carcinomas in Australia, 1985–2002.

Data from Staples, M. P., Elwood, M., Burton, R. C., William, J. L., Marks, R., & Giles, G. G. (2006). Non-melanoma skin cancer in Australia: The 2002 national survey and trends since 1985. *Medical Journal of Australia, 184*, 6–10.

and/or artificial UV radiation in tanning beds (Wu, Han, Li, Li, & Qureshi, 2013).

Trends in the annual incidence rates of basal cell and squamous cell carcinomas of the skin were examined in persons younger than 40 years of age in the predominantly Caucasian population of Olmsted County, Minnesota, during 1976–2003. During the 28-year study period, 417 patients developed basal cell carcinomas and 68 patients developed squamous cell carcinomas. Overall, the age-adjusted incidence of basal cell carcinoma per 100,000 persons was 25.9 for women and 20.9 for men, whereas the incidence of squamous cell carcinoma was approximately 3.9 in men and women. The annual incidence of nonmelanoma skin cancer increased by about 60%, from 18 per 100,000 in 1976–1979 to 29 per 100,000 in 2000–2003.

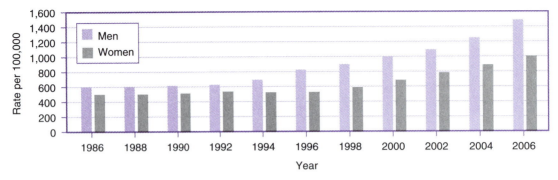

FIGURE 34.6 Trends in the Incidence of Basal Cell Carcinoma in U.S. Men and Women, 1986–2006.

Data from Wu, S., Han, J., Li, W. Q., Li, T., & Qureshi, A. A. (2013). Basal-cell carcinoma incidence and associated risk factors in U.S. women and men. *American Journal of Epidemiology, 178*(6), 890–897.

Notably, this trend was driven largely by the increased annual incidence among young women (13 per 100,000 in 1976–1979 versus 32 per 100,000 in 2000–2003). The investigators speculated that the increased rates of skin cancer among young women of this population may have resulted from increased exposure to solar radiation and/or artificial radiation from tanning beds, or changes in other risk factors for skin cancer such as cigarette smoking (Christenson et al., 2005).

Investigators in Great Britain examined trends in the incidence of basal cell carcinoma of the skin in a primary care population-based cohort study. They identified 11,113 cases from a total of 7.22 million person-years of follow-up data collected between 1996 and 2003. The overall age-adjusted incidence of basal cell carcinoma was 153.9 per 100,000 person-years, and the rate was slightly (~10%) higher in men compared to women. Notably, there was a 3% increase per year across the study period, with the largest increase in incidence seen in the 30–39-year age group (Bath-Hextall, Leonardi-Bee, Smith, Meal, & Hubbard, 2007).

In a longitudinal study of nonmelanoma skin cancer in Denmark, trends in the annual incidence rates of basal cell and squamous cell carcinomas were estimated for the period of 1978–2007. During this 30-year time span, the annual incidence of basal cell carcinomas increased from 27 to 97 cases per 100,000 in women and from 34 to 91 cases per 100,000 in men. Concurrently, the incidence of squamous cell carcinomas increased from 5 to 12 cases per 100,000 in women and from 10 to 19 cases per 100,000 in men. Although increases were noted in all age groups, the rate of increase was greatest among young women. The investigators suggest that these trends may reflect effects of heightened exposure to solar radiation and artificial radiation from tanning beds (Birch-Johansen, Jensen, Mortensen, Olesen, & Kjaer, 2010).

Dutch investigators conducted a longitudinal study of basal cell carcinoma to estimate trends in the incidence rates of basal cell carcinomas by age and gender in the Netherlands. Cases were ascertained from the Eindhoven Cancer Registry in the southeast Netherlands during 1973–2009. During the entire 37-year period, the age-standardized annual rate nearly quadrupled in men (from 40 to 154 per 100,000) and more than quadrupled in women (from 34 to 157 per 100,000). The investigators suggest that heightened exposure to artificial radiation from tanning beds and/or solar radiation may partly explain the increasing trends in basal cell carcinoma of the skin in the Dutch population (Flohil et al., 2013).

In Schleswig-Holstein, the northernmost state of Germany, incidence rates of nonmelanoma skin cancer were estimated during 1998–2000 and later during 2008–2010 to assess the impact of population-based skin cancer screening implemented in the interim. Over the period of study, the incidence of nonmelanoma skin cancer increased by 47% in women (from 81 to 119 cases per 100,000) and by 31% in men (from 111 to 145 cases per 100,000). Increases were noted for all age groups in women and primarily older age groups in men (Eisemann et al., 2013; Katalinic et al., 2003).

Altogether, these findings clearly suggest that the incidence of nonmelanoma skin cancer is increasing not only among the elderly, but also in successive younger generations of several populations. Unless it is reversed by effective preventive measures, the consequences of leisure exposure to UV light portend an impending global epidemic in nonmelanoma skin cancer that will have a huge impact on global health in future years.

▶ Solar Radiation and Nonmelanoma Skin Cancer

The predominant risk factor for nonmelanoma skin cancer is solar radiation. In population studies, the incidence rises with proximity to the equator, where the ultraviolet B (UVB) content of sunlight is greatest.

Fair-skinned individuals have the greatest risk, and susceptibility is increased among individuals with a family history of skin cancer and those who sunburn easily. Individuals with dark skin rarely develop nonmelanoma carcinoma of the skin. The risk for malignant transformation is greatest at sites with the greatest sun exposure. Studies have consistently shown that 70%–90% of basal cell carcinomas arise in sun-exposed skin of the head and neck, particularly the nose. Nevertheless, the risk is also increased for those regions of the skin with intermittent exposure to intense solar radiation (e.g., the trunk and upper portions of the arms and legs) (Armstrong & Kricker, 2001; de Gruijl, 1999; Green & Battistutta, 1990; Miller & Weinstock, 1994; Ridky, 2007).

Types of Solar Radiation

UV radiation is divided into three types based on wavelength. UVA radiation is the longest wavelength, 315–400 nm, and is just slightly shorter than visible light. UVB radiation has a wavelength of 280–315 nm, and UVC, the highest energy radiation, has a wavelength below 280 nm. Each of these forms of UV radiation is harmful to living cells (de Gruijl, 1999).

▶ Risk Factors for Basal Cell Carcinoma of the Skin

Solar Radiation and Basal Cell Carcinoma of the Skin

The evidence-linking basal cell carcinoma of the skin with solar radiation is unequivocal; however, the risk is modified by genetic, phenotypic, and environmental factors (Wong, Strange, & Lear, 2003). Selected studies are discussed in this section.

In an early case–control study of 2654 cases with basal cell carcinomas of the skin and 1938 cancer-free controls, the strongest risk factor was excessive cumulative exposure to solar radiation. Other factors that increased the risk included fair complexion, sensitivity to sunlight and inability to tan, blond hair, blue eyes, increased age, and male gender. Almost all the tumors developed in sun-exposed areas of the skin (Kopf, 1979).

In a Canadian study, 206 male patients with basal cell carcinoma of the skin were compared to 406 age- and gender-matched control subjects without cancer. Significant risk increases were noted for individuals with light, freckled skin who suffered repeat severe sunburn in childhood (Gallagher et al., 1995).

A team of U.S. investigators examined the relation of sun exposure and other factors to the risk of developing basal cell carcinoma of the skin in a prospective cohort of 44,591 predominantly Caucasian U.S. male health professionals, 40–75 years of age and free of cancer at enrollment in 1986. During 8 years of follow-up, 3273 cases of basal cell carcinoma were reported. Significant risk factors included inability to tan (relative risk [RR] = 2.9), cumulative number of blistering sunburns (RR = 2.1 for 10 or more), red hair (RR = 2.4), and living in a region with high solar radiation (RR = 1.5). These findings underscore the major role of sun exposure in the genesis of basal cell skin cancer (van Dam et al., 1999).

Several published epidemiologic investigations have reported an association of *occupational* UV exposure with an increased risk of basal cell carcinoma. To gain a more thorough understanding of this association, investigators in Germany conducted a systematic review of the literature and a meta-analysis of the published risk estimates. Their analysis included data from 24 epidemiologic investigations (19 case–control studies and 5 cohort studies). The combined data revealed a 43% increase in the risk of developing basal cell carcinoma among outdoor workers compared to those with indoor employment (Bauer, Diepgen, & Schmitt, 2011).

Tanning Beds and Basal Cell Carcinoma of the Skin

The use of tanning beds has been consistently found to increase the risk for early development of basal cell carcinoma and other cutaneous malignancies. Selected studies and a meta-analysis of published data are discussed here.

Investigators in Vermont conducted a population-based case–control study that included 603 patients with basal cell carcinoma, 293 patients with squamous cell carcinoma, and 540 control subjects group-matched to the cases by age and gender. The study found that any use of indoor tanning devices was associated with risk increases for both basal cell carcinoma (odds ratio [OR] = 1.5) and squamous cell carcinoma (OR = 2.5). Odds ratios were higher for use initiated before 20 years of age (OR = 1.8 and 3.6 for basal cell and squamous cell carcinomas, respectively), and subjects using indoor tanning devices were more likely to be female and younger than 50 years of age (Karagas et al., 2002).

Investigators in Boston examined exposure to UV light in tanning beds and the risk of developing skin cancer in the Nurses' Health Study (NHS). The study followed 73,494 female nurses for 20 years (from 1989 to 2009) to determine whether the frequency of tanning bed use in young women influenced the incidence rates of skin cancer (basal cell carcinoma, squamous cell carcinoma, and melanoma). During follow-up, 5506 nurses were diagnosed with basal cell carcinoma, 403 with squamous cell carcinoma, and 349 with melanoma. After adjustment for sun exposure and other risk factors, use of tanning beds more than six times per year while attending high school and college increased the risk of developing basal cell carcinoma by 73% (hazard ratio [HR] = 1.73) and, to a lesser extent, squamous cell carcinoma (HR = 1.12) and melanoma (HR = 1.28). The data suggest a greater vulnerability of younger people to the carcinogenic impact of indoor tanning, especially in the development of basal cell carcinoma (Zhang et al., 2012).

Investigators in Connecticut studied the effects of indoor tanning in a case–control study of 376 young patients with basal cell carcinoma and 390 control subjects matched by age and gender. All cases in the study were younger than 40 years of age. Overall, indoor tanning increased the risk of developing basal cell carcinoma by 69%, and the risk increased in a dose–response relationship with the frequency and duration of exposure (Ferrucci et al., 2012).

An international team of investigators recently conducted a systematic review and meta-analysis of the published literature on indoor tanning and non-melanoma skin cancer. They identified 12 published studies with 9328 cases of nonmelanoma skin cancer for analysis. Summary relative risk estimates were elevated for both basal cell carcinoma (RR = 1.29) and squamous cell carcinoma (RR = 1.67). Furthermore, the summary risk estimates were higher among subjects who began using indoor tanning devices before the age of 25 years (RR = 1.40 and RR = 2.02 for basal cell and squamous cell carcinomas, respectively). The evidence suggests that indoor tanning is a significant risk factor for both basal cell and squamous cell carcinomas of the skin, especially when initiated early in life. The results underscore the need for preventive measures aimed at restricting the use of tanning beds among minors (Wehner et al., 2012).

Other Environmental Risk Factors for Basal Cell Carcinoma of the Skin

Environmental factors other than sun exposure may also contribute to the formation of basal cell carcinoma of the skin as well as other cutaneous malignancies. Factors found to increase the risk include immunosuppressive therapy (Stern & Lange, 1990),

intake of psoralens in combination with exposure to UV rays (Stern & Lange, 1988), excessive tanning bed use combined with chronic cigarette smoking and blistering sunburns (Boyd, Shyr, & King, 2002), and chronic exposure to skin irritants such as insecticides, herbicides, petroleum products, and dry-cleaning agents (Gallagher et al., 1995) and arsenic-containing compounds (Hartevelt, Bavinck, Kootte, Vermeer, & Vandenbroucke, 1996). High radiation exposure has also been found to increase the risk; for example, the incidence of skin cancer is significantly increased among atomic bomb survivors (Sadamori, Mine, & Honda, 1991; Yamada et al., 1996).

Chronic arsenic poisoning appears to be a major public health problem. Arsenic exposure may occur through contact with contaminated food, water, or air. Although arsenic is ubiquitous in the environment, its ambient concentration in both food and water may be increased near smelting, mining, or coal-burning establishments. Arsenic tends to accumulate in the skin, and chronic exposure has consistently been found to increase the risk of developing basal cell and squamous cell carcinomas of the skin. Mechanistically, arsenic has been found to amplify the cytotoxicity and mutagenicity of UV radiation. Clinically, patients with arsenic-induced skin cancers are characterized by multiple recurring basal cell and squamous cell carcinomas that occur in areas of the skin usually protected from the sun (Yu, Liao, & Chai, 2006).

▶ Risk Factors for Squamous Cell Carcinoma of the Skin

There is extensive overlap between the risk factors for squamous cell carcinoma and basal cell carcinoma, and certainly, the dominant risk factor for both malignancies is solar radiation. Nevertheless, there are distinct differences in the pathogenesis of these two forms of skin cancer, and comparative studies have elucidated distinct differences in risk depending on the frequency, duration, and type of exposure. Unlike basal cell carcinoma, squamous cell carcinoma of the skin carries a substantial risk of invasion and metastatic spread to other organs, and it often develops from a precursor lesion called *actinic keratosis* (Alam & Ratner, 2001).

Actinic Keratosis and Squamous Cell Carcinoma of the Skin

Actinic keratoses (also called *solar keratoses*) are intraepidermal skin tumors caused by chronic exposure to solar radiation. These scaly lesions are composed of highly keratinized layers of dysplastic cells that occupy the epidermal space without breaching the basement membrane. The prevailing view of actinic keratosis is that it is a precursor lesion that occasionally undergoes malignant transformation to form squamous cell carcinoma. The anatomic distribution of actinic keratosis is therefore synonymous with that of squamous cell carcinoma: Both lesions have a strong predilection for sun-exposed regions of the face, neck, hands, and upper trunk.

Notably, actinic keratosis has the potential to progress to invasive squamous cell carcinoma. However, evidence from several follow-up studies of cases suggests that the risk of progression of actinic keratosis to squamous cell carcinoma is low; in a study of 1689 cases in Australia, the annual risk of progression of individual lesions was approximately 1 per 1000 (Marks, Rennie, & Selwood, 1988). In a more recent study of 169 U.S. male veterans with actinic keratosis, the annual risk of progression was 6 per 1000 (Criscione et al., 2009). Progression of actinic keratosis to squamous cell carcinoma is associated with continuing exposure to solar radiation that elicits erythema, ulceration, thickening, and/or changes in size and shape of the precursor lesion (Feldman & Fleischer, 2011). In a study of 91 patients, the mean time for actinic keratosis to progress to squamous cell carcinoma was 25 months and the range was 2–76 months (Fuchs & Marmur, 2007).

Solar Radiation and Squamous Cell Carcinoma of the Skin

The largest and most comprehensive comparative study of the effects of solar radiation in the development of basal cell and squamous cell carcinomas of the skin is the European study Helios that was conducted in southern Europe. (The Greek term *Helios* means "sun.") Helios was a well-designed case–control investigation of nonmelanocytic skin cancer among different populations from southern Europe. Its primary objective was to clarify similarities and differences in risk factors for the two major forms of skin cancer, basal cell and squamous cell carcinomas. Between 1989 and 1993, investigators in seven regions of southern Europe interviewed 1549 incident cases of basal cell carcinoma, 228 cases of squamous cell carcinoma, and 1795 disease-free controls matched to the cases by age, gender, and location of residence. Data were collected on sun exposure, constitutional factors, and iatrogenic and occupational exposures.

The initial results of the Helios study revealed that both forms of nonmelanoma skin cancer develop primarily in sun-exposed areas of skin on the face, head, arms, legs, and trunk. Pigmentary traits such as red hair and pale eye color as well as a tendency to sunburn were strong and independent indicators of risk for both basal cell carcinoma and squamous cell carcinoma. Self-reported susceptibility to sunburn and resistance to tanning also increased the risk for both types of malignancy (OR = 2.7 for basal cell carcinoma and OR = 2.0 for squamous cell carcinoma). A key finding was that history of sunburns and early age at first sunburn increased the risk for basal cell carcinoma (OR = 1.7) *but not squamous cell carcinoma*. The investigators concluded that basal cell carcinoma and squamous cell carcinoma are influenced by different patterns of exposure to solar radiation: Basal cell carcinoma risk is increased by periods of intense exposure, cumulative episodes of sunburn, and poor ability to tan, whereas squamous cell carcinoma risk is associated with prolonged exposure over time (Zanetti et al., 1996).

A later publication of results from the Helios study provided quantitation of the patterns of exposure to solar radiation associated with the development of basal cell and squamous cell carcinomas. The data revealed a sharp increase in the risk of developing squamous cell carcinoma beginning at a threshold level of 70,000 hours of cumulative sun exposure and maximizing at over 100,000 hours of exposure. In contrast, the risk of developing basal cell carcinoma reached a maximum at 10,000 hours of cumulative sun exposure and declined slightly with higher levels (Rosso et al., 1996) (**FIGURE 34.7**).

Significant associations between cumulative sun exposure and the risk of squamous cell carcinoma of the skin have been observed in other populations. In a population-based case–control study conducted in Australia, investigators compared sun exposure patterns of 132 cases of squamous cell carcinoma with 1031 controls matched by age and gender to the cases. Results revealed increasing risk with higher levels of lifetime sun exposure and a risk maximum (OR = 3.3) at 65,000 hours of exposure. History of blistering sunburns also increased the risk, whereas intermittent weekly sun exposure did not (English et al., 1998).

A case–control study in Florida was designed to investigate patterns and timing of sunlight exposure that influence the development of basal cell and squamous cell carcinomas. The study included 218 cases of basal cell carcinoma, 169 cases of squamous cell carcinoma, and 316 control subjects matched to the cases by age and gender. Results showed that a history

FIGURE 34.7 Risk of Basal Cell and Squamous Cell Carcinomas of the Skin by Cumulative Hours of Sun Exposure.

Data from Rosso, S., Zanetti, R., Martinez, C., Tormo, M. J., Schraub, S., Sancho-Garnier, H., . . . Wechsler, J. (1996). The multicenter south European study 'Helios'. II: Different sun exposure patterns in the aetiology of basal cell and squamous cell carcinomas of the skin. *British Journal of Cancer, 73*(11), 1447–1454.

of blistering sunburn or long-term occupational sun exposure produced similar risk increases (approximately twofold) for both basal cell and squamous cell carcinomas (Iannacone et al., 2012).

To more thoroughly examine the association between occupational sun exposure and the risk of cutaneous squamous cell carcinoma, a team of German investigators conducted a systematic review of the literature and meta-analysis of the published data. The analysis included data from 18 epidemiologic investigations (12 case–control studies and 6 cohort studies). The combined data showed a 77% increase in the risk of developing squamous cell carcinoma among workers who were routinely exposed to solar radiation compared to those employed in indoor occupations (Schmitt, Seidler, Diepgen, & Bauer, 2011).

Other Radiation Exposures and Squamous Cell Carcinoma of the Skin

Sources of radiation other than the sun also increase the risk of developing squamous cell carcinoma of the skin. In a long-term follow-up study of 4799 Swedish patients who had received psoralen and UV A radiation (PUVA) for the treatment of skin disorders, significant risk increases were noted for both men (RR = 5.6) and women (RR = 3.6) compared to the general Swedish population (Lindelöf et al., 1999).

Similar results were observed in a cohort of 1380 psoriasis patients treated with PUVA in Boston. At 25 years of follow-up, only 7% of individuals who underwent fewer than 200 PUVA treatments developed squamous cell carcinoma compared with more than 50% of those who underwent more than 400 treatments (Nijsten & Stern, 2003).

Skin conditions such as psoriasis may also be treated with UVB radiation. In a cohort of 1380

patients followed for up to 25 years, patients who received 300 or more UVB treatments had an approximately 40% increased risk of developing either squamous cell carcinoma or basal cell carcinoma compared to those who received fewer treatments (Lim & Stern, 2005).

Prolonged administration of low-dose ionizing radiation has been used in the treatment of a variety of skin disorders, including eczema, psoriasis, acne vulgaris, and tinea capitis. To examine the effects of therapeutic ionizing radiation on the development of nonmelanoma skin cancer, investigators in New Hampshire conducted a case–control study of 592 cases of basal cell carcinoma, 289 cases of squamous cell carcinoma, and 536 controls matched to the cases by age and gender. Overall, the study revealed elevated risks for both squamous cell carcinoma (OR = 2.94) and basal cell carcinoma (OR = 3.30) confined to the site of radiation exposure (Lichter et al., 2000).

As already noted, the use of artificial devices that emit UV radiation, such as tanning beds, has been found to increase the risk of both squamous cell and basal cell carcinoma of the skin. Based on a meta-analysis of 12 studies, individuals who begin using indoor tanning devices before the age of 25 years increase their risk of developing squamous cell or basal cell carcinoma by 100% and 40%, respectively, compared to nonusers (Wehner et al., 2012).

Other Environmental Risk Factors for Squamous Cell Carcinoma of the Skin

Exposure to arsenic in drinking water and exposure to combustion products have been found to increase the risk of both basal cell carcinoma and squamous cell carcinoma. A biomarker of past arsenic exposure is the concentration in toenail clippings. In a case–control study of skin cancer, arsenic concentrations in toenail clippings from 587 cases with basal cell carcinoma and 284 cases with squamous cell carcinoma were compared with concentrations in clippings from 524 matched controls. Compared to individuals with arsenic concentrations below the median, individuals with concentrations above the 97th percentile were found to have an approximately twofold increase in the risk of developing squamous cell carcinoma and a 44% increase in the risk of developing basal cell carcinoma. Notably, there was a long latency period from exposure to diagnosis; for example, invasive squamous cell carcinoma was diagnosed an average of 20 years after the initial reported exposure to arsenic (Karagas et al., 2001).

Smoking has been linked to certain forms of skin cancer in some studies but not in others. The available evidence on smoking and skin cancer was recently evaluated in a systematic review of the literature and meta-analysis of published risk estimates. Data were analyzed to assess the effects of current smoking on squamous cell carcinoma (six studies) and basal cell carcinoma (16 studies). Smoking was found to increase the risk of developing squamous cell carcinoma (OR = 1.52) but not basal cell carcinoma (Leonardi-Bee, Ellison, & Bath-Hextall, 2012).

▶ Genetics of Nonmelanoma Skin Cancer

The vast majority of basal cell and squamous cell carcinomas of the skin are caused by exposure to UV light. UV radiation, especially UVB, is absorbed by DNA and causes covalent bonding of pyrimidine bases to form dimers. If these dimers are not excised and replaced with normal bases before the DNA is replicated, the daughter cells may carry mutations at those sites that may lead to skin cancer if they disable tumor suppressor genes. Loss of function of mutated tumor–suppressor genes allows uncontrolled cell growth and division that causes tumor formation (Armstrong & Kricker, 2001). Nevertheless, as discussed in the following sections, the spectrum of mutations and genetic alterations and the cellular pathways affected differ between basal cell and squamous cell carcinomas of the skin.

Somatic Mutations in Basal Cell Carcinoma of the Skin

The *Hedgehog* signaling pathway regulates spatial orientation and bilateral development of certain structures and organs during embryogenesis in all vertebrates, including humans. The pathway is called "Hedgehog" because mutated genes of the pathway cause the development of aberrant larvae in drosophila that resemble miniature hedgehogs (Nüsslein-Volhard & Wieschaus, 1980). Recent molecular studies have revealed that mutations in tumor–suppressor genes that encode important proteins of the Hedgehog pathway, PTCH and SMO, are present in about 90% of sporadic (nonheritable) basal cell carcinomas. Such mutations, which are presumably the result of UV radiation, enhance carcinogenesis of basal cells in the epidermis by disrupting the regulation of cell division, transcription, and protein synthesis (De Zwaan & Haass, 2010).

Mutations in the *p53* tumor–suppressor gene are also frequently found in cases of sporadic basal cell carcinoma. Such *p53* mutations often occur together with mutations in the Hedgehog pathway. They typically arise at sites of consecutive pyrimidine DNA sequences, which is indicative of pyrimidine dimer formation due to exposure to UVB radiation (Ling et al., 2001; Rubin, Chen, & Ratner, 2005).

Germline Mutations and Basal Cell Carcinoma of the Skin

Gorlin Syndrome

A rare heritable condition known as Gorlin syndrome (also called nevoid basal cell carcinoma syndrome) is caused by a germline mutation in one allele of the *PTCH1* gene located on the long arm of human chromosome 9. Virtually, all patients with this syndrome develop multiple basal cell carcinomas at an early age, and they may also develop other malignant tumors, including melanoma, medulloblastoma, meningioma, breast cancer, and non-Hodgkin's lymphoma (Gorlin, 2004).

Other Genetic Syndromes and Basal Cell Carcinoma of the Skin

Other rare genetic syndromes have been identified that predispose to multiple basal cell carcinomas of the skin. These include epidermolysis bullosa simplex (Dowling-Meara) and Rombo syndrome, which follow an autosomal dominant inheritance pattern, and Bazex–Dupre–Christol syndrome, which is an X-linked condition. These syndromes involve inheritance of defective genes that cause dysfunction of epidermal basal cells, leading to malignant transformation (NCI, 2014).

Somatic Mutations in Squamous Cell Carcinoma of the Skin

Squamous cell carcinoma of the skin characteristically develops by a multistep model of carcinogenesis. It is likely that the vast majority (~97%) of sporadic cases involve transformation of the precursor lesion, actinic keratosis, to squamous cell carcinoma (Babilas, Landthaler, & Szeimies, 2003; Ortonne, 2002).

A key factor in the development of actinic keratosis is the loss of function of the *p53* tumor–suppressor gene on chromosome 17, which is essential for regulation of the cell cycle. Molecular studies have found *p53* mutations in 75%–80% of actinic keratosis specimens from Caucasians and in more than 90% of cutaneous squamous cell carcinomas. Notably, mutations typically occur at dipyrimidine sites within the gene, implicating dimer formation due to UVB exposure as the mutagenic event. Additional mutations in genes encoding growth factors and DNA repair enzymes likely contribute to the multistep process. Furthermore, actinic keratoses and squamous cell carcinomas are typified by loss of heterozygosity and general chromosomal instability (Boukamp, 2005; Brash et al., 1991, 1996; Ortonne, 2002; Rass, 2005).

Germline Mutations and Squamous Cell Carcinoma of the Skin

Xeroderma Pigmentosum

Xeroderma pigmentosum is a rare genetic syndrome caused by germline mutations that regulate DNA repair. Individuals with this condition are prone to the development of multiple cutaneous malignancies, particularly squamous cell carcinomas, but also melanomas and basal cell carcinomas. The condition was initially described in four young patients by the Hungarian dermatologist Moriz Kaposi in 1874 (Hebra & Kaposi, 1874). A century later, geneticist James Cleaver discovered multiple defects in DNA excision repair genes that caused the syndrome (Cleaver, 1968).

Xeroderma pigmentosum strikes about 1 individual per million in the United States and Europe, but higher frequencies have been observed in some populations (e.g., 1 individual per 22,000 are afflicted in the Japanese population) (Tamura, DiGiovanna, & Kraemer, 2010). Classically, the condition behaves as an autosomal recessive trait whereby full phenotypic expression is manifest when there are genetic defects in both alleles of the affected gene.

The median onset of nonmelanoma skin cancer in patients with xeroderma pigmentosum is under 10 years of age, and more than 50% of affected individuals die before their 40th birthday of other invasive cancers such as malignant melanoma and tumors of the brain and central nervous system (Bradford et al., 2011).

Multiple defects in DNA excision repair genes have been discovered that predispose to xeroderma pigmentosum. Patients with such defects are unable to excise pyrimidine dimers induced by UV radiation in the epidermis of the skin (Cleaver, 1968; States, McDuffie, Myrand, McDowell, & Cleaver, 1998). Consequently, their rates of cutaneous nonmelanoma malignancies and melanoma are 10,000 and 2000 times higher, respectively, than in the general population (DiGiovanna & Kraemer, 2012).

Other Genetic Syndromes and Squamous Cell Carcinoma of the Skin

Several rare genetic syndromes other than xeroderma pigmentosum have been discovered that predispose to the development of squamous cell carcinoma of the skin as well as other malignancies. These include Ferguson–Smith syndrome, various forms of albinism, Rothmund–Thomson syndrome, Fanconi anemia, Zinsser–Cole–Engman syndrome, Bloom syndrome, and Werner syndrome. These syndromes have been linked to a variety of germline mutations that induce chromosomal instability (NCI, 2014).

Genetic Differences in Basal Cell and Squamous Cell Carcinomas of the Skin

There appears to be a clear genetic distinction between basal cell carcinoma and squamous cell carcinoma of the skin. Typically, basal cell carcinomas exhibit a relatively simple genotype characterized by only a few key genetic mutations (e.g., Hedgehog and *p53* mutants). In contrast, although most squamous cell carcinomas do carry *p53* mutations, they tend to be more genetically heterogeneous and characteristically contain mutations of multiple genes and/or other chromosomal aberrations resulting from DNA deletions, additions, and translocations. According to one viewpoint, whereas most basal cell carcinomas develop de novo without evidence of a precursor lesion, the pathogenesis of squamous cell carcinoma of the skin appears to be a multistep process involving the intermediate precancerous lesion, actinic keratosis (Boukamp, 2005).

Immunosuppression and Skin Cancer

Immunosuppression also contributes to the development of nonmelanoma skin cancers. Among solid-organ transplant recipients, the incidence of squamous cell carcinoma is 65–250 times higher and the incidence of basal cell carcinoma is 10 times higher than that observed in the general population. The risks vary with the type of transplant or therapy. For example, heart transplant recipients who require the highest rates of immunosuppression to prevent rejection are at approximately twofold higher risk of developing cutaneous malignancy than liver transplant recipients, in whom much lower levels of immunosuppression are needed to avoid rejection. Furthermore, nonmelanoma skin cancers in solid-organ transplant recipients and chronic lymphocytic leukemia patients occur at a younger age and have a higher risk of recurrence and metastatic spread than the same malignancies in patients with intact immune systems. It is also notable that suppression of the immune system has a greater impact on the development of squamous cell carcinoma than basal cell carcinoma. For example, among transplant patients, the ratio of squamous cell carcinomas to basal cell carcinomas is approximately 2:1, whereas among patients with an intact immune system, the ratio of basal cell carcinomas to squamous cell carcinomas is approximately 4:1 (Glover, Niranjan, Kwan, & Leigh, 1994; Hartevelt, Bavinck, Kootte, Vermeer, & Vandenbroucke, 1990; Jensen et al., 1999; Kaplan & Cook, 2005; Krynitz et al., 2013; Lindelöf, Sigurgeirsson, Gäbel, & Stern, 2000).

Certain infectious agents that cause immune dysfunction are also associated with the development of nonmelanoma skin cancer. In a cohort study conducted in northern California, the incidence of nonmelanoma skin cancer was compared among 6560 HIV-positive subjects and 36,821 HIV-negative subjects monitored during 1996–2008. Results revealed that individuals who were HIV-positive had more than double the risk of developing either basal cell or squamous cell carcinoma of the skin compared to HIV-negative individuals. Furthermore, severely immunocompromised subjects with low CD4 counts (<200 per mL) had more than a fourfold increase in the risk of developing squamous cell carcinoma (Silverberg et al., 2013).

Skin infections by certain strains of human papillomavirus (HPV) have also been linked to the development of nonmelanoma skin cancer. A review of the literature identified 17 studies in which HPV positivity was determined in specimens of squamous cell carcinoma compared to normal skin. Meta-analysis of the data revealed that prior infection with multiple cutaneous HPV strains was associated with a twofold increase in the risk of developing cutaneous squamous cell carcinoma. Analysis of a subset of the data also revealed that among immunocompromised individuals, HPV-positive subjects were three times more likely to develop squamous cell carcinoma than HPV-negative subjects. Based on these results, the investigators suggest that HPV infection may be a cofactor that acts in concert with other factors to heighten the risk of developing cutaneous squamous cell carcinoma (Wang, Aldabagh, Yu, & Arron, 2014).

The increased risk of nonmelanoma skin cancer in immunocompromised patients is influenced by the depletion of Langerhans cells in the epidermis. Immunologic studies suggest that one of the primary roles of these immune cells is to present antigens of invading microbes to regulatory T cells in order to stimulate the immune response. However, some recent studies suggest that the Langerhans cells may, in fact, diminish the immune response under certain conditions, and there is currently hot debate about their specific function in the immune system of the skin (Stoitzner, 2010). Regardless of the exact mechanisms involved, depletion of the Langerhans cell population by immunosuppressive drugs, UV radiation, infection, or other exposures likely plays a critical permissive role in the development of cutaneous squamous cell carcinoma (Gibson, O'Grady, Key, Leader, & Murphy, 1998; Thiers, Maize, Spicer, & Cantor, 1984). Notably, loss of function of the Langerhans cells is associated with chronic inflammation that predisposes to the development of malignancy (Bennett, Robinson, Baron, & Cooper, 2008).

Inflammogenesis of Skin Cancer

Chronic inflammation induced by solar UV radiation and/or other environmental exposures undoubtedly plays a critical role in the genesis of skin cancer. Molecular studies of basal cell carcinomas, squamous cell carcinomas, actinic keratosis, and malignant melanomas have identified a variety of inflammatory factors that stimulate carcinogenesis. These include genes that encode various transcription factors, cytokines, chemokines, and chemokine receptors such as cyclooxygenase-2 (COX-2), prostaglandin E2 (PGE2), nuclear factor kappa B (NF-κB), signal transducer and activator of transcription 3 (STAT3), and hypoxia-inducible factor alpha (HIF-1α). Chronic inflammation stimulates several mechanisms of tumor development, including mutagenesis, mitogenesis, angiogenesis, disruption of apoptosis, immunosuppression, and metastasis. Inflammatory pathways are therefore attractive molecular targets for skin cancer prevention (Maru, Gandhi, Ramchandani, & Kumar, 2014).

Risk of Multiple Basal Cell or Squamous Cell Carcinomas of the Skin

Individuals who develop an initial basal cell or squamous cell carcinoma of the skin are at high risk of developing subsequent skin cancer. In a prospective study of 1805 patients who were diagnosed with an initial basal cell or squamous cell carcinoma of the skin, 35% developed a second skin cancer within 3 years and 50% developed a second skin cancer within 5 years. For both tumor types, the risk was higher among those with severe actinic damage who sunburned easily (Robinson, 1987).

Vitamin D and Skin Cancer

Because vitamin D metabolism is activated in the skin by exposure to sunlight, the level of vitamin D in the blood might be associated with the risk of skin cancer. To test this hypothesis, investigators prospectively evaluated the association between baseline levels of plasma vitamin D [measured as 25(OH)D] and the risk of incident squamous cell carcinoma and basal cell carcinoma among 4641 women from the NHS. During 22 years of follow-up, 510 incident cases of basal cell carcinoma and 75 incident cases of squamous cell carcinoma were reported. The results revealed that compared to individuals with baseline vitamin D levels in the lowest quartile, women in the highest quartile were at increased risk of developing squamous cell carcinoma (OR = 3.77) or basal cell carcinoma (OR = 2.07). These data suggest that a high level of plasma vitamin D may reflect long-term sun exposure and therefore serve as a biomarker of impending nonmelanoma skin cancer (Liang, Nan, Qureshi, & Han, 2012).

Epidemiology of Merkel Cell Carcinoma

Merkel cell carcinoma is a rare and highly aggressive form of skin cancer that develops from specialized cells of the epidermis. Merkel cells are located at terminal nerve endings in the epidermis where they regulate the sensation of touch. They were discovered in 1875 by the German pathologist Friedrick Sigmund Merkel and have since been the subject of considerable controversy concerning their origin. Recently, molecular studies have determined that Merkel cells are specialized epithelial cells that contain mechanoreceptors on their cell membranes, thereby facilitating light touch responses in the skin (Maricich et al., 2009).

Merkel cell carcinoma occurs primarily in elderly adults who are 60–80 years of age. As with other forms of skin cancer (other than melanoma), cases of Merkel cell carcinoma are not routinely reported to tumor registries and, consequently, reliable estimates of incidence are sparse. In a longitudinal study of incident cases identified in the U.S. population through the SEER program of the National Cancer Institute, the annual incidence of Merkel cell carcinoma showed an approximate threefold increase during 1986–2001, from 1.5 to 4.4 cases per million (Hodgson, 2005).

Recent molecular studies conducted by investigators at the University of Pittsburgh identified a polyomavirus in tissues of Merkel cell carcinoma (Feng, Shuda, Chang, & Moore, 2008). Subsequent studies determined that most Merkel cell carcinomas (~80%) contain a mutated polyomavirus gene that causes T cell anergy, depression of the immune system, and disruption of apoptosis (Shuda et al., 2008). Infection of the skin by polyomaviruses and lysogeny of viral DNA with cells in the epidermis is virtually ubiquitous among humans. Although the vast majority of these latent infections are innocuous, malignant transformation does occasionally occur, particularly in viral-infected Merkel cells of older adults with skin damage due to solar radiation and/or immunosuppressive conditions. Compared to the general population, the risk of developing Merkel cell carcinoma is increased 10-fold among organ transplant recipients, 13-fold among patients with HIV disease, and 30-fold among patients with chronic lymphocytic leukemia (Engels, Frisch, Goedert, Biggar, & Miller, 2002; Heath et al., 2008; Penn & First, 1999).

Merkel cell carcinoma typically presents clinically as a small, painless, bluish-red nodule located on the face, neck, hands, or other sun-exposed areas of skin. Nearly half of these tumors develop in the periorbital skin. Unfortunately, most Merkel cell carcinomas have already metastasized at the time of diagnosis; consequently, the prognosis for this form of skin cancer is grim. As with other forms of skin cancer, protection of the skin from damaging solar radiation is essential for prevention (Nghiem & James, 2007).

▶ Environmental Prevention of Skin Cancer

Ultraviolet Radiation and the Ozone Layer

The primary line of defense against harmful rays from the sun is the ozone layer in the stratosphere, 10–50 km above the surface of the earth. Ozone (O_3) forms when molecular oxygen (O_2) in the upper atmosphere absorbs short-wave UVC radiation and decomposes to form singlet oxygen (O), which then reacts with O_2 to form O_3. The O_3 molecules effectively absorb UV radiation up to about 310 nm wavelength; the ozone layer blocks all UVC and most UVB radiation emitted by the sun, thereby protecting life on earth from these damaging rays. In 1995, Paul Crutzen, Mario Molina, and Sherwood Rowland were awarded the Nobel Prize for their pioneering work in atmospheric chemistry that elucidated the formation and decomposition of ozone (Crutzen, Molina, & Rowland, 1995).

The Ozone Hole

The *ozone hole* refers to annual thinning of the ozone layer over Antarctica due to inorganic chlorine molecules that reach the stratosphere (Farman, Gardiner, & Shanklin, 1985). Atmospheric conditions at the earth's poles favor the destruction of ozone by reactive halogen gases. In recent decades, the ozone layer over the South Pole has been depleted by the release of ozone-depleting substances that reach the stratosphere (NASA, 2014) (**FIGURE 34.8**). These substances include chlorofluorocarbons (freons) and bromofluorocarbons (halons) that are widely used in refrigeration. Studies of the mathematical relationship among the thinning of the ozone layer, corresponding increases in UV radiation, and the development of skin cancer suggest that a 1% reduction in ozone concentration will increase UVB radiation exposure by 2%, which would increase the incidence of nonmelanoma skin cancer by 3%–6% (Kripke, 1988). In Australia, where the incidence of nonmelanoma skin cancer is the highest in the world, it is estimated that the ozone layer over Australia has been depleted by 5%–9% since the 1960s (World Meteorological Organization, 1995).

Protecting the Ozone Layer

Accumulating evidence that ozone is being depleted from the earth's stratosphere by man-made substances has stimulated worldwide efforts to protect the ozone layer. The Montreal Protocol is an international treaty designed to protect the ozone layer by phasing out the production of those substances (freons, halons, etc.) responsible for ozone depletion. Because of this international agreement, the ozone hole in Antarctica appears to be slowly recovering (Anderson & Sarma, 2007).

▶ Behavioral Prevention of Skin Cancer

The key to effective primary prevention of skin cancer is protection of the skin from damaging solar radiation. Wearing protective clothing and using sunscreen products with a sun protective factor (SPF) of 30 or higher is highly recommended for all individuals who are routinely exposed to solar radiation, and particularly those with susceptible phenotypes

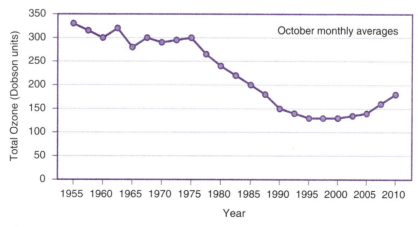

FIGURE 34.8 Depletion of the Ozone Layer Over Halley Bay, Antarctica.

Caption: Data points are 3-year moving averages.

Data from World Meteorological Organization. (1995). *Global ozone research and monitoring project: 1994.* WMO No. 37. Geneva, Switzerland. Retrieved from http://ozonewatch.gsfc.nasa.gov/facts/history.html; National Aeronautics and Space Administration (NASA). (2014). *Ozone hole watch.* Washington, DC. Retrieved from http://ozonewatch.gsfc.nasa.gov/facts/history.html

such as individuals with fair skin and freckles who do not readily tan and who sunburn easily, immunocompromised individuals, genetically predisposed individuals, and individuals with a history of prior skin cancer. Other chronic exposures that damage the skin or cause immunosuppression should also be avoided such as UV radiation from tanning devices, skin irritants, arsenic-containing compounds, and tobacco smoking.

Routine screening for the early detection of actinic keratoses and/or in situ malignancies of the skin is a critical component of effective secondary prevention. The vast majority of skin cancers are curable by early detection and effective therapy. *Mohs surgery* is a highly effective surgical technique that involves intraoperative microscopic examination of serial frozen sections of thin layers of tissue excised from existing lesions. The technique is designed to precisely and completely remove suspicious skin lesions with the objective of obtaining clear surgical margins in order to minimize recurrence.

Former U.S. Surgeon General Boris Lushniak released the *Call to Action to Prevent Skin Cancer* (U.S. Department of Health and Human Services, 2014), a comprehensive plea for increased awareness, policies, and research, with a goal of supporting skin cancer prevention. The five strategic goals of the report are to (1) increase opportunities for sun protection in outdoor settings; (2) provide individuals with the information they need to make informed, healthy choices about UV radiation exposure; (3) promote policies that advance the national goal of preventing skin cancer; (4) reduce harms from indoor tanning; and (5) strengthen research, surveillance, monitoring, and evaluation related to skin cancer prevention.

Despite these recommendations, there is an important caveat to restrictive advice on sun exposure habits designed to reduce the risk of skin cancer. As an example, evidence from a recent epidemiologic study of Swedish women found that those who avoided sun exposure had a twofold increase in all-cause mortality compared to those with high sun exposure, presumably due to their lower levels of vitamin D. The investigators concluded that "following sun exposure advice that is very restrictive in countries with low solar intensity might in fact be harmful to women's health" (Lindqvist et al., 2014).

Maintaining sufficient blood levels of vitamin D (at least 30 ng/mL) is important for prevention of osteoporosis, cardiovascular disease, diabetes, autoimmune disease, and some forms of cancer. More than 90% of the human vitamin D requirement comes from casual exposure to sunlight. Judicious exposure to sunlight (perhaps 10 minutes of exposure two to three times per week) is therefore necessary to meet the body's requirement for vitamin D (Holick, 2002).

References

Alam, M., & Ratner, D. (2001). Cutaneous squamous-cell carcinoma. *New England Journal of Medicine, 344,* 975–983.

Anderson, S. O., & Sarma, K. M. (2007). *Protecting the ozone layer.* London, England: The United Nations History, Earthscan Press.

Armstrong, B. K., & Kricker, A. (2001). The epidemiology of UV induced skin cancer. *Journal of Photochemistry and Photobiology B: Biology, 63,* 8–18.

Arthey, S., & Clarke, V. A. (1995). Suntanning and sun protection: A review of the psychological literature. *Social Science and Medicine, 40,* 265–274.

Australian Institute of Health and Welfare & Cancer Australia. (2008). *Non-melanoma skin cancer: General practice consultations, hospitalization and mortality.* Cancer series no. 43. Cat. no. 39. Canberra, Australia. Retrieved from http://www.aihw.gov.au/WorkArea/DownloadAsset.aspx?id=6442454591

Babilas, P., Landthaler, M., & Szeimies, R. M. (2003). Actinic keratosis. *Hautarzt, 54,* 551–562.

Bath-Hextall, F., Leonardi-Bee, J., Smith, C., Meal, A., & Hubbard, R. (2007). Trends in incidence of skin basal cell carcinoma. Additional evidence from a UK primary care database study. *International Journal of Cancer, 121*(9), 2105–2108.

Bauer, A., Diepgen, T. L., & Schmitt, J. (2011). Is occupational solar ultraviolet irradiation a relevant risk factor for basal cell carcinoma? A systematic review and meta-analysis of the epidemiological literature. *British Journal of Dermatology, 165*(3), 612–625.

Bennett, M. F., Robinson, M. K., Baron, E. D., & Cooper, K. D. (2008). Skin immune systems and inflammation: Protector of the skin or promoter of aging? *Journal of Investigative Dermatology Symposium Proceedings, 13,* 15–19.

Birch-Johansen, F., Jensen, A., Mortensen, L., Olesen, A. B., & Kjaer, S. K. (2010). Trends in the incidence of nonmelanoma skin cancer in Denmark 1978–2007: Rapid incidence increase among young Danish women. *International Journal of Cancer, 127*(9), 2190–2198.

Boukamp, P. (2005). Non-melanoma skin cancer: What drives tumor development and progression? *Carcinogenesis, 26*(10), 1657–1667.

Boyd, A. S., Shyr, Y., & King, L. E., Jr. (2002). Basal cell carcinoma in young women: An evaluation of the association of tanning bed use and smoking. *Journal of the Amercian Academy Dermatology, 46,* 706–709.

Bradford, P. T., Goldstein, A. M., Tamura, D., Khan, S. G., Ueda, T., Boyle, J., … Kraemer, K. H. (2011). Cancer and neurologic degeneration in xeroderma pigmentosum: Long term follow-up characterizes the role of DNA repair. *Journal of Medical Genetics, 48*(3), 168–176.

Brash, D. E., Rudolph, J. A., Simon, J. A., Lin, A., McKenna, G. J., Baden, H. P., … Pontén, J. (1991). A role for sunlight in skin cancer: UV-induced *p53* mutations in squamous cell carcinoma. *Proceedings of the National Academy of Sciences of the United States of America, 88*(22), 10124–10128.

Brash, D. E., Ziegler, A., Jonason, A. S., Simon, J. A., Kunala, S., & Leffell, D. J. (1996). Sunlight and sunburn in human skin cancer: *p53*, apoptosis and tumor promotion. *Journal of Investigative Dermatology Symposium Proceedings, 1*, 136–142.

Byfield, S. D., Chen, D., Yim, Y. M., & Reyes, C. (2013). Age distribution of patients with advanced non-melanoma skin cancer in the United States. *Archives of Dermatologic Research, 305*(9), 845–850.

Christenson, L. J., Borrowman, T. A., Vachon, C. M., Tellefson, M. M., Otley, C. C., Seaver, A. L., & Roenighk, R. K. (2005). Incidence of basal cell and squamous cell carcinomas in a population younger than 40 years. *Journal of the American Medical Association, 294*(6), 681–690.

Cleaver, J. (1968). Defective repair of DNA in xeroderma pigmentosum. *Nature, 218*(5142), 652–656.

Criscione, V. D., Weinstock, M. A., Naylor, M. F., Luque, C., Eide, M. J., & Bingham, S. F., & Department of Veteran Affairs Topical Tretinoin Chemoprevention Trial Group. (2009). Actinic keratoses: Natural history and risk of malignant transformation in the Veterans Affairs Topical Tretinoin Chemoprevention Trial. *Cancer, 115*(11), 2523–2530.

Crutzen, P. J., Molkina, M. J., & Rowland, F. S. (1995). *The Nobel prize in chemistry, 1995*. The Royal Swedish Academy of Sciences. Retrieved from http://www.nobelprize.org /nobel_prizes/chemistry/laureates/1995/illpres/

de Gruijl, F. R. (1999). Skin cancer and solar UV radiation. *European Journal of Cancer, 35*, 2003–2009.

De Zwaan, S. E., & Haass, N. K. (2010). Genetics of basal cell carcinoma. *Australasian Journal of Dermatology, 51*(2), 81–92.

DiGiovanna, J., & Kraemer, K. H. (2012). Shining a light on xeroderma pigmentosum. *Journal of Investigative Dermatology, 132*(3), 785–796.

Eisemann, N., Waldmann, A., Geller, A. C., Weinstock, M. A., Volkmer, B., Greinert, R., … Katalinic, A. (2013). Non-melanoma skin cancer incidence and impact of skin cancer screening on incidence. *Journal of Investigative Dermatology, 134*, 43–50.

Engels, E. A., Frisch, M., Goedert, J. J., Biggar, R. J., & Miller, R. W. (2002). Merkel cell carcinoma and HIV infection. *Lancet, 359*, 497–498.

English, D. R., Armstrong, B. K., Kricker, A., Winter, M. G., Heenan, P. J., & Randel, P. L. (1998). Case-control study of sun exposure and squamous cell carcinoma of the skin. *International Journal of Cancer, 77*, 347–353.

Farman, J. C., Gardiner, B. G., & Shanklin, J. D. (1985). Large losses of total ozone in Antarctica reveal seasonal ClO_x/NO_x interaction. *Nature, 351*, 207–210.

Feldman, S. R., & Fleischer, A. B. (2011). Progression of actinic keratosis to squamous cell carcinoma revisited: Clinical and treatment implications. *Cutis, 87*(4), 201–207.

Feng, H., Shuda, M., Chang, Y., & Moore, P. S. (2008). Clonal integration of a polyomavirus in human Merkel cell carcinoma. *Science, 319*(5866), 1096–1100.

Ferlay, J., Ervik, M., Lam, F., Colombet, M., Mery, L., Piñeros, M., … Bray, F. (2018). *Global cancer observatory: Cancer today*. Lyon, France: International Agency for Research on Cancer. Retrieved from https://gco.iarc.fr/today

Ferrucci, L. M., Cartmel, B., Molinaro, A. M., Leffell, D. J., Bale, A. E., & Mayne, S. T. (2012). Indoor tanning and risk of early-onset basal cell carcinoma. *Journal of the American Academy of Dermatology, 67*(4), 552–562.

Fitzmaurice, C., Akinyemiju, T. F., Al Lami, F. H., Alam, T., Alizadeh-Navaei, R., Allen, C., … Global Burden of Disease Cancer Collaboration. (2018). Global, regional, and national cancer incidence, mortality, years of life lost, years lived with disability, and disability-adjusted life-years for 29 cancer groups, 1990 to 2016: A systematic analysis for the Global Burden of Disease Study. *JAMA Oncology*. Online publication June 02, 2018. doi:10.1001/jamaoncol.2018.2706.

Flohil, S. C., Seubring, I., van Rossum, M. M., Coebergh, J. W., de Vries, E., & Nijsten, T. (2013). Trends in basal cell carcinoma incidence rates: A 37-year Dutch observational study. *Journal of Investigative Dermatology, 133*(4), 913–918.

Fuchs, A., & Marmur, E. (2007). The kinetics of skin cancer: Progression of actinic keratosis to squamous cell carcinoma. *Dermatologic Surgery, 33*(9), 1099–1101.

Gallagher, R. P., Hill, G. B., Bajdik, C. D., Fincham, S., Coldman, A. J., McLean, D. I., & Threlfall, W. J. (1995). Sunlight exposure, pigmentary factors, and risk of nonmelanocytic skin cancer. I. Basal cell carcinoma. *Archives of Dermatology, 131*(2), 157–163.

Gibson, G. E., O'Grady, A., Key, E. W., Leader, M., & Murphy, G. M. (1998). Langerhans cells in benign, premalignant and malignant skin lesions of renal transplant recipients and the effect of retinoid therapy. *Journal of the European Academy of Dermatology and Venereology, 10*(2), 131–136.

Gloster, H. M. Jr., & Neal, K. (2005). Skin cancer in skin of color. *Journal of the American Academy of Dermatology, 55*(5), 741–760.

Glover, M. T., Niranjan, N., Kwan, J. T., & Leigh, I. M. (1994). Non-melanoma skin cancer in renal transplant recipients: The extent of the problem and a strategy for management. *British Journal of Plastic Surgery, 47*(2), 86–89.

Gohara, M. (2015). Skin cancer: An African perspective. *British Journal of Dermatology, 173*(S2), 17–21.

Gorlin, R. J. (2004). Nevoid basal cell carcinoma (Gorlin) syndrome. *Genetics in Medicine, 6*(6), 530–539.

Green, A., & Battistutta, D. (1990). Incidence and determinants of skin cancer in a high-risk Australian population. *International Journal of Cancer, 46*(3), 356–361.

Harris, R. B., Griffith, K., & Moon, T. E. (2001). Trends in the incidence of nonmelanoma skin cancers in southeastern Arizona, 1985–1996. *Journal of the American Academy of Dermatology, 45*(4), 528–536.

Hartevelt, M. M., Bavinck, J. N., Kootte, A. M., Vermeer, B. J., & Vandenbroucke, J. P. (1990). Incidence of skin cancer after renal transplantation in The Netherlands. *Transplantation, 49*(3), 506–509.

Hartevelt, M. M., Bavinck, J. N., Kootte, A. M., Vermeer, B. J., & Vandenbroucke, J. P. (1996). Arsenic in dermatology. *Dermatologic Surgery, 22*, 301–304.

Heath, M., Jaimes, N., Lemos, B., Mostaghimi, A., Wang, L. C., Peñas, P. F., & Nghiem, P. (2008). Clinical characteristics of Merkel cell carcinoma at diagnosis in 195 patients: The AEIOU features. *Journal of the American Academy of Dermatology, 58*, 375–381.

Hebra, F., & Kaposi, M. (1874). On diseases of the skin including exanthemata. Volume III. *The New Sydenham Society, 61*, 252–258.

Hodgson, N. C. (2005). Merkel cell carcinoma: Changing incidence trends. *Journal of Surgical Oncology, 89*(1), 1–4.

Holick, M. F. (2002). Vitamin D: The underappreciated D-lightful hormone that is important for skeletal and cellular health. *Current Opinions in Endocrinology and Diabetes, 9*, 87–98.

Iannacone, M. R., Wang, W., Stockwell, H. G., O'Rourke, K., Giuliano, A. R., Sondak, V. K., … Rollison, D. E. (2012). Patterns and timing of sunlight exposure and risk of basal cell and squamous cell carcinomas of the skin: A case control study. *BMC Cancer, 12*(1), 417. doi:10.1186/1471-2407-12-417.

Ireland National Cancer Registry. (2013). Non-melanoma skin cancer. *Cancer Trends, 20.* Retrieved from http://www.ncri.ie/sites/ncri/files/pubs/CancerTrendsNo.20-NonMelanomaSkinCancer.pdf

Jensen, P., Hansen, S., Møller, B., Leivestad, T., Pfeffer, P., Geiran, O., … Simonsen, S. (1999). Skin cancer in kidney and heart transplant recipients and different long-term immunosuppressive therapy regimens. *Journal of the American Academy of Dermatology, 40*(2 Pt 1), 177–186.

Kaplan, A. L., & Cook, J. L. (2005). Cutaneous squamous cell carcinoma in patients with chronic lymphocytic leukemia. *SKINmed, 4*(5), 300–304.

Karagas, M. R., Stannard, V. A., Mott, L. A., Slattery, M. J., Spencer, S. K., & Weinstock, M. A. (2002). Use of tanning devices and risk of basal cell and squamous cell skin cancers. *Journal of the National Cancer Institute, 94*(3), 224–226.

Karagas, M. R., Stukel, T. A., Morris, J. S., Tosteson, T. D., Weiss, J. E., Spencer, S. K., & Greenberg, E. R. (2001). Skin cancer risk in relation to toenail arsenic concentrations in a US population-based case-control study. *American Journal of Epidemiology, 153*(6), 559–565.

Katalinic, A., Kunze, U., & Schäfer, T. (2003). Epidemiology of cutaneous melanoma and non-melanoma skin cancer in Schleswig-Holstein, Germany: Incidence, clinical subtypes, tumor stages and localization (epidemiology of skin cancer). *British Journal of Dermatology, 149*(6), 1200–1206.

Kopf, A. W. (1979). Computer analysis of 3531 basal cell carcinomas of the skin. *Journal of Dermatology, 6*(5), 267–281.

Kripke, M. L. (1988). Impact of ozone depletion on skin cancers. *Journal of Dermatologic Surgery and Oncology, 14*(8), 853–857.

Krynitz, B., Edgren, G., Lindelöf, B., Baecklund, E., Brattström, C., Wilczek, H., & Smedby, K. E. (2013). Risk of skin cancer and other malignancies in kidney, liver, heart and lung transplant recipients 1970–2008—A Swedish population-based study. *International Journal of Cancer, 132*(6), 1429–1438.

Leonardi-Bee, J., Ellison, T., & Bath-Hextall, F. (2012). Smoking and the risk of non-melanoma skin cancer, systematic review and meta-analysis. *Archives of Dermatology, 148*(8), 939–946.

Liang, G., Nan, H., Qureshi, A. A., & Han, J. (2012). Pre-diagnostic plasma 25-hydroxyvitamin D levels and risk of non-melanoma skin cancer in women. *PLoS One, 7*(4), e35211. doi:10.1371/journal.pone.003521.

Lichter, M. D., Karagas, M. R., Mott, L. A., Spencer, S. K., Stukel, T. A., & Greenberg, E. R. (2000). Therapeutic ionizing radiation and the incidence of basal cell carcinoma and squamous cell carcinoma. The New Hampshire Skin Cancer Study Group. *Archives of Dermatology, 136*(8), 1007–1011.

Lim, J. L., & Stern, R. S. (2005). High levels of ultraviolet B exposure increase the risk of non-melanoma skin cancer in psoralen and ultraviolet A-treated patients. *Journal of Investigative Dermatology, 124*(3), 505–513.

Lindelöf, B., Sigurgeirsson, B., Gäbel, H., & Stern, R. S. (2000). Incidence of skin cancer in 5356 patients following organ transplantation. *British Journal of Dermatology, 143*(3), 513–519.

Lindelöf, B., Sigurgeirsson, B., Tegner, E., Larkö, O., Johannesson, A., Berne, B., … Emtestam, L. (1999). PUVA and cancer risk: The Swedish follow-up study. *British Journal of Dermatology, 141*(1), 108–112.

Lindqvist, P. G., Epstein, E., Landin-Olsson, M., Ingvar, C., Nielsen, K., Stenbeck, M., & Olsson, H. (2014). Avoidance of sun exposure is a risk factor for all-cause mortality: Results from the Melanoma in Southern Sweden cohort. *Journal of Internal Medicine, 176*(1), 77–86.

Ling, G., Ahmadian, A., Persson, A., Undén, A. B., Afink, G., Williams, C., … Pontén, F. (2001). PATCHED and *p53* gene alterations I sporadic and hereditary basal cell cancer. *Oncogene, 20*, 7770–7778.

Maricich, S. M., Wellnitz, S. A., Nelson, A. M., Lesniak, D. R., Gerling, G. J., Lumpkin, E. A., & Zoghbi, H. Y. (2009). Merkel cells are essential for light touch responses. *Science, 324*(5934), 1580–1582.

Marks, R., Rennie, G., & Selwood, T. S. (1988). Malignant transformation of solar keratoses to squamous cell carcinoma. *Lancet, 1*(8589), 795–797.

Maru, G. B., Gandhi, K., Ramchandani, A., & Kumar, G. (2014). The role of inflammation in skin cancer. *Advances in Experimental Medicine and Biology, 816*, 437–469.

Miller, D. L., & Weinstock, M. A. (1994). Nonmelanoma skin cancer in the United States: Incidence. *Journal of the American Academy of Dermatology, 30*, 774–778.

Miller, S. J. (1995). Etiology and pathogenesis of basal cell carcinoma. *Clinics in Dermatology, 13*(6), 527–536.

National Aeronautics and Space Administration (NASA). (2014). *Ozone hole watch*. Washington, DC. Retrieved from http://ozonewatch.gsfc.nasa.gov/facts/history.html

National Cancer Institute. (1996). *SEER rates, 1992–1996*. Bethesda, MD: U.S. Department of Health and Human Services, National Institutes of Health.

National Cancer Institute. (2014). *Genetics of skin cancer*. Bethesda, MD: U.S. Department of Health and Human Services, National Institutes of Health.

Nghiem, P., & James, N. (2007). Merkel cell carcinoma. In K. Wolff, L. A. Goldsmith, S. I. Katz, B. A. Gilchrest, A. S. Paller, & D. J. Leffell (Eds.), *Fitzpatrick's dermatology in general medicine* (7th ed., pp. 1087–1094). New York, NY: McGraw-Hill.

Nijsten, T. E., & Stern, R. S. (2003). The increased risk of skin cancer is persistent after discontinuation of psoralen + ultraviolet A: A cohort study. *Journal of Investigative Dermatology, 121*(2), 252–258.

Nüsslein-Volhard, C., & Wieschaus, E. (1980). Mutations affecting segment number and polarity in drosophila. *Nature, 287*(5785), 795–801.

Ortonne, J. P. (2002). From actinic keratosis to squamous cell carcinoma. *British Journal of Dermatology, 146*(61), 20–23.

Penn, I., & First, M. R. (1999). Merkel's cell carcinoma in organ recipients: Report of 41 cases. *Transplantation, 68*, 1717–1721.

Rass, K. (2005). UV damage and DNA repair in basal cell and squamous cell carcinomas. In J. Reichrath (Ed.), *Molecular mechanisms of basal cell and squamous cell carcinomas* (pp. 18–30). New York, NY: Springer Science.

Ridky, T. W. (2007). Nonmelanoma skin cancer. *Journal of the American Academy of Dermatology, 57*(3), 484–501.

Robinson, J. K. (1987). Risk of developing another basal cell carcinoma. A 5-year prospective study. *Cancer, 60*(1), 118–120.

Rosso, S., Zanetti, R., Martinez, C., Tormo, M. J., Schraub, S., Sancho-Garnier, H., … Wechsler, J. (1996). The multicentre south European study 'Helios'. II: Different sun exposure patterns in the aetiology of basal cell and squamous cell carcinomas of the skin. *British Journal of Cancer, 73*(11), 1447–1454.

Rubin, A. I., Chen, E. H., & Ratner, D. (2005). Basal-cell carcinoma. *New England Journal of Medicine, 353*, 2262–2269.

Sadamori, N., Mine, M., & Honda, T. (1991). Incidence of skin cancer among Nagasaki atomic bomb survivors. *Journal of Radiation Research, 32*(Suppl. 2), 217–225.

Schmitt, J., Seidler, A., Diepgen, T. L., & Bauer, A. (2011). Occupational ultraviolet light exposure increases the risk for the development of cutaneous squamous cell carcinoma: A systematic review and meta-analysis. *British Journal of Dermatology, 164*(2), 291–307.

Shuda, M., Feng, H., Kwun, H. J., Rosen, S. T., Gjoerup, O., Moore, P. S., & Chang, Y. (2008). T antigen mutations are a human tumor-specific signature for Merkel cell polyomavirus. *Proceedings of the National Academy of Sciences of the United States of America, 105,* 16272–16277.

Silverberg, M. J., Leyden, W., Warton, E. M., Quesenberry, C. P., Engels, E. A., & Asgari, M. M. (2013). HIV infection status, immunodeficiency and the incidence of non-melanoma skin cancer. *Journal of the National Cancer Institute, 105*(5), 350–360.

Staples, M., Marks, M., & Giles, G. (1998). Trends in the incidence of non-melanocytic skin cancer (NMSC) treated in Australia 1985–1995. Are primary prevention programs starting to have an effect? *International Journal of Cancer, 78,* 144–148.

Staples, M. P., Elwood, M., Burton, R. C., William, J. L., Marks, R., & Giles, G. G. (2006). Non-melanoma skin cancer in Australia: The 2002 national survey and trends since 1985. *Medical Journal of Australia, 184,* 6–10.

States, J. C., McDuffie, E. R., Myrand, S. P., McDowell, M., & Cleaver, J. E. (1998). Distribution of mutations in the human xeroderma pigmentosum group A gene and their relationships to the functional regions of the DNA damage recognition protein. *Human Mutation, 12*(2), 103–113.

Stern, R. S., & Lange, R. (1990). Incidence of skin cancer after renal transplantation in the Netherlands. *Transplantation, 49,* 506–509.

Stern, R. S., & Lange, R. (1988). Nonmelanoma skin cancer occurring in patients treated with PUVA five to ten years after first treatment. *Journal of Investigative Dermatology, 91*(2), 120–124.

Stoitzner, P. (2010). The Langerhans cell controversy: Are they immunostimulatory or immunoregulatory cells of the skin immune system? *Immunology and Cell Biology, 88,* 348–350.

Tamura, D., DiGiovanna, J. J., & Kraemer, K. H. (2010). Founder mutations in xeroderma pigmentosum. *Journal of Investigative Dermatology, 130*(6), 1491–1493.

Thiers, B. H., Maize, J. C., Spicer, S. S., & Cantor, A. B. (1984). The effect of aging and chronic sun exposure on human Langerhans cell populations. *Journal of Investigative Dermatology, 82*(3), 223–226.

U.S. Department of Health and Human Services. (2014). *The Surgeon General's call to action to prevent skin cancer.* Washington, DC: Author.

van Dam, R. M., Huang, Z., Rimm, E. B., Weinstock, M. A., Spiegelman, D., Colditz, G. A., … Giovannucci, E. (1999). Risk factors for basal cell carcinoma of the skin in men: Results from the health professionals follow-up study. *American Journal of Epidemiology, 150*(5), 459–468.

Wang, J., Aldabagh, B., Yu, J., & Arron, S. T. (2014). Role of human papillomavirus in cutaneous squamous cell carcinoma, a meta-analysis. *Journal of the American Academy of Dermatology, 70*(4), 621–629.

Wehner, M. R., Shive, M. L., Chren, M. M., Han, J., Qureshi, A. A., & Linos, E. (2012). Indoor tanning and non-melanoma skin cancer: Systematic review and meta-analysis. *British Medical Journal, 345,* e5909.

Wong, C. M., Strange, R. C., & Lear, J. T. (2003). Basal cell carcinoma. *British Medical Journal, 327,* 794.

World Meteorological Organization. (1995). *Global ozone research and monitoring project: 1994.* WMO No. 37. Geneva, Switzerland. Retrieved from http://ozonewatch.gsfc.nasa.gov/facts/history.html

Wu, S., Han, J., Li, W. Q., Li, T., & Qureshi, A. A. (2013). Basal-cell carcinoma incidence and associated risk factors in U.S. women and men. *American Journal of Epidemiology, 178*(6), 890–897.

Yamada, M., Kodama, K., Fujita, S., Akahoshi, M., Yamada, S., Hirose, R., & Hori, M. (1996). Prevalence of skin neoplasms among the atomic bomb survivors. *Radiation Research, 146*(2), 223–226.

Yu, H. S., Liao, W. T., & Chai, C. Y. (2006). Arsenic carcinogenesis in the skin. *Journal of Biomedical Science, 13*(5), 657–666.

Zanetti, R., Rosso, S., Martinez, C., Navarro, C., Schraub, S., Sancho-Garnier, H., … Wechsler, J. (1996). The multicentre south European study "Helios." I: Skin characteristics and sunburns in basal cell and squamous cell carcinomas of the skin. *British Journal of Cancer, 73,* 1440–1446.

Zhang, M., Qureshi, A. A., Geller, A. C., Frazier, L., Hunter, D. J., & Han, J. (2012). Use of tanning beds and incidence of skin cancer. *Journal of Clinical Oncology, 30*(14), 1588–1593.

CHAPTER 35

Epidemiology of Classic Sarcoma and Kaposi Sarcoma

▶ Classification of Sarcoma

Classic sarcomas are tumors of connective tissue. These tumors are derived from mesenchymal cells that normally mature into skeletal muscle, smooth muscle, fat, fibrous tissue, bone, and cartilage. They are broadly classified as sarcomas of soft tissue or bone. Sarcomas are named after the cell of origin; those that arise in fat are called liposarcomas, those derived from fibrous tissues are fibrosarcomas, and those that develop in bone are osteosarcomas. Other subtypes include leiomyosarcomas of smooth muscle, rhabdomyosarcomas of skeletal muscle, synovial sarcomas of joint capsule tissues, angiosarcomas of blood vessels, gastrointestinal sarcomas of the gut, chondrosarcomas of cartilage, and Ewing sarcoma of the long bones. Tumors derived from tissues of the peripheral nervous system are also included with the soft-tissue sarcomas, including malignant nerve-sheath tumors (schwannomas) and neurofibromas (Skubitz, 2007).

▶ Global Epidemiology of Sarcoma

Data on sarcomas of bones and soft tissues are conspicuously absent from the global data on cancer routinely reported by the World Health Organization. Although some information is available on Kaposi sarcoma, a tumor derived from blood vessels that is associated with immunosuppression and the epidemic of human immunodeficiency virus (HIV) disease, little is known about the geographic distribution of the more common forms of sarcoma, namely those arising from bone, fat, muscle, and fibrous tissues. Relevant epidemiologic data on these tumors are abstracted primarily from the U.S. Surveillance, Epidemiology, and End Results (SEER) tumor registry and the European Automated Childhood Cancer Information System (ACCIS) database.

▶ Sarcoma in the U.S. Population

In the U.S. population of approximately 310 million people, more than 13,000 individuals are diagnosed with sarcomas every year (2650 with bone tumors and 10,500 with soft-tissue tumors). The annual age-adjusted incidence rates of bone tumors in the U.S. population are about 10 per million in men and 8 per million in women, markedly less than the rates for soft-tissue sarcomas (38 per million in men and 27 per million in women). Nevertheless, among children and adolescents under the age of 20 years, bone sarcomas and soft-tissue sarcomas have relatively similar rates (about 9 per million for bone tumors and 11 per million for soft-tissue tumors), and each type accounts for a significant fraction of all pediatric malignancies.

As shown in **FIGURE 35.1**, the U.S. age distribution of bone sarcomas differs dramatically from that of soft-tissue sarcomas. Nearly 30% of bone sarcomas are diagnosed during childhood and adolescence (under 20 years of age), after which there is a general decline in the number of new cases. The incidence of these tumors peaks during times of rapid growth and development of bones, between the ages of 10 and 15 years for both boys and girls.

In contrast to bone sarcomas, soft-tissue sarcomas are diagnosed at a relatively constant rate throughout the lifespan (**FIGURE 35.1**). This pattern reflects a mixture of age distributions for the various subtypes of soft-tissue sarcomas. For example, rhabdomyosarcomas tend to grow and develop more rapidly and are usually detected before the age of 20 years, whereas liposarcomas, leiomyomas, and gastrointestinal sarcomas are detected more often in adults (Altekruse et al., 2010; Darling, 2007).

In the U.S. population, nearly 1500 men and women die from bone tumors and nearly 4000 die from soft-tissue tumors every year. Similar to the pattern of incidence rates, the overall age-adjusted annual mortality rates for bone tumors (5 per million in men and 4 per million in women) are much lower than the rates for soft-tissue tumors (14 per million in men and 11 per million in women), whereas the pediatric mortality rates are relatively similar (3.5 per million for bone tumors and 4.4 per million for soft-tissue tumors). The U.S. distributions of age at death for bone tumors and soft-tissue tumors are compared in **FIGURE 35.2**. The death curve for bone tumors is bimodal with approximately 29% of deaths occurring in pediatric patients or young adults under the age of 35 years followed by an exponential rise with age and a later peak at 75–84 years. In contrast, the death curve for soft-tissue tumors rises gradually with age and peaks late in life with more than 40% of deaths occurring in the age interval 65–84 years.

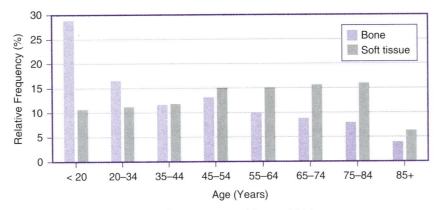

FIGURE 35.1 New Cases of Sarcomas of Bone and Soft Tissue, United States, 2006.

Data from Altekruse, S. F., Kosary, C. L., Krapcho, M., Neyman, N., Aminou, R., Waldron, W., & Edwards, B. K. (2010). *SEER cancer statistics review, 1975–2007*. Bethesda, MD: National Cancer Institute.

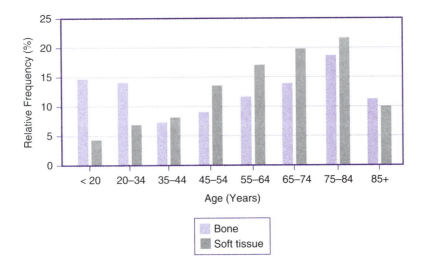

FIGURE 35.2 Deaths from Sarcomas of Bone and Soft Tissue, United States, 2006.

Data from Altekruse, S. F., Kosary, C. L., Krapcho, M., Neyman, N., Aminou, R., Waldron, W., & Edwards, B. K. (2010). *SEER cancer statistics review, 1975–2007*. Bethesda, MD: National Cancer Institute.

It is clear from the preceding discussion that key epidemiologic features of bone tumors and soft-tissue sarcomas differ dramatically for pediatric versus adult populations. In addition to the distributional differences already noted, the histological types of sarcomas that predominate among pediatric patients are replaced by other types among adult patients. Due to these striking distinctions, pediatric and adult sarcomas are discussed separately in the following sections of this chapter.

▶ Epidemiology of Pediatric Sarcomas

Bone Sarcomas in Children and Adolescents

Bone tumors account for slightly more than 6% of all pediatric malignancies. Stiller and colleagues using the ACCIS database reported rates of pediatric bone tumors among European children during 1978–1997. Rates were similar for boys and girls up to 14 years of age (5.5 cases per million), whereas in the older adolescent age group, ages 15–19 years, boys had higher rates than girls (19.3 versus 10.7 cases per million). Combining the rates for these age categories yields estimates of 9.2 cases per million in boys, 6.9 per million in girls, and 8.0 per million for all individuals under 20 years of age. In the European database of 5572 pediatric bone tumors, 52% were classified as osteosarcoma, 34% as Ewing sarcoma, and 6% as chondrosarcoma. No significant time trends were detected (Stiller, Bielack, Jundt, & Steliarova-Foucher, 2006).

Data from the SEER tumor registry in the United States reflect rates of pediatric bone tumors that are similar to the European rates. For the period 1975–1995, the annual incidence of bone tumors was 8.7 per million for individuals under the age of 20 years, and boys had higher annual rates than girls (9.4 versus 7.9 cases per million). As in Europe, no significant time trends were observed in the U.S. annual rates. **FIGURE 35.3** shows the age distribution of bone tumors diagnosed among U.S. children. Clearly, onset peaks at age 15 years, coinciding with the growth spurt during adolescence (Gurney, Swensen, & Bulterys, 1999; Gurney, Young, Roffers, Smith, & Bunin, 1999).

Of the approximately 700 bone tumors diagnosed among children and adolescents in the United States every year, about 56% are classified as osteosarcoma, 34% as Ewing sarcoma, and 6% as chondrosarcoma. Osteosarcomas arise most often in the metaphyseal zones near the extremities of elongating long bones (femur, tibia, and humerus), whereas Ewing sarcoma is more likely to develop in the marrow of bones of the central axis (pelvis, rib cage, ischium, sternum). Osteosarcoma occurs at approximately the same rate in African-American and Caucasian children, whereas the rate of Ewing sarcoma is about six times higher in Caucasians. The relative paucity of Ewing sarcoma in children of African descent is consistent in populations other than the United States (Parkin, Stiller, Draper, & Bieber, 1988).

Subtypes of Pediatric Bone Sarcomas

Osteosarcoma

Osteosarcoma is the most common primary malignant tumor of bone among children and adolescents, accounting for 3%–4% of all malignancies in individuals less than 20 years of age. Approximately 400

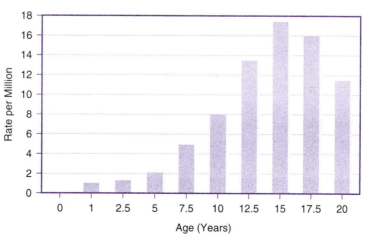

FIGURE 35.3 Age Distribution of Bone Sarcomas in Children and Adolescents, United States.

Data from Gurney, J. G., Swensen, A. R., & Bulterys, M. (1999). Chapter VIII. Malignant bone tumors. In L. A. G. Ries, M. A. Smith, J. G. Gurney, M. Linet, T. Tamra, J. L. Young, & G. R. Bunin (Eds.), *Cancer incidence and survival among children and adolescents: United States SEER program 1975–1995* (pp. 99–110, NIH Pub. No. 99-4649). Bethesda, MD: National Cancer Institute, SEER Program.

cases are diagnosed each year in the United States, most (~75%) in children and adolescents. Osteosarcomas are characterized by the production of immature bone (osteoid) by the malignant cells. The most common anatomic sites of origin are the femur, tibia, and humerus bones (Kumar, Abbas, & Aster, 2014).

Ewing Sarcoma. Nearly a century ago, James Ewing first described the pathologic features of the tumor that bears his name (Ewing, 1921). *Ewing sarcoma* is characterized as an undifferentiated tumor of the diaphyses of long bones of the extremities. In contrast to osteosarcoma, Ewing sarcoma is sensitive to radiation. As discussed in the following section, such tumors are now identified by karyotypic studies that reveal the presence of reciprocal chromosomal translocations involving the Ewing sarcoma gene (*EWSR-1*) on chromosome 22. Ewing sarcomas also occasionally arise in soft tissues. Ewing sarcoma is the second most common bone tumor among children and adolescents, accounting for more than one-third of bone sarcomas and about 2% of all malignancies in individuals less than 20 years of age. Although the peak incidence of Ewing sarcoma occurs during adolescence, molecularly confirmed cases have been discovered in adults as old as 80 years (Kumar et al., 2014).

Chondrosarcoma. Chondrosarcomas account for about 6% of bone tumors that occur in children and adolescents. These cartilaginous tumors occur more often in adults and are discussed in a later section of this chapter.

Cytogenetics of Pediatric Bone Sarcomas

Certain types of bone sarcomas have similar (nonrandom) patterns of chromosomal translocations and aberrations. For example, nearly all cases of Ewing sarcoma demonstrate one of several reciprocal chromosomal translocations involving break points within the Ewing sarcoma gene (*EWSR-1*) located on the long arm of chromosome 22. Such translocations create chimeric fusion proteins with oncogenic potential. About 95% of the *EWSR-1* translocations reposition a portion of the *EWSR-1* gene very near the Friend leukemia integration (*FLI-1*) locus on chromosome 11. The *FLI-1* gene encodes a protein involved in the regulation of cellular proliferation and differentiation. The chimeric fusion proteins encoded by *EWSR-1* and *FLI-1* reciprocal translocations stimulate tumorigenesis of bone (Ewing sarcoma); translocations of the *EWSR-1* gene to other loci have also been found in

association with other types of sarcomas (e.g., myxoid liposarcoma). It is likely that these proteins act as transcription activators, deregulating genes associated with cell signaling, proliferation, angiogenesis, apoptosis, tissue invasion, and metastasis; consequently, they provide potential targets for molecular therapy (Delaney, Hornicek, Lessnick, & Mankin, 2010; Ladanyi, 1995).

Unlike Ewing sarcoma, osteosarcomas *do not* consistently manifest specific chromosomal translocations or molecular defects; rather, they tend to have a complex karyotype. Nevertheless, osteosarcomas do develop in association with certain *rare* genetic anomalies. Specifically, osteosarcomas are a component of the profile of malignancies that develop in hereditary retinoblastoma, Li–Fraumeni syndrome, and Rothmund–Thomson syndrome.

Hereditary retinoblastoma is caused by a genetic mutation in the retinoblastoma gene (*Rb1*). When the mutant *Rb1* gene is present, carriers invariably develop retinoblastoma in either one or both eyes. Treatment usually involves enucleation of the afflicted eye combined with external beam radiotherapy. Abramson and colleagues studied 817 patients who were treated for bilateral retinoblastoma during childhood. Among survivors, the cumulative risk of subsequently developing a second primary malignancy was found to cumulate at about 1% per year, reaching 53% at 50 years of age. Among the 180 second primary tumors reported, 60 were bone tumors, 36 of which developed in the skull and facial bones and 24 in bones of the extremities outside of the field of radiation. Soft-tissue sarcomas of the head and neck (*n* = 60) and brain tumors (*n* = 12) also developed at high rates among survivors (Abramson & Frank, 1998). Other studies suggest that the onset of osteosarcoma following radiotherapy occurs earlier in bones within the field of radiation, possibly due to radiation-induced mutations in the second (normal) *Rb1* gene (Chauveinc et al., 2001). There is controversy as to whether the development of osteosarcoma in retinoblastoma survivors is due to the *Rb1* gene defect, radiotherapy for retinoblastoma, or the combination of both factors.

Li–Fraumeni syndrome carries a high risk for sarcomas, brain tumors, breast cancer, leukemia, lymphoma, and adrenal cortical carcinoma. This syndrome is caused by a genetic mutation in either of two tumor–suppressor genes, *p53* or *CHEK2*. Individuals who inherit a defective *p53* or *CHEK2* gene have an approximately 85% lifetime risk of developing one or more of the malignancies characteristic of Li–Fraumeni syndrome. Among women with the syndrome, the lifetime risk approaches 100% due to their inordinately high risk of developing premenopausal breast cancer (Li et al., 1998).

Rothmund–Thomson syndrome is an extraordinarily rare genetic disorder caused by an autosomal recessive gene defect in the helicase gene (*RECQL-4*) located on the long arm of chromosome 8. DNA helicases are enzymes that unwind DNA and are involved in many basic cellular processes (DNA replication, transcription, translation, recombination, and repair, and ribosome biogenesis). Homozygous carriers of two mutant copies of the gene have early photosensitivity and develop a skin rash known as *poikiloderma*, juvenile cataracts, and skeletal anomalies. Most individuals with this syndrome develop osteosarcomas early in life (Leonard, Craft, Moss, & Malcolm, 1996; Wang et al., 2003).

Soft-Tissue Sarcomas in Children and Adolescents

Soft-tissue sarcomas account for approximately 7.4% of all childhood tumors. In the United States, the annual incidence of soft-tissue sarcomas in individuals under 20 years of age is 11 per million. Annual rates are about 20% higher in boys than girls (12.2 versus 10.3 per million). Of the approximately 900 soft-tissue sarcomas that develop in children and adolescents in the United States every year, about 41% are rhabdomyosarcomas of skeletal muscle and 24% are sarcomas of fibrous tissues. Other types such as histiocytomas, synovial sarcomas, and liposarcomas occur less frequently. **FIGURE 35.4** shows the age distribution of soft-tissue tumors diagnosed in the U.S. pediatric population. The early peak in the age distribution of soft-tissue sarcomas is due to the early onset of rhabdomyosarcomas followed by a nadir

and then escalating rates of fibrosarcoma, synovial sarcoma, and other forms. Rare cases of congenital fibrosarcoma have also been reported. No notable ethnic differences have been observed in the pediatric rates of the various histologic subtypes of soft-tissue sarcomas. Nor have there been trends in the annual rates over the past several decades (Gurney et al., 1999).

Subtypes of Pediatric Soft-Tissue Sarcomas

Rhabdomyosarcoma. *Rhabdomyosarcoma* is the most common pediatric solid tumor, accounting for more than half of soft-tissue sarcomas and approximately 4% of all malignancies among individuals under 20 years of age. Rhabdomyosarcomas arise from primitive cells that are the precursors of striated skeletal muscle. They predominantly arise in soft tissues of the head, neck, genitourinary tract, and extremities. These tumors are divisible into two main histologic types, embryonal rhabdomyosarcoma and alveolar rhabdomyosarcoma. In embryonal rhabdomyosarcomas, which are more common in children, the malignant cells resemble embryonal cells of a typical embryo at 6–8 weeks of development. In alveolar rhabdomyosarcomas, which are more common in older children and teenagers, the malignant cells resemble pulmonary alveolar cells of the embryo at 10–12 weeks of development.

Fibrosarcoma. Fibrosarcomas are diagnosed more often in adults, but they also occur among children and adolescents and account for 20%–30% of bone tumors among individuals under 20 years of age. Tumors in this category arise from fibroblasts, the

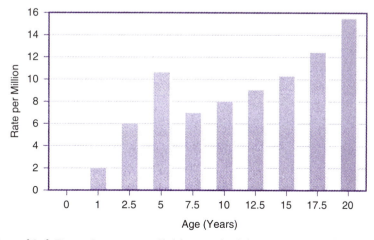

FIGURE 35.4 Age Distribution of Soft-Tissue Sarcomas in Children and Adolescents, United States.

Data from Gurney, J. G., Swensen, A. R., & Bulterys, M. (1999). Malignant bone tumors. In L. A. G. Ries, M. A. Smith, J. G. Gurney, M. Linet, T. Tamra, J. L. Young, & G. R. Bunin (Eds.), *Cancer incidence and survival among children and adolescents: United States SEER program 1975–1995* (pp. 111–122, NIH Pub. No. 99-4649). Bethesda, MD: National Cancer Institute, SEER Program.

precursor cells of collagen-rich connective tissues. Fibrosarcomas are most often discovered in the soft connective tissues of the trunk and extremities, but they also occasionally develop from fibroblasts of the long bones (Cordon-Cardo, 1997).

Rare cases of fibrosarcoma discovered at birth or shortly thereafter have been reported in the literature. Such *congenital fibrosarcomas* usually involve the extremities and are characterized by sheets of anaplastic spindle-shaped tumor cells and abundant deposition of collagen. They are slow growing, and although they invade other contiguous tissues, including bone, they do not readily metastasize to distant anatomic sites (Balsaver, Butler, & Martin, 1967; Exelby, Knapper, Huvos, & Beattie, 1973).

Synovial Sarcoma. *Synovial sarcomas* account for about 15%–20% of soft-tissue tumors in children and adolescents. These tumors arise most often in the soft tissues near the large joints of the arm (elbow) and leg (knee) but can also occur at many other anatomic sites. Histologically, the tumors are composed of two cell types, spindle cells and epithelial cells; consequently, these tumors reflect a *biphasic* pattern of growth. Synovial sarcomas are characterized by a signature chromosomal translocation involving chromosome 18 and the X chromosome, which is discussed in the following section.

Alveolar Soft-Part Sarcoma. Alveolar soft-part sarcoma is a very rare type of soft-tissue sarcoma that arises mainly in children and adolescents. These tumors are usually slow growing but tend to be highly angiogenic. They are characterized by intensive ingrowth of new blood vessels (angiogenesis), thereby facilitating dissemination of tumor cells into the bloodstream. Tumor cells often metastasize to the lungs and the brain. Alveolar soft-part sarcomas most often arise in muscles and soft tissues of the thigh or leg but can also develop from connective tissues at other anatomic sites. Histologically, the tumor cells grow in a pattern resembling pulmonary alveolar cells, leading to the name *alveolar soft-part sarcoma* (Christopherson, Foote, & Stewart, 1952).

Cytogenetics of Pediatric Soft-Tissue Sarcomas

As with pediatric bone sarcomas, the various forms of soft-tissue sarcomas that are diagnosed in children and adolescents are characterized by certain cytogenetic abnormalities. *Rhabdomyosarcomas* often show deletions of the short arm of chromosome 11 and loss of tumor–suppressor genes, or reciprocal translocations involving the *FKHR* gene on chromosome 13 and the *PAX* genes on chromosomes 1 and 2. The *FKHR* gene regulates transcription and the *PAX* genes help regulate cell differentiation during embryogenesis. The chimeric fusion protein (called *FOX01*) encoded by the translocated gene has oncogenic potential resulting in the development of rhabdomyosarcomas consisting of cells with characteristics of pulmonary alveolar cells (Barr, 1997).

Some fibrosarcomas also involve reciprocal translocations of specific genes on specific chromosomes that result in the expression of chimeric fusion proteins with oncogenic potential. For example, congenital fibrosarcomas that are present at birth are characterized by a translocation gene product of the *ETV6* gene on chromosome 12 and the *NTRK3* gene on chromosome 13. These genes are intricately involved in the regulation of DNA mitosis and cell differentiation (Knezevich et al., 1998).

Synovial sarcoma is also characterized by the presence of a chimeric fusion protein that results from a reciprocal translocation. In this tumor, the *SYT* gene of the long arm of chromosome 18 is translocated in close proximity to one of three closely related genes (*SSX1*, *SSX2*, or *SSX4*) located on the X chromosome. The *SYT* gene is a transcription activator whereas the *SSX* genes are transcription repressors. The resulting chimeric fusion protein can produce one of two patterns of growth in the development of synovial sarcomas, a monophasic pattern of spindle cell growth or a biphasic pattern involving both spindle cells and epithelial cells (Clark et al., 1994).

Karyotypic and molecular studies have also revealed a characteristic reciprocal translocation and fusion protein in *alveolar soft-parts sarcoma*. The translocation involves chromosome 17 and the X chromosome, creating a fusion of the *TFE3* and *ASPA* genes and the corresponding chimeric fusion protein that enhances transcription of other genes with oncogenic potential (Ladanyi et al., 2001).

In summary, reciprocal chromosomal translocations constitute most specific genetic alterations associated with pediatric sarcomas. As noted for pediatric sarcomas of both bone and soft tissues, many specific reciprocal chromosomal translocations have been identified and the chimeric fusion proteins encoded by the translocated genes characterized. It is likely that these proteins act as transcription activators—deregulating genes associated with sarcoma development. Thus, in addition to providing specific and sensitive diagnostic markers, such molecules provide potential targets for therapy with monoclonal antibodies (Ladanyi, 1995; Ladanyi & Bridge, 2000).

▶ Epidemiology of Adult Sarcomas

Although some reciprocal chromosomal translocations and genetic aberrations have been identified in adult sarcomas, most such tumors *do not* manifest characteristic genetic anomalies. As with other adult forms of cancer, adult sarcomas are characterized by several critical interrelated biological mechanisms, including overexpression of oncogenes and/or underexpression of tumor–suppressor genes due to mutagenic and/or epigenetic effects, sustained uncontrolled cell division, angiogenesis, dysregulated apoptosis, immunosuppression, metastatic spread, and invasive potential of tumor cells. Dysregulation of the inflammatory cascade may be an important trigger and promoter of all these biological mechanisms.

Bone Sarcomas in Adults

After adolescence, the relative frequency of primary bone tumors gradually declines throughout the lifespan (**FIGURE 35.1**). There are four main subtypes of adult sarcomas of bone: osteosarcoma, chondrosarcoma, Ewing sarcoma, and giant cell sarcoma. Each subtype is discussed separately.

Osteosarcoma

Although about 75% of *osteosarcomas* are diagnosed in children and adolescents, such tumors are occasionally discovered in adults. Among adult cases, males exceed females (a 35% male excess was observed in one series of 47 cases diagnosed after 40 years of age) and tumors most often involve the lower limbs (55% of cases) or the axial skeleton (38% of cases) (Carsi & Rock, 2002).

Unlike other tumors of bone, osteosarcomas are characterized by the formation of osteoid matrix by tumor cells (Kumar et al., 2014). Characteristic cytogenetic or molecular aberrations have not been discovered in studies of osteosarcoma tissues; however, as already discussed in the section of this chapter on pediatric bone tumors, osteosarcomas are a component of the profile of malignancies that develop in rare genetic syndromes such as hereditary retinoblastoma, Li–Fraumeni syndrome, and Rothmund–Thomson syndrome.

Chondrosarcoma

Chondrosarcomas are tumors that produce hyaline cartilage. Most chondrosarcomas (80%–90% of cases) arise de novo in older adults in the sixth or seventh decade of life without any evidence of premalignancy. Such tumors predominantly arise in and around the pelvis and scapula, although any site of cartilage formation may be involved (Azzarelli et al., 1986). Although chondrosarcomas do not ordinarily manifest specific cytogenetic abnormalities, one rare subtype, *extraskeletal myxoid chondrosarcoma*, is defined by the presence of a fusion gene between the orphan nuclear receptor *CHN1/NR4A3* and one of several partners, most commonly the Ewing sarcoma gene, *EWSR-1*.

About 10%–20% of chondrosarcomas develop in young adults due to malignant transformation of benign neoplasms within bones (osteochondromas) or exterior to bones (enchondromas). Certain hereditary conditions such as Ollier disease (multiple enchondromatosis) or Maffucci syndrome (multiple enchondromas and hemangiomas) predispose to the development of chondrosarcoma (Kumar et al., 2014).

Hereditary multiple exostoses are a rare genetic disorder in which multiple bony spurs (also known as exostoses or osteochondromas) develop on the bones of a child. Approximately 90% of cases with this disorder are due to inheritance of either of two mutated tumor–suppressor genes, *EXT1* or *EXT2*. These genes normally encode protein components of heparan sulfate proteoglycans that are essential for normal cartilage development; mutant forms cause uncontrolled proliferation and lack of differentiation of chondrocytes, sometimes resulting in the development of chondrosarcoma.

Ewing Sarcoma. Ewing sarcoma rarely develops in adults over the age of 25 years. Nevertheless, adult cases that have been reported in the literature invariably demonstrate one of the reciprocal translocations of the Ewing sarcoma gene (*EWSR-1*) that characterize pediatric cases. Such tumors diagnosed in adults show a propensity for rapid metastatic spread and poor survival (Baldini et al., 1999)

Giant Cell Tumor of Bone. *Giant cell tumors of bone*, also known as *osteoclastomas*, constitute about 5% of adult bone tumors. These tumors are characterized by the presence of large (giant) multinucleated osteoclasts (cells that resorb bone matrix) admixed with spindle-shaped fibroblasts. Giant cell tumors are usually benign but can be locally aggressive. They most commonly arise in the epiphyses (growth plates) of long bones with diagnosis in the third or fourth decade of life (Mendenhall, Zlotecki, Scarborough, Gibbs, & Mendenhall, 2006).

Normal osteoclasts are large cells in bone that contain 15–20 closely packed nuclei and cytoplasm with abundant vacuoles and vesicles. The primary function of osteoclasts is to resorb bone matrix. It is notable that osteoclasts are derived from mononuclear cells (macrophages) of the blood rather than progenitor cells of bone (Walker, 1972, 1973).

Osteoclast formation requires a ligand called *RANKL (receptor activator for nuclear factor κB ligand)* that activates the receptor for nuclear factor κB (RANK). Activation of nuclear factor κB by RANKL induces the differentiation and maturation of osteoclasts from mononuclear cells (macrophages) in hematopoietic tissues. Tight homeostatic regulation of these molecules is critical for normal osteoclast development and activity because overexpression of RANKL has been found to be associated with the development of giant cell tumors of bone (Mendenhall et al., 2006; Thomas & Skubitz, 2009).

Soft-Tissue Sarcomas in Adults

Soft-tissue sarcomas occur with regular, albeit low, frequency throughout the lifespan (**FIGURE 35.1**). Subtypes are classified by the cell and/or anatomic site of origin: liposarcoma (adipocytes), leiomyosarcoma (smooth muscle), gastrointestinal stromal tumors (intestinal stroma), and angiosarcoma (blood or lymphatic vessels). *Malignant fibrous histiocytomas* are heterogeneous sarcomas consisting of histiocytic cells and fibroblasts. *Kaposi sarcoma*, a malignancy arising from lymphatic endothelium, is named after Moritz Kaposi (1837–1902), a Hungarian dermatologist who first described its features and symptoms (Kaposi, 1872).

Liposarcoma

Lipomas are *benign* tumors composed of adipose tissue that arise most often in the subcutaneous tissues of the neck, trunk, and extremities. They are the most common form of soft-tissue tumor, with an estimated prevalence of about 1%. Lipomas have no metastatic potential, distinguishing them from liposarcomas, which are malignant neoplasms that can invade other tissues. Lipomas are typically diagnosed in adults ages 40–60 years of age, but occasionally they are discovered in children (Bancroft, Kransdorf, Peterson, & O'Connor, 2006; Kumar et al., 2014).

Whether lipomas are *premalignant* tumors is controversial, because malignant transition of lipoma to liposarcoma has not been definitively demonstrated in humans. Nevertheless, liposarcomas are clearly derived from adipocytes (fat cells) and are often composed of cell populations containing both normal and malignant adipocytes.

Liposarcomas are the most common histological type of sarcoma found in adults. These malignant tumors comprise more than 20% of all adult sarcomas. In contrast to lipomas, which usually develop in subcutaneous fat, liposarcomas typically arise in deep-seated fat of muscle or other tissues. Liposarcomas are extraordinarily heterogeneous and can be histologically characterized by the mixtures of cells they contain. For example, myxoid liposarcoma is characterized by malignant adipocytes in various stages of differentiation (Kumar et al., 2014).

Leiomyosarcoma

Uterine fibroids (*uterine leiomyomas*) are the most common of all tumors in women. These benign tumors are typically discovered during the reproductive years, with a prevalence of about 30%. They originate from cells in the smooth muscle layer of the uterus (the myometrium). Most uterine fibroid tumors are asymptomatic and harmless, but they can enlarge causing pain, discomfort, and urinary incontinence, in which case they are usually surgically excised by hysterectomy (Wallach & Vlahos, 2004).

The malignant version of leiomyoma is *leiomyosarcoma*. These malignant tumors can arise from smooth muscle anywhere in the body, most commonly in the uterus, stomach and intestinal tract, blood vessels, and skin. Leiomyosarcomas comprise 5%–10% of all soft-tissue sarcomas in adults. Whether benign leiomyomas undergo malignant transformation to leiomyosarcoma is controversial. Nevertheless, cases have been reported in which malignant transformation has apparently been observed over time (Indraccolo, Luchetti, & Indraccolo, 2008). It is noteworthy that uterine leiomyomas are often surgically removed, thereby negating the chance of malignant transformation.

Gastrointestinal Stromal Tumors

Sarcomas arising from connective (mesenchymal) tissues in the wall of the stomach or other gastrointestinal organs are called *gastrointestinal stromal tumors (GISTs)*. Tran and colleagues utilized the U.S. SEER database to characterize distributional features of GISTs in the U.S. population during 1992–2000.

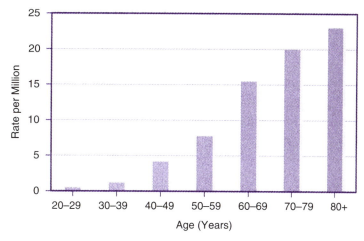

FIGURE 35.5 Age-Specific Incidence of Gastrointestinal Stromal Tumors (GISTs), United States, 1992–2006.

Data from Tran, T., Davila, J. A., & El-Serag, H. B. (2005). The epidemiology of malignant gastrointestinal stromal tumors: An analysis of 1,458 cases from 1992 to 2000. *American Journal of Gastroenterology, 100,* 162–168.

During this period, 1458 cases were reported, 54% in men and 46% in women. Tumors were distributed throughout the gastrointestinal tract—51% in the stomach, 36% in the small intestine, 7% in the colon, 5% in the rectum, and 1% in the esophagus. Estimates of the annual age-adjusted incidence rates were 8.3 per million in men, 5.7 per million in women, and 6.8 per million overall. As shown in **FIGURE 35.5**, GISTs are predominantly a malignancy of old age and are rarely diagnosed before the age of 40 years. Peak onset occurs in the eighth decade of life (Tran, Davila, & El-Serag, 2005).

GISTs apparently arise from the interstitial cells of Cajal, cells that serve as electrical pacemakers and generate spontaneous electrical slow waves and smooth muscle contractions (peristalsis) in the walls of the gastrointestinal tract (Connolly, Gaffney, & Reynolds, 2003; Sanders, Koh, & Ward, 2006). Such cells have morphological characteristics like fibroblasts and express specific tyrosine kinase receptors on their cell membranes that control differentiation and maturation (Lorincz et al., 2008).

Angiosarcoma

Angiosarcoma is an uncommon subtype of soft-tissue sarcoma that can arise from the endothelial cells that line blood vessels (hemangiosarcoma) or lymphatic vessels (lymphangiosarcoma). These tumors occasionally develop in the scalp or face of older adults or in patients who have undergone radiation therapy for dermatitis or other conditions. An association with lymphedema, a complication of mastectomy for breast cancer, has also been noted. In addition, angiosarcoma of the liver has been etiologically linked to at least three chemical carcinogens: arsenic in

arsenical pesticides, thorotrast (a radioactive contrast medium used prior to 1950), and polyvinyl chloride (an alkylating agent and gas used in the manufacture of plastic). Important studies of environmental risk factors for adult sarcomas are discussed later in this chapter.

Malignant Fibrous Histiocytoma

Malignant fibrous histiocytoma is a rare type of soft-tissue sarcoma that is discovered most often in the elderly, usually between the ages of 50 and 70 years. Histologically, such tumors consist of a mixture of histiocytes (cells derived from tissue macrophages or monocytes) and fibroblasts (cells of mesenchymal lineage). Based on early pathologic investigations, this tumor was initially characterized as the most common sarcoma in late adult life (O'Brien & Stout, 1964); however, in more recent studies, most of such tumors have been reclassified as poorly differentiated liposarcomas or leiomyosarcomas. In a population-based study of malignant fibrous sarcoma in Sweden, the annual incidence rate was estimated at only 4.2 per million (Rööser, Willén, Gustafson, Alvegård, & Rydholm, 1991).

Dermatofibrosarcoma Protuberans

Dermatofibrosarcoma protuberans is a rare form of fibrosarcoma that arises from the dermis (the layer of skin between the epidermis and subcutaneous tissue). This tumor can infiltrate contiguous tissues but rarely metastasizes to distant sites. Dermatofibrosarcoma protuberans is cytogenetically defined by a translocation of chromosomes 17 and 22 in which a collagen promoter gene (*COL1A1*) is juxtaposed to the platelet-derived growth factor (*PDGF*) gene, resulting in constitutive production of PDGF. This scenario creates an autocrine loop in which PDGF stimulates PDGF receptors of tumor cells, promoting their perpetual growth and survival. Monoclonal antibodies directed against the PDGF receptor have shown some benefit in the treatment of patients with this tumor (Patel et al., 2008).

Desmoid Tumor

Desmoid tumors are benign slow-growing tumors without metastatic potential. Histologically, these tumors resemble fibrosarcomas. Although most cases are sporadic, desmoid tumors develop in about 10%–15% of patients with familial adenomatous polyposis (FAP) or Gardner's syndrome (adenomatous polyposis coli) in which multiple adenomatous polyps and malignant adenocarcinomas develop in the colon. This syndrome is caused by inheritance of an autosomal dominant mutant *APC* (adenomatous polyposis coli) gene on chromosome 5.

An investigative team in London conducted a meta-analysis of desmoid tumors among patients with FAP. Desmoid tumors developed in 559 (12%) of 4625 FAP patients. Peak onset was in the second and third decades, and 80% of tumors were diagnosed by age 40 years. Having a family history of desmoid tumors conferred a sevenfold increase in the risk, suggesting the existence of modifier genes (Sinha, Tekkis, Gibbons, Phillips, & Clark, 2010).

Cytogenetics of Soft-Tissue Adult Sarcomas

Although not as common as in pediatric sarcomas, nonrandom genetic abnormalities have been discovered in some soft-tissue sarcomas in adults. For example, translocation of the CCAAT-enhanced binding protein (*CEBP*) gene on chromosome 12 to chromosome 16 is characteristic of *myxoid liposarcoma*. The *CEBP* gene encodes a factor that is critical for normal differentiation of adipocytes, and its translocation creates a chimeric fusion protein that interferes with differentiation and leads to cancer development (Adelmant, Bilbert, & Freytag, 1998; Turc-Carel et al., 1986). A second molecular transcription factor, peroxisome proliferator-activator receptor gamma (*PPAR-γ*), is also often overexpressed in malignant liposarcoma cells (Tontonoz et al., 1997). Cytogenetic studies of liposarcomas have also revealed the presence of ring or giant-marker chromosomes derived from the short arm of chromosome 12 with

amplification of specific oncogenes in this region (Coindre et al., 2003).

The existing scientific literature reflects highly variable and inconsistent cytogenetic and molecular genetic changes in *leiomyosarcoma*. Wang and colleagues reviewed the karyotypes of 100 leiomyosarcomas and found no consistent aberrations at the chromosomal level. Because the most frequent chromosomal deletions were detected in the long arms of chromosomes 10 and 13, regions where tumor–suppressor genes *PTEN* and *Rb* reside, the investigators concluded that loss of function of tumor–suppressor genes and/or activation of oncogenes associated with such changes are likely involved in the development of leiomyosarcoma (Wang, Lu, Fisher, Bridge, & Shipley, 2001).

Approximately 95% of GISTs have been found to carry mutant forms of an important tyrosine kinase receptor gene called *c-KIT*. The *c-KIT* receptor facilitates differentiation and maturation of stem cells into hematopoietic cells and several other cell lineages. It was first identified in the laboratories of the German biochemist Axel Ullrich (Yarden et al., 1987). Mutations in *c-KIT* cause overexpression of tyrosine kinase receptors in the cell membrane resulting in unregulated phosphorylation and disruption of communication pathways inside the cell. Constitutive expression of mutant forms of *c-KIT* therefore leads to malignant transformation and the development of GISTs (as well as testicular seminoma, malignant melanoma, and myeloid leukemia). Notably, a monoclonal antibody directed against the *c-KIT* protein has been found effective in the treatment of GISTs (Edling & Hallberg, 2007; Joensuu et al., 2001).

Cytogenetic studies of *angiosarcomas* reflect considerable heterogeneity and no consistent pattern of chromosomal or genetic aberrations. Literature reports based on limited sample sizes have revealed karyotypes with gains or losses of many different chromosomal regions without a common chromosomal profile (Baumhoer, Gunawan, Becker, & Füzesi, 2005). One recent study reported a reciprocal chromosomal translocation involving chromosomes 1 and 21 in a 79-year-old woman with a primary bone angiosarcoma. Although the biological significance of this translocation is unclear, it could involve abnormal expression of the gene for colony stimulating factor (*CSF-1*), which is located on chromosome 1 (Dunlap, Magenis, Davis, Himoe, & Mansoor, 2009).

Some genetic syndromes are associated with the development of soft-tissue sarcoma in adults. *Neurofibromatosis type 1*, or *von Recklinghausen disease*, is a rare autosomal dominant condition caused by mutation in the *NF1* gene located on chromosome 17. The *NF1* gene encodes the protein neurofibromin, which is essential for the development of fibrous nerve sheaths. Patients with this genetic disorder have a high incidence of benign schwannomas and neurofibromas as well as an increased risk of developing malignant peripheral nerve-sheath tumors (malignant schwannomas and neurofibrosarcomas).

Neurofibromatosis type 2, also a rare autosomal dominant disorder, is caused by mutation in the *NF2* gene located on chromosome 22, which is essential for development of myelin nerve sheaths. This syndrome is associated with the development of meningiomas as well as schwannomas of cranial nerves, especially the vestibular nerve.

Gardner syndrome is an autosomal dominant disorder caused by mutation of the APC gene located on the long arm of chromosome 5. Carriers of the mutant *APC* gene develop multiple polyps throughout the colon; without total colectomy, the probability of transformation to colon cancer is virtually 100%. Approximately 15%–20% of afflicted individuals also develop other extracolonic tumors such as osteomas, fibromas, desmoid tumors, and thyroid cancer (Gardner, 1951; Johnson, Gilbert, Zimmermann, & Watne, 1972; Markowitz & Bertagnolli, 2009).

Environmental Risk Factors for Adult Sarcoma

Ionizing Radiation

There is consistent evidence that radiation exposure increases the risk of developing both bone and soft-tissue sarcomas. The association was first observed by the German physician Dr. A. Beck, who commented on the unusually high incidence of sarcomas in patients who had previously been irradiated for tuberculosis arthritis (Beck, 1922). Subsequently in the United States, Martland and Humphreys reported finding 42 bone sarcomas in 1468 female watch-dial painters exposed to radioactive luminous paint, an incidence proportion of 2.8% (Martland & Humphreys, 1929). Several more reports of excess rates of bone sarcomas soon appeared in the literature, most notably a report from investigators at Memorial Sloan-Kettering Hospital in New York City describing 50 cases of radiation-induced osteogenic sarcoma identified during 1931–1970 (Arlen et al., 1971).

Postradiation sarcomas arise more often in bones than soft tissues, perhaps due to the greater absorption of radioactivity by bone (Robinson, Neugut, & Wylie, 1988). Nevertheless, excess rates of soft-tissue

sarcomas have been observed subsequent to certain types of radiotherapy. For example, investigators in Sweden observed a 90% excess of soft-tissue sarcomas among 122,991 women treated for breast cancer from 1958 to 1992 (standardized incidence ratio = 1.9). Furthermore, 63% of the reported sarcomas developed in the exposed region of the irradiated breast or the ipsilateral arm. Among the 116 sarcomas detected, there were 40 angiosarcomas and 76 sarcomas of other subtypes. In substudies of these tumors, angiosarcomas were found to develop in association with lymphedema of the ipsilateral axilla and arm (Karlsson, Holmberg, Samuelsson, Johansson, & Wallgren, 1998).

Chemical and Occupational Exposures

Some epidemiologic studies have noted increases in the risk of developing soft-tissue or bone sarcomas among individuals with certain occupational exposures (e.g., sawdust and wood dust, cutting oils [solvents], arsenicals, phenoxy herbicides, chlorophenols, and dioxins). However, results are inconsistent from study to study, which is most likely due to the use of occupation as a proxy for exposure to broad classes of chemicals and the lack of precise information on the type, concentration, and duration of specific chemical exposures. Furthermore, inconsistencies in study results may also reflect different disease etiologies for sarcoma subtypes (Hoppin et al., 1999).

Various implant materials, including chromium, nickel, cobalt, titanium, and polyethylene, are also suspected risk factors, though epidemiologic evidence for causation is lacking. It is obvious that more precise measures of environmental exposures are needed in order to accurately quantify the risk.

Angiosarcoma of the liver is an unfortunate human model for both radiation and chemical carcinogenesis. This rare tumor has been found in excess among patients exposed to thorotrast (a radioactive contrast medium used in the past for imaging studies), workers exposed to polyvinyl chloride as a solution or gas where plastics are manufactured, and individuals exposed to arsenic in arsenical pesticides. Selected studies are discussed here.

Between September 1967 and December 1973, four cases of angiosarcoma of the liver were diagnosed among men employed in the polyvinyl–chloride polymerization section of the BF Goodrich manufacturing plant near Louisville, Kentucky. This section of the plant began operations in 1938. It employed 270 people and produced polyvinyl chloride as well as a variety of copolymers by polymerization of vinyl-chloride monomers. All four men had worked continuously in the section for at least 14 years prior to onset of illness and had worked directly in various phases of the polymerization process. None of the patients gave a history of prolonged alcohol use or exposure to hepatotoxins outside the workplace. In particular, none had ever had exposure to thorium dioxide (thorotrast) or to arsenic, two materials known specifically to induce hepatic angiosarcoma in humans (Creech & Johnson, 1974).

Subsequent studies in Australia, Italy, Germany, and the United Kingdom also revealed that polyvinyl–chloride workers were at increased risk for the development of hepatic angiosarcoma (Mundt et al., 2000). In 1983, a team of international investigators charted the latency periods from time of exposure to vinyl-chloride monomers or thorotrast to time of death due to angiosarcoma of the liver. Exposure to thorotrast occurred during 1928–1955 and exposure to polyvinyl chloride occurred during 1940–1970. Among 101 men exposed to thorotrast who later died from liver angiosarcoma, the median latency period from exposure to death was 22 years. Among 95 men exposed to polyvinyl chloride who later died from liver angiosarcoma, the median latency period was substantially longer at 29 years. The investigators suggest that their results reflect different mechanisms of radiation versus chemical carcinogenesis (Spirtas et al., 1983).

Boffetta and colleagues conducted a meta-analysis of cancer mortality and exposure to polyvinyl chloride using data from eight published studies, two multi-center cohorts, and six smaller studies. They found an increase in the standardized mortality ratio (SMR) due to soft-tissue sarcoma (SMR = 2.52), the predominant cell type being angiosarcoma. Their results also showed a significant increase in mortality due to primary liver cancer (SMR = 2.96), although there was significant heterogeneity among studies (Boffetta, Matisane, Mundt, & Dell, 2003).

All known cases of angiosarcoma that have developed from exposure to vinyl-chloride monomers were in workers who were regularly exposed to very high levels for many years. Most of these workers cleaned accretions in reactors, a practice that has now been replaced by automated high-pressure water jets. Other epidemiologic studies have demonstrated that the risk of developing hepatic angiosarcoma is also significantly increased with exposure to thorium dioxide (thorotrast) or arsenical pesticides (Falk, Caldwell, Ishak, Thomas, & Popper, 1981; Falk, Telles, Ishak, Thomas, & Popper, 1979).

Rous Sarcoma Virus

In the early 1900s, Dr. Peyton Rous reported a series of experiments with chicken sarcoma at Rockefeller University in New York City. He found that by injecting cell-free extracts derived from chicken sarcoma into healthy Plymouth Rock chickens, he could transfer the tumor from one chicken to another. Rous found that extracts of tumors that passed through a Berkefeld filter (which did not allow passage of bacteria) could transfer the sarcoma to other chickens. This was the first demonstration of an oncogenic virus and heralded the beginning of the field of cancer virology. Rous was awarded the Nobel Prize for his discoveries in 1966 (Rous, 1910, 1911; Rous & Huggins, 1966).

Later studies revealed that the transmissible Rous sarcoma virus (RSV) was a retrovirus containing RNA rather than DNA and that the transforming region of the virus was an oncogene (named *SRC* for *sarcoma*) (Crawford & Crawford, 1961; Oppermann, Levinson, Varmus, Levintow, & Bishop, 1979; Stehelin, Fujita, Padgett, Varmus, & Bishop, 1977). During the 1970s, J. Michael Bishop and Harold Varmus directed a series of studies showing that the SRC gene encodes a constitutively active form of the enzyme tyrosine kinase that stimulates carcinogenesis, a discovery for which they received the Nobel Prize in 1989 (Bishop & Varmus, 1989). Although the RSV that causes sarcomas in chickens was the first tumor virus found to cause solid tumors, the only virus now known to cause sarcoma in humans is human herpes virus 8 (HHV-8), which causes the development of Kaposi sarcoma.

Kaposi Sarcoma

Kaposi sarcoma is a tumor that *sometimes* develops in individuals who are severely immunocompromised. It was originally described in 1872 by Dr. Moritz Kaposi, a Hungarian dermatologist practicing at the University of Vienna (Kaposi, 1872). Before the epidemic of acquired immune deficiency syndrome (AIDS) in the 1980s, Kaposi sarcoma was practically unheard of in populations of developed nations. Only rare cases were reported, most occurring in organ transplant patients who received cyclosporin or other immunosuppressive drugs to prevent transplant rejection. But following the onset of the AIDS epidemic, the incidence of Kaposi sarcoma increased more than 1000-fold in those subgroups at high risk for HIV. The main subgroups are homosexual and bisexual men, intravenous drug abusers, and sexually promiscuous men and women.

Due to its prevalence in individuals who are immunodeficient, Kaposi sarcoma became widely known as one of the defining conditions of AIDS during the 1980s. The etiologic agent of AIDS is HIV, and AIDS is now appropriately called HIV disease. The causal RNA retrovirus, later named the HIV, was first isolated in France in 1983 by Françoise Barré-Sinoussi and colleagues in the laboratory of Luc Montaignier (Barré-Sinoussi et al., 1983). The same virus was also isolated from several AIDS patients by Robert Gallo and colleagues at the National Institutes of Health and by Jay Levy and colleagues in San Francisco (Gallo et al., 1984; Levy et al., 1984). Shortly thereafter, Montaignier's group isolated a closely related virus in West African patients. The original virus was designated HIV-1 and the West African virus HIV-2.

Although associated with HIV disease, Kaposi sarcoma is actually caused by another virus, human herpes virus 8 (HHV-8). The two viruses, HIV-2 and HHV-8, are endemic in sub-Saharan Africa, and it is in the populations of this region that Kaposi sarcoma is now the leading cause of cancer death among men.

Discovery of Human Herpes Virus 8 (HHV-8)

In 1994, Yuan Chang, Patrick Moore, and Ethel Cesarman at Columbia University in New York isolated a novel herpes virus from the tumor cells of a Kaposi sarcoma. They later sequenced the virus and identified it as the eighth human herpes virus; hence, it was given the name HHV-8. This virus has since been found in all Kaposi sarcomas tested and is considered the cause of the disease. In infected lymphatic endothelial cells, HHV-8 incorporates genes from the host DNA into its own DNA, thus avoiding detection and destruction by the immune system. This process leads to active proliferation and immortalization of infected cells, resulting in the development of Kaposi sarcoma (Cesarman, Chang, Moore, Said, & Knowles, 1995; Chang et al., 1994; Moore & Chang, 1995).

Pathologic Features of Kaposi Sarcoma

Despite its name, Kaposi sarcoma does not arise from connective tissue and is therefore *not* a true sarcoma; rather, Kaposi sarcoma arises from the endothelial cells that line lymphatic vessels. The tumor is characterized by the formation of vascular channels engorged with red blood cells, giving it a dark red papular appearance. Such papules may be solitary or multifocal (Cancian, Hansen, & Boshoff, 2013).

The tumor cells of Kaposi sarcoma are spindle-shaped cells characteristic of fibroblasts in connective tissue. Detection of proteins such as latency-associated nuclear antigen (LANA) that are specific for HHV-8 in tumor cells confirms the diagnosis of Kaposi sarcoma (Moore et al., 1996). Kaposi sarcoma is typically found on the skin, but metastatic spread to other sites is common, especially the mouth, the gastrointestinal tract, and the respiratory tract. Kaposi sarcoma is associated with significant morbidity and mortality worldwide (Parkin, Bray, Ferlay, & Pisani, 2005).

Transmission of HHV-8

Herpes viruses can be transmitted by intimate sexual contact and by transplantation of contaminated organs. In sub-Saharan Africa, where high rates of HHV-8 prevail, Kaposi sarcoma is the most common of all cancers. As with other herpes viral infections, HHV-8 may persist in a dormant state for many years, only to be reactivated by conditions of severe immunosuppression such as HIV disease. Active HHV-8 infection specifically initiates and promotes malignant transformation of the lymphatic endothelium in the genesis of Kaposi sarcoma.

Global Burden of Kaposi Sarcoma

During 2018, 41,799 new cases of Kaposi sarcoma were diagnosed in the world population (28,248 in men and 13,551 in women) and 19,902 individuals died from the disease (13,117 men and 6785 women). Approximately 84% of all cases and 94% of all deaths occurred in sub-Saharan Africa, where HIV-2 is endemic, and there is limited access to therapy. Kaposi sarcoma was the leading cause of cancer deaths among men in the Southeastern African nations of Malawi, Mozambique, Uganda, and Zambia. In this region, average incidence rates (~10 and ~5 per 100,000 in men and women, respectively) and mortality rates (~6 per 100,000 in men and ~3 per 100,000 in women) were 10- to 400-fold higher than in other regions of the world. Malawi had the highest incidence and mortality rates of Kaposi sarcoma in the world in 2018 (36 per 100,000 and 23 per 100,000, respectively) yielding a mortality/incidence ratio of 0.64. By comparison, the incidence among U.S. men was 0.57 per 100,000 and the mortality was 0.04 per 100,000, yielding a mortality/incidence ratio of 0.07 (**FIGURE 35.6**) (Bray et al., 2018; Ferlay et al., 2018).

Seropositivity rates for HHV-8 coincide closely with the high rates of Kaposi sarcoma in sub-Saharan Africa. Co-infection by HIV is also prominent in these same African populations. It is noteworthy that there are marked ethnic differences in the rates of Kaposi

Estimated age-standardized incidence rates (World) in 2018, kaposi sarcoma, males, all ages

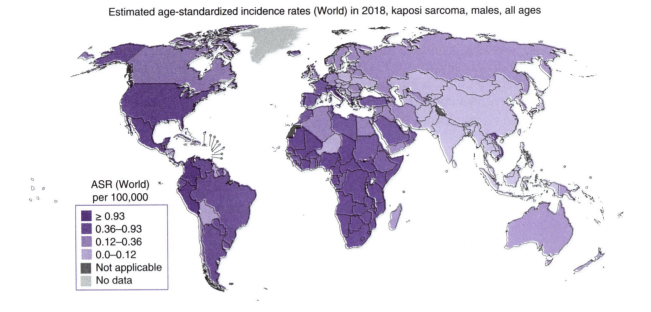

Estimated age-standardized mortality rates (World) in 2018, kaposi sarcoma, males, all ages

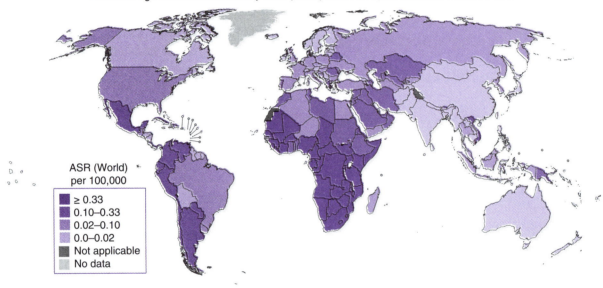

FIGURE 35.6 Global Incidence and Mortality Rates of Kaposi Sarcoma in African Men, 2018.

Caption: ASR: Rates per 100,000 are age-standardized to the world population, 2000–2025.

Reproduced with permission from Ferlay, J., Ervik, M., Lam, F., Colombet, M., Mery, L., . . . Bray, F. (2018). *Global cancer observatory: Cancer today.* Lyon, France: International Agency for Research on Cancer. Available from: https://gco.iarc.fr/today, accessed [09 October 2018].

sarcoma. For example, individuals of Asian descent rarely develop the disease, even those with HIV infection. Such ethnic disparities may reflect differences in the rates of HIV and HHV-8 co-infection (Parkin et al., 2005).

During 2008–2018, the global incidence of Kaposi sarcoma in men *increased* from 0.5 to 0.7 per 100,000 while the global mortality *decreased* from 0.4 to 0.3 per 100,000. These changes reflect some progress in the treatment of HIV disease but an absence of progress in curbing the transmission of HIV (Bray et al., 2018; Ferlay et al., 2010, 2013, 2018).

Subtypes of Kaposi Sarcoma

Several subtypes of Kaposi sarcoma have been defined. The main ones are as follows:

- *Classic Kaposi sarcoma* is a rare and relatively indolent form affecting elderly men from the Mediterranean coastal region or of Eastern European descent.
- *Endemic Kaposi sarcoma* is a moderately aggressive form found predominantly in young individuals from sub-Saharan Africa. It is *not* associated with HIV disease.

- *Transplant-related Kaposi sarcoma* is a rare form that develops in organ transplant patients who receive powerful immunosuppressive drugs such as cyclosporine.
- *AIDS-related Kaposi sarcoma* is a highly aggressive form and is one of the defining components of AIDS (HIV disease).

Impact of AIDS on Kaposi Sarcoma

A team of investigators spearheaded by Denis Burkitt investigated the geographic distributions of Kaposi sarcoma, non-Hodgkin's lymphoma, and Burkitt's lymphoma in populations of sub-Saharan Africa *prior to the AIDS epidemic*. High cumulative rates of Kaposi sarcoma (exceeding 6 per 1000 in men ages birth–64 years) were found in equatorial Africa whereas the rates were low (nearly zero) in Northern and Southern regions. Rates were up to 10-fold higher in men than women, and in certain populations, such as in Uganda and Zaire, the estimated cumulative rates of Kaposi sarcoma (approximately 15 per 1000) were like those for common malignancies of the Western world (e.g., colon cancer). These rates are hundreds of times higher than rates of Kaposi sarcoma reported for the populations of England and the United States in the pre-AIDS era. The authors noted the discovery of the etiologic viral agent of Kaposi sarcoma (HHV-8) in 1994 and suggested that the geographic and gender-related distribution of Kaposi sarcoma "may possibly mirror the distribution of the virus prior to the advent of AIDS" (Cook-Mozaffari, Newton, Beral, & Burkitt, 1998).

Before the epidemic of AIDS, Kaposi sarcoma was rare in Western countries, comprising only 0.3% of all cancers in men and 0.1% in women in the United States and Europe. During the 1970s, the cumulative (lifetime) incidence rates averaged less than 0.5 per 100,000 in U.S. men and less than 0.1 per 100,000 in U.S. women. Cases were occasionally discovered in older people of Mediterranean or Eastern European descent, often with a family history of the disease, and in immuno-suppressed organ transplant recipients (Biggar, Horm, Fraumeni, Greene, & Goedert, 1984; Parkin et al., 2005).

Following the onset of the HIV epidemic, rates of Kaposi sarcoma increased dramatically among men in developed nations. In the United States, the annual incidence rates peaked in 1989 at 9.6 per 100,000 (**FIGURE 35.7**). Since that time, rates have declined to pre-AIDS levels, presumably in response to effective combined chemotherapy for HIV disease by highly active antiretroviral therapy (HAART) (Stebbing & Portsmouth, 2003).

Remarkably, the AIDS epidemic has had a negligible impact on the rates of Kaposi sarcoma in the U.S. female population (**FIGURE 35.7**). Although this may reflect their relatively low rates of HIV and HHV-8 co-infection, another possibility is that there are other risk factors to which women are not ordinarily exposed. For example, use of amyl nitrites has been explored as a cofactor in the development of Kaposi sarcoma among AIDS patients (Fung & Tran, 2006).

In central Africa, post-AIDS rates of Kaposi sarcoma have continued to increase in populations with high endemic rates and little access to effective therapy, such as in Uganda, Malawi, Zimbabwe, and Swaziland. Indeed, Kaposi sarcoma is now the most common cancer in men and the second most common cancer in women in many nations of sub-Saharan Africa (Parkin et al., 2005).

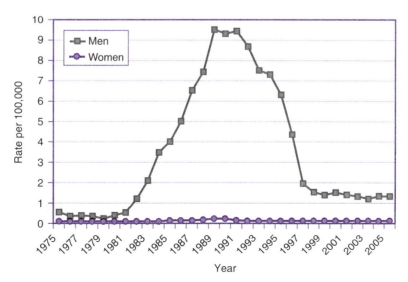

FIGURE 35.7 Age-Adjusted Annual Incidence of Kaposi Sarcoma by Gender, United States, 1975–2005.

Data from Altekruse, S. F., Kosary, C. L., Krapcho, M., Neyman, N., Aminou, R., Waldron, W., & Edwards, B. K. (2010). *SEER cancer statistics review, 1975–2007*. Bethesda, MD: National Cancer Institute.

▶ Cyclooxygenase-2 in Sarcomas

As in many other forms of cancer, the overexpression of cyclooxygenase-2 (COX-2) has been found to be a prominent feature of pediatric sarcomas. At the University of Cincinnati in the United States, Dickens and colleagues evaluated COX-2 expression in a series of 59 pediatric sarcomas using immunohistochemical analysis and cDNA microarray analysis. Tumor specimens included rhabdomyosarcoma, osteosarcoma, and Ewing sarcoma. Expression of COX-2 was detected in 83% of tumors by immunohistochemistry and in 89% of tumors by microarray analysis. In samples of normal osteocytes from nonmalignant bone and muscle tissues, no COX-2 expression was detected. The investigators suggest that COX-2 inhibitors should be tested in the treatment of pediatric sarcomas (Dickens, Kozielski, Khan, Forus, & Cripe, 2002).

At Helsinki University in Finland, Lassus and colleagues evaluated COX-2 expression by immunohistochemistry in 103 specimens of adult soft-tissue sarcomas. They found COX-2 expression in 50 of the 103 tumors (49%) and in all 10 biphasic synovial sarcomas in the sample. They noted that COX-2 was expressed primarily by epithelial cells and in cells proximal to necrotic areas. The investigators concluded that COX-2 expression is associated with epithelial differentiation and tumor necrosis (Lassus et al., 2005).

At the University of Naples in Italy, Rossiello and colleagues evaluated COX-1 and COX-2 in tissues of Kaposi sarcoma using immunohistochemistry and Western blot analysis. They investigated 35 cases of classic Kaposi sarcoma and 27 cases of epidemic Kaposi sarcoma. The results revealed that both COX-1 and COX-2 were overexpressed by tumor cells of all cases; furthermore, COX overexpression was detected in early and late stages of tumor progression, suggesting that the COX enzymes are involved in the pathogenesis of Kaposi sarcoma (Rossiello et al., 2007).

▶ Prevention and Control of Kaposi Sarcoma

In developed nations, most cases of Kaposi sarcoma are diagnosed in patients with HIV/AIDS. Taking measures to avoid HIV infection could therefore prevent the vast majority of Kaposi sarcoma cases in these populations. Currently, there is no effective vaccine against either HIV or HHV-8. Consequently,

prevention depends on reducing the chance of infection by avoiding unprotected sex with HIV carriers and abstaining from injecting recreational drugs because hypodermic needles may be contaminated.

The successful prevention and control of HIV/AIDS depends on interrupting transmission of the virus. The main features of prevention are avoiding sexual contact with any HIV-infected individual, avoiding use of injectable drugs, avoiding contact with contaminated bodily fluids, and practicing universal precautions (for healthcare workers). All blood products and blood donors should be carefully screened to avoid contamination. Accurate information about HIV/AIDS prevention and control should be disseminated to the general public, preferably before sexual activity begins.

Most HIV infections are acquired through unprotected sexual activity between partners, one of whom has HIV. The primary mode of HIV infection worldwide is through sexual contact between members of the opposite sex. The male latex condom, if used correctly without oil-based lubricants, is the single most effective available technology to reduce the sexual transmission of HIV and other sexually transmitted infections. Studies on couples where one partner is infected show that with consistent condom use, HIV-infection rates for the uninfected partner are below 1% per year (Cayley, 2004).

Antiretroviral treatment of infected patients has been found to significantly reduce the sexual transmission of HIV by reducing the level of virus in bodily fluids. In a recent multicenter study conducted in Botswana, Brazil, India, Kenya, Malawi, South Africa, Thailand, Zimbabwe, and the United States, 1763 couples discordant for HIV positivity were randomly assigned to either a treatment group where the HIV-positive partner received antiretroviral drugs immediately or a control group where no drug was given. Out of 28 HIV infections that developed among study participants who were HIV-negative at baseline, 27 developed among members of the untreated couples. The early preventive treatment therefore led to a 96% reduction in HIV transmission to HIV-negative partners, strong evidence of the value of early intervention with antiretroviral therapy in such couples (Cohen et al., 2011).

Healthcare workers should follow universal precautions to reduce their risk of exposure to contaminated blood. These precautions include wearing gloves, masks, protective eyewear or shields, and gowns or aprons that prevent exposure of the skin or mucous membranes to blood-borne pathogens. Frequent and thorough washing of the skin immediately after being contaminated with blood or other bodily fluids reduces the chance of infection. Sharp objects like needles, scalpels, and glass must be carefully disposed of to prevent needle stick injuries with contaminated items (Kerr, Kimber, Debeck, & Wood, 2007).

Injection of illicit drugs using contaminated needles and syringes is a major mode of HIV transmission among intravenous drug abusers. Harm reduction strategies such as needle-exchange programs have been used with some success in reducing rates of HIV infection associated with intravenous drug abuse (Wodak & Cooney, 2006).

In the past, transfusions of contaminated blood and clotting factors were responsible for some HIV infections. As a result of improved HIV testing in blood banks, there is now a very low risk of HIV infection from blood products in the United States and most developed nations. Some poorer countries have not yet developed high-quality screening programs of blood and blood products, leading to a higher risk of HIV infection with transfusion. The World Health Organization (WHO) has developed an integrated strategy for the provision of safe blood and blood products and safe, efficacious blood transfusion for all member nations (WHO, 2010).

To avoid mother-to-child transmission, HIV-infected mothers are encouraged to avoid breastfeeding their infant and instead use replacement feeding that is acceptable, feasible, affordable, sustainable, and safe. However, if replacement feeding is unavailable, exclusive breastfeeding is recommended during the first month of life and then should be discontinued as soon as possible (WHO, 2006).

One way to change risky behavior is health education. Several studies have shown the positive impact of culturally adapted educational programs advocating cautious sexual behavior. In 2010, a United Nations AIDS Inter-Agency Task Team encouraged more research on the actual implementation of sex-education programs (such as teacher training, access to related services through schools and the community, or parental attitudes to HIV and AIDS education), and more longitudinal studies on the deeper complexities of the relationship between education and HIV prevention and control (Lakhanpal & Ram, 2008; Rindermann & Meisenberg, 2009).

▶ Prevention and Treatment of Other Sarcomas

Only a few modifiable risk factors are known for other types of sarcoma, so population-based preventive strategies are generally absent. Exposure to excess radiation should be avoided and care should be taken to minimize exposure to environmental pollutants such as polyvinyl chloride, sawdust and wood dust, cutting oils (solvents), arsenicals, phenoxy herbicides, chlorophenols, and dioxins. It is also advisable to consider surgical removal of benign lesions that have potential for malignant transformation, in particular lipomas and leiomyomas.

The development of optimal treatment strategies for sarcoma is complicated by the large number of subtypes, the heterogeneity in their biological behavior, and the small number of patients with particular subtypes enrolled in trials. However, exciting new research has identified molecular markers for some sarcomas, particularly those in children, and such molecules are natural targets for therapy with monoclonal antibodies.

References

Abramson, D. H., & Frank, C. M. (1998). Second nonocular tumors in survivors of bilateral retinoblastoma: A possible age effect on radiation-related risk. *Ophthalmology, 105*(4), 573–580.

Adelmant, G., Bilbert, J. D., & Freytag, S. O. (1998). Human translocation liposarcoma-CCAAT/enhancer binding protein (C/EBP) homologous protein (TLS-CHOP) oncoprotein prevents adipocyte differentiation by directly interfering with C/EBPβ function. *Journal of Biological Chemistry, 273*, 15574–15581.

Altekruse, S. F., Kosary, C. L., Krapcho, M., Neyman, N., Aminou, R., Waldron, W., & Edwards, B. K. (2010). *SEER cancer statistics review, 1975–2007*. Bethesda, MD: National Cancer Institute.

Arlen, M., Higinbotham, N. L., Huvos, A. G., Marcove, R. C., Miller, T., & Shah, I. C. (1971). Radiation-induced sarcoma of bone. *Cancer, 28*, 1087–1099.

Azzarelli, A., Gennari, L., Quagliuolo, V., Bonfanti, G., Cerasoli, S., & Bufalino, R. (1986). Chondrosarcoma: 55 unreported cases: Epidemiology, surgical treatment and prognostic factors. *European Journal of Surgical Oncology, 12*(2), 165–168.

Baldini, E. H., Demetri, G. D., Fletcher, C. D., Foran, J., Marcus, K. C., & Singer, S. (1999). Adults with Ewing's sarcoma/primitive neuroectodermal tumor: Adverse effect of older age and primary extraosseous disease on outcome. *Annals of Surgery, 230*(1), 79–86.

Balsaver, A. M., Butler, J. J., & Martin, R. G. (1967). Congenital fibrosarcoma. *Cancer, 20*, 1607–1616.

Bancroft, L. W., Kransdorf, M. J., Peterson, J. J., & O'Connor, M. I. (2006). Benign fatty tumors: Classification, clinical course, imaging appearance, and treatment. *Skeletal Radiology, 35*(10), 719–733.

Barr, F. G. (1997). Molecular genetics and pathogenesis of rhabdomyosarcoma. *Journal of Pediatric Hematology/Oncology, 19*, 483–491.

Barré-Sinoussi, F., Chermann, J. C., Rey, F., Nugeyre, M. T., Chamaret, S., Gruest, J., … Montagnier, L. (1983). Isolation of a T-lymphotropic retrovirus from a patient at risk for acquired immune deficiency syndrome (AIDS). *Science, 220,* 868–871.

Baumhoer, D., Gunawan, B., Becker, H., & Füzesi, L. (2005). Comparative genomic hybridization in four angiosarcomas of the female breast. *Gynecologic Oncology, 97,* 348–352.

Beck, A. (1922). Zur Frage des Rontgensarkoms, zugleich ein Beitrag zur Pathogenese des Sarkoms. *Münchener medizinische Wochenschrift, 69,* 623–625.

Biggar, R. J., Horm, J., Fraumeni, J. F., Jr., Greene, M. H., & Goedert, J. J. (1984). Incidence of Kaposi's sarcoma and mycosis fungoides in the United States including Puerto Rico, 1973–81. *Journal of the National Cancer Institute, 73*(1), 89–94.

Bishop, J. M., & Varmus, H. E. (1989). The Nobel prize in physiology or medicine, 1989. Retrieved from www.nobelprize.org /nobel_prizes/medicine/laureates/1989/press.html

Boffetta, P., Matisane, L., Mundt, K. A., & Dell, L. D. (2003). Meta-analysis of studies of occupational exposure to vinyl chloride on relation to cancer mortality. *Scandinavian Journal of Work, Environment and Health, 29,* 220–229.

Bray, F., Ferlay, J., Soerjomataram, I., Siegel, R. L., Torre, L. A., & Jemal, A. (2018). Global cancer statistics 2018: GLOBOCAN estimates of incidence and mortality worldwide for 36 cancers in 185 countries. *CA: A Cancer Journal for Clinicians, 68*(6), 394–424.

Cancian, L., Hansen, A., & Boshoff, C. (2013). Cellular origin of Kaposi's sarcoma and Kaposi's sarcoma–associated herpesvirus-induced cell reprogramming. *Trends in Cell Biology, 23*(9), 421–432.

Carsi, B., & Rock, M. G. (2002). Primary osteosarcoma in adults older than 40 years. *Clinical Orthopaedics and Related Research, 397,* 53–61.

Cayley, W. E., Jr. (2004). Effectiveness of condoms in reducing heterosexual transmission of HIV. *American Family Physician, 70*(7), 1268–1269.

Cesarman, E., Chang, Y., Moore, P. S., Said, J. W., & Knowles, D. M. (1995). Kaposi's sarcoma–associated herpesvirus-like DNA sequences in AIDS-related body-cavity-based lymphomas. *New England Journal of Medicine, 332*(18), 1186–1191.

Chang, Y., Cesarman, E., Pessin, M. S., Lee, F., Culpepper, J., Knowles, D. M., & Moore, P. S. (1994). Identification of herpesvirus-like DNA sequences in AIDS-associated Kaposi's sarcoma. *Science, 266,* 1865–1869.

Chauveinc, L., Mosseri, V., Quintana, E., Desjardins, L., Schlienger, P., Doz, F., & Dutrillaux, B. (2001). Osteosarcoma following retinoblastoma: Age at onset and latency period. *Ophthalmic Genetics, 22*(2), 77–88.

Christopherson, W. M., Foote, F. W., & Stewart, F. W. (1952). Alveolar soft part sarcomas: Structurally characteristic tumors of uncertain histogenesis. *Cancer, 5,* 100–111.

Clark, J., Rocques, P. J., Crew, A. J., Gill, S., Shipley, J., Chan, A. L., … Cooper, C. S. (1994). Identification of novel genes, *SYT* and *SSX,* involved in the t(X;18)(p11.2;q11.2) translocation found in human synovial sarcoma. *Nature Genetics, 7,* 502–508.

Cohen, M. S., Chen, Y. Q., McCauley, M., Gamble, T., Hosseinipour, M. C., Kumarasamy, N., … Fleming, T. R. (2011). Prevention of HIV-1 infection with early antiretroviral therapy. *New England Journal of Medicine, 365,* 493–505.

Coindre, J. M., Mariani, O., Chibon, F., Maira, O., Somerhausen, N. A., Favre-Guilevin, E., … Aurias, A. (2003). Most malignant fibrous histiocytomas developed in the retroperitoneum are dedifferentiated liposarcomas: A review of 25 cases initially diagnosed as malignant fibrous histiocytoma. *Modern Pathology, 16*(3), 256–262.

Connolly, E., Gaffney, E., & Reynolds, J. (2003). Gastrointestinal stromal tumors. *British Journal of Surgery, 90,* 1178–1186.

Cook-Mozaffari, P., Newton, R., Beral, V., & Burkitt, D. P. (1998). The geographical distribution of Kaposi's sarcoma and of lymphomas in Africa before the AIDS epidemic. *British Journal of Cancer, 78*(11), 1521–1528.

Cordon-Cardo, C. (1997). Sarcomas of the soft tissues and bone. In V. T. DeVita, Jr. (Ed.), *Cancer principles and practice of oncology* (pp. 1731–1782). New York, NY: Lippincott-Raven.

Crawford, L. V., & Crawford, E. M. (1961). The properties of Rous sarcoma virus purified by density gradient centrifugation. *Virology, 13,* 227–232.

Creech, J. L., Jr., & Johnson, M. N. (1974). Angiosarcoma of the liver in the manufacture of polyvinyl chloride. *Journal of Occupational Medicine, 16,* 150–151.

Darling, J. (2007). A different view of sarcoma statistics. *Electronic Sarcoma Update Newsletter, 4*(6).

Delaney, T. F., Hornicek, F. J., Lessnick, S. L., & Mankin, H. J. (2010). Epidemiology, pathology, and molecular genetics of the Ewing sarcoma family of tumors. *UpToDate,* Version 18.3. Retrieved from www.uptodate.com/contents/epidemiology -pathology-and-molecular-genetics-of-the-ewing-sarcoma -family-of-tumors

Dickens, D. S., Kozielski, R., Khan, J., Forus, A., & Cripe, T. P. (2002). Cyclooxygenase-2 expression in pediatric sarcomas. *Pediatric and Developmental Pathology, 5*(4), 356–364.

Dunlap, J. B., Magenis, R. E., Davis, C., Himoe, E., & Mansoor, A. (2009). Cytogenetic analysis of a primary bone angiosarcoma. *Cancer Genetics and Cytogenetics, 194*(1), 1–3.

Edling, C. E., & Hallberg, B. (2007). c-Kit-a hematopoietic cell essential receptor tyrosine kinase. *International Journal of Biochemistry and Cell Biology, 39*(11), 1995–1998.

Ewing, J. (1921). Diffuse endothelioma of bone. *Proceedings of the New York Pathological Society, 21,* 17–24.

Exelby, P. R., Knapper, W. H., Huvos, A. G., & Beattie, E. J., Jr. (1973). Soft-tissue fibrosarcoma in children. *Journal of Pediatric Surgery, 8*(3), 415–420.

Falk, H., Caldwell, G. G., Ishak, K. D., Thomas, L. B., & Popper, H. (1981). Arsenic-related hepatic angiosarcoma. *American Journal of Industrial Medicine, 2*(1), 43–50.

Falk, H., Telles, N. C., Ishak, K. G., Thomas, L. B., & Popper, H. (1979). Epidemiology of thorotrast-induced hepatic angiosarcoma in the United States. *Environmental Research, 18*(1), 65–73.

Ferlay, J., Ervik, M., Lam, F., Colombet, M., Mery, L., Piñeros, M., … Bray, F. (2018). *Global cancer observatory: Cancer today.* Lyon, France: International Agency for Research on Cancer. Retrieved from https://gco.iarc.fr/today

Ferlay, J., Shin, H.-R., Bray, F., Forman, D., Mathers, C., & Parkin, D. M. (2010). Estimates of worldwide burden of cancer in 2008: GLOBOCAN 2008. *International Journal of Cancer, 127*(12), 2893–2917.

Ferlay, J., Soerjomataram, I., Ervik, M., Dikshit, R., Eser, S., Mathers, C., … Bray, F. (2013). *GLOBOCAN 2012 v1.0. Cancer incidence and mortality worldwide: IARC CancerBase No. 11* [Internet]. Lyon, France: International Agency for Research on Cancer. Retrieved from http://globocan.iarc.fr

Fung, H. L., & Tran, D. C. (2006). Effects of inhalant nitrites on VEGF expression: A feasible link to Kaposi's sarcoma? *Journal of Neuroimmune Pharmacology, 1*(3), 317–322.

Gallo, R. C., Salahuddin, S. Z., Popovic, M., Shearer, G. M., Kaplan, M., Haynes, B. F., … Safai, B. (1984). Frequent detection and isolation of cytopathic retroviruses (HTLV-III) from patients with AIDS and at risk for AIDS. *Science, 224*(4648), 500–503.

Gardner, E. J. (1951). A genetic and clinical study of intestinal polyposis, a predisposing factor for carcinoma of the colon and rectum. *American Journal of Human Genetics, 3*(2), 167–176.

Gurney, J. G., Swensen, A. R., & Bulterys, M. (1999). Chapter VIII. Malignant bone tumors. In L. A. G. Ries, M. A. Smith, J. G. Gurney, M. Linet, T. Tamra, J. L. Young, & G. R. Bunin (Eds.), *Cancer incidence and survival among children and adolescents: United States SEER program 1975–1995* (pp. 99–110, NIH Pub. No. 99-4649). Bethesda, MD: National Cancer Institute, SEER Program.

Gurney, J. G., Young, J. L., Roffers, S. D., Smith, M. A., & Bunin, G. R. (1999). Chapter IX. Soft tissue sarcomas. In L. A. G. Ries, M. A. Smith, J. G. Gurney, M. Linet, T. Tamra, J. L. Young, & G. R. Bunin (Eds.), *Cancer incidence and survival among children and adolescents: United States SEER program 1975–1995* (pp. 111–122, NIH Pub. No. 99-4649). Bethesda, MD: National Cancer Institute, SEER Program.

Hoppin, J. A., Tolbert, P. E., Flanders, W. D., Zhang, R. H., Daniels, D. S., Ragsdale, B. D., & Brann, E. A. (1999). Occupational risk factors for sarcoma subtypes. *Epidemiology, 10*(6), 300–306.

Indraccolo, U., Luchetti, G., & Indraccolo, S. R. (2008). Malignant transformation of uterine leiomyomata. *European Journal of Gynaecological Oncology, 29*(5), 543–534.

Joensuu, H., Roberts, P. J., Sarlomo-Rikala, M., Andersson, L. C., Tervahartiala, P., Tuveson, D., … Demetri, G. D. (2001). Effect of the tyrosine kinase inhibitor STI571 in a patient with a metastatic gastrointestinal stromal tumor. *New England Journal of Medicine, 344*(14), 1052–1056.

Johnson, J. G., Gilbert, E., Zimmermann, B., & Watne, A. L. (1972). Gardner's syndrome, colon cancer, and sarcoma. *Journal of Surgical Oncology, 4*(4), 354–362.

Kaposi, M. (1872). Idiopathisches multiples pigmentsarkom der haut. *Archiv für Dermatologie und Syphilis, 4*, 265–273.

Karlsson, P., Holmberg, E., Samuelsson, A., Johansson, K. A., & Wallgren, A. (1998). Soft tissue sarcoma after treatment for breast cancer—A Swedish population-based study. *European Journal of Cancer, 34*(13), 2068–2075.

Kerr, T., Kimber, J., Debeck, K., & Wood, E. (2007). The role of safer injection facilities in the response to HIV/AIDS among injection drug users. *Current HIV/AIDS Reports, 4*(4), 158–164.

Knezevich, S. R., Garnett, M. J., Pysher, T. J., Beckwith, J. B., Grundy, P. E., & Sorensen, P. H. (1998). *ETV6-NTRK3* gene fusions and trisomy 11 establish a histogenetic link between mesoblastic nephroma and congenital fibrosarcoma. *Cancer Research, 58*, 5046–5048.

Kumar, V., Abbas, A. K., & Aster, J. C. (2014). *Robbins and Cotran pathologic basis of disease* (9th ed.). Philadelphia, PA: Mosby & Saunders.

Ladanyi, M. (1995). The emerging molecular genetics of sarcoma translocations. *Diagnostic Molecular Pathology, 4*(3), 162–173.

Ladanyi, M., & Bridge, J. A. (2000). Contribution of molecular genetic data to the classification of sarcomas. *Human Pathology, 31*, 532–538.

Ladanyi, M., Lui, M. Y., Antonescu, C. R., Krause-Boehm, A., Meindl, A., Argani, P., … Bridge, J. (2001). The der(17)t(X;17)(p11;q25) of human alveolar soft part sarcoma fuses the *TFE3* transcription factor gene to *ASPL*, a novel gene at 17q25. *Oncogene, 20*(1), 48–57.

Lakhanpal, M., & Ram, R. (2008). Educational attainment and HIV/AIDS prevalence: A cross-country study. *Economics of Education Review, 27*, 14–21.

Lassus, P., Ristimaki, A., Huuhtanen, R., Tukiainen, E., Asko-Seljavaara, S., Andersson, L. C., … Bohling, T. (2005). Cyclooxygenase-2 expression in human soft-tissue sarcomas is related to epithelial differentiation. *Anticancer Research, 25*, 2669–2674.

Leonard, A., Craft, A. W., Moss, C., & Malcolm, A. J. (1996). Osteogenic sarcoma in the Rothmund-Thomson syndrome. *Medical and Pediatric Oncology, 26*(4), 249–253.

Levy, J. A., Hoffman, A. D., Kramer, S. M., Landis, J. A., Shimabukuro, J. M., & Oshiro, L. S. (1984). Isolation of lymphocytopathic retroviruses from San Francisco patients with AIDS. *Science, 225*(4664), 840–842.

Li, F. P., Fraumeni, J. F., Jr., Mulvihill, J. J., Blattner, W. A., Dreyfus, M. G., Tucker, M. A., & Miller, R. W. (1998). A cancer family syndrome in twenty-four kindreds. *Cancer Research, 48*(18), 5358–5362.

Lorincz, A., Redelman, D., Horvath, V. J., Bardsley, M. R., Chen, H., & Ordog, T. (2008). Progenitors of interstitial cells of Cajal in the postnatal murine stomach. *Gastroenterology, 134*, 1083–1093.

Markowitz, S. D., & Bertagnolli, M. M. (2009). Molecular basis of colorectal cancer. *New England Journal of Medicine, 361*(25), 2449–2460.

Martland, H., & Humphries, R. E. (1929). Osteogenic sarcoma in dial painters using luminous paint. *Archives of Pathology, 7*, 406–417.

Mendenhall, W. M., Zlotecki, R. A., Scarborough, M. T., Gibbs, P. C., & Mendenhall, N. P. (2006). Giant cell tumor of bone. *American Journal of Clinical Oncology, 29*(1), 96–99.

Moore, P. S., & Chang, Y. (1995). Detection of herpesvirus-like DNA sequences in Kaposi's sarcoma in patients with and without HIV infection. *New England Journal of Medicine, 332*(18), 1181–1185.

Moore, P. S., Gao, S. J., Dominguez, G., Cesarman, E., Lungu, O., Knowles, D. M., … Chang, Y. (1996). Primary characterization of a herpesvirus agent associated with Kaposi's sarcoma. *Journal of Virology, 70*(1), 549–558.

Mundt, K. A., Dell, L. D., Austin, R. P., Luippold, R. S., Noess, R., & Bigelow, C. (2000). Historical cohort study of 10,109 men in the North American vinyl chloride industry, 1942–1972. Update of cancer mortality to 31 December. *Occupational and Environmental Medicine, 57*, 774–781.

O'Brien, J. E., & Stout, A. P. (1964). Malignant fibrous xanthomas. *Cancer, 17*, 1445–1455.

Oppermann, H., Levinson, A. D., Varmus, H. E., Levintow, L., & Bishop, J. M. (1979). Uninfected vertebrate cells contain a protein that is closely related to the product of the avian sarcoma virus transforming gene (src). *Proceedings of the National Academy of the Sciences of the United States of America, 76*(4), 1804–1808.

Parkin, D. M., Bray, F., Ferlay, J., & Pisani, P. (2005). Global cancer statistics, 2002. *CA: A Cancer Journal for Clinicians, 55*, 74–108.

Parkin, D. M., Stiller, C. A., Draper, G. J., & Bieber, C. A. (1988). The international incidence of childhood cancer. *International Journal of Cancer, 42*, 511–520.

Patel, K. U., Szabo, S. S., Hernandez, V. S., Prieto, V. G., Abruzzo, L. V., Lazar, A. J. F., & López-Terrada, D. (2008). Dermatofibrosarcoma protuberans COL1A1-PDGFB fusion is identified in virtually all dermatofibrosarcoma protuberans cases when investigated by newly developed multiplex reverse transcription polymerase chain reaction and fluorescence in situ hybridization assays. *Human Pathology, 39*(2), 184–193.

Rindermann, H., & Meisenberg, G. (2009). Relevance of education and intelligence at the national level for health: The case of HIV and AIDS. *Intelligence, 37*, 383–395.

Robinson, E., Neugut, A. I., & Wylie, P. (1988). Clinical aspects of postirradiation sarcomas. *Journal of the National Cancer Institute, 80*, 233–240.

Rööser, B., Willén, H., Gustafson, P., Alvegård, T. A., & Rydholm, A. (1991). Malignant fibrous histiocytoma of soft tissue. A population-based epidemiologic and prognostic study of 137 patients. *Cancer, 67*(2), 499–505.

Rossiello, L., Ruocco, E., Signoriello, G., Micheli, P., Rienzo, M., Napoli, C., & Rossiello, R. (2007). Evidence of COX-1 and COX-2 expression in Kaposi's sarcoma tissues. *European Journal of Cancer, 43*(8), 1232–1241.

Rous, P. (1910). A transmissable avian neoplasm. *Journal of Experimental Medicine, 12*, 696–705.

Rous, P. (1911). A sarcoma of the fowl transmissible by an agent separable from the tumor cells. *Journal of Experimental Medicine, 13*, 397–399.

Rous, P., & Huggins, C. B. (1966). The Nobel prize in physiology or medicine, 1966. Retrieved from http://www.nobelprize.org/nobel_prizes/medicine/laureates/1966/

Sanders, K., Koh, S., & Ward, S. (2006). Interstitial cells of Cajal as pacemakers in the gastrointestinal tract. *Annual Review of Physiology, 68*, 307–343.

Sinha, A., Tekkis, P. P., Gibbons, D. C., Phillips, R. K., & Clark, S. K. (2010). Risk factors predicting desmoid occurrence in patients with familial adenomatous polyposis: A meta-analysis. *Colorectal Disease, 13*, 1222–1229.

Skubitz, K. M. (2007). Sarcoma. *Mayo Clinic Proceedings, 82*(11), 1409–1432.

Spirtas, R., Beebe, G., Baxter, P., Dacey, F., Faber, M., Falk, H., … Stafford, J. (1983). Angiosarcoma as a model for comparative carcinogenesis. *Lancet, 322*(8347), 456.

Stebbing, J., & Portsmouth, B. (2003). How does HAART lead to the resolution of Kaposi's sarcoma? *Journal of Antimicrobial Chemotherapy, 51*(5), 1095–1098.

Stehelin, D., Fujita, D. J., Padgett, T., Varmus, H. E., & Bishop, J. M. (1977). Detection and enumeration of transformation-defective strains of avian sarcoma virus with molecular hybridization. *Virology, 76*(2), 675–684.

Stiller, C. A., Bielack, S. S., Jundt, G., & Steliarova-Foucher, E. (2006). Bone tumours in European children and adolescents, 1978–1997. Report from the Automated Childhood Cancer Information System project. *European Journal of Cancer, 42*(13), 2124–2135.

Thomas, D. M., & Skubitz, T. (2009). Giant-cell tumour of bone. *Current Opinion in Oncology, 21*, 338–344.

Tontonoz, P., Singer, S., Forman, B. M., Sarraf, P., Fletcher, J. A., Fletcher, C. D., … Spiegelman, B. M. (1997). Terminal differentiation of human liposarcoma cells induced by ligands for peroxisome proliferator-activated receptor gamma and the retinoid X receptor. *Proceedings of the National Academy of the Sciences of the United States of America, 94*(1), 237–241.

Tran, T., Davila, J. A., & El-Serag, H. B. (2005). The epidemiology of malignant gastrointestinal stromal tumors: An analysis of 1,458 cases from 1992 to 2000. *American Journal of Gastroenterology, 100*, 162–168.

Turc-Carel, C., Limon, J., Dal Cin, P., Rao, U., Karakousis, C., & Sandberg, A. A. (1986). Cytogenetic studies of adipose tissue tumors. II. Recurrent reciprocal translocation t(12:16) (q13;p11) in myxoid liposarcomas. *Cancer Genetics and Cytogenetics, 23*(4), 291–299.

Walker, D. G. (1972). Congenital osteopetrosis in mice cured by parabiotic union with normal siblings. *Endocrinology, 91*(4), 916–920.

Walker, D. G. (1973). Osteopetrosis cured by temporary parabiosis. *Science, 180*(88), 875.

Wallach, E. E., & Vlahos, N. F. (2004). Uterine myomas: An overview of development, clinical features, and management. *Obstetrics and Gynecology, 104*, 393–406.

Wang, L. L., Gannavarapu, A., Kozinetz, C. A., Moise, L., Levy, M. L., Lewis, R. A., … Zackai, E. H. (2003). Association between osteosarcoma and deleterious mutations in the RECQL4 gene in Rothmund-Thomson syndrome. *Journal of the National Cancer Institute, 95*(9), 669–674.

Wang, R., Lu, Y. J., Fisher, C., Bridge, J. A., & Shipley, J. (2001). Characterization of chromosome aberrations associated with soft-tissue leiomyosarcomas by twenty-four-color karyotyping and comparative genomic hybridization analysis. *Genes, Chromosomes and Cancer, 31*, 54–64.

Wodak, A., & Cooney, A. (2006). Do needle syringe programs reduce HIV infection among injecting drug users: A comprehensive review of the international evidence. *Substance Use and Misuse, 41*(6–7), 777–813.

World Health Organization. (2006). *HIV and infant feeding technical consultation, consensus statement.* Geneva, Switzerland: Author.

World Health Organization. (2010). *Screening donated blood for transfusion-transmissible infections: Recommendations.* Geneva, Switzerland: Author.

Yarden, Y., Kuang, W. J., Yang-Feng, T., Coussens, L., Munemitsu, S., Dull, T. J., … Ullrich, A. (1987). Human proto-oncogene c-kit: A new cell surface receptor tyrosine kinase for an unidentified ligand. *EMBO Journal, 6*(11), 3341–3351.

© Andrew Brookes/Getty Images

CHAPTER 36

Epidemiology of Lymphoma: Non-Hodgkin's Lymphoma, Hodgkin's Lymphoma, and Multiple Myeloma

▶ Classification of Lymphoma

The World Health Organization categorizes lymphomas into three broad groups: non-Hodgkin's lymphoma (NHL), Hodgkin's lymphoma, and multiple myeloma. NHLs show considerable heterogeneity and are divisible into those arising from B cells or T cells. This chapter focuses primarily on the epidemiology of NHL with brief sections devoted to Hodgkin's lymphoma and multiple myeloma.

Lymphomas are malignancies that can arise in the lymphocytes of lymphoid tissue anywhere in the body, most commonly within lymph nodes. Hodgkin's lymphoma, which is distinguishable by the presence of multinucleated Reed–Sternberg cells, constitutes 10%–15% of all lymphomas (Reed, 1902). Multiple myeloma, a neoplasm of plasma cells, constitutes 15%–20% of lymphomas. The remaining 65%–75% of lymphomas, the NHLs, arise at various stages in the maturation of B lymphocytes or T lymphocytes. According to classification schemes currently used in clinical practice, NHLs can be subdivided into a bewildering array of subtypes. In most populations, 80%–90% of NHLs are derived from the B-cell lineage (Harris et al., 1999).

Lymphomas are cohesive malignancies (solid tumors) composed primarily of lymphocytes. Their origin, usually in lymph nodes, may involve an arrest in differentiation of immature lymphocytes, or alternatively, retrodifferentiation of mature lymphocytes. In either case, there is sustained unrelenting proliferation of the transformed cells. As with other malignancies, the initiation, growth, development, and metastatic spread of lymphomas involves various cellular and genetic processes, including mutagenesis, mitogenesis, angiogenesis, aberrant apoptosis, immunosuppression, and metastasis.

Lymphocytes arise from hematopoietic stem cells of the bone marrow. The B lymphocytes mature and differentiate in the lymph nodes, whereas T lymphocytes do so in the thymus gland. The different types of lymphocytes display specific cell surface receptors and have characteristic morphological features and distinct functions in the immune system. For example, the maturation, differentiation, and proliferation of T lymphocytes spawn at least three distinct subpopulations: antigen-presenting T cells (also called helper T cells), suppressor T cells, and killer T cells.

With appropriate stimulation by helper T cells, mature B lymphocytes differentiate into plasma cells that secrete antibodies directed against specific antigens recognized as foreign to the human immune system. Malignancies of plasma cells are called *myelomas*, and because neoplasms of plasma cells usually involve multiple anatomic sites throughout the skeletal system and sometimes soft tissues, the condition is commonly called *multiple myeloma*.

▶ Epidemiology of Non-Hodgkin's Lymphoma

Global Burden of Non-Hodgkin's Lymphoma

During 2018, 509,590 new cases of NHL were diagnosed in the world population (284,713 in men and 224,877 in women) and 248,724 individuals died from the disease (145,969 men and 102,755 women). The age-adjusted incidence rate was 6.7 per 100,000 in men and 4.7 per 100,000 in women, and the age-adjusted mortality rate was 3.3 per 100,000 in men and 2.0 per 100,000 in women). In the past decade, 2008–2018, the annual incidence rates of NHL increased by approximately 11% in men and women whereas the mortality rates have remained relatively stable (Bray et al., 2018; Ferlay, Shin, Forman, Mathers, & Parkin, 2010).

Incidence rates of NHL vary widely and tend to be higher in populations of developed nations (**FIGURE 36.1**). As in other years, the 2018 rates were high in North America, Western Europe, and Australia/New Zealand (~10 per 100,000) and low in India and China (~3 per 100,000) (Ferlay et al., 2013, 2018). High rates were also observed in some populations residing in the tropical zone of Africa, partly due to the high incidence of Burkitt's lymphoma, a particularly aggressive form of B-cell lymphoma that develops primarily in children. Of further note is that T-cell lymphomas are most common in Japan and the Caribbean (Shipp, Mauch, & Harris, 1997). Caution is advised, however, in drawing epidemiologic conclusions based on the wide variability in international rates because many nations do not have population-based cancer registries, and reporting may therefore be incomplete.

Mortality rates were highest in the populations of the Middle East and Africa (4–6 per 100,000) and lowest in India, China, and Eastern Asia (1–2 per 100,000) (Figure 36.1). In African populations where mortality is high, the available healthcare resources are generally inadequate for effective treatment. Nevertheless, relatively high death rates from NHL are also evident in the populations of many developed nations. For example, mortality rates in men of the United States,

Canada, and Australia (3.6–3.9 per 100,000) were higher than in most other nations (Ferlay et al., 2018).

Global Patterns and Trends of Non-Hodgkin's Lymphoma

The global burden of NHL has steadily increased in the 21st century (**FIGURE 36.2**). During 1990–2018, the annual number of new cases more than doubled (from 230,000 to 509,590), and the annual number of deaths increased by 97% (from 126,000 to 248,724) (Bray et al., 2018; Ferlay et al., 2010, 2013, 2018; Fitzmaurice, 2017, 2018; Parkin, Bray, Ferlay, & Pisani, 2005; Parkin, Pisani, & Ferlay, 1999a, 1999b; World Health Organization, 2008).

The rising absolute number of new cases and deaths from NHL is partially due to increasing longevity and growth of the world population. These demographic forces have resulted in more individuals living to later ages when the risk of death from lymphoma is highest. As shown in **FIGURE 36.3**, lymphoma onset rises with age, and nearly 75% of deaths occur after the age of 65 years (Altekruse et al., 2010). Nevertheless, as discussed in the following sections of this chapter, other factors have also contributed to the rising global burden of NHL.

Non-Hodgkin's Lymphoma in the United States

In nations with population-based cancer registries, marked increases were observed in the annual incidence rates of NHL during the later decades of the 20th century. For example, in the United States, the incidence doubled for both men and women during 1970–1995 (**FIGURE 36.4**). The rising incidence rates during this time period were consistent in men and women of all ethnicities and age groups except for the very young (Devesa & Fears, 1992). Subsequently, during 1995–2015, the rates stabilized and appeared to have declined slightly in women (Altekruse et al., 2010; Noone et al., 2018).

Several factors have contributed to the increasing trends in NHL in populations of the United States and other developed nations. In particular, escalations in the incidence among young adult males and (to a lesser extent) females occurred following the onset of the acquired immune deficiency syndrome (AIDS) epidemic in 1981 (Hartge, Devesa, & Fraumeni, 1994). With the discovery of the human immunodeficiency virus (HIV), which is considered the causative agent of AIDS, this syndrome is currently referred to as *HIV disease* (Barré-Sinoussi et al., 1983; Gallo et al., 1983).

Estimated age-standardized incidence rates (World) in 2018, non-Hodgkin lymphoma, both sexes, all ages

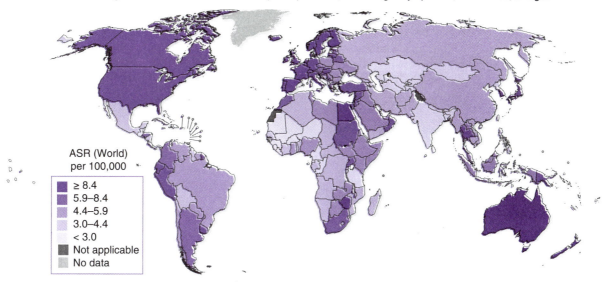

Estimated age-standardized mortality rates (World) in 2018, non-Hodgkin lymphoma, both sexes, all ages

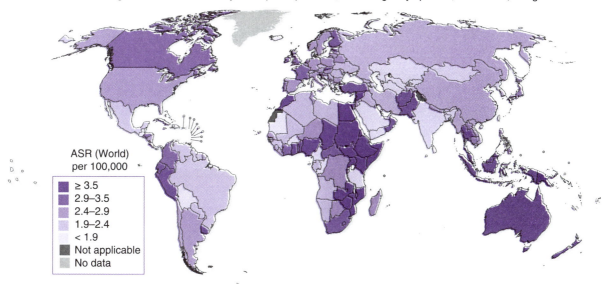

FIGURE 36.1 Global Incidence and Mortality Rates of Non-Hodgkin's Lymphoma, 2018.

Caption: ASR: Rates per 100,000 are age-standardized to the world population, 2000–2025.

Reproduced with permission from Ferlay, J., Ervik, M., Lam, F., Colombet, M., Mery, L., Piñeros, M., . . . Bray, F. (2018). *Global cancer observatory: Cancer today*. Lyon, France: International Agency for Research on Cancer. Retrieved from https://gco.iarc.fr/today, accessed [09 October 2018].

Other factors that have contributed to the rising incidence of NHL include improvements in the detection and reporting of lymphomas and refinements in the classification system of lymphoproliferative disorders, resulting in the diagnosis of relatively more cases of NHL. For example, certain extranodal lymphoproliferative conditions and T-cell neoplasms are now recognized and classified as NHL. Although stomach and skin remain the most common extranodal sites, primary disease in the brain has sharply increased (Groves, Linet, Travis, & Devesa, 2000). Furthermore, the incidence of NHL is also increased among cancer patients treated by chemotherapy and among subjects undergoing heart or kidney transplants, all of whom

experience immunosuppression (Banks, 1992; Müller, Ihorst, Mertelsmann, & Engelhardt, 2005). Despite these coincident trends, a large portion of the increase in NHL during the later 20th century remains to be explained.

As shown in Figure 36.4, the annual incidence of NHL in the United States increased until about 1995, but then subsequently declined. This pattern coincides with a decline in the development of HIV disease due to primary preventive measures and/or use of highly active antiretroviral therapy that inhibits progression of HIV infection to active disease (Eltom, Jemal, Mbulaiteye, Devesa, & Biggar, 2002). Nevertheless, the incidence of NHL *not* related to HIV disease is continuing to

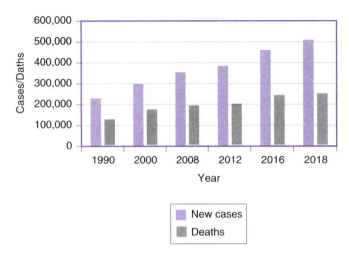

FIGURE 36.2 Global Trends of Non-Hodgkin's Lymphoma, 1990–2018.

Data from Bray, F., Ferlay, J., Soerjomataram, I., Siegel, R. L., Torre, L. A., & Jemal, A. (2018). Global cancer statistics 2018: GLOBOCAN estimates of incidence and mortality worldwide for 36 cancers in 185 countries. *CA: A Cancer Journal for Clinicians, 68*(6), 394–424; Ferlay, J., Shin, H. R., Forman, D., Mathers, C., & Parkin, D. M. (2010). Estimates of worldwide burden of cancer in 2008. *International Journal of Cancer, 127*(12), 2893–2917; Ferlay, J., Soerjomataram, I., Ervik, M., Dikshit, R., Eser, S., Mathers, C., . . . Bray, F. (2013). *GLOBOCAN 2012 v1.0. Cancer incidence and mortality worldwide: IARC CancerBase No. 11* [Internet]. Lyon, France: International Agency for Research on Cancer. Retrieved from http://globocan.iarc.fr; Parkin, D. M., Bray, F., Ferlay, J., & Pisani, P. (2005). Global cancer statistics, 2002. *CA: A Cancer Journal for Clinicians, 55*, 74–108; Parkin, D. M., Pisani, P., & Ferlay, J. (1999a). Estimates of the worldwide incidence of 25 major cancers in 1990. *International Journal of Cancer, 80*(6), 827–841; Parkin, D. M., Pisani, P., & Ferlay, J. (1999b). Global cancer statistics. *CA: A Cancer Journal for Clinicians, 49*(1), 33–64; World Health Organization. (2008). *World cancer report 2008*. Lyon, France: International Agency for Research on Cancer; Fitzmaurice, C., Allen, C., Barber, R. M., Barregard, L., Bhutta, Z. A., Brenner, H., . . . Global Burden of Disease Cancer Collaboration. (2017). Global, regional, and national cancer incidence, mortality, years of life lost, years lived with disability, and disability-adjusted life-years for 32 cancer groups, 1990–2015: A systematic analysis for the Global Burden of Disease Study. *JAMA Oncology, 3*(4), 524–548. Fitzmaurice, C., Akinyemiju, T. F., Al Lami, F. H., Alam, T., Alizadeh-Navaei, R., Allen, C., . . . Global Burden of Disease Cancer Collaboration. (2018). Global, regional, and national cancer incidence, mortality, years of life lost, years lived with disability, and disability-adjusted life-years for 29 cancer groups, 1990–2016: A systematic analysis for the Global Burden of Disease Study. *JAMA Oncology*. Online publication. doi:10.1001/jamaoncol.2018.2706.

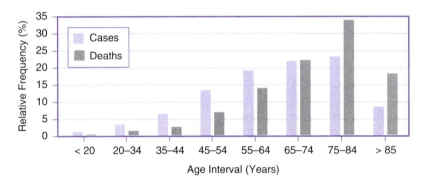

FIGURE 36.3 Age-Specific Frequencies of New Cases and Deaths: Non-Hodgkin's Lymphoma.

Data from Altekruse, S. F., Kosary, C. L., Krapcho, M., Neyman, N., Aminou, R., Waldron, W., . . . Edwards, B. K. (2010). *SEER cancer statistics review, 1975–2007*. Bethesda, MD: National Cancer Institute.

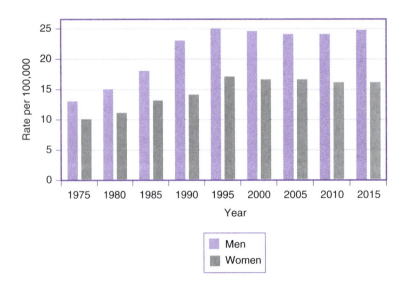

FIGURE 36.4 Annual Incidence Rates of Non-Hodgkin's Lymphoma, United States, 1970–2010.

Caption: Rates are age-standardized to the U.S. population of 2000.

Data from Altekruse, S. F., Kosary, C. L., Krapcho, M., Neyman, N., Aminou, R., Waldron, W., . . . Edwards, B. K. (2010). *SEER cancer statistics review, 1975–2007*. Bethesda, MD: National Cancer Institute; Noone, A. M., Howlader, N., Krapcho, M., Miller, D., Brest, A., Yu, M., . . . Cronin, K. A. (Eds.). (2018). *SEER cancer statistics review, 1975–2015*. Bethesda, MD: National Cancer Institute. Retrieved from https://seer.cancer.gov/csr/1975_2015/.

increase, particularly among older men and women. It is well known that old age is accompanied by decreased immune function (immunosuppression) and higher susceptibility to infection, conditions that may heighten the risk of developing lymphoma as well as other malignancies (Fisher & Fisher, 2004; Müller et al., 2005).

Gender and Ethnic Differences in Non-Hodgkin's Lymphoma

In the U.S. population, more than 21,000 individuals died from NHL each year during 2003–2007. The age-adjusted mortality rate was 6.9 per 100,000 per year and the median age at death was 75 years of age. Death rates were 60% higher for men than women (8.7 vs. 5.5) and higher among Caucasians (9.1 in men and 5.7 in women) compared to other ethnicities (5.8 in men and 4.1 in women) (Altekruse et al., 2010).

During 2003–2007, the age-adjusted incidence rate of NHL was 19.6 per 100,000 per year. Incidence rates were 43% higher in men than women (23.6 vs. 16.5 per 100,000), and higher in Caucasians (24.6 in men and 17.2 in women) than other ethnic groups (16.2 in men and 12.1 in women). American Indians and Alaska natives had the lowest rates (12.5 in men and 10.6 in women) (Altekruse et al., 2010).

Risk Factors for Non-Hodgkin's Lymphoma

Multiple viruses and bacteria have been found in association with the development of NHL (Alexander, Mink, Adami, Chang, et al., 2007; Fisher & Fisher, 2004; Melbye, Ekström Smedby, & Trichopoulos, 2008; Müller et al., 2005). These infectious agents appear to be associated with two principal biological phenomena involved in the genesis of this malignancy: immunosuppression and antigenic stimulation. Immunosuppression can be incited not only by microbes but also by powerful drugs routinely used in transplant therapy. Indeed, the combination of drug-induced immunosuppression and heightened antigenic stimulation through reactivation of latent Epstein–Barr virus (EBV) infection appears to markedly accelerate lymphomagenesis. Selected microbes and conditions and their effects on the pathogenesis of NHL are discussed in the following sections.

Genetics of Non-Hodgkin's Lymphoma

Family studies suggest that genetic susceptibility has a modest influence on the development of NHL. For example, the presence of one or more first-degree relatives (parents, siblings, and offspring) afflicted with a hematopoietic malignancy has been found to increase the risk of developing NHL by two- to fourfold (Linet & Pottern, 1992; Zhu et al., 1998). Nevertheless, it is not clear whether familial clustering is truly attributable to genetic predisposition or rather to similar environmental exposures. Furthermore, familial lymphomas account for less than 5% of all cases, and it is unlikely that hereditary factors per se played a substantial role in the increasing trend in NHL in the United States and other populations.

Primary congenital immunodeficiency is a rare condition that results in the absence of specific types of immunoglobulins in the immune system. This disorder arises due to point mutations in the genes controlling immunoglobulin formation, most of which are located on chromosomes 2, 14, and 22. When congenital immunodeficiency is present, the risk of developing lymphoma is high, up to 25% by the age of 25 years. This condition also shortens the lifespan considerably, because most afflicted patients die before the age of 50 years. Certain other genetic syndromes also increase the risk of developing lymphoma. These include ataxia telangiectasia, a condition marked by DNA repair defects and impaired cell-mediated immunity; Wiscott–Aldrich syndrome, a rare X-linked condition characterized by eczema, thrombocytopenia (low platelets), immunodeficiency, and bloody diarrhea; and the X-linked lymphoproliferative syndrome characterized by fatal or near-fatal infectious mononucleosis due to EBV and immunoglobulin deficiency in childhood (Filipovich, Mathur, Kamat, & Shapiro, 1992).

Lymphomas are genetically characterized by the presence of chromosomal translocations, which are usually balanced reciprocal recombinations that involve a switch of DNA between two chromosomes. Such chromosomal rearrangements are *not* heritable and are thought to occur during immune reactions against various infectious agents, particularly EBV. Rearrangements often involve the immunoglobulin genes of B cells or the receptor genes of T cells (Tycko & Sklar, 1990). At the molecular level, such translocations induce neoplastic development by either activating tumor oncogenes or inactivating tumor suppressor genes. The most common translocations found in NHLs involve juxtaposition of genes that regulate transcription to regions of chromosome 14 that control promotion and enhancement elements of highly active immunoglobulin genes. In studies of lymphoma karyotypes, chromosomal translocations have been detected in up to 90% of NHLs (Grogan & Miller, 1995; Offit, Wong, Filippa, Tao, & Chaganti, 1991; Vega & Medeiros, 2003; Ye, 2000).

HIV Disease and Non-Hodgkin's Lymphoma

Following the onset of the AIDS epidemic and the discovery of HIV in the early 1980s, population registries were established in many countries in order to monitor the number of new cases and evaluate the impact of widespread efforts to control the epidemic. Analysis of the HIV/AIDS registry data has helped elucidate important clues regarding the genesis of NHL.

In 1999, a team of Italian investigators reported findings on the association of lymphoma and HIV disease based on registry data from the United States, Europe, and Australia. The study involved the analysis of datasets developed by linking registries of AIDS patients with population-based cancer registries. During 1988–1997, AIDS surveillance data from 17 Western European countries revealed that more than 7000 cases involved NHL as the AIDS-defining illness, and during the 1990s, NHL was the AIDS-defining condition in approximately 5% of cases. Among adults with HIV/AIDS, the relative risks for NHL ranged from 15 for low-grade disease (confined to one lymph node) to 400 for high-grade disease (affecting multiple nodes and/or sites). The relative risk (RR) of Hodgkin's lymphoma among individuals with HIV/AIDS was also increased (RR = 10). The extraordinarily high risk for the development of NHL among individuals who are HIV-seropositive has led to its recognition as an AIDS-defining condition (Dal Maso & Franceschi, 2003; Franceschi, Dal Maso, & La Vecchia, 1999).

The HIV-associated NHLs are invariably derived from B lymphocytes, and more than 80% originated at extranodal sites, most commonly in the brain and central nervous system. These lymphomas usually present as high-grade malignancies, with 60%–70% being metastatic at the time of diagnosis. An Australian case–control study identified the duration of immunosuppression and the degree of B-cell stimulation as primary risk factors (Grulich et al., 2000). Although sequences of the HIV genome have never been found incorporated into the DNA of lymphoma cells, it is notable that EBV is often present in tumor tissues and/or the cerebral spinal fluid of cases. It has thus been suggested that interactions involving co-infection with EBV and/or other viruses predispose to the development of NHL through immunosuppression and impairment of cell-mediated immunity in patients with HIV disease (Biggar, Frisch, Engels, & Goedert, 2001; Cinque et al., 1993).

Immunosuppression and Non-Hodgkin's Lymphoma

Immunosuppression has consistently been found to be a strong risk factor in the development of NHL. Individuals with drug-induced immunodeficiency for the purpose of suppressing posttransplant organ rejection or treating autoimmune conditions or resulting from sustained chemotherapy for cancer are among those at high risk. Enormous increases in RR (more than 100-fold) have been observed in organ transplant patients who receive sustained aggressive immunosuppressive regimens (Opelz & Henderson, 1993). As with HIV/AIDS patients, active infection with EBV is a common finding in posttransplant patients (Cleary, Chao, Warnke, & Sklar, 1984; Kinlen, 1992; Purtilo, 1980). Furthermore, a striking feature of some posttransplant patients who receive aggressive therapy is the short interval from the time of transplant to the diagnosis of malignancy, often within 6 months (Swinnen et al., 1990). Such rapidly evolving tumors have a predilection for the brain and are associated with sustained immunosuppression and active EBV infection (Palackdharry, 1994).

Molecular studies suggest that three host-factors interact to increase the risk of developing NHL in immunosuppressed individuals: active EBV infection, defects in immunoregulation and production of inflammatory cytokines, and genetic defects precipitating abnormal immunoglobulin and T-cell receptor gene rearrangement. Both congenital and acquired immunodeficiencies appear to have common features that predispose to chronic antigenic stimulus of B lymphocytes and the development of NHL (Filipovich et al., 1992).

Autoimmune Disease and Non-Hodgkin's Lymphoma

The risk of developing NHL is also increased in patients with autoimmune conditions such as rheumatoid arthritis, systemic lupus erythematosus, Sjogren's syndrome, and celiac disease (Harris, Cooke, Thompson, & Waterhouse, 1967; Kamel, van de Rijn, Hanasono, & Warnke, 1995; Pettersson, Pukkala, Teppo, & Friman, 1992). Although such conditions are conventionally treated with immunosuppressive drugs, persistent inflammation appears to have a dominant etiologic role in the genesis of lymphoma. For example, Baecklund and colleagues demonstrated a 25-fold increase in the risk of developing NHL among patients with highly inflammatory rheumatoid arthritis compared to a similar group with low inflammation, after adjustment for treatment (Baecklund, Ekbom, Sparén, Feltelius, & Klareskog, 1998).

EBV and Burkitt's Lymphoma

EBV is a member of the herpes family of viruses. The virus is ubiquitous in the human population. Following infection in childhood, EBV persists in a dormant state as an episomal plasmid in B lymphocytes in 80%–90% of adults. When the first exposure to EBV occurs in adolescence, up to 50% of individuals manifest *infectious mononucleosis*. If an EBV-positive individual experiences sustained immunosuppression (as in HIV disease or posttransplant immunosuppressive therapy), the EBV plasmid can transform into active virus and resume proliferation in B lymphocytes. Such activity markedly heightens the risk of developing NHL (Alexander, Mink, Adami, Chang, et al., 2007; Fisher & Fisher, 2004; Müller et al., 2005).

In populations residing in the tropical zone of Africa, a form of childhood B-cell lymphoma called *Burkitt's lymphoma* is endemic. This tumor typically arises in the jaw bones. Burkitt's lymphoma is named after the British investigator Denis Burkitt, who studied its epidemiology and etiology in the children of New Guinea and sub-Saharan Africa. Burkitt's lymphoma develops in children in these geographic regions with a startlingly high incidence rate, accounting for up to 25% of all childhood malignancies (Burkitt, 1958, 1983).

In pathologic studies of Burkitt's lymphoma ascertained from the endemic areas of Africa and New Guinea, EBV is detected in nearly 100% of cases. Epstein and colleagues first detected EBV in a lymphoma specimen taken from a child in New Guinea, providing the first example of a tumor-related virus (Epstein, Achong, & Pope, 1967). Most cases also have a medical history of malaria and have been found to have elevated levels of antibodies against both EBV and the malarial parasite *Plasmodium falciparum* (Carpenter et al., 2008). Burkitt initially noted the geographic clustering of EBV and malarial infection and suggested that the convergence of these two infectious agents in the same host predisposes to the development of B-cell lymphoma (Burkitt, 1971, 1983).

A defining cytogenetic feature of nearly all cases of Burkitt's lymphoma is the presence of a chromosomal translocation involving the *c-myc* gene. The *c-myc* gene, which is normally located on the long arm of chromosome 8, encodes a protein that is essential for the regulation of transcription and expression of many other genes. Translocations of the *c-myc* gene to positions very near the heavy chain immunoglobulin loci on chromosome 14 have been found in approximately 80% of cases of Burkitt's lymphoma, and translocations of *c-myc* to immunoglobulin loci on chromosomes 2 and 12 are present in the remaining 20% of cases. These *c-myc* translocations result in hyperactivity of immunoglobulin genes and overproliferation of B cells, leading to the development of lymphoma. Transformation to malignancy involves the perpetual proliferation of B lymphocytes involving dysregulation of mitosis, differentiation, apoptosis, and cell adhesion (Blum, Lozanski, & Byrd, 2004; Ferry, 2006).

It is obvious from the preceding discussion that the pathogenesis of Burkitt's lymphoma is complex, often involving the interaction of at least three factors: EBV infection, malarial infection, and chromosomal translocation involving the *c-myc* gene. A stepwise process has been proposed in which EBV and malaria may depress the regulatory function of T cells, leading to unbridled proliferation of B cells with the *c-myc* translocation (de Thé, 1993).

The clinical variants of Burkitt's lymphoma include endemic, sporadic, and immunodeficiency-related disease. Endemic Burkitt's lymphoma occurs in young African children, aged 4–7 years, with a male-to-female ratio of 2:1. The incidence is about 13 per 100,000 in children of endemic areas such as New Guinea and sub-Saharan Africa, more than 50 times higher than in U.S. children. The tumors characteristically involve the jaw bone but can also arise in the gastrointestinal and/or urogenital tract (Ferry, 2006). EBV is present in nearly all cases, and high levels of antibodies against both EBV and *Plasmodium falciparum* have been found to increase the risk by fivefold (Carpenter et al., 2008). As initially suggested by Denis Burkitt, the immunosuppressive effect of chronic malarial infection predisposes the host to EBV-induced proliferation and malignant transformation of B lymphocytes (Burkitt, 1983).

Sporadic Burkitt's lymphoma occasionally develops in children *without* geographic or temporal clustering. The gastrointestinal tract, particularly around the ileocecal valve, is the most common anatomic site of involvement. EBV is present in only 10%–30% of sporadic tumors (Ferry, 2006).

Immunodeficiency-associated Burkitt's lymphoma occurs in association with HIV/AIDS, organ transplant, and congenital immunodeficiency. Burkitt's lymphoma accounts for 30%–40% of NHL in patients with HIV disease and is estimated to be 1000 times more common in such patients than in the general population. Analogous to malaria, HIV infection and other immunosuppressive conditions lead to EBV-induced proliferation and malignant transformation of B lymphocytes (Ferry, 2006).

Human T-Cell Lymphotropic Virus and Lymphoma

In 1974, Japanese investigators discovered a rare form of T-cell leukemia in two Japanese adults (Yodoi, Takatsuki, & Masuda, 1974). Further investigation soon identified a cluster of 16 patients with lymphoma or leukemia arising from T lymphocytes in the population living on the islands off the southern coast of Japan (Takatsuki, Uchiyama, Sagawa, & Yodoi, 1977; Uchiyama, Yodoi, Sagawa, Takatsuki, & Uchino, 1977). Shortly thereafter, in the laboratories of Dr. Robert Gallo at the U.S. National Institutes of Health, an RNA retrovirus was identified in malignant T cells of tumor specimens and named *human T-cell lymphotropic virus* (*HTLV-1*) (Poiesz et al., 1980). In studies conducted by Japanese investigators, T-cell-specific antibodies were detected in 76 of 80 patients (95%) with T-cell leukemia/lymphoma and 26% of healthy adults from endemic areas (Hinuma et al., 1981; Yoshida, Miyoshi, & Hinuma, 1982).

Subsequent epidemiologic investigations have confirmed the presence of high seroprevalence rates of HTLV-1 in populations of Southern Japan (30%), the Caribbean (7%), New Guinea (5%), and Central Africa (3%). In endemic regions, adult T-cell lymphomas and leukemias account for more than 50% of all lymphoid malignancies (Manns & Blattner, 2003).

Seropositivity for HTLV-1 develops early in life because of vertical transmission from mother to child during delivery or breastfeeding. The virus can also be transmitted sexually and through transfusion of contaminated blood. With sustained infection beginning in childhood, the cumulative lifetime risk of developing T-cell lymphoma/leukemia approaches 5% (Cleghorn et al., 1995). Carriers of HTLV-1 apparently manifest progressive immunosuppression and uncontrolled proliferation of infected helper T cells that can eventually lead to the development of adult T-cell lymphoma or leukemia (Takatsuki, 2005).

Helicobacter pylorus and Non-Hodgkin's Lymphoma

Helicobacter pylorus (*H. pylorus*) is a flagellated bacterium that infects the gastric mucosa. This unusual bacterium was discovered by Australian investigators Barry Marshall and Robin Warren in 1982, in recognition of which they were awarded the 2005 Nobel Prize in Physiology or Medicine (Marshall & Warren, 2005). It is estimated that more than 50% of the world's population harbor *H. pylori* in their upper gastrointestinal tract (Pounder & Ng, 1995).

Since its discovery, numerous investigations have examined linkages between *H. pylori* and human disease. Chronic colonization of the gastric mucosa by *H. pylori* is associated with chronic gastritis and the development of peptic ulcer disease, gastric adenocarcinoma, and gastric lymphoma arising in mucous-associated lymphoid tissue (gastric MALT lymphoma) (Isaacson & Spencer, 1995; Kusters, van Vliet, & Kuipers, 2006).

The evidence linking chronic *H. pylori* infection to the genesis of gastric lymphoma is compelling. In a study conducted in London, Wotherspoon and colleagues detected *H. pylori* in 101 of 110 cases with primary gastric MALT lymphoma and suggested that infection-induced gastritis provides the background lymphoid tissue in which NHL develops (Wotherspoon, Ortiz-Hidalgo, Falzon, & Isaacson, 1991).

At Stanford University in California, Parsonnet and colleagues conducted a nested case–control study to evaluate the potential role of *H. pylorus* in the development of non-Hodgkin's gastric lymphoma. (In a nested study design, the cases accrue over time in a specific cohort after collection of baseline data, and matched controls are ascertained from the same cohort.) The investigators compared baseline *H. pylori* seropositivity in 33 patients who developed gastric NHL to controls matched 4:1 to the cases on age, gender, and time of serum collection. Results revealed more than a sixfold increase in the risk of developing gastric lymphoma related to baseline *H. pylori* seropositivity. The median interval between serum collection for *H. pylori* testing and onset of gastric lymphoma was 14 years, suggesting a long-term process of carcinogenesis (Parsonnet et al., 1994).

Subsequent in vitro experiments have demonstrated that malignant B cells proliferate only after T-cell-specific activation by *H. pylori* (Hussell, Isaacson, Crabtree, & Spencer, 1993). In clinical studies, antibiotic therapy directed against *H. pylori* infection produced regression of low-grade gastric lymphoma (Wotherspoon et al., 1993). These findings support a model of chronic *H. pylori* infection, chronic inflammation, and T-cell-modulated antigenic stimulation of B-cell proliferation in the pathogenesis of gastric MALT lymphoma (Wotherspoon, 1998).

Human Herpes Virus 8

Human herpes virus 8 (HHV-8), also called *Kaposi's sarcoma-associated herpes virus (KSHV)*, was discovered by Yuan Chang, Patrick Moore, and colleagues at Columbia University in 1994 (Chang et al., 1994). This virus has been detected in most patients with primary effusion lymphoma, a rare B-cell lymphoma seen almost exclusively in HIV-positive patients (Cesarman, Chang, Moore, Said, & Knowles, 1995). Such patients often present with dual EBV and HHV-8 infection; therefore, delineation of the etiologic role of each virus is difficult. Primary effusion lymphomas appear to involve monoclonal expansion of viral-infected cells (Judde et al., 2000).

Hepatitis C Virus and Non-Hodgkin's Lymphoma

Approximately 300 million people worldwide are infected with *hepatitis C virus (HCV)*, a single-strand RNA virus. The seroprevalence of HCV is high in certain populations of Asia and Africa (3%) and low in most developed countries (1%). Although not known to be oncogenic, HCV has immunomodulatory effects and has been shown to replicate in peripheral blood mononuclear cells.

Although HCV is a major etiologic factor in the development of hepatocellular carcinoma, its role in the development of NHL is less clear. Early molecular studies detected anti-HCV antibodies in sera and HCV RNA sequences in biopsy specimens from some patients with B-cell NHL (Luppi et al., 1998; Silvestri et al., 1996). A systematic review of HCV seroprevalence among NHL patients revealed high rates in some populations (Southern and Eastern Europe, Japan, and Southern United States) but not in others (Northern Europe, Northern United States, Canada, and certain Asian countries) (Negri, Little, Boiocchi, La Vecchia, & Franceschi, 2004). Nevertheless, in a pooled analysis of 48 studies of B-cell NHL, HCV infection was present in 13% of 5542 patients; based on meta-analysis of 10 studies that included estimates of the odds ratio (OR), the overall risk was increased more than 10-fold (combined OR = 10.8) (Gisbert, García-Buey, Pajares, & Moreno-Otero, 2003). In a subsequent meta-analysis of 23 studies of HCV and NHL, HCV-seropositive subjects were nearly six times more likely to develop NHL than HCV-seronegative subjects (combined OR = 5.7) (Matsuo et al., 2004).

Despite the increase in lymphoma risk with HCV exposure suggested by meta-analyses, it is noteworthy that some studies *do not* reflect an association between HCV and NHL. For example, in a prospective study of 48,420 persons in northern California, serological evidence of HCV infection was *totally absent* in all 57 patients who developed NHL (Rabkin et al., 2002). And in Thailand, a nation with a relatively high prevalence of HCV, no link was found between HCV infection and NHL (Udomsakdi-Auewarakul, Auewarakul, Sukpanichnant, & Muangsup, 2000). Furthermore, in a U.S. study of 304,411 adults with AIDS, standardized incidence ratios of NHL by grade were *inversely* related to the prevalence rates of HCV infection (Engels et al., 2002). These disparities among study results may have multiple causes, including genetic, cultural, and/or environmental differences in populations; variation in HCV strains; and the different methods used for the diagnosis of lymphoma and/or assessment of HCV seropositivity (Alexander, Mink, Adami, Chang, et al., 2007).

Simian Virus 40 and Non-Hodgkin's Lymphoma

Millions of people worldwide were inadvertently exposed to live *simian virus 40 (SV40)* between 1955 and 1963 through immunization with SV40-contaminated polio vaccines. This virus is known to induce malignancies in laboratory animals, including primary brain cancer, bone cancer, mesothelioma, and lymphoma. Recent molecular studies have shown that SV40 DNA is present in a significant fraction (~40%) of tumor specimens from patients with NHL (Shivapurkar et al., 2002; Vilchez et al., 2002).

Butel and colleagues studied SV40 seropositivity in malignant lymphoid tissues from 156 patients with NHL (76 HIV-positive patients and 78 HIV-negative patients), in nonmalignant lymphoid samples from 107 patients without tumors, and in colorectal tumors from 54 patients. Polymerase chain reaction and Southern blot hybridization techniques were used to detect the DNA sequences of SV40. Specific SV40 DNA sequences were detected in 64 specimens (42%) from lymphoma patients compared to *none* of the nonmalignant lymphoid specimens or colorectal tumors (Butel, Vilchez, Jorgensen, & Kozinetz, 2003). Furthermore, a retrospective study in Japan demonstrated a fourfold increase in the odds of detecting SV40 sequences in large B-cell lymphomas (19%) compared to controls (4.7%), suggesting that SV40 may be a candidate etiologic factor for lymphoma (Nakatsuka et al., 2003).

The findings of SV40 DNA sequences in human lymphoma prompted population-based studies in Denmark and the United States that compared cancer incidence rates in cohorts of children with and without exposure to the (allegedly) contaminated Salk polio vaccine. Fortunately, these studies found *no* increase in cancer rates associated with exposure (Carroll-Pankhurst et al., 2001; Engels et al., 2003).

Not all studies have found an association between SV40 and lymphoma. For example, a Spanish study that used enzyme immunoassay to detect antibodies to SV40 in sera from 520 patients with NHL and 587 matched controls actually found a higher frequency of SV40 seropositivity among the controls than cases (9.5% versus 5.9%) (de Sanjose et al., 2003). In addition, a molecular study that assessed SV40 antibody reactivity found no significant difference in the frequency of seropositivity between serum samples from

724 cases of NHL and 622 matched controls (Engels et al., 2004). Given these contrasting results, it seems advisable to clarify the differences in studies of SV40 DNA sequences and seropositivity through additional investigations.

Other Pathogens and Non-Hodgkin's Lymphoma

Borrelia burgdorferi is a small spirochete that can be transmitted to humans by the bite of an infected tick. Systemic human infection with this microorganism (borreliosis) causes skin rash, arthritis, and neurologic deficits, a clinical picture commonly referred to as Lyme disease. Recently, infection with *B. burgdorferi* has been linked to lymphoproliferative conditions, which have been known to evolve into primary cutaneous B-cell lymphomas. Most of these observations have come from European countries, with little evidence of such an association in North America (Cerroni, Zochling, Putz, & Kerl, 1997; Garbe, Stein, Dienemann, & Orfanos, 1991; Jelic & Filipovic-Ljeskovic, 1999; Willemze et al., 1997).

Mantle cell lymphoma, a B-cell malignancy arising in the mantle zone of lymph nodes, has also been found in association with borreliosis. Schöllkopf and colleagues conducted a Danish–Swedish case–control study of 3055 patients with NHL and 3187 population controls to evaluate the association of lymphoma subtypes with *B. burgdorferi*. History of tick bite or *Borrelia* infection was ascertained through personal interviews and enzyme-linked immunosorbent assay serum analyses for antibodies against *B. burgdorferi*. Self-reported history of *B. burgdorferi* infection (OR = 2.5) and seropositivity for anti-*Borrelia* antibodies (OR = 3.6) were both found to increase the risk of mantle cell lymphoma, suggesting that *B. burgdorferi* infection predisposes to the development of this malignancy (Schöllkopf et al., 2008).

Other infectious agents have also been found in association with B-cell lymphomas. *Mediterranean lymphoma* is an unusual B-cell lymphoma that arises in small intestinal MALT. Early-stage disease regresses with antibiotic treatment, suggesting a bacterial etiology. In a recent small series, five of seven tumor specimens of Mediterranean lymphoma tested positive for the intestinal bacteria *Campylobacter jejuni* (Lecuit et al., 2004).

Ocular adnexal lymphoma, a rare form of lymphoma that arises in the conjunctival membranes of the eye socket, also shows an association with an infectious microbe. In a molecular study of ocular adnexal lymphoma samples, 32 of 40 tumors (80%) carried *Chlamydia psittaci* DNA, whereas all specimens were negative for *Chlamydia trachomatis* and *Chlamydia pneumoniae*. This observation suggests that *Chlamydia psittaci* infection predisposes to the development of ocular adnexal lymphoma (Ferreri et al., 2004).

Clearly, the number of pathogens involved in the genesis of immunoproliferative lymphoid neoplasms is growing. As a rule, these infectious agents appear to enhance the initiation and promotion of malignancy by antigenic stimulation of B cells coupled with immunosuppression of T cells.

Pesticide and Insecticide Exposures in Non-Hodgkin's Lymphoma

Several cohort and case–control studies have evaluated exposure to pesticides, insecticides, and/or herbicides as risk factors in the development of NHL. In general, nonsignificant findings have been reported.

For example, Blair and colleagues studied a U.S. cohort of 52,393 licensed pesticide applicators and 32,345 spouses and found *no* significant associations between lymphoma mortality with the number of years handling pesticides or any other measure of exposure. The overall mortality due to NHL in the cohort showed no difference from the general population (standardized mortality ratio = 1.0) (Blair et al., 2005). Several other cohort studies also evaluated the risk of developing NHL among persons employed in occupations involving potential exposure to pesticides, herbicides, and/or insecticides. Studies of occupational cohorts of farmers, pesticide-manufacturing workers, and pesticide applicators from Italy, Iceland, Sweden, Norway, Canada, and Australia have yielded mixed and generally nonsignificant results (Alexander, Mink, Adami, Chang, et al., 2007).

Meta-analyses of published studies of agricultural workers reflect the inconsistency in results. In an analysis of 14 studies that evaluated cancer risk among farmers, the combined estimate of NHL risk was not significant (Blair, Zahm, Pearce, Heineman, & Fraumeni, 1992). Subsequently, a meta-analysis of 36 studies found a weak positive association overall (RR = 1.10); however, there was significant heterogeneity among studies, and the directional change in risk differed for case–control studies (RR = 1.19) and cohort studies (RR = 0.95) (Khuder, Schaub, & Keller-Byrne, 1998).

Thus, although a few studies suggest there may be an increased risk of NHL in occupations with heightened exposure to pesticides and related compounds, technical difficulties inherent in assessment of the intensity and duration of exposure limit any interpretation of causality. Studies that infer exposure based on occupation or job title have many limitations, most notably the lack of detailed information regarding exposure to specific environmental factors for each individual. Furthermore, complete information on other potential exposures or confounding factors is often missing or not collected. Results of these studies therefore reflect a general lack of consistent evidence to support an etiologic link between pesticide/herbicide/insecticide exposure and the development of NHL (Alexander, Mink, Adami, Chang, et al., 2007; Fisher & Fisher, 2004; Müller et al., 2005).

Other Chemical Exposures and Non-Hodgkin's Lymphoma

Studies of chemical workers have also failed to delineate consistent associations with NHL. Studies of workers potentially exposed to petroleum products, solvents, trichloroethylene, asbestos, occupational dusts, and other chemicals have generally been negative or inconclusive. Thus, as with pesticides and herbicides, epidemiologic investigations have not clearly identified specific occupational exposures to specific chemicals that increase the risk of developing NHL (Alexander, Mink, Adami, Chang, et al., 2007; Figgs, Dosemeci, & Blair, 1995).

Hair Dye and Non-Hodgkin's Lymphoma

Hair dyes contain compounds that are mutagenic and carcinogenic in animals. Numerous human studies have therefore evaluated the relationship between exposure to these compounds and the risk of developing malignant neoplasms, including NHL. Based on a meta-analysis of 14 studies, Takkouche and colleagues reported a significant increase in the risk among ever users of hair dye compared to never users (combined RR = 1.23). However, there was significant heterogeneity among studies, and the risk estimate derived from case–control studies (RR = 1.27) was higher than that from cohort studies (RR = 1.10). Thus, differential recall between cases and controls may have contributed to the elevated risk estimates in the case–control studies. Furthermore, dose–response relationships have not been consistently observed between lymphoma risk and the duration of use (Takkouche, Etminan, & Montes-Martinez, 2005).

Ultraviolet Radiation and Non-Hodgkin's Lymphoma

Zheng and colleagues speculated that sun exposure might increase the risk of developing NHL on the following grounds: The incidence of NHL has increased in parallel with that of cutaneous melanoma; antecedent

skin cancer increases the risk of developing NHL; sun exposure has immunosuppressive effects; and the risk of NHL increases with immunosuppression (Zheng et al., 1992). In support of this hypothesis, Cartwright and colleagues reported a significant positive correlation between the incidence rates of NHL and non-melanocytic skin cancer among nine cancer registries worldwide (Cartwright, McNally, & Staines, 1994).

In opposition to this hypothesis, three case–control studies of NHL and sun exposure found significant *inverse* relationships (Armstrong & Kricker, 2007). Thus, the data on individual sun exposure and risk of NHL are more consistent with a *protective* than a causal effect of sun exposure. Furthermore, in a geographic study of annual mortality rates reported during 1970–1989 for economic regions within the United States, the mortality rates due to NHL showed a significant *inverse* association with average levels of UV exposure, whereas the rates for melanoma increased with exposure (Hartge, Devesa, Grauman, Fears, & Fraumeni, 1996).

Because these studies were not powered to examine lymphoma subtypes, it is noteworthy that some molecular investigations have found indirect evidence linking sun exposure to the development of *cutaneous* NHLs. For example, McGregor and colleagues examined the type and frequency of *p53* gene mutations in a series of 55 cases of primary cutaneous lymphoma and found 14 separate *p53* mutations with a mutation spectrum characteristic of DNA damage caused by ultraviolet B radiation. These mutations were most evident in the progression of a type of cutaneous T-cell lymphoma known as *mycosis fungoides* (McGregor et al., 1999). Well-designed epidemiologic studies that are powered to examine lymphoma by subtype should help resolve the present conflicting results on sun exposure and NHL.

Tobacco, Alcohol, and Non-Hodgkin's Lymphoma

Tobacco and tobacco metabolites are known to be carcinogenic; however, there is little scientific evidence to support an association between tobacco use and the development of NHL. Zahm and colleagues examined smoking and NHL in a combined analysis of data from three population-based case–control studies conducted in four Midwestern states in the United States. Data on smoking and other variables were available for 1177 cases and 3625 controls. Overall, there was no association between smoking and the risk of developing NHL (OR = 1.0) and no clear dose–response relationships were evident (Zahm, Weisenburger, Holmes, Cantor, & Blair, 1997).

In a subsequent meta-analysis, Morton and colleagues examined the association between cigarette smoking and subtypes of NHL using data collected through the International Lymphoma Epidemiology Consortium (InterLymph). The database included information on smoking and other variables for 6594 cases and 8892 controls ascertained in nine case–control studies conducted in the United States, Europe, and Australia. Overall, smoking was associated with only a slight increase in the risk (OR = 1.07). Among subtypes of NHL, only follicular lymphoma was associated with current smoking (OR = 1.31); however, the test for trend with pack-years of smoking was not significant. Risk estimates for other subtypes ranged from 0.79 to 1.11 and were nonsignificant (Morton, Hartge, et al., 2005). These and many other epidemiologic investigations do not provide consistent evidence that tobacco exposure has a role in the genesis of NHL.

Several studies have detected a weak *inverse* association between alcohol consumption and the risk of developing NHL. Morton and colleagues examined the relationship in a pooled analysis of nine case–control studies conducted in the United States, Great Britain, Sweden, and Italy. Data on alcohol intake and other variables were available for 6492 cases and 8683 controls. Overall, the results suggested that people who drank alcohol had a slightly lower risk than nondrinkers (OR = 0.83), and current drinkers had a lower risk (OR = 0.73) than former drinkers (OR = 0.95). The investigators suggest the need for additional investigations to determine whether confounding by lifestyle factors or immunomodulatory effects by alcohol are responsible for this association (Morton, Zheng, et al., 2005).

Dietary Factors and Non-Hodgkin's Lymphoma

Nutritional studies of NHL reflect mixed results for most dietary factors investigated. One possible exception is fish consumption, which shows a weak *inverse* association with the risk of developing NHL in several studies. For example, in a U.S. study of 1418 cases and 4202 controls, intake in the highest quartile compared to the lowest quartile reduced the risk by 29% (Fritschi, Ambrosini, Kliewer, Johnson, & Canadian Cancer Registries Epidemiologic Research Group, 2004). Nevertheless, observed risk reductions do not reach statistical significance in all studies (Fernandez, Chatenoud, La Vecchia, Negri, & Franceschi, 1999); additional investigations are needed to clarify if high fish consumption has preventive value.

Blood Transfusions and Non-Hodgkin's Lymphoma

Interest in blood transfusion and its relation to NHL spiked after three prospective cohort studies reported increases in the risk of developing NHL following transfusion. Cerhan and colleagues initially investigated this association in a prospective cohort of 37,337 older women in Iowa. Baseline information was collected in 1986, and after 5 years of follow-up, a total of 68 cases of NHL were detected. Women who reported ever receiving a blood transfusion were at increased risk of developing NHL (RR = 2.2) (Cerhan et al., 1993). In a subsequent study of the same cohort of women after 12 years of follow-up resulting in detection of 229 cases of NHL, a significant risk increase (RR = 1.6) was again observed among women reporting a history of blood transfusion (Cerhan et al., 2001).

Shortly after publication of the initial findings from the Iowa cohort, Blomberg and colleagues reported similar increases in the risk of developing NHL associated with a history of blood transfusion in two Swedish cohorts (Blomberg, Möller, Olsson, Anderson, & Jonsson, 1993), and Memon and Doll found a greater than twofold increase in mortality due to NHL among subjects who had received perinatal transfusions in a cohort of 13,000 Britons (Memon & Doll, 1994). Moreover, several biological mechanisms seemed plausible to explain transfusion-related lymphoma development, including oncogenic virus transmission, transfusion-induced immunosuppression, and engraftment of malignant lymphoma cells from donors (Chow & Holly, 2002).

Nevertheless, five subsequent case–control studies have since revealed inconsistent results with only one showing a significant positive association. Thus, the association between blood transfusion and development of NHL remains to be clarified. As has been pointed out, future studies should be designed to collect more detailed information on the exposure variable, including the type and amount of transfusion products received by each subject. Similarly, such studies should be powered to facilitate risk estimates for lymphoma subtypes (Chow & Holly, 2002).

Breast Implants and Non-Hodgkin's Lymphoma

Anaplastic large cell lymphoma is a rare T-cell lymphoma typically seen in children and young adults. Such tumors are seldom detected in breast tissues. Nevertheless, published case reports of primary anaplastic large cell lymphoma arising in the fibrous capsules of breast implants have produced speculation that breast prostheses may increase the risk of developing this rare tumor (Bishara, Ross, & Sur, 2009).

To determine if the risk of developing anaplastic large cell lymphoma is related to breast implants, investigators in Amsterdam conducted a matched case–control study among women in the Netherlands. Cases and controls were ascertained from the population-based nationwide pathology registry. Eleven cases were identified who had been diagnosed with primary anaplastic large cell lymphoma of the breast during 1990–2006. Cases were age-matched to controls with other histologic types of breast lymphomas in an overall ratio of about 3:1. Among the 11 cases, 5 had received breast prostheses for cosmetic purposes 1–23 years prior to diagnosis, whereas among the 35 control patients, only one had received a breast implant. The odds ratio linking the development of anaplastic large cell lymphoma to breast prostheses was markedly increased and statistically significant (OR = 18.2, $P < 0.01$). Although these preliminary findings suggest an association between breast implants and the subsequent development of anaplastic large cell lymphoma of the breast, even women with implants have an exceedingly low *absolute risk* (de Jong et al., 2008).

Epidemiology of Hodgkin's Lymphoma

Hodgkin's lymphoma is a B-cell lymphoma that is defined by the presence of morphologically altered immune cells called Reed–Steinberg cells. In nations with population-based tumor registries, Hodgkin's lymphoma accounts for less than 15% of all lymphomas (Altekruse et al., 2010).

The disease is named after Thomas Hodgkin, who first described elemental clinical features of lymphoid malignancies in 1832 (Hodgkin, 1832). The Reed–Sternberg cell is named after Dorothy Reed and Carl Sternberg, who discovered it in the malignant lymphoid tissues of patients with Hodgkin's lymphoma more than a century ago (Reed, 1902; Sternberg, 1898). These giant multinucleate tumor cells sometimes have the unusual appearance of "owl eyes" peering out from the microscopic field due to the presence of a double nucleus (Lukes & Collins, 1975).

Because of the coexpression of markers of several different cell types in Hodgkin's lymphoma tissues, the cellular origin of Reed–Sternberg cells remained enigmatic for many decades. Nevertheless, isolation of these cells by microscopic laser dissection and gene amplification by polymerase chain reaction have clarified their derivation through the presence of immunoglobulin gene rearrangements. Thus, nearly a century after their discovery, Reed–Sternberg cells have been definitively characterized as transformed lymphocytes arising from B cells in the germinal centers of lymph nodes (Bräuninger et al., 1997; Kanzler, Küppers, Hansmann, & Rajewsky, 1996; Küppers et al., 1994).

Global Burden of Hodgkin's Lymphoma

Worldwide, 79,990 new cases of Hodgkin's lymphoma were diagnosed in 2018 and 26,167 people died from the disease. Of these, 46,559 cases (58%) and 15,770 deaths (60%) occurred in men. Age-adjusted incidence and mortality rates for men (1.1 per 100,000 and 0.4 per 100,000) were higher than for women (0.8 per 100,000 and 0.2 per 100,000) (Ferlay et al., 2018; Fitzmaurice et al., 2018).

Worldwide estimates of the annual number of deaths from Hodgkin's lymphoma have remained relatively stable during 1990–2018. Each year, 25,000–30,000 individuals die from the disease in an approximate 2:1 ratio of men to women (Fitzmaurice et al., 2017, 2018; Ferlay et al., 2010, 2013, 2018; Parkin, Bray, Ferlay, & Pisani, 2001; Parkin et al., 1999a, 1999b, 2005).

Incidence rates of Hodgkin's lymphoma tend to be higher in developed countries than developing countries. In 2018, rates exceeded 2 per 100,000 for the United States and Canada, Australia/New Zealand, and most nations of Western Europe and Scandinavia compared to rates less than 1 per 100,000 for China, India, and most nations of Southeast Asia and sub-Saharan Africa (Ferlay et al., 2018).

Mortality rates of Hodgkin's lymphoma show a different pattern than the incidence rates. In 2018, rates exceeded 0.5 per 100,000 in North and Central Africa, the Middle East, Northern Asia, and the Russian Federation compared to rates less than 0.5 in North America, Europe, China, and Australia/New Zealand. Disparities in incidence and mortality likely reflect underdiagnosis and lack of access to therapy in underserved populations.

Ethnic Differences and Trends in Hodgkin's Lymphoma in the United States

Based on data from the SEER program of the U.S. National Cancer Institute, 8490 new cases of Hodgkin's lymphoma were diagnosed in 2010 and 1320

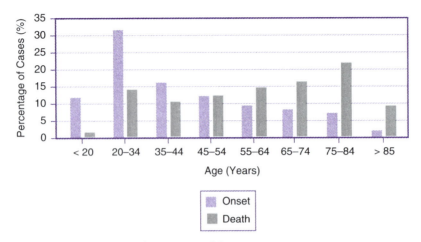

FIGURE 36.5 Age Distributions of Hodgkin's Lymphoma, United States.

Data from Altekruse, S. F., Kosary, C. L., Krapcho, M., Neyman, N., Aminou, R., Waldron, W., . . . Edwards, B. K. (2010). *SEER cancer statistics review, 1975–2007*. Bethesda, MD: National Cancer Institute.

individuals died from the disease. The highest annual incidence rates were observed among Caucasians (3.2 per 100,000 in men and 2.5 per 100,000 in women) and the lowest were among Asian/Pacific Islanders (1.5 per 100,000 in men and 1.1 per 100,000 in women). During the time period 1998–2007, incidence rates increased among U.S. men and women by about 2% per year. Nevertheless, during the same period, mortality rates declined, and 5-year survival rates now exceed 90% for patients who are diagnosed without distant metastasis (Altekruse et al., 2010).

Pathology of Hodgkin's Lymphoma

Classical Hodgkin's lymphoma always arises in lymph nodes and is classified into four subtypes. The most common of these is the *nodular sclerosing* type in which the affected lymph nodes are largely replaced by fibrotic tumor nodules. The second most common is the *mixed cellularity* subtype in which affected lymph nodes are infiltrated by inflammatory cells without fibrosis. *Lymphocyte-rich* and *lymphocyte-depleted* subtypes are rare forms (Lukes & Collins, 1975).

Recent molecular studies show that the malignant cells of Hodgkin's lymphoma often carry incapacitating mutations of the immunoglobulin genes (Bräuninger et al., 1997; Kanzler et al., 1996; Küppers et al., 1994). Furthermore, approximately 40% of Hodgkin's lymphomas are positive for EBV, and EBV-positive tumors typically carry mutations that induce aberrant signal transduction and render immunoglobulin genes ineffectual. These molecular findings suggest that viral proteins may induce mutational events in tumor suppressor genes and/or interfere with apoptosis and other processes that restrict cancer development (Bräuninger et al., 2006; Melbye, Hjalgrim, & Adami, 2008).

Genetic studies have found markedly higher concordance rates of Hodgkin's lymphoma among monozygous (identical) twins than dizygous twins, and risk increases have been observed in association with several antigens of the human leukocyte antigen (HLA) locus. Although these studies suggest that genetic variability at the HLA locus may influence the development of Hodgkin's lymphoma, it is noteworthy that familial Hodgkin's disease accounts for less than 5% of cases (Cartwright & Watkins, 2004).

Unlike NHL, which shows an exponential increase in age-specific incidence, Hodgkin's lymphoma has a bimodal age of onset distribution with an early peak (15–34 years of age) and a late peak (over 55 years of age). For example, in the United States during 2003–2007, 44% of cases were diagnosed before age 35 years and 28% were diagnosed at 55 years or older. Similarly, the distribution of deaths by age also shows an early peak at 20–34 years and a late peak at 75–84 years (**FIGURE 36.5**) (Altekruse et al., 2010).

▶ Risk Factors for Hodgkin's Lymphoma

Despite differences in their age distributions, the profile of factors that increase the risk of developing Hodgkin's lymphoma is like that of NHL. Risk factors include male gender, family history, recent history of infectious mononucleosis or active infection with EBV, a weakened immune system due to HIV disease or use of immunosuppressive drugs, and the presence of somatic mutations and/or gene rearrangements that cause dysfunction of immunoglobulins. Nevertheless, as discussed in the following section, genetic factors have now been identified that specifically increase the risk of developing Hodgkin's lymphoma in young adults. Interestingly, one such factor is linked to the development of multiple sclerosis, an autoimmune inflammatory disease that leads to demyelination of the axons of nerves.

Genetic Predisposition to Hodgkin's Lymphoma

Comparison of the frequencies of concordance/discordance among monozygous and dizygous twins provides strong evidence that genetic factors influence the early development of Hodgkin's lymphoma. Mack and colleagues conducted a long-term follow-up study of 432 sets of twins in which one twin had developed Hodgkin's lymphoma prior to 50 years of age, in order to evaluate the concordance/discordance of Hodgkin's lymphoma in monozygous versus dizygous twins. After an average of 14 years of follow-up, both twins developed Hodgkin's lymphoma in 10 of 179 pairs of monozygous twins (5.5%) compared to none of 187 pairs of dizygous twins. The investigators estimated that Hodgkin's lymphoma in one monozygous twin increased the risk of disease in the second twin nearly 100-fold and concluded that genetic factors play a significant role in the development of this malignancy (Mack et al., 1995).

Hodgkin's Lymphoma and Multiple Sclerosis

Case reports of familial clusters of multiple sclerosis and Hodgkin's lymphoma in young adults prompted a large investigation of this familial association in Denmark. Using Danish population-based registries, Hjalgrim and colleagues identified 11,790 patients with multiple sclerosis and estimated the incidence of Hodgkin's lymphoma in 19,599 of their first-degree relatives. Reciprocally, they also identified 4381 patients with Hodgkin's lymphoma and estimated the incidence of multiple sclerosis in 7388 of their first-degree relatives. Results revealed a significant increase in the risk of developing Hodgkin's lymphoma among the relatives of patients with multiple sclerosis (RR = 1.40) and a significant risk increase for multiple sclerosis among relatives of patients with Hodgkin's lymphoma (RR = 1.93). Based on these results, the investigators suggested that "a common genetic and/or immunologic predisposition to the two diseases may be mediated through interaction with environmental risk factors such as EBV infection" (Hjalgrim et al., 2004).

Recently, a genome-wide association study was conducted by a team of investigators in London for the purpose of identifying genetic polymorphisms associated with Hodgkin's lymphoma. In the investigation,

single nucleotide polymorphisms (SNPs) were compared among 2024 cases with Hodgkin's lymphoma and 1853 controls without disease. Findings revealed that susceptibility to Hodgkin's lymphoma was significantly elevated by a genetic variant of the eomesodermin (*EOMES*) gene on chromosome 3. This specific *EOMES* variant is known to disrupt cell-mediated immunity, and most notably, the same *EOMES* variant has also been found to heighten predisposition to multiple sclerosis. Thus, a specific genetic polymorphism of the *EOMES* gene appears to heighten susceptibility to both multiple sclerosis and Hodgkin's lymphoma in young adults (Frampton et al., 2013).

▶ Epidemiology of Multiple Myeloma

Multiple myeloma, also known as *plasma cell myeloma*, is a malignancy of plasma cells, which are B lymphocytes that produce antibodies. In this disease, collections of neoplastic plasma cells accumulate in bones and the bone marrow, causing bone lesions and interfering with the production of normal blood cells. Because *multiple* anatomic sites are usually involved in the same patient, the name *multiple myeloma* is appropriate. Characteristic signs and symptoms include hypercalcemia, renal failure, anemia, and bone lesions (Raab, Podar, Breitkreutz, Richardson, & Anderson, 2009).

Multiple myeloma develops from B lymphocytes that have migrated from the germinal centers of lymph nodes to other tissues. It is thus classified as a type of lymphoma. Cytogenetic features of multiple myeloma are like those of other B-cell lymphomas. Chromosomal translocations involving the immunoglobulin genes of chromosomes 2, 14, and 22 are often involved in the transformation of normal B cells to myeloma cells. For example, translocations and gene rearrangements involving the heavy chain immunoglobulin locus on chromosome 14 are found in approximately 50% of cases (Kyle & Rajkumar, 2004).

Global Burden of Multiple Myeloma

The annual numbers of cases of multiple myeloma and attributable deaths have more than doubled in the world population in the past three decades. In 2018, 159,985 new cases were diagnosed and 106,105 people died from multiple myeloma compared to 57,000 cases and 45,000 deaths in 1990 (Ferlay et al., 2010, 2013, 2018; Parkin et al., 1999a, 1999b). These increases are primarily due to increasing longevity, because diagnosis is rare prior to age

40 years, and nearly 95% of cases are diagnosed in individuals of 65 years and older.

Ethnic and Gender Differences in Multiple Myeloma

Striking ethnic differences are evident in U.S. rates of multiple myeloma. In particular, African-American men and women have the highest reported annual rates of multiple myeloma in the world (14.3 cases per 100,000 in men and 10.0 cases per 100,000 in women), more than double the rates found among Caucasians (6.7 per 100,000 in men and 4.1 per 100,000 in women) (**FIGURE 36.6**).

In search of an explanation for the high multiple myeloma rates among African Americans, studies were designed to elucidate possible genetic susceptibility. These early studies targeted the HLA locus on chromosome 6; in 1983, Leech and colleagues identified an HLA gene (*HLA-Cw2*) associated with excess risk among African-American cases (Leech, Brown, & Scharifeld, 1985; Leech et al., 1983). Subsequently, a larger study was conducted to further evaluate associations between myeloma risk and genotypes of the HLA locus. The study examined frequencies of *HLA-Cw2* and several other HLA antigens in 46 African-American cases and 88 controls, and 85 Caucasian cases and 122 controls. Findings revealed that the presence of *HLA-Cw2* significantly increased the risk in both African Americans (RR = 5.7) and Caucasians (RR = 2.6), suggesting that *HLA-Cw2* may contribute to the increased incidence among African Americans (Pottern et al., 1992).

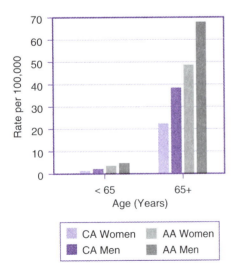

FIGURE 36.6 Annual Incidence of Multiple Myeloma by Age, Gender, and Race, United States.

Caption: CA = Caucasian American, AA = African American.

Data from Altekruse, S. F., Kosary, C. L., Krapcho, M., Neyman, N., Aminou, R., Waldron, W., ... Edwards, B. K. (2010). *SEER cancer statistics review, 1975–2007*. Bethesda, MD: National Cancer Institute.

As with other types of lymphoma, significant increases in the risk of developing multiple myeloma have been observed among patients with AIDS and certain other infectious conditions. Risk increases have been noted in cohorts of AIDS patients in the United States, Puerto Rico, and Australia (Goedert et al., 1998; Grulich, Wan, Law, Coates, & Kaldor, 1999). In a national Swedish cohort, the risk of multiple myeloma was significantly increased among individuals with hepatitis C infection (Duberg et al., 2005). In other studies, risk increases have been reported among relatives of myeloma patients, and a modest relationship has been observed between obesity and myeloma development (Alexander, Mink, Adami, Cole, et al., 2007).

Monoclonal gammopathy of undetermined significance (MGUS) refers to the presence of a high concentration of a specific monoclonal immunoglobulin protein in the blood. Such monoclonal proteins are sometimes called *paraproteins*. Patients with MGUS have been found to have a markedly increased risk of developing multiple myeloma.

In a series of 241 patients diagnosed with MGUS at the Mayo Clinic, 94 patients (39%) developed myeloma during 25 years of follow-up (Kyle et al., 2004). In a larger series of 1384 patients with MGUS, 115 patients progressed to multiple myeloma in 11,009 person-years of follow-up, and the RR of developing multiple myeloma was increased by 25-fold compared to the general population. These patients developed multiple myeloma or a related disorder at a rate of 1% per year, and the initial concentration of serum monoclonal protein was found to be a significant predictor of progression (Kyle et al., 2002). The prevalence rates of MGUS in population surveys have a pattern like the incidence rates of multiple myeloma in the U.S. population: African Americans have twofold higher rates than Caucasians (8.4% versus 3.6%), and men have higher rates than women (4.0% versus 2.7%) (Cohen, Crawford, Rao, Pieper, & Currie, 1998; Kyle et al., 2006).

In a landmark study of MGUS, Landgren and colleagues followed 77,469 adults enrolled in the nationwide population-based Prostate, Lung, Colorectal, and Ovarian (PLCO) Cancer Screening Trial. During the study, 71 subjects developed multiple myeloma; serum samples had been collected from them 2–10 years prior to diagnosis. Notably, MGUS was present in 100% of patients at least 2 years prior to the diagnosis of multiple myeloma, and the concentration of monoclonal protein was found to be a significant predictor of progression. Based on these results, the investigators concluded that, "monoclonal gammopathy of undetermined significance (MGUS) is a premalignant plasma cell proliferative disorder associated with a life-long risk of progression to multiple myeloma" (Landgren et al., 2009).

▶ Waldenström's Macroglobulinemia

Waldenström's macroglobulinemia is a rare condition characterized by a monoclonal gammopathy of immunoglobulin M (IgM) plus infiltration of the bone marrow by plasma cells derived from a single clone of B lymphocytes (Kumar, Abbas, & Aster, 2014). This condition was named after the Swedish physician Jan Gosta Waldenström, who first described two patients with the condition in 1944 (Waldenström, 1944). Though similar in some respects to myeloma, Waldenström's macroglobulinemia rarely causes bone lesions and is now classified as a form of low-grade NHL.

A team of investigators at the U.S. National Cancer Institute investigated associations between Waldenström's macroglobulinemia and chronic immunostimulatory conditions in a cohort of 4 million male veterans who received health care in Veteran's Administration (VA) hospitals during 1969–1996. Data on each subject were ascertained from computerized medical records maintained in the VA medical system. During an average follow-up of 12 years, a total of 361 cases of Waldenström's macroglobulinemia were identified, yielding an age-standardized incidence of 0.34 cases per 100,000 person-years. Disease risk was significantly elevated in individuals with autoimmune conditions (RR = 2.2), hepatitis (RR = 3.4), HIV disease (RR = 12.1), or rickettsiosis (RR = 3.4), a zoonotic infection transmitted by ticks and fleas. These results suggest that chronic immune stimulation plays an important role in the etiology and pathogenesis of Waldenström's macroglobulinemia (Koshiol, Gridley, Engels, McMaster, & Landgren, 2008).

In addition to chronic immune stimulation, most patients with Waldenström's macroglobulinemia have been found to carry chromosomal defects. Deletion of the long arm of chromosome 6 (6q deletion) is the most commonly observed cytogenetic abnormality. In a U.S. study, bone marrow samples from 38 patients were examined by fluorescence in situ hybridization (FISH), and 6q deletions were detected in 21 of the 38 specimens (55%) (Schop et al., 2006). Subsequently, in a larger international study of 102 patients, 6q deletions were detected in 54% of bone marrow specimens and were found to be associated with a worsened prognosis (Ocio et al., 2007).

In summary, the general epidemiologic features of Waldenström's macroglobulinemia are like those of other forms of lymphoma. The trisomic combination of immunosuppression, chronic antigenic stimulation, and specific chromosomal aberrations stimulate the terminal differentiation of plasma cells that subsequently invade and proliferate uncontrollably in the bone marrow.

▶ Models of Pathogenesis of Lymphoma

Biological mechanisms responsible for the genesis of lymphoma are variable and complex, and although some events and interactions have been elucidated, much remains to be discovered. In many patients, lymphomagenesis appears to involve chronic antigenic stimulation by one or more infectious agents in combination with chromosomal translocations, somatic mutations, gene rearrangements, and/or epigenetic changes that cause dysregulation and/or hyperactivity of immunoglobulin genes. Although the exact sequence of molecular events is unknown, the end result is the perpetual proliferation of lymphocytes characteristic of lymphoid malignancy. Imbalance in the function of T and B lymphocytes appears to be an important stimulus. For example, drug-induced immunosuppression of T cells in conjunction with active EBV infection and B-cell response has been found to rapidly accelerate the genesis of lymphoma in posttransplant patients and those with HIV disease. The complex nature of lymphomagenesis is perhaps best illustrated by endemic Burkitt's lymphoma, a B-cell malignancy that involves a trisomy of risk factors (chronic EBV and malarial infection in combination with chromosomal translocation of the *c-myc* oncogene to a position very near one of the immunoglobulin loci) (de Thé, 1993; Ferry, 2006; Küppers, 2005).

▶ Prevention of AIDS-Related Lymphoma

Primary prevention of AIDS-related lymphomas depends largely upon avoiding HIV infection (Thun, DeLancey, Center, Jemal, & Ward, 2010). Preventive behaviors include sexual abstinence, monogamous sex with an uninfected partner, regular condom use, and abstinence from injection drug use. Similar precautions are recommended for individuals who are HIV-positive to prevent infecting others and avoid other sexually transmitted and blood-borne diseases. Screening of high-risk individuals to identify HIV seropositivity is therefore imperative for control of AIDS and AIDS-related conditions, including lymphoma.

Tertiary Prevention of Lymphoma in AIDS Patients

Key measures of immunosuppression and disease progression in patients with AIDS include the CD4 and CD8 lymphocyte counts and the viral load. In particular, severe immunosuppression reflected by a very low CD4 count is a major risk factor for the development of AIDS-related lymphoma.

In recent years, a variety of antiretroviral drugs have been developed for the treatment of patients with AIDS. In randomized clinical trials conducted in several countries, antiretroviral drugs taken in combination have proved superior to single-drug regimens in reducing the HIV viral load and improving the CD4 lymphocyte count. Such multidrug therapy is called *highly active antiretroviral therapy (HAART)*. Furthermore, following the introduction of HAART, the incidence of AIDS-related lymphoma has dramatically declined.

An example of the chemopreventive value of HAART against lymphoma development comes from the Swiss HIV Cohort Study. In this investigation, 12,959 people with HIV disease were followed during 1984–2006 to assess the long-term impact of HAART compared to single-drug regimens. For the entire cohort, 429 cases of NHL were detected in 75,222 person-years of observation. Patients receiving HAART contributed 36,787 person-years in the study. The annual incidence of NHL in the cohort peaked during pre-HAART years, 1993–1995 (13.6 per 1000 person-years), and reached a nadir during post-HAART years, 2002–2006 (1.8 per 1000 person-years). After adjustment for age, baseline CD4 count, and other variables, HAART was found to reduce the risk of developing NHL by 76% (hazard ratio = 0.74). Furthermore, the reduction in risk has been sustained up to 10 years after initiation of HAART, even among patients with a low-baseline CD4 count. These findings support the efficacy of HAART regardless of immune impairment at initiation of treatment. The investigators concluded that "although it was already clear that HAART prevents [non-Hodgkin's lymphoma] through improvement of immune status, this study shows that HAART avoids the majority of non-Hodgkin's lymphoma], even among the most severely immunosuppressed individuals" (Polesel et al., 2008).

▶ Summary

In many nations of the world, particularly those with population-based cancer registries, incidence rates of NHL, Hodgkin's lymphoma, and multiple myeloma have risen steadily in the past three decades. These upward trends reflect increases in three immunological states: immunosuppression due to primary or acquired immunodeficiency, chronic antigenic stimulation, and disruption of normal lymphocyte function and proliferation. Other contributing factors include heightened rates of immune dysfunction in aging populations and improvements in the detection and reporting of these malignancies.

Rates of lymphoma are high in patients with acquired immunosuppression due to HIV infection, in posttransplant patients treated with immunosuppressive drugs, and in patients with autoimmune conditions or cancer who received immunosuppressive chemotherapy. Heightened antigenic stimulation often involves active infection by ubiquitous microbes such as EBV and *H. pylori* in a genetically susceptible host. Genetic errors in immunoglobulin genes due to somatic mutations and gene rearrangements are characteristic of many lymphomas, and such mutations have been found to induce aberrant signal transduction and render immunoglobulin genes ineffectual. Exposure to other exogenous factors such as agrichemicals, ultraviolet radiation, and allogeneic blood transfusions may also heighten the risk.

Prevention involves avoidance or elimination of factors known to cause immunodeficiency and/or that inordinately heighten the antigenic response. Screening high-risk groups for the presence of HIV and *H. pylori* are advisable measures for lymphoma control. As pointed out in a review of NHL, "Interdisciplinary collaborations are needed to investigate the broad scope of factors that may alter individual susceptibility and promote lymphoid malignancies" (Fisher & Fisher, 2004).

Therapy for Lymphoma

Results of clinical trials suggest that the addition of monoclonal antibodies to regimens of conventional chemotherapeutic agents has significantly improved the survival rates for patients with NHL. A variety of monoclonal antibodies are under study, many of which target cell-membrane receptors of lymphocytes. One example is rituximab, which specifically targets the CD20 receptors of B lymphocytes. Addition of rituximab to conventional therapeutic regimens significantly improves survival in patients with CD20-positive B-cell lymphoma (Plosker & Figgitt, 2003).

References

Alexander, D. D., Mink, P. J., Adami, H. O., Chang, E. T., Cole, P., Mandel, J. S., & Trichopoulos, D. (2007). The non-Hodgkin lymphomas: A review of the epidemiologic literature. *International Journal of Cancer, 120*(S12), 1–39.

Alexander, D. D., Mink, P. J., Adami, H. O., Cole, P., Mandel, J. S., Oken, M. M., & Trichopoulos, D. (2007). Multiple myeloma: A review of the epidemiologic literature. *International Journal of Cancer, 120*(S12), 40–61.

Altekruse, S. F., Kosary, C. L., Krapcho, M., Neyman, N., Aminou, R., Waldron, W., … Edwards, B. K. (2010). *SEER cancer statistics review, 1975–2007*. Bethesda, MD: National Cancer Institute.

Armstrong, B. K., & Kricker, N. (2007). Sun exposure and non-Hodgkin lymphoma. *Cancer Epidemiology, Biomarkers and Prevention, 16*(3), 396–400.

Baecklund, E., Ekbom, A., Sparén, P., Feltelius, N., & Klareskog, L. (1998). Disease activity and risk of lymphoma in patients with rheumatoid arthritis: Nested case-control study. *British Medical Journal, 317*, 180–181.

Banks, P. M. (1992). Changes in diagnosis of non-Hodgkin's lymphomas over time. *Cancer Research, 52*, 5453s.

Barré-Sinoussi, F., Chermann, J. C., Rey, F., Nugeyre, M. T., Chamaret, S., Gruest, J., … Montagnier, L. (1983). Isolation of a T-lymphotropic retrovirus from a patient at risk for acquired immune deficiency syndrome (AIDS). *Science, 220*, 868–870.

Biggar, R. J., Frisch, M., Engels, E. A., & Goedert, J. J. (2001). Risk of T-cell lymphomas in persons with AIDS. *Journal of Acquired Immune Deficiency Syndromes, 26*, 371–376.

Bishara, M. R., Ross, C., & Sur, M. (2009). Primary anaplastic large cell lymphoma of the breast arising in reconstruction mammoplasty capsule of saline filled breast implant after radical mastectomy for breast cancer: An unusual case presentation. *Diagnostic Pathology, 2*(4), 11.

Blair, A., Sandler, D. P., Tarone, R., Lubin, J., Thomas, K., Hoppin, J. A., … Alavanja, M. C. (2005). Mortality among participants in the agricultural health study. *Annals of Epidemiology, 15*, 279–285.

Blair, A., Zahm, S. H., Pearce, N. E., Heineman, E. F., & Fraumeni, J. F. (1992). Clues to cancer etiology from studies of farmers. *Scandinavian Journal of Work, Environment and Health, 18*, 209–215.

Blomberg, J., Möller, T., Olsson, H., Anderson, H., & Jonsson, M. (1993). Cancer morbidity in blood recipients—Results of a cohort study. *European Journal of Cancer, 29A*, 2101–2105.

Blum, K. A., Lozanski, G., & Byrd, J. C. (2004). Adult Burkitt leukemia and lymphoma. *Blood, 104*, 3009–3020.

Bray, F., Ferlay, J., Soerjomataram, I., Siegel, R. L., Torre, L. A., & Jemal, A. (2018). Global cancer statistics 2018: GLOBOCAN estimates of incidence and mortality worldwide for 36 cancers in 185 countries. *CA: A Cancer Journal for Clinicians, 68*(6), 394–424.

Bräuninger, A., Küppers, R., Strickler, J. G., Wacker, H. H., Rajewsky, K., & Hansmann, M. L. (1997). Hodgkin's and Reed–Sternberg cells in lymphocyte predominant Hodgkin's disease represent clonal populations of germinal center-derived tumor B cells. *Proceedings of the National Academy of Sciences of the United States of America, 94*, 9337–9342.

Bräuninger, A., Schmitz, R., Bechtel, D., Renné, C., Hansmann, M. L., & Küppers, R. (2006). Molecular biology of Hodgkin's and Reed/Sternberg cells in Hodgkin's lymphoma. *International Journal of Cancer, 118*(8), 1853–1861.

Burkitt, D. (1958). A sarcoma involving the jaws in African children. *British Journal of Surgery, 46*(197), 218–223.

Burkitt, D. P. (1971). Epidemiology of Burkitt's lymphoma. *Proceedings of the Royal Society of Medicine, 64*(9), 909–910.

Burkitt, D. P. (1983). The discovery of Burkitt's lymphoma. *Cancer, 51*, 1777–1786.

Butel, J. S., Vilchez, R. A., Jorgensen, J. L., & Kozinetz, C. A. (2003). Association between SV40 and non-Hodgkin's lymphoma. *Leukemia and Lymphoma, 44*(Suppl. 3), S33–S39.

Carpenter, L. M., Newton, R., Casabonne, D., Ziegler, J., Mbulaiteye, S., Mbidde, E., … Beral, V. (2008). Antibodies against malaria and Epstein-Barr virus in childhood Burkitt lymphoma: A case-control study in Uganda. *International Journal of Cancer, 122*(6), 1319–1323.

Carroll-Pankhurst, C., Engels, E. A., Strickler, H. D., Goedert, J. J., Wagner, J., & Mortimer, E. A., Jr. (2001). Thirty-five year mortality following receipt of SV40-contaminated polio vaccine during the neonatal period. *British Journal of Cancer, 85*(9), 1295–1297.

Cartwright, R., McNally, R., & Staines, A. (1994). The increasing incidence of non-Hodgkin's lymphoma (NHL): The possible role of sunlight. *Leukemia and Lymphoma, 14*, 387–394.

Cartwright, R. A., & Watkins, G. (2004). Epidemiology of Hodgkin's disease: A review. *Hematological Oncology, 22*, 11–26.

Cerhan, J. R., Wallace, R. B., Dick, F., Kemp, J., Parker, A. S., Zheng, W., … Folsom, A. R. (2001). Blood transfusions and risk of non-Hodgkin's lymphoma subtypes and chronic lymphocytic leukemia. *Cancer Epidemiology, Biomarkers and Prevention, 10*(4), 361–368.

Cerhan, J. R., Wallace, R. B., Folsom, A. R., Potter, J. D., Munger, R. G., & Prineas, R. J. (1993). Transfusion history and cancer risk in older women. *Annals of Internal Medicine, 119*, 8–15.

Cerroni, L., Zochling, N., Putz, B., & Kerl, H. (1997). Infection by *Borrelia burgdorferi* and cutaneous B-cell lymphoma. *Journal of Cutaneous Pathology, 24*, 457–461.

Cesarman, E., Chang, Y., Moore, P. S., Said, J. W., & Knowles, D. M. (1995). Kaposi's sarcoma–associated herpesvirus-like DNA sequences in AIDS-related body-cavity-based lymphomas. *New England Journal of Medicine, 332*(18), 1186–1191.

Chang, Y., Cesarman, E., Pessin, M. S., Lee, F., Culpepper, J., Knowles, D. M., & Moore, P. S. (1994). Identification of herpesvirus-like DNA sequences in AIDS-associated Kaposi's sarcoma. *Science, 266*(5192), 1865–1869.

Chow, E. J., & Holly, E. A. (2002). Blood transfusions and non-Hodgkin's lymphoma. *Epidemiology Reviews, 24*(2), 269–279.

Cinque, P., Brytting, M., Vago, L., Castagna, A., Parravicini, C., Zanchetta, N., … Linde, A. (1993). Epstein-Barr virus DNA in cerebrospinal fluid from patients with AIDS-related primary lymphoma of the central nervous system. *Lancet, 342*(8868), 398–401.

Cleary, M. L., Chao, J., Warnke, R., & Sklar, J. (1984). Immunoglobulin gene rearrangement as a diagnostic criterion of B-cell lymphoma. *Proceedings of the National Academy of Sciences of the United States of America, 81*, 593–597.

Cleghorn, F. R., Manns, A., Falk, R., Hartge, P., Hanchard, B., Jack, N., … Blattner, W. (1995). Effect of human T-lymphotropic virus type I infection on non-Hodgkin's lymphoma incidence. *Journal of the National Cancer Institute, 87*(13), 1009–1014.

Cohen, H. J., Crawford, J., Rao, M. K., Pieper, C. F., & Currie, M. S. (1998). Racial differences in the prevalence of monoclonal gammopathy in a community-based sample of the elderly. *American Journal of Medicine, 104,* 439–444.

Dal Maso, L., & Franceschi, S. (2003). Epidemiology of non-Hodgkin lymphomas and other haemolymphopoietic neoplasms in people with AIDS. *Lancet Oncology, 4*(2), 110–119.

de Jong, D., Vasmel, W. L. E., de Boer, J. P., Verhave, G., Barbé, E., Casparie, M. K., & van Leeuwen, F. E. (2008). Anaplastic large-cell lymphoma in women with breast implants. *Journal of the American Medical Association, 300*(17), 2030–2035.

de Sanjose, S., Shah, K. V., Domingo-Domenech, E., Engels, E. A., de Sevilla, A. F., Alvaro, T., … Viscidi, R. P. (2003). Lack of serological evidence for an association between simian virus 40 and lymphoma. *International Journal of Cancer, 104,* 522–524.

de Thé, G. (1993). The etiology of Burkitt's lymphoma and the history of the shaken dogmas. *Blood Cells, 19,* 667–673.

Devesa, S. S., & Fears, T. (1992). Non-Hodgkin's lymphoma time trends, United States and international data. *Cancer Research, 52,* 5432s–5440s.

Duberg, A. S., Nordstrom, M., Torner, A., Reichard, O., Strauss, R., Janzon, R., … Ekdahl, K. (2005). Non-Hodgkin's lymphoma and other nonhepatic malignancies in Swedish patients with hepatitis C virus infection. *Hepatology, 41,* 652–659.

Eltom, M. A., Jemal, A., Mbulaiteye, S. M., Devesa, S. S., & Biggar, R. J. (2002). Trends in Kaposi's sarcoma and non-Hodgkin's lymphoma incidence in the United States from 1973 through 1998. *Journal of the National Cancer Institute, 94*(16), 1204–1210.

Engels, E. A., Frisch, M., Lubin, J. H., Gail, M. H., Biggar, R. J., & Goedert, J. J. (2002). Prevalence of hepatitis C virus infection and risk for hepatocellular carcinoma and non-Hodgkin lymphoma in AIDS. *Journal of Acquired Immune Deficiency Syndromes, 31,* 536–541.

Engels, E. A., Katki, H. A., Nielsen, N. M., Winther, J. F., Hjalgrim, H., Gjerris, F., … Frisch, M. (2003). Cancer incidence in Denmark following exposure to poliovirus vaccine contaminated with simian virus 40. *Journal of the National Cancer Institute, 95*(7), 532–539.

Engels, E. A., Viscidi, R. P., Galloway, D. A., Carter, J. J., Cerhan, J. R., … Hartge, P. (2004). Case-control study of Simian Virus 40 and non-Hodgkin lymphoma in the United States. *Journal of the National Cancer Institute, 96*(18), 1368–1374.

Epstein, M. A., Achong, B. G., & Pope, J. H. (1967). Virus in cultured lymphoblasts from a New Guinea Burkitt lymphoma. *British Medical Journal, 2*(5547), 290–291.

Ferlay, J., Ervik, M., Lam, F., Colombet, M., Mery, L., Piñeros, M., … Bray, F. (2018). *Global cancer observatory: Cancer today.* Lyon, France: International Agency for Research on Cancer. Retrieved from https://gco.iarc.fr/today

Ferlay, J., Shin, H. R., Forman, D., Mathers, C., & Parkin, D. M. (2010). Estimates of worldwide burden of cancer in 2008. *International Journal of Cancer, 127*(12), 2893–2917.

Ferlay, J., Soerjomataram, I., Ervik, M., Dikshit, R., Eser, S., Mathers, C., … Bray, F. (2013). *GLOBOCAN 2012 v1.0. Cancer incidence and mortality worldwide: IARC CancerBase No. 11* [Internet]. Lyon, France: International Agency for Research on Cancer. Retrieved from http://globocan.iarc.fr

Fernandez, E., Chatenoud, L., La Vecchia, C., Negri, E., & Franceschi, S. (1999). Fish consumption and cancer risk. *American Journal of Clinical Nutrition, 70*(1), 85–90.

Ferreri, A. J. M., Guidoboni, M., Ponzoni, M., De Conciliis, C., Dell'Oro, S., Fleischhauer, K., … Dolcetti, R. (2004). Evidence for an association between *Chlamydia psittaci* and ocular adnexal lymphomas. *Journal of the National Cancer Institute, 96,* 586–594.

Ferry, J. A. (2006). Burkitt's lymphoma: Clinicopathologic features and differential diagnosis. *Oncologist, 11*(4), 375–383.

Figgs, L. W., Dosemeci, M., & Blair, A. (1995). United States non-Hodgkin's lymphoma surveillance by occupation 1984–1989: A twenty-four state death certificate study. *American Journal of Industrial Medicine, 27,* 817–835.

Filipovich, A. H., Mathur, A., Kamat, D., & Shapiro, R. S. (1992). Primary immunodeficiencies: Genetic risk factors for lymphoma. *Cancer Research, 52,* 5465s–5467s.

Fisher, S. G., & Fisher, R. I. (2004). The epidemiology of non-Hodgkin's lymphoma. *Oncogene, 23,* 6524–6534.

Fitzmaurice, C., Akinyemiju, T. F., Al Lami, F. H., Alam, T., Alizadeh-Navaei, R., Allen, C., … Global Burden of Disease Cancer Collaboration. (2018). Global, regional, and national cancer incidence, mortality, years of life lost, years lived with disability, and disability-adjusted life-years for 29 cancer groups, 1990–2016: A systematic analysis for the Global Burden of Disease Study. *JAMA Oncology.* Online publication. doi:10.1001/jamaoncol.2018.2706

Fitzmaurice, C., Allen, C., Barber, R. M., Barregard, L., Bhutta, Z. A., Brenner, H., … Global Burden of Disease Cancer Collaboration. (2017). Global, regional, and national cancer incidence, mortality, years of life lost, years lived with disability, and disability-adjusted life-years for 32 cancer groups, 1990–2015: A systematic analysis for the Global Burden of Disease Study. *JAMA Oncology, 3*(4), 524–548.

Frampton, M., da Silva Filho, M. I., Broderic, P., Thomsen, H., Forsti, A., Vijayakrishnan, J., … Houlston, R. S. (2013). Variation at 3p24.1 and 6q23.3 influences the risk of Hodgkin's lymphoma. *Nature Communications, 4,* 2549. doi:10.1038/ncomms3549.

Franceschi, S., Dal Maso, L., & La Vecchia, C. (1999). Advances in the epidemiology of HIV-associated non-Hodgkin's lymphoma and other lymphoid neoplasms. *International Journal of Cancer, 83*(4), 481–485.

Fritschi, L., Ambrosini, G. L., Kliewer, E. V., Johnson, K. C., & Canadian Cancer Registries Epidemiologic Research Group. (2004). Dietary fish intake and risk of leukaemia, multiple myeloma, and non-Hodgkin lymphoma. *Cancer Epidemiology, Biomarkers and Prevention, 13*(4), 532–537.

Gallo, R. C., Sarin, P. S., Gelmann, E. P., Robert-Guroff, M., Richardson, E., Kalyanaraman, V. S., … Popovic, M. (1983). Isolation of human T-cell leukemia virus in acquired immune deficiency syndrome (AIDS). *Science, 220*(4599), 865–867.

Garbe, C., Stein, H., Dienemann, D., & Orfanos, C. E. (1991). *Borrelia burgdorferi*–associated cutaneous B cell lymphoma: Clinical and immunohistologic characterization of four cases. *Journal of the American Academy of Dermatology, 24,* 584–590.

Gisbert, J. P., García-Buey, L., Pajares, J. M., & Moreno-Otero, R. (2003). Prevalence of hepatitis C virus infection in B cell non-Hodgkin's lymphoma: Systematic review and meta-analysis. *Gastroenterology, 125,* 1723–1732.

Goedert, J. J., Cote, T. R., Virgo, P., Scoppa, S. M., Kingma, D. W., Gail, M. H., … Biggar, R. J. (1998). Spectrum of AIDS-associated malignant disorders. *Lancet, 351,* 1833–1899.

Grogan, T., & Miller, T. (1995). Natural history and pre-treatment evaluation of non-Hodgkins lymphomas. In C. M. Haskell (Ed.), *Cancer treatment* (pp. 979–1005). Philadelphia, PA: W. B. Saunders.

Groves, F. D., Linet, M. S., Travis, L. B., & Devesa, S. S. (2000). Cancer surveillance series: Non-Hodgkin's lymphoma incidence by histologic subtype in the United States from 1978 through 1995. *Journal of the National Cancer Institute, 92,* 1240–1251.

Grulich, A. E., Wan, X., Law, M. G., Coates, M., & Kaldor, J. M. (1999). Risk of cancer in people with AIDS. *AIDS, 13,* 839–843.

Grulich, A. E., Wan, X., Law, M. G., Milliken, S. T., Lewis, C. R., Garsia, R. J., … Kaldor, J. M. (2000). B-cell stimulation and prolonged immune deficiency are risk factors for non-Hodgkin's lymphoma in people with AIDS. *AIDS, 14,* 133–140.

Harris, N. L., Jaffe, E. S., Diebold, J., Flandrin, G., Muller-Hermelink, H. K., Vardiman, J., … Bloomfield, C. D. (1999). World Health Organization classification of neoplastic diseases of the hematopoietic and lymphoid tissues: Report of the Clinical Advisory Committee meeting—Airlie House, Virginia, November 1997. *Journal of Clinical Oncology, 17*(12), 3835–3849.

Harris, O. D., Cooke, W. T., Thompson, H., & Waterhouse, J. A. H. (1967). Malignancy in adult coeliac disease and idiopathic steatorrhoea. *American Journal of Medicine, 42,* 899–912.

Hartge, P., Devesa, S. S., & Fraumeni, J. F., Jr. (1994). Hodgkin's and non-Hodgkin's lymphomas. *Cancer Surveys, 19–20,* 423–453.

Hartge, P., Devesa, S. S., Grauman, D., Fears, T. R., & Fraumeni, J. F., Jr. (1996). Non-Hodgkin's lymphoma and sunlight. *Journal of the National Cancer Institute, 88,* 298–300.

Hinuma, Y., Nagata, K., Hanaoka, M., Nakai, M., Matsumoto, T., Kinoshita, K. I., … Miyoshi, I. (1981). Adult T-cell leukemia: Antigen in an ATL cell line and detection of antibodies to the antigen in human sera. *Proceedings of the National Academy of Sciences of the United States of America, 78*(10), 6476–6480.

Hjalgrim, H., Rasmussen, S., Rostgaard, K., Nielsen, N. M., Koch-Henriksen, N., Munksgaard, L., … Melbye, M. (2004). Familial clustering of Hodgkin lymphoma and multiple sclerosis. *Journal of the National Cancer Institute, 96,* 780–784.

Hodgkin, T. (1832). On some morbid experiences of the absorbent glands and spleen. *Medico-Chirurgical Transactions, 17,* 69–97.

Hussell, T., Isaacson, P. G., Crabtree, J. E., & Spencer, J. (1993). The response of cells from low-grade B-cell gastric lymphomas of mucosa-associated lymphoid tissue to *Helicobacter pylori*. *Lancet, 342,* 571–574.

Isaacson, P. G., & Spencer, J. (1995). The biology of low grade MALT lymphoma. *Journal of Clinical Pathology, 48*(5), 395–397.

Jelic, S., & Filipovic-Ljeskovic, I. (1999). Positive serology for Lyme disease borrelias in primary cutaneous B-cell lymphoma: A study in 22 patients: Is it a fortuitous finding? *Hematological Oncology, 17,* 107–116.

Judde, J. G., Lacoste, V., Briere, J., Kassa-Kelembho, E., Clyti, E., Couppie, P., … Gessain, A. (2000). Monoclonality or oligoclonality of human herpesvirus 8 terminal repeat sequences in Kaposi's sarcoma and other diseases. *Journal of the National Cancer Institute, 92,* 729–736.

Kamel, O. W., van de Rijn, M., Hanasono, M. M., & Warnke, R. A. (1995). Immunosuppression-associated lymphoproliferative disorders in rheumatic patients. *Leukemia and Lymphoma, 16,* 363.

Kanzler, H., Küppers, R., Hansmann, M. L., & Rajewsky, K. (1996). Hodgkin's and Reed–Sternberg cells in Hodgkin's disease represent the outgrowth of a dominant tumor clone derived from (crippled) germinal center B cells. *Journal of Experimental Medicine, 184,* 1495–1505.

Khuder, S. A., Schaub, E. A., & Keller-Byrne, J. E. (1998). Meta-analyses of non-Hodgkin's lymphoma and farming.

Scandinavian Journal of Work, Environment and Health, 24, 255–261.

Kinlen, L. (1992). Immunosuppressive therapy and acquired immunological disorders. *Cancer Research, 52,* 5474s–5476s.

Koshiol, J., Gridley, G., Engels, E., McMaster, M., & Landgren, O. (2008). Chronic immune stimulation and subsequent Waldenström macroglobulinemia. *Archives of Internal Medicine, 168*(17), 1903–1909.

Kumar, V., Abbas, A. K., & Aster, J. C. (2014). *Robbins and Cotran pathologic basis of disease* (9th ed.). Philadelphia, PA: Mosby & Saunders.

Küppers, R. (2005). Mechanisms of B-cell lymphoma pathogenesis. *Nature Reviews Cancer, 5*(4), 251–262.

Küppers, R., Rajewsky, K., Zhao, M., Simons, G., Laumann, R., Fischer, R., & Hansmann, M. L. (1994). Hodgkin's disease: Hodgkin's and Reed–Sternberg cells picked from histological sections show clonal immunoglobulin gene rearrangements and appear to be derived from B cells at various stages of development. *Proceedings of the National Academy of Sciences of the United States of America, 91,* 10962–10966.

Kusters, J. G., van Vliet, A. H. M., & Kuipers, E. J. (2006). Pathogenesis of *Helicobacter pylori* infection. *Clinical Microbiology Reviews, 19*(3), 449–490.

Kyle, R. A., & Rajkumar, S. V. (2004). Multiple myeloma. *New England Journal of Medicine, 351*(18), 1860–1873.

Kyle, R. A., Therneau, T. M., Rajkumar, S. V., Larson, D. R., Plevak, M. F., & Melton, L. J., III. (2004). Long-term follow-up of 241 patients with monoclonal gammopathy of undetermined significance: The original Mayo Clinic series 25 years later. *Mayo Clinic Proceedings, 79,* 859–866.

Kyle, R. A., Therneau, T. M., Rajkumar, S. V., Larson, D. R., Plevak, M. F., Offord, J. R., … Melton, L. J., III. (2006). Prevalence of monoclonal gammopathy of undetermined significance. *New England Journal of Medicine, 354,* 1362–1369.

Kyle, R. A., Therneau, T. M., Rajkumar, S. V., Offord, J. R., Larson, D. R., Plevak, M. F., & Melton, L. J., III. (2002). A long-term study of prognosis in monoclonal gammopathy of undetermined significance. *New England Journal of Medicine, 346,* 564–569.

Landgren, O., Kyle, R. A., Pfeiffer, R. M., Katzmann, J. A., Caporaso, N. E., Hayes, R. B., … Rajkumar, S. V. (2009). Monoclonal gammopathy of undetermined significance (MGUS) consistently precedes multiple myeloma: A prospective study. *Blood, 113*(22), 5412–5417.

Lecuit, M., Abachin, E., Martin, A., Poyart, C., Pochart, P., Suarez, F., … Lortholary, O. (2004). Immunoproliferative small intestinal disease associated with *Campylobacter jejuni*. *New England Journal of Medicine, 350,* 239–248.

Leech, S. H., Brown, R., & Scharifeld, M. S. (1985). Genetic studies in multiple myeloma: Immunoglobulin allotype associations. *Cancer, 5,* 1473–1476.

Leech, S. H., Bryan, C. F., Elston, R. C., Rainey, J., Bickers, J. N., & Pelias, M. Z. (1983). Genetic studies in multiple myeloma: Association with HLA-Cw5. *Cancer, 51,* 1408–1411.

Linet, M. S., & Pottern, L. M. (1992). Familial aggregation of hematopoietic malignancies and risk of non-Hodgkin's lymphoma. *Cancer Research, 52S,* 5468–5473.

Lukes, R. J., & Collins, R. D. (1975). New approaches to the classification of the lymphomata. *British Journal of Cancer, Suppl. 2,* 1–28.

Luppi, M., Longo, G., Ferrari, M. G., Barozzi, P., Marasca, R., Morselli, M., … Torelli, G. (1998). Clinico-pathological characterization of hepatitis C virus-related B-cell non-Hodgkin's lymphomas without symptomatic cryoglobulinemia. *Annals of Oncology, 9*, 495–498.

Mack, T. M., Cozen, W., Shibata, D. K., Weiss, L. M., Nathwani, B. N., Hernandez, A. M., … Rappaport, E. B. (1995). Concordance for Hodgkin's disease in identical twins suggesting genetic susceptibility to the young-adult form of the disease. *New England Journal of Medicine, 332*, 413–419.

Manns, A., & Blattner, W. A. (2003). The epidemiology of the human T-cell lymphotropic virus type I and type II: Etiologic role in human disease. *Transfusion, 31*(1), 67–75.

Marshall, B. J., & Warren, R. J. (2005). *The Nobel prize in physiology or medicine, 2005.* Retrieved from www.mja.com.au/journal/2005/183/11/2005-nobel-prize-physiology-or-medicine

Matsuo, K., Kusano, A., Sugumar, A., Nakamura, S., Tajima, K., & Mueller, N. E. (2004). Effect of hepatitis C virus infection on the risk of non-Hodgkin's lymphoma: A meta-analysis of epidemiological studies. *Cancer Science, 95*, 745–752.

McGregor, J. M., Crook, T., Fraser-Andrews, E. A., Rozycka, M., Crossland, S., Brooks, L., & Whittaker, S. J. (1999). Spectrum of *p53* gene mutations suggests a possible role for ultraviolet radiation in the pathogenesis of advanced cutaneous lymphomas. *Journal of Investigative Dermatology, 112*(3), 317–321.

Melbye, M., Ekström Smedby, K.,•& Trichopoulos, D. (2008). Non-Hodgkin lymphoma. In H.-O. Adami, D. Hunter & D. Trichoupoulos (Eds.), *Textbook of cancer epidemiology* (pp. 535–555). Oxford, UK: Oxford University Press.

Melbye, M., Hjalgrim, H., & Adami, H.-O. (2008). Hodgkin's lymphoma. In H.-O. Adami, D. Hunter & D. Trichopoulos (Eds.), *Textbook of cancer epidemiology* (pp. 520–534). Oxford, UK: Oxford University Press.

Memon, A., & Doll, R. (1994). A search for unknown blood-borne oncogenic viruses. *International Journal of Cancer, 58*, 366–368.

Morton, L. M., Hartge, P., Holford, T. R., Holly, E. A., Chiu, B. C., Vineis, P., … Zheng, T. (2005). Cigarette smoking and risk of non-Hodgkin lymphoma: A pooled analysis from the International Lymphoma Epidemiology Consortium (InterLymph). *Cancer Epidemiology, Biomarkers and Prevention, 14*, 925–933.

Morton, L. M., Zheng, T., Holford, T. R., Holly, E. A., Chiu, B. C., Costantini, A. S., … InterLymph Consortium. (2005). Alcohol consumption and risk of non-Hodgkin lymphoma: A pooled analysis. *Lancet Oncology, 6*, 469–476.

Müller, A. M. S., Ihorst, G., Mertelsmann, R., & Engelhardt, M. (2005). Epidemiology of non-Hodgkin's lymphoma (NHL): Trends, geographic distribution, and etiology. *Annals of Hematology, 84*, 1–12.

Nakatsuka, S., Liu, A., Dong, Z., Nomura, S., Takakuwa, T., Miyazato, H., & Aozasa, K. (2003). Simian virus 40 sequences in malignant lymphomas in Japan. *Cancer Research, 63*, 7606–7608.

Negri, E., Little, D., Boiocchi, M., La Vecchia, C., & Franceschi, S. (2004). B-cell non-Hodgkin's lymphoma and hepatitis C virus infection: A systematic review. *International Journal of Cancer, 111*, 1–8.

Noone, A. M., Howlader, N., Krapcho, M., Miller, D., Brest, A., Yu, M., … Cronin, K. A. (Eds.). (2018). *SEER cancer statistics review, 1975–2015.* Bethesda, MD: National Cancer Institute. Retrieved from https://seer.cancer.gov/csr/1975_2015/

Ocio, E. M., Schop, R. F. J., Gonzalez, B., Van Wier, S. A., Hernandez-Rivas, J. M., Gutierrez, N. C., … Fonseca, R. (2007). 6q deletion in Waldenström macroglobulinemia is associated with features of adverse prognosis. *British Journal of Haematology, 136*(1), 80–86.

Offit, K., Wong, G., Filippa, D. A., Tao, Y., & Chaganti, R. S. (1991). Cytogenetic analysis of 434 consecutively ascertained specimens of non-Hodgkin's lymphoma: Clinical correlations. *Blood, 77*(7), 1508–1515.

Opelz, G., & Henderson, R. (1993). Incidence of non-Hodgkin lymphoma in kidney and heart transplant recipients. *Lancet, 342*(8886–8887), 1514–1516.

Palackdharry, C. S. (1994). The epidemiology of non-Hodgkin's lymphoma: Why the increased incidence? *Oncology, 8*(8), 67–73; discussion 73–78.

Parkin, D. M., Bray, F., Ferlay, J., & Pisani, P. (2001). Estimating the world cancer burden, GLOBOCAN 2000. *International Journal of Cancer, 94*, 153–156.

Parkin, D. M., Bray, F., Ferlay, J., & Pisani, P. (2005). Global cancer statistics, 2002. *CA: A Cancer Journal for Clinicians, 55*, 74–108.

Parkin, D. M., Pisani, P., & Ferlay, J. (1999a). Estimates of the worldwide incidence of 25 major cancers in 1990. *International Journal of Cancer, 80*(6), 827–841.

Parkin, D. M., Pisani, P., & Ferlay, J. (1999b). Global cancer statistics. *CA: A Cancer Journal for Clinicians, 49*(1), 33–64.

Parsonnet, J., Hansen, S., Rodriguez, L., Gelb, A. B., Warnke, R. A., Jellum, E., … Friedman, G. D. (1994). *Helicobacter pylori* infection and gastric lymphoma. *New England Journal of Medicine, 330*, 1267–1271.

Pettersson, T., Pukkala, E., Teppo, L., & Friman, C. (1992). Increased risk of cancer in patients with systemic lupus erythematosus. *Annals of the Rheumatic Diseases, 51*(4), 437–439.

Plosker, G. L., & Figgitt, D. P. (2003). Rituximab: A review of its use in non-Hodgkin's lymphoma and chronic lymphocytic leukaemia. *Drugs, 63*(8), 803–843.

Poiesz, B. J., Ruscetti, F. W., Gazdar, A. F., Bunn, P. A., Minna, J. D., & Gallo, R. C. (1980). Detection and isolation of type C retrovirus particles from fresh and cultured lymphocytes of a patient with cutaneous T-cell lymphoma. *Proceedings of the National Academy of Sciences of the United States of America, 77*, 7415–7419.

Polesel, J., Clifford, G., Rickenbach, M., Dal Maso, L., Battegay, M., Bouchardy, C., … the Swiss HIV Cohort Study. (2008). Non-Hodgkin's lymphoma incidence in the Swiss HIV Cohort Study before and after highly active antiretroviral therapy. *AIDS, 22*(2), 301–306.

Pottern, L. M., Gart, J. J., Nam, J. M., Dunston, G., Wilson, J., Greenberg, R., … Schwartz, A. G. (1992). HLA and multiple myeloma among black and white men: Evidence of a genetic association. *Cancer Epidemiology, Biomarkers and Prevention, 1*(3), 177–182.

Pounder, R. E., & Ng, D. (1995). The prevalence of *Helicobacter pylori* infection in different countries. *Alimentary Pharmacology and Therapeutics, 9 Suppl. 2*, 33–39.

Purtilo, D. T. (1980). Epstein–Barr virus–induced oncogenesis in immune-deficient individuals. *Lancet, 1*, 300–303.

Raab, M. S., Podar, K., Breitkreutz, I., Richardson, P. G., & Anderson, K. C. (2009). Multiple myeloma. *Lancet, 374*(9686), 324–339.

Rabkin, C. S., Tess, B. H., Christianson, R. E., Wright, W. E., Waters, D. J., Alter, H. J., & Van Den Berg, B. J. (2002). Prospective study of hepatitis C viral infection as a risk factor for subsequent B-cell neoplasia. *Blood, 99*, 4240–4242.

Reed, D. (1902). On the pathological changes in Hodgkin's disease, with special reference to its relation to tuberculosis. *Johns Hopkins Hospital Reports, 10*, 133–196.

Schöllkopf, C., Melbye, M., Munksgaard, L., Smedby, K. E., Rostgaard, K., Glimelius, B., … Hjalgrim, H. (2008). *Borrelia* infection and risk of non-Hodgkin lymphoma. *Blood, 111*(12), 5524–5529.

Schop, R. F., Van Wier, S. A., Xu, R., Ghobrial, I., Ahmann, G. J., Greipp, P. R., … Fonseca, R. (2006). 6q deletion discriminates Waldenström macroglobulinemia from IgM monoclonal gammopathy of undetermined significance. *Cancer Genetics and Cytogenetics, 169*(2), 150–153.

Shipp, M. A., Mauch, P. M., & Harris, N. L. (1997). Non-Hodgkin's lymphomas. In V. DeVita, Jr., S. Hellman & S. A. Rosenberg (Eds.), *Cancer principles and practice of oncology* (Vol. 3, pp. 2165–2220). Philadelphia, PA: Lippincott-Raven.

Shivapurkar, N., Harada, K., Reddy, J., Scheuermann, R. H., Xu, Y., McKenna, R. W., … Gazdar, A. F. (2002). Presence of simian virus 40 DNA sequences in human lymphomas. *Lancet, 359*, 851–852.

Silvestri, F., Pipan, C., Barillari, G., Zaja, F., Fanin, R., Infanti, L., … Baccarani, M. (1996). Prevalence of hepatitis C virus infection in patients with lymphoproliferative disorders. *Blood, 87*(10), 4296–4301.

Sternberg, C. (1898). Uber eine eigenartige unter dem Bilde der Pseudoleukamie verlaufende Tuberculose des lymphatischen Apparates. *Zeitschrift fuer Heilkunde, 19*, 21–90.

Swinnen, L., Costanzo-Nordin, M. R., Fisher, S. G., O'Sullivan, E. J., Johnson, M. R., Heroux, A. L., … Fisher, R. I. (1990). Increased incidence of lymphoproliferative disorder after immunosuppression with the monoclonal antibody OKT3 in cardiac-transplant recipients. *New England Journal of Medicine, 323*(25), 1723–1728.

Takatsuki, K. (2005). Discovery of adult T-cell leukemia. *Retrovirology, 2*, 16.

Takatsuki, K., Uchiyama, T., Sagawa, K., & Yodoi, J. (1977). Adult T cell leukemia in Japan. In S. Seno, F. Takaku & S. Irino (Eds.), *Topics in hematology* (pp. 73–77). Amsterdam, Netherlands: Excerpta Medica.

Takkouche, B., Etminan, M., & Montes-Martinez, A. (2005). Personal use of hair dyes and risk of cancer: A meta-analysis. *Journal of the American Medical Association, 293*, 2516–2525.

Thun, M. J., DeLancey, J. O., Center, M. M., Jemal, A., & Ward, E. M. (2010). The global burden of cancer: Priorities for prevention. *Carcinogenesis, 31*(1), 100–110.

Tycko, B., & Sklar, J. (1990). Chromosomal translocations in lymphoid neoplasia: A reappraisal of the recombinase model. *Cancer Cells, 2*(1), 1–8.

Uchiyama, T., Yodoi, J., Sagawa, K., Takatsuki, K., & Uchino, H. (1977). Adult T-cell leukemia: Clinical and hematologic features of 16 cases. *Blood, 50*, 481–492.

Udomsakdi-Auewarakul, C., Auewarakul, P., Sukpanichnant, S., & Muangsup, W. (2000). Hepatitis C virus infection in patients with non-Hodgkin lymphoma in Thailand. *Blood, 95*, 3640–3641.

Vega, F., & Medeiros, L. J. (2003). Chromosomal translocations involved in non-Hodgkin lymphomas. *Archives of Pathology and Laboratory Medicine, 127*(9), 1148–1160.

Vilchez, R. A., Madden, C. R., Kozinetz, C. A., Halvorson, S. J., White, Z. S., Orgensen, J. L., … Butel, J. S. (2002). Association between simian virus 40 and non-Hodgkin lymphoma. *Lancet, 359*, 817–823.

Waldenström, J. (1944). Incipient myelomatosis or "essential" hyperglobulinemia with fibrinogenopenia—A new syndrome? *Acta Medica Scandinavica, 117*, 216–247.

Willemze, R., Kerl, H., Sterry, W., Berti, E., Cerroni, L., Chimenti, S., … Meijer, C. J. L. M. (1997). EORTC classification for primary cutaneous lymphomas: A proposal from the Cutaneous Lymphoma Study Group of the European Organization for Research and Treatment of Cancer. *Blood, 90*, 354–371.

World Health Organization. (2008). *World cancer report 2008.* Lyon, France: International Agency for Research on Cancer.

Wotherspoon, A. C. (1998). *Helicobacter pylori* infection and gastric lymphoma. *British Medical Bulletin, 54*(1), 79–85.

Wotherspoon, A. C., Doglioni, C., Diss, T. C., Pan, L., Moschini, A., de Boni, M., & Isaacson, P. G. (1993). Regression of primary low-grade B-cell gastric lymphoma of mucosa-associated lymphoid tissue type after eradication of *Helicobacter pylori*. *Lancet, 342*, 575–577.

Wotherspoon, A. C., Ortiz-Hidalgo, C., Falzon, M. R., & Isaacson, P. G. (1991). *Helicobacter pylori*–associated gastritis and primary B-cell gastric lymphoma. *Lancet, 338*, 1175–1176.

Ye, B. H. (2000). Role of BCL-6 in the pathogenesis of non-Hodgkin's lymphoma. *Cancer Investigation, 18*, 356–365.

Yodoi, J., Takatsuki, K., & Masuda, T. (1974). Letter: Two cases of T-cell chronic lymphocytic leukemia in Japan. *New England Journal of Medicine, 290*(10), 572–573.

Yoshida, M., Miyoshi, I., & Hinuma, Y. (1982). Isolation and characterization of retrovirus from cell lines of human adult T-cell leukemia and its implication in the disease. *Proceedings of the National Academy of Sciences of the United States of America, 79*(6), 2031–2035.

Zahm, S. H., Wiesenberger, D. D., Holmes, F. F., Cantor, K. P., & Blair, A. (1997). Tobacco and non-Hodgkin's lymphoma: Combined analysis of three case-control studies (United States). *Cancer Causes and Control, 8*, 159–166.

Zheng, T., Mayne, S. T., Boyle, P., Holford, T. R., Liu, W. L., & Flannery, J. (1992). Epidemiology of non-Hodgkin lymphoma in Connecticut. 1935–1988. *Cancer, 70*, 840–849.

Zhu, K., Levine, R. S., Gu, Y., Brann, E. A., Hall, I., Caplan, L. S., & Baum, M. K. (1998). Non-Hodgkin's lymphoma and family history of malignant tumors in a case-control study (United States). *Cancer Causes and Control, 9*, 77–82.

CHAPTER 37

Epidemiology of Leukemia

▶ Classification of Leukemia

Leukemia arises in the bone marrow from cell lineages that form the immune cells that circulate in the blood. The three basic types of immune cells are myelocytes, lymphocytes, and monocytes. Leukemias are therefore broadly categorized as either myelocytic, lymphocytic, or monocytic. A further classification is based on whether disease follows a rapidly fatal course in a matter of weeks if left untreated (acute leukemia) or persists over a period of years (chronic leukemia).

The term *leukemia*, which means "white blood," was first used by the famous German pathologist Rudolph Virchow in describing the predominance of circulating white blood cells versus red blood cells that often exists in patients with leukemia. As pointed out by Stanley Robbins and Ramzi Cotran in their classic text, leukemias are best characterized by diffuse replacement of bone marrow by proliferating leukemic cells, abnormal forms of malignant cells circulating in the blood, and infiltrates of leukemic cells in various anatomic sites such as the liver, spleen, lymph nodes, and elsewhere (Kumar, Abbas, & Aster, 2014; Robbins & Cotran, 1979).

Standard nomenclature for the leukemias is given in **TABLE 37.1**. The six basic types are acute and chronic forms of lymphocytic leukemia, myelocytic leukemia, and monocytic leukemia. Each can be further subdivided according to the morphology of the

TABLE 37.1 Classification of Leukemias

Type of Leukemia	Common Characteristics
Acute lymphocytic leukemia (ALL)	Predominant type in children, usually B-cell origin, T-cell origin is rare
Chronic lymphocytic leukemia (CLL)	Predominant type in adults, usually B-cell origin, T-cell origin is rare
Acute myelocytic leukemia (AML)	Occurs in young adults, usually myelocyte (granulocyte) origin
Chronic myelocytic leukemia (CML)	Adult leukemia of granulocytes due to translocation (Philadelphia chromosome)
Acute monocytic leukemia	Less common adult leukemia of monocyte origin
Chronic monocytic leukemia	Rare adult leukemia of monocyte origin

Data from Vardiman, J. W., Thiele, J., Arber, D. A., Brunning, R. D., Borowitz, M. J., Porwit, A., . . . Bloomfield, C. D. (2009). The 2008 revision of the World Health Organization (WHO) classification of myeloid neoplasms and acute leukemia. *Blood, 114*(5), 937–951.

cell of origin and staining characteristics of cells. For example, when cells are routinely stained with hematoxylin and eosin dye, the cells are identifiable as neutrophils (neutral stain), basophils (blue stain), or eosinophils (red stain). Cell types can also be molecularly characterized by the presence of cell membrane receptors. Such receptors are used to differentiate T- and B-lymphocytic leukemias. Rare forms of leukemia have also been identified such as histiocytic or hairy-cell leukemia (derived from monocytes and macrophages) and erythroleukemia, in which most tumor cells are of erythropoietic lineage (Vardiman et al., 2009).

Hematopoiesis

Immune cells of the blood are continuously being formed in the bone marrow. They originate from progenitor (stem) cells and undergo tightly regulated differentiation into the various lineages of immune cell populations. It is estimated that more than *1 trillion* new cells are produced daily to maintain homeostasis in the peripheral circulation. Hematopoietic stem cells reside in the bone marrow and have the unique ability to differentiate into all the mature cell types that circulate in the blood (**FIGURE 37.1**). There are differences of opinion regarding the cell of origin of monocytes, which are not shown in the diagram. The conventional view is that monocytes arise from myeloid precursors; however, some studies suggest that monocytes are derived from stem cells that are distinct from the myeloid lineage. Macrophages (also called phagocytes) develop from circulating monocytes that migrate into tissues of the body (Dale, Boser, & Liles, 2008; Vardiman et al., 2009).

Production of red and white blood cells is regulated with extreme precision in the human body. A plethora of growth factors, hormones, and transcription factors are involved in the differentiation and maturation of progenitor cells. For example, erythropoietin secreted by the kidneys stimulates the formation of red blood cells, and thrombopoietin stimulates the formation of blood platelets.

In children, hematopoiesis occurs in the marrow of the long bones such as the femur and tibia. In adults, it occurs mainly in the pelvis, cranium, vertebrae, and sternum. Differentiation and maturation of progenitor cells begin in the bone marrow and continue throughout the life cycle of immune cells. Cells of the immune system enter the blood and lymphatic systems through an extensive plexus of fenestrated capillaries that anastomose with the bone marrow. Lymphocytes differentiate into T lymphocytes in the thymus whereas the final maturation of B lymphocytes occurs in the lymph nodes.

Pathogenesis of Leukemia

Leukemia refers to immature immune cells in the bone marrow that are undergoing uncontrolled proliferation. Without treatment, the expanding clone of leukemic cells replaces other cell populations in the bone marrow, blood, and lymph. Cytogenetic/genetic analyses of leukemia tissues often reveal the presence of reciprocal chromosomal translocations, chromosomal deletions, and/or DNA point mutations. Reciprocal exchanges of DNA between chromosomes can form hybrid genes that encode chimeric fusion proteins that deregulate critical cellular processes such as mitosis, apoptosis, and angiogenesis. Chromosomal deletions

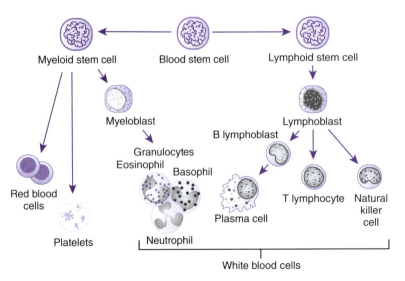

FIGURE 37.1 Hematopoiesis.

can silence tumor–suppressor genes that regulate these same processes. Point mutations may also be involved as well as epigenetic modifications in the expression of proto-oncogenes or tumor–suppressor genes. Such genetic errors can be acquired at any time during the lifespan, and some undoubtedly occur during early growth and development, perhaps even in utero during embryogenesis. Inherited genetic defects are uncommon. Various models have been proposed suggesting that two or more DNA errors are required to form a leukemic clone of cells. Endogenous hormones may also play a role in leukemogenesis, particularly

cortisol, which culls populations of immature immune cells by inducing apoptosis (Vardiman et al., 2009).

▶ Global Epidemiology of Leukemia

FIGURE 37.2 shows the global patterns of leukemia incidence and mortality based on data collected by the World Health Organization (WHO) in 2018 (Ferlay et al., 2018). Average incidence rates are relatively high (7.5 per 100,000) in developed areas such as the United

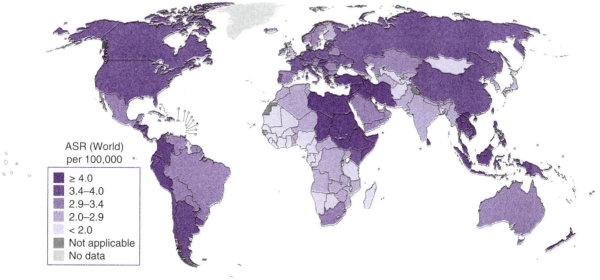

FIGURE 37.2 Global Incidence and Mortality Rates of Leukemia, 2018.

Caption: ASR: Rates per 100,000 are age-standardized to the world population, 2000–2025.

States, Western Europe, Scandinavia, and Australia/ New Zealand compared to developing nations such as India, China, and those in sub-Saharan Africa where the rates are lower (4.0 per 100,000) (Bray et al., 2018). Underreporting may partially account for such differences, particularly in nations without population-based cancer registries.

In contrast to the global pattern of incidence, high annual mortality rates (4–5 per 100,000) were found in several nations of Northeastern Africa (Libya, Egypt, Sudan, Ethiopia, and Somalia) and the Middle East (Iran, Iraq, Syria, Jordan, Israel, and Turkey). Males living in Gaza (Palestine) had the highest mortality rate from leukemia in the world in 2018 (8.5 per 100,000). In those populations where mortality is exceptionally high, the available health-care resources are generally inadequate for effective treatment. Nevertheless, relatively high death rates from leukemia are also evident in the populations of many developed nations, including the United States. According to the latest WHO/International Agency for Research on Cancer (IARC) data from 2008, 2012, and 2018 and data from the Global Burden of Disease Study in 2016, leukemias in children and adults now cause more than 300,000 deaths every year, approximately 3.2% of all cancer deaths (Bray et al., 2018; Ferlay, Shin, Forman, Mathers, & Parkin, 2010; Ferlay et al., 2013, 2018; Fitzmaurice et al., 2018).

The global numbers of leukemia cases and deaths steadily increased during 1990–2018 (**FIGURE 37.3**).

Over the entire time span, the annual number of new cases increased by 75% (from 250,000 to 437,000) and the annual number of deaths increased by 68% (from 184,000 to 310,000). During 2018, 249,454 cases and 179,518 deaths occurred in men and 187,579 cases and 129,488 deaths occurred in women. In contrast to the substantial increases in the annual numbers of cases and deaths, the annual incidence and mortality rates of leukemia have remained fairly constant, e.g., during 2008–2018, the annual age-adjusted incidence rate in men increased about 3% and the rate in women remained the same. As in past years, the age-adjusted incidence and mortality rates in men in 2018 (6.1 per 100,000 and 4.2 per 100,000) were more than 40% higher than women (4.3 per 100,000 and 2.8 per 100,000) (Bray et al., 2018; Ferlay et al., 2010, 2013, 2018; Fitzmaurice et al., 2017, 2018; Parkin, Bray, Ferlay, & Pisani, 2005; Parkin, Pisani, & Ferlay, 1999a,1999b).

The rising absolute number of leukemia cases and deaths is largely due to increasing longevity and growth of the world population. These demographic factors have resulted in more individuals living to later ages when the risk of death from leukemia is highest. **FIGURE 37.4** shows the age distribution of new cases and deaths based on data from the United States collected during 2003–2007 (43,050 cases and 21,840 deaths). Leukemia onset shows an early peak during childhood and then rises throughout the lifespan, with more than 70% of deaths occurring after the age of 65 years (Altekruse et al., 2010).

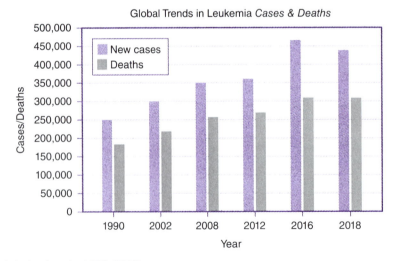

FIGURE 37.3 Global Trends in Leukemia, 1990–2018.

Data from Bray, F., Ferlay, J., Soerjomataram, I., Siegel, R. L., Torre, L. A., & Jemal, A. (2018). Global cancer statistics 2018: GLOBOCAN estimates of incidence and mortality worldwide for 36 cancers in 185 countries. *CA: A Cancer Journal for Clinicians, 68*(6), 394–424; Ferlay, J., Shin, H. R., Forman, D., Mathers, C., & Parkin, D. M. (2010). Estimates of worldwide burden of cancer in 2008. *International Journal of Cancer, 127*(12), 2893–2917; Ferlay, J., Soerjomataram, I., Ervik, M., Dikshit, R., Eser, S., Mathers, C., ... Bray, F. (2013). *GLOBOCAN 2012 v1.0. Cancer incidence and mortality worldwide: IARC CancerBase No. 11* [Internet]. Lyon, France: International Agency for Research on Cancer. Retrieved from http://globocan.iarc.fr; Parkin, D. M., Bray, F., Ferlay, J., & Pisani, P. (2001). Estimating the world cancer burden, GLOBOCAN 2000. *International Journal of Cancer, 94*, 153–156; Parkin, D. M., Bray, F., Ferlay, J., & Pisani, P. (2005). Global cancer statistics, 2002. *CA: A Cancer Journal for Clinicians, 55*, 74–108; Parkin, D. M., Pisani, P., & Ferlay, J. (1999a). Estimates of the worldwide incidence of 25 major cancers in 1990. *International Journal of Cancer, 80*(6), 827–841; Parkin, D. M., Pisani, P., & Ferlay, J. (1999b). Global cancer statistics. *CA: A Cancer Journal for Clinicians, 49*(1), 33–64; World Health Organization. (2008). *World cancer report.* Geneva, Switzerland; Fitzmaurice, C., Allen, C., Barber, R. M., Barregard, L., Bhutta, Z. A., Brenner H, ... Global Burden of Disease Cancer Collaboration (2017). Global, regional, and national cancer incidence, mortality, years of life lost, years lived with disability, and disability-adjusted life-years for 32 cancer groups, 1990 to 2015: A systematic analysis for the Global Burden of Disease Study. *JAMA Oncology, 3*(4), 524–548. Fitzmaurice, C., Akinyemiju, T. F., Al Lami, F. H., Alam, T., Alizadeh-Navaei, R., Allen, C., ... Global Burden of Disease Cancer Collaboration (2018). Global, regional, and national cancer incidence, mortality, years of life lost, years lived with disability, and disability-adjusted life-years for 29 cancer groups, 1990 to 2016: A systematic analysis for the Global Burden of Disease Study. *JAMA Oncology.* Published online June 02, 2018. doi:10.1001/jamaoncol.2018.2706.

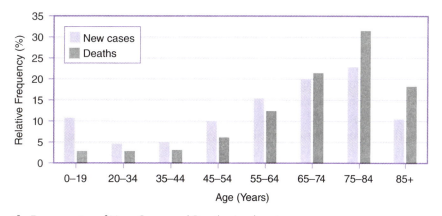

FIGURE 37.4 Age-Specific Frequencies of New Cases and Deaths: Leukemia.

Data from Altekruse, S. F., Kosary, C. L., Krapcho, M., Neyman, N., Aminou, R., Waldron, W., … Edwards, B. K. (2010). *SEER cancer statistics review, 1975–2007*. Bethesda, MD: National Cancer Institute.

TABLE 37.2 Relative Subtypes of Leukemia in the World Population, 2016			
Type of Leukemia	**Males (%)**	**Females (%)**	**All (%)**
Acute Lymphocytic	44,000 (24.2)	32,000 (23.9)	76,000 (24.1)
Chronic Lymphocytic	61,000 (33.5)	45,000 (33.6)	106,000 (33.5)
Acute Myeloid	58,000 (31.9)	45,000 (33.6)	103,000 (32.6)
Chronic Myeloid	19,000 (10.4)	14,000 (10.4)	33,000 (10.4)
Total	182,000	134,000	316,000

Caption: 150,000 cases of leukemia diagnosed in 2018 were unclassified.

Data from Fitzmaurice, C., Akinyemiju, T. F., Al Lami, F. H., Alam, T., Alizadeh-Navaei, R., Allen, C., … Global Burden of Disease Cancer Collaboration (2018). Global, regional, and national cancer incidence, mortality, years of life lost, years lived with disability, and disability-adjusted life-years for 29 cancer groups, 1990 to 2016: A systematic analysis for the Global Burden of Disease Study. *JAMA Oncology*. Published online June 02, 2018. doi:10.1001/jamaoncol.2018.2706.

▶ Incidence and Mortality of Leukemia Subtypes

A total of 316,000 cases of leukemia were categorized by subtype in the *Global Burden of Disease Study* of 2016. The cases of each subtype are shown for males and females in **TABLE 37.2**. The relative frequencies of the four subtypes were remarkably similar for males and females. Chronic lymphocytic leukemia and acute myeloid leukemia each accounted for approximately 33% of cases, and acute lymphocytic leukemia and chronic myeloid leukemia accounted for 24% and 10% of cases, respectively. The male to female ratio was also similar for each subtype ranging from 1.29 for acute myeloid leukemia to 1.38 for acute lymphocytic leukemia. Based on the pooled data across all subtypes, 57.6% of cases were diagnosed in males and 42.4% in females for an overall male to female ratio of 1.36.

The annual age-adjusted mortality rate was highest for acute myeloid leukemia (1.6 per 100,000 in males and 1.0 per 100,000 in females) and the lowest for chronic myeloid leukemia (0.4 per 100,000 in males and 0.3 per 100,000 in females) (Fitzmaurice et al., 2018).

▶ Trends in Leukemia Incidence and Survival

A team of Italian investigators examined trends in the age-standardized annual mortality rates for leukemia based on death certificate data collected by the World Health Organization during 1960–1997. Data were available for the European Union (consisting of 27 member nations) and other developed regions of the world. In the European Union, the peak rates for children up to 14 years of age were observed in 1960–1964, after which mortality decreased more than 70%, reaching a nadir of 1.2 per 100,000 in males and 0.9 per 100,000 in females in 1995–1997. Substantial decreases in mortality were also noted for young and middle-aged adults, aged 15–44 years (40%) and 45–59 years (25%), but not for older age groups. The observed decline in leukemia mortality over the 35-year calendar period corresponds to nearly 250,000 saved lives. Leukemia mortality rates in the United States and Japan started from different values, but trends were like those of the European Union in the late 1990s, indicating that the impact of therapeutic advancements has been comparable in developed areas of the world. In Eastern Europe, however, the declines in leukemia mortality occurred later and were appreciably smaller (Levi, Lucchini, Negri, Barbui, & La Vecchia, 2000).

Investigators at the University of Minnesota examined time trends in the annual age-specific incidence rates of different types of leukemia in the U.S. population during 1973–1998. Their analysis was based on 66,404 leukemia cases identified by the Surveillance, Epidemiology, and End Results (SEER) program of the U.S. National Cancer Institute. In analyses by subtype of leukemia, significant increases were observed for acute lymphocytic leukemia in all age groups except individuals over 65 years of age. Among children and adolescents under 20 years of age, the annual incidence rate of acute lymphocytic leukemia increased by 1.1% per year. Notably, 5-year survival improved by about 15% in younger age groups, presumably because of improved regimens of chemotherapy; however, there was little improvement in survival for older individuals, and survival actually worsened for elderly African Americans (Xie, Davies, Xiang, Robison, & Ross, 2003).

▶ Pediatric Leukemia: Trends in Incidence and Mortality

Approximately 11% of all cases of leukemia are diagnosed in children and adolescents under the age of 20 years. The profile of pediatric leukemia is distinctly different from that in adults. *Acute lymphocytic leukemia* accounts for approximately 75% of cases among children and adolescents younger than 15 years of age, and more than 80% of cases for children younger than 10 years of age. In contrast, the relative frequency of acute lymphocytic leukemia declines dramatically with age, and other types account for 75% of leukemias diagnosed after the age of 50 years.

FIGURE 37.5 shows the age-specific annual incidence of childhood leukemia in U.S. children and adolescents up to 19 years of age. There is a sharp peak for ages 2–3 years (96 cases per million), after which the incidence declines. The incidence of the predominant subtype in children, acute lymphocytic leukemia, also peaks in 2-year-olds, at 83 per million (Smith, Gloeckler-Ries, Gurney, & Ross, 1999).

In developed nations, the annual death rate from leukemia in children has fallen by more than 50% in the past three decades. This favorable downward trend in mortality has occurred even though the incidence of childhood leukemia has *increased* more than 30% over the same time period (Smith et al., 2010). For example, during 1975–1995, the incidence among U.S. children under age 15 years increased steadily by about 0.9% per year as the mortality rate fell by 2.4% per year (Ries, 1999; Ries et al., 1998; Smith et al., 1999). Similar trends have been noted in Europe; for example, during 1970–1999, the incidence of childhood leukemia increased by an average of 1.4% per

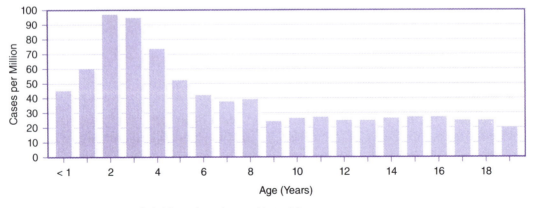

FIGURE 37.5 Age-Specific Incidence of Childhood Leukemia, United States.

Data from Smith, M. A., Gloeckler-Ries, L. A., Gurney, J. G., & Ross, J. A. (1999). Leukemia. In L. A. G. Ries, M. A. Smith, J. G. Gurney, M. Linet, T. Tamra, J. L. Young, & G. R. Bunin (Eds.), *Cancer incidence and survival among children and adolescents: United States SEER program 1975–1995* (pp. 17–34, NIH Pub. No. 99–4649). Bethesda, MD: National Cancer Institute, SEER Program.

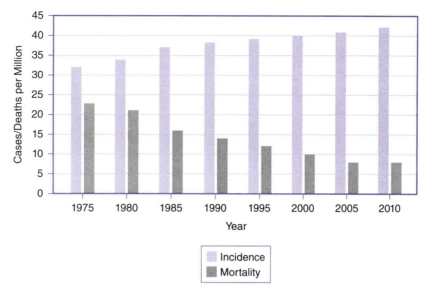

FIGURE 37.6 Incidence and Mortality Trends in Pediatric Leukemia, United States, 1975–2010.

Data from Ries, L. A. G., Kosary, C. L., Hankey, B. F., Miller, B. A., Clegg, L., & Edwards, B. K. (Eds.). (1998). *SEER cancer statistics review 1973–1996.* Bethesda, MD: National Cancer Institute; Ries, L. A. G. (1999). Childhood cancer mortality. In L. A. G. Ries, M. A. Smith, J. G. Gurney, M. Linet, T. Tamra, J. L. Young, & G. R. Bunin (Eds.), *Cancer incidence and survival among children and adolescents: United States SEER program 1975–1995* (pp. 165–170; NIH Pub. No. 99-4649). Bethesda, MD: National Cancer Institute, SEER Program; Smith, M. A., Gloeckler-Ries, L. A., Gurney, J. G., & Ross, J. A. (1999). Leukemia. In L. A. G. Ries, M. A. Smith, J. G. Gurney, M. Linet, T. Tamra, J. L. Young, & G. R. Bunin (Eds.), *Cancer incidence and survival among children and adolescents: United States SEER program 1975–1995* (pp. 17–34; NIH Pub. No. 99-4649). Bethesda, MD: National Cancer Institute, SEER Program; Smith, M. A., Seibel, N. L., Seibel, N. L., Altekruse, S. F., Ries, L. A. G., Melbert, D. L., ... Reaman, G. H. (2010). Outcomes for children and adolescents with cancer: Challenges for the twenty-first century. *Journal of Clinical Oncology, 28*(15), 2625–2634.

year whereas the overall mortality rate declined by nearly 60% (Shah & Coleman, 2007). Declines in mortality have been noted for boys and girls of all ages. The inverse trends in the incidence and mortality rates for U.S. children under 15 years of age are shown for the period 1975–2010 in **FIGURE 37.6**.

The falling leukemia mortality in children of developed nations reflects a marked increase in survival due to rapid detection coupled with improved therapy. In the United States, the 5-year survival rate for children who developed acute lymphocytic leukemia increased from 61% in 1975–1978 to 89% in 1999–2002 (**FIGURE 37.7**). As stated by Malcolm Smith and colleagues at the U.S. National Cancer Institute, "the improvement in survival for children with acute lymphocytic leukemia over the past 35 years is one of the great success stories of clinical oncology" and reflects the therapeutic benefit of combination chemotherapy, radiation therapy, and bone marrow transplantation (Smith et al., 2010).

Despite the obvious benefit of early detection and effective therapy in some parts of the world, survival remains poor for children who develop leukemia in less-developed nations. For example, the 5-year survival rate for children stricken with leukemia who live in the Philippines is only 33% compared to nearly 90% for afflicted children of the same ethnicity in the United States. Such differences highlight the deficiencies in pediatric cancer care and the need for major improvements in diagnostic and treatment facilities in developing countries (Redaniel et al., 2010).

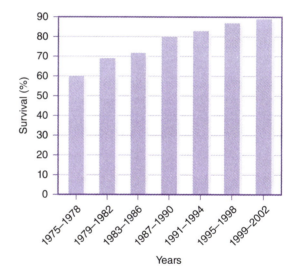

FIGURE 37.7 Acute Lymphocytic Leukemia: Five-Year Survival in Children, United States, 1975–2002.

Data from Smith, M. A., Seibel, N. L., Seibel, N. L., Altekruse, S. F., Ries, L. A. G., Melbert, D. L., ... Reaman, G. H. (2010). Outcomes for children and adolescents with cancer: Challenges for the twenty-first century. *Journal of Clinical Oncology, 28*(15), 2625–2634.

Pediatric Leukemia: Risk Factors

Leukemia is the most common cancer in children and has been intensively investigated using molecular, genetic, clinical, and epidemiologic techniques. Nevertheless, except for ionizing radiation, rare genetic syndromes, and certain chemotherapeutic drugs that are implicated in a small fraction of cases, causal factors for most cases are obscure and the etiology remains enigmatic.

Gender and Ethnic Differences of Childhood Leukemia

Marked gender and ethnic differences have been noted in the incidence rates of pediatric acute lymphocytic leukemia. For children under 15 years of age, boys have about 1.2 times higher risk than girls, and Caucasians have about twice the risk of African Americans. Such differences are not spurious, because they have persisted for several decades (Harris, Harrell, Patil, & Al-Rashid, 1987; Smith et al., 1999).

Reasons for these gender and ethnic differences are speculative. The recently proposed *adrenal hypothesis* relates the higher leukemia risk in children of higher socioeconomic classes to their relatively low exposure to infectious viruses and bacteria during the early years of life. Presumably, the risk of acute lymphocytic leukemia is *reduced* when childhood infections during infancy induce the hypothalamic-pituitary-adrenal axis to secrete high levels of plasma cortisol. Corticosteroids are known to regulate the maturation and proliferation of B lymphocytes by stimulating apoptosis, and high levels may eliminate leukemic cells and/or progenitor B lymphocytes with leukemogenic potential. Furthermore, early infection and heightened cortisol secretion may favor the maturation and proliferation of T lymphocytes that secrete *anti-inflammatory* rather than *proinflammatory* cytokines, thereby reducing the risk of leukemogenesis (Schmiegelow, Vestergaard, Nielsen, & Hjalgrim, 2008).

Familial Associations of Childhood Leukemia

Some studies have noted an association between childhood leukemia and the presence of autoimmune conditions among relatives. A team of investigators in Paris designed a case–control study to assess the relationship between childhood leukemia and a family history of autoimmune conditions such as type 1 diabetes mellitus, thyroid disease, and rheumatoid arthritis. Family histories of autoimmune disease in first- and second-degree relatives were ascertained for 279 incident cases of acute leukemia and 285 controls matched by age, gender, and ethnicity. The study revealed a significant association between familial autoimmune disease and the risk of leukemia (odds ratio [OR] = 1.7). The relationship was stronger for autoimmune thyroid conditions such as Grave's disease or Hashimoto's thyroiditis (OR = 3.5) but diminished for other types of thyroid diseases (goiter or adenoma). These results suggest that a family history of autoimmune thyroid disease may be associated

with childhood acute leukemia (Perillat-Menegaux et al., 2003).

Investigators at the University of Montreal in Quebec explored genetic polymorphisms of the P-450 enzyme system to determine potential associations of xenobiotic-metabolizing enzymes and the risk of developing childhood leukemia. They compared polymorphisms among 177 children with acute lymphocytic leukemia to 304 controls matched by age and gender. The results revealed increased odds ratios for individuals carrying the null polymorphism of the glutathione-S transferase gene (*GSTM-1*) (OR = 1.8) or the *CYP-1A1-2A* allele (OR = 1.7). Furthermore, the odds of disease were higher for individuals carrying both genotypes (OR = 3.3). The investigators suggest that these findings have biological plausibility in that the *CYP-1A1-2A* enzyme activates polycyclic aromatic compounds that are not metabolized for excretion by individuals with the null *GSTM-1* genotype (Krajinovic, Labuda, Richer, Karimi, & Sinnett, 1999).

Genetic Syndromes and Childhood Leukemia

The risk of developing acute lymphocytic leukemia is increased in subjects with certain rare genetic syndromes and conditions. These include Down syndrome, Bloom syndrome, Shwachman syndrome, ataxia telangiectasia, neurofibromatosis, and Fanconi anemia.

Down syndrome (trisomy 21) markedly increases the risk of developing acute leukemia. The syndrome is named after the British physician John Langdon Down, who first described it in 1866 (Down, 1866). The genetic anomaly identified as an extra 21st chromosome was discovered by the French pediatrician/cytogeneticist Jérôme Lejeune in 1959 (Lejeune, 1959).

Down syndrome is a chromosomal condition caused by the presence of an extra copy of genetic material on the 21st chromosome, either in whole (trisomy 21) or in part (when due to translocations). In addition to its characteristic phenotypic, mental, and cognitive features, Down syndrome carries a high risk for development of leukemia. In particular, the risk of acute lymphoblastic leukemia is elevated at least 10-fold and the risk of acute myelogenous leukemia is increased at least 50-fold in patients with Down syndrome, perhaps due to overexpression of proto-oncogenes on the extra 21st chromosome (Hasle, Clemmensen, & Mikkelsen, 2000).

Bloom syndrome (congenital telangiectatic erythema) is a rare autosomal recessive disorder characterized by telangiectasia (clusters of small cutaneous dilated blood vessels or spider veins), photosensitivity, growth deficiency of prenatal onset, variable degrees of immunodeficiency, and increased susceptibility to various forms of cancer, including leukemia. The New York dermatologist David Bloom first described the syndrome in 1954 (Bloom, 1954). Approximately 20% of patients with Bloom syndrome develop specific malignancies (acute leukemia, lymphoma, and/or gastrointestinal adenocarcinoma). Cancer risk in such patients is increased 150–300 times compared to the general population (German, 1993).

Bloom syndrome is caused by a mutation of a tumor–suppressor gene designated *BLM* (short for Bloom) traced to the long arm of chromosome 15. The protein encoded by the normal gene has DNA helicase activity and functions in the maintenance of genomic stability. Mutant forms of *BLM* increase the exchange of DNA during mitosis (sister chromatid exchange) and chromosomal instability, which are presumably responsible for the characteristic phenotypic abnormalities and cancer predisposition (Cheok et al., 2005).

Shwachman–Bodian–Diamond syndrome is a rare autosomal recessive disorder caused by a mutated gene, *SBDS*, on the long arm of chromosome 7. The *SBDS* gene appears to help regulate RNA metabolism and ribosomal assembly of proteins in the cell. Individuals homozygous for the mutant *SBDS* gene typically manifest exocrine pancreatic dysfunction, skeletal anomalies, anemia, neutropenia, and progressive bone marrow failure that may transform to acute myelogenous leukemia (Bodian, Sheldon, & Lightwood, 1964; Popovic et al., 2002; Shwachman, Diamond, Oski, & Khaw, 1964).

Ataxia telangiectasia is a rare autosomal recessive disorder caused by a mutant gene (*ATM*) located on the long arm of chromosome 11 that is critical for regulating checkpoints during cell division and for repairing errors in DNA replication. This condition is characterized by lack of coordination and cognitive control, immune deficiency, and telangiectasia (clusters of small dilated blood vessels), particularly in the sclera of the eye. Patients who are homozygous recessive for the *ATM* mutation have an approximate risk of 1% per year of developing either leukemia or lymphoma (Canman & Lim, 1998).

Neurofibromatosis type 1 (von Recklinghausen's disease) is a rare autosomal dominant disorder characterized by the development of multiple fibromas (neurofibromas) of the skin, brain, and other anatomic sites. The rare disorder was first described by the German physician Friedrich von Recklinghausen in 1882. The syndrome is due to a mutant autosomal dominant gene called *NF1* located on the long arm of chromosome 17. The mutant gene encodes a protein called neurofibromin that regulates cell division of fibrous nerve sheaths (Boyd, Korf, & Theos, 2009).

In addition to causing neurofibromas, mutant forms of *NF1* also increase the risk of developing leukemia and lymphoma. Stiller and colleagues at Oxford quantified the risk among 58 subjects with neurofibromatosis type 1 based on data ascertained from the National Registry of Childhood Tumors in Great Britain. Over the 17-year study period, 12 cases of acute lymphocytic leukemia (relative risk [RR] = 5.4), 5 cases of non-Hodgkin's lymphoma (RR = 10.0), and 5 cases of myelomonocytic leukemia (RR = 221) were detected among the 58 patients with neurofibromatosis type 1 (Stiller, Chessells, & Fitchett, 1994). These results suggest that the *NF1* gene has pleiotropic impact on the regulation of hematopoiesis.

Fanconi anemia is a rare autosomal recessive genetic disorder named after the Swiss pediatrician Guido Fanconi, who initially described it (Fanconi, 1927). Fanconi anemia is caused by mutations in any of 13 different genes that encode proteins involved in the regulation of DNA repair during replication. One of these genes is the well-known breast cancer susceptibility gene, *BRCA-2*. Up to 75% of patients have congenital defects, commonly short stature, and developmental disabilities and abnormalities at various anatomic sites. Approximately 20% of patients develop some form of cancer, the most common of which is *acute myelocytic leukemia*, and 90% suffer myelodysplasia with bone marrow failure by the age of 40 years. The median age at death for patients with Fanconi anemia is about 40 years (D'Andrea, 2010).

Drugs and Childhood Leukemia

Certain chemotherapeutic agents have been found to heighten the risk of leukemia development in children and adults. For example, the compound *epipodophyllotoxin* (etoposide and teniposide) has been linked to the development of acute myeloid leukemia. This compound interferes with the function of topoisomerases, enzymes that unwind and wind DNA for transcription and replication. Investigators at St. Jude Children's Research Hospital in Memphis, Tennessee, examined the effects of epipodophyllotoxin therapy among 734 consecutive children with acute lymphoblastic leukemia who attained completed remission and received continuation (maintenance) treatment according to specific schedules of epipodophyllotoxin administration. After 6 years of follow-up, secondary acute myelocytic leukemia was diagnosed in 21 of the 734 patients, yielding a cumulative risk of 3.8%. Within subgroups receiving higher dosages of epipodophyllotoxin, the cumulative risk increased to more than 12%. In comparative groups not treated with epipodophyllotoxin, the highest cumulative risk was 1.6%. The results indicate that maintenance therapy with epipodophyllotoxin stimulates leukemogenesis of myelocytic cells (Pui et al., 1991).

Radiation and Childhood Leukemia

The Life Span Study was initiated in 1950 to monitor the impact of radiation exposure among survivors of the atomic bomb explosions in Japan during World War II. As of the year 2000, 204 leukemia deaths had occurred among 49,204 survivors who received a bone marrow radiation dose of at least 0.005 Gy, constituting an excess of 94 cases (46%) attributable to radiation from the atomic bomb explosions. The dose response pattern in excess number of observed deaths reflects a nonlinear pattern; however, even at low doses in the range of 0.2–0.5 Gy, the leukemia risk is elevated (**FIGURE 37.8**). Risk increases have been noted for acute lymphocytic leukemia in children and acute and chronic myelocytic leukemia in adults, but not other types (Preston et al., 1994, 2004).

A recent population-based study found a marked increase in the rates of leukemia among children in Southern Iraq during the period 1993–2007. Investigators from the University of Basrah in Iraq and the University of Washington in Seattle analyzed leukemia registry data collected at Ibn Ghazwan Hospital in Basrah to evaluate leukemia trends since 1993. Annual leukemia incidence rates were estimated from 698 cases diagnosed in children aged 14 years or younger. The annual incidence (cases per 100,000) increased dramatically during the period of study, from 2.6 in 1993 to 6.9 in 2007, peaking at 12.2 in 2006. Estimates for the final 3 years of the study are more than double the rates in the European Union or the United States (Hagopian et al., 2010).

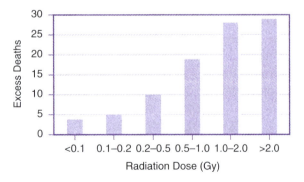

FIGURE 37.8 Dose Response of Excess Leukemia Deaths and Radiation Exposure Among Atomic Bomb Survivors.

Data from Smith, M. A., Seibel, N. L., Seibel, N. L., Altekruse, S. F., Ries, L. A. G., Melbert, D. L., ... Reaman, G. H. (2010). Outcomes for children and adolescents with cancer: Challenges for the twenty-first century. *Journal of Clinical Oncology, 28*(15), 2625–2634.

These results have led to speculation that heightened exposure to chemical warfare agents since 2003, in particular benzene and depleted uranium dust, may be responsible for the increased incidence of childhood leukemia, although additional investigations will be needed to definitively establish an etiologic link (Greiser & Hoffman, 2010).

Seasonal Onset of Acute Lymphocytic Leukemia

Acute lymphocytic leukemia is characterized by quick onset with rapid transition from good health to life-threatening disease, particularly in children. Typically, a newfound bleeding diathesis leads to the diagnosis by discovery of lymphoblasts in the peripheral blood and bone marrow. Due to its acute nature, onset of this form of leukemia has been examined for seasonal periodicity by several investigators, in the hope of elucidating etiologic factors.

Investigators at the University of Nebraska examined month-of-onset of successive cases of acute lymphocytic leukemia diagnosed during 1971–1980 in the Midwestern United States. They detected significant peaks in early winter and late summer coinciding with peak rates of influenza and hay fever from ragweed pollen, respectively (Harris & Al-Rashid, 1984). Subsequently, these same investigators examined all cases of acute lymphocytic leukemia reported in the U.S. SEER database during 1973–1980 and found that in eight of nine SEER locations, the pattern of onset fits a trimodal pattern with peaks in winter, spring, and summer, coinciding with seasonal elevations in the rates of allergenic and infectious diseases that are capable of promoting lymphocytic proliferation and transformation (Harris et al., 1987).

Investigators in the United Kingdom found a 40% excess of acute lymphocytic leukemia cases diagnosed in summer months compared to winter months based on analysis of data from the East Anglian Cancer Registry collected during 1971–1994. Seasonal patterns were not evident for other forms of leukemia. The authors suggest the data are most compatible with an infectious etiology of acute lymphocytic leukemia (Badrinath, Day, & Stockton, 1997).

Despite these results, many other investigators have *not* found evidence of seasonality in the onset of acute lymphocytic leukemia. In an attempt to resolve the question, Gao and colleagues conducted an extensive analysis of reported data on 27,000 cases from 11 countries over a wide range of latitudes. Although there was evidence of seasonal peaks and valleys in certain populations, no consistent pattern of seasonality emerged by latitude, and the investigators concluded that seasonal influences are not likely to be of major etiologic importance (Gao, Chia, & Machin, 2007).

Cytogenetics of Pediatric Leukemia

Cytogenetic abnormalities are characteristic of pediatric acute lymphocytic leukemia. Karyotypic studies of the chromosomes reveal translocations, inversions, or deletions of chromosomes in the lymphoblasts of approximately 90% of cases. Approximately 40% of karyotypes are pseudodiploid (46 chromosomes with structural or numeric abnormalities), 35%–45% are hyperdiploid (47 or more chromosomes), less than 10% are hypodiploid (fewer than 46 chromosomes), and 10%–15% are diploid (46 chromosomes without detectable abnormalities) (Pui, Relling, & Downing, 2004).

Reciprocal translocations are the most common structural chromosomal aberrations found in acute lymphocytic leukemia. The first translocation discovered in pediatric acute lymphocytic leukemia was t(9;22), a reciprocal translocation involving juxtaposition of the *BCR* gene on chromosome 9 to the promoter region of the *ABL* gene on chromosome 22. The altered chromosome 22 produced by this translocation is called the *Philadelphia chromosome* because it was discovered by investigators at the University of Pennsylvania and the Fox-Chase Cancer Research Institute in Philadelphia (Nowell & Hungerford, 1960). The resulting hybrid gene, *BCR-ABL*, encodes a chimeric fusion protein that stimulates the intracellular *RAS* signal transduction pathway, leading to uncontrolled proliferation of lymphocytes and myelocytes. The Philadelphia chromosome, which is found in about 5% of pediatric acute lymphocytic leukemia cases, is the defining genetic signature of chronic myelocytic (granulocytic) leukemia in adults (Kurzrock, Kantarjian, Druker, & Talpaz, 2003).

An exciting development in leukemia research was the discovery of the *TEL-AML1* fusion gene created by the t(12;21) translocation, which is found in approximately 25% of cases of acute lymphocytic leukemia. The *TEL* gene appears to repress transcription of the *AML1* gene, thereby inhibiting normal differentiation of B lymphocytes (Golub et al., 1995). In addition to somatic rearrangements of the *TEL* gene, germline *TEL* mutations have also been discovered in pediatric acute lymphocytic leukemia that are associated with a relatively poor prognosis (Rubnitz et al., 1997, 2008).

The t(1;19) translocation is detected in 15%–25% of pediatric acute lymphocytic leukemia cases. This translocation fuses the *E2A* gene on chromosome 19 with the *PBX1* gene on chromosome 1, producing a hybrid gene that encodes a chimeric fusion protein, *E2A-PBX1*, that serves as a transcription activator of several other genes (Pui et al., 1994).

The most common chromosomal deletion found in pediatric acute lymphocytic leukemia involves loss of a portion of the short arm of chromosome 9. Such deletions are found in about 11% of cases and are associated with poor survival (Heerema et al., 1999).

In 35%–45% of young patients with acute lymphocytic leukemia, tumor cells manifest extrachromosomes (hyperdiploidy) without apparent structural abnormalities. Chromosome 21 is the most frequently detected "extra" chromosome (Down syndrome or trisomy 21). In addition, about 5% of patients manifest hypodiploidkaryotypes characterized by the loss of certain chromosomes. An important finding is that the chromosomal pattern detected in the karyotype of children with leukemia is often an accurate predictor of survival. For example, patients with normal or hyperdiploid karyotypes respond better to treatment and have longer survival than those with translocations, deletions, or hypodiploidy (Bloomfield et al., 1986).

Genome-wide association studies of single nucleotide polymorphisms and targeted genetic polymorphism studies have also identified germline (inherited) mutations associated with the development and progression of pediatric acute lymphocytic leukemia. These include point mutations in the *TEL* gene and the *ARID5B* gene, both of which regulate transcription in embryonic development and during cell growth and differentiation (Healy, Richer, Bourgey, Kritikou, & Sinnett, 2010; Rubnitz et al., 2008).

▶ Adult Leukemia

The relative incidence of myelocytic leukemia compared to lymphocytic leukemia increases with age and is the prominent form of leukemia in adults. In adults over the age of 50 years, approximately 60% of leukemias arise from myelocytes and 40% from lymphocytes. Leukemias diagnosed in adults (20 years or older) account for nearly 90% of all cases.

The genesis of myelocytic leukemia is like that of lymphocytic leukemia. Progenitor (stem) cells in the bone marrow appear to become "frozen" at a particular stage of differentiation, giving rise to a proliferative clone of leukemic cells (myeloblasts). The expanding clone of leukemic cells interrupts normal hematopoiesis, leading to neutropenia, anemia, and thrombocytopenia. Epidemiologic features of the major subtypes of adult leukemias are discussed in the following sections.

Acute Myelocytic Leukemia

Acute myelocytic (myelogenous) leukemia accounts for about 25% of adult leukemias. Several subtypes of this form of leukemia have been defined based on cellular morphology, the degree of maturation, staining characteristics, and cytogenetic findings. Following an early peak during the first year of life, the incidence of acute myelocytic leukemia remains low until age 40 years, after which it increases exponentially with age. Most cases are diagnosed after age 60 years, and the median onset is about 65 years of age (**FIGURE 37.9**) (Gurney, Severson, Davis, & Robison, 1995).

Worldwide, acute myelocytic leukemia causes nearly 65,000 deaths per year, approximately 25% of all deaths attributable to leukemia. The incidence is highest in developed countries such as the United States, Australia, and nations in Western Europe. In the United States, nearly 12,000 men and women were diagnosed with acute myelocytic leukemia in 2006; the average age-adjusted annual incidence during 1975–2003 was 3.4 per 100,000. No significant time trends have been noted in the past few decades (American Cancer Society, 2005; Ries et al., 2003). The higher rates in developed countries partially reflect greater longevity because the elderly are at greatest risk (Figure 37.9).

Acute myelocytic leukemia shows a clear male predominance. For example, the 2006 age-adjusted rate in U.S. men (4.6 per 100,000) was about 50% higher than in women (3.0 per 100,000). The annual mortality rate was also higher in men (3.5 per 100,000) than in women (2.2 per 100,000). Survival dramatically declines with later onset of acute myelocytic leukemia. The 5-year survival rate for individuals diagnosed before age 50 years is 50% compared to only 5% for individuals diagnosed at 65 years or older (Altekruse et al., 2010).

Acute Myelocytic Leukemia: Risk Factors

Acute myelocytic leukemia is the most common type of all leukemias, yet the known risk factors account for only a small fraction of cases. One relatively common

feature of this disease is the presence of cytogenetic abnormalities, which are found in up to 80% of cases. These include translocations, trisomic conditions, and other chromosomal deletions and aberrations.

The most common translocations found in acute myelocytic leukemia are t(8;21) and t(15;17). Both translocations create chimeric fusion proteins that promote leukemogenesis of immature myelocytes by deregulating nuclear binding factors and gene expression (Lavau & Dejean, 1994; McNeil et al., 1999). Significant advances have been made in the treatment of acute myelocytic leukemia with the introduction of new chemotherapeutic regimens that target specific cytogenetic markers of leukemia subtypes (Bloomfield et al., 1998).

In addition to chromosomal aberrations, some point mutations and epigenetic alterations have also been found in association with leukemia development. In England, Bowen and colleagues used polymerase chain reaction technology to examine allelic frequencies of genes encoding carcinogen-metabolizing enzymes of the P-450 enzyme system among 447 cases of acute myelocytic leukemia. They found that a variant form of the *CYP1A1* gene was associated with an increase in risk (OR = 2.36). The investigators suggest that the *CYP1A1-2B* allele may predispose to the development of certain subtypes of acute myelocytic leukemia by catalyzing the formation of carcinogenic polycyclic aromatic hydrocarbons or other reactive compounds (Bowen et al., 2003).

Epigenetic silencing of tumor–suppressor genes and/or amplification of proto-oncogenes may also contribute to leukemogenesis. For example, hypermethylation of the *p15-INK4B* gene, a negative cell cycle regulator of myelocytes, has been identified in a significant fraction of cases (Christiansen, Andersen, & Pedersen-Bjergaard, 2003).

As with other forms of leukemia, the risk of developing acute myelocytic leukemia is increased by radiation exposure. The most notable example is among survivors of the atomic bomb explosions in Japan,

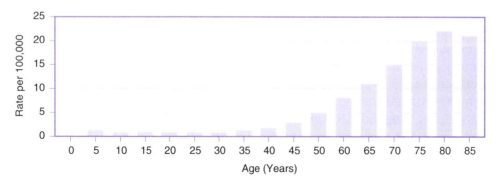

FIGURE 37.9 Age-Specific Incidence of Acute Myelocytic Leukemia.

Data from Deschler, B., & Lübbert, M. (2006). Acute myeloid leukemia: Epidemiology and etiology. *Cancer, 107*, 2099–2107.

who were found to have a fourfold increase in the risk with a peak 5–7 years after exposure (Preston et al., 1994). Excess rates of acute myelocytic leukemias have also been observed secondary to therapeutic radiation exposure (Kossman & Weiss, 2000).

Excess rates of acute myelocytic leukemia have been observed secondary to intensive chemotherapy for other forms of cancer. For example, alkylating agents such as cyclophosphamide and topoisomerase inhibitors such as epipodophyllotoxin have both been reported to significantly increase the risk (Le Beau, Albain, et al., 1986; Le Beau, Pettenati, et al., 1986; Pui et al., 1991). A team of Swedish investigators examined the rate of secondary leukemia in a cohort of 115 patients who received chemotherapy for other malignancies. In patients primarily treated with alkylating agents, the risk increased by approximately 1% per year over 8 years of follow-up, and in those receiving both alkylating agents and topoisomerase inhibitors, the risk increased more than 100-fold. These investigators point out that secondary development of acute myelocytic leukemia "has become the most serious long-term complication of cancer therapy" (Pedersen-Bjergaard et al., 1993).

Certain chemicals have also been implicated as risk factors for acute myelocytic leukemia, including benzene, embalming fluids (formalin), ethylene oxides, and herbicides (Deschler & Lübbert, 2006; Savitz & Andrews, 1997). Furthermore, chronic cigarette smoking has been found to increase the risk of certain subtypes of acute myelocytic leukemia (Pogoda, Preston-Martin, Nichols, & Ross, 2002).

Myelodysplastic Syndrome (Preleukemia)

It has long been recognized that individuals who develop acute myelocytic leukemia often manifest a prodromal period of anemia, myelocytic dysplasia, and abnormal erythropoiesis (red blood cell production). The first description of *preleukemia* was published in 1953 by Block and colleagues, who characterized the transformation of myelodysplasia to acute myelocytic leukemia among 12 patients (Block, Jacobson, & Bethard, 1953). In 1976, a French-American-British team of physicians and researchers defined refractory anemia in combination with myelocytic dysplasia as the *myelodysplastic syndrome.*

It is now recognized that the myelodysplastic syndrome actually consists of a diverse collection of hematological conditions characterized by various degrees of anemia, dysplasia of myeloid cells, neutropenia, and other symptoms. *Myeloid dysplasia* refers to abnormal differentiation and maturation of myeloid progenitor (stem) cells, resulting in alterations in their size, shape, organization, and function. Often, myeloid dysplasia is accompanied by excessive proliferation (hyperplasia) of deranged myelocytes.

Myeloid dysplasia is invariably associated with anemia due to ineffectual erythropoiesis and the lack of production of functional red blood cells. Over time, the disease worsens, and patients develop refractory anemia, neutropenia, and thrombocytopenia. In about 30% of cases, the condition eventually transforms into acute myelocytic leukemia.

In recent years, cytogenetic, morphological, and clinical data have been reassessed to create more accurate prognostic categories of the myelodysplastic syndrome. In general, patients are classified according to the type and severity of cytopenia, the fraction of myeloblasts in the bone marrow, the appearance of multiple cytogenetic aberrations, and the likelihood of developing acute myelocytic leukemia within 1 year. In the most severe form, patients have refractory anemia and pancytopenia, 21%–30% of cells in the bone marrow are myeloblasts, and the chance of transformation to acute myelocytic leukemia is very high, about 40% per year (Greenberg et al., 1997).

The incidence and prevalence rates of myelodysplastic disease have not been accurately quantified in most populations. This paucity of epidemiologic data reflects the absence of population-based screening and early detection programs, plus inconsistencies in the diagnosis and classification of disease. Nevertheless, small regional studies have provided some initial estimates and suggest that the incidence is increasing, particularly among the elderly. In a study conducted in the population of Düsseldorf in Germany during 1986–1990, the annual incidence for all ages was 3.9 per 100,000 in men and 4.3 per 100,000 in women. The peak rates occurred after 70 years of age, 33.9 per 100,000 in men and 18.0 per 100,000 in women. Among 1759 cases, 82% were diagnosed after age 50 years, and the median age of onset was 71 years. Studies in other centers found similar patterns of onset as well as increasing numbers of cases, largely reflecting improvements in geriatric disease detection and medical care (Aul, Giagounidis, & Germing, 2001).

Certain cytogenetic abnormalities are regularly found in myeloblasts of patients with the myelodysplastic syndrome. The most common abnormality is deletion of the long arm of chromosome 5 (also called 5q– syndrome), initially discovered in 1974 (Van den Berghe et al., 1974). More recent studies have identified genes encoding colony-stimulating factors and receptors (*GM-CSF, CSF-1, FMS*) and interleukin genes (*IL-3, IL-4, IL-5*) that regulate hematopoiesis, which are lost in the 5q– syndrome (Bunn, 1986; Le Beau, Albain, et al., 1986; Le Beau, Pettenati, et al., 1986; van

Leeuwen, Martinson, Webb, & Young, 1989). Several cytogenetic findings have been linked to the prognosis of myelodysplastic disease and/or conversion to acute myelocytic leukemia. For example, cases with single abnormalities of the long arm of chromosome 1 experience poor survival, and those with trisomy 8 have a high risk of malignant transformation; in contrast, patients with deletions in the short arm of chromosome 12 show relatively good survival. Clinical studies of cases reveal that cytogenetic features, the proportion of bone marrow myeloblasts, and hemoglobin and blood platelet levels are the main prognostic factors of survival and transformation to acute leukemia (Solé et al., 2000).

The risk factors for myeloid dysplasia are synonymous with those for acute myelocytic leukemia: exposure to ionizing radiation, benzene-containing compounds, alkylating agents and topoisomerase inhibitors used in cancer therapy, and immunosuppressive drugs used in organ transplantation (Aul et al., 2001).

Chronic Myelocytic (Granulocytic) Leukemia

Chronic myelocytic (granulocytic) leukemia is defined by the presence of the Philadelphia chromosome, which is caused by a reciprocal translocation involving juxtaposition of the *BCR* gene on chromosome 9 to the promoter region of the *ABL* gene on chromosome 22, designated t(9;22). The resulting hybrid gene, *BCR-ABL*, encodes a chimeric fusion protein that stimulates the intracellular *RAS* signal transduction pathway, leading to uncontrolled proliferation of myelocytes and other immune cells (Kurzrock et al., 2003). The Philadelphia chromosome was introduced earlier in this chapter in the section on pediatric leukemia, because it was first discovered in cells of a pediatric leukemia patient by investigators in Philadelphia (Nowell & Hungerford, 1960).

Chronic myelocytic leukemia is characterized by increased proliferation of granulocytes of all types in the bone marrow. Basophils and eosinophils are virtually always increased. Presence of the Philadelphia chromosome identified by cytogenetic or genetic analysis of tumor cells validates the diagnosis (Savage, Szydlo, & Goldman, 1997). This form of leukemia may persist in a chronic phase for many years, but eventually terminates in a blast crisis with widespread metastatic spread of myeloblasts and lymphoblasts and short survival (Kantarjian et al., 1988).

Chronic myelocytic leukemia is most commonly diagnosed in middle-aged and older adults and accounts for approximately 15%–20% of adult leukemias. The only definitive risk factor for this form of leukemia is ionizing radiation. Among survivors of the atomic bomb blasts in Japan who have been followed for more than half a century, the cumulative incidence of chronic myelocytic leukemia is about sevenfold higher than in the general population (Preston et al., 1994).

Radiotherapy has also been linked to the development of chronic myelocytic leukemia. Preston-Martin and colleagues conducted a case–control study of radiation exposure in 136 cases diagnosed in Los Angeles hospitals during 1979–1985 and 136 neighborhood controls. ORs were estimated by the cumulative level of bone marrow exposure to radiotherapy. Results revealed a dose response in the risk with increasing radiation dose maximizing at OR = 2.4 for the highest cumulative dose (at least 2000 mrads) (Preston-Martin, Thomas, Yu, & Henderson, 1989).

Chronic Lymphocytic Leukemia

Chronic lymphocytic leukemia is typified by excess proliferation of small but well-differentiated (mature) lymphocytes in the bone marrow and peripheral blood. In most cases, the vast majority (98%) of malignant lymphocytes are B cells. Leukemic cells are, on average, smaller but otherwise morphologically like normal lymphocytes. Furthermore, the cells from most patients have membrane receptors, antigens, and immunoglobulins that are characteristic of mature B lymphocytes. However, they are functionally deficient and incapable of mounting an immune response. Hence, patients with chronic lymphocytic leukemia are predisposed to a variety of infectious conditions.

Chronic lymphocytic leukemia is a disease of older adults, with nearly 90% of cases diagnosed after the age of 55 years. The condition often takes years to progress, and patients are usually monitored for clinical and hematologic changes before initiation of treatment. However, transformation of the chronic form to an acute blast crisis carries a high risk of death.

In the United States, approximately 15,000 new cases were diagnosed in 2010 and more than 4000 deaths were attributed to chronic lymphocytic leukemia. Annual incidence rates per 100,000 were higher in men than women (5.7 versus 3.0) and were highest in Caucasians (6.1 in men and 3.2 in women) and lowest in Asians and Pacific Islanders (1.3 in men and 0.7 in women). Annual death rates were also highest in Caucasians (2.1 in men and 1.0 in women) and lowest in Asians and Pacific Islanders (0.4 in men and 0.1 in women). Five-year survival approaches 80% for Caucasians but is less than 70% for African Americans (Altekruse et al., 2010).

Certain ethnic groups have been found to have high incidence and prevalence rates of chronic lymphocytic leukemia. For example, relatively high rates have been reported for Ashkenazi Jews in Israel compared to other ethnic groups (Bartal, Bentwich, Manny, & Izak, 1978). The relative importance of genetic and environmental factors is currently being explored in comparative studies of different ethnic groups. However, in an investigation of 302 cases of B-cell chronic lymphocytic leukemia, ethnicity per se had no discernible effects on the biological and clinical behavior of the disease (Shvidel, Shtarlid, Klepfish, Sigler, & Berrebi, 1998).

Chronic Lymphocytic Leukemia: Risk Factors

Familial history is one of the strongest risk factors for the development of chronic lymphocytic leukemia. Studies of monozygous and dizygous twins, siblings, and pedigrees with multiple generations have established that close relatives of probands (index cases) are at high risk. For example, in a Swedish study of 14,336 first-degree relatives of 5918 probands with chronic lymphocytic leukemia and 28,876 first-degree relatives of 11,778 control subjects, first-degree relatives of the probands were found to have a 7.5-fold increase in the risk of also developing chronic lymphocytic leukemia (Goldin, Pfeiffer, Li, & Hemminki, 2004). Genome-wide association studies and linkage studies are currently being conducted to elucidate the genes responsible for the increase in familial risk of chronic lymphocytic leukemia (Goldin & Caporaso, 2007).

Chromosomal abnormalities are well documented in chronic lymphocytic leukemia. The most common of these is an interstitial deletion of the long arm of chromosome 13, which has been found in approximately 50% of cases. Other common cytogenetic findings include specific deletions of the long arm of chromosome 11 (20%), trisomy 12 (15%), specific deletions of the long arm of chromosome 6 (10%), and specific deletions of the short arm of chromosome 17 (5%) (Stilgenbauer, Dohner, & Lichter, 1993). Such nonrandom chromosomal deletions and aberrations may confer selective advantage to B lymphocytes by inactivation of tumor–suppressor genes, or conversely, by amplifying the expression of proto-oncogenes.

Point mutations and epigenetic changes that alter gene expression without changing the nucleotide sequence may also be involved in the genesis of chronic lymphocytic leukemia. For example, hypermethylation and epigenetic silencing of the death-associated protein kinase (*DAPK1*) gene, which regulates apoptosis, has been noted in a large kindred affected with chronic lymphocytic leukemia (Plass, Byrd, Raval, Tanner, & De La Chapelle, 2007).

Despite compelling evidence that ionizing radiation causes most forms of leukemia, including acute lymphocytic leukemia, most studies of chronic lymphocytic leukemia have not detected risk increases with radiation exposure. These results have led some expert committees to conclude that ionizing radiation is not a significant risk factor for chronic lymphocytic leukemia (United Nations Scientific Committee on the Effects of Atomic Radiation, 2000). However, it has also been pointed out that methodological difficulties such as lack of statistical power and limited duration of follow-up have hampered efforts to detect an association (Richardson, Wing, Schroeder, Schmitz-Feuerhake, & Hoffmann, 2005).

Data are limited on the association of specific chemical exposures and the development of chronic lymphocytic leukemia. Although some individual studies suggest risk increases associated with certain occupational exposures (e.g., agrichemicals, petroleum, and rubber), there is little consistency of results from study to study (Linet et al., 2007).

Agent Orange has been linked to the genesis of several lymphoproliferative disorders, including chronic lymphocytic leukemia. The compound was widely used during the Vietnam War as a defoliant. It is a 50:50 mixture of two phenoxyl herbicides, 2,4-dichlorophenoxyacetic acid (2,4-D) and 2,4,5-trichlorophenoxyacetic acid (2,4,5-T). Agent Orange was manufactured by U.S. chemical companies and given its name because it was shipped to Vietnam in orange-striped 55-gallon barrels. The 2,4,5-T used to produce Agent Orange was later discovered to be contaminated with 2,3,7,8-tetrachlorodibenzodioxin, an extremely toxic dioxin compound.

Investigators at the Ohio State University examined computerized patient treatment files collected by the Veteran's Administration (VA) hospital system to estimate incidence rates of various malignancies among the 3.7 million U.S. veterans treated in VA hospitals during 1970–1982. During this period, 31,835 hematopoietic and lymphatic cancers were diagnosed in the VA user sample. Compared to the general U.S. population, the VA sample showed risk increases in lymphocytic leukemia (RR = 1.54), granulocytic leukemia (RR = 1.23), and monocytic leukemia (RR = 1.51). Risk increases were also noted for Hodgkin's disease (RR = 1.93), non-Hodgkin's lymphoma (RR = 1.20), and multiple myeloma (RR = 1.51). Notably, the risk of developing either leukemia or lymphatic cancer was approximately 70% higher among Vietnam-era veterans than other veterans in the sample (Namboodiri & Harris, 1991).

In 2002, the U.S. Institute of Medicine issued an update in a series of consensus reports examining the impact of chemical defoliants, including Agent Orange, on human health. The combined evidence was found sufficient to support an association between exposure to herbicides sprayed during the Vietnam War and the risk of developing chronic lymphocytic leukemia in veterans who served in Vietnam. Other Institute of Medicine consensus reports document significant associations between herbicide exposure and the development of Hodgkin's lymphoma or non-Hodgkin's lymphoma in Vietnam War veterans (Institute of Medicine, 2003).

Chronic Lymphocytic Leukemia: Survival

A devastating event in patients with chronic lymphocytic leukemia is the abrupt conversion of a chronic, relatively indolent disease into an acute, decompensated, accelerated phase with a marked increase in lymphoblasts in both the bone marrow and the peripheral circulation. As with other forms of leukemia, the blast crisis of chronic leukemia is associated with short survival, often just a few weeks. As described in the next few paragraphs, certain genetic and cytogenetic markers have been found to predict accelerated progression of chronic lymphocytic leukemia and transition into a blast crisis.

Although it seems paradoxical, a *less favorable* clinical course of chronic lymphocytic leukemia is *inversely* correlated with the presence of somatic mutations in the gene that encodes the heavy-chain variable region of immunoglobulins. Patients with the nonmutated immunoglobulin gene have a more aggressive course and shorter survival than patients with mutated genes (Van Bockstaele, Verhasselt, & Philippe, 2009).

Molecular investigations have identified an important protein, ZAP-70, that also has prognostic significance in chronic lymphocytic leukemia. The ZAP-70 protein is a tyrosine kinase encoded by a gene located on the long arm of chromosome 2. It is an integral component in cell signaling by T lymphocytes; however, the gene can also be expressed in B lymphocytes. Notably, patients who are *positive* for ZAP-70 progress about twice as rapidly as patients who are *negative* (Orchard, Ibbotson, Best, Parker, & Oscier, 2006). Gene expression profiles and clinical studies show that ZAP-70 positivity is highly correlated with the nonmutated immunoglobulin subtype, suggesting that both biomarkers influence adverse survival by the same biological mechanism (Klein et al., 2001; Rosenwald et al., 2001).

In general, the appearance of multiple chromosomal aberrations in leukemic cells (e.g., chromosomal deletions and trisomy) has been found to herald poor prognosis and an impending blast crisis in patients with chronic lymphocytic leukemia. Nevertheless, there is a lack of consistency of results from different centers, and additional investigations are needed to clarify the prognostic value of genetic and cytogenetic biomarkers.

Hairy-Cell Leukemia

Hairy-cell leukemia is an uncommon hematological malignancy characterized by the accumulation of abnormal B lymphocytes in the bone marrow and peripheral circulation. Hairy-cell leukemia is rare, with an annual incidence of 3 cases per million in U.S. men and 0.6 cases per million in U.S. women. It is usually classified as a subtype of chronic lymphoid leukemia. Fewer than 2000 new cases are diagnosed annually in North America and Western Europe combined. Hairy-cell leukemia was first identified and pathologically characterized by Bertha Bouroncle and colleagues at the Ohio State University in 1958 (Bouroncle, Wiseman, & Doan, 1958; Vardiman et al., 2009).

Due to the rare nature of this form of leukemia, only limited data are available regarding its genesis. Nevertheless, at least 12 cases of familial hairy-cell leukemia have been published, and afflicted relatives have been found to have certain human leukocyte antigen (HLA) haplotypes in common (Gramatovici, Bennett, Hiscock, & Grewal, 1993). The role of the HLA locus in the genesis of hairy-cell leukemia is as yet undetermined (Cannon, Mobarek, Wegge, & Tabbara, 2008; Villemagne, Bay, Tournilhac, Chaleteix, & Travade, 2005).

In 2003, the Institute of Medicine announced there was sufficient evidence in the published literature to support an association between exposure to herbicides (such as Agent Orange) and the development of chronic B-cell leukemia, including hairy-cell leukemia (Institute of Medicine, 2003).

Monocytic Leukemia

Monocytic leukemia arises from the monocytic lineage of immune cells. Monocytes are produced in the bone marrow from hematopoietic stem cell precursors called monoblasts. Monocytes circulate in the bloodstream for 1–3 days after which they migrate into tissues throughout the body. In the tissues, monocytes mature into highly specialized macrophages that avidly engulf and digest foreign bodies, necrotic cells, damaged or infected cells, and proteins and other debris from injured cells. The diagnosis of acute monocytic leukemia is confirmed when more than 20% of immune cells of the bone marrow are myeloblasts (Dale et al., 2008; Vardiman et al., 2009).

As in other forms of leukemia, there is an increased risk of monocytic leukemia in subjects with rare genetic disorders that impact on cell division, DNA repair, apoptosis, and angiogenesis. These include Down syndrome, Fanconi anemia, Bloom syndrome, ataxia telangiectasia, and neurofibromatosis. Environmental risk factors for monocytic leukemia are like those for myelocytic leukemia and include exposure to ionizing radiation, pesticides and herbicides, alkylating agents, and topoisomerase inhibitors.

Most cases of monocytic leukemia are diagnosed in adults, usually after the age of 50 years. The disease usually presents as an acute leukemia and may develop after exposure to ionizing radiation, herbicides and pesticides, or certain chemotherapeutic agents, particularly epipodophyllotoxins and anthracyclines (Vardiman et al., 2009). *Chronic monocytic leukemia* is extraordinarily rare; only a small number of cases have been reported in the literature (Bearman, Kjeldsberg, Pangalis, & Rappaport, 1981).

Monocytic leukemia is characterized by specific chromosomal abnormalities. The most common of these involve deletions of portions of the long arm of chromosome 11 or a reciprocal translocation, t(9:11), involving chromosomes 9 and 11. These genetic rearrangements involve the *MLL* locus that encodes a methyltransferase involved in regulation of transcription (Dewald, Morrison-DeLap, Schuchard, Spurbeck, & Pierre, 1983; Guenther et al., 2005). A second translocation, t(8;16), found in some monocytic leukemia cases creates a transfusion protein that promotes leukemogenesis of immature monocytes and myelocytes by deregulating nuclear binding factors and gene expression (Borrow et al., 1996). In addition,

mutations and duplications have been observed in the *Flt3* tumor–suppressor gene in approximately 40% of cases (Liu, Yu, Jia, Zhang, & Guo, 2007).

Monocytic leukemia does occasionally occur in children, most often in those less than 2 years of age. The incidence in U.S. children under the age of 15 years ranges from 4.8 to 6.6 cases per million; however, in children with Down syndrome (trisomy 21), the relative risk of monocytic leukemia is increased 150-fold for ages 1–4 years (Hasle et al., 2000).

▶ Prevention and Control of Leukemia

The development of leukemia is influenced by many risk factors, including inherited disorders, behavioral factors (tobacco smoking), environmental factors (exposure to radiation and toxic chemicals), chemotherapy, immune system deficiencies, and infectious agents. Other than avoidance of tobacco and high-dose radiation, no specific lifestyle changes can be recommended that are proven to lower the risk.

Many forms of leukemia can be successfully treated with chemotherapy and radiation. Bone marrow and stem cell transplants are reserved for patients who do not respond to other forms of therapy. Recent advances have been made in treating specific types of leukemia using targeted immunotherapy with monoclonal antibodies in combination with radiation and chemotherapy.

References

Altekruse, S. F., Kosary, C. L., Krapcho, M., Neyman, N., Aminou, R., Waldron, W., … Edwards, B. K. (2010). *SEER cancer statistics review, 1975–2007*. Bethesda, MD: National Cancer Institute.

American Cancer Society. (2005). *Cancer facts and figures, 2005*. Atlanta, GA: Author.

Aul, C., Giagounidis, A., & Germing, U. (2001). Epidemiological features of myelodysplastic syndromes: Results from regional cancer surveys and hospital-based statistics. *International Journal of Hematology, 73*(4), 405–410.

Badrinath, P., Day, N. E., & Stockton, D. (1997). Seasonality in the diagnosis of acute lymphocytic leukaemia. *British Journal of Cancer, 75*(11), 1711–1773.

Bartal, A., Bentwich, Z., Manny, N., & Izak, G. (1978). Ethical and clinical aspects of chronic lymphocytic leukemia in Israel. *Acta Hematologica, 60*, 161–171.

Bearman, R. M., Kjeldsberg, C. R., Pangalis, G. A., & Rappaport, H. (1981). Chronic monocytic leukemia in adults. *Cancer, 48*, 2239–2255.

Block, M., Jacobson, L. O., & Bethard, W. F. (1953). Preleukemic acute human leukemia. *Journal of the American Medical Association, 152*, 1018–1028.

Bloom, D. (1954). Congenital telangiectatic erythema resembling lupus erythematosus in dwarfs; probably a syndrome entity. *American Journal of Diseases of Children, 88*(6), 754–758.

Bloomfield, C. D., Goldman, A. I., Alimena, G., Berger, R., Borgstrom, G. H., Brandt, L., … Garson, O. M. (1986). Chromosomal abnormalities identify high-risk and low-risk patients with acute lymphoblastic leukemia. *Blood, 67*(2), 415–420.

Bloomfield, C. D., Lawrence, D., Byrd, J. C., Carroll, A., Pettenati, M. J., Tantravahi, R., … Mayer, R. J. (1998). Frequency of prolonged remission duration after high-dose cytarabine intensification in acute myeloid leukemia varies by cytogenetic subtype. *Cancer Research, 58*(18), 4173–4179.

Bodian, M., Sheldon, W., & Lightwood, R. (1964). Congenital hypoplasia of the exocrine pancreas. *Acta Paediatrica, 53*, 282–293.

Borrow, J., Stanton, V. P., Jr., Andresen, J. M., Becher, R., Behm, F. G., Chaganti, R. S. K., … Housman, D. E. (1996). The translocation t(8;16)(p11;p13) of acute myeloid leukaemia fuses a putative acetyltransferase to the CREB–binding protein. *Nature Genetics, 14*, 33–41.

Bouroncle, B. A., Wiseman, B. K., & Doan, C. A. (1958). Leukemic reticuloendotheliosis. *Blood, 13*, 609–630.

Bowen, D. T., Frew, M. E., Rollinson, S., Roddam, P. L., Dring, A., Smith, M. T., … Morgan, G. J. (2003). *CYP1A1*2B* (Val) allele is overrepresented in a subgroup of acute myeloid leukemia patients with poor-risk karyotype associated with

NRAS mutation, but not associated with *FLT3* internal tandem duplication. *Blood, 101*, 2770–2774.

Boyd, K. P., Korf, B. R., & Theos, A. (2009). Neurofibromatosis type 1. *Journal of the American Academy of Dermatology, 61*(1), 1–14.

Bray, F., Ferlay, J., Soerjomataram, I., Siegel, R. L., Torre, L. A., & Jemal, A. (2018). Global cancer statistics 2018: GLOBOCAN estimates of incidence and mortality worldwide for 36 cancers in 185 countries. *CA: A Cancer Journal for Clinicians, 68*(6), 394–424.

Bunn, H. F. (1986). 5q- and disordered haematopoiesis. *Clinics in Haematology, 15*(4), 1023–1035.

Canman, C. E., & Lim, D. S. (1998). The role of ATM in DNA damage responses and cancer. *Oncogene, 17*(25), 3301–3308.

Cannon, T., Mobarek, D., Wegge, J., & Tabbara, I. A. (2008). Hairy cell leukemia: Current concepts. *Cancer Investigation, 26*(8), 860–865.

Cheok, C. F., Bachrati, C. Z., Chan, K. L., Ralf, C., Wu, L., & Hickson, I. D. (2005). Roles of the Bloom's syndrome helicase in the maintenance of genome stability. *Biochemical Society Transactions, 33*, 1456–1459.

Christiansen, D. H., Andersen, M. K., & Pedersen-Bjergaard, J. (2003). Methylation of *p15INK4B* is common, is associated with deletion of genes on chromosome arm 7q and predicts a poor prognosis in therapy-related myelodysplasia and acute myeloid leukemia. *Leukemia, 17*(9), 1813–1819.

D'Andrea, A. D. (2010). Susceptibility pathways in Fanconi's anemia and breast cancer. *New England Journal of Medicine, 362*(20), 1909–1919.

Dale, D. C., Boser, L., & Liles, W. C. (2008). The phagocytes: Neutrophils and monocytes. *Blood, 112*(4), 935–945.

Deschler, B., & Lübbert, M. (2006). Acute myeloid leukemia: Epidemiology and etiology. *Cancer, 107*, 2099–2107.

Dewald, G. W., Morrison-DeLap, S. J., Schuchard, K. A., Spurbeck, J. L., & Pierre, R. V. (1983). A possible specific chromosome marker for monocytic leukemia: Three more patients with t(9;11)(p22;q24) and another with t(11;17)(q24;q21), each with acute monoblastic leukemia. *Cancer Genetics and Cytogenetics, 8*(3), 203–212.

Down, J. L. H. (1866). Observations on an ethnic classification of idiots. *Clinical Lecture Reports, London Hospital, 3*, 259–262.

Fanconi, G. (1927). Familiäre, infantile perniciosähnliche Anämie (perniziöses Blutbild und Konstitution). *Jahrbuch für Kinderheilkunde und physische Erziehung, Wien, 117*, 257–280.

Ferlay, J., Ervik, M., Lam, F., Colombet, M., Mery, L., Piñeros, M., … Bray, F. (2018). *Global cancer observatory: Cancer today.* Lyon, France: International Agency for Research on Cancer. Retrieved from https://gco.iarc.fr/today

Ferlay, J., Shin, H. R., Forman, D., Mathers, C., & Parkin, D. M. (2010). Estimates of worldwide burden of cancer in 2008. *International Journal of Cancer, 127*(12), 2893–2917.

Ferlay, J., Soerjomataram, I., Ervik, M., Dikshit, R., Eser, S., Mathers, C., … Bray, F. (2013). *GLOBOCAN 2012 v1.0. Cancer incidence and mortality worldwide: IARC CancerBase No. 11* [Internet]. Lyon, France: International Agency for Research on Cancer. Retrieved from http://globocan.iarc.fr

Fitzmaurice, C., Akinyemiju, T. F., Al Lami, F. H., Alam, T., Alizadeh-Navaei, R., Allen, C., … Global Burden of Disease Cancer Collaboration. (2018). Global, regional, and national cancer incidence, mortality, years of life lost, years lived with disability, and disability-adjusted life-years for 29 cancer groups, 1990 to 2016: A systematic analysis for the Global Burden of Disease Study. *JAMA Oncology.* Online publication. doi:10.1001/jamaoncol.2018.2706.

Fitzmaurice, C., Allen, C., Barber, R. M., Barregard, L., Bhutta, Z. A., Brenner H, … Global Burden of Disease Cancer Collaboration. (2017). Global, regional, and national cancer incidence, mortality, years of life lost, years lived with disability, and disability-adjusted life-years for 32 cancer groups, 1990 to 2015: A systematic analysis for the Global Burden of Disease Study. *JAMA Oncology, 3*(4), 524–548.

Gao, F., Chia, K. S., & Machin, D. (2007). On the evidence for seasonal variation in the onset of acute lymphoblastic leukemia (ALL). *Leukemia Research, 31*(10), 1327–1338.

German, J. (1993). Bloom syndrome: A mendelian prototype of somatic mutational disease. *Medicine (Baltimore), 72*(6), 393–406.

Goldin, L., Pfeiffer, R. M., Li, X., & Hemminki, K. (2004). Familial risk of lymphoproliferative tumors in families of patients with chronic lymphocytic leukemia: Results from the Swedish Family-Cancer Database. *Blood, 104*, 1850–1854.

Goldin, L. R., & Caporaso, N. E. (2007). Family studies in chronic lymphocytic leukaemia and other lymphoproliferative tumours. *British Journal of Haematology, 139*(5), 774–779.

Golub, T. R., Barker, G. F., Bohlander, S. K., Hiebert, S. W., Ward, D. C., Bray-Ward, P., … Gilliland, D. G. (1995). Fusion of the *TEL* gene on 12p13 to the *AML1* gene on 21q22 in acute lymphoblastic leukemia. *Proceedings of the National Academy of Sciences of the United States of America, 92*(11), 4917–4921.

Gramatovici, M., Bennett, J. M., Hiscock, J. G., & Grewal, K. D. (1993). Three cases of familial hairy cell leukemia. *American Journal of Hematology, 42*(4), 337–339.

Greenberg, P., Cox, C., LeBeau, M. M., Fenaux, P., Morel, P., Sanz, G., … Bennett, J. (1997). International scoring system for evaluating prognosis in myelodysplastic syndromes. *Blood, 89*(6), 2079–2088.

Greiser, E., & Hoffman, W. (2010). Questionable increase of childhood leukemia in Basrah, Iraq. *American Journal of Public Health, 100*(9), 1556–1557.

Guenther, M. G., Jenner, R. G., Chevalier, B., Nakamura, T., Croce, C. M., Canaani, E., & Young, R. A. (2005). Global and Hox-specific roles for the *MLL1* methyltransferase. *Proceedings of the National Academy of Sciences of the United States of America, 102*(24), 8603–8608.

Gurney, J. G., Severson, R. K., Davis, S., & Robison, L. L. (1995). Incidence of cancer in children in the United States. Sex-, race-, and 1-year age-specific rates by histologic type. *Cancer, 75*, 2186–2195.

Hagopian, A., Lafta, R., Hassan, J., Davis, S., Mirick, D., & Takaro, T. (2010). Trends in childhood leukemia in Basrah, Iraq, 1993–2007. *American Journal of Public Health, 100*(6), 1081–1087.

Harris, R. E., & Al-Rashid, R. A. (1984). Seasonal variation in the incidence of childhood acute lymphocytic leukemia in Nebraska. *Nebraska Medical Journal, 69*, 192–198.

Harris, R. E., Harrell, F. E., Jr., Patil, K. D., & Al-Rashid, R. (1987). The seasonal risk of pediatric/juvenile acute lymphocytic leukemia in the USA. *Journal of Chronic Diseases, 40*, 915–924.

Hasle, H., Clemmensen, I. H., & Mikkelsen, M. (2000). Risks of leukaemia and solid tumours in individuals with Down's syndrome. *Lancet, 355*(9199), 165–169.

Healy, J., Richer, C., Bourgey, M., Kritikou, E. A., & Sinnett, D. (2010). Replication analysis confirms the association of *ARID5B* with childhood B-cell acute lymphoblastic leukemia. *Haematologica, 95*(9), 1608–1611.

Heerema, N. A., Sather, H. N., Sensel, M. G., Liu-Mares, W., Lange, B. J., Bostrom, B. C., … Uckun, F. M. (1999). Association of chromosome arm 9p abnormalities with adverse risk in childhood acute lymphoblastic leukemia: A report from the Children's Cancer Group. *Blood, 94*(5), 1537–1544.

Institute of Medicine. (2003). *Veterans and Agent Orange: Update 2002.* Washington, DC: Institute of Medicine of the National Academies, U.S. National Academy of Science.

Kantarjian, H., Dixon, D., Keating, M., Talpaz, M., Walters, R., McCredie, K., & Freireich, E. (1988). Characteristics of accelerated disease in chronic myelogenous leukemia. *Cancer, 61*(7), 1441–1446.

Klein, U., Tu, Y., Stolovitzky, G. A., Mattioli, M., Cattoretti, G., Husson, H., … Dalla-Favera, R. (2001). Gene expression profiling of B cell chronic lymphocytic leukemia reveals a homogeneous phenotype related to memory B cells. *Journal of Experimental Medicine, 194*, 1625–1638.

Kossman, S. E., & Weiss, M. A. (2000). Acute myelogenous leukemia after exposure to strontium-89 for the treatment of adenocarcinoma of the prostate. *Cancer, 88*, 620–624.

Krajinovic, M., Labuda, D., Richer, C., Karimi, S., & Sinnett, D. (1999). Susceptibility to childhood acute lymphoblastic leukemia: Influence of *CYP1A1, CYP2D6, GSTM1*, and *GSTT1* genetic polymorphisms. *Blood, 93*(5), 1496–1501.

Kumar, V., Abbas, A. K., & Aster, J. C. (2014). *Robbins and Cotran pathologic basis of disease* (9th ed.). Philadelphia, PA: Mosby & Saunders.

Kurzrock, R., Kantarjian, H. M., Druker, B. J., & Talpaz, M. (2003). Philadelphia chromosome-positive leukemias: From basic mechanisms to molecular therapeutics. *Annals of Internal Medicine, 138*(10), 819–830.

Lavau, C., & Dejean, A. (1994). The t(15;17) translocation in acute promyelocytic leukemia. *Leukemia, 8*(10), 1615–1621.

Le Beau, M. M., Albain, K. S., Larson, R. A., Vardiman, J. W., Davis, E. M., Blough, R. R., … Rowley, J. D. (1986). Clinical and cytogenetic correlations in 63 patients with therapy-related myelodysplastic syndromes and acute nonlymphocytic leukemia: Further evidence for characteristic abnormalities of chromosomes no. 5 and 7. *Journal of Clinical Oncology, 4*, 325–345.

Le Beau, M. M., Pettenati, M. J., Lemons, R. S., Diaz, M. O., Westbrook, C. A., Larson, R. A., … Rowley, J. D. (1986). Assignment of the *GM-CSF, CSF-1,* and *FMS* genes to human chromosome 5 provides evidence for linkage of a family of genes regulating hematopoiesis and for their involvement in the deletion (5q) in myeloid disorders. *Cold Spring Harbor Symposia on Quantitative Biology, 51*(Pt 2), 899–909.

Lejeune, J. (1959). Le mongolisme. Premier example d'aberration autosomique humaine. *Annales de Genetique, 1*, 41–49.

Levi, F., Lucchini, F., Negri, E., Barbui, T., & La Vecchia, C. (2000). Trends in mortality from leukemia in subsequent age groups. *Leukemia, 14*(11), 1980–1985.

Linet, M. S., Schubauer-Berigan, M. K., Weisenburger, D. D., Richardson, D. B., Landgren, O., Blair, A., … Dores, G. M. (2007). Chronic lymphocytic leukaemia: An overview of aetiology in light of recent developments in classification and pathogenesis. *British Journal of Haematology, 139*(5), 672–686.

Liu, H., Yu, H., Jia, H. Y., Zhang, W., & Guo, C. J. (2007). Detection of *FLT3* gene mutation in hematologic malignancies and its clinical significance. *Zhongguo Shi Yan Xue Ye Xue Za Zhi, 15*(4), 709–713.

McNeil, S., Zeng, C., Harrington, K. D., Hiebert, S., Lian, J. B., Stein, J. L., … Stein, G. S. (1999). The t(8;21) chromosomal translocation in acute myelogenous leukemia modifies intranuclear targeting of the AML1/CBFa2 transcription factor. *Proceedings of the National Academy of Sciences, 96*(26), 14882–14887.

Namboodiri, K. K., & Harris, R. E. (1991). Hematopoietic and lymphoproliferative cancer among male veterans using the Veterans Administration Medical System. *Cancer, 68*(5), 1123–1130.

Nowell, P., & Hungerford, D. (1960). A minute chromosome in chronic granulocytic leukemia. *Science, 132*, 1497.

Orchard, J., Ibbotson, R., Best, G., Parker, A., & Oscier, D. (2006). ZAP-70 in B cell malignancies. *Leukemia and Lymphoma, 46*(12), 1689–1698.

Parkin, D. M., Bray, F., Ferlay, J., & Pisani, P. (2001). Estimating the world cancer burden, GLOBOCAN 2000. *International Journal of Cancer, 94*, 153–156.

Parkin, D. M., Bray, F., Ferlay, J., & Pisani, P. (2005). Global cancer statistics, 2002. *CA: A Cancer Journal for Clinicians, 55*, 74–108.

Parkin, D. M., Pisani, P., & Ferlay, J. (1999a). Estimates of the worldwide incidence of 25 major cancers in 1990. *International Journal of Cancer, 80*(6), 827–841.

Parkin, D. M., Pisani, P., & Ferlay, J. (1999b). Global cancer statistics. *CA: A Cancer Journal for Clinicians, 49*(1), 33–64.

Pedersen-Bjergaard, J., Philip, P., Larsen, S. O., Andersson, M., Daugaard, G., Ersbøll, J., … Osterlind, K. (1993). Therapy-related myelodysplasia and acute myeloid leukemia. Cytogenetic characteristics of 115 consecutive cases and risk in seven cohorts of patients treated intensively for malignant diseases in the Copenhagen series. *Leukemia, 7*(12), 1975–1986.

Perillat-Menegaux, P., Clave, J., Auclerc, M. F., Baruchel, A., Leverger, G., Nelken, B., … Hémon, D. (2003). Family history of autoimmune thyroid disease and childhood acute leukemia. *Cancer Epidemiology, Biomarkers and Prevention, 12*(1), 60–63.

Plass, C., Byrd, J. C., Raval, A., Tanner, S. M., & De La Chapelle, A. (2007). Molecular profiling of chronic lymphocytic leukaemia: Genetics meets epigenetics to identify predisposing genes. *British Journal of Haematology, 139*, 744–752.

Pogoda, J. M., Preston-Martin, S., Nichols, P. W., & Ross, R. K. (2002). Smoking and risk of acute myeloid leukemia: Results from a Los Angeles County case-control study. *American Journal of Epidemiology, 155*, 546–553.

Popovic, M., Goobie, S., Morrison, J., Ellis, L., Ehtesham, N., Richards, N., … Rommens, J. M. (2002). Fine mapping of the locus for Shwachman–Diamond syndrome at 7q11, identification of shared disease haplotypes, and exclusion of *TPST1* as a candidate gene. *European Journal of Human Genetics, 10*(4), 250–258.

Preston, D. L., Kusumi, S., Tomonaga, M., Izumi, S., Ron, E., Kuramoto, A., … Mabuchi, K. (1994). Cancer incidence in atomic bomb survivors. Part III. Leukemia, lymphoma and multiple myeloma, 1950–1987. *Radiation Research, 137*(2 Suppl.), S68–S97.

Preston, D. L., Pierce, D. A., Shimizu, Y., Cullings, H. M., Fujita, S., Funamoto, S., & Kodama, K. (2004). Effect of recent atomic bomb survivor dosimetry changes on cancer mortality risk estimates. *Radiation Research, 162*, 377–389.

Preston-Martin, S., Thomas, D. C., Yu, M. C., & Henderson, B. E. (1989). Diagnostic radiography as a risk factor for chronic myeloid and monocytic leukaemia (CML). *British Journal of Cancer, 59*(4), 639–644.

Pui, C. H., Raimondi, S. C., Hancock, M. L., Rivera, G. K., Ribeiro, R. C., Mahmoud, H. H., … Behm, F. G. (1994). Immunologic, cytogenetic, and clinical characterization of childhood acute lymphoblastic leukemia with the t(1;19) (q23; p13) or its derivative. *Clinical Oncology, 12*(12), 2601–2606.

Pui, C. H., Relling, M. V., & Downing, J. R. (2004). Acute lymphoblastic leukemia. *New England Journal of Medicine, 350*, 1535–1548.

Pui, C. H., Ribeiro, R. C., Hancock, M. L., Rivera, G. K., Evans, W. E., Raimondi, S. C., ... Crist, W. M. (1991). Acute myeloid leukemia in children treated with epipodophyllotoxins for acute lymphoblastic leukemia. *New England Journal of Medicine, 325*, 1682–1687.

Redaniel, M. T., Laudico, A., Miraol-Lumague, M. R., Alcasabas, A. P., Pulte, D., & Brenner, H. (2010). Geographic and ethnic differences in childhood leukaemia and lymphoma survival: Comparisons of Philippine residents, Asian Americans and Caucasians in the United States. *British Journal of Cancer, 103*, 149–154.

Richardson, D. B., Wing, S., Schroeder, J., Schmitz-Feuerhake, I., & Hoffmann, W. (2005). Ionizing radiation and chronic lymphocytic leukemia. *Environmental Health Perspectives, 113*, 1–5.

Ries, L. A. G. (1999). Childhood cancer mortality. In L. A. G. Ries, M. A. Smith, J. G. Gurney, M. Linet, T. Tamra, J. L. Young, & G. R. Bunin (Eds.), *Cancer incidence and survival among children and adolescents: United States SEER program 1975–1995* (pp. 165–170, NIH Pub. No. 99-4649). Bethesda, MD: National Cancer Institute, SEER Program.

Ries, L. A. G., Kosary, C. L., Hankey, B. F., Miller, B. A., Clegg, L., & Edwards, B. K. (Eds.). (1998). *SEER cancer statistics review 1973–1996.* Bethesda, MD: National Cancer Institute.

Ries, L. A. G., Kosary, C. L., Hankey, B. F., Miller, B. A., Clegg, L., & Edwards, B. K. (Eds.). (2003). *SEER cancer statistics review, 1975–2000.* Bethesda, MD: National Cancer Institute.

Robbins, S. L., & Cotran, R. S. (1979). *Pathologic basis of disease* (2nd ed.). Philadelphia: W. B. Saunders.

Rosenwald, A., Alizadeh, A. A., Widhopf, G., Simon, R., Davis, R. E., Yu, X., ... Staudt, L. M. (2001). Relation of gene expression phenotype to immunoglobulin mutation genotype in B cell chronic lymphocytic leukemia. *Journal of Experimental Medicine, 194*, 1639–1647.

Rubnitz, J. E., Downing, J. R., Pui, C. H., Shurtleff, S. A., Raimondi, S. C., Evans, W. E., ... Behm, F. G. (1997). *TEL* gene rearrangement in acute lymphoblastic leukemia: A new genetic marker with prognostic significance. *Journal of Clinical Oncology, 15*(3), 1150–1157.

Rubnitz, J. E., Wichlan, D., Devidas, M., Shuster, J., Linda, S. B., Kurtzberg, J., ... Children's Oncology Group. (2008). Prospective analysis of *TEL* gene rearrangements in childhood acute lymphoblastic leukemia: A Children's Oncology Group study. *Journal of Clinical Oncology, 26*(13), 2186–2191.

Savage, D. G., Szydlo, R. M., & Goldman, J. M. (1997). Clinical features at diagnosis in 430 patients with chronic myeloid leukaemia seen at a referral centre over a 16-year period. *British Journal of Haematology, 96*(1), 111–116.

Savitz, D. A., & Andrews, K. W. (1997). Review of epidemiologic evidence on benzene and lymphatic and hematopoietic cancers. *American Journal of Industrial Medicine, 31*, 287–295.

Schmiegelow, K., Vestergaard, T., Nielsen, S. M., & Hjalgrim, H. (2008). Etiology of common childhood acute lymphoblastic leukemia: The adrenal hypothesis. *Leukemia, 22*, 2137–2141.

Shah, A., & Coleman, M. P. (2007). Increasing incidence of childhood leukaemia: A controversy re-examined. *British Journal of Cancer, 97*(7), 1009–1012.

Shvidel, L., Shtarlid, M., Klepfish, A., Sigler, E., & Berrebi, A. (1998). Epidemiology and ethnic aspects of B cell chronic lymphocytic leukemia in Israel. *Leukemia, 12*, 1612–1617.

Shwachman, H., Diamond, L. K., Oski, F. A., & Khaw, K. T. (1964). The syndrome of pancreatic insufficiency and bone marrow dysfunction. *Journal of Pediatrics, 65*, 645–663.

Smith, M. A., Gloeckler-Ries, L. A., Gurney, J. G., & Ross, J. A. (1999). Leukemia. In L. A. G. Ries, M. A. Smith, J. G. Gurney, M. Linet, T. Tamra, J. L. Young, & G. R. Bunin (Eds.), *Cancer incidence and survival among children and adolescents: United States SEER program 1975–1995* (pp. 17–34, NIH Pub. No. 99-4649). Bethesda, MD: National Cancer Institute, SEER Program.

Smith, M. A., Seibel, N. L., Seibel, N. L., Altekruse, S. F., Ries, L. A. G., Melbert, D. L., ... Reaman, G. H. (2010). Outcomes for children and adolescents with cancer: Challenges for the twenty-first century. *Journal of Clinical Oncology, 28*(15), 2625–2634.

Solé, F., Espinet, B., Sanz, G. F., Cervera, J., Calasanz, M. J., Luño, E., ... Woessner, S. (2000). Incidence, characterization and prognostic significance of chromosomal abnormalities in 640 patients with primary myelodysplastic syndromes. *British Journal of Haematology, 108*, 346–356.

Stilgenbauer, S., Dohner, H., & Lichter, P. (1993). Genomic aberrations in B-cell chronic lymphocytic leukemia. In B. Cheson (Ed.), *Chronic lymphocytic leukemia* (2nd ed., pp. 353–376). New York, NY: Marcel Dekker.

Stiller, C. A., Chessells, J. M., & Fitchett, M. (1994). Neurofibromatosis and childhood leukaemia/lymphoma: A population-based UKCCSG study. *British Journal of Cancer, 70*(5), 969–972.

United Nations Scientific Committee on the Effects of Atomic Radiation. (2000). Annex I. Epidemiological evaluation of radiation-induced cancer. In *Sources and effects of ionizing radiation* (pp. 297–431). New York, NY.

Van Bockstaele, F., Verhasselt, B., & Philippe, J. (2009). Prognostic markers in chronic lymphocytic leukemia: A comprehensive review. *Blood Reviews, 23*(1), 25–47.

Van den Berghe, H., Cassiman, J. J., David, G., Fryns, J. P., Michaux, J. L., & Sokal, G. (1974). Distinct haematological disorder with deletion of long arm of no. 5 chromosome. *Nature, 251*(5474), 437–438.

van Leeuwen, B. H., Martinson, M. E., Webb, G. C., & Young, I. G. (1989). Molecular organization of the cytokine gene cluster, involving the human *IL-3, IL-4, IL-5,* and *GM-CSF* genes, on human chromosome 5. *Blood, 73*, 1142–1148.

Vardiman, J. W., Thiele, J., Arber, D. A., Brunning, R. D., Borowitz, M. J., Porwit, A., ... Bloomfield, C. D. (2009). The 2008 revision of the World Health Organization (WHO) classification of myeloid neoplasms and acute leukemia. *Blood, 114*(5), 937–951.

Villemagne, B., Bay, J. O., Tournilhac, O., Chaleteix, C., & Travade, P. (2005). Two new cases of familial hairy cell leukemia associated with HLA haplotypes A2, B7, Bw4, Bw6. *Leukemia and Lymphoma, 46*(2), 243–245.

World Health Organization. (2008). *World cancer report.* Geneva, Switzerland: Author.

Xie, Y., Davies, S. M., Xiang, Y., Robison, L. L., & Ross, J. A. (2003). Trends in leukemia incidence and survival in the United States (1973–1998). *Cancer, 97*(9), 2229–2235.

© Andrew Brookes/Getty Images

CHAPTER 38

Epidemiology of Brain Tumors: Glioma, Meningioma, Acoustic Neuroma, and Pituitary Tumors

▶ Global Epidemiology of Brain Tumors

According to sequential reports from the World Health Organization (WHO), the incidence and mortality of tumors of the brain and central nervous system (CNS) are rising. Since 1990, reported new cases and deaths have more than doubled in both men and women (**FIGURE 38.1**). In 2018, brain and CNS tumors were diagnosed in 296,851 individuals (162,534 in men and 134,217 in women) and caused 241,037 deaths (133,843 in men and 105,194 in women). By comparison, 127,000 new cases were detected and 95,000 individuals died of brain/CNS tumors in 1990 (Bray et al., 2018; Ferlay, Shin, Forman, Mathers, & Parkin, 2010; Ferlay et al., 2013; Fitzmaurice et al., 2017, 2018; Parkin, Bray, Ferlay, & Pisani, 2005; Parkin, Pisani, & Ferlay, 1999a, 1999b; Parkin, Whelan, Ferlay, Teppo, & Thomas, 2002).

Corresponding to the increasing numbers of cases and deaths, the annual age-standardized incidence and mortality rates have both increased approximately 30% in the 21st century. These increases are due in large part to the widespread use of advanced neuroimaging (computerized tomography and magnetic resonance imaging) and other diagnostic techniques (e.g., stereotactic biopsy) resulting in earlier and more accurate detection of brain tumors (Bray et al., 2018; Ferlay et al., 2010, 2013, 2018; Parkin et al., 1999a, 1999b, 2002, 2005).

In 2018, the global incidence was higher in men than women (3.9 per 100,000 versus 3.1 per 100,000) and higher in developed countries (5.0 per 100,000 in men and 4.0 per 100,000 in women) than in developing countries (2.4 per 100,000 in men and 1.7 per 100,000 in women). Incidence rates were relatively high (exceeding 5 per 100,000) in developed nations such as the United States, Western European and Scandinavian countries, Brazil, Argentina, the Russian Federation, and Australia/New Zealand compared to developing nations such as India and those in sub-Saharan Africa, where the rates were lower, ranging from 1 to 2 per 100,000. The highest incidence rates were observed in Latvia (10.6 and 9.6 per 100,000 for men and women, respectively) and rates exceeding 6 per 100,000 were observed in several other countries in the North Central region of Europe (Bray et al., 2018; Ferlay et al., 2018) (**FIGURE 38.2**).

Global patterns of incidence and mortality are similar. Nations with high incidence rates also had high mortality rates. Men had higher mortality than

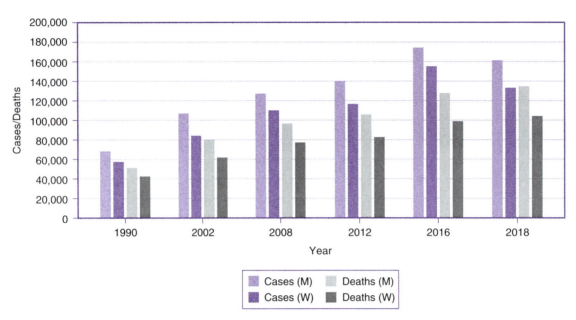

FIGURE 38.1 Global Trends in Malignant Tumors of the Brain and Nervous System, 1990–2018.

Data from Ferlay, J., Shin, H. R., Forman, D., Mathers, C., & Parkin, D. M. (2010). Estimates of worldwide burden of cancer in 2008. *International Journal of Cancer, 127*(12), 2893–2917; Ferlay, J., Soerjomataram, I., Ervik, M., Dikshit, R., Eser, S., Mathers, C., . . . Bray, F. (2013). *GLOBOCAN 2012 v1.0. Cancer incidence and mortality worldwide: IARC CancerBase No. 11* [Internet]. Lyon, France: International Agency for Research on Cancer. Retrieved from http://globocan.iarc.fr; Parkin, D. M., Bray, F., Ferlay, J., & Pisani, P. (2001). Estimating the world cancer burden, GLOBOCAN 2000. *International Journal of Cancer, 94,* 153–156; Parkin, D. M., Bray, F., Ferlay, J., & Pisani, P. (2005). Global cancer statistics, 2002. *CA: A Cancer Journal for Clinicians, 55,* 74–108; Parkin, D. M., Pisani, P., & Ferlay, J. (1999a). Estimates of the worldwide incidence of 25 major cancers in 1990. *International Journal of Cancer,* (6), 827–841; Parkin, D. M., Pisani, P., & Ferlay, J. (1999b). Global cancer statistics. *CA: A Cancer Journal for Clinicians, 49*(1), 33–64; Fitzmaurice, C., Allen, C., Barber, R. M., Barregard, L., Bhutta, Z. A., Brenner, H., . . . Global Burden of Disease Cancer Collaboration. (2017). Global, regional, and national cancer incidence, mortality, years of life lost, years lived with disability, and disability-adjusted life-years for 32 cancer groups, 1990 to 2015: A systematic analysis for the Global Burden of Disease Study. *JAMA Oncology, 3*(4), 524–548. Fitzmaurice, C., Akinyemiju, T. F., Al Lami, F. H., Alam, T., Alizadeh-Navaei, R., Allen, C., . . . Global Burden of Disease Cancer Collaboration (2018). Global, regional, and national cancer incidence, mortality, years of life lost, years lived with disability, and disability-adjusted life-years for 29 cancer groups, 1990 to 2016: A systematic analysis for the Global Burden of Disease Study. *JAMA Oncology.* Published online June 02, 2018. doi:10.1001/jamaoncol.2018.2706.

women (3.2 versus 2.3 per 100,000), and the mortality/incidence ratio was approximately 20% higher in developing nations than in developed nations (0.0.87 versus 0.73).

Schwartzbaum and colleagues reported a four-fold difference in the incidence of primary malignant brain tumors between countries with a high incidence (e.g., Canada, Australia, New Zealand, Denmark, Finland, and the United States) and countries with a low incidence (e.g., India and the Philippines). Such differences are difficult to interpret because diagnostic practices, access to and quality of care, and completeness of reporting differ widely worldwide (Fisher, Schwartzbaum, Wrensch, & Wiemels, 2007; Schwartzbaum, Fisher, Aldape, & Wrensch, 2006).

▶ Brain Tumors in the United States

Based on recent data from the Surveillance, Epidemiology, and End Results (SEER) program of the U.S. National Cancer Institute and the Central Brain Tumor Registry of the United States (CBTRUS), approximately 22,000 new cases of primary malignant brain tumors are diagnosed every year in the United States, and more than 13,000 deaths are attributed to such tumors. During the past two decades, the age-adjusted annual incidence rate in the United States declined slightly from 7.0 cases per 100,000 in 1990 to 6.5 cases per 100,000 during 2000–2015 (Altekruse et al., 2010; CBTRUS, 2008; Horner et al., 2009; Noone et al., 2018).

Annual incidence and mortality rates in the United States have been relatively stable since 2000. Age-adjusted incidence and mortality rates are consistently higher for men (7.6 and 5.4 per 100,000) than women (5.5 and 3.5 per 100,000); however, survival differs dramatically by histology and age. For example, patients with aggressive malignant gliomas, such as glioblastoma multiforme, have very poor survival rates (only about 3% survive 5 years) whereas patients with low-grade gliomas have 5-year survival rates exceeding 70% (Noone et al., 2018).

As shown in **FIGURE 38.3**, the relative frequencies of newly diagnosed cases of malignant brain tumors and attributable deaths both show early peaks during adolescence. A disturbing fact is that brain cancer is the leading cause of cancer mortality among people under the age of 35 years (Bondy et al., 2008). As discussed in a separate section of this chapter, the histological profile of pediatric brain tumors differs markedly from that in adults. Following the early peak, incidence and mortality accelerate rapidly with age among adults (Altekruse et al., 2010; CBTRUS, 2008; Horner et al., 2009).

Estimated age-standardized incidence rates (World) in 2018, brain, nervous system, both sexes, all ages

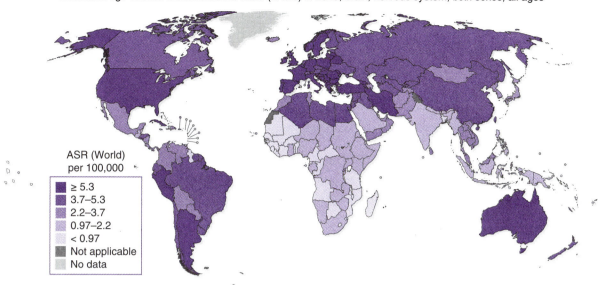

Estimated age-standardized mortality rates (World) in 2018, brain, nervous system, both sexes, all ages

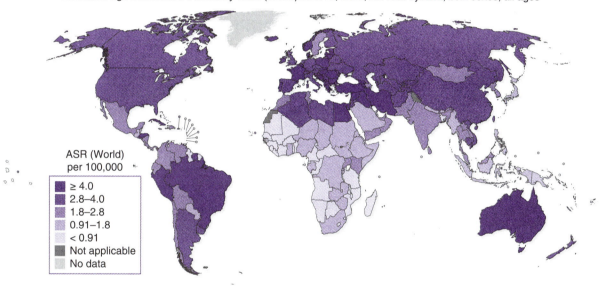

FIGURE 38.2 Global Incidence and Mortality Rates of Brain Tumors, 2018.

Caption: ASR: Rates per 100,000 are age-standardized to the world population, 2000–2025.

Reproduced with permission from Ferlay, J., Ervik, M., Lam, F., Colombet, M., Mery, L., Piñeros, M., . . . Bray, F. (2018). *Global cancer observatory: Cancer today*. Lyon, France: International Agency for Research on Cancer. Retrieved from https://gco.iarc.fr/today, accessed [09 October 2018].

▶ Classification of Brain Tumors

As pointed out by Stanley Robbins and Ramzi Cotran in their classic textbook of pathology, "the term brain tumor should be restricted only to neoplasms arising from any of the constituent cells within brain substance, neuroglial cells, neurons, cells of the blood vessels and connective tissues" (Kumar, Abbas, & Aster, 2014; Robbins & Cotran, 1979). It is also important to note that metastatic tumors from other primary anatomic sites account for 25%–30% of all intracranial tumors.

The classification of primary brain tumors is based on the cell of origin. Tumors arising from glial cells (neuroglia) are called gliomas, those arising from neurons are called neuromas or neuroblastomas, and tumors arising from meningeal cells are called meningiomas. The most common types of primary brain tumors that develop in adults are gliomas, meningiomas, pituitary gland tumors, acoustic neuromas, and lymphomas (**TABLE 38.1**). These five cell types constitute approximately 90% of all primary brain tumors, with gliomas and meningiomas accounting for approximately two-thirds of all tumors that arise in the brain.

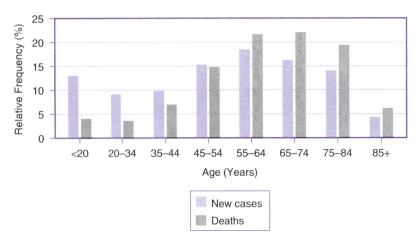

FIGURE 38.3 Age-Specific Frequency of New Cases and Deaths: Malignant Tumors of the Brain and Nervous System, United States.

Data from Altekruse, S. F., Kosary, C. L., Krapcho, M., Neyman, N., Aminou, R., Waldron, W., … Edwards, B. K. (2010). *SEER cancer statistics review, 1975–2007*. Bethesda, MD: National Cancer Institute.

TABLE 38.1 Profile of Brain Tumors, United States

Classification of Primary Brain Tumors	Relative Frequency (%)
Neuroepithelial tumors (Glioma)	33
Meningeal tumors (Meningioma)	34
Sellar tumors (Pituitary Gland)	12
Nerve tumors (Acoustic Neuroma)	9
Embryonal tumors (Medulloblastoma)	1
Lymphomas	3
Other or unclassified	8
Total	100

Total sample size = 158,088 Tumors

Data from Centralized Brain Tumor Registry of the United States. *CBTRUS statistical report: Primary brain and central nervous system tumors diagnosed in eighteen states in 2004–2006*. Hinsdale, IL: Author. Retrieved from http://www.cbtrus.org

Gliomas account for more than one-third of primary brain tumors in adults. Gliomas develop from neuroepithelial cells. There are several types of gliomas. One type, the astrocytoma, arises from star-shaped cells called astrocytes and can grow anywhere in the brain or spinal cord. In adults, astrocytomas most often arise in the cerebrum, the largest part of the brain that fills most of the upper skull. Glioblastoma

multiforme is an especially aggressive form of astrocytoma. Gliomas are diagnosed about twice as frequently in men compared to women.

Meningiomas also account for more than one-third of adult brain tumors. Meningiomas develop from the meninges, the protective membrane covering the brain directly underneath the skull. These tumors are usually benign and grow very slowly. Indeed, meningiomas rarely metastasize to other tissues, and symptoms such as headache, visual impairment, and focal seizures are due to compression of surrounding tissues by the expanding tumor in the confined intracranial vault. In contrast to gliomas, which predominate in men, meningiomas are diagnosed about twice as frequently in women compared to men. As discussed in the section on risk factors, gliomas and meningiomas have distinctly different sets of risk factors.

Schwannomas are benign tumors that develop from Schwann cells in the peripheral nervous system. Schwann cells are named after the German physiologist Theodor Schwann, who first described them in 1838 (Aszmann, 2000). These cells produce the myelin that covers and protects the peripheral or cranial nerve fibers connected with the brain. Acoustic neuromas are a type of schwannoma that arise from the Schwann cells that wrap around the acoustic nerve between the brain and the ear. Acoustic neuromas account for most of the brain tumors that arise in and around the cranial nerves.

Tumors arising from tissues and structures within the bony compartment called the sella turcica in the center of the brain are called *sellar tumors*. Sellar tumors usually develop from the pituitary gland. Less common types of primary brain tumors include primary lymphomas that develop from collections of lymphocytes within the brain, vascular tumors, germ cell tumors, sarcomas, and tumors of the pineal gland.

Cell of Origin of Glioma

Glioma is a cancer that arises from the glial cells (glia) of the brain. These cells were first described by the famous German pathologist Rudolph Virchow, who named them *nervenkitt* (nerve glue) or glia (Virchow, 1846, 1854). Glial cells outnumber neurons by about 9:1, but most are unable to generate action potentials or communicate by electrical signaling. Glia are crudely divisible by size into macroglia and microglia.

Macroglia are further categorized as astrocytes and oligodendrocytes. Astrocytes nurture and support neurons, and their tentacle-like processes encircle and envelop the synapses between nerve cells, supplying energy and oxygen necessary for the transmission of nerve impulses. Astrocytes also modulate the neuronal influx and efflux of important ions such as calcium, sodium, potassium, and chloride, and serve as a conduit for waste disposal. As such, they are often juxtaposed between cerebral blood vessels and neurons, and they provide biochemical support to endothelial cells of the blood–brain barrier (**FIGURE 38.4**).

Oligodendrocytes are macroglia that produce and secrete myelin, the insulatory material of neurons. A single oligodendrocyte can extend its tentacle-like processes to scores of axons, wrapping a sheath of myelin around each axon.

Small glial cells (microglia) protect the brain against invading microbes through immunosurveillance and innate immune reactions, and they assist in wound healing following traumatic injury to neurons. Microglia develop from hematopoietic stem cells rather than the neuroepithelium (Kimelberg, Jalonen, & Walz, 1993; Pollard & Earnshaw, 2008; Purves et al., 2008).

Glia were once believed to be relatively passive cells whose only purpose was to support the function of neurons. Nevertheless, in recent years, certain macroglia (particularly astrocytes) have been found to act in a partnering role with neurons in the processes of signal transduction and neurotransmission. Specifically, astrocytes are now known to play a very active role in modulating signal propagation and synaptic action by controlling the uptake of neurotransmitters at or near the synaptic cleft, and some are even capable of secreting neurotransmitters. For example, astrocytes are activated by elevated levels of calcium ions and have been found to secrete the neurotransmitter glutamate as partners in the neuronal response to excitation (Araque, Parpura, Sanzgiri, & Haydon, 1999; Santello & Volterra, 2008).

Because cancer involves uncontrolled cell division, it is important to realize that glia *do* retain the ability to undergo cell division in adulthood, whereas neurons do not. Following injury due to trauma or

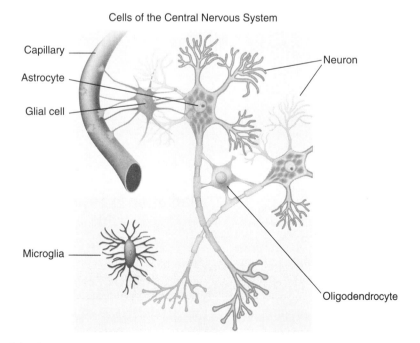

Cells of the Central Nervous System

Capillary
Astrocyte
Glial cell
Neuron
Microglia
Oligodendrocyte

FIGURE 38.4 Astrocyte of the Brain.

stroke, there is often profound proliferation of glial cells (gliosis) at or near the site of injury.

Types of Glioma

Glioma tumors are further classified by glial cell type into astrocytomas, glioblastomas multiforme, oligodendrogliomas, ependymomas, and mixed gliomas. *Glioblastoma multiforme* is the most common and most aggressive type of glioma. Patients diagnosed with glioblastoma have a median survival time of less than 1 year. Approximately 50%–60% of gliomas are classified as glioblastoma. These tumors develop from cells of the cerebral white matter and tend to grow rapidly and become very large before producing symptoms that lead to diagnosis. The cell of origin of glioblastoma multiforme has long been the subject of controversy and debate. The current view is that glioblastoma arises from pluripotent neural progenitor (stem) cells in the subventricular zone of the mature brain (Quigley, Post, & Ehrlich, 2007).

Astrocytomas account for 20%–30% of all gliomas. These tumors arise from astrocytes or their precursor cells. As their name implies, astrocytes are star-shaped cells that perform multiple functions, including support of endothelial cells of the blood–brain barrier, provision of nutrients and energy to neurons and maintenance of their ionic balance, and repair of nerve tissues following traumatic injury. The cytoplasm of astrocytes is densely populated with mitochondria and other organelles. These cells are highly branched, and their cellular processes envelop the synapses of nerve cells to facilitate transport of glucose for energy and ions (principally calcium) to stimulate neurotransmission. Furthermore, astrocytes have been found capable of communicating with neurons by calcium-modulated release of the neurotransmitter glutamate (Santello & Volterra, 2008).

Ependymomas account for about 6% of all gliomas. They arise from the layer of neuroepithelial cells that line both the hollow cavities of the brain and the canal containing the spinal cord. Within the brain, ependymomas most often arise from the floor of the fourth ventricle, situated in the lower back portion of the brain.

Oligodendrogliomas account for less than 5% of all gliomas. They arise from the oligodendrocytes, glial cells that are primarily responsible for laying down myelin around axons of neurons.

Microglia are the predominant immune cells of the brain that normally function in a protective role against foreign microbes and agents. Paradoxically, these cells are often abundant in and around developing gliomas, particularly astrocytomas, and they may release growth-promoting factors that actually accelerate tumor development and progression (Graeber, Scheithauer, & Kreutzberg, 2002).

Risk Factors for Glioma

Gliomas account for about 75% of all *malignant* brain tumors that develop in adults. This figure excludes meningiomas, which are invariably benign. Only a few risk factors for glioma have been identified and corroborated through independent investigation. Established risk factors include exposure to high-dose ionizing radiation, chronic immunosuppression, and certain rare genetic syndromes. Studies of other factors, including nonionizing radiation from cellular telephones, viral and microbial agents, household chemicals, nutritional factors, and certain environmental toxins, have thus far yielded equivocal results (Fisher et al., 2007; Schwartzbaum et al., 2006).

Gender Difference in Gliomas

Gliomas are detected about 1.5 times more often in men than in women, and reciprocally, meningiomas develop about 1.5 times more often in women. These gender differences may reflect the influence of hormones. To clarify associations of reproductive factors and glioma risk in women, Whelan and colleagues conducted a case–control study of 371 female glioma cases ascertained from hospitals and clinics in four Midwestern states and 527 controls randomly selected from licensed drivers and Health Care Finance Administration enrollees. All cases were confirmed by pathology. Compared with women who never breastfed, women who breastfed for 18 months or more were at increased risk (odds ratio [OR] = 1.8), and women who used estrogen replacement therapy had a decreased glioma risk compared to nonusers (OR = 0.7). These results suggest that estrogens may provide a modest degree of protection against the development of malignant gliomas (Huang et al., 2004).

Radiation Exposure and Brain Tumors

There is consistent evidence from several prospective epidemiologic investigations showing that high exposure to ionizing radiation increases the risk of developing glioma and other tumors of the brain. Sources of radiation include therapeutic and diagnostic medical procedures, occupational exposures as in uranium mining and radiology, atmospheric testing of nuclear weapons, natural sources, industrial accidents, and atomic bomb explosions.

In a study of mortality among U.S. physicians over a 50-year period, Matanoski and colleagues found two- to threefold increases in brain cancer mortality among cohorts of radiologists from the 1920s and 1930s compared to cohorts of other physicians (Matanoski, Seltser, Sartwell, Diamond, & Elliott, 1975). Subsequent studies have also noted increases in the incidence of brain tumors among physicians and radiologists (Andersen et al., 1999; Yoshinaga, Mabuchi, Sigurdson, Doody, & Ron, 2004).

A team of investigators characterized the incidence of brain tumors among atomic bomb survivors in Hiroshima and Nagasaki as a function of radiation dose. Tumors diagnosed between 1958 and 1995 among 80,160 atomic bomb survivors were ascertained using the Hiroshima and Nagasaki tumor registries, medical records, and death certificates. Malignant neoplasms were confirmed by pathology. Results revealed a significant dose response in risk with increasing radiation exposure. (Each additional sievert of radiation increased the risk by 20%). The investigators concluded that even moderate doses of radiation (<1 sievert) increase the risk of developing nervous system tumors (Preston et al., 2002; United Nations, 2000).

Several epidemiologic studies provide strong evidence that childhood exposure to ionizing radiation for the treatment of benign diseases increases the risk of developing a brain tumor later in life. In a study conducted in New York City, a cohort of 2224 children given X-ray treatment and a matched cohort of 1380 given topical medications for ringworm of the scalp (*tinea capitis*) during 1940–1959 were followed over nearly four decades to determine the comparative incidence of brain tumors. The average dose of ionizing radiation administered was 1.4 Gy. Sixteen intracranial tumors were detected in the irradiated cohort (7 brain cancers, 4 meningiomas, and 5 acoustic neuromas) compared to 1 acoustic neuroma in the control cohort. The standardized incidence ratio for brain cancer was 3.0, and the irradiated children also had

excess incidence rates of other tumors, including basal cell carcinomas of the skin and tumors of the thyroid and parotid glands (Shore, Albert, & Pasternack, 1976; Shore, Moseson, Harley, & Pasternack, 2003).

In Israel, a team of investigators studied the relationship between radiotherapy in childhood for tinea capitis and the development of tumors of the brain and nervous system. A total of 10,834 children received ionizing radiation during 1948 and 1960 and were followed for 30 years or more. Sixty neural tumors developed in the cohort of irradiated children, a rate of 1.8 per 10,000 person-years of follow-up. Compared with a matched population control group of 10,834 nonirradiated subjects and a second control group of 5392 nonirradiated siblings of the irradiated children, the cumulative risk of neural tumors was increased more than eightfold (relative risk [RR] = 8.4) (**FIGURE 38.5**). Risk increases were noted for meningiomas (RR = 9.5), gliomas (RR = 2.6), and nerve sheath tumors (RR = 18.8). The investigators found significant risk increases at exposure levels of 1–2 Gy, and they were also able to demonstrate a significant dose response in the risk with increasing exposure to ionizing radiation (Ron et al., 1988). In a subsequent investigation of these same cohorts after a median follow-up of 40 years, similar risk increases and dose responses were observed, prompting the investigators to conclude that "brain and meninges tissues are highly sensitive to radiation carcinogenesis" (Sadetzki et al., 2005).

Investigators in Sweden examined the risk of brain tumors in two cohorts containing a total of 28,008 children who received ionizing radiation therapy for hemangioma (a benign tumor of blood vessels). The average dose of radiation was low (7 cGy), but there was wide variation in exposure (up to 11.5 Gy). These cohorts were followed using the Swedish Cancer Register for detection of intracranial tumors during the period 1958–1993. For both cohorts, a total of 86 individuals developed brain tumors compared to

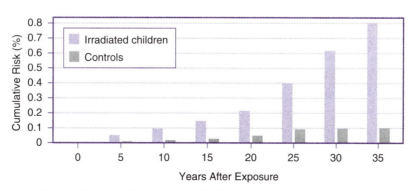

FIGURE 38.5 Cumulative Risk of Neural Tumors After Radiation for Tinea Capitis.

Data from Ron, E., Modan, B., Boice, J. D. Jr., Alfandary, E., Stovall, M., Chetrit, A., & Katz, L. (1988). Tumors of the brain and nervous system after radiotherapy in childhood. *New England Journal of Medicine, 319*(16), 1033–1039.

61 expected, yielding a standardized incidence ratio of 1.42. The excess relative risk increased by 2.7 per unit (Gy) of radiation exposure, suggesting a cause and effect dose–response relationship between the absorbed dose of ionizing radiation and brain tumor development. The findings also suggested that the risk was higher with exposure to ionizing radiation during infancy (Karlsson et al., 1998).

The development of a new primary neoplasm has long been recognized as a possible late effect of curative therapy involving ionizing radiation in combination with chemotherapy for an original childhood cancer. The Childhood Cancer Survivor Study (CCSS) is a large, retrospective cohort study of long-term survivors of childhood cancer. Participants were ascertained from 26 centers in the United States and Canada. To quantify the relative impact of radiation, chemotherapy, and other factors, Neglia and colleagues conducted a nested case–control study of secondary primary neoplasms of the brain and nervous system in the CCSS cohort of 14,361 5-year survivors of childhood cancers (leukemia or primary brain tumors). Each patient with a second primary was matched to four control subjects who had not developed a second primary by age, gender, and time since the original cancer diagnosis. Detailed information on the dose of ionizing radiation and the types and dosages of chemotherapeutic agents were ascertained from the medical records, and conditional logistic regression was used to estimate ORs. A total of 40 gliomas and 66 meningiomas were detected in the cohort. The median interval from the original diagnosis to detection was shorter for gliomas (9 years) than meningiomas (17 years). Radiation exposure was associated with increased risk of glioma (OR = 6.78) and meningioma (OR = 9.94), and there was a significant dose response in risk with increasing dosage of ionizing radiation. After adjustment for radiation dose, chemotherapeutic agents were *not* found to be associated with the risk of developing a subsequent primary brain tumor. The investigators concluded that exposure to radiation therapy is the most important risk factor for the development of a new primary brain tumor. They also noted that irradiation during infancy carries the highest risk for the development of a subsequent glioma (Neglia et al., 2006).

Mobile Phones and Brain Tumors

Mobile (cellular) phones have become an integral part of modern telecommunications and are now routinely used by nearly 4.6 billion people throughout the world. Since these devices are low-powered radio-frequency transmitters, several expert groups have expressed concerns about the health and safety of low-level exposure to radio-frequency electromagnetic fields with long-term mobile phone use (WHO, 2014). Consequently, an international case–control study, INTERPHONE, was launched to investigate possible associations between mobile phone use and the development of brain tumors. The study included interviews with 2708 patients with glioma, 2409 patients with meningioma, and matched controls ascertained from 13 countries. The results actually showed that regular mobile phone use was associated with a *decrease* in the odds ratios for both glioma (OR = 0.81) and meningioma (OR = 0.79). ORs were less than 1.0 for all deciles of lifetime number of phone calls and nine deciles of cumulative call time. However, in the 10th decile of "recalled" cumulative call time (51,640 hours), the OR was significantly increased for glioma (OR = 1.40) but not for meningioma (OR = 1.15). However, the investigators state that "there were implausible values of reported use in this group." Although they could not rule out an effect at the highest exposure level, biases and error prevented a causal interpretation (INTERPHONE Study Group, 2010).

Several investigators have analyzed subsets of the INTERPHONE database. For example, investigators in Sweden examined detailed information on mobile phone use among 371 cases of glioma and 273 cases of meningioma compared to 574 control subjects matched by age, gender, and residential area. For regular mobile phone use, the odds ratios were reduced for both glioma (OR = 0.8) and meningioma (OR = 0.7), and no increases in risk were observed for any type or anatomic location of brain tumor after more than 10 years of exposure. The authors concluded that "the data do not support the hypothesis that mobile phone use is related to an increased risk of glioma or meningioma" (Lönn, Ahlbom, Hall, Feychting, & Swedish INTERPHONE Study Group, 2005).

Other investigators examined the use of mobile phones and the risk of *acoustic neuromas* because of the proximity of the ipsilateral acoustic nerve to the handset. In a case–control study conducted in four Nordic countries and the United Kingdom, 678 cases of acoustic neuroma were compared to 3553 controls. In the pooled dataset, there was no overall association between regular mobile phone use and the risk of acoustic neuroma (OR = 0.9); furthermore, subgroup analyses by duration of use, lifetime cumulative hours of exposure, total number of calls made, and type of mobile phone failed to reveal significant associations. Interestingly, the risk of acoustic neuroma development on the *same* side of the head as reported phone use was increased with use for 10 years or more (OR = 1.8); but reciprocally, the risk to the *opposite* side decreased by a corresponding amount, making interpretation difficult (Schoemaker et al., 2005).

It is important to note that case–control studies are prone to differential reporting bias whereby the cases (with disease) may report differently than the controls (without disease). Thus, in case–control studies of self-reported environmental exposures that are perceived by the general public to present a health risk, such bias may artificially increase the risk.

Allergy, Asthma, and Glioma

Hochberg, Toniolo, Cole, and Salcman (1990) conducted a case–control study of 160 patients with brain tumors ascertained from hospitals in Boston, Massachusetts; Providence, Rhode Island; and Baltimore, Maryland. Controls were 128 healthy persons who were friends of the cases. Their results suggested an inverse association between the development of glioblastoma and susceptibility to allergies (OR = 0.60).

Subsequently, several other epidemiologic studies examined the association between allergic conditions such as asthma and the development of brain tumors, and most of these investigations also found an inverse association (Schwartzbaum et al., 2003). To quantify the risk and check for heterogeneity among studies, Linos and colleagues identified eight observational studies that examined associations between atopic diseases (asthma, eczema, hay fever, or allergy) and glioma or meningioma and performed a meta-analysis by pooling estimates according to the inverse of their variances. Their analysis involved 3450 patients with gliomas and 1070 patients with meningiomas. Pooled estimates revealed that the risk of glioma development was significantly reduced for each atopic condition (RR = 0.61 for allergy, RR = 0.68 for asthma, and RR = 0.69 for eczema). There was no association between atopic disease and the risk of meningioma. The investigators concluded that there is a strong inverse association between atopic disease and the development of glioma that is not likely explainable by methodological bias (Linos, Raine, Alonso, & Michaud, 2007).

More recently, Chen et al. (2010) identified four additional published studies for inclusion in a meta-analysis to evaluate the association between allergic conditions and glioma risk. Their analysis was based on 12 studies (10 case–control and 2 cohort studies) containing 6408 glioma patients and a total of 61,090 participants. Compared to subjects without allergies, those with reported allergic conditions had a 40% reduced risk of glioma (pooled OR = 0.60). The risk reductions were consistent for specific conditions (OR = 0.70 for asthma, OR = 0.69 for eczema, and OR = 0.78 for hay fever).

Although the results of these meta-analyses show consistency of effects, it has been pointed out that in most of the studies, spouses or close relatives were often called upon to provide information about the medical histories of patients with brain tumors; therefore, the inverse association with allergic conditions may be an artifact of general underreporting of asthmatic conditions for cases. In a novel investigation, Schwartzbaum and colleagues attempted to rule out such reporting bias by examining the distributions of asthma and allergy-related genetic polymorphisms in 111 patients with glioblastoma multiforme and 421 controls. Like other studies, their results revealed that *self-reported* history of allergic conditions reduced the risk of glioma development (OR = 0.64). But what is most important about this study is that the risk was independently modified by single nucleotide polymorphisms related to asthma susceptibility (interleukin-4 receptor a and interleukin-13), and these genetic effects could not have been influenced by reporting bias. Specifically, genetic polymorphisms that heighten asthma risk were found to reduce the risk of glioma development and vice versa. For example, interleukin-4 receptor a polymorphisms, which are known to decrease the risk of asthma, were found to increase the risk of glioma (OR = 1.61), and an interleukin-13 polymorphism that is known to increase the risk of asthma was found to decrease glioma risk (OR = 0.56). The investigators suggest that because germline mutations were used as biomarkers of susceptibility to asthma and allergic conditions, these results cannot be attributed to recall bias. As such, these findings tend to validate the inverse associations between adult glioma and self-reported histories of allergies that have been consistently observed in epidemiologic research over the past 20 years (Schwartzbaum et al., 2005, 2006).

Nonsteroidal Anti-Inflammatory Drugs and Glioma

Evidence from epidemiologic and experimental studies suggests that use of nonsteroidal anti-inflammatory drugs (NSAIDs) reduces the risk of a number of malignant neoplasms, including cancers of the colon, breast, prostate, and lung (Harris, 2009). These results prompted an investigation of the association between use of aspirin and other NSAIDs and risk of adult glioblastoma multiforme. The association was evaluated among 236 incident cases and 401 population-based controls frequency-matched on age, gender, and ethnicity from the San Francisco Bay Area Adult Glioma Study. Cases (or proxies) and controls were interviewed in person between 1997 and 2000. Cases with glioblastoma multiforme reported less use of at least 600 pills of all types of NSAIDs combined during the 10-year prediagnostic period than did controls (OR = 0.53). Findings were consistent for aspirin (OR = 0.51), ibuprofen (OR = 0.41), and naproxen or other NSAIDs (OR = 0.34). Eliminating participants who initiated NSAID use within 2 years of diagnosis yielded similar results. These findings show an inverse association between NSAID use and the risk of developing glioblastoma multiforme. The authors suggest the need for further studies to determine whether NSAIDs might be effective in the inhibition of glioma development or progression (Sivak-Sears, Schwartzbaum, Miike, Moghadassi, & Wrensch, 2004).

U.S. Study of Brain Tumors

A team of U.S. investigators conducted a comprehensive multicenter study of adult brain tumors to identify, compare, and quantify the risk factors for glioma, meningioma, and acoustic neuroma (Inskip et al., 2001). The study included 782 brain tumor cases and 799 controls ascertained from medical centers in Phoenix, Arizona; Brigham and Women's Hospital in Boston, Massachusetts; and Western Pennsylvania Hospital in Pittsburgh. Cases included 489 patients with gliomas, 197 patients with meningiomas, and 96 patients with acoustic neuromas. The controls were ascertained from the same hospitals with matching to the cases on gender, race, age, and location of residence. Data were collected by research nurses using standardized questionnaires. Furthermore, blood samples were collected to explore associations of germline mutations and polymorphisms with the development of brain tumors.

The study found no evidence of higher brain tumor risk among people who use handheld cellular phones compared to those who did not use them. The risk of developing brain tumors did not increase with increasing years of use or average minutes of use per day, nor did brain tumors among cellular phone users occur more often than expected on the side of the head on which people reported using their phone. There was no evidence for an increased risk of any of the three major categories of tumors (glioma, meningioma, or acoustic neuroma) among persons who used cellular telephones 60 or more minutes per day, or regularly for up to 5 years (Inskip et al., 2001).

There was evidence that people with a history of allergies or autoimmune diseases were at reduced risk for developing glioma. Allergies evaluated included asthma, eczema, hay fever, and allergies to medicine, insects, food, and chemicals. Autoimmune diseases included rheumatoid arthritis, lupus erythematosus, multiple sclerosis, diabetes, and pernicious anemia. The reduced risk associated with history of allergies was specific for gliomas (OR = 0.67), but there was no significant association between history of allergies and risk of meningioma or acoustic neuroma. History of autoimmune disease, however, was associated with a reduced risk of both glioma (OR = 0.49) and meningioma (OR = 0.59). The exact nature of the immunological basis for these associations remains to be determined (Brenner et al., 2002).

Genetic data from the study were also examined to determine effects of polymorphisms in glutathione S-transferase and the cytochrome P450 system, two families of genes involved in the metabolism of solvents that may play a role in the development of brain tumors. One polymorphism of *GSTP1* was found associated with an 80% increase in glioma risk, but results for other polymorphisms were indeterminate (De Roos et al., 2003).

Genetic Anomalies and Brain Tumors

A few genetic syndromes have been found that heighten the risk of developing a brain tumor. These include neurofibromatosis 1 and 2, tuberous sclerosis, retinoblastoma, Li–Fraumeni syndrome, Turcot's syndrome, and Cowden syndrome. These genetic syndromes are caused by heritable mutations in certain tumor suppressor genes that are critical to the processes of normal cell division and function. Furthermore, certain brain tumors such as retinoblastoma and oligodendroglioma are also characterized by specific gene mutations or chromosomal deletions.

Neurofibromatosis Types 1 and 2

Neurofibromatosis type 1 (von Recklinghausen's disease) is a rare autosomal dominant disorder first described by the German physician Friedrech von Recklinghausen in 1882. This condition is characterized by the development of multiple fibromas (neurofibromas) of the skin, brain, and other anatomic sites. Some patients also develop gliomas of the optic nerve. The syndrome is due to a mutant autosomal dominant gene called *NF1* located on the long arm of chromosome 17.

The gene encodes a protein called neurofibromin that regulates cell division of fibrous nerve sheaths. Mutant forms of *NF1* result in the development of neurofibromas (Boyd, Korf, & Theos, 2009).

Neurofibromatosis type 2 is a rare autosomal dominant disorder caused by a mutation of a tumor suppressor gene called *NF2* located on the long arm of chromosome 22. The gene encodes a protein called *merlin* that is essential for the formation of the myelin sheaths of nerves. Mutant forms of *NF2* result in the development of *schwannomas* of the vestibular branch of the eighth cranial nerve as well as tumors of other cranial nerves. Furthermore, approximately 50% of *NF2* mutant carriers develop meningiomas (Asthagiri et al., 2009).

Li–Fraumeni Syndrome

Li–Fraumeni syndrome is a rare autosomal dominant hereditary disorder (Li & Fraumeni, 1969). The syndrome is linked to germline mutations of the *p53* tumor suppressor gene located on the short arm of chromosome 17. Such mutations can be inherited or arise de novo early in embryogenesis or in one of the parents' germ cells (Varley, 2003). Patients who carry the *p53* mutant gene are at risk for a wide range of malignancies, including breast cancer, brain tumors, acute leukemia, soft tissue and bone sarcomas, and adrenal cortical carcinoma. A genetic variant of the Li–Fraumeni syndrome may be due to a mutation of another gene called *CHEK2* located on the long arm of chromosome 22 (Bell et al., 1999). Mutant forms of *CHEK2* lead to dysfunctional DNA repair during cell division, thereby increasing the risk of certain malignancies. However, there is controversy about whether *CHEK2* mutations cause a similar profile of cancer as *p53* mutations in the Li–Fraumeni syndrome (Evans, Birch, & Narod, 2008).

Turcot's Syndrome

Turcot's syndrome is a rare genetic disorder characterized clinically by the concurrence of a primary brain tumor and multiple colorectal adenomas. The condition is caused by mutations in the *APC* gene located on chromosome 5 or mismatch repair genes on chromosomes 2 and 3. The *APC* gene plays a critical role in several cellular processes, and the mismatch repair genes are responsible for the detection and repair of errors that occur during DNA replication. Mutant forms of these genes cause adenomatous polyps of the colon and medulloblastomas of the cerebellum (Hamilton et al., 1995). Mutations of the *APC* gene and the mismatch repair genes also cause familial adenomatous polyposis (FAP) and other hereditary colon cancer syndromes.

Tuberous Sclerosis

Tuberous sclerosis is a rare genetic disorder that causes development of nonmalignant fibromas in the brain and other anatomic sites, including the kidneys, heart, eyes, lungs, and skin. This condition is caused by mutations in either of two tumor suppressor genes, *TSC1* or *TSC2*, located on chromosomes 9 and 16, respectively. These genes encode two proteins, *hamartin* and *tuberin*, that regulate cell proliferation and differentiation. Mutant forms of *TSC1* and *TSC2* result in the development of giant cell astrocytomas, fibrous cortical tumors in the brain, and subependymal tumors in the walls of the ventricles of the brain (Yates, 2006).

Cowden Syndrome

Cowden syndrome (also known as *multiple hamartoma syndrome*) is a rare autosomal dominant inherited disorder characterized by multiple tumor-like growths called hamartomas and an increased risk of certain forms of cancer. The characteristic hamartomas of Cowden syndrome are small, noncancerous growths that are most commonly found on the skin and mucous membranes (such as the lining of the mouth and nose), but they can also occur in the intestinal tract and other parts of the body. This syndrome is caused by a mutant gene known as *PTEN* located on the long arm of chromosome 10. The *PTEN* gene encodes a protein known as *phosphatase and tensin homolog* that helps regulate normal cell division and growth. Mutant forms of *PTEN* result in the development of hamartomas and increase the risk of developing thyroid cancer, breast cancer, and endometrial cancer. In addition, individuals with Cowden syndrome sometimes develop slow-growing benign tumors of the cerebellum (Eng, 1998).

Retinoblastoma

Retinoblastoma is a rare malignant tumor that arises from the retinal cells of the eye. In a study of U.S. SEER data for 1975–2004, the age-adjusted annual rate of retinoblastoma for males and females was 12 cases per million. Most cases occurred in children (~90% before 5 years of age), and about one-third of cases developed bilateral disease in the first 2 years of life (Broaddus, Topham, & Sigh, 2009).

Retinoblastomas are caused by mutations of the retinoblastoma gene (*Rb1*) located on the short arm of chromosome 13. The *Rb1* gene was discovered by a team of investigators in 1986 (Dryja, Friend, & Weinberg, 1986). In its nonmutated form, *Rb1* encodes a tumor suppressor protein that regulates DNA replication during cell division. Mutations in *Rb1* cause retinoblastoma of the eye, and occasionally malignant tumors of the pineal gland (Du & Pogoriler, 2006; Parsam, Kannabiran, Honavar, Vemuganti, & Ali, 2009).

In 1971, Alfred Knudson hypothesized that retinoblastoma arises from two mutational events. In the heritable form, a mutated *Rb1* gene is inherited from one parent and the second occurs in somatic cells of the retina. In the nonheritable form, both *Rb1* mutations occur in somatic cells of the retina (Knudson, 1971). The *Rb1* gene was the first tumor suppressor gene ever discovered, and Knudson's two-hit mutation theory of retinoblastoma has been generalized as the *two-hit somatic mutation theory of cancer.*

The original multi-hit theory of cancer was proposed by Carl Nordling (1953), who stated that

the cancerous cell contains not one but a number of mutated genes. The occurrence of such accumulations of mutations may be expected to increase according to a certain exponent of age as well as according to the increase of cell proliferation. (pp. 68–72)

▶ Oligodendroglioma

Oligodendrogliomas are believed to originate from the oligodendrocytes of the brain or their precursor cells. These tumors constitute less than 5% of all malignant brain tumors. A common genetic structural deformity found in oligodendroglioma is codeletion of chromosomal arms 1p and 19q. In fact, this striking feature is considered the "genetic signature" of oligodendroglioma. In a recent study, 1p loss was present in 35 of 42 tumors (83%), 9q loss was present in 28 of 39 tumors (72%), both 1p and 9q losses were present in 27 of 39 tumors (69%), and at least one deletion was present in all tumors. Such deletions may silence the expression of important tumor suppressor genes such as the *CAMTA1* gene, a transcription regulator on chromosome 1 (Barbashina, Salazar, Holland, Rosenblum, & Ladanyi, 2005).

Cellular Signaling Pathways and Brain Tumors

Genetic alterations found to be associated with the development of brain tumors tend to disrupt cellular signaling pathways that regulate key processes

of carcinogenesis such as cell division, DNA repair, angiogenesis, and apoptosis. Expression of growth factors such as epidermal growth factor (*EGFR*), protein kinase activators (*RAS*), vascular endothelial growth factor (*VEGF*), and/or inactivation of tumor suppressor genes such as *p53*, *Rb1*, and *PTEN* are currently under intense investigation to elucidate mechanisms of carcinogenesis. Elucidation of such mechanisms could obviously reveal targets for effective molecular therapy.

As pointed out by many investigators, inflammation is a powerful contributing factor to the development of cancer, including brain tumors (Harris, 2009; Kaluz & Van Meir, 2011). For example, glioblastoma multiforme tissues are characterized by the presence of immune cell infiltrates and the expression of inflammatory cytokines. In a study of the immunohistochemistry of 47 glioblastomas, 35 tumors (74.4%) stained positive for cyclooxygenase-2 (COX-2), the rate-limiting enzyme of the prostaglandin inflammatory cascade, and tumors with a high rate of proliferation tended to have greater COX-2 expression (Prayson, Castilla, Vogelbaum, & Barnett, 2002).

Many studies have implicated hypoxia (lack of oxygen) and sustained activation of hypoxia inducible factor (HIF-1) as key events in carcinogenesis. It is therefore noteworthy that *HIF-1* can be induced by factors other than hypoxia, primarily proinflammatory mediators such as interleukin-1b and NF-κB. According to one model of glioblastoma development, activation of *HIF-1* is sustained by an autocrine loop that involves the protein kinase (*RAS*) cascade and amplified expression of interleukin-1b (Kaluz & Van Meir, 2011; Sharma, Dixit, Koul, Mehta, & Sen, 2010).

▶ Risk Factors for Meningiomas

Intracranial meningiomas account for more than one-third of all brain tumors. Although most meningiomas are benign (~95%), their expansion in the closed cranial vault can produce serious neurological symptoms and even death.

Meningiomas arise from cells of the meninges, the membranous tissue that covers the surface of the brain beneath the skull. Meningeal membranes also line the ventricles of the brain and cover certain structures and glands within the brain such as the pineal gland and the thalamus. The exact cell of origin is thought to be the arachnoid cap cell, a progenitor (stem) cell of mature meningeal tissue (Bondy et al., 2008).

Meningiomas are diagnosed roughly twice as often in women compared to men. In the United States, the age-adjusted rates of meningioma are 8.4 per 100,000

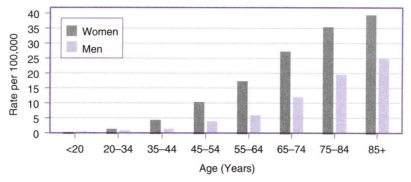

FIGURE 38.6 Age-Specific Incidence of Meningioma, United States, 2002–2006.

Data from Central Brain Tumor Registry of the United States. (2010). CBTRUS *statistical report: Primary brain and central nervous system tumors diagnosed in eighteen states in 2002–2006.* Hinsdale, IL: Author; Wiemels, J., Wrensch, M., & Claus, E. B. (2010). Epidemiology and etiology of meningioma. *Journal of Neurooncology, 99*(3), 307–314.

in women and 3.6 per 100,000 in men. In contrast to gliomas, which can occur in children, meningiomas are infrequently diagnosed before the age of 20 years, and the age-specific incidence rises steadily throughout the adult life span (**FIGURE 38.6**).

As with malignant gliomas of the brain, ionizing radiation is the major environmental risk factor for meningioma. Several studies have consistently found that exposure to high doses of ionizing radiation markedly elevates the risk of developing meningioma. For example, in the well-known cohort study of 10,834 Israeli children who received ionizing radiation to the scalp for the treatment of tinea capitis (ringworm) during 1948–1960, the risk of subsequent development of meningioma over 40 years of follow-up was increased nearly 10-fold (RR = 9.5). The mean latency period from radiation exposure to detection was 36 years, reflecting the extremely slow growth of most meningiomas (Ron et al., 1988; Sadetzki et al., 2005). It is also notable that multiple sources of radiation have been found to increase the risk of meningioma development, including radiation therapy for certain intracranial malignancies such as lymphoma and leukemia (Neglia et al., 2006), and full mouth dental X-rays (Longstreth et al., 2004).

The excess female risk for meningioma compared to males has been linked to reproductive factors and hormone (estrogen) exposure. Women have more than a threefold higher incidence than men during the reproductive years, and a few epidemiologic studies have linked exogenous estrogens to the relatively high female risk. In the Nurses' Health Study, current use of exogenous estrogens was found to increase the risk in both premenopausal women (RR = 2.48) and postmenopausal women (RR = 1.86) (Jhawar, Fuchs, Colditz, & Stampfer, 2003). In the INTERPHONE case–control study of brain tumors, an increased risk of meningioma was observed among postmenopausal women who had ever received hormone replacement therapy (OR = 1.7) (Wigertz et al., 2008). In a retrospective cohort study of the Mayo Clinic database,

the incidence of meningioma among women who received hormone replacement therapy was more than twofold higher than among women with no exposure (865 versus 366 per 100,000, adjusted OR = 2.2) (Blitshteyn, Crook, & Jaeckle, 2008). To clarify the effects of estrogen and other hormones on the pathogenesis of meningioma, it is suggested that future studies incorporate information on both hormonal exposures and the molecular expression of hormone receptors in meningeal tumor tissues (Wiemels, Wrensch, & Claus, 2010).

Although epidemiologic studies have consistently found that allergic conditions reduce the risk of developing *glioma*, it is unclear whether these conditions influence *meningioma* development. To help clarify the issue, Schoemaker et al. (2005) conducted a pooled analysis of two population-based case–control studies of meningioma and allergic conditions. The analysis included 475 cases and 1716 controls ascertained during 2001–2004 in the United Kingdom. The analysis revealed that meningioma risk was significantly reduced by individual allergic conditions, including asthma (OR = 0.85), hay fever (OR = 0.81), and eczema (OR = 0.72). Interestingly, the risk reductions were greatest among children with allergic conditions (OR = ~0.50) whereas the estimates of risk were close to unity for adults (Schoemaker et al., 2005).

Familial clustering of meningioma is uncommon, although some studies suggest that relatives of affected cases are at increased risk. For example, Malmer and colleagues examined the risk to relatives of index cases of meningioma (probands) ascertained through the Swedish National Cancer Registry and found a twofold increase in the risk among first-degree relatives compared to unrelated spouses (OR = 2.2) (Malmer, Henriksson, & Gronberg, 2003). In a similar analysis incorporating data from both the Swedish and Norwegian Registry databases, Hemminiki and colleagues also found an increase in meningioma risk among offspring of probands (OR = 1.6) (Hemminki,

Tretli, Sundquist, Johannesen, & Granstrom, 2009). Although these results suggest the existence of genetic factors that heighten susceptibility to meningioma development, at present, no linkage and/or segregation studies of familial meningioma have been reported (Wiemels et al., 2010).

As already noted, the currently available evidence suggests that certain risk factors for meningioma are like those for breast cancer (e.g., exposure to exogenous estrogens). Furthermore, several studies have demonstrated that breast cancer and meningioma develop in the *same* patient more often than expected. For example, in a study of second primary tumors that developed among women with either a first primary breast cancer or meningioma, the risk was increased for breast cancer after meningioma (RR = 1.54), and reciprocally, for meningioma after breast cancer (RR = 1.64). The investigators concluded that shared risk factors may account for this association (Custer, Koepsell, & Mueller, 2002).

In a genome-wide association study designed to examine single nucleotide polymorphisms (SNPs) in genes that regulate DNA repair, several polymorphisms were identified that were significantly associated with meningioma. Notably, three of these genetic variants were in a gene called *BRIP1* that is also associated with breast cancer. The *BRIP1* gene interacts with the breast cancer gene, *BRCA1*, in the repair of DNA double-strand breaks. This finding suggests that the association between meningioma and breast cancer may be due to shared genetic susceptibility (similar polymorphisms in DNA repair genes) in addition to shared environmental risk factors (estrogen replacement therapy) (Bethke et al., 2008).

Pituitary Tumors

Pituitary gland tumors account for about 15% of intracranial tumors in adults and 11% in children. These tumors are usually benign but can secrete excessive amounts of prolactin or growth hormone. Furthermore, enlargement of the pituitary gland in the confined bony compartment in the center of the brain, the *sella turcica*, can produce compressive injury and also result in substantial morbidity. The etiology of pituitary tumors is largely unknown.

Schoemaker and Swerdlow (2009) conducted a population-based case–control study in Southeast England to examine potential risk factors for pituitary tumors. Data on medical and reproductive history, female hormones, and cigarette smoking were collected by personal interview from 299 cases and 630 controls aged 18–59 years. Tumor risk was reduced in subjects reporting a past diagnosis of hay fever (OR = 0.7) but not asthma or eczema. Among women, certain features of menopause were found to increase the risk. Women who underwent surgical menopause within 1 year of diagnosis or experienced menopause before the age of 40 years were found to be at markedly increased risk (OR = 6.7 and OR = 7.5, respectively). The effect of early menopause remained when evaluating menopausal status 10 years before diagnosis. The risk was also increased among women who delivered their first child before the age of 20 years compared with nulliparous women (OR = 3.4). No significant associations were observed for ever use of oral contraceptives, hormone replacement therapy, cigarette smoking, past head injury, or past diagnosis of epilepsy. This study suggests an elevated risk of pituitary tumors in relation to surgically induced menopause, early postmenopausal age, and young age at first childbirth, and possibly a reduced risk with allergic conditions such as hay fever. Reasons for these associations need further investigation, but among women, abrupt or early changes in the hormonal milieu appear to play a role in the genesis of pituitary tumors (Schoemaker & Swerdlow, 2009).

An international team of researchers based in Finland examined three clusters of familial pituitary adenomas using chip-based technologies to characterize germline mutations. Within these families, mutant forms of the aryl hydrocarbon receptor interacting protein (*AIP*) gene were identified by linkage and segregation analysis in those individuals who developed pituitary adenomas. The aryl hydrocarbon receptor activates certain genes of the P450 system involved in a variety of metabolic pathways, including xenobiotic and drug metabolism. In a series of pituitary adenomas ascertained from cases in Northern Finland, the investigators found that two *AIP* mutations accounted for 16% of all pituitary adenomas and 40% of pituitary adenomas diagnosed in patients under the age of 35 years. Based on these results, they suggest that inherited tumor susceptibility due to low penetrance genes, such as *AIP*, may be more common than previously thought (Vierimaa et al., 2006).

Primary Lymphoma of the Brain

Immunosuppressed patients have an inordinately high risk of developing a primary lymphoma of the brain. Patients with progressive human immunodeficiency virus (HIV) infection complicated by Epstein–Barr virus (EBV) reactivation and posttransplant patients receiving powerful immunosuppressive drugs are at greatest risk.

▸ Brain Tumors in Children

The profile of brain tumors that occur in children and adolescents up to 19 years of age differs markedly from that in adults. More than 70% of childhood tumors are malignant gliomas arising from astrocytes, oligodendrocytes, ependymoma cells, or primitive neuroectoderm cells. Pituitary tumors account for about 11% of childhood tumors and are more commonly found in late adolescence. Meningiomas, which account for about 34% of adult brain tumors, comprise only about 4% of childhood brain tumors. The remaining histological types (neuroblastomas, nerve sheath tumors, germ cell tumors) each account for less than 5% of childhood tumors (CBTRUS, 2010).

Medulloblastomas are derived from progenitor (stem) cells of the neuroectoderm and are often referred to as *primitive neuroectodermal tumors (PNET)*. Medulloblastomas are one type of PNET that are found near the midline of the cerebellum. These tumors are more common in children under the age of 5 years. They tend to grow rapidly and often block drainage of the cerebral spinal fluid, causing symptoms associated with increased intracranial pressure. Medulloblastoma cells can spread (metastasize) to other areas of the central nervous system, especially around the spinal cord.

Nonrandom patterns of chromosomal deletions and aberrations have been discovered in several histologic types of childhood brain tumors. These findings suggest that the loss or inactivation of tumor suppressor genes are critical events in tumorigenesis. For example, deletions and aberrations involving chromosome 17 are characteristic cytogenetic findings in medulloblastoma cells. Elucidation of key cellular events that are disrupted by such genetic changes is critical to finding molecular targets for effective therapeutic intervention (Biegel, 1999).

In the United States, the annual incidence of childhood brain tumors "jumped" from 2.3 cases per 100,000 in 1975 to 3.2 cases per 100,000 in 1985, and since that time the rates have remained relatively stable. Malcolm Smith and colleagues at the National Cancer Institute attributed this rapid increase to improved detection of brain tumors with the advent of magnetic resonance imaging (MRI) during the early 1980s. There have also been refinements in the pathological classification of brain tumors due to improved neurosurgical techniques for obtaining biopsy specimens of brain tumors (Smith, Freidlin, Ries, & Simon, 1998).

As pointed out by an Ohio pediatrician, Dr. Arthur Varner:

In the report by Smith et al., the authors' conclusion is that the increasing incidence of brain tumors in children is best explained by a "jump model" with the optimum point of change being around 1985, the time of rapidly increasing availability of MRI. The authors discount environmental factors, since the change seemed to occur rapidly. (Smith et al., 1998; Varner, 1999)

Nevertheless, as noted by Dr. Varner, an abrupt change in drug use among children *did occur* at that time, namely, a large fraction of parents switched their children from pediatric aspirin to acetaminophen due to concern about aspirin as a potential cause of Reye's syndrome, and this led to a rapid and substantial decline in the use of pediatric aspirin in the early 1980s. According to U.S. marketing data for the period 1979–1985, annual purchases of pediatric aspirin declined from 600 million pills in 1979 to less than 200 million pills in 1985, coincident with a marked increase in sales of acetaminophen products (Arrowsmith, Kennedy, Kuritsky, & Faich, 1987). Varner (1999) states that "the anti-inflammatory effects of aspirin, as opposed to acetaminophen, may have been an unrecognized protective factor in the development of brain tumors, as has been demonstrated for other cancers." Indeed, it is now well known that aspirin and other NSAIDs have chemopreventive activity against many solid tumors through inhibition of the COX-2 prostaglandin inflammatory cascade, whereas acetaminophen is *not* a COX-2 inhibitor (Harris, 2009). Furthermore, recent molecular studies have shown that the tumor cells of high-grade gliomas and medulloblastomas diagnosed in children markedly overexpress COX-2 and related inflammatory cytokines (Bodey, Siegel, & Kaiser, 2006).

▸ Therapeutic Approaches to Glioma and Other Brain Tumors

Diagnosis of Brain Tumors

Brain tumors can present clinically by a myriad of neurological signs and symptoms such as headache, nausea, vomiting, altered consciousness, visual disturbances, impaired hearing, loss of smell, emotional changes, paralysis, and other losses of function. Radiologically, these neoplasms present as masses with partial contrast enhancement due to limited disruption of the blood–brain barrier. Noninvasive, high-resolution techniques, such as computed tomography (CT) scans and especially

MRI, have enhanced the detection of brain tumors. Histologically, malignant tumors are classified and staged based on the morphology and staining characteristics of tumor cells, nuclear atypia, and mitotic activity.

Prognosis of Malignant Brain Tumors

In general, the prognosis for a patient diagnosed with a malignant brain tumor such as glioma is quite poor. Of 10,000 Americans diagnosed each year with malignant gliomas, only about 50% are alive 1 year after diagnosis, and survival drops to less than 25% after 2 years. Glioblastoma has a 14-month median survival after diagnosis. Tumor histology and grade are important prognostic factors. For example, patients diagnosed with anaplastic astrocytoma typically survive 3 or more years.

Van Meir and colleagues (2010) have recently published an excellent review of exciting new advances in neuro-oncology with emphasis on malignant glioma. They state that

> … new discoveries are being made in basic and translational research, which are likely to improve this situation further in the next 10 years. These include agents that block one or more of the disordered tumor proliferation signaling pathways, and that overcome resistance to already existing treatments. Targeted therapies such as antiangiogenic therapy with antivascular endothelial growth factor antibodies (bevacizumab) are finding their way into clinical practice. Large-scale research efforts are ongoing to provide a comprehensive understanding of all the genetic alterations and gene expression changes underlying glioma formation. These have already refined the classification of glioblastoma into four distinct molecular entities that may lead to different treatment regimens. The role of cancer stem-like cells is another area of active investigation. There is definite hope that by 2020, new cocktails of drugs will be available to target the key molecular pathways involved in gliomas and reduce their mortality and morbidity, a positive development for patients, their families, and medical professionals alike. (pp. 166–193)

References

Altekruse, S. F., Kosary, C. L., Krapcho, M., Neyman, N., Aminou, R., Waldron, W., … Edwards, B. K. (2010). *SEER cancer statistics review, 1975–2007*. Bethesda, MD: National Cancer Institute.

Andersen, A., Barlow, L., Engeland, A., Kjærheim, K., Lynge, E., & Pukkala, E. (1999). Work-related cancer in the Nordic countries. *Scandinavian Journal of Work, Environment and Health, 25*(Suppl. 2), 1–116.

Araque, A., Parpura, V., Sanzgiri, R. P., & Haydon, P. G. (1999). Tripartite synapses: Glia, the unacknowledged partner. *Trends in Neuroscience, 22*(5), 208–215.

Arrowsmith, J. B., Kennedy, D. L., Kuritsky, J. N., & Faich, G. A. (1987). National patterns of aspirin use and Reye's syndrome reporting, United States, 1980–1985. *Pediatrics, 79*, 858–863.

Asthagiri, A. R., Parry, D. M., Butman, J. A., Kim, H. J., Tsilou, E. T., Zhuang, Z., & Lonser, R. R. (2009). Neurofibromatosis type 2. *Lancet, 373*(9679), 1974–1986.

Aszmann, O. C. (2000). The life and work of Theodore Schwann. *Journal of Reconstructive Microsurgery, 16*(4), 291–295.

Barbashina, V., Salazar, P., Holland, E. C., Rosenblum, M. K., & Ladanyi, M. (2005). Allelic losses at 1p36 and 19q13 in gliomas: Correlation with histologic classification, definition of a 150-kb minimal deleted region on 1p36, and evaluation of *CAMTA1* as a candidate tumor suppressor gene. *Clinical Cancer Research, 11*(3), 1119–11128.

Bell, D. W., Varley, J. M., Szydlo, T. E., Kang, D. H., Wahrer, D. C., Shannon, K. E., … Haber, D. A. (1999). Heterozygous germ line *hCHK2* mutations in Li-Fraumeni syndrome. *Science, 286*, 2528–2531.

Bethke, L., Murray, A., Webb, E., Schoemaker, M., Muir, K., McKinney, P., … Houlston, R. (2008). Comprehensive analysis of DNA repair gene variants and risk of meningioma. *Journal of the National Cancer Institute, 100*, 270–276.

Biegel, J. A. (1999). Cytogenetics and molecular genetics of childhood brain tumors. *Oncology, 1*, 139–151.

Blitshteyn, S., Crook, J. E., & Jaeckle, K. A. (2008). Is there an association between meningioma and hormone replacement therapy? *Journal of Clinical Oncology, 26*, 279–282.

Bodey, B., Siegel, S. E., & Kaiser, H. E. (2006). Cyclooxygenase-2 (COX-2) overexpression in childhood brain tumors. *In Vivo, 20*(4), 519–525.

Bondy, M. L., Scheurer, M. E., Malmer, B., Barnholtz-Sloan, J. S., Davis, F. G., Il'yasova, D., … Brain Tumor Epidemiology Consortium. (2008). Brain tumor epidemiology: Consensus from the brain tumor epidemiology consortium. *Cancer, 113*(Suppl. 7), 1953–1968.

Boyd, K. P., Korf, B. R., & Theos, A. (2009). Neurofibromatosis type 1. *Journal of the American Academy of Dermatology, 61*(1),1–14.

Bray, F., Ferlay, J., Soerjomataram, I., Siegel, R. L., Torre, L. A., & Jemal, A. (2018). Global cancer statistics 2018: GLOBOCAN estimates of incidence and mortality worldwide for 36 cancers in 185 countries. *CA: A Cancer Journal for Clinicians, 68*(6), 394–424.

Brenner, A. V., Linet, M. S., Fine, H. A., Shapiro, W. R., Selker, R. G., Black, P. M., & Inskip, P. D. (2002). History of allergies and autoimmune diseases and risk of brain tumors in adults. *International Journal of Cancer, 99*, 252–259.

Broaddus, E., Topham, A., & Sigh, A. D. (2009). Incidence of retinoblastoma in the USA: 1975–2004. *British Journal of Ophthalmology, 93*, 21–23.

Central Brain Tumor Registry of the United States. (2008). *Statistical report: Primary brain tumors in the United States, 2000–2004*. Hinsdale, IL: Author.

Central Brain Tumor Registry of the United States. (2010). *Statistical report: Primary brain and central nervous system tumors diagnosed in 18 states in 2002–2006.* Hinsdale, IL: Author.

Chen, C., Xu, T., Chen, J., Zhou, J., Yan, Y., Lu, Y., & Wu, S. (2010). Allergy and risk of glioma: A meta-analysis. *European Journal of Neurology, 18*(3), 387–395.

Custer, B. S., Koepsell, T. D., & Mueller, B. A. (2002). The association between breast carcinoma and meningioma in women. *Cancer, 94,* 1626–1635.

De Roos, A. J., Rothman, N., Inskip, P. D., Linet, M. S., Shapiro, W. R., Selker, R. G., … Bell, D. A. (2003). Genetic polymorphisms in *GSTM1, -P1, -T1* and *CYP2E1* and the risk of adult brain tumors. *Cancer Epidemiology, Biomarkers and Prevention, 12,* 14–27.

Dryja, T. P., Friend, S., & Weinberg, R. A. (1986). Genetic sequences that predispose to retinoblastoma and osteosarcoma. *Symposium on Fundamental Cancer Research, 39,* 115–119.

Du, W., & Pogoriler, J. (2006). Retinoblastoma family genes. *Oncogene, 25*(38), 5190–5200.

Eng, C. (1998). Genetics of Cowden syndrome: Through the looking glass of oncology. *International Journal of Oncology, 12*(3), 701–710.

Evans, D. G., Birch, J. M., & Narod, S. A. (2008). Is *CHEK2* a cause of the Li–Fraumeni syndrome? *Journal of Medical Genetics, 45,* 63–64.

Ferlay, J., Ervik, M., Lam, F., Colombet, M., Mery, L., Piñeros, M., … Bray, F. (2018). *Global cancer observatory: Cancer today.* Lyon, France: International Agency for Research on Cancer. Retrieved from https://gco.iarc.fr/today

Ferlay, J., Shin, H. R., Forman, D., Mathers, C., & Parkin, D. M. (2010). Estimates of worldwide burden of cancer in 2008. *International Journal of Cancer, 127*(12), 2893–2917.

Ferlay, J., Soerjomataram, I., Ervik, M., Dikshit, R., Eser, S., Mathers, C., … Bray, F. (2013). *GLOBOCAN 2012 v1.0. Cancer incidence and mortality worldwide: IARC CancerBase No. 11* [Internet]. Lyon, France: International Agency for Research on Cancer. Retrieved from http://globocan.iarc.fr

Fisher, J. L., Schwartzbaum, J. A., Wrensch, M., & Wiemels, J. L. (2007). Epidemiology of brain tumors. *Neurologic Clinics, 25,* 867–890.

Fitzmaurice, C., Akinyemiju, T. F., Al Lami, F. H., Alam, T., Alizadeh-Navaei, R., Allen, C., … Global Burden of Disease Cancer Collaboration. (2018, June). Global, regional, and national cancer incidence, mortality, years of life lost, years lived with disability, and disability-adjusted life-years for 29 cancer groups, 1990 to 2016: A systematic analysis for the Global Burden of Disease Study. *JAMA Oncology.* Online Publication. doi:10.1001/jamaoncol.2018.2706.

Fitzmaurice, C., Allen, C., Barber, R. M., Barregard, L., Bhutta, Z. A., Brenner, H., … Global Burden of Disease Cancer Collaboration. (2017). Global, regional, and national cancer incidence, mortality, years of life lost, years lived with disability, and disability-adjusted life-years for 32 cancer groups, 1990 to 2015: A systematic analysis for the Global Burden of Disease Study. *JAMA Oncology, 3*(4), 524–548.

Graeber, M. B., Scheithauer, B. W., & Kreutzberg, G. W. (2002). Microglia in brain tumors. *Glia, 40*(2), 252–259.

Hamilton, S. R., Liu, B., Parsons, R. E., Papadopoulos, N., Jen, J., Powell, S. M., … Kinzler, K. W. (1995). The molecular basis of Turcot's syndrome. *New England Journal of Medicine, 332,* 839–847.

Harris, R. E. (2009). Cyclooxygenase-2 (COX-2) blockade in the chemoprevention of cancers of the colon, breast, prostate, and lung. *Inflammo-Pharmacology, 17,* 1–13.

Hemminki, K., Tretli, S., Sundquist, J., Johannesen, T. B., & Granstrom, C. (2009). Familial risks in nervous-system tumours: A histology-specific analysis from Sweden and Norway. *Lancet Oncology, 10,* 481–488.

Hochberg, F., Toniolo, P., Cole, P., & Salcman, M. (1990). Non-occupational risk indicators of glioblastoma in adults. *Journal of Neuro-Oncology, 8,* 55–60.

Horner, M. J., Ries, L. A. G., Krapcho, M., Neyman, N., Aminou, R., Howlader, N., … Edwards, B. K. (Eds.). (2009). *SEER cancer statistics review, 1975–2006.* Bethesda, MD: National Cancer Institute.

Huang, K., Whelan, E. A., Ruder, A. M., Ward, E. M., Deddens, J. A., Davis-King, K. E., … Brain Cancer Collaborative Study Group. (2004). Reproductive factors and risk of glioma in women. *Cancer Epidemiology, Biomarkers and Prevention, 13*(10), 1583–1588.

Inskip, P. D., Tarone, R. E., Hatch, E. E., Wilcosky, T. C., Shapiro, W. R., Selker, R. G., … Linet, M. S. (2001). Cellular telephone use and brain tumors. *New England Journal of Medicine, 344,* 79–86.

INTERPHONE Study Group. (2010). Brain tumour risk in relation to mobile telephone use: Results of the INTERPHONE international case–control study. *International Journal of Epidemiology, 39*(3), 1–20.

Jhawar, B. S., Fuchs, C. S., Colditz, G. A., & Stampfer, M. J. (2003). Sex steroid hormone exposures and risk for meningioma. *Journal of Neurosurgery, 99,* 848–853.

Kaluz, S., & Van Meir, E. G. (2011). At the crossroads of cancer and inflammation: *RAS* rewires an HIF-driven IL-1 autocrine loop. *Journal of Molecular Medicine, 89,* 91–94.

Karlsson, P., Holmberg, E., Lundell, M., Mattsson, A., Holm, L. E., & Wallgren, A. (1998). Intracranial tumors after exposure to ionizing radiation during infancy: A pooled analysis of two Swedish cohorts of 28,008 infants with skin hemangioma. *Radiation Research, 150,* 357–364.

Kimelberg, H. K., Jalonen, T., & Walz, W. (1993). Regulation of the brain microenvironment: Transmitters and ions. In S. Murphy (Ed.), *Astrocytes: Pharmacology and function* (pp. 193–222). San Diego, CA: Academic Press.

Knudson, A. G. (1971). Mutation and cancer: Statistical study of retinoblastoma. *Proceedings of the National Academy of Sciences of the United States of America, 68*(4), 820–823.

Kumar, V., Abbas, A. K., & Aster, J. C. (2014). *Robbins and Cotran pathologic basis of disease* (9th ed.). Philadelphia, PA: Mosby & Saunders.

Li, F. P., & Fraumeni, J. F. (1969). Soft-tissue sarcomas, breast cancer, and other neoplasms. A familial syndrome? *Annals of Internal Medicine, 71*(4), 747–752.

Linos, E., Raine, T., Alonso, A., & Michaud, D. (2007). Atopy and risk of brain tumors: A meta-analysis. *Journal of the National Cancer Institute, 99,* 1544–1550.

Longstreth, W. T., Jr., Phillips, L. E., Drangsholt, M., Koepsell, T. D., Custer, B. S., Gehrels, J. A., & Belle, G. (2004). Dental X-rays and the risk of intracranial meningioma: A population-based case–control study. *Cancer, 100,* 1026–1034.

Lönn, S., Ahlbom, A., Hall, P., Feychting, M., & Swedish Interphone Study Group. (2005). Long-term mobile phone use and brain tumor risk. *American Journal of Epidemiology, 161*(6), 526–535.

Malmer, B., Henriksson, R., & Gronberg, H. (2003). Familial brain tumours—Genetics or environment? A nationwide cohort study of cancer risk in spouses and first-degree relatives of brain tumour patients. *International Journal of Cancer, 106,* 260–263.

Matanoski, G. M., Seltser, R., Sartwell, P. E., Diamond, E. L., & Elliott, E. A. (1975). The current mortality rates of radiologists and other physician specialists: Specific causes of death. *American Journal of Epidemiology, 101*, 199–210.

Neglia, J. P., Robison, L. L., Stovall, M., Liu, Y., Packer, R. J., Hammond, S., … Inskip, P. D. (2006). New primary neoplasms of the central nervous system in survivors of childhood cancer: A report from the Childhood Cancer Survivor Study. *Journal of the National Cancer Institute, 98*(21), 1528–1537.

Noone, A. M., Howlader, N., Krapcho, M., Miller, D., Brest, A., Yu, M., … Cronin, K. A. (2018). *SEER Cancer Statistics Review, 1975–2015*, Bethesda, MD: National Cancer Institute.

Nordling, C. O. (1953). A new theory on the cancer-inducing mechanism. *British Journal of Cancer, 7*, 68–72.

Parkin, D. M., Bray, F., Ferlay, J., & Pisani, P. (2005). Global cancer statistics, 2002. *CA: A Cancer Journal for Clinicians, 55*, 74–108.

Parkin, D. M., Pisani, P., & Ferlay, J. (1999a). Estimates of the worldwide incidence of 25 major cancers in 1990. *International Journal of Cancer, 80*(6), 827–841.

Parkin, D. M., Pisani, P., & Ferlay, J. (1999b). Global cancer statistics, 1990. *CA: A Cancer Journal for Clinicians, 49*(1), 33–64.

Parkin, D. M., Whelan, S. L., Ferlay, J., Teppo, L., & Thomas, D. B. (2002). *Cancer incidence in five continents* (vol. 5). Lyon, France: IARC Press.

Parsam, V. L., Kannabiran, C., Honavar, S., Vemuganti, G. K., & Ali, M. J. (2009). A comprehensive, sensitive and economical approach for the detection of mutations in the *RB1* gene in retinoblastoma. *Journal of Genetics, 88*(4), 517–527.

Pollard, W., & Earnshaw, W. C. (2008). *Cell biology*. Philadelphia, PA: Saunders Elsevier.

Prayson, R. A., Castilla, E. A., Vogelbaum, M. A., & Barnett, G. H. (2002). Cyclooxygenase-2 (COX-2) expression by immunohistochemistry in glioblastoma multiforme. *Annals of Diagnostic Pathology, 6*(3), 148–153.

Preston, D. L., Ron, E., Yonehara, S., Kibuke, T., Fjuii, H., Kishikawa, M., … Mabuchi, K. (2002). Tumors of the nervous system and pituitary gland associated with atomic bomb radiation exposure. *Journal of the National Cancer Institute, 94*, 1555–1563.

Purves, D., Augustine, G. J., Fitzpatrick, D., Hall, W. C., LaMantia, A., McNamara, J. O., & White, L. E. (2008). *Neuroscience*. Sunderland, MA: Sinauer Associates.

Quigley, M. R., Post, C., & Ehrlich, G. (2007). Some speculation on the origin of glioblastoma. *Neurosurgery Review, 30*, 16–21.

Robbins, S. L., & Cotran, R. S. (1979). *Pathologic basis of disease* (2nd ed.). Philadelphia: W. B. Saunders.

Ron, E., Modan, B., Boice, J. D., Jr., Alfandary, E., Stovall, M., Chetrit, A., & Katz, L. (1988). Tumors of the brain and nervous system after radiotherapy in childhood. *New England Journal of Medicine, 319*(16), 1033–1039.

Sadetzki, S., Chetrit, A., Freedman, L., Stovall, M., Modan, B., & Novikov, I. (2005). Long-term follow-up for brain tumor development after childhood exposure to ionizing radiation for tinea capitis. *Radiation Research, 163*, 424–432.

Santello, M., & Volterra, A. (2008). Synaptic modulation by astrocytes via Ca(2+)-dependent glutamate release. *Neuroscience, 158*(1), 253–259.

Schoemaker, M. J., & Swerdlow, A. J. (2009). Risk factors for pituitary tumors: A case-control study. *Cancer Epidemiology, Biomarkers and Prevention, 18*(5), 1492–1500.

Schoemaker, M. J., Swerdlow, A. J., Ahlbom, A., Auvinen, A., Blaasaas, K. G., Cardis, E., … Tynes, T. (2005). Mobile phone use and risk of acoustic neuroma: Results of the Interphone case–control study in five North European countries. *British Journal of Cancer, 93*, 842–848.

Schwartzbaum, J., Ahlbom, A., Malmer, B., Lönn, S., Brookes, A. J., Doss, H., … Feychting, M. (2005). Polymorphisms associated with asthma are inversely related to glioblastoma multiforme. *Cancer Research, 65*, 6459–6465.

Schwartzbaum, J., Fonsson, F., Ahlbom, A., Preston-Martin, S., Lönn, S., Söderberg, K. C., & Feychting, M. (2003). Cohort studies of association between self-reported allergic conditions, immune-related diagnoses and glioma and meningioma risk. *International Journal of Cancer, 106*(3), 423–428.

Schwartzbaum, J. A., Fisher, J. L., Aldape, K. D., & Wrensch, M. (2006). Epidemiology and molecular pathology of glioma. *Nature Clinical Practice Neurology, 2*, 494–503.

Sharma, V., Dixit, D., Koul, N., Mehta, V., & Sen, E. (2010). *RAS* regulates interleukin-1β-induced HIF-1α transcriptional activity in glioblastoma. *Journal of Molecular Medicine, 89*(1), 1–14.

Shore, R. E., Albert, R. E., & Pasternack, B. S. (1976). Follow-up study of patients treated by X-ray epilation for tinea capitis; Resurvey of post-treatment illness and mortality experience. *Archives of Environmental Health, 31*(1), 21–28.

Shore, R. E., Moseson, M., Harley, N., & Pasternack, B. S. (2003). Tumors and other diseases following childhood X-ray treatment for ringworm of the scalp (tinea capitis). *Health Physics, 85*(4), 404–408.

Sivak-Sears, N. R., Schwartzbaum, J. A., Miike, R., Moghadassi, M., & Wrensch, M. (2004). Case-control study of use of nonsteroidal antiinflammatory drugs and glioblastoma multiforme. *American Journal of Epidemiology, 159*, 1131–1139.

Smith, M. A., Freidlin, B., Ries, L. A., & Simon, R. (1998). Trends in reported incidence of primary malignant brain tumors in children in the United States. *Journal of the National Cancer Institute, 90*(17), 1269–1277.

United Nations. (2000). *Scientific Committee on the Effects of Atomic Radiation Sources and Effects of Ionizing Radiation: UNSCEAR 2000 report to the general assembly, with scientific annexes*. New York, NY. Retrieved from http://www.unscear.org/unscear/en/publications/2000_1.html

Van Meir, E. G., Hadjipanayis, C. G., Norden, A. D., Shu, H. K., Wen, P. Y., & Olson, J. J. (2010). Exciting new advances in neuro-oncology: The avenue to a cure for malignant glioma. *CA: A Cancer Journal for Clinicians, 60*, 166–193.

Varley, J. M. (2003). Germline *TP53* mutations and Li-Fraumeni syndrome. *Human Mutation, 21*(3), 313–320.

Varner, A. (1999). Letter to the editor: Re: Trends in reported incidence of primary malignant brain tumors in children in the United States. *Journal of the National Cancer Institute, 91*(11), 973.

Vierimaa, O., Georgitsi, M., Lehtonen, R., Vahteristo, P., Kokko, A., Raitila, A., … Aaltonen, L. A. (2006). Pituitary adenoma p redisposition caused by germ line mutations in the *AIP* gene. *Science, 312*, 1228–1230.

Virchow, R. (1846). Ueber das granulirte aussehen der wandungen der gehirnventrikel. *Allgemeine Zeitschrift Fur Psychiatrie, 3*, 242–250.

Virchow, R. (1854). Ueber das ausgebreitete Vorkommen einer dem Nervenmark analogen substanz in den tierischen Geweben. *Virchows Archive Fur Pathologische Anatomie, 6*, 562.

World Health Organization. (2014). *Electromagnetic fields and public health: Mobile phones.* Geneva, Switzerland: Author. Retrieved from http://www.who.int/mediacentre/factsheets/fs193/en/

Wiemels, J., Wrensch, M., & Claus, E. B. (2010). Epidemiology and etiology of meningioma. *Journal of Neuro-Oncology, 99*(3), 307–314.

Wigertz, A., Lonn, S., Hall, P., Auvinen, A., Christensen, H. C., Johansen, C., … Feychting, M. (2008). Reproductive factors and risk of meningioma and glioma. *Cancer Epidemiology, Biomarkers and Prevention, 17*, 2663–2670.

Yates, J. R. (2006). Tuberous sclerosis. *European Journal of Human Genetics, 14*(10), 1065–1073.

Yoshinaga, S., Mabuchi, K., Sigurdson, A. J., Doody, M. M., & Ron, E. (2004). Cancer risks among radiologists and radiologic technologists: Review of epidemiologic studies. *Radiology, 233*, 313–321.

Epidemiology of Chronic Respiratory, Metabolic, and Musculoskeletal Diseases

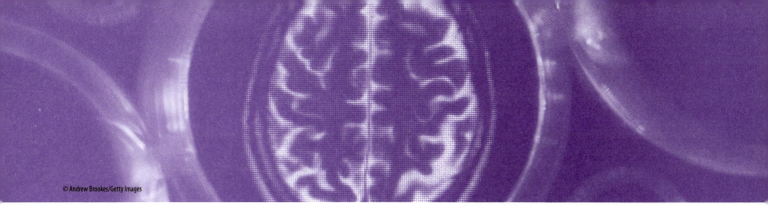

CHAPTER 39

Epidemiology of Chronic Obstructive Pulmonary Disease

▶ Introduction

*C*hronic Obstructive Pulmonary Disease (COPD) is a progressive debilitating lung disease that afflicts more than 300 million individuals and causes nearly 3.2 million deaths annually in the world population. This chronic lung disease is currently the third leading cause of death among all diseases and is responsible for enormous disability accounting for about 3% of the total *disability-adjusted life years* (DALY). The pathogenesis of COPD is primarily a consequence of persisting inhalation of tobacco smoke and/or polluted air with superimposed respiratory infections.

▶ Anatomy and Function of the Lungs

The human lungs are paired organs that perform the cardinal function of exchanging carbon dioxide in the blood for oxygen in inspired air. The left lung is divided into two lobes and the right lung into three lobes. Together, they contain approximately 1500 miles of airways and 300–500 million alveoli where the carbon dioxide and oxygen exchange occurs. The total surface area of adult human lungs is approximately 70 square meters (roughly the same area as one side of a tennis court). If all the capillary vessels that envelop the alveoli were unwound and laid end to end, they would extend for more than

600 miles (Robbins & Cotran, 1979; Weinberger, 2004).

Inspired air is conducted into the lungs through the trachea, the bronchi, and the bronchioles (**FIGURE 39.1**). This *conducting zone* is not involved in gas exchange and is reinforced with cartilage to maintain patency for the inhalation and exhalation of air. Its function is to warm the inspired air to 37°C and humidify the air. Small projections known as *cilia* effectively cleanse inspired air by wave-like motions that propel foreign material back into the larger bronchi and trachea where the cough reflex completes the expulsion. Furthermore, mucus-secreting cells and immune cells line the airways and help protect the lungs by trapping viruses, bacteria, pollen, dust, and other foreign material.

Exchange of gases occurs in the *respiratory zone*, which consists of respiratory bronchioles, the alveolar ducts, and the alveoli (Figure 39.1). The alveolar epithelium is a continuous layer of cells consisting of two principal cell types: *Type I pneumocytes* that cover 95% of the alveolar surface and granular *Type II pneumocytes* that secrete *pulmonary surfactant* (the major lubricant in the lungs) and are involved in repairing damage to the alveoli. Type I pneumocytes interface with the endothelial cells lining the pulmonary capillaries to facilitate the diffusion of carbon dioxide and oxygen across the alveolar-capillary membrane.

Total lung capacity ranges between 4 and 6 L and is contingent upon age, height, weight, and gender. On average, females have 20%–25% less capacity

539

Conducting Zone

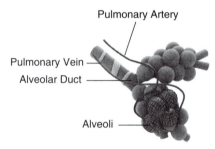

Respiratory Zone

FIGURE 39.1 Diagram of Human Lungs.
© Sebastian Kaulitzki/Shutterstock.

than males. The typical adult resting respiratory rate is 10–20 breaths per minute, and with each breath about 500 mL of air is exchanged (the *tidal volume)*. Nevertheless, the lungs have a tremendous reserve volume and the amount of air that can be exchanged by *forced* inspiration and expiration is about 4 L (the *vital capacity*). The average human breathes approximately 11,000 L of air containing 2.31 L of oxygen per day (Weinberger, Cockrill, & Mandel, 2018a).

▶ Diagnosis of COPD

COPD actually refers to the presence of either of two conditions, emphysema or chronic bronchitis, which may exist simultaneously or separately in a given individual. The diagnosis of COPD is initially suggested by chronic repeated episodes of dyspnea (shortness of breath), wheezing, and coughing with or without mucous production.

In emphysema uncompromised by chronic bronchitis, the patient is typically barrel-chested and dyspneic with obviously prolonged expiration due to

air trapping in the lungs. Significant weight loss is a common presenting symptom. Such patients remain well oxygenated and are thus referred to as *pink puffers*. Pathologically, the lungs are characterized by permanent enlargement of the air spaces distal to the terminal bronchioles accompanied by significant destruction of the alveolar walls.

Chronic bronchitis is clinically defined as persistent cough with sputum production for at least 3 months in at least 2 consecutive years. This condition in its pure form involves chronic bacterial or viral infection and inflammation of the lungs. Patients characteristically are obese and may be *cyanotic* and *hypercapnic* due to lack of oxygen and excess carbon dioxide in the blood, respectively. Due to the bluish tinge of skin and lips from cyanosis and fluid retention from congestive right heart failure (*cor pulmonale*), such patients are referred to as *blue bloaters*. The classic signs and symptoms of patients with emphysema versus chronic bronchitis are compared in **TABLE 39.1**.

The diagnosis of COPD is confirmed using spirometry, a test that measures the ratio of the forced expiratory volume of air in 1 second by the patient (FEV1) to the forced vital capacity of the lungs (FVC). Ratios less than 0.70 are diagnostic of COPD. Radiographic images of the lungs may aid in the diagnosis, and biopsy specimens are sometimes ascertained to microscopically assess the degree of alveolar destruction in emphysema. The stages of COPD based upon post-spirometry values measured after administration of a bronchodilator (e.g., a beta 2 agonist) are shown in **TABLE 39.2**.

It is important to realize that emphysema and chronic bronchitis are often superimposed in the same patient. Indeed, the coexistence of both conditions in the same individual is the rule rather than the exception. However, chronic bronchitis is diagnosed according to clinical parameters (productive cough for 3 months in 2 consecutive years). Consequently, chronic bronchitis is easier to diagnose giving rise to higher prevalence rates. Nevertheless, pathologic studies of biopsy specimens from COPD patients with stage III or stage IV disease invariably reflect the presence of components of *both* emphysema and chronic bronchitis (Weinberger, Cockrill, & Mandel, 2018b).

▶ Age Distribution of COPD

The onset of COPD (chronic bronchitis and/or emphysema) increases exponentially with age in both men and women. The age-specific prevalence of COPD estimated from a random sample of the general population

TABLE 39.1 Emphysema versus Chronic Bronchitis

Pink Puffer	Blue Bloater
No bronchitis	Bronchitis, cough, mucous, infection
Barrel chest	No barrel chest
Early dyspnea	Late dyspnea
Hyperventilation	Cyanosis
Adequate oxygenation	Hypercapnia
Hunched over	Cor pulmonale, CHF
Weight loss	Obesity

TABLE 39.2 Stages of COPD

Stage of COPD	Symptoms	Spirometry
Stage I: Mild	Shortness of breath (SOB), cough	FEV1/FVC < 0.70 FEV1 < 80%
Stage II: Moderate	SOB, cough, sputum	FEV1/FVC < 0.70 FEV1 < 80%
Stage III: Severe	SOB, fatigue, cough, sputum	FEV1/FVC < 0.70 FEV < 50%
Stage IV: Very severe	SOB, cyanosis, respiratory failure	FEV1/FVC < 0.70 FEV1 < 30%

of England ($n = 10,750$) is shown in **FIGURE 39.2**. Note that after age 55 years, the prevalence in men is approximately double that in women (e.g., 12% of men over 75 years have COPD compared to 6% in women) (Nacul, Soljak, & Meade, 2007). This marked gender difference primarily reflects the greater rates of smoking among men (as discussed in the section on COPD risk factors). The age distribution of COPD differs markedly from that of asthma, which is similar for men and women and actually declines in the later years of life.

▶ Global Burden of COPD

In 2015, 3.19 million individuals died of COPD and there were approximately 175 million individuals living with symptomatic COPD in the world population. The global number of COPD deaths in 2015 is significantly higher than previous estimates from 1990, 2000, and 2010 that range from 2.8 to 3.0 million. Paradoxically, the age-adjusted mortality rate of COPD declined more than 40% during 1990–2015, but this favorable trend was counteracted by growth and aging of the world population resulting in more older individuals contracting and dying from COPD than ever before (Burney, Patel, Newson, Minelli, & Naghavi, 2015; GBD 2015 Chronic Respiratory Disease Collaborators, 2017).

It is notable that previous estimates of the global prevalence of COPD exceed 300 million. The lower estimate of 175 million prevalent cases in 2015 is based upon a more restrictive diagnostic threshold

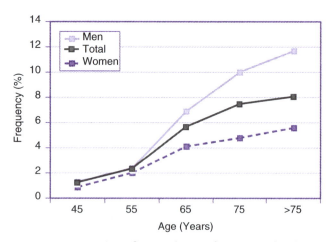

FIGURE 39.2 Age-Specific Prevalence of COPD, England, 2005.

Data from Nacul, L. C., Soljak, M., & Meade, T. (2007). Model for estimating the population prevalence of chronic obstructive pulmonary disease: Cross sectional data from the Health Survey for England. *Population Health Metrics* 5(8):1478–1482.

for COPD that detects "symptomatic disease." As discussed later in this chapter, COPD is often underdiagnosed, particularly among young people with mild disease in the absence of evaluation of lung function by spirometry. The currently recommended criterion for diagnosing COPD is a ratio of FEV1 to FVC < 0.70 after bronchodilation (see Table 39.2).

The global burden of COPD is increasing, especially in developing countries where there is high exposure to the two major risk factors, tobacco smoke and air pollution. More than 90% of COPD deaths occur in low- and middle-income nations where billions of people are exposed daily to high concentrations of indoor air pollution from heat and cooking sources, and nearly 50% of adults are exposed to tobacco smoke either by active or passive smoking (Gordon, Bruce, & Grigg, 2014; Liu et al., 2017; Zeng et al., 2016).

FIGURE 39.3 shows the worldwide distribution of age-adjusted mortality rates from COPD for individuals 40 years or older based on data from 2010 (Burney et al., 2016). Mortality rates from COPD in high-risk populous nations such as India and China exceed 300 per 100,000 in contrast to rates under 50 per 100,000 in developed countries of Western Europe and Scandinavia where air pollution has been curbed by environmental protection, and smoking rates have been reduced due to successful programs of tobacco control.

Most patients suffer from COPD for many years with severe disability and diminished quality of life. The rapidly rising prevalence, morbidity, and mortality due to COPD, particularly in developing countries, are generating enormous healthcare costs worldwide.

DALY is a measure that combines the years of life lost due to premature death and disability from disease (*DALY = YLL + YDL, where YLL = years of life lost due to premature death and YDL = years of life lost due to severe disability*). The global pattern of DALY for COPD is like the global pattern of COPD mortality in Figure 39.3. High DALY rates are present in nations of Eastern Europe and Southern Asia (China and India) where smoking rates are high, particularly among men. Other exposures (e.g., pollution from burning biomass for heat and cooking) also contribute significantly to the DALY from COPD in the populations of developing countries (see discussion of risk factors for COPD). Globally, COPD accounts for about 3% of the total DALY due to all diseases (GBD 2015 Chronic Respiratory Disease Collaborators, 2017; López-Campos, Ruiz-Ramos, & Soriano, 2016).

▶ Trends in Mortality Rates of COPD: United States and Western Europe

Mortality rates of COPD appear to be changing in certain populations of the world. In the United States, age-adjusted COPD mortality rates in men increased during 1970–2000 and then declined during 2000–2015, whereas in women, the mortality rates increased during 1970–2000 and then plateaued (Ford, 2015) (**FIGURE 39.4**). Similar trends are evident among men and women in the developed nations of Western Europe where COPD mortality rates are declining in men but not in women leading to convergence of male and female mortality (López-Campos, Ruiz-Ramos, & Soriano, 2014). The predominant risk factor for COPD in developed nations is cigarette smoking. These trends in COPD mortality are thus largely explainable by the declining rates of smoking in men versus slightly increasing rates in women. Nevertheless, there is some evidence suggesting that women may have heightened susceptibility to cigarette smoke or other sources of lung pollution compared to men. Further investigations are needed to better understand and quantify the potential role of occupational and environmental exposures in contributing to the mortality of COPD among women (Sørheim et al., 2010).

▶ Pathogenesis of COPD

COPD is initiated by inflammation, usually due to chronic exposure of the airways by tobacco smoke and or densely polluted air (**FIGURE 39.5**). Inflammation triggers chemotaxis and infiltration of the bronchioles and alveoli by macrophages and neurophils. These

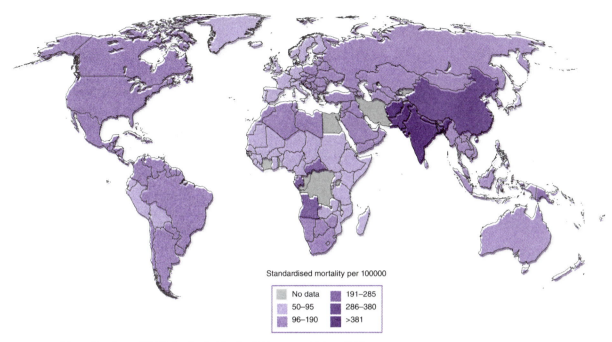

FIGURE 39.3 Mortality from COPD for Individuals 40 Years or Older, 2010.

Reproduced with permission of the © ERS 2018: *European Respiratory Journal* May 2015, 45(5):1239–1247; doi: 10.1183/09031936.00142414.

Age adjusted mortality rates among U.S. adults ≥ 25 years of age.

FIGURE 39.4 Trends in COPD Mortality, United States, 1970–2015.

Data from Ford, E. S. (2015). Trends in mortality from COPD among adults in the United States. *Chest, 148*(4), 962–970; National Vital Statistics System, Centers for Disease Control, Atlanta, Georgia.

cells of the innate immune system secrete cytokines and enzymes such as collagenase, elastase, and matrix metalloproteinases that in turn biodegrade elastin, collagen, and other proteins leading to the loss of alveolar wall integrity and enlargement of the alveolar air spaces. These features are the pathological hallmarks of *emphysema.*

Tobacco smoke also stimulates metaplastic and dysplastic changes in the mucous secreting cells (goblet cells) that line the bronchioles. Hypersecretion of mucous by goblet cells coupled with infiltration of the bronchioles by mononuclear leukocytes (white blood

cells) leads to occlusion, infection, and narrowing of the airways. These features are the pathological hallmarks of *chronic bronchitis.*

It is estimated that in at least half of COPD cases, these processes are triggered by exposure to the thousands of noxious chemicals in tobacco smoke and the deposition of tobacco residue (tar) in the lungs (Marsh, Aldington, Shirtcliffe, Weatherall, & Beasley, 2006). Inflammation ensues with the influx of inflammatory cells leading to the pathologic changes characteristic of both emphysema and chronic bronchitis. Additionally, increased oxidative stress caused by the free

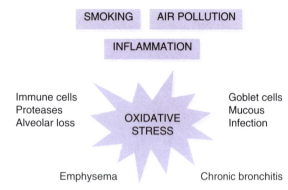

FIGURE 39.5 Pathogenesis of COPD.
© Jones & Bartlett Learning.

radicals in tobacco smoke and the oxidants released by cells of the immune system produce necrosis and apoptosis of exposed cells. Both emphysematous destruction and small airway inflammation are often found in combination in individual patients, leading to the spectrum that is known as COPD. When emphysema is moderate or severe, loss of elastic recoil, rather than bronchiolar disease, is the mechanism of airflow limitation. In contrast, when emphysema is mild and chronic bronchitis is the dominant component of disease, bronchiolar abnormalities are most responsible for the deficit in lung function.

Tobacco Use and COPD

The predominant etiologic agent in the genesis of both emphysema and chronic bronchitis is cigarette smoking (or any other form of smoking tobacco). Nevertheless, there is substantial international variation in death rates possibly reflecting smoking behavior, type and processing of tobacco, pollution, climate, respiratory management, and genetic factors.

In order to examine the prevalence of COPD in developing and middle-income nations, an international team of investigators from five participating centers in Latin America initiated the Latin American Project for the Investigation of Obstructive Lung Disease (PLATINO). Centers in major metropolitan cities of Brazil, Chile, Mexico, Uruguay, and Venezuela contributed patients for the study. A total of 5315 adults aged 40 years or older were sampled with approximately similar numbers of individuals representing each site. The presence of COPD was defined as lung function less than 70% of normal based upon spirometry. Prevalence estimates of COPD ranged from 7.8% in Mexico to 19.7% in Uruguay. The investigators suggested that the high COPD prevalence in the Uruguay sample may be related to not only high rates of smoking but also high altitude and the lower oxygen content of ambient air. They also noted that the health

burden of COPD was greater than previously realized (Menezes et al., 2005).

Halbert and colleagues conducted a review and meta-analysis of studies reporting prevalence estimates of COPD. Their study included population-based prevalence estimates of COPD, chronic bronchitis, and/or emphysema reported during 1990–2004. A total of 101 estimates based upon sample populations from 28 countries were ascertained from 67 published reports for analysis. The pooled estimates of prevalence were 7.6% for COPD ($n = 37$ studies), 6.4% for chronic bronchitis ($n = 38$ studies), and 1.8% for emphysema (8 studies). Restriction of data to only cases confirmed by spirometry yielded a prevalence estimate of 8.9%. Subgroup analyses showed that the prevalence rates were highest in smokers (15.4%) and individuals over 65 years of age (14.2%). Rates were also higher in men than women (9.8% vs. 5.6%) and higher in urban populations compared to rural or mixed populations (10.2% vs. 6.4%). The investigators noted the presence of significant heterogeneity among the reported estimates that was incompletely explained by sampling differences in age and smoking (Halbert et al., 2006).

Recently, the Global Obstructive Lung Disease Initiative (GOLD) was initiated by the World Health Organization (WHO) in collaboration with the Global Alliance Against Respiratory Diseases (GARD) in order to raise awareness of the increasing burden of COPD, implement programs of prevention to decrease morbidity and mortality, and promote further COPD research (Rabe et al., 2007). Subsequently, the Burden of Obstructive Lung Disease (BOLD) initiative was developed by GOLD primarily to estimate the worldwide prevalence of COPD and its risk factors using standardized methods (Buist et al., 2005). These methods were developed in conjunction with PLATINO conducted in five Latin American countries (Menezes et al., 2005).

An early report based upon 12 participating centers in the BOLD initiative examined the prevalence of COPD among 9425 adults aged 40 years or more. Centers representing China, Turkey, Austria, South Africa, Iceland, Germany, Poland, Norway, Canada, the United States, Australia, and the Philippines were included in the study. At least 600 participants were recruited per center and the diagnosis of COPD was confirmed by spirometry. Logistic regression analysis was used to estimate adjusted odds ratios (ORs) for COPD associated with 10-year age increments and 10-pack-year increments of smoking. The prevalence of stage II or higher COPD was 11.8% in men, 8.5% in women, and 10.1% overall. The risk of COPD increased by 94% for each 10-year age increment and the smoking-related risk of COPD increased by 28% in women and 16% in men for each 10-pack-year increment of smoking. Heterogeneity of smoking effects was observed in women but not in men, leading the investigators to suggest the need to study factors other than smoking in order to implement primary and secondary policies of prevention (Buist et al., 2007).

The *Obstructive Lung Disease in Northern Sweden (OLIN) Study* was designed to determine the cumulative incidence of COPD in cohorts of subjects with respiratory symptoms. Two methods of COPD diagnosis were compared, the British Thoracic Society (BTS) criteria and the GOLD criteria. The GOLD criteria use a lower threshold of lung dysfunction (FEV1/FVC < 0.70) for detection of COPD than the BTS criterion (FEV1/FVC < 0.70 and FVE1 < 80% of normal). The final cohort included 1109 men and women from Northern Sweden who completed technically adequate spirometric pulmonary function tests. The 10-year cumulative incidence was 8.2% by BTS criteria and 13.5% by GOLD criteria. The incidence of COPD increased with age and intensity of smoking but did not differ by gender or heredity (familial predisposition). The ORs for chronic smokers compared to never smokers did not differ appreciably for the BTS (OR = 5.4) and GOLD criteria (OR = 4.6). Results using the more liberal GOLD criteria indicate that 50% of chronic smokers eventually develop COPD (Lindberg et al., 2005; Lundbäck et al., 2003).

As part of the Copenhagen Heart Study in Denmark, a population sample of 8045 men and women aged 30–60 years with normal lung function at baseline was followed for 25 years to determine changes in lung function by spirometry and mortality due to COPD. Among chronic smokers, 36% developed COPD compared to only 8% among nonsmokers. The OR for developing clinically significant (stage II or higher) COPD was 6.3 for continuous smokers compared to never smokers. Smoking cessation during the follow-up period markedly decreased the risk of developing COPD (e.g., approximately 12% of early quitters developed COPD). During the follow-up period, 100 of the 109 deaths from COPD occurred among individuals who were smokers (Løkke, Lange, Scharling, Fabricius, & Vestbo, 2006).

The Rotterdam study was designed to examine the incidence of COPD and the risk associated with aging and smoking in a prospective cohort of men and women in the Netherlands. In the study cohort, 7983 participants aged 55 years or older at baseline were followed on average for 11 years. During 70,209 person-years of observation, 648 incident cases of COPD were detected by spirometry reports. The diagnosis of COPD was based upon spirometry values indicative of at least stage II disease (FEV1/FVS < 0.70 and FEV1 < 80% of normal value). The incidence of COPD for the entire cohort was 9.2 cases per 1000 person-years. Crude incidence rates were higher in men than women (14.4 vs. 6.2 per 1000 person-years) and higher in smokers than never smokers (12.8 vs. 3.9 per 1000 person-years). As shown in **FIGURE 39.6**, age-gender-adjusted estimates of the hazard ratio (relative risk) increased dramatically with pack-years of smoking, e.g., 10-pack-years of smoking increased the risk nearly fourfold and 50-pack-years of smoking increased the risk nearly ninefold. These results underscore the etiologic link between smoking and the development of COPD. Nevertheless, as the van Durme et al. (2009) point out:

> *Incident COPD cases were also detected among male and especially female never smokers, indicating that—besides active smoking—other environmental exposures such as passive smoking, occupational exposures, and (outdoor and indoor) air pollution might contribute to the development of COPD.* (pp. 368–377)

Environmental Tobacco Smoke and COPD

A few epidemiologic studies have examined the risk of developing COPD in individuals exposed to environmental tobacco smoke (ETS). Jaakkola reviewed the results of three case–control studies and three cohort studies, all of which found significant increases in the risk of developing COPD in elderly nonsmoking individuals who reported chronic exposure to ETS (Jaakkola, 2006). Estimates of relative risk for the highest exposure levels ranged from 1.7 to 5.6 and 4 of the studies found a significant dose response in COPD risk with increasing duration of ETS exposure. The biological effects of ETS are like those of mainstream smoke and individuals with chronic heavy exposure should be considered at increased risk for the development of COPD.

Indoor Air Pollution and COPD

Recent estimates from the World Health Organization suggest that nearly 3 billion people, almost half of the world population, are continually exposed to biomass smoke from the combustion of solid fuels such as wood and coal (WHO, 2006). In many regions of Africa, Central America, and Asia, most rural homes use solid fuel as the primary cooking and heating fuel.

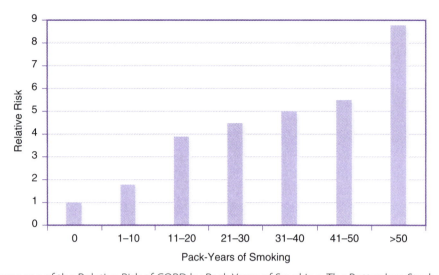

FIGURE 39.6 Dose Response of the Relative Risk of COPD by Pack-Years of Smoking: The Rotterdam Study.

Data from van Durme, Y. M., Verhamme, K. M., Stijnen, T., van Rooij, F. J., Van Pottelberge, G. R., Hofman, A., … Brusselle, G. G. (2009). Prevalence, incidence, and lifetime risk for the development of COPD in the elderly: The Rotterdam study. *Chest, 135,* 368–377.

Because of their routine cooking and other domestic activities, women in these households tend to have far greater exposure to indoor air pollution than men.

Epidemiologic evidence has accrued regarding the risk of COPD associated with chronic exposure to biomass smoke. Kurmi and colleagues conducted a review and meta-analysis of 23 epidemiologic investigations in order to quantify the risk associated with indoor air pollution. These studies included population samples from China, Turkey, Saudi Arabia, Spain, Columbia, and Mexico. Despite heterogeneity among study designs and population samples, chronic exposure to biomass smoke significantly increased the risk of developing COPD (OR = 2.8) and chronic bronchitis (OR = 2.3) compared to no exposure. Chronic indoor exposure to wood smoke conferred the highest risk (OR = 4.5) although chronic exposure to biomass smoke from other types of fuel (coal, charcoal, straw, and dung) also produced significant risk increases (Kurmi, Sample, Simkhada, Smith, & Ayers, 2010).

In a separate meta-analysis, Hu and colleagues analyzed data from 15 studies including population samples from China, India, Nepal, Turkey, Pakistan, Saudi Arabia, Spain, Brazil, Columbia, Bolivia, and Mexico. Overall, chronic exposure to biomass smoke significantly increased the risk of developing COPD in both women (OR = 2.7) and men (OR = 4.3) and in cigarette smokers (OR = 4.4) and nonsmokers (Hu et al., 2010).

Air Pollution and COPD

In their comprehensive textbook on the pathogenesis of disease, Stanley Robbins and Ramzi Cotran provide an excellent discussion of air pollution and the lung disorders collectively called *pneumoconiosis*. Numerous studies have shown that air contaminants that are present in the atmospheric environment of the industrialized world are capable of provoking lung dysfunction and respiratory ailments including COPD. Hundreds of millions of tons of air pollutants are discharged each year from the combustion of gasoline and fossil fuels, in both developed and developing nations. As quoted from Robbins and Cotran (1979) on environmental pathology:

> To be found in city air are variable mixtures of carbon, sulfur, and nitrogen oxides; organic residues containing tars and aldehydes (some of which may be potentially carcinogenic); the vaporized metals and acids emitted by industry and gasoline engines; and all manner of organic and inorganic dust. (pp. 521–560)

The authors go on to point out that "*cigarette smoking potentiates or exaggerates the effects of air contamination*" (Robbins & Cotran, 1979). Repeated inhalation of coal dust or other carbon particles leads to the deposition of these materials throughout the respiratory bronchioles and alveolar spaces producing carbon pigmentation of the lungs known as *pulmonary anthracosis*. Many other small particles that enter the airways, both organic and inorganic, can also lead to pneumoconiosis (e.g., silicosis is a particularly severe form of pneumoconiosis resulting from the inhalation of silica dust).

In general, pneumoconiosis is characterized by the accumulation of such particles within the macrophages of the lungs accompanied by irritation, inflammation, and the release of destructive enzymes and reactive oxygen species that result in cell necrosis and, subsequently, pulmonary fibrosis. These same processes are integral to the development of chronic bronchitis, emphysema, and COPD. Hence, rates of COPD are high among those individuals exposed to high levels of coal dust, silica dust, and other types of air pollution.

The etiologic role of coal mine dust in the pathogenesis of debilitating pneumoconiosis and *black lung disease* is a well-known phenomenon. Albeit, exposure to coal dust also heightens the risk of COPD. Studies of the relation between COPD and exposure to respirable coal mine dust have been carried out in Britain, the United States, Italy, and Germany (Coggon & Taylor, 1998).

In an investigation of coal miners versus telecommunications workers in South Wales, more of the miners reported symptoms of chronic bronchitis than controls (31% vs. 5%) and 20% of the miners had lower than normal forced expiratory volumes compared to 10% of controls. Differences were apparent for both smokers and nonsmokers (Lloyd, Gauld, & Soutar, 1986).

Lewis and colleagues compared spirometry measures of FEV1 (forced expiratory lung volume in one second) in 1286 coal miners with 567 men in other occupations sampled from the East Midlands of England. After adjustment for age, height, and smoking, the mean FEV1 was 155 mL lower in the miners, suggesting that they were developing higher rates of COPD (Lewis, Bennett, Richards, & Britton, 1996).

An important body of work on coal miners and COPD was conducted in the British Pneumoconiosis Field Research (PFR) program conducted by the Institute of Occupational Medicine. This series of investigations was based on data for more than 30,000 miners at 24 collieries in Great Britain. In an analysis of 3380 of these miners who either smoked cigarettes or were nonsmokers, the cumulative exposure to coal dust over 10 years was assessed and related to the risk of 4 end points: FEV1 < 80%; symptoms of chronic bronchitis; symptoms of chronic bronchitis and FEV1 < 80%; and FEV1 < 65%. In both smokers and nonsmokers, ORs for all end points increased by approximately twofold with high cumulative exposure to coal dust (Marine, Gurr, & Jacobsen, 1988).

The U.S. National Study of Coal Workers' Pneumoconiosis (SCWP) examined risk factors for COPD including coal dust exposure in miners from 31 nationally distributed collieries. Data were collected on chest radiographs, spirometric measures of lung function, details of clinical symptoms, and smoking habits of the miners. In a study of 7139 miners, linear regression was used to relate pulmonary function to cumulative coal dust exposure. After adjustment for age, height, mine location, and smoking, exposure to coal dust was associated with significantly lower FEV1 values (Attfield & Hodous, 1992).

Italian investigators reported the results of an 11-year follow-up study of Sardinian coal miners. Analysis of 909 miners who had worked in the mines for more than 2 years revealed declining FEV1 function and more frequent onset of chronic bronchitis with increasing exposure to coal dust (Carta, Aru, Barbieri, Vataneo, & Casula, 1996).

Oxman and colleagues described a study of 544 miners who worked in a colliery at Recklinghausen in Germany. Analysis of cross-sectional data revealed a significant negative association between coal dust exposure and FEV1 (Oxman et al., 1993).

Due to their increased exposure to silica dust, gold miners have been studied to assess their risk of developing COPD and silicosis. Such studies have examined the level of silica dust and the severity of COPD in postmortem lung specimens. In a review of studies of South African gold miners, the incidence of chronic bronchitis was found to increase with increasing exposure to silica dust, and individuals in jobs with high exposure to silica dust for 20 years or more exhibited significantly more extensive lung damage from emphysema than individuals with low exposure (Hnizdo & Vallyathan, 2003).

In general, findings from SCWP and PFR and other studies of miners are similar in demonstrating increased rates of COPD and significant loss of pulmonary function in miners who are chronically exposed to coal mine dust or silica dust. Clearly, occupational mining dust is an important cause of COPD.

As opposed to studies of high-risk groups such as miners who are exposed to inordinately high levels of occupational dust, investigations of the health effects of air pollution in the general population are more complex due to difficulties in obtaining accurate measures of exposure to relatively low levels of contamination over long periods of time. Two U.S. studies, the *Harvard Six Cities Study* and the *American Cancer Society Study*, have attempted to examine the contribution of air pollution to overall morbidity and mortality.

The Harvard Six Cities Study was designed to evaluate effects of air pollution on the mortality among cohorts of adults sampled from Watertown, Massachusetts; Kingston and Harriman, Tennessee; Steubenville, Ohio; Portage, Wyocena, and Pardeeville, Wisconsin; and Topeka, Kansas. A total of 8111 adults

25–74 years of age were followed for 14–16 years to determine associations of mortality with the level of air pollution. Each participant reported their age, gender, weight, height, education level, smoking history, occupational exposures, and medical history at baseline. Concentrations of total suspended particulate matter, sulfur dioxide, ozone, and suspended sulfates were measured in each community at a centrally located air-monitoring station. Based on proportional hazards (Cox) general linear regression, smoking had the strongest association with mortality. Nevertheless, after adjustment for smoking and other health risk factors, the city-specific all-cause mortality rates were positively associated with the average levels of air pollutants (hazard ratio = 1.26). Increasing levels of air pollution, particularly involving fine particulates and sulfates, were associated with higher mortality from lung cancer and cardiopulmonary disease (Dockery et al., 1993).

The American Cancer Society Study examined effects of particulate air pollution using ambient air pollution data from 151 U.S. metropolitan areas and risk–factor information for 552,138 adults who resided in these areas. Participants in the study completed a risk–factor questionnaire to ascertain detailed information on age, gender, smoking, and other risk factors. Exposure to sulfate and fine-particulate air pollution (primarily from fossil fuel combustion) was estimated from national databases. Relationships of air pollution to all-cause mortality and mortality from lung cancer and cardiopulmonary disease were examined by multivariate analysis controlling for smoking and other risk factors. All-cause mortality in the most polluted areas was 15% higher than in the least polluted areas and exposure to high levels of particulate air pollution significantly increased mortality due to lung cancer and cardiopulmonary disease (Pope et al., 1995).

Subsequent analyses of the data from the Harvard Six Cities Study and the American Cancer Society Study of air pollution and mortality were conducted by a team of investigators in order to check the original findings. Collectively, this *reanalysis* of the data from these two studies confirmed the original results and provided evidence that exposure to high concentrations of sulfur dioxide in addition to fine particulates and sulfates heightens the mortality risk (Krewski et al., 2003).

The exhaust from motor vehicles is a significant source of air pollution, contributing nitrogen oxides, carbon monoxide, benzene, and other volatile organic compounds to the ambient air near high-traffic roadways. Evidence is emerging from epidemiologic investigations linking exposure to motor vehicle exhaust near high-volume traffic roads with adverse health effects including COPD. Novel experimental designs are necessary to accrue such evidence as illustrated by the following investigation.

Lindgren and colleagues conducted a geographical study of COPD and traffic-related air pollution in Southern Sweden. Exposures were measured as the volume of traffic per minute and the concentration of nitrogen oxide compounds in ambient air. Cases were identified by self-report in a sample of 9319 individuals aged 18–77 years. Individuals were linked by geocoded residential addresses to a Swedish road database and an emission database of nitrogen oxide concentrations in ambient air for the region. The study found that living within 100 meters of a high-traffic road (>10 cars per minute) significantly increased the risk of COPD (OR = 1.64). There was also a significant positive dose response of the level of nitrogen oxide concentration and COPD risk (OR = 1.55 for the highest concentration) (Lindgren et al., 2009).

α₁ Antitrypsin Deficiency and COPD

The best documented genetic risk factor for COPD is α_1 antitrypsin deficiency, a relatively rare condition that is present in only 1%–2% of patients with mild to moderate COPD. Nevertheless, up to 50% of patients over 40 years of age with severe (stage IV) COPD have been found to have α_1 antitrypsin deficiency. As pointed out by Graham Devereux in his review of COPD: *"Detection of such cases identifies family members who will require genetic counseling and patients who might be suitable for future potential treatment with α_1 antitrypsin replacement"* (Devereux, 2006).

The glycoprotein α_1 antitrypsin is responsible for inhibiting collagenase, elastase, and other proteases derived from leukocytes, particularly in the alveoli of the lungs. If α_1 antitrypsin is deficient or absent, there is uncontrolled degradation of alveolar proteins such as elastase and collagen resulting in the accelerated development of emphysema.

The inheritance pattern of alleles is codominant, and since the gene for α_1 antitrypsin is highly polymorphic, some rare genotypes (e.g., ZZ) result in extremely low concentrations of active α_1 antitrypsin (10%–20% of normal) whereas other genotypes may result in intermediate levels. With severe α_1 antitrypsin deficiency, progression of COPD can be rapid, particularly in combination with cigarette smoking (Devereux, 2006; Robbins & Cotran, 1979).

Underdiagnosis of COPD

Several studies suggest that COPD is often underdiagnosed, particularly among those individuals with mild disease. Two sets of criteria have been used by clinicians to confirm the presence of COPD: the BTS and the GOLD criteria. The GOLD criteria shown earlier in Table 39.2 use a lower threshold of lung dysfunction (FEV1/FVC < 0.70) for detection of COPD than the BTS criterion (FEV1/FVC < 0.70 and FVE1 < 80% of normal). Consequently, application of the GOLD criteria detects higher incidence and prevalence rates of COPD.

The *OLIN Study* was designed to compare the BTS and GOLD guidelines for COPD detection in cohorts of subjects ascertained from Northern Sweden. Subjects enrolled for study already had clinical respiratory symptoms (e.g., persistent cough, wheezing, shortness of breath, and sputum production) but had not undergone spirometric testing. Among 1236 patients, 14% of patients had COPD by the GOLD criterion compared to only 8.2% by the BTS criterion, an absolute difference of more than 5% (Lindberg, Bjerg, Ronmark, Larsson, & Lundback, 2006).

Many other investigations also reveal that COPD is underdiagnosed, particularly among those patients with mild disease. In a review and meta-analysis of data on the diagnosis and prevalence of COPD, Halbert and colleagues noted significant heterogeneity due to differences in diagnostic methodology. Their analysis is based upon 37 prevalence estimates ascertained from 62 published studies. Notably, the application of spirometric criteria resulted in nearly a twofold higher prevalence estimate compared with either patient-reported or physician-diagnosed COPD (9.2% vs. 4.9% and 5.2%, respectively). These findings suggest the need for standardization of diagnostic measures of COPD in subsequent epidemiologic investigations. Spirometric evaluation of patients using the GOLD criteria has been adopted as an epidemiologic case definition by the BOLD initiative and PLATINO. Widespread application of a valid and reproducible method of COPD diagnosis is critical to gain a better understanding of the global burden of COPD (Halbert et al., 2006).

Population Attributable Fraction: Smoking and COPD

The *population attributable fraction* (*PAF*) is the fraction of a disease that can be attributed to a particular risk factor. The PAF is calculated in various ways; for example, if the relative risk (*RR*) and the frequency of the risk factor (*f_e*) are known, then

$$PAF = \frac{f_e(RR-1)}{\left[f_e(RR-1)+1\right]}$$

If the incidence rate of disease for individuals who are exposed to a risk factor (I_E) and individuals who are not exposed to the risk factor (I_{NE}) are known, then

$$PAF = \frac{f_e\left(I_E - I_{NE}\right)}{\left[f_e\left(I_E - I_{NE}\right)+\left(1-f_e\right)I_{NE}\right]}$$

For example, if the RR of COPD among chronic smokers is 5 and the prevalence of chronic smoking is 40%, the PAF = 61.5%.

Estimates of the fraction of COPD attributable to cigarette smoking vary widely, ranging from 40% to 90% depending on the population under study, the detail of smoking exposure, and the diagnostic criteria that are used. A review of estimates from recent studies suggests that the PAF from smoking is approximately 50% with up to 20% of cases due to other sources of pollution such as biomass smoke from cooking and heating in poorly ventilated dwellings (Marsh et al., 2006).

It is best to keep in mind that the strength of risk factors and corresponding estimates of PAF may vary widely depending upon the population under study and the exposure frequencies. As an example, in a report based on the Chinese Epidemiologic Survey of COPD in 20,245 adults aged 40 years or older, 86.2% of 1024 smokers who developed COPD were men, whereas 69.4% of 644 nonsmokers who developed COPD were women. Furthermore, the prevalence of smoking in men (74.3%) was nearly seven times higher than in women (11.3%). Thus, factors other than cigarette smoke (e.g., smoke from burning coal and biomass in poorly ventilated dwellings) appear to have a significant impact on the development of COPD, particularly among Chinese women (Zhou et al., 2009).

Pneumonia and COPD

In the normal lung, three major defense mechanisms maintain a sterile microenvironment that is free of bacterial and viral contamination. The cough reflex, cilia of the bronchial tree, and immune cells of the lung parenchyma (Kupffer cells) are all instrumental in preventing lower respiratory infections. In the setting of COPD, these mechanisms are compromised and bacterial or viral infection of the lower respiratory tree (pneumonia) is a common comorbidity that exacerbates the disease. In COPD, the lungs become susceptible to repeated acute airway mucosal infections with viruses and bacterial pathogens leading to episodes of increased inflammation and more severe symptoms. A variety of pathogens have been implicated including bacteria (Hemophilus, Streptococcus, Staphylococcus, and Pseudomonas) and viruses (rhinoviruses, influenza viruses, coronaviruses, and respiratory syncytial virus) (Alfredo et al., 2007; Sethi, 2010). In a study of 65 patients hospitalized due to exacerbation of COPD symptoms, most patients (78%) had viral and/or bacterial infection and patients with bacterial and viral co-infection exhibited the greatest impairment of lung function (Papi et al., 2006).

HIV and COPD

Some studies have noted a possible link between HIV infection and the development and progression of COPD. In a recent meta-analysis including 30 studies and 151,686 participants, the odds of having COPD were 14% higher in HIV-infected individuals than in HIV-negative controls (Bigna, Kenne, Asangbeh, & Sibetcheu, 2018).

Lung Cancer and COPD

The dominant risk factor for both lung cancer and COPD is chronic tobacco smoking. Furthermore, the impaired lung function of COPD patients may also increase their lung cancer risk. Swedish investigators studied the association of COPD and lung cancer in a large cohort of individuals (*n* = 176,997) for whom spirometry measurements were available at baseline. The stage of COPD was determined using the GOLD criteria for spirometric measures of lung function. During 1971–2001, 834 incident cases of lung cancer were detected in the cohort through linkage with the Swedish National Cancer Registry. As shown in **FIGURE 39.7**, the RR of lung cancer is significantly increased in patients with COPD and more severe disease accentuates the risk (Purdue et al., 2007).

Case Fatality of COPD Exacerbation

COPD is a progressive debilitating condition in which patients often experience exacerbations of lung obstruction, infection, and damage. Such episodes require hospitalization and may result in respiratory failure and death. In a meta-analysis of more than 57,000 COPD patients hospitalized for severe COPD exacerbation, the in-hospital case fatality was nearly 10% and the cumulative case fatality increased to over 40% after 2 years of follow-up (**FIGURE 39.8**). The investigators concluded that severe exacerbation of COPD has a high case-fatality rate and is a major cause of death in this disease (Hoogendoorn, Hoogenveen, Rutten-van Mölken, Vestbo, & Feenstra, 2011).

Prevention of COPD

As with all smoking-related diseases, the key to primary prevention is complete abstinence from

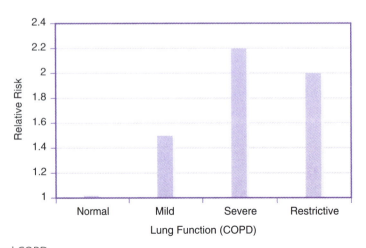

FIGURE 39.7 Lung Cancer and COPD.

Data from Purdue, M. P., Gold, L., Järvholm, B., Alavanja, M. C. R., Ward, M. H., & Vermeulen, R. (2007). Impaired lung function and lung cancer incidence in a cohort of Swedish construction workers. *Thorax, 62,* 51–56.

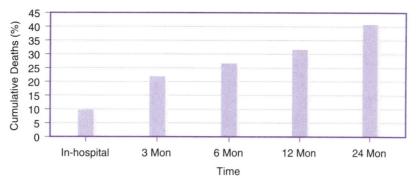

FIGURE 39.8 COPD Case Fatality.

Data from Hoogendoorn, M., Hoogenveen, R. T., Rutten-van Mölken, M. P., Vestbo, J., & Feenstra, T. L. (2011). Case fatality of COPD exacerbations: A meta-analysis and statistical modelling approach. *European Respiratory Journal, 37*, 508–515.

tobacco use. As elaborated earlier in this text, educational efforts must be initiated early in life to prevent young individuals from taking up the smoking habit. Effective educational programs have produced impressive results in some nations (e.g., smoking rates have declined dramatically in certain developed countries such as the United States and the United Kingdom). Furthermore, many countries and local jurisdictions throughout the world have successfully implemented laws requiring indoor workplaces and public places to be smoke free. Nevertheless, it is startling that nearly one-third of adults in the world population continue to smoke tobacco (WHO, 2008b). Recently, an international program of tobacco control titled the *Tobacco Free Initiative (TFI)* was ratified and implemented through the auspices of WHO to curb the epidemic of tobacco-related diseases throughout the world (WHO, 2009a, 2009b, 2009c, 2015).

A key component of effective COPD prevention is the early detection of mild symptoms when the disease process is reversible and lung function can be restored to normal. A positive development is the adoption of standardized measures of lung function based upon spirometry (e.g., the GOLD criteria for detection and staging of COPD). Certainly, there is strong evidence that smoking cessation effectively reduces the risk of COPD progression in patients with mild disease. In nonsmokers with early symptoms, the source of pollution and lung irritation should be identified and steps taken for remediation.

▶ Smoking Cessation in COPD Patients

Though smoking cessation is the single most important behavioral change to prevent COPD or reduce its progression, intensive intervention involving counseling, pharmacotherapy, or both is usually required to successfully motivate an individual to quit smoking. The *Lung Health Study* was designed to examine the impact of a smoking cessation program in middle-aged patients with asymptomatic airway obstruction (mild COPD). Patients enrolled in the study ($n = 5887$) were randomized to receive intensive intervention versus usual care to help them quit smoking. Ten clinical centers located in the United States and Canada enrolled patients for study. The intervention was a 10-week smoking cessation program that included a strong physician message and 12 group sessions using behavior modification and nicotine gum, plus either *ipratropium* or a placebo inhaler. The vital status of each patient was followed up to 14.5 years to determine progression/regression of their lung disease and mortality due to cardiovascular disease, lung cancer, or pulmonary disease. After 5 years of follow-up, 21.7% of patients who received the special intervention had stopped smoking compared to 5.4% of patients receiving usual care. After 14.5 years of follow-up, all-cause mortality was reduced by about 15% in the intervention group compared to the usual care group. Notably, the death rate from respiratory diseases other than lung cancer was significantly less in the intervention group than the usual care group (0.56 vs. 1.08 per 1000 person-years). These results demonstrate that an intensive smoking cessation program can produce significant reduction in all-cause mortality in people with mild to moderate airway obstruction (Anthonisen et al., 2005).

Several randomized trials have focused on effects of smoking cessation interventions to reduce the progression of COPD. Strassmann and colleagues conducted a meta-analysis of six such trials to evaluate smoking cessation counseling with or without pharmacotherapy or nicotine replacement among 7372 COPD patients. Their analysis showed that intervention involving counseling plus nicotine replacement had the greatest effect on prolonged abstinence rates.

Compared to usual care, patients receiving treatment were five times more likely to sustain smoking cessation (Strassmann et al., 2009).

Control of Air Pollution

Chronic exposure to high concentrations of indoor or outdoor air pollution increases the risk of developing COPD. Outdoor pollution is mainly due to the combustion of fossil fuel for heating, industry, and transport. Motor vehicle exhaust is a primary source. Indoor pollution arises from the combustion of biomass (e.g., wood and coal) for cooking and heating.

In many nations, outdoor pollution has been greatly reduced by switching from coal to cleaner burning fuels such as oil and gas and by the elimination of poorly controlled incinerators. Emission of toxic chemicals in motor vehicle exhaust has been reduced through the use of catalytic converters and air injection systems and development of more efficient engines. In many developed countries, progress in improving air quality and reducing motor vehicle emissions has been maintained as a result of national clean air acts (US EPA, 2017).

Control of indoor pollutants is by ventilation, removal of the source of pollution, improved cooking and heating devices, and behavioral adjustments to avoid exposure. In many nations, new laws have been passed and are being strictly enforced to prohibit smoking in public buildings and regulate the content of toxic and polluting substances in building materials (WHO, 2018). Special efforts must be taken to reduce lung damage in individuals with extreme occupational exposure to air pollutants (e.g., miners, foundry workers, and textile mill workers). Air quality in these environments can be improved using filtration and purification systems that cleanse the air supply and mobile positive-pressure face mask filters that protect the individual (US EPA, 2018).

Global Alliance Against Chronic Respiratory Diseases

WHO has launched a comprehensive international program GARD with the purpose of integrating the collective knowledge of national and international organizations, institutions, and agencies to implement an effective global strategy for the prevention, detection, treatment, and monitoring of chronic respiratory diseases such as COPD and asthma. Detailed discussion of the objectives of GARD, its structure, member nations and organizations, an overview of chronic respiratory diseases, and the proposed framework for action can be found on the WHO GARD website (WHO, 2010).

References

Alfredo, P., Gaetano, C., Paolo, C., Marco, C., Johnston, S. L., & Alberto, P. (2007). Pathophysiology of viral-induced exacerbations of COPD. *International Journal of Chronic Obstructive Pulmonary Disease, 2*(4), 477–483.

Anthonisen, N. R., Skeans, M. A., Wise, R. A., Manfreda, J., Kanner, R. E., Connett, R. E., & Lung Health Study Research Group. (2005). The effects of a smoking cessation intervention on 14.5-year mortality: A randomized clinical trial. *Annals of Internal Medicine, 142*, 233–239.

Attfield, M. D., & Hodous, T. K. (1992). Pulmonary function of US coal miners related to dust exposure estimates. *The American Review of Respiratory Disease, 145*, 605–609.

Bigna, J. J., Kenne, A. M., Asangbeh, S. L., & Sibetcheu, A. T. (2018). Prevalence of chronic obstructive pulmonary disease in the global population with HIV: A systematic review and meta-analysis. *The Lancet Global Health, 6*(2), 193–202.

Buist, A. S., McBurnie, M. A., Vollmer, W. M., Gillespie, S., Burney, P., Mannino, D. M., ... BOLD Collaborative Research Group. (2007). International variation in the prevalence of COPD (The BOLD study): A population-based prevalence study. *Lancet, 370*(9589), 741–750.

Buist, A. S., Vollmer, W. M., Sullivan, S. D., Weiss, K. B., Lee, T. A., Menezes, A. M. B., ... Burney, P. G. J. (2005). The burden of lung disease initiative (BOLD): Rational and design. *COPY, 2*, 277–283.

Burney, P. G. J., Patel, J., Newson, R., Minelli, C., & Naghavi, M. (2015). Global and regional trends in chronic obstructive pulmonary disease mortality 1990–2010. *The European Respiratory Journal, 45*(5), 1239–1247.

Carta, P., Aru, G., Barbieri, M. T., Vataneo, G., & Casula, D. (1996). Dust exposure, respiratory symptoms, and longitudinal decline in lung function in young coal miners. *Occupational and Environmental Medicine, 53*, 312–319.

Coggon, D., & Taylor, A. N. (1998). Coal mining and chronic obstructive pulmonary disease: A review of the evidence. *Thorax, 53*, 398–407.

Devereux, G. (2006). ABC of chronic obstructive pulmonary disease. Definition, epidemiology, and risk factors. *BMJ, 332*(7550), 1142–1144.

Dockery, D. W., Pope, C. A., Xu, X., Spengler, J. D., Ware, J. H., Fay, M. E., ... Speizer, F. E. (1993). An association between air pollution and mortality in six U.S. cities. *New England Journal of Medicine, 329*, 1753–1759.

Ford, E. S. (2015). Trends in mortality from COPD among adults in the United States. *Chest, 148*(4), 962–970.

GBD 2015 Chronic Respiratory Disease Collaborators. (2017). Global, regional, and national deaths, prevalence, disability-adjusted life years, and years lived with disability for chronic obstructive pulmonary disease and asthma, 1990–2015: A systematic analysis for the Global Burden of Disease Study 2015. *The Lancet Respiratory Medicine, 5*(9), 691–706.

Gordon, S. B., Bruce, N. G., & Grigg, J. (2014). Respiratory risks from household air pollution in low and middle income countries. *Lancet Respiratory Medicine, 2*(10), 823–860.

Halbert, R. J., Natoli, J. L., Gano, A., Badamgarav, E., Buist, A. S., & Mannino, D. M. (2006). Global burden of COPD: Systematic review and meta-analysis. *The European Respiratory Journal, 28*, 523–532.

Hoogendoorn, M., Hoogenveen, R. T., Rutten-van Mölken, M. P., Vestbo, J., & Feenstra, T. L. (2011). Case fatality of COPD exacerbations: A meta-analysis and statistical modelling approach. *European Respiratory Journal, 37*, 508–515.

Hnizdo, E., & Vallyathan, V. (2003). Chronic obstructive pulmonary disease due to occupational exposure to silica dust: A review of epidemiological and pathological evidence. *Occupational and Environmental Medicine, 60*(4), 237–243.

Hu, G., Zhou, Y., Tian, J., Yao, W., Li, J., Li, B., & Ran, P. (2010). Risk of COPD from exposure to biomass smoke. *Chest, 138*(1), 20–31.

Jaakkola, M. S. (2006). Environmental tobacco smoke and health in the elderly. *European Respiratory Journal, 19*(1), 172–181.

Krewski, D., Burnett, R., Goldberg, M., Hoover, B. K., Siemiatycki, J., Jerrett, M., … White, W. (2003). Overview of the reanalysis of the Harvard Six Cities Study and American Cancer Society Study of particulate air pollution and mortality. *Journal of Toxicology Environmental Health, 66*(15), 1507–1552.

Kurmi, O. P., Sample, S., Simkhada, P., Smith, W. C. S., & Ayers, J. G. (2010). COPD and chronic bronchitis risk of indoor air pollution from solid fuel: A systematic review and meta-analysis. *Thorax, 65*, 221–228.

Lewis, S., Bennett, J., Richards, K., & Britton, J. (1996). A cross sectional study of the independent effect of occupation on lung function in British coal miners. *Occupational and Environmental Medicine, 53*, 125–128.

Lindberg, A., Bjerg, A., Ronmark, E., Larsson, L. G., & Lundback, B. (2006). Prevalence and underdiagnosis of COPD by disease severity and the attributable fraction of smoking. Report from the Obstructive Lung Disease in Northern Sweden Studies. *Respiratory Medicine, 100*, 264–272.

Lindberg, A., Jonsson, A. C., Rönmark, E., Lundgren, R., Larsson, L. G., & Lundbäck, B. (2005). Ten-year cumulative incidence of COPD and risk factors for incident disease in a symptomatic cohort. *Chest, 127*(5), 1544–1552.

Lindgren, A., Stroh, E., Montnémery, P., Nihlén, U., Jakobsson, K., & Axmon, A. (2009). Traffic-related air pollution associated with prevalence of asthma and COPD/chronic bronchitis. A cross-sectional study in Southern Sweden. *International Journal of Health Geographics, 8*(2), 1476–1480.

Liu, S., Zhang, M., Yang, L., Li, Y., Wang, L., Huang, Z., … Zhou, M. (2017). Prevalence and patterns of tobacco smoking among Chinese adult men and women: Findings of the 2010 national smoking survey. *Journal of Epidemiology and Community Health, 71*(2), 154–161.

Lloyd, M. H., Gauld, S. J., & Soutar, C. A. (1986). Respiratory ill health among coal miners and telecommunication workers in South Wales. *British Journal of Industrial Medicine, 43*, 177–181.

Løkke, A., Lange, P., Scharling, H., Fabricius, P., & Vestbo, J. (2006). Developing COPD: A 25 year follow up study of the general population. *Thorax, 61*, 935–939.

López-Campos, J. L., Ruiz-Ramos, M., & Soriano, J. B. (2014). Mortality trends in chronic obstructive pulmonary disease in Europe, 1994–2010: A joinpoint regression analysis. *The Lancet Respiratory Medicine, 2*(1), 54–62.

López-Campos, J. L., Ruiz-Ramos, M., & Soriano, J. B. (2016). Global burden of COPD. *Respirology, 21*(1), 14–23.

Lundbäck, B., Lindberg, A., Lindström, M., Rönmark, E., Jönsson, E., Larsson, L.G., … Larsson, K. (2003). Obstructive lung disease in Northern Sweden Studies. Not 15 but 50% of smokers develop COPD? Report from the Obstructive Lung Disease in Northern Sweden Studies. *Respiratory Medicine, 97*, 115–122.

Marine, W. M., Gurr, D., & Jacobsen, M. (1988). Clinically important effects of dust exposure and smoking in British coal miners. *The American Review of Respiratory Disease, 137*, 106–112.

Marsh, S., Aldington, S., Shirtcliffe, P., Weatherall, M., & Beasley, R. (2006). Smoking and COPD: What really are the risks? *The European Respiratory Journal, 28*, 883–884.

Menezes, A. M., Padilla, R. P., Jardim, J. R., Muino, A., Lopez, M. V., Valdivia, G., … PLATINO Team. (2005). Chronic obstructive pulmonary disease in five Latin American cities (the PLATINO study): A prevalence study. *Lancet, 366*, 1875–1881.

Nacul, L. C., Soljak, M., & Meade, T. (2007). Model for estimating the population prevalence of chronic obstructive pulmonary disease: Cross sectional data from the Health Survey for England. *Population Health Metrics, 5*(8) doi:10.1186/1478-7954-5-8.

Oxman, A. D., Muir, D. C. F., Shannon, H. S., Stock, S. R., Hnizdo, E., & Lange, H. J. (1993). Occupational dust exposure and chronic obstructive pulmonary disease. *The American Review of Respiratory Disease, 148*, 38–48.

Papi, A., Bellettato, C. M., Braccioni, F., Romagnoli, M., Casolari, P., Caramori, G., … Johnston, S. L. (2006). Infections and airway inflammation in chronic obstructive pulmonary disease severe exacerbations. *American Journal of Respiratory and Critical Care Medicine, 173*(10), 1114–1121.

Pope, C. A., Thun, M. J., Namboodiri, M. M., Dockery, D. W., Evans, J. S., Speizer, F. E., & Heath, C. W. (1995). Particulate air pollution as a predictor of mortality in a prospective study of US adults. *American Journal of Respiratory and Critical Care Medicine, 151*(3), 669–674.

Purdue, M. P., Gold, L., Järvholm, B., Alavanja, M. C. R., Ward, M. H., & Vermeulen, R. (2007). Impaired lung function and lung cancer incidence in a cohort of Swedish construction workers. *Thorax, 62*, 51–56.

Quaderi, S. A., & Hurst, J. R. (2018). The unmet global burden of COPD. *Global Health Epidemiology and Genomics, 3*, e4. doi:10.1017/gheg.2018.1.

Rabe, K. F., Hurd, S., Anzueto, A., Barnes, P. J., Buist, S. A., Calverley, P., … Zielinski, J. (2007). Global initiative for chronic obstructive lung disease. Global strategy for the diagnosis, management, and prevention of chronic obstructive pulmonary disease: GOLD executive summary. *American Journal of Respiratory and Critical Care Medicine, 176*, 532–555.

Robbins, S. L., & Cotran, R. S. (1979). Environmental pathology. In S. L. Robbins & R. S. Cotran (Eds.), *Pathologic basis of disease* (pp. 521–560). Philadelphia, PA: W B Saunders Company.

Sethi, S. (2010). Infection as a comorbidity of COPD. *The European Respiratory Journal, 35*(6),1209–1215.

Sørheim, I. C., Johannessen, A., Gulsvik, A., Bakke, P. S., Silverman, E. K., & DeMeo, D. L. (2010). Gender differences in

COPD: Are women more susceptible to smoking effects than men? *Thorax, 65,* 480–485.

Strassmann, R., Bausch, B., Spaar, A., Kleijnen, J., Braendli, O., & Puhan, M. A. (2009). Smoking cessation interventions in COPD: A network meta-analysis of randomised trials. *European Respiratory Journal, 34*(3), 634–640.

United States Environmental Protection Agency. (2017). *Summary of the Clean Air Act.* US EPA, Research Triangle Park, North Carolina. Retrieved from www.EPA.gov clean air act

United States Environmental Protection Agency, US EPA. (2018). *Managing air quality—Control strategies to achieve air pollution reduction.* US EPA, Research Triangle Park, North Carolina. Retrieved from www.epa.gov/air-quality-management-process

van Durme, Y. M., Verhamme, K. M., Stijnen, T., van Rooij, F. J., Van Pottelberge, G. R., Hofman, A., … Brusselle, G. G. (2009). Prevalence, incidence, and lifetime risk for the development of COPD in the elderly: The Rotterdam study. *Chest, 135,* 368–377.

Weinberger, S. E., Cockrill, B. A., & Mandel, J. (2018a). Pulmonary anatomy and physiology: The basics. In *Principles of pulmonary medicine* (7th ed., pp. 1–18). Amsterdam, Netherlands: Elsevier, Inc.

Weinberger, S. E., Cockrill, B. A., & Mandel, J. (2018b). Chronic obstructive pulmonary disease. In *Principles of pulmonary medicine* (7th ed., pp. 93–112). Amsterdam, Netherlands: Elsevier, Inc.

World Health Organization. (2006). *Fuel for life-household energy and health.* Geneva, Switzerland: World Health Organization.

World Health Organization. (2008a). *The global burden of disease: Update 2004.* Geneva, Switzerland: World Health Organization.

World Health Organization. (2008b). *WHO Report on the global tobacco epidemic, 2008: The MPOWER package.* Geneva, Switzerland: World Health Organization.

World Health Organization. (2009a). *WHO Report on the global tobacco epidemic, 2009.* Geneva, Switzerland: World Health Organization.

World Health Organization. (2009b). *Disease and injury country estimates. Death and DALY estimates for 2004 by cause for WHO Member States (Persons, all ages).* Geneva, Switzerland: World Health Organization.

World Health Organization. (2009c). *Global surveillance, prevention and control of chronic respiratory diseases; A comprehensive approach.* Geneva, Switzerland: World Health Organization.

World Health Organization. (2010). *Global alliance against chronic diseases, action plan, 2008–2013.* Geneva, Switzerland: World Health Organization.

World Health Organization. (2015). *WHO global report on trends in prevalence of tobacco smoking 2015.* Geneva, Switzerland: World Health Organization. Retrieved from http://www.who.int/iris/handle/10665/156262

World Health Organization. (2018). *Clean air for health: Geneva action agenda.* Geneva, Switzerland: World Health Organization. Retrieved from www.who.int/phe/news/clean-air-for-health/en

Zeng, J., Yang, S., Wu, L., Wang, J., Wang, Y., Liu, M., … He, Y. (2016). Prevalence of passive smoking in the community population aged 15 years and older in China: A systematic review and meta-analysis. *BMJ Open, 6*(4), e009847. doi:10.1136/bmjopen-2015-009847.

Zhou, Y., Wang, C., Yao, W., Chen, P., Kang, J., Huang, S., … Ran, P. (2009). COPD in Chinese nonsmokers. *European Respiratory Journal, 33*(3), 509–518.

CHAPTER 40
Epidemiology of Asthma

▶ Clinical Diagnosis of Asthma

Asthma is a chronic restrictive inflammatory disease of the upper airways that usually first presents during childhood or adolescence. Though this disease has some similarities with other chronic inflammatory lung diseases, asthma has distinct clinical and epidemiologic characteristics that clearly differentiate it from the two primary conditions of chronic obstructive pulmonary disease (COPD), chronic bronchitis and emphysema.

In contrast to COPD, which impacts smaller ciliated bronchioles and alveoli in the lower airways, the pathophysiological effects of asthma are localized in the upper airways including the trachea, bronchi, and larger bronchioles. These upper airway structures are lined by non-ciliated squamous epithelium that is hyperresponsive to inhaled allergens or other stimuli in the asthmatic patient. Consequently, bronchioles

of the upper airways become persistently inflamed and narrowed due to edema, mucus production, and smooth muscle remodeling (**FIGURE 40.1**).

A further distinction from COPD and other chronic diseases is that asthma onset usually occurs early in life and the prevalence declines in adulthood. Characteristic patterns of onset during the lifespan are shown for males and females in **FIGURE 40.2**. Note that the prevalence is higher in males during childhood and adolescence, but then becomes higher in females during adulthood (Senthilselvan, Lawson, Rennie, & Dosman, 2003).

Early clinical signs of asthma include chronic rhinitis and conjunctivitis, coughing, wheezing, shortness of breath, chest tightness, and acute episodes of respiratory distress provoked by allergenic stimuli, infection, respiratory irritants, exposure to cold air, exercise, emotional stress, and drugs (Higgins, 1974). Pathologically, the bronchi and bronchioles are often occluded

Normal bronchiole

Asthmatic bronchiole

FIGURE 40.1 Comparison of Normal and Asthmatic Bronchiole.

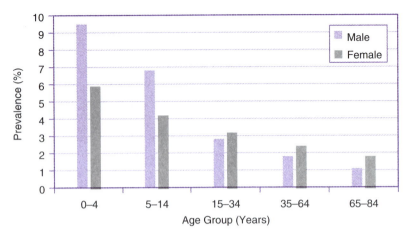

FIGURE 40.2 Prevalence of Asthma by Age.

Rates for 65–84 years were estimated by linear regression.

Data from Senthilselvan, A., Lawson, J., Rennie, D. C., & Dosman, J. A. (2003). Stabilization of an increasing trend in physician-diagnosed asthma prevalence in Saskatchewan, 1991 to 1998. *Chest, 124*(2), 438–448.

by thick mucous plugs laden with inflammatory eosinophilic cells and containing characteristic crystalline microscopic structures called Curschmann's spirals and Charcot-Leyden crystals (Sakula, 1986).

In the asthmatic patient, spirometry testing classically reveals that lung dysfunction is partially reversible by administration of a short-acting beta-agonist such as *albuterol*. Spirometry measures the maximal volume of air forcibly exhaled after maximal inhalation (the forced vital capacity, *FVC*) and the volume of air expired during the first second (*FEV1*). When the prebronchodilation and postbronchodilation spirometry values are compared, improved values of 12% or more plus a normal *FEV1/FVC* ratio suggest the presence of restrictive lung disease, a.k.a., asthma (American Thoracic Society, 1991, 1995; Bye, Kerstein, & Barsh, 1992).

Asthma can also be detected by a *peak flow meter*, a handheld device that measures expiratory air pressure. Classically, peak expiratory flow that varies by more than 20% before and after bronchodilation indicates the presence of asthma. Other tests are sometimes used to confirm the diagnosis. The *exhaled nitric oxide test* measures the level of nitric oxide in exhaled air. High levels reflect inflammation in the upper airways and the presence of asthma.

Global Burden of Asthma

In 2015, 397,000 people died from asthma in the world population, a 26.7% reduction from the 541,000 asthma-related deaths in 1990. In contrast, the number of prevalent cases of asthma in 2015 was 12.6% higher than in 1990 (358 million versus 318 million). Asthma afflicts females more often than males (190

million versus 168 million prevalent cases) but the age-adjusted mortality is higher in males than females (6.7 versus 5.6 per 100,000) (Soriano et al., 2017).

Review of published studies of the global burden of asthma reveal wide discrepancies in the estimates of deaths and prevalent cases. As pointed out by *Global Burden of Disease (GBD)* investigators,

> *for many countries in the world that do not have functional vital registration systems, we had to rely on death estimates of all chronic respiratory diseases from verbal autopsy studies because these studies cannot distinguish between asthma, COPD, or other chronic respiratory diseases. Initiatives to strengthen vital registration systems are key to improving population health measurement because verbal autopsy can only identify a restricted set of diseases.* (pp. 691–706)

Global Studies of Asthma in Children and Adults

Two large multinational studies have been conducted to assess the global prevalence of asthma in the world population: The *International Study of Asthma and Allergies in Childhood* (ISAAC) and the *European Community Respiratory Health Survey* (ECRHS I and ECRHS II).

Asthma in Children

The *ISAAC* was initiated in 1991. This ongoing study uses standardized methodology and testing to assess the prevalence and severity of asthma, rhinitis and eczema in children, elucidate risk factors, evaluate the impact of therapy, and provide a framework for future etiological research of these conditions (Asher et al., 1995).

Phase I of ISAAC assessed the prevalence of asthmatic symptoms in young children aged 6–7 years (*n* = 257,800 subjects from 91 centers in 38 countries) and older children aged 13–14 years (*n* = 463,801 subjects from 155 centers in 56 countries). Population samples of about 3000 children were studied from each center. Participating centers in ISAAC represented most regions of the world. The results of phase I of ISAAC revealed wide geographic variation in the rates of asthmatic symptoms (e.g., prevalence estimates for "*wheeze in the last 12 months*" ranged from 2.1% to 32.2%). The highest estimates in both young and older children were observed in English-speaking and Latin American countries (ISAAC, 1998a). Examination of comorbidity data from phase I of ISAAC also revealed significant positive correlations between prevalence estimates for asthma, rhinoconjunctivitis, and atopic eczema (ISAAC, 1998b).

▶ Asthma in Adults

The initial phase of the ECRHS I was designed to assess the prevalence and geographical variation in asthma, allergy, and allergic sensitization in adults living primarily in European countries. In this large survey, data were collected from about 140,000 adults aged 10–44 years from 22 countries. Clinical procedures included administration of a detailed questionnaire to ascertain information about symptoms and risk factors, administration of a quality of life questionnaire, collection of blood specimens to measure IgE-specific antibodies against common aeroallergens, and lung function testing by spirometry. Asthma prevalence varied widely, ranging from 2.0% to 11.9%. Prevalence estimates were lower in Eastern and Southern Europe and higher in Western (English-speaking) European nations (Heinrich et al., 2002).

Comparison of the findings of ISAAC and the ECRHS revealed strong positive correlations between the prevalence data for children and adults from countries represented in both surveys. While there were differences in the absolute levels of prevalence, the geographical patterns from the two studies showed good agreement, thereby validating results (Pearce, Douwes, & Beasley, 2000; Pearce, Pekkanen, & Beasley, 1999)

▶ Global Initiative for Asthma

The *Global Initiative for Asthma* (GINA) Program was established in 1989 to increase awareness among government and public health officials, healthcare workers, and the general population about the rising global burden of asthma. Recently, GINA commissioned an investigative team headed by Dr. Richard Beasley of New Zealand to examine data from ISAAC and ECRHS and summarize findings (Masoli, Fabian, Holt, Beasley, & GINA Program, 2004).

A composite map of the worldwide prevalence of asthma based on the GINA investigation is shown in **FIGURE 40.3**. Relatively, high prevalence estimates (>10%) are apparent in the United States, Canada, Great Britain, Australia, Brazil, and Peru, whereas much lower estimates (<5%) are noted for the large populations of China, India, and the Russian Federation. Based upon these data, it was estimated that at least 300 million people currently suffer from asthma in the world population (Masoli et al., 2004).

Important conclusions drawn from the GINA investigation and the more recent GBD Study include the following: (1) asthma currently affects more than 358 million people worldwide, (2) international patterns are not fully explained by current knowledge, (3) the prevalence of asthma is increasing in children and adults, and with increasing urbanization, even steeper increases are projected in the coming decades, (4) persons suffering from asthma do not have access to the appropriate medications in many regions of the world, (5) asthma causes approximately 400,000 deaths per year worldwide, many of which are due to suboptimal long-term medical care and lack of access to emergency services during the final attack of *status asthmaticus*, (6) economic costs of asthma are considerable and significantly more resources are needed in order to make appropriate long-term pharmacologic therapy available to asthmatic patients, and (7) more resources are also needed to reduce air pollution from smoking, motor vehicle exhaust, and other environmental sources that may exacerbate asthmatic attacks.

A widely used measure of the health burden of disease is the disability-adjusted years of life lost (*DALY = YLL + YDL where YLL = years of life lost due to premature death and YDL = years of life lost due to severe disability*). **FIGURE 40.4** shows the global DALY rates for asthma (WHO, 2009). Obviously, the geographic pattern of DALY rates differs dramatically from the pattern of prevalence rates in Figure 40.2 (e.g., DALY rates are highest in nations with low prevalence or that lack standardized data, particularly in Africa). The GINA investigators estimated that 15 million DALY were lost due to asthma in 2004, which reflects the rising prevalence and inadequate access to long-term therapy and emergency treatment, particularly in

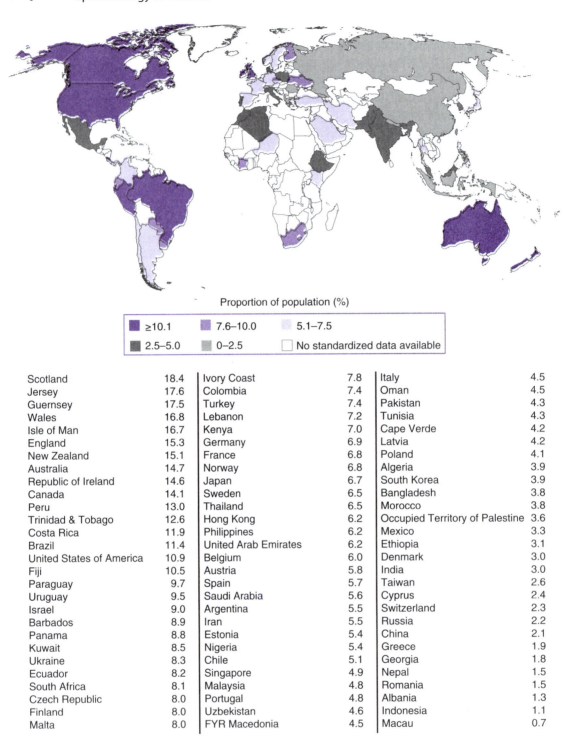

Proportion of population (%)

≥10.1	7.6–10.0	5.1–7.5
2.5–5.0	0–2.5	No standardized data available

Scotland	18.4	Ivory Coast	7.8	Italy	4.5
Jersey	17.6	Colombia	7.4	Oman	4.5
Guernsey	17.5	Turkey	7.4	Pakistan	4.3
Wales	16.8	Lebanon	7.2	Tunisia	4.3
Isle of Man	16.7	Kenya	7.0	Cape Verde	4.2
England	15.3	Germany	6.9	Latvia	4.2
New Zealand	15.1	France	6.8	Poland	4.1
Australia	14.7	Norway	6.8	Algeria	3.9
Republic of Ireland	14.6	Japan	6.7	South Korea	3.9
Canada	14.1	Sweden	6.5	Bangladesh	3.8
Peru	13.0	Thailand	6.5	Morocco	3.8
Trinidad & Tobago	12.6	Hong Kong	6.2	Occupied Territory of Palestine	3.6
Costa Rica	11.9	Philippines	6.2	Mexico	3.3
Brazil	11.4	United Arab Emirates	6.2	Ethiopia	3.1
United States of America	10.9	Belgium	6.0	Denmark	3.0
Fiji	10.5	Austria	5.8	India	3.0
Paraguay	9.7	Spain	5.7	Taiwan	2.6
Uruguay	9.5	Saudi Arabia	5.6	Cyprus	2.4
Israel	9.0	Argentina	5.5	Switzerland	2.3
Barbados	8.9	Iran	5.5	Russia	2.2
Panama	8.8	Estonia	5.4	China	2.1
Kuwait	8.5	Nigeria	5.4	Greece	1.9
Ukraine	8.3	Chile	5.1	Georgia	1.8
Ecuador	8.2	Singapore	4.9	Nepal	1.5
South Africa	8.1	Malaysia	4.8	Romania	1.5
Czech Republic	8.0	Portugal	4.8	Albania	1.3
Finland	8.0	Uzbekistan	4.6	Indonesia	1.1
Malta	8.0	FYR Macedonia	4.5	Macau	0.7

FIGURE 40.3 Worldwide Prevalence of Asthma.

Data from GINA, Global Burden of Asthma, 2004–2005

underdeveloped countries (Masoli et al., 2004). Similar findings were observed in the GBD Study of 2015 in which asthma accounted for 26.1 million DALY, approximately 1.1% of the total DALY from all diseases (Soriano et al., 2017).

The findings from ISAAC and the ECRHS suggest that the prevalence of asthma is rising in many countries throughout the world; indeed, there is widespread concern that asthma may reach epidemic proportions in the coming years (Eder & Ege, 2006). However, part of the observed increase may be attributed to greater awareness of asthmatic conditions and higher detection rates in the populations under study. Furthermore, population-based studies have not been conducted in many nations and the global picture is far from complete.

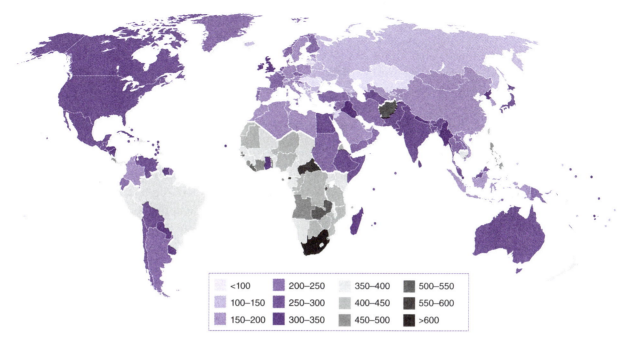

FIGURE 40.4 Disability-Adjusted Life Years, Asthma, 2004.

Values are Disability-adjusted life years per 100,000 individuals.

Reproduced from World Health Organization. *The global burden of disease: 2004*. Available at www.who.int/evidence/bod

▶ The Hygiene Hypothesis of Asthma

In 1989, a brief report was published in the *British Medical Journal* by David P. Strachan that suggested allergic diseases are prevented by infection in early childhood transmitted by unhygienic exposure to older siblings or acquired prenatally from mothers infected by contact with older children. Strachan presented evidence for this hypothesis from a prospective study of 17,414 British children born in 1958 and followed to age 23 years. Prevalence estimates of hay fever during the past 12 months were obtained for the birth cohort when subjects were 11 and 23 years of age. Prevalence estimates of hay fever by number of older siblings at ages 11 and 23 years are shown in Figure 40.4. Clearly, the prevalence of hay fever decreases with increasing number of older siblings. A similar trend was also noted for eczema during the first year of life (declining prevalence with increasing number of older siblings). Strachan interpreted these interesting findings to mean that exposure of younger children to infectious agents already contracted by older children in the family conferred protection against the development of allergic conditions such as eczema, hay fever, and asthma.

Strachan's *hygiene hypothesis* has been the subject of intense immunological and epidemiologic research. The theory has been used to infer that the increased incidence of allergic diseases in industrialized nations is due to decreases in infectious diseases with immunization and antibiotics, decreases in family size, and increases in certain allergenic and inflammatory stimuli.

If it is indeed true that exposure to infectious agents, symbiotic microorganisms (e.g., gut flora or probiotics), and parasites increases resistance to the development of allergic diseases such as eczema, hay fever, and asthma, then the important question becomes, *what is the biological mechanism*?

One proposed mechanism is that early exposure to certain infectious agents induces homeostatic balance between subsets of circulating T lymphocytes. Specifically, early infection may increase the population of T helper lymphocytes of the innate immune system (Th-1 cells) to counterbalance T helper cells of the acquired immune system (Th-2 cells). Alternative mechanisms have also been suggested (e.g., perhaps the developing immune system must receive stimuli from infectious agents, symbiotic bacteria, and parasites in order to develop regulatory T lymphocytes that suppress both the innate and the acquired immune response, thereby reducing inflammation and atopic reactions) (Bufford & Gern, 2005). As discussed in the following section, several risk factors, including both allergens and infectious agents, have been found to increase the risk of asthma development. The emerging epidemiology indicates important effects of genotype by environment interactions in the pathogenesis of asthma.

▶ Risk Factors of Asthma

Combinations of risk factors have been found to significantly heighten the risk of developing asthma. For example, many asthmatic patients report genetic or familial predisposition coupled with environmental exposure to inhaled substances that provoke allergic reactions or irritate the upper airways. Examples of environmental factors that may stimulate asthmatic attacks include indoor allergens (tobacco smoke, house dust mites, pet dander, cockroach allergens, biomass smoke), outdoor allergens (pollen, mold, motor vehicle exhaust), infectious agents (particularly respiratory rhinoviruses), chemical irritants in the workplace, cold air, emotional stress, physical exercise, drugs and drug interactions, and certain foods and food additives. Key studies of some of these factors are discussed in the following paragraphs.

▶ Atopy and Asthma

Atopy refers to the production of specific antibodies belonging to the IgE class of immunoglobulins in response to common environmental allergens. Atopic allergic reactions are often the major culprits that initiate asthma in the upper airways. As shown in **FIGURE 40.5**, allergenic stimuli induce Th2 cells to secrete an array of cytokines (Interleukins 4, 5, 9, and 13) that stimulate large B lymphocytes of the immune system (known as plasma cells) to synthesize and release E-type immunoglobulins (IgE). In turn, IgE antibodies activate receptors on the cell membranes of mast cells in the upper airways leading to the release of highly inflammatory substances such as histamines, leukotrienes prostaglandins, chemokines cytokines, and heparin. Inflamed tissues are infiltrated by macrophages and eosinophilic cells of the immune system that also elaborate cytokines and actively participate in the inflammatory process. Release of destruction

enzymes by these immune cells causes necrosis and shedding of the bronchial epithelium and secretion of mucin resulting in the development of characteristic mucous plugs of the disease. This combination of immune-modulated events causes remodeling and constriction of the upper airways and restriction of airflow both into and out of the lungs. Atopy can be assessed by skin prick testing as well as total serum IgE (Amin, 2012; Hiemstra, McCray, & Bals, 2015; Holgate & Polosa, 2006; Wegmann, 2009).

Leukotrienes are lipid compounds synthesized from arachidonic acid that sustain the allergic inflammatory response in patients with chronic asthma. The biosynthesis of leukotrienes is catalyzed by 5-lipoxygenase (5-LOX) and 5-lipoxygenase activating protein (FLAP) in response to persisting allergic stimuli. Specific leukotrienes (e.g., cysteinyl leukotrienes and leukotriene B4) expressed by mast cells perpetuate inflammation, edema, and obstruction of the upper airways by enhancing vascular permeability, mucus production, and smooth muscle constriction (Hallstrand & Henderson, 2010).

Many allergens have been indicted in the genesis of atopic asthma. Sources include pollen, pet dander, dust mites, cockroaches, mice, molds, environmental tobacco smoke, and biomass smoke. However, definitive evidence of cause and effect has been difficult to ascertain. Epidemiologic studies of childhood asthma are complicated by the young age of target populations, profound genetic and environmental differences, and difficulty in accurately measuring exposure to specific allergens using standardized methods. Perhaps because of these problematic issues, high environmental levels of offending allergens have not been consistently found to increase the risk of asthma development (Pearce et al., 2000). Selected studies are discussed in the following paragraphs.

Sporik and colleagues examined a cohort of 67 British children from 1978 to 1989 to determine the relation of house dust mite antigen and the

FIGURE 40.5 The Atopic Inflammatory Response.

development of asthma. During 11 years of follow-up, 17 children developed asthma, 16 of whom were sensitized to dust mite allergens. Among the 50 children who did not develop asthma, 19 were atopic. Among children exposed to high levels of dust mites in the home before age 1 year, the relative risk of asthma development was 4.8. Based on these observations, it was concluded that exposure to house dust mites early in childhood is a strong determinant of subsequent asthma development (Sporik, Holgate, Platts-Mills, & Cogswell, 1990).

The German *Multicenter Allergy Study* was designed to examine exposure to dust mites and cat allergens and asthma development in a prospective birth cohort of 1314 children enrolled in five German cities. Periodic measurements of indoor allergen exposure and specific IgE antibodies to food and inhalant allergens were available for 939 children who were followed to the age of 7 years. The overall prevalence of asthma in the study was 6.1%. The study demonstrated a clear association between allergen exposure during infancy and subsequent sensitization. The association became apparent at the age of 3 years and was stronger at 7 years of age. Furthermore, there was a strong association between immune sensitization and the development of asthma. Nevertheless, levels of allergen exposure measured in the home at 6 months were *not* associated with asthma development (Lau et al., 2000).

In the *Asthma Multicenter Infant Cohort Study* of 1000 newborns conducted by investigators in the United Kingdom and Spain, allergens were measured in the homes of 3-month-old babies followed by skin prick testing at 6 years of age. Exposure to cat allergens but not dust mites increased sensitization to skin testing (OR = 4.4) and the risk of asthma (OR = 2.6) (Torrent et al., 2007).

Huss and colleagues conducted skin tests in 1041 children aged 5–12 years with *mild to moderate* asthma to determine allergenic risk factors. They also tested for specific allergens in the home environments. Data were obtained from eight North American cities participating in the *U.S. Childhood Asthma Management Program*. Children living in homes with high levels of dust mites or cockroaches were more likely to have positive skin tests than children with no exposure (OR = 9.0 and 2.2, respectively). Sensitization was also related to serum IgE and the total number of positive skin tests (Huss et al., 2001).

Despite observed inconsistencies in the association between environmental measures of allergy exposure and asthma development, there is consensus that high levels of individual sensitization responses

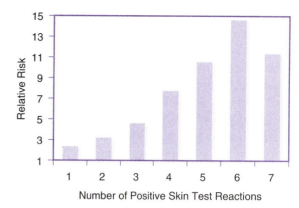

FIGURE 40.6 Dose Response of Asthma Risk and Positive Skin Test Reactions.

Data from Pearce, N., Pekkanen, J., & Beasley, R. (1999). How much asthma is really attributable to atopy? *Thorax, 54,* 268–272.

measured by skin prick or IgE level significantly increase the risk. In a review and meta-analysis of available studies on skin prick testing, various measures of testing revealed a striking dose response between the relative risk of asthma and the number of positive tests. As shown in **FIGURE 40.6**, the risk of asthma increases by more than 10-fold for individuals with five or more positive skin test reactions to a variety of common allergens (Pearce et al., 1999). A similar though less dramatic dose response has been reported between the risk of asthma and the level of total serum IgE (Burrows, Halonen, Lebowitz, Knudson, & Barbee, 1982; Sears et al., 1991).

ISAAC utilized standardized methodology to study asthma and allergy in children aged 8–12 years on a global basis. Thirty study centers in 22 countries enrolled subjects from environments reflecting a wide range of living conditions from rural Africa to urban Europe. Data were collected by parental questionnaires (*n* = 54,439), skin prick testing (*n* = 31,759), and measurements of allergen-specific IgE in serum (*n* = 8951). The prevalence of current "wheeze" varied widely from 0.8% in Ecuador to 25.6% in Brazil and the fraction of individuals with current wheeze attributable to atopy ranged from 0% in Turkey to 93.8% in China. The prevalence of wheeze and fraction of wheeze attributable to atopy (skin test reactivity) were positively correlated with gross national income per capita (i.e., sensitivity rates increased with increasing income per capita). The ISAAC investigators concluded from these results that the link between atopic sensitization and asthmatic symptoms in children differs markedly between populations and increases with economic development (Weinmayr et al., 2007).

While most asthmatic cases are diagnosed in childhood, adult onset constitutes a significant fraction of disease, perhaps up to one-third in some populations. In the *ECRHS*, associations of specific types of allergic rhinitis and bronchial hyper-responsiveness were examined in 3719 *adults* followed over nine years. In subjects with allergic rhinitis, the risk of developing bronchial hyper-responsiveness was markedly increased in individuals sensitized to cat allergens (OR = 7.9) or dust mites (OR = 2.8) (Shaaban et al., 2007).

The totality of current evidence therefore suggests that sensitization to certain allergens plays a significant role in the development of asthma in both children and adults. Nevertheless, as demonstrated by the results of ISAAC, there is marked variability among populations in the prevalence of atopic asthma (Weinmayr et al., 2007). Asthma development appears to be a complex, interactive process involving the interaction of several environmental and genetic factors (National Heart, Lung, Blood Institute, 2007).

▶ Respiratory Viruses and Asthma

Respiratory viruses have been found to influence the development of childhood asthma. In particular, the onset of asthma in children is often preceded by severe infection due to respiratory viruses, particularly respiratory syncytial virus (RSV) and rhinoviruses.

Early studies linked seasonal viral infections to the subsequent development of asthma (Aberg, 1989; Anderson, Bailey, & Bland, 1981). More recently, Wu and colleagues studied the relationship of winter virus infections during infancy and the development of childhood asthma in over 95,000 U.S. infants born between 1995 and 2000. Subjects were enrolled for study through the Tennessee Medicaid program. The risk of developing asthma tracked with the timing of infant birth and the winter virus peak. Infants born 4 months prior to the winter virus peak had a 29% increase in the odds of developing asthma compared to infants born 12 months prior to the peak. The results suggest that winter viral infection during infancy is a risk factor for the subsequent development of asthma (Wu et al., 2008).

Investigators at the University of Arizona conducted a prospective study of 880 U.S. children who were enrolled at birth and followed for the development of lower respiratory tract infections in the first 3 years of life and then evaluated for the presence or absence of physician-diagnosed asthma at ages 6 and 11 years. At age 6, physician-diagnosed asthma was present in 13.6% of children with a history of early pneumonia compared to 4.6% of subjects with no history of lung infection (OR = 3.3). At 11 years of age, 25.6% of children in the early pneumonia group had developed asthma compared to 11% in the reference group (OR = 2.2). Furthermore, lung function was significantly compromised in the asthmatic group but showed significant improvement with administration of the beta-blocker, *albuterol*. These findings suggest that early childhood pneumonia is an important risk factor for asthma (Castro-Rodríguez et al., 1999).

Sigurs and colleagues studied asthma development in a cohort of 47 Swedish children who were hospitalized with bronchiolitis during infancy due to RSV. The rate of asthma development in the RSV bronchiolitis cohort was compared to a matched control group of 93 disease-free infants. All children were evaluated at age 7 years by physical examinations, skin prick tests, and serum IgE tests for common food and pet allergens. The cumulative prevalence of asthma in the RSV group was 30% compared to 3% in the control group. The odds ratio of asthma development in children who were hospitalized for RSV bronchiolitis as infants compared to controls was 12.7. Furthermore, allergenic responses to common foods and allergens were also heightened with RSV exposure (OR = 2.4). These results indicate that early exposure to RSV serves as a strong stimulus for subsequent asthma development (Sigurs, Bjarnason, Sigurbergsson, & Kjellman, 2000).

Jackson and colleagues studied 259 U.S. children from birth to 6 years of age to assess the etiology and timing of specific *wheezing* viral respiratory infections in relation to the development of asthma. Viral etiology was determined by multiplex reverse transcriptase polymerase chain reaction in cultured specimens ascertained by nasal lavage. Viral etiologies were identified in 90% of the respiratory infections and the risk of asthma development increased following early infection by RSV (OR = 2.6), rhinovirus (OR = 9.8), or combined infection (OR = 10). Nearly 90% of children who developed rhinovirus infection with wheezing before 3 years of age subsequently developed asthma by the age of 6 years (Jackson et al., 2008).

▶ Environmental Tobacco Smoke and Asthma

Investigators at the California Environmental Protection Agency conducted a meta-analysis of 37 epidemiologic investigations of environmental tobacco smoke and asthma. Across all studies, maternal smoking increased asthma risk by 60% and household exposure increased the risk by 45% (Dunn and Zeise, 1997; Dunn, Zeise, & Waller, 1997).

These findings provide compelling evidence that environmental tobacco smoke increases the risk of asthma in children (Cook & Strachan, 1999; Strachan & Cook, 1998). Nevertheless, heterogeneity of study designs and lack of control for potential confounders has produced some inconsistencies in the evidence.

Vork and colleagues used meta-regression analysis to synthesize data from 38 epidemiologic studies that adjusted effects of environmental tobacco smoke for history of atopy. Their primary objective was to elucidate consistent patterns of risk by eliminating potential sources of bias and confounding. Increased summary estimates of relative risk (RR) were observed for both *prevalent asthma* and *incident asthma* with exposure to environmental tobacco smoke from any source (RR = 1.48 and 1.21, respectively) and from maternal smoking (RR = 1.29 and 1.24, respectively). Stratification of the data by age revealed differences in the relative risk estimates for young children aged 5 years or less (RR = 1.05) versus older children aged 6–18 years (RR = 1.33). These findings suggest that the duration of exposure to environmental tobacco smoking is an important factor in the genesis of asthma (Vork, Broadwin, & Blaisdell, 2007).

▶ Atopy, Environmental Tobacco Smoke, and Asthma

Jaakkola and colleagues examined the joint effect of genetic propensity to asthma and exposure to environmental tobacco smoke in a prospective population-based study of 2531 children born in Oslo, Norway. Data were collected on health and environmental exposures at the time of birth and after 6, 18, 24, and 48 months of follow-up. Parental atopy was defined as a history of maternal or paternal asthma or hay fever and exposure to environmental tobacco smoke was defined as smokers in the household. Parental atopy independently increased the risk of asthma (OR = 1.67) whereas exposure to environmental tobacco smoke *per se* had no effect. Notably, parental atopy *plus* exposure to environmental tobacco smoke produced a stronger effect than either risk factor alone (OR = 2.68). The results suggest a joint effect of parental atopy and exposure to environmental tobacco smoke in the development of asthma in young children (Jaakkola, Naftad, & Magnus, 2001).

▶ Food Allergy and Asthma

Investigators in Chicago, Illinois, conducted a nested case–control study of 201 children with asthma and 366 children of similar age without asthma to determine the relationship between food allergies and physician-diagnosed asthma. Food allergies to common foods (egg, sesame, peanut, soy, milk, shrimp, walnut, codfish, and wheat) were determined following ingestion of specific foods using skin prick testing and serum IgE. Logistic regression was used to estimate odds ratios with adjustment for other factors including sensitization to common aeroallergens. The presence of symptomatic food allergies significantly increased the risk of asthma in younger children (OR = 5.3) and older children (OR = 4.9). Effects of specific allergies to milk, eggs, and peanuts were also statistically significant. The results suggest that symptomatic food allergies significantly increase the risk of asthma development in children (Schroeder et al., 2009). Furthermore, they provide corroboration of earlier findings suggesting that specific allergies (e.g., milk, eggs, and peanuts) enhance the genesis of asthma (Kulig, Bergmann, Tacke, Wahn, & Guggenmoos-Holzmann, 1998; Leung, Lam, Chan, Li, & Tang, 2002; Penard-Morand et al., 2005).

▶ Asthma and Obesity

As elaborated elsewhere in this text, obesity is a major cause of morbidity and mortality worldwide. Life-threatening and debilitating sequelae of this condition include cardiovascular disease, diabetes, and malignancy. Furthermore, the obesity epidemic continues to expand, threatening to envelop virtually all populations of the planet. Due to parallel increases in the rates of obesity and asthma over time, scientific interest has recently focused on a potential etiologic link between excess adiposity and the development of asthma.

Several prospective studies have examined the associations between weight gain, obesity, and the development of asthma in children. The *Children's Health Study* enrolled 3792 school-age children from 12 Southern California communities to examine obesity and asthma. All children were asthma-free at baseline. Participants were examined annually from 1993 to 1998. Body mass was determined by height and weight measurements, and incident cases of asthma were detected based upon symptoms and lung function tests. Over 4 years of follow-up, 288 new cases of asthma were detected in the cohort. The risk of incident asthma was significantly higher among children who were obese (RR = 1.6); overweight boys were at higher risk (RR = 2.06) than overweight girls (RR = 1.25). Effects of excess weight were strongest in those individuals without detectable allergies (RR = 1.77). The authors concluded that increased body weight was associated with increased risk of asthma development, particularly in boys and in non-allergic children (Gilliland et al., 2003).

Flaherman and Rutherford examined obesity and physician-diagnosed asthma in children using meta-analysis. Twelve cohort studies met inclusion criteria for the study. Combined results from four studies revealed that high body mass during middle childhood increased the risk of subsequent asthma development (RR = 1.5). Combined results from nine studies also revealed a modest effect of high birth weight on the risk of developing asthma (RR = 1.2). The results indicate that children with high body weight either at birth or later in childhood are at increased risk for the subsequent development of asthma. The authors suggest several potential mechanisms including diet, gastroesophageal reflux, mechanical effects of obesity, atopy, and hormonal influences (Flaherman & Rutherford, 2006). In addition, adipocytes engorged with triglycerides are induced to secrete a variety of inflammatory cytokines (adipokines) that may influence asthma risk.

Obesity has been determined to be a risk factor for asthma development in adults as well as children. Swedish investigators examined risk factors for incident asthma, including obesity, in a case–control study of 309 adults with asthma and a similar number of age- and gender-matched controls. Compared to subjects with optimal body mass (BMI: 20–24.9), obese men and women (BMI > 30) had similar increases in the risk of developing asthma (OR = 3.3 and 3.0, respectively). These estimates retained statistical significance after adjustment for other significant risk factors including hay fever, family history of asthma, allergic sensitization, and smoking (Rönmark, Andersson, Nyström, Forsberg, Järvholmand, & Lundbäck, 2005).

Beuther and Sutherland explored the relationship between obesity and asthma in adults using meta-analysis. Seven prospective epidemiologic investigations involving 333,102 subjects met inclusion criteria for the study. Compared with normal weight (BMI < 25), being overweight (BMI: 25–29.9) or obese (BMI > 30) increased the odds of incident asthma (OR = 1.38 and 1.92, respectively). Estimates were similar for men and women and there was a significant dose response in the risk with increasing body mass. The investigators concluded that being overweight or obese increases the risk of asthma development in adults (Beuther & Sutherland, 2007).

Asthma and Household Cleaning Products

Some studies have examined the effects of cleaning solutions and sprays used in the home. In *ECRHS*, frequent household exposure to cleaning sprays and solutions more than doubled the relative risk of developing asthma (RR = 2.4) (Zock et al., 2007). Likewise, of the environments of healthcare professionals found

increased odds of developing asthma with exposure to aerosolized irritants such as cleaning solvents and there was a significant dose response between reported asthma and the length of time on the job (e.g., OR = 4.1 for >27 years) (Delclos et al., 2007).

Drug-Induced Asthma

The link between asthma, nasal polyposis, and aspirin sensitivity was first reported by Widal in 1922. Nearly half a century later, Samter and Beers further characterized this condition, which typically involves the progressive development of chronic rhinitis, asthma, nasal polyposis, and hypersensitivity to aspirin in young adults (Samter & Beers, 1968). Reactions to aspirin in such patients can produce severe asthma attacks and episodes of anaphylaxis. The disorder is often called *Samter's triad*.

Investigators in Finland conducted a postal survey of 4300 Finnish adults, aged 18–64 years, to assess the prevalence of asthma and its risk factors. Respondents included 1408 men and 1694 women. The prevalence of reported physician-diagnosed asthma in the sample was 4.6%. Reported aspirin intolerance more than doubled the odds of developing asthma (OR = 2.2). Other significant risk factors included allergic rhinitis (OR = 3.9), nasal polyposis (OR = 3.9), and familial history of asthma (OR = 2.5). Samter's triad was present in 4.3% of subjects who reported they had physician-diagnosed asthma (Hedman, Kaprio, Poussa, & Nieminen, 1999).

Published estimates of the prevalence of aspirin sensitivity among asthmatic patients vary widely ranging from 4% to 44%. In a comprehensive review of the literature, Jenkins and colleagues pooled data from 21 randomized clinical trials of asthmatic patients in which sensitivity to asthma was determined by oral provocation testing and by verbal history. Based upon provocation testing, the pooled prevalence of aspirin sensitivity among asthmatic patients was 21% in adults and 5% in children. These values are markedly higher than estimates based on verbal history (3% in adults and 2% in children). These results suggest that many asthmatic patients may be unaware of their sensitivity to aspirin (Jenkins, Costello, & Hodge, 2004).

In a retrospective review of 208 patients who underwent sinus surgery for chronic rhinosinusitis, Samter's triad was present in 10 patients (4.8%). Subgroup analyses showed that aspirin hypersensitivity was present in 25.6% of patients with both nasal polyps and asthma, and 16.9% of patients with asthma (Kim & Kountakis, 2007).

Sensitivity to aspirin, ibuprofen, and other non-steroidal anti-inflammatory drugs (NSAIDs) may be largely due to their impact on the biosynthesis of prostaglandins versus leukotrienes. The NSAIDs reduce inflammation by specifically inhibiting cyclooxygenase, the rate-limiting enzyme of the prostaglandin cascade, thereby shunting conversion of arachidonic acid to leukotrienes rather than prostaglandins. Exposure of the upper airways to certain leukotrienes (e.g., leukotriene B-4) can produce inflammatory responses that lead to the development of asthma (Leff, 2000).

▶ Vaccination and Childhood Asthma

In recent years, the prevalence of asthma has risen dramatically throughout the world, most notably in developed countries. In most cases, asthma is diagnosed in childhood and adolescence, often during the first 6 years of life. Since childhood immunization is routinely practiced in the industrialized world, the emerging burden of asthma in children has prompted studies of a possible etiologic link with immunization.

To resolve the question, investigators in Israel conducted a meta-analysis of studies of immunization and asthma. The study included seven studies of pertussis vaccination ($n = 186,663$ children) and five studies of bacillus Calmette-Guérin (BCG) vaccination ($n = 41,479$ children). Pertussis vaccine is directed against *Bordetella pertussis,* the bacterium that causes whooping cough, and BCG is a vaccine consisting of attenuated human tubercle bacilli. No statistically significant associations were detected in the meta-analysis. Thus, the currently available data from observational studies do not support a link between either BCG or pertussis vaccine and the risk of asthma development in childhood (Balicer, Grotto, Mimouni, & Mimouni, 2007).

▶ Genetics of Asthma

Expression of the asthmatic phenotype depends not only on the environment but also on the underlying genetic predisposition. It is the combination of these influences that ultimately determines whether asthma develops in a given individual. Therefore, in considering the origins of asthma and the development of effective interventions for prevention and therapy, contributions of genes, environments, and genotype × environment interactions need to be accurately identified and quantified. Genome-wide association studies of single nucleotide polymorphisms (SNPs) and genetic linkage studies of affected relatives within kindreds have been used to explore the human genome for genes that increase susceptibility to asthma and atopy.

A recent review of nearly 500 genetic studies revealed that 25 "true" susceptibility genes have been discovered that increase susceptibility to asthma or atopy in six or more populations (Ober & Hoffjan, 2006). Nevertheless, the effects of single genes appear to be small and contingent upon the environment and population studied, thereby reflecting the importance of gene–environment and gene–gene interactions. Simple inheritance patterns of asthma susceptibility genes have not been identified; rather, the inheritance of susceptibility genes and their translation to the asthmatic phenotype is that of a complex polygenic disorder.

The *GABRIEL* Project is a multidisciplinary study initiated in 2006 to identify genetic and environmental causes of asthma in the European community. The project is led by an international team of 164 scientists from 19 countries in Europe, along with other groups in the United Kingdom, Canada, and Australia. Using the latest research techniques across a variety of disciplines, including genetics, epidemiology, and immunology, this team is currently investigating representative population samples of asthmatic patients and control subjects from these locations to identify key factors in the development of asthma.

Members of the GABRIEL Consortium recently conducted a large genome-wide association study of 10,365 cases with physician-diagnosed asthma and 16,110 unaffected controls matched on ancestry. A total of 582,892 SNPs were determined for each subject in the study. The study was powered to detect the statistical significance of odds ratios in the range of 1.1–1.2. Small effects of a few genes were found with known biological effects on inflammatory interleukins and their receptors and regulatory T cells of the acquired immune system. Only one genetic locus, *HLA-DR* of the major histocompatibility gene, was found to have a genome-wide association with total serum IgE concentration. The investigators concluded that "*asthma is genetically heterogeneous*" wherein a few common alleles increase genetic susceptibility by influencing components of the adaptive immune system and inflammatory damage to the upper airways (Moffatt et al., 2010).

A novel discovery in the field of asthma research involves the *YKL-40* protein, which belongs to a family of enzymes known as chitinases. These enzymes are produced in humans as an innate immune response to *chitin* exposure. Chitin is a long-chain polysaccharide that serves as an armor or cell wall for fungi and arthropods, including all crustaceans and insects. Interestingly, chitin is found in insects such as dust mites and cockroaches that are known to provoke allergenic responses, and animal studies have shown that chitinase is a powerful stimulant of allergic reactions and inflammation (e.g., Reese et al., 2007). Subsequently, in human studies of the U.S. *Hutterite* population, subjects with asthma or broncho-hyper-responsiveness were found to have significantly elevated levels of *YKL-40* compared to subjects without asthma (the Hutterite population is a small genetically isolated religious community of European descent now residing in South Dakota and other locations in the United States). Further studies of asthma in the Hutterite population and in other population samples have revealed that differences in *YKL-40* and asthma susceptibility are genetically determined. Specifically, a variant of the promoter region of the *CHI3L1* gene on chromosome 1 that encodes *YKL-40* significantly increases serum levels of the protein and confers greater susceptibility to asthma and broncho-hyper-responsiveness (Ober et al., 2008). Thus, genetic variation at the *YKL-40* locus may play an important role in determining the risk of asthma development in response to chitin exposure.

Preventing Asthma Progression: Avoidance of Environmental Tobacco Smoke

Chilmonczyk and colleagues examined the association of environmental tobacco smoke, urinary levels of cotinine (a nicotine metabolite), and exacerbations of disease in 199 children with asthma. Serum theophylline levels were used to adjust for confounding due to disease management. Median urinary cotinine levels increased according to reported exposure to environmental tobacco smoke (5.6 ng per ml for no exposure, 13.1 ng per ml for primarily maternal exposure, and 55.8 ng per ml for maternal exposure plus other significant exposure). Children with high exposure to environmental tobacco smoke (based on either reported exposure or the level of urinary cotinine) had approximately twice the risk of experiencing acute exacerbation compared to those with low exposure. Furthermore, spirometry measures of lung function decreased significantly with increasing exposure (Chilmonczyk et al., 1993).

Gerald and colleagues conducted a randomized clinical trial to assess the effects of reducing exposure to environmental tobacco smoke in children with asthma. Children were randomized to receive either supervised asthma therapy with counseling to avoid exposure to environmental tobacco smoke or usual care without counseling. Children whose exposure decreased had fewer hospitalizations and emergency room visits and they were 48% less likely to experience an episode of poor asthma control (Gerald et al., 2009). These results underscore the importance of making sure that asthmatic children avoid any exposure to environmental tobacco smoke.

Risk Factors for Fatal Asthma Attack

Status asthmaticus is a medical emergency in which severe airway obstruction and asthmatic symptoms persist despite the administration of standard therapy. This condition can present with little warning and progress rapidly to asphyxiation. Patients who have frequent and severe symptoms (wheezing, coughing, chest tightness, shortness of breath) are at greatest risk of having a fatal asthma attack. Two patterns of fatal asthma attacks have been observed: *slow onset* in which death occurs after disease progression over days or weeks, and *rapid onset* in which death occurs within a few hours of the exacerbation of symptoms. Slow onset prior to *status asthmaticus* is characterized by eosinophilic inflammation and obstruction of airway lumens by tenacious mucus plugs and desquamated epithelium; whereas rapid onset fatal asthma is mainly due to smooth muscle bronchospasm and neutrophil invasion of the upper airways. Patients at high risk require special education on avoidance of exacerbating stimuli and intensified therapy for maintaining patency of the airways (Higgins, 2003; Papiris, Kotanidou, Malagari, & Roussos, 2002).

Therapy for the Asthmatic Patient

Though asthma is an incurable condition, symptoms can be controlled reasonably well using inhaled beta-blockers such as *albuterol* for relief of acute attacks and inhaled corticosteroids such as *budesonide* for long-term maintenance therapy. Inhaled corticosteroids are the preferred class of long-term medications to manage persistent asthma in both children and adults. Numerous studies in asthmatic children have established that inhaled corticosteroids reduce the frequency of asthmatic attacks, improve pulmonary function, improve quality of life, enhance exercise tolerance, and reduce hospitalizations (Rachelefsy, 2009).

Treatment protocols should be individualized to proactively monitor and manage symptoms and prevent attacks. In children with asthma, handheld spray devices efficiently deliver regulated aerosolized doses of these drugs into the upper airways in order to prevent asthmatic attacks and maintain air flow. Identification and avoidance of specific triggers of asthmatic attacks is a critical component of asthma management. Such stimuli are variable from person to person and may include smoke, mold, dust mites, pollen, pet dander, exercise, food allergies, respiratory infection, and other environmental factors. The GINA is an international organization of healthcare professionals and public health officials committed to reducing the burden of asthma worldwide. The recent GINA publication entitled "*Global Strategy for Asthma Management and Prevention*" presents evidence-based guidelines for asthma management and prevention (GINA, 2011).

▶ ## Summary

According to an Expert Panel Report of the National Heart Lung and Blood Institute,

Asthma is a chronic inflammatory disorder of the airways in which many cell and cellular elements play a role: in particular, mast cells, eosinophils, T lymphocytes, macrophages, neutrophils, and epithelial cells. In susceptible individuals, this inflammation causes recurrent episodes of wheezing, breathlessness, chest tightness, and coughing, particularly at night or in the early morning. These episodes are usually associated with widespread but variable airflow obstruction that is often reversible either spontaneously or with treatment. The inflammation also causes an associated increase in the existing bronchial hyper-responsiveness to a variety of stimuli. Reversibility of airflow limitation may be incomplete in some patients with asthma. (National Heart, Lung, Blood Institute, 2007)

Asthma is clearly a multifactorial disease. Several important risk factors have been identified including environmental allergens, respiratory viruses, environmental tobacco smoke, and obesity. Genetic predisposition appears to be polygenic and the transition of susceptible genotype to asthmatic phenotype appears to be highly dependent upon interactions with environmental factors. In the asthmatic patient, allergenic and environmental triggers of exacerbation and attacks must be avoided. Therapeutic approaches are currently available that allow most asthmatic patients to enjoy a high quality of life. Elucidation of causative genotype by environmental interactions in future studies will be of benefit in the prevention and reversal of the asthmatic process.

References

Aberg, N. (1989). Birth season variation in asthma and allergic rhinitis. *Clinical and Experimental Allergy, 19*, 643–648.

American Thoracic Society. (1991). Lung function testing: Selection of reference values and interpretative strategies. *The American Review of Respiratory Disease, 144*, 1202–1018.

American Thoracic Society. (1995). Standardization of spirometry: Update. *American Journal of Respiratory and Critical Care Medicine, 152*, 1107–1036.

Amin, K. (2012). The role of mast cells in allergic inflammation. *Respiratory Medicine, 106*(1), 9–14.

Anderson, H. R., Bailey, P. A., & Bland, J. M. (1981). The effect of birth month on asthma, eczema, hayfever, respiratory symptoms, lung function, and hospital admissions for asthma. *International Journal of Epidemiology, 10*, 45–51.

Asher, M. I., Keil, U., Anderson, H. R., Beasley, R., Crane, J., Martinez, F., … Stewart, A. W. (1995). International study of asthma and allergies in childhood (ISAAC): Rationale and methods. *The European Respiratory Journal, 8*, 483–491.

Balicer, R. D., Grotto, I., Mimouni, M., & Mimouni, D. (2007). Is childhood vaccination associated with asthma? A meta-analysis of observational studies. *Pediatrics, 120*(5), e1269–e1277.

Beuther, D. A., & Sutherland, E. R. (2007). Overweight, obesity, and incident asthma. *American Journal of Respiratory and Critical Care Medicine, 175*, 661–666.

Bufford, J. D., & Gern, J. E. (2005). The hygiene hypothesis revisited. *Immunology and Allergy Clinics of North America, 25*(2), 247–262.

Burrows, B., Halonen, M., Lebowitz, M. D., Knudson, R. J., & Barbee, R. A. (1982). The relationship of serum immunoglobulin E, allergy skin tests, and smoking to respiratory disorders. *The Journal of Allergy and Clinical Immunology, 70*, 199–204.

Bye, M. R., Kerstein, D., & Barsh, E. (1992). The importance of spirometry in the assessment of childhood asthma. *American Journal of Diseases of Children, 146*, 977–978.

Castro-Rodríguez, J. A., Holberg, C. J., Wright, A. L., Halonen, M., Taussig, L. M., … Martinez, F. D. (1999). Association of radiologically ascertained pneumonia before age 3 yr with asthma like symptoms and pulmonary function during childhood: A prospective study. *American Journal of Respiratory and Critical Care Medicine, 159*(6), 1891–1897.

Chilmonczyk, B. A., Salmun, L. M., Megathlin, K. N., Neveux, L. M., Palomaki, G. E., Knight, G. J., … Haddow, J. E. (1993). Association between exposure to environmental tobacco smoke and exacerbations of asthma in children. *The New England Journal of Medicine, 328*, 1665–1669.

Cook, D. G., & Strachan, D. P. (1999). Health effects of passive smoking-10: Summary of effects of parental smoking on the respiratory health of children and implications for research. *Thorax, 54*(4), 357–366.

Delclos, G. L., Gimeno, D., Arif, A. A., Burau, K. D., Carson, A., Lusk, C., … Antó, J. M. (2007). Occupational risk factors and asthma among health care professionals. *American Journal of Respiratory and Critical Care Medicine, 175*, 667–675.

Dunn, A., & Zeise, L. (Eds.). (1997). *Health effects of exposure to environmental tobacco smoke.* Sacramento, CA: California Environmental Protection Agency.

Dunn, A., Zeise, L., & Waller, K. (1997). Developmental toxicity II: Postnatal manifestations. In A. Dunn & L. Zeise (Eds.) *Health effects of exposure to environmental tobacco smoke* (pp. 4-1-4-48). Sacramento, CA: California Environmental Protection Agency.

Eder, W., & Ege, M. J. (2006). The asthma epidemic. *The New England Journal of Medicine, 355*, 2226–2235.

Flaherman, V., & Rutherford, G. W. (2006). A meta-analysis of the effect of high weight on asthma. *Archives of Disease in Childhood, 91*, 334–339.

Gerald, L. B., Gerald, J. K., Gibson, L., Patel, K., Zhang, S., & McClure, L. A. (2009). Changes in environmental tobacco smoke exposure and asthma morbidity among urban school children. *Chest, 135*(4), 911–916.

Gilliland, F. D., Berhane, K., Islam, T., McConnell, R., Gauderman, W. J., Gilliland, S. S., … Peters, J. M. (2003). Obesity and the risk of newly diagnosed asthma in school-age children. *American Journal of Epidemiology, 158*(5), 406–415.

Global Initiative for Asthma (GINA). (2011). Global Strategy for Asthma Management and Prevention. NHLBI/WHO workshop report. Washington, DC: National Institutes of Health, National Heart, Lung and Blood Institute.

Hallstrand, T. S., & Henderson, W. R. (2010). An update on the role of leukotrienes in asthma. *Current Opinion in Allergy and Clinical Immunology, 10*(1), 60–66.

Hedman, J., Kaprio, J., Poussa, T., & Nieminen, M. M. (1999). Prevalence of asthma, aspirin intolerance, nasal polyposis and chronic obstructive pulmonary disease in a population-based study. *International Journal of Epidemiology, 28*, 717–722.

Heinrich, J., Richter, K., Frye, C., Meyer, I., Wölke, G., Wjst, M., … Wichmann, H. E. (2002). European community respiratory health survey in adults (ECRHS). *Pneumologie, 56*(5), 297–303.

Hiemstra, P. S., McCray, P. B., & Bals, R. (2015). The innate immune function of airway epithelial cells in inflammatory lung disease. *The European Respiratory Journal, 45*(4), 1150–1162.

Higgins, I. T. T. (1974). *Epidemiology of chronic respiratory disease. A literature review.* EPA-650/1-74-007. Washington, DC: Environmental Protection Agency.

Higgins, J. C. (2003). The 'crashing asthmatic.' *American Family Physician, 67*(5), 997–1004.

Holgate, S. T., & Polosa, R. (2006). The mechanisms, diagnosis, and management of severe asthma in adults. *Lancet, 368*, 780–793.

Huss, K., Adkinson, N. F., Eggleston, P. A., Dawson, C., Van Natta, M. L., & Hamilton, R. G. (2001). House dust mite and cockroach exposure are strong risk factors for positive allergy skin test responses in the Childhood Asthma Management Program. *Journal of Allergy and Clinical Immunology, 107*(1), 48–54.

ISAAC. (1998a). Worldwide variations in the prevalence of asthma symptoms: The International Study of Asthma and Allergies in Childhood (ISAAC). The International Study of Asthma and Allergies in Childhood (ISAAC) Steering Committee. *The European Respiratory Journal, 12*, 315–335.

ISAAC. (1998b). Worldwide variation in prevalence of symptoms of asthma, allergic rhinoconjunctivitis, and atopic eczema: ISAAC. The International Study of Asthma and Allergies in Childhood (ISAAC) Steering Committee. *Lancet, 351*, 1225–1232.

Jaakkola, J. J. K., Naftad, P., & Magnus, P. (2001). Environmental tobacco smoke, parental atopy, and childhood asthma. *Environmental Health Perspectives, 109*, 579–582.

Jackson, D. J., Gangnon, R. E., Evans, M. D., Roberg, K. A., Anderson, E. L., Pappas, T. E., … Lemanske, R. F., Jr. (2008). Wheezing rhinovirus illnesses in early life predict asthma development in high-risk children. *American Journal of Respiratory and Critical Care Medicine, 178*, 667–672.

Jenkins, C., Costello, J., & Hodge, L. (2004). Systematic review of prevalence of aspirin induced asthma and its implications for clinical practice. *BMJ, 328*(7437), 434–437.

Kim, J. E., & Kountakis, S. E. (2007). The prevalence of Samter's triad in patients undergoing functional endoscopic sinus surgery. *Ear, Nose, & Throat Journal, 86*(7), 396–399.

Kulig, M., Bergmann, R., Tacke, U., Wahn, U., & Guggenmoos-Holzmann, I. (1998). Long-lasting sensitization to food during the first two years precedes allergic airway disease. The MAS Study Group, Germany. *Pediatric Allergy and Immunology, 9*, 61–67.

Lau, S., Illi, S., Sommerfeld, C., Niggemann, B., Bergmann, R., von Mutius, E., & Wahn, U. (2000). Early exposure to house-dust mite and cat allergens and development of childhood asthma: A cohort study. Multicentre Allergy Study Group. *Lancet, 356*, 1392–1397.

Leff, A. R. (2000). Role of leukotrienes in bronchial hyperresponsiveness and cellular responses in airways. *Thorax, 55*, S32–S37.

Leung, T. F., Lam, C. W., Chan, I. H., Li, A. M., & Tang, N. L. (2002). Sensitization to common food allergens is a risk factor for asthma in young Chinese children in Hong Kong. *Journal of Asthma, 39*, 523–529.

Masoli, M., Fabian, D., Holt, S., Beasley, R., & Global Initiative for Asthma (GINA) Program. (2004). The global burden of asthma: Executive summary of the GINA Dissemination Committee Report. *Allergy, 59*, 469–478.

Moffatt, M. F., Gut, I. F., Dmeenais, F., Strachan, D. P., Bouzigon, E., Heath, S., … WOCM for the GABRIEL Consortium. (2010). A large-scale, consortium-based genomewide association study of asthma. *The New England Journal of Medicine, 363*, 1211–1221.

National Heart, Lung, Blood Institute. (2007). *National Asthma Education and Prevention Program. Expert panel report 3: Guidelines for the diagnosis and management of asthma.* Washington, DC: U.S. Department of Health and Human Services, National Institutes of Health.

Ober, C., & Hoffjan, S. (2006). Asthma genetics 2006: The long and winding road to gene discovery. *Genes and Immunity, 7*, 95–100.

Ober, C., Tan, Z., Sun, Y., Possick, J. D., Pan, L., Nicolae, R., … Chupp, G. L. (2008). Effect of variation in *CHI3L1* on serum YKL-40 level, risk of asthma, and lung function. *The New England Journal of Medicine, 358*, 1682–1691.

Papiris, S., Kotanidou, A., Malagari, K., & Roussos, C. (2002). Clinical review: Severe asthma. *Crit Care, 6*(1), 30–44.

Pearce, N., Douwes, J., & Beasley, R. (2000). Is allergen exposure the major primary cause of asthma? *Thorax, 55*, 424–431.

Pearce, N., Pekkanen, J., & Beasley, R. (1999). How much asthma is really attributable to atopy? *Thorax, 54*, 268–272.

Pearce, N., Sunyer, J., Cheng, S., Chinn, S., Bjorksten, B., Burr, M., … Burney, P. (2000). Comparison of asthma prevalence in the ISAAC and the ECRHS. ISAAC Steering Committee and the European Community Respiratory Health Survey. International Study of Asthma and Allergies in Childhood. *European Respiratory Journal, 16*(3), 420–426.

Penard-Morand, C., Raherison, C., Kopferschmitt, C., Caillaud, D., Lavaud, F., Charpin, D., … Annesi-Maesano, I. (2005). Prevalence of food allergy and its relationship to asthma and allergic rhinitis in schoolchildren. *Allergy, 60,* 1165–1171.

Rachelefsy, G. (2009). Inhaled corticosteroids and asthma control in children: Assessing impairment and risk. *Pediatrics, 123*(1), 353–366.

Reese, T. A., Liang, H. E., Tager, A. M., Luster, A. D., Van Rooijen, N., Voehringer, D., & Locksley, R. M. (2007). Chitin induces accumulation in tissue of innate immune cells associated with allergy. *Nature, 447,* 92–96.

Robbins, S. L., & Cotran, R. S. (1979). Chapter 18. The respiratory system. In *Pathologic basis of disease* (2nd ed., pp. 818–881). Philadelphia, PA: W.B. Saunders Company.

Rönmark, E., Andersson, C., Nyström, L., Forsberg, B., Järvholmand, B., & Lundbäck, B. (2005). Obesity increases the risk of incident asthma among adults. *European Respiratory Journal, 25*(2), 282–288.

Sakula, A. (1986). Charcot-Leyden crystals and Curschmann spirals in asthmatic sputum. *Thorax, 41,* 503–507.

Samter, M., & Beers, R. F. (1968). Intolerance to aspirin. Clinical studies and consideration of its pathogenesis. *Annals of Internal Medicine, 68*(5), 975–983.

Schroeder, A., Kumar, R., Pongracic, J. A., Sullivan, C. L., Caruso, D. M., Costello, J., … Wang, X. (2009). Food allergy is associated with an increased risk of asthma. *Clinical and Experimental Allergy, 39*(2), 261–270.

Sears, M. R., Burrows, B., Flannery, E. M., Herbison, G. P., Hewitt, C. J., & Holdaway, M. D. (1991). Relation between airway responsiveness and serum IgE in children with asthma and in apparently normal children. *The New England Journal of Medicine, 325,* 1067–1071.

Senthilselvan, A., Lawson, J., Rennie, D. C., & Dosman, J. A. (2003). Stabilization of an increasing trend in physician-diagnosed asthma prevalence in Saskatchewan, 1991 to 1998. *Chest, 124*(2), 438–448.

Shaaban, R., Zureik, M., Soussan, D., Antó, J. M., Heinrich, J., Janson, C., … Leynaert, B. (2007). Allergic rhinitis and onset of bronchial hyperresponsiveness: A population-based study. *American Journal of Respiratory and Critical Care Medicine, 176,* 659–666.

Sigurs, N., Bjarnason, R., Sigurbergsson, F., & Kjellman, B. (2000). Respiratory syncytial virus bronchiolitis in infancy is an important risk factor for asthma and allergy at age 7. *American Journal of Respiratory and Critical Care Medicine, 161*(5), 1501–1507.

Soriano, J. B., Abajobir, A. A., Abate, K. H., Abera, S. F., Agrawal, A., Ahmed, M. B., … Vos, T. (2017). Global, regional, and national deaths, prevalence, disability-adjusted life years, and years lived with disability for chronic obstructive pulmonary disease and asthma, 1990–2015: A systematic analysis for the Global Burden of Disease Study 2015. *The Lancet Respiratory Medicine, 5*(9), 691–706.

Sporik, R., Holgate, S. T., Platts-Mills, T. A. E., & Cogswell, J. J. (1990). Exposure to house-dust mite allergen (Der p1) and the development of asthma in childhood. A prospective study. *The New England Journal of Medicine, 323,* 502–507.

Strachan, D. P. (1989). Hay fever, hygiene and household size. *BMJ, 299*(6710), 1259–1260.

Strachan, D. P., & Cook, D. G. (1998). Parental smoking and childhood asthma: Longitudinal and case-control studies. *Thorax, 53*(3), 204–212.

Torrent, M., Sunyer, J., Garcia, R., Harris, J., Iturriaga, M. V., Puig, C., … Cullinan, P. (2007). Early-life allergen exposure and atopy, asthma, and wheeze up to 6 years of age. *American Journal of Respiratory and Critical Care Medicine, 176,* 446–453.

Vork, K. L., Broadwin, R. L., & Blaisdell, R. J. (2007). Developing asthma in childhood from exposure to secondhand tobacco smoke: Insights from a meta-regression. *Environmental Health Perspectives, 115*(10), 1394–1400.

Wegmann, M. (2009). Th2 cells as targets for therapeutic intervention in allergic bronchial asthma. *Expert Review of Molecular Diagnostics, 9*(1), 85–100.

Weinmayr, G., Weiland, S. K., Björkstén, B., Brunekreef, B., Büchele, G., Cookson, W. O. C., … Wong, G. W., and the ISAAC Phase Two Study Group. (2007). Atopic sensitization and the international variation of asthma symptom prevalence in children. *American Journal of Respiratory and Critical Care Medicine, 176,* 565–574.

WHO. (2009). *Death and DALY estimates for 2004 by cause for WHO Member States (Persons, all ages)*. Geneva: World Health Organization.

Widal, M. F. (1922). Anaphylaxie et idiosyncrasie. *La Presse médicale, 119,* 48–51.

Wu, P., Dupont, W. D., Griffin, M. R., Carroll, K. N., Mitchel, E. F., Gebretsadik, T., & Hartert, T. V. (2008). Evidence of a causal role of winter virus infection during infancy in early childhood asthma. *American Journal of Respiratory and Critical Care Medicine, 11,* 1123–1129.

Zock, J. P., Plana, E., Jarvis, D., Antó, J. M., Kromhout, H., Kennedy, S. M., … Torén, K. (2007). The use of household cleaning sprays and adult asthma: An international longitudinal study. *American Journal of Respiratory and Critical Care Medicine, 176,* 735–741.

CHAPTER 41

Epidemiology of Diabetes Mellitus

Susanne K. Scott and Randall E. Harris

▶ Introduction

Diabetes mellitus is a complex chronic metabolic disease characterized by high fasting blood glucose. The two major forms of diabetes, type 1 and type 2, arise by different mechanisms. Elevated blood glucose, or hyperglycemia, arises when insulin, a key hormone produced by the beta (β) cells of the *islets of Langerhans* of the pancreas, is either no longer secreted (diabetes type 1) or no longer able to adequately facilitate glucose entry into the cells for energy production (diabetes type 2).

Because of its unprecedented global impact since the early 1980s, diabetes may be incorrectly labeled or considered only a contemporary disease. This is largely due to its strong association with prominent features of modern-day lifestyle, primarily increasing caloric intake and decreasing physical activity, which have contributed to an equally alarming global increase in the prevalence of obesity. The historical written record that describes the medical condition of diabetes, however, has a cross-cultural lineage spanning thousands of years.

▶ Historical Summary of Diabetes Mellitus

Diabetes mellitus has an ancient recorded history dating to 5th century BC Indian texts. The earliest description of cases included thirst, emaciation, and excessive output of sweet urine (Eknoyan & Nagy, 2005). Ancient Egyptian documents (Buqrat, 460 BC, and Papyrus of Ebers, *circa* 1550 BC) described excessive urine output but without reference to sweet urine (Ali, Anwar, Ahmed, & Chand, 2006). The Chinese (Huang Ti's Canon of Medicine, *Nei Ching Su Wen*, revised during 475–221 BC, and Chang Chung-Ching, 229 AD) described classic diabetes mellitus in much the same way as the Indian Hindus, who most likely observed patients with type 2 diabetes, linking the disease with risk factors such as socioeconomic status ("*the rich*"), excess calories ("*large quantities*"), and simple carbohydrates ("*rice, cereal, sweets*") (Eknoyan & Nagy, 2005; Guthrie & Humphreys, 1988; Henschen, 1969).

While Demetrius of Apamea (*circa* first or 2nd century BC) has been credited with coining the term "diabetes," which derives from Greek origins and means "to siphon" (Henschen, 1969), Aretaeus of Cappadocia (*circa* 81–138 AD) first clinically described diabetes (Ali et al., 2006; Kirchof, Popat, & Malowany, 2008) and wrote of a "cure" in his book entitled *Therapeutics of Chronic Diseases* (Henschen, 1969).

Aretaeus, and later, Galen of Pergamum (*circa* 129–200 AD), whose experiments on dogs showed the kidneys to be the source of urine, considered diabetes to be a rare disease of the kidneys (Gemmill, 1972). Both men, however, never commented on the sweetness of urine, leading one to question whether it was *diabetes insipidus*, commonly caused by antidiuretic hormone (ADH) deficiency, and not *diabetes mellitus* that they were describing (Henschen, 1969). For the half-century following Galen, Greek physicians cited Galen's descriptive, theoretical, and etiologic work on diabetes, and contributed new medical literature focusing primarily on treatments that included medicinal herbs, wines, and bloodletting (Christopoulou-Aletra & Papavramidou, 2008).

Early historical writings show that tasting urine was the first diagnostic diabetes test. The early Egyptians, Indians, and Asians noted the sweet taste of urine from patients, and Chang Chung-Ching (229 AD) stated that "*the urine was so sweet that the dogs liked it.*" Hindu medical textbooks from the 5th century described sweet honey and sugarcane urine of patients (Guthrie & Humphreys, 1988). Theodore Protospatharios (630 AD) recommended examining the residue of heated of urine as a diagnostic test (Henschen, 1969).

Like the Indian Hindus centuries before, the Iranian physician Avicenna (980–1037), the Swiss physician Paracelsus (1493–1541), and the Italian anatomist Morgagni (1635–1683) all described the urine of patients as tasting sweet. Paracelsus concluded that diabetes was caused by salt deposition in the kidneys, which led to *polydipsia* (excessive thirst) and *polyuria* (excessive urine). He based this on the observation that an unknown white substance remained after evaporating urine from diabetic patients (Ali et al., 2006; Pickup & William, 1997).

In 1674, the English physician Thomas Willis (1621–1675) tasted the urine of afflicted patients and gave the disease the name diabetes *mellitus*, meaning honey sweet (Eknoyan & Nagy, 2005), which he differentiated from *diabetes insipidus* in his classic work, *Pharmaceutice Rationalis*. A century passed before Robert Wyatt in 1774 and Mathew Dobson in 1776 showed that the sweetness in urine was accompanied by sugar in the blood (Eknoyan & Nagy, 2005).

In the 19th and early 20th centuries, the first quantitative clinical and diagnostic tools were developed to test for elevated sugar in the urine (*glycosuria*) and blood (*hyperglycemia*). In addition, French, Italian, German, and American researchers studied and experimented on the liver, digestive system, and pancreas. Diabetologist Apollinaire Bouchardat (1806–1886) noticed the disappearance of glycosuria among food-rationed diabetics in Paris during the Franco-Prussian War. He subsequently treated diabetic patients with fasting and low carbohydrate diets. Bouchardat also observed that weight reduction and exercise improved metabolism and he is credited with developing the paradigm of patient education and personal responsibility for

diabetic control (Chast, 2000). The discovery of insulin in 1921 by Canadian scientists Frederick Banting, Charles Best, John James Rickard Macleod, and James Collip forever transformed type 1 diabetes from a rare and fatal disease to one where prolonged survival was possible (Gale, 2002).

▶ Role of Insulin in Diabetes

Carbohydrate is the preferred source of energy for the human body. Glucose, a monosaccharide, is the basic unit of complex carbohydrates and is the primary sugar metabolized for energy. The cellular use of carbohydrate for energy depends upon multiple factors including the digestive breakdown of complex carbohydrates to glucose, the absorption of glucose through the small intestine, and the transport of glucose via the portal circulation to the cells that use it. Glucose uptake occurs first in the liver where excess glucose is packaged and stored in limited quantities as glycogen before systemic distribution to the rest of the tissues of the body.

Insulin is synthesized and secreted by the beta (β) cells of the endocrine pancreas within specialized areas called the *islets of Langerhans*. Insulin release into the bloodstream is rapidly triggered in response to increased blood glucose, for example, after a carbohydrate-rich meal. In turn, insulin induces glucose uptake for energy production in muscle cells and storage in fat cells.

Glucose enters most cells of the body through facilitated diffusion via a family of transmembrane proteins called glucose transporters (Gould & Holman, 1993). Some cells, specifically those of striated muscle (myocytes) and fat (adipocytes), require insulin to facilitate glucose uptake, whereas others such as neurons, retinal cells, red blood cells, and kidney cells do not. Insulin-stimulated cellular uptake of glucose is initiated when insulin binds to insulin-specific receptors located within the plasma membrane of target cells (Shepherd & Kahn, 1999).

Glucose transporter 4 (GLUT-4) is the gateway for insulin-mediated cellular glucose uptake (Shepherd & Kahn, 1999). Once insulin binds with the insulin receptor, a cascade of physiologic intracellular signaling events unfolds, including translocation of GLUT-4 from a nonactivated state within cytoplasmic vesicles to insertion within the plasma membrane, where cellular uptake of glucose then proceeds (Czech & Corvera, 1999; Kandror & Pilch, 1996; Pessin, Thurmond, Elmendorf, Coker, & Okada, 1999). The process is depicted in **FIGURE 41.1**.

FIGURE 41.1 Effects of Insulin on Glucose Uptake and Metabolism.

Diabetes mellitus is a disease state of persistent inappropriate excess blood glucose (hyperglycemia) caused by the inability of *endogenous* insulin to adequately mediate glucose uptake for the target cells that require it. Reasons for inadequate insulin action may include lack of insulin production by the β-cells of the pancreas (insulin insufficiency) and reduced, downregulated, or dysregulated insulin receptor signaling (insulin resistance).

▶ Diagnosis of Diabetes

Several blood glucose tests are available and recommended for the diagnosis of diabetes. A diagnosis is made when the blood glucose exceeds a clinically identified threshold level or diagnostic cut point for the particular test in use (**TABLE 41.1**). A repeat confirmatory same-test is recommended on a subsequent day for a definitive diagnosis (American Diabetes Association, 2010).

Fasting Plasma Glucose Test

The fasting plasma glucose test is currently considered the diagnostic test of choice over other available tests, such as the hemoglobin A1c and the 2-hour post-load plasma glucose test, primarily due to the ease, convenience, speed, patient acceptability, cost, reproducibility, and reduced intraindividual variation of the test. According to the American Diabetes Association, the fasting blood glucose is also able to predict microvascular complications to a similar degree as the complex and more expensive 2-hour post-load plasma glucose tolerance test (American Diabetes Association, 2010).

As the name implies, a minimal overnight 8-hour fast is required prior to the test, and a diagnosis of diabetes is made when the fasting blood glucose is 126 mg/dL or greater.

Oral Glucose Tolerance Test

The oral glucose tolerance test is considered the *gold standard* of diagnostic tests for diabetes; however, it is more complex and expensive than other tests, and also requires fasting for at least 8 hours prior to testing (National Institute of Diabetes and Digestive and Kidney Diseases, NIDDK, 2008). To obtain the glucose tolerance for a patient, the fasting blood glucose is measured at baseline, and a standard dose of glucose is then given (75 g) and plasma glucose is measured 2 hours later. A fasting level of 126 mg/dL or higher and a post-load level of 200 mg/dL is diagnostic of diabetes.

Random Blood Test

A random blood glucose test may be used as a screening test if diabetic symptoms are present. This test assumes a nonfasted state and therefore allows for higher glucose values. A test result of 200 mg/dL or higher warrants further testing using one of the clinically recommended diagnostic blood glucose tests (NIDDK, 2008).

Hemoglobin A1c Test (HbA1c)

Hemoglobin A1c (HbA1c) is the newest blood test recommended for diagnosing diabetes (American Diabetes Association, 2010). It assesses average

TABLE 41.1 Diagnostic Tests for Diabetes

Diagnostic Test	Normal	Prediabetes	Diabetes
Fasting glucose (mg/dL)	<100	100–125	>126
Glucose tolerance (mg/dL)	<140	140–199	>200
Random blood test (mg/dL)	<140	140–100	>200
Hemoglobin A1c	<6.0%	6.0%–6.5%	>6.5%

glucose levels over a 2–3-month period. Fasting is not required for the test. Traditionally, HbA1c is used by diabetics to monitor blood glucose levels. In this capacity, the level of HbA1c can be used as an indicator of treatment effectiveness. A diagnosis of diabetes is made when the HbA1c is 6.5% or higher. The HbA1c test quantifies the percentage of hemoglobin (the oxygen carrying molecule of the red blood cell) that has been bound by glucose within the 120-day life span of the red blood cell (Kilpatrick, 2000). The nonenzymatic binding of glucose to hemoglobin is called *glycosylation* or *glycation*. The higher the blood glucose, the higher the level of glycated hemoglobin (Gomero et al., 2008).

Types of Diabetes

There are two major types of diabetes mellitus (types 1 and 2), which are differentiated, in large part, by their underlying etiologies. In type 1 diabetes, the pancreas no longer produces insulin, primarily due to autoimmune destruction of the β-cells. Type 1 diabetes is therefore characterized as *insulin dependent*. It develops primarily in children and accounts for about 5%–10% of all diabetics.

In classic type 2 diabetes, insulin is still produced and secreted, but because of *insulin resistance* of target cells coupled with relative *insulin insufficiency*, blood glucose is not adequately controlled. Type 2 diabetes develops primarily in adults and accounts for 90%–95% of all diabetics. Conditions that lead to ineffective insulin action are likely influenced by various combinations of underlying genetic, inherited, congenital, acquired, and/or environmental factors.

A third type, gestational diabetes, is diagnosed during pregnancy (Homko, 2010). Pregnancy increases the metabolic workload of the maternal pancreas and heightens both insulin resistance and insulin insufficiency.

Other etiologic forms of diabetes are due to rare genetic defects of the β-cells and defects in insulin action, signaling, or secretion. Diabetes can also be caused by diseases of the exocrine pancreas such as cystic fibrosis, endocrinopathies (e.g., Cushing syndrome), certain infections (e.g., congenital rubella and cytomegalovirus), certain medications (chemotherapeutics and glucocorticoids), as well as rare autoimmune disorders and genetic syndromes, such as Down syndrome or Prader–Willi syndrome (NIDDK, 2010).

Global Pandemic of Diabetes Mellitus

The beginning of the 21st century marked a profound increase in the global burden of diabetes, which is now described as a pandemic (Narayan et al., 2006). While heightened levels of obesity and greater longevity are clearly important determinants of this worldwide phenomenon, the web of causation is complex and involves multiple factors including fetal and childhood growth and development, maternal biology and influence, genetics, nutrition, urbanization, automation, perceptions of weight gain, changes in food costs, greater access to foods high in fat and calories, and proclivity to lack of exercise through a sedentary lifestyle. As pointed out by Dr. Lucy Candib (2007) in her essay on diabetes and obesity in vulnerable populations,

> *The strategy with the most powerful long-term effect in curtailing the escalation is reduction in the prevalence of obesity. [Nevertheless] The merger of many interacting forces conjoined in creating this global phenomenon calls for explanatory models and ways of thinking that go beyond traditional singular notions of causality.* (pp. 541–556)

▶ Global Prevalence of Diabetes

Diabetes mellitus is currently the most frequently diagnosed of non-communicable diseases and the fastest-growing chronic disease in the world (Gupta & Kumar, 2008; Sudagani & Hitman, 2005). According to survey data from the 221 member nations and territories of the International Diabetes Federation (IDF), 451 million adults aged 18–99 years of age had diabetes in 2017, an increase of 58% from the estimated 285 million adults with diabetes in 2010, and more than 2.6 times the estimated 171 million adults with diabetes in 2000 (Cho et al., 2018; IDF, Diabetes Atlas, 2006, 2010, 2017).

Across *all* age groups, the worldwide prevalence of diabetes has more than tripled in the 21st century, rising from 2.8% in 2000 to 8.6% in 2017 (Cho et al., 2018; IDF Diabetes Atlas, 2010). The greatest increase in prevalence has occurred among the elderly, rising from <5% in 1970 to nearly 18% in 2017 for adults 65 years or older (**FIGURE 41.2**).

Since 2015, investigators of the IDF have gathered information to estimate not only the prevalence of diabetes, but also the fraction of cases that remain undiagnosed. It is remarkable that during 2017, nearly half of all people living with diabetes in the world population were undiagnosed. The absence of screening for diabetes is particularly dire in low-income populations where more than 75% of cases remain undiagnosed, and even in many highly developed nations, it is estimated that more than one-third of diabetics are undiagnosed (Cho et al., 2018).

The global pandemic of diabetes is largely due to type 2 diabetes that predominantly strikes in adulthood. In 1995, survey data from 188 member nations of the World Health Organization (WHO) revealed that 4.0% of adults aged 20 years or older had diabetes (King, Aubert, & Herman, 1998). In 2010, IDF investigators analyzed survey data from 216 member nations and territories and found that 6.6% of adults aged 20–79 years had diabetes (IDF Atlas, 2010). In that same year, an independent team of investigators found a similar prevalence of 6.4% based on analysis of population surveys from 91 countries (Shaw, Sicree, & Zimmit, 2010). During 2017, IDF investigators reported prevalence estimates of 8.4% in women and 8.9% in men aged 18–99 years (Cho et al., 2018).

These data reflect an alarming 4% annual increase in the worldwide prevalence of adult diabetes over the past 22 years. If this steep trajectory continues, the worldwide number of diabetics is expected to exceed 400 million by 2025 and will surpass 693 million by 2045, essentially quadrupling the absolute number of diabetics during the past half-century (Cho et al., 2018; Hossain, Kawar, & El Nahas, 2007; Shaw et al., 2010; Wild, Roglic, Green, Sicree, & King, 2004).

The international survey data show wide variation in the prevalence of adult diabetes among countries (**FIGURE 41.3**). Most notably, the Republic of Nauru, an island nation in Micronesia in the southwest Pacific, had the highest prevalence in 2010 (nearly 31%) while the Republic of Rwanda, located in the East-Central African highlands, had the lowest (about 1%). The prevalence was also high (>15%) in several other island nations of Micronesia and in nations bordering the Persian Gulf such as the United Arab Emirates and Saudi Arabia (Naeem, 2015). In Egypt, the prevalence of type 2 diabetes has risen above 15% for adults aged 20–79 years (Hegazi, El-Gamal, Abdel-Hady, & Hamdy, 2015). In China, a nationally representative sample found that over 92 million adults had diabetes in 2008 (9.7% of the adult population) and 148 million had prediabetes (15.5% of the adult population) (Yang et al., 2010). In the Western hemisphere, recent prevalence estimates exceed 9% for the populations of

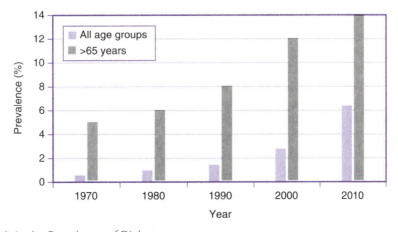

FIGURE 41.2 Global Trends in the Prevalence of Diabetes.

Data from World Health Organization, 1970–2010. IDF Diabetes Atlas, 4th ed.; Cho, N. H., Shaw, J. E., Karuranga, S., Huang, Y., da Rocha Fernandes, J. D., Ohlrogge, A. W., & Malanda, B. (2018). IDF Diabetes Atlas: Global estimates of diabetes prevalence for 2017 and projections for 2045. *Diabetes Research and Clinical Practice, 138,* 271–281.

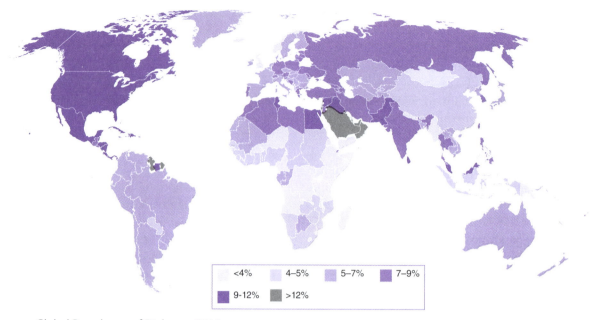

FIGURE 41.3 Global Prevalence of Diabetes, 2010.
Reproduced from World Health Organization. *The global burden of disease: 2010.* Available at www.who.int/evidence/bod

Mexico, Canada, and the United States (IDF Diabetes Atlas, 2010, 2017).

The global pattern of prevalent diabetes is similar to that of obesity and energy consumption. Nations where the prevalence is high have a greater burden of obesity (>30%) and higher levels of energy intake per capita (>3200 kcals per day); reciprocally, nations in which the prevalence is low have less obesity (<15%) and consume less energy (<2800 kcals per day). The data suggest that diabetes is uncommon in developing countries where a traditional lifestyle has been preserved, whereas communities that have undergone westernization and urbanization are at higher risk (Hossain et al., 2007).

The accelerating worldwide prevalence of diabetes has occurred in concert with changes in population dynamics and demography. In particular, more people are living beyond the age of 65 years when the diabetic risk is high (Wild et al., 2004), and many nations are experiencing urbanization, or the migration of their populations from rural areas to cities (Candib, 2007). In particular, the increasing prevalence of type 2 diabetes is closely linked to the upsurge in obesity (Hossain et al., 2007; Sobngwi et al., 2004).

▶ Distribution of Diabetes by Gender and Age

Investigators of the IDF recently compiled data from population samples in 221 countries and territories to estimate the age-gender-specific prevalence of diabetes. The importance of age is illustrated in **FIGURE 41.4**. The prevalence increases exponentially with age reaching maximums of approximately 20% in men at age 65 years and 19% in women at age 70 years. Prevalence estimates are higher for men than women until age 75 and then become slightly higher in elderly women compared to men (Cho et al., 2018). The observed gender difference late in life is most likely due to the combined effects of there being more elderly women than men in most populations and the increasing prevalence of diabetes in the upper age brackets (Wild et al., 2004).

▶ Global Deaths Attributable to Diabetes

The global death toll from diabetes is trending upward in the 21st century, increasing from 3.2 million in the year 2000 to 5.0 million in 2017 (**FIGURE 41.5**). Likewise, the proportionate mortality of diabetes increased from 6% to nearly 10% during the same period (Cho et al., 2018; Roglic & Unwin, 2005, 2010).

It is important to realize that global estimates of disease mortality are primarily based upon the underlying causes of death abstracted from death certificates. Since diabetes is a major risk factor for other life-threatening events such as heart attack and stroke and since vital statistics based on death certificates are not available in some underdeveloped nations,

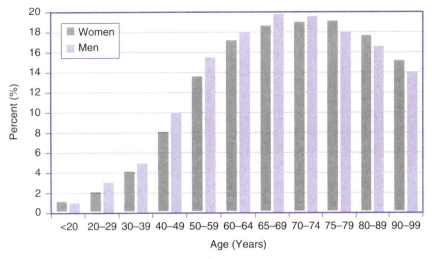

FIGURE 41.4 Age-Gender-Specific Prevalence of Diabetes Mellitus.

Data from Cho, N. H., Shaw, J. E., Karuranga, S., Huanga, Y., da Rocha Fernandes, J. D., Ohlrogge, A. W., & Malanda, B. (2018). IDF Diabetes Atlas: Global estimates of diabetes prevalence for 2017 and projections for 2045. *Diabetes Research and Clinical Practice, 138*, 271–281.

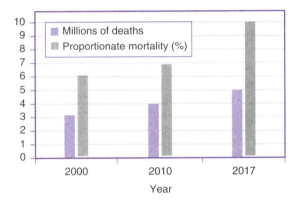

FIGURE 41.5 Diabetes Mellitus: Global Deaths and Proportionate Mortality 2000–2017.

Data from Roglic, G., & Unwin, N. (2005). Global mortality attributable to diabetes: Time for a realistic estimate. *Diabetes Voice, 50*(1), 33–34; Roglic, G., & Unwin, N. (2010). Mortality attributable to diabetes: Estimates for the year 2010. *Diabetes Research and Clinical Practice, 87*, 15–19; Cho, N. H., Shaw, J. E., Karurangaa, S., Huanga, Y., da Rocha Fernandesa, J. D., Ohlroggea, A. W., & Malandaa, B. (2018). IDF Diabetes Atlas: Global estimates of diabetes prevalence for 2017 and projections for 2045. *Diabetes Research and Clinical Practice, 138*, 271-281.

many investigators believe that the number of deaths attributable to diabetes based on vital statistics may be grossly underestimated.

To correct for potential under-reporting, WHO investigators Gojka Roglic and Nigel Unwin used census data for the world population of 2000 together with cause-specific mortality rates reported by WHO and estimates of the risk of death in diabetics versus nondiabetics derived from the literature to recalculate the deaths attributable to diabetes. They found that in 2000, 3.2 million people died from diabetes, approximately 6% of all-cause mortality for that year. Their estimates, which are approximately 10% higher than those based on death certificates, are likely to be a more accurate reflection of the death toll from diabetes (Roglic & Unwin, 2005).

In a subsequent investigation using similar methods, Roglic and Unwin calculated the number of deaths attributable to diabetes among adults aged 20–79 years for the world population of 2010 and populations residing in selected countries and geographic regions. They estimated that 3.96 million deaths were attributable to diabetes in 2010, or approximately 6.8% of all-cause global mortality. The highest number of deaths attributable to diabetes occurred in countries with the largest populations: approximately 1 million deaths in India, 575,000 in China, 231,000 in the United States, and 182,000 in the Russian Federation. Estimates of relative mortality attributable to diabetes varied widely among regions, ranging from 6% in Africa to 15.7% in North America. Estimates were also calculated for 2007 and compared with those for 2010. In the 3-year time span, the overall number of deaths attributable to diabetes increased by 5.5%. The largest increases in relative mortality were found in North America (29%), Southeast Asia (12%), and the Western Pacific (11%) (Roglic & Unwin, 2010).

The most recent estimates of deaths from diabetes and proportionate mortality reported by investigators of the IDF include individuals aged 18–99 years. Of the 5.0 million deaths from diabetes in 2017, 4 million occurred among people living in low- and middle-income countries, and in low-income countries, 73% of the diabetes-related deaths occurred before the age of 60 years. The results indicate that diabetes is a leading cause of premature death worldwide, and the death toll is expected to rise further, particularly in developing countries where the prevalence is increasing and access to health care is limited (Cho et al., 2018; Roglic & Unwin, 2010).

▶ Disability-Adjusted Life Years for Diabetes

The disability-adjusted life years (DALY) lost from diabetes measures the years of life lost due to premature death (YLL) plus the years lost to severe disability (YLD), DALY = YLL + YLD. National estimates of DALYs due to diabetes reported by WHO are shown in **FIGURE 41.6**. High DALYs are evident in many developing nations of Africa, the Middle East, Asia, the southwest Pacific, Central America, and South America. In nations with high DALYs (>600 per 100,000), populations are migrating from rural areas to cities (urbanization) leading to lifestyle modifications (high caloric diet and sedentary lifestyle) favoring positive energy balance, excessive weight gain, and the genesis of type 2 diabetes (Sobngwi et al., 2004). Of the 5 million annual deaths attributable to diabetes, nearly two-thirds occur in developing countries where 80% of the world population lives. It is in these nations that the general lack of access to effective sustained therapy for diabetes results in not only premature death, but also high disability.

▶ Burden of Diabetes in the United States

The prevalence of diabetes across all age groups has risen more than fivefold in the United States in the past half century, from less than 2% during 1965–1975

to 9.4% in 2015 (**FIGURE 41.7**). The greatest absolute increase occurred among the elderly; for example, the prevalence of diabetes increased from approximately 8% to over 20% for adults 65 years and older during 1980–2015 (CDC, 2010; Mokdad et al., 2001, 2000; National Diabetes Statistics Report, 2017).

Due to the absence of national screening programs, many Americans who have elevated blood glucose are not aware that they have diabetes. In recent years, fasting blood glucose and hemoglobin A1c have been tested in population samples to derive estimates of the prevalence of individuals with undetected diabetes. Based on these estimates, 30.2 million adults had diabetes in 2015 (14.9 million women and 15.3 million men), 23.0 million had physician-diagnosed diabetes (11.7 million women and 11.3 million men), and 7.2 million had undiagnosed diabetes (3.1 million women and 4.0 million men) (CDC, 2010, 2017). These data suggest that about 1 in 4 individuals with diabetes is unaware they have the disease. There is obviously an urgent need to institute broad scale screening programs in order to identify and treat individuals with type 2 diabetes who are currently unaware of their condition.

Investigators at the National Institute of Diabetes and Digestive and Kidney Disease (NIDDK) reported similar findings for adults based upon analysis of data from the National Health and Nutrition Examination Surveys (NHANES) of 1988–2006. They examined the prevalence of diabetes diagnosed by elevated hemoglobin A1c (6.5% or higher) among probability samples

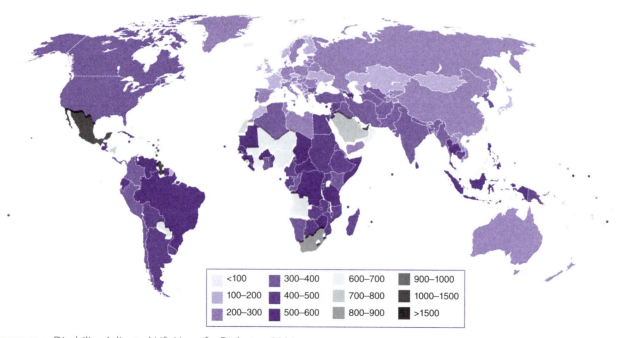

<100	300–400	600–700	900–1000
100–200	400–500	700–800	1000–1500
200–300	500–600	800–900	>1500

FIGURE 41.6 Disability-Adjusted Life Years for Diabetes, 2004.

Values are Disability-Adjusted Life Years per 100,000 individuals.

Reproduced from World Health Organization. *The global burden of disease: 2004.* Available at www.who.int/evidence/bod

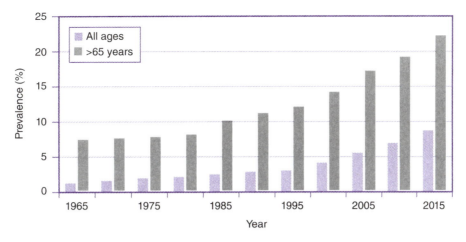

FIGURE 41.7 Prevalence of Diabetes in the United States, 1965–2015.

Data from U.S. National Health and Nutrition Survey (NHANES), 1960–2010; Centers for Disease Control and Prevention. (2010). *National Center for Chronic Disease Prevention and Health Promotion.* Division of Diabetes Translation; National Diabetes Statistics Report, 2017.

of U.S. adults aged 20 and over, and estimated the fraction of diabetics who remained undiagnosed. The age-standardized prevalence of *physician-diagnosed* diabetes increased from 5.3% to 7.6% (43%) during this time span, whereas the prevalence of *undiagnosed* diabetics declined from 2.1% to 1.6%. While gender differences were not apparent, standardized estimates of prevalence were nearly twice as high in Hispanics and African Americans as in Caucasians.

Investigators at the Centers for Disease Control (CDC) used data from the National Health Interview Surveys of 1984–2000 to project the lifetime risk of diabetes by age, gender, and ethnicity for the cohort born in 2000 in the United States. The estimated lifetime risk of developing diabetes was 32.8% in men and 38.5% in women. Hispanic men and women had the highest lifetime risks, 45.4% and 52.5%, respectively. In addition, the life span of a person diagnosed with diabetes at age 40 was found to be 11 years shorter (for men) and 14 years shorter (for women) than disease-free individuals (Narayan, Boyle, Thompson, Sorensen, & Williamson, 2003).

Overall, these results underscore the continuing rise in the incidence and prevalence of diabetes among U.S. adults in this century, particularly among Hispanics and African Americans; they also suggest that 20%–25% of diabetics remain undiagnosed (Cowie et al., 2010). Clearly, diabetes has reached epidemic proportions in the U.S. population.

▶ Mortality from Diabetes in the United States

Concurrent with the dramatic increase in the prevalence of diabetes in the United States during the past three decades, the death toll has also accelerated.

According to vital statistics abstracted from death certificates in 2005, diabetes contributed to more than 233,000 deaths and was directly responsible for more than 75,000 deaths. The relative mortality (percentage of all deaths) due to diabetes in that year reached a peak at 3.1% (Kung, Hoyert, Xu, & Murphy, 2008). During 2015, diabetes contributed to 253,000 deaths and was the underlying cause of death listed on 79,500 death certificates (CDC, 2010, 2017; Murphy et al., 2017). By comparison, in 1980, diabetes was responsible for 36,000 deaths and the relative mortality was 1.8% (Rogot, Sorlie, Johnson, Glover, & Makus, 1985). Estimates of relative mortality reflect a fourfold increase in deaths from diabetes since 1960 (**FIGURE 41.8**).

A number of studies suggest that diabetes is likely to be under-reported as the main cause of death or a contributing factor on death certificates. Investigators at the CDC used data from the 1986 *National Mortality Followback Survey* to estimate the frequency that diabetes was recorded on the death certificates of diabetics. They examined death certificates of 2766 decedents who were diabetic in life and found that diabetes was recorded on 38.2% of certificates and 9.6% as the underlying cause of death. The investigators concluded that diabetes is usually not listed on the death certificate and is more likely to be recorded for older patients with long-standing disease or comorbid conditions (Bild & Stevenson, 1992).

A research team from the University of Michigan examined the frequency of reported diabetes on the death certificates of 540 decedents with known diabetes. Subjects were enrolled in the *Translating Research into Action for Diabetes Study* (TRIAD), a multicenter prospective study of nearly 12,000 participants with diabetes. Diabetes was recorded on 39% of death certificates and as the underlying cause of death for only 10% of decedents. The investigators

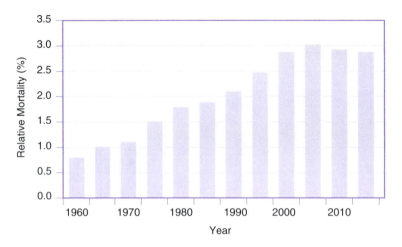

FIGURE 41.8 Relative Mortality of Diabetes in the United States, 1960–2015.

Data from U.S. National Health and Nutrition Survey (NHANES), 1960–2010; Centers for Disease Control and Prevention. (2010). *National Center for Chronic Disease Prevention and Health Promotion*. Division of Diabetes Translation; Murphy, S. L., Xu, J., Kochanek, K. D., Curtin, S. C., & Arias, E. (2017). Deaths: Final data for 2015. *National Vital Statistics Reports, 66*(6).

concluded that vital statistics based on death certificates markedly underestimate the prevalence of diabetes among decedents (McEwen et al., 2006).

Investigators at the University of California in San Diego examined reporting of diabetes on the death certificates of 3209 decedents who were enrolled in the *Rancho Bernardo* cohort in 1972–1974 and followed to 2003. Of those who died, 378 had a history of diabetes but only 168 (44%) had diabetes reported anywhere on the death certificate. Diabetes was approximately twice as likely to be reported on the death certificates of diabetics who died of cardiovascular causes compared with other causes, reflecting increased recognition that diabetes is a major cardiovascular risk factor (Cheng, Wingard, Kritz-Silverstein, & Barrett-Connor, 2008).

▶ Population-Based Models of Diabetes

In type 1 diabetes, the pancreas no longer produces insulin, primarily due to autoimmune destruction of the β-cells. With classical type 2 diabetes, insulin is still produced and secreted, but because of insulin resistance of target cells coupled with relative insulin insufficiency, blood glucose is not adequately controlled. All conditions that lead to ineffective insulin action are likely influenced by various combinations of underlying genetic, congenital, acquired, and/or environmental factors and their interactions. In addition, the temporal sequence of these conditions and the cause and consequence pathways to the onset of diabetes add to the heterogeneity and complexity surrounding the pathogenesis of diabetes.

Etiologic complexities of diabetes are illustrated by a brief summary of hypothetical population-based models that seek to explain the origin of the global pandemic of diabetes. Neel's *thrifty genotype hypothesis* implicates the evolutionary selection of "*thrifty genes*," which facilitate efficient storage of fat during times of nutritional abundance, and which helped hunter–gatherer populations survive times of famine and food scarcity (Neel, 1962). Neel postulated that the genetic selection that served human populations so well in the past has been "*rendered detrimental by progress*." In other words, an abundance of food and calories that are perpetually available will inevitably lead to obesity and obesity-related chronic diseases, such as type 2 diabetes.

Various mechanisms have been advanced to explain the link between excess caloric intake, obesity, and type 2 diabetes. Adipose tissue clearly plays a central role in pathogenesis since it is the chief reservoir for the storage of body fat and an essential regulatory organ in maintaining energy homeostasis. The "energy storage capacity" of adipose tissue is restricted by the size, number, and metabolic integrity of adipocytes. Several investigators therefore suggest that type 2 diabetes is the result of the inability of the adipocyte population to expand and undergo sufficient cellular differentiation to accommodate excess calories (Danforth, 2000; Leonhardt, Hanefeld, Schneider, & Haller, 1972; Scott, Rabito, Butler, & Harris, 2004). A corollary to the *energy storage capacity hypothesis* is that unremitting caloric surplus is complicated by the failure of adipocytes to maintain protection against lipotoxicity. Protective factors include enhanced proliferation of adipocytes (lipogenesis) and secretion of protective adipokines such as leptin and adiponection. Leptin has been found to suppress appetite and induce fatty acid oxidation thereby reducing toxicity from the accumulation of fat, ceramide, and cholesterol in skeletal muscle, liver, and other tissues, and adiponection has anti-inflammatory, pro-angiogenic, and anti-apoptotic properties. Conversely, when the energy storage capacity of the adipocyte population is surpassed, protection against lipotoxicity is severely compromised due to secretion of excessive inflammatory adipokines such as resistin coupled with rising concentrations of circulating triglycerides and fatty acids. These are key factors in the development of not only insulin resistance, but also β-cell insufficiency and depletion due to the heightened demand for insulin (Bays, Mandarino, & DeFronzo, 2004; Frühbeck, Gomez-Ambrosi, Muruzabai, & Burrell, 2001; Petersen & Shulman, 2006; Unger & Scherer, 2010; Willett, Manson, & Liu, 2002).

Other models have been proposed in which nutritional conditions in the prenatal and postnatal environments influence the later development of type 2 diabetes. The *thrifty phenotype hypothesis*, also known as the *fetal origins hypothesis*, proposes that poor nutritional conditions during fetal development lead to intrauterine growth restriction and produce phenotypic changes such as low birth weight and body size, lowered metabolism, and altered glucose-insulin metabolism that are adapted for nutritional scarcity later in life (Barker, 1997; Hales & Barker, 1992). If, during postnatal growth and development of the child, the nutritional environment then becomes plentiful, inappropriate (accelerated) growth trajectory may occur, thereby resulting in the development of chronic health conditions later in life.

A variation of the fetal origins hypothesis is the theory of *metabolic programming* in which adaptation of the fetus to nutritional stress at a sensitive period of development leads to permanent changes in physiology and metabolism (Lucas, 1991). Animal studies have shown that maternal malnutrition during fetal development results in permanent effects in the offspring, including reduced pancreatic islet vascularization, size and function, and heightened insulin resistance, lending some support to the concept of metabolic programming (Patel, Srinivasan, & Aalinkeel, 2000).

Human studies also suggest that long-term postnatal development may be modified by metabolic experiences in utero. For example, Silverman and colleagues found that the offspring of diabetic mothers is more likely to become obese and develop impaired glucose tolerance than controls (Silverman, Metzger, Cho, & Loeb, 1995; Silverman, Rizzo, Cho, & Metzger, 1998). Dabelea and colleagues compared siblings born

before and after their mother developed diabetes in 19 families ascertained from the Pima Indian tribe residing in Arizona. This special population has one of the highest rates of type 2 diabetes in the world. The study revealed that siblings born *after* their mothers were diagnosed with diabetes were three times more likely to develop type 2 diabetes and have higher body mass than siblings born before. Results suggest that the diabetic intrauterine environment conveys a high risk for the development of diabetes and obesity to offspring (Dabelea et al., 2000).

Obviously, these proposed models and mechanisms are not mutually exclusive and may interact to heighten the risk of developing insulin resistance and glucose intolerance. Such models provide a template for continuing investigation of the genetic, endocrine, metabolic, and morphological changes that underlie the etiopathogenesis of type 2 diabetes.

▶ The Health Impact of Diabetes

Diabetes has been found to increase the risk of developing a variety of comorbid conditions. Compared to nondiabetic subjects, diabetics have two- to fourfold higher rates of ischemic heart disease, stroke, and hypertension and five- to tenfold higher rates of blindness, kidney disease, neuropathy, and amputation. When comparing people with and without diabetes, the death rate among men is almost double (1.9), while among women it is 2.6 (Lee, Cheung, Cape, & Zinman, 2000). Furthermore, persons with diabetes suffer disproportionately from physical and cognitive disability and have twice the risk of developing dementia in old age compared to nondiabetics (Engelgau et al., 2004).

Although diabetes is among the top 10 leading causes of death in the United States and the fastest-growing non-communicable disease in the world, the onset of type 2 diabetes can often go undetected for years before a medical diagnosis is made (Gregg et al., 2004; Harris, Klein, Welborn, & Knuiman, 1992). In many developing countries, up to 90% of people with adult-onset diabetes are undiagnosed. In China, roughly 6 out of 10 diabetics are undiagnosed. Lack of public awareness and diagnostic opportunities are cited as reasons for the high percentage of undiagnosed diabetes in poor and developing countries (IDF Diabetes Atlas, 2010). Even in developed countries such as the United States, up to 30% of diabetes cases are undiagnosed (Gregg et al., 2004). This is because hyperglycemia, similar to hypertension, often lacks clinical signs and symptoms. The following paragraphs discuss the pathogenesis of conditions that commonly arise in diabetics and which contribute significantly to their high rates of morbidity and mortality.

Diabetic Ketoacidosis

Diabetic ketoacidosis is a life-threatening phenomenon that occurs in individuals with severe hyperglycemia (blood glucose levels exceeding 250 mg/dL). Most patients who develop ketoacidosis have poorly controlled type 1 (insulin-dependent) diabetes mellitus, and about one-fifth of cases are first-time presenters with newly diagnosed disease. Nevertheless, varying degrees of ketoacidosis has been increasingly recognized among patients with type 2 diabetes. Poor patient education is an important determinant of this catastrophic event (Eledrisi, Alshanti, Shah, Brolosy, & Jaha, 2006; Kitabchi, Umpierrez, Murphy, & Kreisberg, 2006; Kitabchi & Wall, 1999).

Ketoacidosis results from an extension of normal physiological mechanisms that compensate for starvation. Normally, in the fasting state, there is a transition of metabolism from glycolysis (breakdown of glycogen) to lipolysis (breakdown of fat) for energy. Free fatty acids are released by adipocytes (fat cells) and transported to the liver bound to albumin. There they are broken down into acetate which is transformed into ketoacids (acetoacetate and beta-hydroxybutyrate). The ketoacids are then exported from the liver to peripheral tissues (notably brain and muscle) where they can be oxidized. Diabetic ketoacidosis represents a derangement of the above mechanism in diabetics with markedly elevated levels of blood glucose (hyperglycemia). Despite vast amounts of circulating glucose, it cannot be used as an energy source owing to lack of insulin. Ketogenic pathways are thus maximally activated, and the supply of ketones exceeds peripheral utilization. Ketone bodies are acidic and high concentrations lower blood pH leading to ketoacidosis. During ketosis, a relatively small amount of acetone is produced, thus giving the breath of ketotic patients a typical "fruity" smell. The high blood glucose also induces profound osmotic diuresis and dehydration resulting in deficits in key electrolytes such as sodium, potassium, chloride, phosphate, magnesium, and calcium.

Case-fatality rates among patients who develop diabetic ketoacidosis vary widely, ranging from 1% to 10%. Such variation is likely due to patients presenting at different stages of the process and/or differences in management. Causes of death in such patients include acute myocardial infarction, stroke, septic shock, profound acidosis of arterial blood, and cerebral edema. Patient management involves suppression of ketosis by administration of insulin, fluid resuscitation, and restoration of electrolyte balance in the blood, plus treatment of any coexisting conditions (Eledrisi et al., 2006; Kitabchi et al., 2006; Kitabchi & Wall, 1999).

Microvascular Complications of Diabetes

Undetected or uncontrolled type 2 diabetes often results in silent pathology that can do irreparable damage at the *microvascular* (small blood vessel) level, causing irreversible consequences to health and quality of life such as diabetic retinopathy and blindness, diabetic nephropathy and kidney failure, and/or diabetic neuropathy and amputation (Fowler, 2008; Moss, Klein, & Klein, 1991). Primary pathogenic mechanisms include increased intracellular oxidative stress, increased proinflammatory activity, and the accelerated formation of advanced glycation end-products (AGEs), which are a class of complex reactive compounds that alter the structural properties of tissue proteins (Brownlee, 2005; Hatfield & Mulfinger, 2005). Unlike most cells that can control the concentration of intracellular glucose, susceptible cell types, specifically capillary endothelieal cells in the retina, mesangial cells in the renal glomeruli, and neurons/schwann cells in the peripheral nerves, are unprotected from extracellular glycemic exposure (Brownlee, 2005). Population-based studies have shown that by the time type 2 diabetes is diagnosed, over 20% of patients already have diabetic retinopathy and 10% have nephropathy (Harris et al., 1992; Klein, Klein, Moss, & Demets, 1988). Diabetes is, in fact, a leading cause of these devastating conditions and they account for much of the economic burden associated with the disease (WHO Expert Consultation, 2004).

Macrovascular Complications of Diabetes

Extended duration of undiagnosed or uncontrolled hyperglycemia increases the risk for macrovascular (large blood vessel) complications (Fowler, 2008; Stratton et al., 2001; Younis, Broadbent, Vora, & Harding, 2003). For example, there is a twofold increase in overall premature mortality, a fourfold increase in deaths due to cardiovascular disease (CVD), and a fourfold increase in stroke deaths among diabetics compared to nondiabetics (USPTFS, 2008). In addition, CVD is the primary cause of death among both type 1 and type 2 diabetics, eventually killing one out of every two patients (Fowler, 2008; Wingard & Barrett-Conner, 1995).

While persistent hyperglycemia *per se* has been implicated in the microvascular complications of diabetes, mechanisms related to atherogenesis and the development of atherosclerotic plaque in blood vessels are typically invoked to explain the macrovascular complications of diabetes. For example, both in vitro and in vivo (animal) studies suggest that insulin-resistant adipocytes (fat cells) increase the *free fatty acid flux* by releasing large quantities of free fatty acids into the blood that are subsequently oxidized in the mitochondria of the vascular endothelium resulting in overproduction of reactive oxygen species (Brownlee, 2005; Petersen & Shulman, 2006). Indeed, endothelial injury resulting from increased oxidative stress is one of the primary triggers in the *response to injury hypothesis of atherogenesis* (Libby, 2002; Libby, Ridker, & Hansson, 2009; Ross, 1999; Ross & Glomset, 1976).

The *response to injury hypothesis of atherogenesis* proposes that initial injury (mechanical, chemical, oxidative, immune reactive, or infectious) to the endothelial cells causes their release of cytokines and other proinflammatory and vasoactive compounds (Ross, 1999; Ross & Glomset, 1976). These molecular events initiate a complex inflammatory cascade leading to the formation and development of atherosclerotic plaque (atherogenesis). For example, expression of *vascular cellular adhesion molecule-1 (VCAM-1)* by endothelial cells mediates the adhesion of monocytes, lymphocytes, and other immune cells to the vascular epithelium in the early stages of atherogenesis (Ley & Huo, 2001). Sustained atherogenesis and the development of atherosclerotic plaque in blood vessels are the underlying cause of the majority of deaths from cardiovascular diseases.

It is important to realize that hyperglycemia and insulin resistance often go unrecognized for many years in adults and, as a consequence, the presence of microvascular and macrovascular complications is a near certainty when type 2 diabetes is finally diagnosed (Sheehy et al., 2010). In contrast, the prominent clinical signs and symptoms of type 1 diabetes usually lead to a prompt diagnosis, and with effective treatment (insulin replacement) and glycemic control, the risk of long-term sequelae can be ameliorated (Moore, Gregory, Kumah-Crystal, & Simmons, 2009). Albeit, diabetic children are more sensitive to insulin deficiency than adults and are thus at higher risk for the rapid and catastrophic development of ketoacidosis, which is associated with significant mortality, even in countries with well-developed healthcare systems (Dahlquist & Kallen, 2005).

Epidemiology of Type 1 Diabetes

Type 1 diabetes, previously called *insulin-dependent diabetes mellitus* or *juvenile-onset diabetes*, is characterized by a lack of endogenous insulin production. It is the major form of diabetes in children and young adults and accounts for 5%–10% of all diabetics. In patients without insulin, glucose is not able to enter into the cells that require insulin-mediated glucose uptake. This can lead to dangerously high levels of blood glucose and life-threatening *diabetic ketoacidosis* (metabolic acidosis caused by the by-products of fatty acid oxidation accumulating in the blood). Because glucose is available for energy but cannot be used by the cells that require insulin's action, the phrase *starvation amidst plenty* has been linked with type 1 diabetes. Type 1 diabetes is diagnosed with a recommended blood sugar test, coupled with auto-antibody assessment, and/or the presence of classic signs and symptoms such as *ketonuria* (ketones in the urine), excessive thirst, persistent hunger, unexplained weight loss, and excessive urination.

There are two subforms of type 1 diabetes. *Type 1a* is caused by autoimmune destruction of the β-cells of the pancreas, confirmed by the presence of β-cell autoantibodies, while *type 1b* is nonautoimmune pancreatic β-cell destruction that is *idiopathic* or of unknown origin. Serum autoantibodies reactive against the pancreatic β-cells are detectable in approximately 90% of patients diagnosed with type 1 diabetes. The process of autoimmune destruction occurs in the genetically susceptible and has a rather long latency period, as a large proportion of β-cells must be destroyed before signs and symptoms of type 1 diabetes occurs (American Diabetes Association, 2010; Eisenbarth & McCulloch, 2010).

Rising Incidence of Type 1 Diabetes

The global incidence of type 1 diabetes has increased markedly in the past 50 years, especially among children under 5 years of age (Bingley & Gale, 1989; Eurodiab ACE Study Group, 2000; Gale, 2002; Gillespie et al., 2004; Krolewski, Warram, Rand, & Kahn, 1987; Onkamo, Vaananen, Karvonen, & Tuomilehto, 1999; Patterson et al., 2009). Significant increases

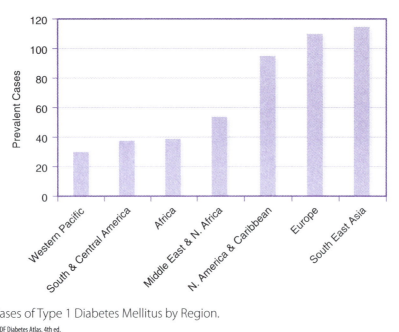

FIGURE 41.9 Prevalent Cases of Type 1 Diabetes Mellitus by Region.

Data from World Health Organization, 1970–2010. IDF Diabetes Atlas, 4th ed.

have been documented in Finland, England, Norway, Israel, Austria, and several other countries. In Finland, which has one of the world's highest rates, the annual incidence has more than tripled since 1953, from 12 per 100,000 to current levels of approximately 40 per 100,000 (Patterson et al., 2009; Tuomilehto et al., 1995). Globally, the average annual rate of increase is approximately 3%. Furthermore, there are no signs that the trend is abating. According to the International Diabetes Federation, 76,000 children under the age of 15 developed type 1 diabetes in 2010, and 480,000 children are currently living with the disease, approximately 115,000 in Southeast Asia, 110,000 in Europe, and 95,000 in North America (**FIGURE 41.9**) (IDF Diabetes Atlas, 2010; McCarty & Zimmet, 1994; Sudagani & Hitman, 2005).

In a recent worldwide study covering the period 1990–1999, investigators of the *Diabetes Mondiale Project (DIAMOND)* examined the incidence of type 1 diabetes in children up to 15 years of age from 114 populations in 112 centers and 57 countries. A total of 43,013 cases were diagnosed in study populations containing a total of 84 million children. For the decade, the average annual increase in the incidence of type 1 diabetes was 2.8%. The observed rate of increase was slightly higher during 1995–1999 compared to 1990–1994 (3.4% vs. 2.4%). High rates of increase were notable in Europe (3.2%), Asia (4.0%), and North America (5.3%). Annual rates varied widely by nation from 0.1 per 100,000 in China and Venezuela to 39.9 per 100,000 in Finland. The U.S. annual rate was approximately 17 per 100,000. Based on these results, the investigators concluded that "*the constantly increasing*

incidence of type 1 diabetes over such a short period of time cannot be explained by shifts in genetic susceptibility alone," and they stressed the need to search for causative agents in the environment or genetic by environmental interactions (DIAMOND, 2006; Karvonen et al., 2000).

Epidemiologic studies also indicate that the greatest increase in incidence is occurring in previously low-prevalence geographic areas. For example, Patterson and colleagues examined trends in the incidence of type 1 diabetes during 1989–2003 in 20 population-based registries in 17 European countries. Estimates were based upon 29,311 new cases diagnosed in children before their 15th birthday. The overall annual increase in the incidence of type 1 diabetes during this time period was 3.9%. Greater rates of increase were observed in younger age groups, 5.4% for ages 0–4 years, 4.3% for ages 5–9 years, and 2.9% for ages 10–14 years. The median annual rate was approximately 11 per 100,000, but rates varied widely, from 5.2 per 100,000 in Poland to 39.9 per 100,000 in Finland. Other Scandinavian countries also had high annual rates (e.g., 25.8 per 100,000 in Sweden and 21.1 per 100,000 in Norway); however, the former communist bloc countries in Eastern Europe, specifically Poland, Romania, the Czech Republic, and Slovakia, have experienced the most rapid rates of increase. By 2020, the total number of new annual cases of type 1 diabetes in Europe is expected to rise to 24,400 from the 15,000 new cases estimated in 2005, with incident cases doubling among children under 5 years of age. Among youngsters under age 15, the number of existing European cases in 2020 is expected to rise to 160,000 from 94,000 (Patterson et al., 2009).

In the search for causative agents responsible for the rise in type 1 diabetes in the past half-century, many environmental factors have been studied which could trigger autoimmune responses responsible for the destruction of pancreatic β-cells of the islets of Langerhans. Enteric viruses, dietary proteins such as those found in milk or wheat, reduced exposure to sunshine or reduced intake of vitamin D, organic pollutants and other toxins, perinatal exposures to toxic contaminants, and increasing obesity levels among children have all been implicated as possible environmental triggers; nevertheless, definitive proof of causation remains elusive (Gale, 2002, 2005).

A number of hypotheses have been proposed to explain the rise in type 1 diabetes. The *hygiene hypothesis*, initially proposed to explain the concurrent patterns of asthma and allergy (Strachan, 1989), suggests that exposure to a wide range of infectious agents in childhood is necessary for successful maturation of the innate immune system; and in the absence of such exposure, cell-mediated immunity becomes more robust, thereby predisposing to type 1 diabetes and other autoimmune diseases. According to this hypothesis, improved hygienic conditions during childhood may have contributed to the rising incidence of type 1 diabetes (Kolb & Elliot, 1994). The *accelerator hypothesis* initially proposed by Wilkin suggests that metabolic overload of pancreatic β-cells brought about by accelerated growth during childhood, insulin resistance, and fat accumulation leads to their destruction through apoptosis and autoimmune reactions (Fourlanos, Harrison, & Colman, 2008; Wilkin, 2001).

There is also speculation and some evidence suggesting that environmental changes have induced a transition to earlier onset in a relatively constant pool of genetically susceptible individuals resulting in an increase in the incidence of type 1 diabetes in younger but not older age groups (Gale, 2002, 2005). Nevertheless, application of a population-based genetic model involving increasing penetrance of alleles conferring susceptibility through environmental changes was found incompatible with the Finnish data on type 1 diabetes (Pitkäniemi, Onkamo, Tuomilehto, & Arjas, 2004).

▶ # Risk Factors for Type 1 Diabetes

Risk factors for type 1 diabetes include genetic propensity and family history, environmental and/or dietary

factors or triggers, ethnoracial distribution, and geography. Albeit, definitive linkages between these factors and molecular mechanisms of pathogenesis have not been fully clarified and remain under intense study.

Genetics of Type 1 Diabetes

A modest genetic risk of developing type 1 diabetes has been confirmed by twin studies and family studies. Disease concordance rates are several-fold higher in monozygous (identical) twins than dizygous twins (maximum concordance estimates, 70% vs. 13%, respectively). Furthermore, among monozygous twin pairs with only one twin affected, the nondiabetic twins show a high prevalence (up to 76%) of anti-islet β-cell autoantibodies. However, the absolute risk attributable to genetics per se is small since only 10%–15% of cases have an affected first degree relative and the risk to offspring with an affected parent or sibling is less than 10% (American Diabetes Association, 2010; Redondo et al., 1999; Warram, Krolewski, & Kahn, 1988).

Multiple polymorphisms of genes in both the major and nonmajor histocompatibility complexes located on chromosome 6 have been found to influence the risk of type 1 diabetes. For example, certain alleles of the major histocompatibility complex (also called human leukocyte antigen, HLA) appear to modulate the risk. Specifically, HLA-DR3/4 and HLA-DQ8 have been found to significantly increase progression to type 1 diabetes (Barker et al., 2004; Pietropaolo & Trucco, 2003). Such alleles presumably encode antigens that predispose to autoimmune destruction of β-cells in the pancreas by killer T lymphocytes. The prevalence of susceptibility genes varies by ethnic origin and this may explain, in part, why type 1 diabetes is common in some countries such as Finland and Sardinia, but relatively rare in countries such as China and Mexico (Eisenbarth & McCulloch, 2010).

Environmental Factors and Type 1 Diabetes

In addition to genetic and familial predisposition, viral exposures, particularly to mumps, Coxsackie virus B, Epstein-Barr virus, congenital rubella syndrome, and cytomegaloviruses have been implicated as possible triggers for β-cell autoimmunity, but it is unclear whether they are necessary or sufficient to cause type 1 diabetes (Dorman, LaPorte, & Songer, 2003). Such triggers may contribute directly to immune activation by inciting cross-reactivity against pancreatic islet proteins bearing a similar structure or indirectly by inciting the production of proinflammatory cytokines that injure pancreatic islet tissue (Gregory et al., 2010). Dietary factors in early life have also been hypothesized to influence the development of type 1 diabetes, particularly cow's milk (Yoon, 1990). One proposed mechanism is that early introduction of β lactoglobulin in cow's milk triggers antibodies that interfere with T cell regulation and induce immune reactions against the pancreatic β-cells (Goldfarb, 2008).

The wide geographic variation in type 1 diabetes has been well documented by large prospective studies and surveillance surveys (IDF Diabetes Atlas, 2010). Moreover, some studies also show seasonal variation in the onset of type 1 diabetes (Eurodiab ACE Study Group, 2000; Levy-Marchal, Patterson, & Green, 1995; McKinney, 2001; Ye, Chen, Ashkenazi, & Laron, 1998). For example, a large study of 31,091 cases from 105 centers worldwide found significant seasonality in the diagnosis of type 1 diabetes in 42 of the locations. The incidence among children, particularly boys, from birth to 14 years, was typically higher in the winter months and lower in the summer depending on geographic location and latitude (Moltchanova, Schreier, Lammi, & Karvonen, 2009). These results suggest there may be significant variability in the environmental triggers of type 1 diabetes, perhaps related to certain viral or bacterial infections being more prevalent in the winter months.

Ethnic Disparities in Type 1 Diabetes

Although epidemiologic features of type 1 diabetes, such as gender distribution and peak age at onset, are relatively similar across populations, the global variation in the incidence of type 1 diabetes is greater than any other chronic disease that affects children (Dorman et al., 2003). For example, children in Finland and Sardinia are nearly 400 times more likely to develop diabetes than children in the People's Republic of China. Profound changes have also been observed in migrant populations (e.g., the incidence of type 1 diabetes is four times greater among Chinese children living in Hong Kong compared with those who live in China) (Yang et al., 1998).

Marked ethnic differences are also apparent in the United States. Whereas Asians, Hispanics, and African Americans are at relatively high risk for type 2 diabetes, Caucasians have the highest risk for the development of type 1 diabetes. Multiple factors (e.g., genetic susceptibility, family history, and certain environmental triggers) may contribute to the increased risk for developing type 1 diabetes among Caucasians (Lambert et al., 2004).

Type 1 Diabetes in Sardinia

One notable epidemiologic observation is the high incidence of type 1 diabetes in Sardinia (an island 120 miles off the west coast of Italy) compared to continental Italy. In fact, Sardinia has one of the highest incidence rates in the world (approximately 39 cases per 100,000 among children under 15 years of age) which is nearly seven times higher than in comparable regions on the west coast of Italy (Casu, Pascutto, Bernardinelli, the Sardinian IDDM Epidemiology Study Group, & Songini, 2004). Sardinia is therefore a *hot spot* for the development of islet cell autoimmunity and type 1 diabetes and, as a consequence, epidemiologic studies of the Sardinian population have intensified.

Recent studies of Sardinian children have focused on an increasing trend in the prevalence of obesity and related conditions. In a sample of 1000 children aged 6–10 years attending primary schools in the capital city, Cagliari, the observed prevalence of obesity increased by age and lower socioeconomic status. The prevalence of obesity was 23% at age 10 compared to 14% at age 6; and in the lowest socioeconomic class, the prevalence was 26.5% in boys and 23.6% in girls. The authors concluded that obesity is becoming a serious social health problem among the youth of Sardinia (Sanna, Soro, & Calo, 2006).

Cambuli and colleagues studied insulin resistance and other clinical features of 104 obese children ascertained from a pediatric obesity clinic in Cagliari, Sardinia, in comparison to 54 children of normal weight. At baseline, the overweight and obese children had significantly *higher* blood levels of insulin, triglycerides, and leptin, and significantly *lower* levels of HDL-cholesterol and adiponectin than normal weight children. The average insulin resistance of the overweight and obese children was nearly twofold higher than normal weight children. Furthermore, after 1 year of intervention (diet and exercise), values for overweight/obese children who lost weight tended to normalize. In particular, baseline levels of adiponectin in the overweight/obese children increased by nearly threefold following intervention. The results indicate that dietary and physical intervention has benefit for overweight and obese children and suggest that adiponectin has potential as a biomarker of metabolic overload (Cambuli et al., 2008).

Other factors may also be at work in causing the increased incidence of type 1 diabetes among the children of Sardinia. For example, the time frame of major reductions in parasitic diseases and the eradication of polio, malaria, and tuberculosis in Sardinia coincide closely with increases in atopic and immunomediated diseases (type 1 diabetes, multiple sclerosis, Crohn's disease, celiac disease) (Casu et al., 2004). These trends are consistent with the *hygiene hypothesis*, which proposes that the absence of immunogenic stimuli early in life may heighten the risk of developing autoimmune diseases (Strachan, 1989). Furthermore, the Sardinian population has been described as a *genetic isolate* and certain genes that predispose to diabetes or other autoimmune conditions may have reached high frequencies due to natural selection and/or inbreeding.

Type 1 Diabetes and Multiple Sclerosis in Sardinia

In addition to having high rates of type 1 diabetes, the Sardinian population also has higher incidence and prevalence rates of multiple sclerosis than other European and Italian populations (Rosati et al., 1996). Since both conditions involve autoimmune reactions (destruction of neurons in multiple sclerosis and pancreatic β-cells in diabetes), they may have genetic and/or environmental risk factors in common.

Morrosu and colleagues at the University of Cagliari therefore designed studies to elucidate familial and genetic associations between type 1 diabetes and multiple sclerosis in the Sardinian population. They first conducted a cohort study to examine the incidence of type 1 diabetes in 1090 individuals with multiple sclerosis and their parents ($n = 2180$) and siblings ($n = 3300$). All participants were ascertained at the Multiple Sclerosis Clinic in Cagliari. Type 1 diabetes developed five times more often in patients with multiple sclerosis than in the general population, and the presence of familial multiple sclerosis increased the odds of developing type 1 diabetes more than threefold (OR = 3.4). In a subsequent investigation, the same investigators compared *human leukocyte antigen (HLA)* genotypes in 1052 patients with type 1 diabetes, 1049 patients with multiple sclerosis, and 1917 control subjects. Susceptibility to both disorders was associated with common variants of the *HLA-DRB1* and *HLA-DQB1* loci, but coinheritance of these alleles could only partially explain the increase in diabetes among patients with multiple sclerosis. The results suggest that in the high-risk Sardinian population, HLA and non-HLA genetic factors and/or unknown environmental factors contribute significantly to the association of both type 1 diabetes and multiple sclerosis (Marrosu et al., 2002, 2004).

Obesity and Type 1 Diabetes Mellitus

The role of obesity in the pathogenesis of type 1 diabetes is controversial. To clarify the presence and strength of the association, Veberteen and colleagues conducted a meta-analysis of BMI and type 1 diabetes. They identified eight case–control studies and one cohort study involving 2658 cases for analysis. Of the nine studies, seven reported finding a significant association between a measure of increased body mass and type 1 diabetes. Overall, the odds of developing type 1 diabetes increased by twofold in obese children compared to normal weight children (OR = 2.03) and the risk increased by 1.25 per unit increase in BMI. The authors concluded that "*our systematic review indicates a likely association between childhood obesity, or higher BMI, and subsequent increased risk of childhood-onset type 1 diabetes*" (Verbeeten, Elks, Daneman, & Ong, 2011).

▶ Birth Weight and Type 1 Diabetes

Finnish children reportedly have the highest incidence of type 1 diabetes in the world, exceeding 40 cases per 100,000 in the 1990s. Recently, investigators at the National Public Health Institute in Helsinki examined incidence trends in type 1 diabetes during 1980–2005. During this time period, 10,737 children under 15 years of age were diagnosed with type 1 diabetes, and the average age-standardized incidence was 42.9 cases per 100,000 per year. Notably, the incidence more than doubled in the 25-year period, from 31.4 per 100,000 in 1980 to 64.2 per 100,000 in 2005. The greatest rate of increase (4.7% per year) occurred in children under 5 years of age (Harjutsalo, Sjöberg, & Tuomilehto, 2008). The frequency of overweight or obese children aged 5–15 years also increased during the same time period, from 9.5% in the mid-1980s to 20% in 2005. It is also noteworthy that the average birth weight in Finland actually *declined* during this time, suggesting that early postnatal weight gain may play a more significant role in the genesis of type 1 diabetes (Kautiainen, Rimpelä, Vikat, & Virtanen, 2002; Salo, 2006).

Birth weight and weight gain during the first postnatal year have been examined as risk factors for type 1 diabetes in a number of epidemiologic studies. To clarify their effects, Harder and colleagues conducted a meta-analysis of 12 published studies of birth weight and type 1 diabetes involving 2,398,150 children, 7491 of whom had type 1 diabetes. Results indicate that each 1000 g increase in birth weight increases the risk by 7%. Furthermore, patients with type 1 diabetes gained significantly more weight during the first year of life than controls. The authors concluded that birth weight and particularly early weight gain are significant risk factors for the development of type 1 diabetes (Harder et al., 2009).

Accelerator Hypothesis of Type 1 Diabetes

Though the existing epidemiologic evidence supports a positive association between childhood obesity and type 1 diabetes, definitive proof of cause and effect is lacking. The *accelerator hypothesis* of Wilkin proposes that type 1 and type 2 diabetes are both triggered by insulin resistance that heightens apoptosis (programmed death) and immune-mediated destruction of the β-cells of the pancreas (Wilkin, 2001). Conceivably, excessive weight gain during the early years of life and particularly during the pubertal growth spurt could heighten the vulnerability of hyperfunctioning β-cells to such processes.

Nevertheless, some studies have failed to find an association between insulin resistance and obesity in type 1 diabetics. In a clinical investigation of premenopausal women, Greenfield and colleagues compared insulin resistance and other factors in 10 women with type 1 diabetes to 10 women without disease who were matched to the cases on body mass index. Though insulin sensitivity was significantly reduced in the diabetic women compared to controls, the two groups had similar levels of lipids, androgens, energy expenditure, physical activity, blood pressure, and abdominal adiposity. Thus, the study, albeit small, demonstrated insulin resistance among premenopausal women with type 1 diabetes that appeared to be unrelated to abdominal obesity, lipids, or androgens (Greenfield, Samaras, & Chisholm, 2002).

Furthermore, genetic linkages have not been substantiated by studies using specific markers of type 1 and type 2 diabetes. For example, in a genetic study of single nucleotide polymorphisms covering 12 gene regions associated with type 2 diabetes among 7606 type 1 diabetics and 8218 controls without diabetes, there were no convincing genetic linkages between type 1 and type 2 diabetes or interactions of these regions with other factors including autoantibody status and the major HLA class II genotypes (Raj et al., 2009).

Treatment for Type 1 Diabetes

Though there is no treatment that can cure type 1 diabetes, insulin replacement by daily injection or other methods can effectively maintain blood glucose levels within normal limits (McCulloch, 2010). Timing and dosing of exogenous insulin in relation to dietary patterns and activity levels are necessary to avoid hyperglycemia and life-threatening diabetic ketoacidosis and dangerously low blood glucose levels called *hypoglycemia* that can lead to diabetic coma. For the type 1 diabetic, lifelong daily insulin replacement and glucose monitoring are required to maintain proper blood glucose levels and minimize the complications that can arise from hyperglycemia or hypoglycemia.

Prediabetes

Prediabetes is defined as impaired fasting glucose and/or impaired glucose tolerance. In this condition, blood glucose is higher than normal, but not high enough to be diagnosed with type 2 diabetes. It is likely to be a metabolic state, where in order to maintain normal blood glucose levels, the pancreatic β-cells secrete excess insulin in response to increasing insulin resistance (Wang et al., 2010). A fasting plasma glucose test between 100 and 126 mg/dL indicates the prediabetic state of *impaired fasting glucose*. If the oral glucose tolerance test is used, a 2-hour 75 g post-load plasma glucose level between 140 and 200 mg/dL is indicative of prediabetes and *impaired glucose tolerance*. According to the American Diabetes Association, a hemoglobin A1c test of 5.7%–6.4% reflects an increased risk for developing type 2 diabetes and is also categorized as a prediabetic state (ADA, 2010). An estimated 344 million adults were living with impaired glucose tolerance in 2010, a worldwide prevalence of 7.9% (IDF Diabetes Atlas, 2010). Several studies conducted in a wide range of populations provide clear evidence that prediabetes is a significant risk factor for the development of type 2 diabetes and microvascular and macrovascular disease.

A recent example comes from the *Strong Heart Study*, a population-based longitudinal study of American Indians. In this investigation, 1677 subjects who were nondiabetic at baseline were followed over a median of 7.8 years to determine the effects of prediabetes and other risk factors on the relative risk of developing type 2 diabetes. Compared to men and women with normal glucose tolerance, diabetes incidence was more than twofold higher among gender-stratified prediabetics, even after adjusting for age, body mass index, waist circumference, albuminuria, smoking, family history of diabetes, and quartiles of physical activity. Overall, the incidence of diabetes among individuals with either impaired fasting glucose and/or impaired glucose tolerance was 66.1 per 1000 person-years, 2.35-fold higher than normotensive individuals. The investigators concluded that prediabetic status is an independent predictor of conversion to type 2 diabetes (Wang et al., 2010).

Gerstein and colleagues examined the association of prediabetes with type 2 diabetes in a meta-analysis of prospective cohort studies published from 1979 to 2004 (comprised of 30,000 individuals and representing a broad range of ethnicities and countries). Estimates of the annual incidence of type 2 diabetes among prediabetics ranged from 5% to 10%. Overall, the annual incidence of type 2 diabetes was 7.0% for individuals with impaired fasting glucose, 6.1% for individuals with impaired glucose tolerance, and 14% for those with both conditions. Compared to normotensive individuals, the relative risk was fivefold higher in subjects with impaired fasting glucose, sevenfold higher in subjects with impaired glucose tolerance, and more than 12-fold higher in subjects with both conditions. These results indicate that impaired fasting glucose and/or impaired glucose tolerance are predictive of impending type 2 diabetes and suggest that dysglycemia is progressive and time-dependent (Gerstein et al., 2007).

▶ Type 2 Diabetes

In type 2 diabetes (also called *non-insulin-dependent diabetes* or *adult-onset diabetes*), which represents approximately 90%–95% of all cases of diabetes, insulin is still produced and secreted by the pancreas but its impact on glucose uptake is ineffectual. Elevated blood glucose occurs when there is a mismatch between the amount of insulin that is produced and secreted by the β-cells of the pancreas and the amount needed to maintain normal blood glucose levels. This mismatch is caused by target tissue insulin resistance, relative insulin insufficiency, or both (NIDDK, 2008).

Although insulin resistance can be caused by genetic syndromes, primary target cell defects, autoantibodies to insulin, or accelerated insulin degradation (Reaven, 1995), the most common cause of insulin resistance is relative weight gain or obesity. Excess energy beyond the body's capacity to store it appears to attenuate insulin-mediated cellular glucose uptake and to suppress energy uptake, initially within muscle cells (which have limited glycogen storage capacity) and later within the primary site of excess energy storage, the adipocytes (which have abundant storage capacity for excess calories from protein, carbohydrate, and alcohol that are converted and stored as triacylglycerol). Diminished energy uptake likely occurs through physiologic decreases in the number of insulin receptors and down-regulation or inhibition of target cell insulin receptor signaling (Olatunbosun & Dagogo-Jack, 2010).

▶ Risk Factors for Type 2 Diabetes

The known major risk factors for type 2 diabetes include family history, age, ethnicity, obesity, and prediabetes. Family history generally reflects genetic propensity as well as the shared environment, cultural practices, and behaviors of family members. Family history is one of the strongest predictors of type 2 diabetes. The risk of developing diabetes is doubled if one first degree relative (parent or sibling) has the disease and is increased over fourfold if two or more first degree relatives have the disease (Valdez, Yoon, Liu, & Khoury, 2007). Nevertheless, the profound increase in diabetes incidence and prevalence within the past several decades rules out a genetic basis for the excess burden of the disease, and points to insidious environmental factors that most likely play a permissive role in the etiology of diabetes.

Genetics of Type 2 Diabetes

The β3 *adrenoreceptor gene* on the short arm of chromosome 8 encodes a protein that modulates fat metabolism and thermogenesis (conversion of energy to heat). This gene is expressed primarily in fat and muscle cells. One specific mutation of the β3 adrenoreceptor gene called *TRP64ARG* is almost four times more common in Pima Indians living in Arizona than Caucasians of European descent, and nearly twice as common in other groups at high risk for diabetes such as African Americans and Mexican Americans (Walston et al., 1995). Notably, the Arizona Pimas have one of the highest rates of type 2 diabetes in the world (as discussed in the section of this chapter on dietary fat and type 2 diabetes). The mutated TRP64ARG gene (which involves a single amino acid substitution of arginine for tryptophan) has been found to enhance lipolysis in adipose tissue and reduce thermogenesis in muscle and has also been associated with heightened insulin resistance in obese and high-risk subgroups (Zhan & Ho, 2005). Thus, the high gene frequency of the TRP64ARG mutation may be partially responsible for the extraordinarily high rates of type 2 diabetes in the Pima Indians of Arizona as well as heightened rates in other high-risk populations.

Other genes have also been identified that increase the risk of insulin resistance and development of type 2 diabetes. The *calpain-10 gene (CAPN10)* located on the long arm of chromosome 2 encodes a protease that influences both insulin secretion and insulin action, and single nucleotide polymorphisms of this gene have been noted that increase insulin resistance and the risk of developing type 2 diabetes in several populations (Lynn et al., 2002).

A syndrome known as *maturity onset of diabetes in the young (MODY)* shows autosomal dominant inheritance and is characterized by onset of type 2 diabetes *without* β-cell autoantibodies in one or more family members under the age of 25 years. Gene variants of *hepatocyte nuclear factor* genes (HNF-1α, HNF-4α, and HNF-1β), the *glucokinase* gene (GCK), and the *peroxisome proliferator-activated receptor-g gene (PPARg)* have been linked to this syndrome.

These genetic variants may contribute significantly to the risk of type 2 diabetes conferring insulin resistance of liver, muscle, and fat and/or deficiencies in insulin secretion. It is likely that in the near future additional studies of the human genome will lead to the discovery of many more gene variants that influence the risk of type 2 diabetes (McCulloch, 2004). As pointed out by Hansen and Pederson in their review of the genetics of type 2 diabetes, "*the results of these efforts are likely to be the platform for major progress in the development of personalized antidiabetic drugs with higher efficacy and few side effects*" (Hansen & Pederson, 2005).

Obesity and Type 2 Diabetes

Obesity is the strongest modifiable predictor of type 2 diabetes. Maintaining a healthy weight or losing a moderate amount of excess weight have both been shown to improve metabolic health (Colditz, Willett, Rotnitzky, & Manson, 1995; Klein et al., 2004; NHLBI, 1998; Tremblay et al., 1999; Truesdale, Stevens, & Cai, 2005; Willett, Dietz, & Colditz, 1999). In the *Health Professionals Follow-up Study*, a team of U.S. investigators prospectively examined associations between changes in body weight and body fat distribution measured during 1986–1996 and the subsequent development of diabetes during 1996–2000 among 22,171 men aged 40–75 years. Results showed that weight gain was monotonically related to the risk of diabetes, with an average risk increase of 7.3% per kg of weight gain. Compared to men with stable weight, those who gained at least 6 kg more than doubled their risk of developing diabetes (RR = 2.1); and reciprocally, those who lost at least 6 kg reduced their risk by 50%. Similar results were seen using waist circumference to evaluate body mass. Of all cases of incident diabetes in the cohort, 56% were attributable to a weight gain of 7 kg or greater, whereas only 20% of cases were attributable to a 2.5 cm increase in waist circumference (Koh-Banerjee et al., 2004).

The cause and effect relationship between obesity and type 2 diabetes is dramatically illustrated for U.S. men and women in **FIGURE 41.10**. Relative risk estimates are abstracted from the *U.S. Health Professionals Follow-up Study* for men (Chan, Rimm, Colditz, Stampfer, & Willett, 1994) and the *Nurses' Health Study* for women (Colditz et al., 1995). Compared with a BMI of 21, the relative risk of developing type 2 diabetes rises exponentially with increasing BMI. The relative risk rises to more than 40 for gravidly obese men and more than 90 for gravidly obese women, and furthermore, multifold risk elevations are notable even for modest increases in body mass.

Obesity disproportionately affects African Americans, Hispanics, American Indians, and Pacific Islanders, all of whom are at higher risk for

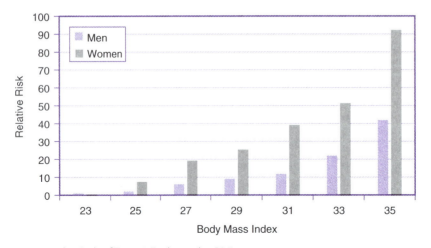

FIGURE 41.10 Dose Response in the Risk of Type 2 Diabetes by BMI.

Data from Chan, J. M., Rimm, E. B., Colditz, G. A., Stampfer, M. J., & Willett, W. C. (1994). Obesity, fat distribution, and weight gain as risk factors for clinical diabetes in men. *Diabetes Care, 17*(9), 961–969; Colditz, G. A., Willett, W. C., Rotnitzky, A., & Manson, J. E. (1995). Weight gain as a risk factor for clinical diabetes mellitus in women. *Annals of Internal Medicine, 122,* 481–486.

developing type 2 diabetes compared to Caucasians. Asians, on the other hand, also have a higher risk for type 2 diabetes than Caucasians, but at a lower BMI and fat mass compared to other ethnoracial groups (Shai et al., 2006). This may be due to their decreased storage capacity. For example, Mott et al. (1999) evaluated body fat and age in a sample of healthy New York City volunteers ($n = 1324$) of four ethnic groups, aged 20 and older. Using a four-compartment model of body composition which included measures of body volume, total body water, total body bone mineral mass, and body weight, Asian men and women had mean lower fat mass at every decade of age compared to Caucasians, African Americans, and Puerto Ricans. In another study, Pan et al. (2004) consistently found higher prevalence rates of hypertension, diabetes, and hyperuricemia in Taiwanese compared to African Americans or Caucasians by level of BMI.

Dietary Factors and Diabetes Risk

Dietary factors have also been found to influence the risk of developing type 2 diabetes. In particular, the glycemic index, glycemic load, type of fat, type of carbohydrate, dietary fiber, magnesium, and an emerging potential risk factor, high fructose corn syrup, have all been investigated in experimental and epidemiologic studies.

Glycemic Index and Type 2 Diabetes

The glycemic index is a measure of postprandial increase in blood glucose due to intake of a specific food relative to that induced by glucose per se. Use of the glycemic index in evaluating risk of diabetes, and perhaps just as important, its clinical application in diabetes management, has proven to be reproducible. Numerous studies have also shown that the glycemic index is predictable in the context of mixed meals, which was an early criticism (Wolever et al., 1994).

The glycemic index was developed in 1981 by David Jenkins and associates at St. Michael's Hospital in Toronto, Canada. Jenkins realized that carbohydrate exchange lists do not account for the physiological effects of foods and that the type of carbohydrate as well as other dietary factors influence postprandial glycemia. Jenkins and his team sought a valid measure of the conversion of carbohydrates to glucose that could be effectively used in the dietary management of diabetes to maintain good glucose control (Jenkins et al., 1981).

Using groups of 5–10 normal weight, nondiabetic men and women, Jenkins introduced 62 individual foods and glucose (controlling for total carbohydrate quantity by standardizing to 50 g) in random order, after overnight fasts, and using specified mean protocols. Subsequent glucose tolerance tests were conducted and the glycemic index value for each food was calculated as the area under the 2-hour blood glucose response curve expressed as a percentage of the appropriate mean glucose tolerance test value (Jenkins et al., 1981). In simple terms, "*glycemic index is a concept that ranks foods on the basis of their acute glycemic impact (relative to glucose = 100)*" (Brand-Miller, 1994).

Dietary studies have revealed wide variability in the glycemic index based on the type of carbohydrate. In general, simple carbohydrates (e.g., sugars) have higher values than complex carbohydrates (starches). However, there are numerous exceptions to these general rules and many factors can influence the glycemic index of food including variety, processing, and preparation, as well as the precise mixture of liquid, fat, protein, fiber, and carbohydrate ingested. Inverse relationships have been observed between the glycemic indices of foods and their content of fat, protein, and dietary fiber. Some experts in the field of human nutrition advise that while the glycemic index is a valid and useful concept, application and interpretation in dietary studies are "*deceptively complex*" (Wolever, 1997).

A modification of the *glycemic index* that takes into account the amount of carbohydrate ingested is called the *glycemic load*. The glycemic load of food adjusts the glycemic index of carbohydrate for the content of carbohydrate the food contains based on the formula, *glycemic load = glycemic index × total carbohydrate content (g)/(100)*. Several large prospective cohort studies have found positive associations between the glycemic index or the glycemic load and the risk of type 2 diabetes.

Jenkin's glycemic index and the related measurement, the glycemic load, have been widely used in epidemiologic and clinical investigations. In 1997, an expert committee of the Food and Agricultural Organization and the WHO endorsed the use of the glycemic index to classify carbohydrate-rich foods and help guide food choices (Foster-Powell, Holt, & Brand-Miller, 2002). Nevertheless, considerable controversy exists as to the value of the glycemic index or the glycemic load in predicting the development of certain conditions such as type 2 diabetes and/or guiding dietary choices in patients with disease.

Hodge and colleagues examined associations of type 2 diabetes with the glycemic index and other dietary factors in a prospective cohort of 36,787 men and women aged 40–69 years from Melbourne,

Australia. During four years of follow-up, 365 cases were identified among 31,641 participants. High levels of the dietary glycemic index were found to increase the risk (OR = 1.32 per 10-unit increase). Risk increases were also observed for high intakes of white bread (OR = 1.37 for the highest versus lowest quartiles) and starch (OR = 1.47 per 100 g per day) whereas risk reductions were observed for higher intakes of magnesium, total carbohydrates, and sugars. These associations were attenuated with adjustment for measures of obesity. Intake of fiber was not associated with diabetes in the study. The investigators concluded that reducing the glycemic index by decreasing intake of white bread while maintaining a high carbohydrate diet may reduce the risk of developing type 2 diabetes (Hodge, English, O'Dea, & Giles, 2004).

Collaborators from the Shanghai Cancer Institute in China and Vanderbilt and UCLA in the United States studied associations of the glycemic index and glycemic load with type 2 diabetes in a cohort of 64,227 Chinese women with no history of diabetes at baseline. After 4.6 years (297,755 person-years) of follow-up, 1608 incident cases of type 2 diabetes were detected. Relative risk estimates for the highest versus the lowest quintile were 1.21 for the glycemic index, 1.34 for the glycemic load, 1.28 for carbohydrate intake, and 1.78 for rice intake. The investigators concluded that high intake of foods with a high glycemic index or a high glycemic load, especially rice, the main carbohydrate source in the target population, increased the risk of developing type 2 diabetes (Villegas et al., 2007).

Krishnan and colleagues examined associations of the glycemic index and cereal fiber with type 2 diabetes among 59,000 women of the *Black Women's Health Study* who were disease-free at baseline. During 8 years of follow-up, 1938 cases of type 2 diabetes were detected. Women with a high glycemic index (highest quintile) had an increase in the relative risk (RR = 1.23) whereas those with a high intake of cereal fiber had a decrease in risk (RR = 0.82). Associations were strongest for leaner women with BMI < 25, RR = 1.91 for high glycemic index, and RR = 0.41 for high cereal fiber intake. The investigators concluded that increasing cereal fiber in the diet may be effective in reducing the risk of type 2 diabetes (Krishnan et al., 2007).

Barclay and colleagues conducted a systematic review and meta-analysis of 37 prospective cohort studies of associations of the glycemic index and the glycemic load with type 2 diabetes and other chronic diseases. The adjusted relative risks in comparisons of the highest with the lowest quintiles were RR = 1.40

for the glycemic index and RR = 1.27 for the glycemic load. Furthermore, significant increases in risk associated with high glycemic indices were also noted for other chronic diseases including coronary heart disease (RR = 1.25) and gallbladder disease (RR = 1.26). Mechanisms by which high glycemic index diets contribute to the development of type 2 diabetes include insulin resistance of target cells due to persistent glycemic exposure and accelerated pancreatic β-cell insufficiency due to a chronically higher insulin demand per quantity of carbohydrate (Barclay et al., 2008).

Dietary Fiber and Type 2 Diabetes

Some epidemiologic studies have found that certain types of dietary fiber protect against the development of type 2 diabetes. Selected investigations plus a meta-analysis of dietary fiber and diabetes are discussed in the following paragraphs.

Meyer and colleagues conducted a cohort study of total dietary fiber, soluble dietary fiber, carbohydrates, fruits, and vegetables, refined grains, magnesium, and the glycemic index in 35,988 older women from Iowa. During 6 years of follow-up, 1141 cases of type 2 diabetes were reported. Strong inverse associations were observed for high versus low intakes of whole grain (RR = 0.79), total dietary fiber (RR = 0.78), and magnesium (RR = 0.67). Intakes of total carbohydrates, refined grains, fruits and vegetables, and soluble fiber and the glycemic index were unrelated to diabetes risk. The authors concluded that "*these data support a protective role for grains (particularly whole grains), cereal fiber, and dietary magnesium in the development of diabetes in older women*" (Meyer et al., 2000).

Stevens and colleagues studied associations of the glycemic index, the glycemic load, and types of dietary fiber with type 2 diabetes among 12,251 adults aged 45–64 years enrolled in the *Atherosclerosis Risk in Communities (ARIC)* observational cohort. After 9 years of follow-up, a total of 1447 cases of type 2 diabetes were reported. A significant risk reduction was observed for high versus low intake of cereal fiber among Caucasians (RR = 0.75) but the reduction among African Americans (RR = 0.86) did not reach statistical significance. The authors concluded that cereal fiber may have a protective role against type 2 diabetes in Caucasians and suggested the need for more studies of African Americans (Stevens et al., 2002).

A team of investigators in Helsinki conducted a cohort study of fiber and whole-grain intake among 2286 men and 2030 women, aged 40–69 years, ascertained through the *Finland Nationwide Health Registry*. During the 10-year follow-up period, type 2 diabetes was diagnosed in 54 men and 102 women. In comparisons of highest versus lowest quartiles, risk reductions were observed for consumption of whole grain (RR = 0.65) and cereal fiber (RR = 0.39) (Montonen, Kneckt, Järvinen, Aromaa, & Reunanen, 2003).

Schulze and colleagues conducted a prospective cohort study of dietary fiber, magnesium, and type 2 diabetes among 9702 men and 15,365 women, aged 35–65 years, enrolled in the *European Prospective Investigation of Cancer and Nutrition, Potsdam*. During 176,117 person-years of follow-up, they observed 844 incident cases of type 2 diabetes. High intake of cereal fiber was inversely associated with the risk of diabetes (RR = 0.72 for highest vs. lowest quintile) whereas no associations were found for vegetable fiber, fruit fiber, or magnesium. Furthermore, in a meta-analysis of nine cohort studies, high cereal fiber intake was also found to reduce the risk (combined RR = 0.67 for the highest versus lowest quintile) but there were no significant effects of fruit or vegetable fiber. The authors also conducted a meta-analysis of eight studies of magnesium and type 2 diabetes, in which they found a significant overall risk reduction for high versus low intake (combined RR = 0.77) (Schulze et al., 2007).

Dietary fiber consists of both soluble and insoluble forms. Soluble fiber has been shown to inhibit macronutrient absorption, reduce postprandial glucose responses, and beneficially influence blood lipids (Torsdottir, Alpsten, Holm, Sandberg, & Tölli, 1991; Weickert & Pfeiffer, 2008). Nevertheless, it is primarily insoluble (cereal) fiber that has consistently been found associated with reduced diabetes risk (Weickert et al., 2005). The biological mechanism by which insoluble fiber protects against diabetes is unknown; however, in a small dietary intervention study, the administration of insoluble cereal fiber to overweight and obese women was found to improve insulin sensitivity (Weickert et al., 2006).

Magnesium and Type 2 Diabetes

As noted in the above discussion, several epidemiologic studies of type 2 diabetes have included investigation of effects of magnesium intake. Furthermore, a meta-analysis of eight studies by Schulze and colleagues found an overall risk reduction of 23% with high magnesium intake (Schulze et al., 2007). One notable investigation of magnesium and type 2 diabetes involved 85,060 women enrolled in the *Nurses' Health Study* and 42,872 men enrolled in the *Health Professionals' Follow-up Study*. After 18 years of follow-up in women and 12 years of follow-up in men, 4085 female cases and 1333 male cases of type 2 diabetes

were documented. After adjusting for age, BMI, physical activity, family history of diabetes, smoking, alcohol consumption, and history of hypertension and hypercholesterolemia, the relative risk of type 2 diabetes among those in the highest compared to the lowest quintile of total magnesium intake was similarly reduced in both women (RR = 0.66) and men (RR = 0.67). Furthermore, the risk reductions retained statistical significance after further adjustment for dietary variables including glycemic load, polyunsaturated fat, trans fat, cereal fiber, and processed meat in multivariate models, and the estimates were stable for subgroups of BMI, physical activity, and family history of diabetes. These findings suggest that magnesium has significant chemo-preventive activity against the development of type 2 diabetes and prompted the authors to state that "*this study supports the dietary recommendation to increase consumption of major food sources of magnesium such as whole grains, nuts, and green leafy vegetables*" (Lopez-Ridaura et al., 2004).

Several mechanisms have been proposed to explain the beneficial effects of magnesium in protecting against the development of type 2 diabetes. Intracellular magnesium is a critical cofactor for several enzymes in carbohydrate metabolism, and deficiencies may trigger insulin resistance by interfering with intracellular insulin signaling (Takaya, Higashino, & Kobayashi, 2004; Tosiello, 1996).

Dietary Fat and Type 2 Diabetes

Dietary fat has also been implicated as a potential risk factor for type 2 diabetes. However, it is difficult to separate effects of dietary fat *per se* from effects that are related to obesity and increased BMI, which are powerful risk factors in the development of type 2 diabetes (see Figure 41.10).

In nutritional studies, it is important to stratify the types of fat, as specific fatty acids appear to have differential effects on the genesis of type 2 diabetes. Furthermore, results may differ substantially for men and women and for ethnically distinct populations. Obviously, such studies are limited by the survey instrument, the imprecision of self-reported dietary questionnaires, and the interrelatedness of the various dietary factors, especially dietary fat and total calories. Indeed, marked inconsistencies in reported findings on dietary fat as well as other components of diet have led to substantial controversy regarding the benefit or detriment of certain combinations of dietary fat and carbohydrates for the prevention and/or therapy of type 2 diabetes. Selected studies of this controversial issue are described in the following paragraphs.

International correlation and comparative studies show that populations consuming diets with a higher proportion of fat have higher prevalence rates of type 2 diabetes (Feskens et al., 1995; Fujimoto, 1996). However, such population comparisons have limited value in testing for cause and effect and are subject to the *ecological fallacy* whereby within-population heterogeneity is not considered.

A few longitudinal and cohort studies have examined the association of dietary fat and the incidence of diabetes. In the *Zutphen Study* conducted in the Netherlands, fat and cholesterol intake were studied in 394 nondiabetic men, aged 50–70 years, during 1960–1970. Diabetic status was confirmed in 1970 by oral glucose tolerance tests. Positive associations were noted between abnormal glucose tolerance and the intake of saturated fat and cholesterol whereas negative associations were observed for the intake of pectin and sugar products (Feskens & Kromhout, 1990).

The Pima Indians of Arizona have the highest reported incidence and prevalence rates of type 2 diabetes in the United States. In 1978, the age-gender adjusted incidence of diabetes was 26.5 per 1000, nearly 20-fold higher than U.S. Caucasian populations. Adult Pima Indians typically develop diabetes early in adulthood (mean onset is 36 years), which puts them at extraordinarily high risk of developing major complications including hypertension, kidney failure, and cardiovascular disease (Knowler, Bennett, Hamman, & Miller, 1978). The *traditional diet* of the Mexican Pima Indians consists of 8%–12% fat, 70%–80% carbohydrate, and 12%–18% protein. In contrast, the modern-day diet of Pima Indians who migrated to Arizona has changed dramatically and is comprised of approximately 50% carbohydrate, 40% fat, and 10% protein (Arizona Department of Health Services, 2004).

In a longitudinal study conducted during 1982–1992, 200 healthy nondiabetic subjects from the Pima Indian population of Arizona were evaluated for diabetes yearly using oral glucose tolerance tests. Among the 87 women and 113 men, type 2 diabetes developed in 38 subjects (24 women and 14 men). The average follow-up time for these subjects was 5.3 years. Percentage of body fat and waist-to-hip circumference were strong predictors of developing type 2 diabetes, increasing the risk by 8-fold and 12-fold, respectively, in comparisons of the 90th and 10th percentiles. Low glucose sensitivity (abnormal glucose tolerance) was the strongest single risk factor for the development of type 2 diabetes (RR = 31.1) and the effects of obesity were attenuated in models containing measures of insulin resistance. Based on these results, the authors suggest that insulin resistance and glucose tolerance

worsen as a result of increasing obesity, aging, and/or other factors (Lillioja et al., 1993).

Additional studies have compared lifestyles and rates of diabetes in the Pima Indians of Arizona versus Mexico. This comparison evaluates the impact of a dramatic change in diet in populations with roughly equivalent gene pools. Ravussin, Valencia, Esparza, Bennett, and Schulz (1994) traveled to a remote mountainous area of northwestern Mexico to assess the clinical characteristics of 19 women (mean age, 36 years) and 16 men (mean age, 48 years) of the Mexican Pima Indian tribe. Measurements of weight, height, body fat, blood pressure, plasma glucose, cholesterol, and hemoglobin A1c were taken for comparison with matched controls of the Arizona Pima population. The matching ratio of Arizona Pimas to Mexican Pimas was 10:1. Arizona Pimas were 40% heavier (90.2 vs. 64.2 kg) with 34% higher BMI (33.4 vs. 24.9) and plasma cholesterol (174 vs. 146 mg/dL) than Mexican Pimas. Only 2 of 19 women (11%) and 1 of 16 men (6%) in the sample of Mexican Pimas had diabetes, contrasting with prevalences of 37% and 54% in men and women of the Arizona Pimas. Based on these findings, the Ravussin and Smith (2002) suggest,

> *despite a similar potential genetic predisposition to these conditions, a traditional lifestyle, characterized by a diet including less animal fat and more complex carbohydrates and by greater energy expenditure in physical labor, may protect against the development of diabetes and related diseases.* (pp. 363–378)

The *Colorado San Luis Valley Study* was designed to examine the diets of 1317 Mexican Americans and the development of diabetes and glucose intolerance. All subjects were disease-free at baseline. Levels of dietary fat and carbohydrate in 70 individuals who developed type 2 diabetes and 171 individuals who developed glucose intolerance were compared to 1076 control subjects who remained disease-free during 4 years of follow-up. Diabetic status was established by an oral glucose tolerance test for each subject. The odds ratios for a 40 g per day increase in fat intake were 1.51 for type 2 diabetes and 1.62 for glucose intolerance, suggesting that high-fat, low carbohydrate diets increase the risk of developing type 2 diabetes (Marshall, Hamman, & Baxter, 1991).

In the *Nurses' Health Study*, associations of types of dietary fat with the risk of type 2 diabetes were examined among 84,302 women aged 34–59 years at baseline. During 14 years of follow-up, 2507 cases of type 2 diabetes were documented. In multivariate models that adjusted for energy intake, percentages of energy from protein and specific fatty acids and BMI, intakes of total fat, saturated fat, and monounsaturated fat were not associated with diabetes risk. However, for a 5% increase in energy from polyunsaturated fat, the risk *decreased* by 37% (RR = 0.67), and for a 2% increase in energy from trans fat, the risk increased by 39% (RR = 1.39). The findings suggest that in women, trans-fatty acids increase the risk and polyunsaturated fatty acids are protective, while other types of fat are neutral (Salmeron et al., 2001).

In the *Health Professional's Follow-Up Study*, associations of dietary fats and meat intake with the risk of type 2 diabetes were examined among 42,504 men aged 40–75 years at baseline. The results revealed increased risks for high intake of total fat (RR = 1.27) and saturated fat (RR = 1.34). However, these risks disappeared after adjustment for BMI. There were no associations of diabetes risk with oleic acid, trans-fatty acid, long chain *n*-3 polyunsaturated fat, or a-linolenic acid. Frequent consumption of processed meat was associated with an increase in the risk (RR = 1.46) and high intake of linoleic acid reduced the risk in some subgroups. These findings implicate high intake of processed meat as a risk factor and suggest that the effects of fat intake in men may not be independent of body mass (van Dam, Willett, Rimm, Stampfer, & Hu, 2002).

A number of randomized dietary intervention studies have been conducted to compare the impact of various nutritional approaches for patients with type 2 diabetes. Two basic dietary therapies have been compared in such studies, diets low in saturated fat and high in carbohydrates versus diets high in monounsaturated fat. In a recent meta-analysis of nine such studies, diets high in monounsaturated fat produced significantly greater net reductions in fasting plasma triacylglycerol (19%) and very low-density lipoprotein cholesterol (22%) than low saturated fat, high carbohydrate diets. Findings suggest that compared with a high carbohydrate diet, a diet rich in monounsaturated fat improves the glycemic and lipoprotein profiles and provides significant benefit for diabetic patients (Garg, 1998).

High Fructose Corn Syrup and Type 2 Diabetes

High fructose corn syrup has recently attracted attention as a potential risk factor in the development of type 2 diabetes, possibly through its effects on weight gain and obesity. For example, during the time period 1970–1990, the consumption of high fructose corn syrup increased more than 1000%, far exceeding the changes in intake of any other food or food groups.

High fructose corn syrup, which is a mixture of primarily fructose and sucrose (usually 55% and 42%, respectively), is currently the sole caloric sweetener of soft drinks, and its increasing use has occurred in close parallel with the rising prevalence of obesity and type 2 diabetes in the United States (Bray, Nielsen, & Popkin, 2004).

Although the data are sparse, recent short-term studies suggest that overconsumption of fructose-laden sweeteners may have a detrimental impact on glucose metabolism. Swarbrick and colleagues investigated the metabolic effects of consuming fructose-sweetened beverages for 10 weeks in seven overweight or obese women under energy-balanced conditions. The intervention diet supplied 25% of energy from fructose. Fructose consumption significantly increased blood concentrations of fasting glucose, postprandial triacylglycerol (the storage form of fat), and apolipoprotein-B (the integral protein of the low-density lipoprotein that transports cholesterol to tissues) while decreasing insulin response (Swarbrick et al., 2008).

In a small clinical trial, Stanhope and colleagues administered fructose or glucose in beverages providing 25% of energy requirements over 10 weeks to overweight or obese men and women. Fifteen subjects received fructose and 17 subjects received glucose. Although both groups had similar weight gains during the study, visceral adipose volume was significantly increased *only* in the fructose-treated group. Also, fructose increased hepatic de novo lipogenesis and postprandial triglyceride levels as well as blood concentrations of apolipoprotein-B and LDL cholesterol. Furthermore, fasting plasma glucose and insulin levels *increased* whereas insulin sensitivity *decreased* with fructose but not glucose consumption. Based on these results, the authors suggest that high dietary fructose specifically increases lipogenesis, promotes dyslipidemia, decreases insulin sensitivity, and increases visceral adiposity in overweight or obese adults (Stanhope et al., 2009). This is perhaps one of the first studies to show selective adipose deposition based on the type of monosaccharide.

These early studies therefore suggest that consuming a high level of fructose (e.g., by drinking beverages sweetened with high fructose corn syrup) may increase the risk of developing insulin resistance and type 2 diabetes. Unlike glucose, fructose does not stimulate insulin secretion or leptin release, and since these hormones are critical in the regulation of food intake and body weight, sweeteners with high levels of fructose may promote increased energy uptake and weight gain (Bray et al., 2004). Nevertheless, additional well-designed long-term studies are needed to confirm these early observations.

Ethnic Disparities in Type 2 Diabetes

Type 2 diabetes disproportionately affects Asians, Hispanics, Native Americans, Pacific Islanders, and African Americans (IDF Diabetes Atlas, 2010; NIDDK, 2008). As discussed earlier in the section on risk factors, obesity increases the risk of diabetes and is the strongest modifiable predictor of type 2 diabetes. Nevertheless, diabetes risk is modified by ethnicity, and paradoxically, Asians, although phenotypically leaner on average than members of most other ethnic groups, have been found to be at high risk for developing type 2 diabetes at relatively low levels of body mass (Lauderdale & Rathouz, 2000).

For example, Shai and colleagues found that ethnicity significantly modified the effects of body mass on the risk of diabetes in a multiethnic cohort study conducted as a part of the *U.S. Nurses' Health Study*. They studied associations between measures of body mass (BMI and BMI gain) and the risk of diabetes in 78,419 middle-aged female nurses who were healthy at baseline and followed for up to 20 years during 1980–2000. Compared to Caucasians, the BMI and age-adjusted relative risks for type 2 diabetes were 34% and 86% higher among Hispanics and African Americans, respectively. The relative risk, however, was 126% higher among Asian women, who also exhibited the *lowest* mean baseline BMI and lowest mean BMI gain. For each 5 kg weight gain, the risk of diabetes increased by 84% for Asians, 38% for African Americans, 37% for Caucasians, and 4% for Hispanics. Controlling for additional factors including energy and alcohol intake, exercise, and smoking status did not appreciably alter the relative risks (Shai et al., 2006).

Similar results have been observed by other investigators and there is general consensus that Asian men and women have higher risks of developing type 2 diabetes at lower BMIs than other ethnoracial groups (Bei-Fan & the Cooperative Meta-analysis Group on Obesity in China, 2003; Deurenberg-Yap & Deurenberg, 2003; Misra, 2003; Pan et al., 2004). Although Asians have a very low prevalence of obesity, they are still at higher risk for developing type 2 diabetes compared to Caucasians, and Asians are at highest risk for type 2 diabetes at any given level of BMI, compared to Caucasian Americans, African Americans, and Hispanic Americans (Shai et al., 2006). The physiological basis for this ethnic differential in risk may relate to body composition and the distribution of body fat. For example, some studies suggest that persons of Asian origin have a higher percentage of body fat and/or a higher level of visceral or abdominal fat at the same level of BMI than control subjects of other ethnicities (Deurenberg-Yap & Deurenberg, 2003; Tanaka, Horimai, & Katsukawa, 2003).

In the United States, obesity and diabetes statistics have become less transparent with respect to certain minority groups. Specifically, the aggregation of data for Asian and Pacific Islander populations in government reports and some epidemiologic studies conceals important differences in the prevalence of obesity (Harrison et al., 2005; NIDDK, 2008). This is probably an attempt to overcome statistical problems associated with small sample sizes. At issue is a significant underestimation of the prevalence of obesity among Pacific Islanders, shown clearly in a recent study of childhood obesity among Asians and Pacific Islanders. In this study of children aged 9–17 years old, the obesity prevalence among the aggregated Asian/Pacific Islander group was 13%. However, once the data were disaggregated, the Asian obesity prevalence was 12.1%, while among the Pacific Islanders, the prevalence was threefold higher at nearly 36% (Shabbir, Kwan, Wang, Shih, & Simon, 2010). As in children, adult Pacific Islanders (to include Native Hawaiian, Guamanian, Samoan, Tahitian, and others) exhibit one of the highest obesity levels of all ethnic groups, while Asians, which include Southeast Asian subgroups, Asian Indian, Chinese, Japanese, Korean, and Filipino, have the lowest (WHO, 2004).

Although Asians are purported to represent approximately 95% of the entire Asian/Pacific Islander category, the relative proportions of Asians and Pacific Islanders for any particular study may differ. Aggregating Asian and Pacific Islander data makes it difficult to identify the relative contribution of obesity (or other risk factors) to the risk of diabetes for each group, and to adequately compare estimates across studies or evaluate trends over time. Obviously, aggregating data across ethnic groups or BMI categories results in diabetes statistics that fail to discern important differences in the burden of disease. Rather than aggregating these two highly dissimilar populations, oversampling of each may provide more accurate and precise estimates per group and improve public health analytic and intervention efforts (Brown & Rother, 2010).

▶ The Metabolic Syndrome (Syndrome X)

The recognition of constellations of clinical entities that predispose individuals to subsequent more gravid conditions has become increasingly important in developing effective multidisciplinary therapeutic strategies. Such is the case for the *metabolic syndrome or syndrome X*. According to the National Cholesterol Education Program's Adult Treatment Panel III Report, the constellation of symptoms defining the metabolic syndrome consists of abdominal obesity (increased waist circumference), atherogenic dyslipidemia (increased triglycerides and decreased HDL-cholesterol), hypertension, insulin resistance (impaired glucose uptake in the presence of normal or elevated insulin levels), a proinflammatory state (elevated C-reactive protein), and a prothrombotic state (increased plasminogen activator inhibitor). The clinical diagnosis is made when any three of these conditions exist in the same individual (Grundy et al., 2004).

Certain components of the metabolic syndrome were described by Dr. Gerald Phillips of Columbia University in New York. His definition included glucose intolerance, hyperinsulinemia, hypercholesterolemia, hypertriglyceridemia, and hypertension in association with obesity, aging, and an elevation in the ratio of estrogen to testosterone (Phillips, 1977). Dr. Gerald Reaven of Stanford University described a similar constellation of symptoms and ascribed the predominant underlying condition to be "insulin resistance" (Reaven, 1988).

There is debate regarding whether obesity and/or insulin resistance cause the metabolic syndrome or if they are consequences of other metabolic abnormalities. One pathogenic sequence involves the development of obesity and excess adiposity; subsequently, adipocytes that have reached their threshold of fat storage respond by secreting inflammatory substances called adipokines that interfere with the insulin-driven glucose transport system (Unger, 2003; Unger & Scherer, 2010). A number of markers of systemic inflammation, including C-reactive protein, are often increased in individuals with the metabolic syndrome, as are fibrinogen, interleukin 6 (IL–6), and tumor necrosis factor-alpha (TNFα). Two prominent adipokines that may be involved in insulin resistance are leptin and resistin, both of which have been observed to increase in association with obesity and insulin resistance (Degawa-Yamauchi et al., 2003). However, other investigators have not observed this association and in fact have noted *decreased* levels of resistin associated with obesity (Nagaev & Smith, 2001). Additional studies will be needed to clarify the role of specific adipokines in the pathogenesis of insulin resistance.

In 2002, members of the *National Cholesterol Education Program Expert Panel on Detection, Evaluation and Treatment of High Blood Cholesterol in Adults* analyzed data from the *Third Nutrition Examination Survey (NHANES III)* to determine the prevalence and other characteristics of the metabolic syndrome. Estimates of prevalence were obtained from a cross-sectional survey of a nationally representative sample of 8814 men and women of the United States collected during 1988–1994. The age-adjusted prevalence of the metabolic syndrome for this time frame was 23.7%. Estimates were similar for men and women but varied by ethnicity (e.g., Mexican Americans had a higher prevalence [31.9%] than Caucasian Americans [23.8%] or African Americans [21.9%]). The prevalence increased with age to levels greater than 40% for individuals aged 60 years or older. Extrapolating to data from the 2000 U.S. census, the investigators estimated that approximately 47 million adults in the United States met the criteria for the metabolic syndrome during 1988–1994 (Ford, Giles, & Dietz, 2002).

In a subsequent analysis of NHANES data ($n = 3423$) for the time period 2003–2006, approximately 34% of U.S. adults met the criteria for the metabolic syndrome. Prevalence estimates increased with age reaching levels higher than 50% for men and women 60 years and older. The survey reflects a marked increase (from 24% to 34%) in the prevalence of the metabolic syndrome among U.S. adults during the past two decades; currently, it is estimated that nearly one-third of U.S. adults (66 million) are afflicted by the metabolic syndrome (Ervin, 2009).

Estimates from the United States, Western Europe, Japan, Australasia, and elsewhere suggest that 75% of patients with prediabetes and 86% of patients diagnosed with type 2 diabetes also have the metabolic syndrome (Grundy, 2006). In fact, some investigators suggest that without treatment, virtually all patients with the syndrome will progress to type 2 diabetes. A number of studies have shown that the metabolic syndrome as well as its individual components are predictive of the development of type 2 diabetes (Hanley et al., 2005; Hanson, Imperatore, Bennett, & Knowler, 2002; Laaksonen et al., 2002; Lorenzo et al., 2003). But whether the syndrome itself is a better predictor than the sum of its individual components is controversial and remains under study.

The metabolic syndrome also increases the risk of developing coronary heart disease, myocardial infarction, and stroke. In an analysis of 10,357 adults participating in the Third NHANES, presence of the metabolic syndrome doubled the risk of myocardial infarction (OR = 2.0) and stroke (OR = 2.2) in both men and women (Ninomiya et al., 2004).

In the international INTERHEART Study, 26,903 subjects from 52 centers worldwide were classified according to criteria of the IDF into cases with the metabolic syndrome and controls not meeting the criteria. Presence of the metabolic syndrome more than doubled the risk of myocardial infarction (OR = 2.2) and estimated risk increases were similar by region and ethnic group. Overall, the metabolic syndrome accounted for approximately 17% of the risk of developing myocardial infarction (Mente et al., 2010).

In a meta-analysis of 21 prospective studies, individuals with the metabolic syndrome compared to those without had increases in mortality from any cause (RR = 1.35), cardiovascular disease (RR = 1.74), coronary heart disease (RR = 1.53), and stroke (RR = 1.76) (Galassi, Reynolds, & He, 2006). While the underlying physiology and even the defining clinical components of the metabolic syndrome remain subjects of hot debate, it is undeniable that the complex of obesity, insulin resistance, hypertension, hyperlipidemia, and impaired glucose metabolism known as the *metabolic syndrome* markedly heightens the risk of type 2 diabetes and catastrophic thrombotic cardiovascular outcomes such as myocardial infarction and stroke.

Gestational Diabetes

Gestational diabetes mellitus refers to hyperglycemia that arises during pregnancy. During 2017, International Federation of Diabetes (IDF) investigators estimated that 21.3 million live births (16.2%) were negatively affected by hyperglycemia during pregnancy. Of these, 18.4 million cases (86%) were due to gestational diabetes in the mother.

There is considerable variation in the prevalence of gestational diabetes both among and within countries. In a comprehensive review of 77 studies, median estimates of prevalence ranged from 5.8% in Europe to 12.9% in the Middle East and North Africa, and estimates were influenced by the intensity of screening, diagnostic criteria and inherent characteristics of the study populations. Risk factors for gestational diabetes include advanced maternal age, obesity, abdominal adiposity, genetic predisposition, sedentary lifestyle, and parity. Furthermore, the risk of type 2 diabetes increases dramatically in women with a history of gestational diabetes (e.g. relative risk estimates ranging from 3 up to 47 have been reported) (Zhu & Zhang, 2016).

Gestational diabetes is detected in approximately 200,000 pregnant women annually in the United States, or about 7.5% of pregnancies (Homko, 2010;

IADPSG, 2010; IDF Diabetes Atlas, 2010). Gestational diabetes disproportionately occurs in ethnic groups at high risk for developing type 2 diabetes, such as women of Hispanic, Asian, American Indian/Pacific Islander, and African-American origin (Dabelea et al., 2005; Lawrence, Contreras, Chen, & Sacks, 2008).

Although the *prevalence* of gestational diabetes remained stable from 1999 to 2005 in the United States, there are indications that the *incidence* has risen. For example, Lawrence and colleagues noted that among all the deliveries at Kaiser Permanente hospitals in Southern California, 10% involved women with pre-existing diabetes in 1999, which doubled to 21% by 2005 (Lawrence et al., 2008). Congenital malformations, spontaneous abortion, and *macrosomia* (excessive birth weight) are three major pregnancy complications associated with pregestational diabetes. In addition to fetal risk, the health consequences of diabetes, retinopathy, nephropathy, neuropathy, and cardiovascular disease are all accentuated by pregnancy (Leary, Pettitt, & Jovanivic, 2010). Women with a history of gestational diabetes mellitus are at a two- to threefold elevated risk for developing type 2 diabetes (Kim, Newton, & Knopp, 2002).

Type 2 Diabetes in Children and Adolescents

Type 2 diabetes is becoming more common in children and adolescents, and in some ethnic pediatric populations it is more common than type 1 diabetes (American Diabetes Association, 2010). Obesity is the primary risk factor for type 2 diabetes and the global increases in the prevalence of overweight and obese individuals over the past 60 years are inexorably linked to the increase in type 2 diabetes. Calorically, dense and nutritionally poor food and drink choices coupled with increased sedentary behaviors and decreases in physical activity are implicated as the primary behavioral culprits. Environmental factors are thought to influence behaviors in children. These include parental lifestyle and guidance, the built environment, safety factors, school policies on physical education, access to healthier food choices, value-driven trends in the cost:size ratio of energy-dense fast foods, and inappropriate marketing to children.

Double Diabetes

Differentiating type 1 from type 2 diabetes is complicated by an entity known as *double diabetes*, also coined 1.5 diabetes, type 3 diabetes, LADY (latent autoimmune diabetes in youth), or LADA (latent autoimmune diabetes in adulthood) (Kroner, 2009; Pozzilli & Buzzetti, 2007). This *hybrid* form of diabetes can present clinically as type 2 diabetes, but observed markers of autoimmunity to pancreatic β-cells are also evident. Double diabetes can also present clinically as type 1 diabetes with either a concomitant underlying insulin resistance syndrome or acquired insulin resistance due to a long-term chronic positive energy balance coupled with tight exogenous insulin-mediated glucose control. Indeed, 20%–30% of type 1 diabetic patients receiving insulin replacement therapy subsequently become overweight or obese thereby predisposing them to insulin resistance (McCulloch, 2010; Moore et al., 2009; Nadeau et al., 2010).

▶ Economic Impact of Diabetes

The predicted healthcare burden and profound economic implications of the long-term management of diabetes is staggering and unsustainable. Worldwide, the annual estimated cost is $490 billion in U.S. dollars (IDF Diabetes Atlas, 2010). After adjusting for age and gender differences, the average U.S. medical expenditure among diabetics living in the United States in 2007 was 2.3 times higher than what expenditures would have been in the absence of diabetes, at a total cost of $174 billion dollars annually (USPTFS, 2008). In addition, nearly one out of five healthcare dollars in the United States is spent on the care of diabetic patients (Permutt, Wasson, & Cox, 2005). Clearly, the cost of effective treatment and management has outstripped the resources of healthcare systems worldwide, underscoring the critical need for more cost-effective strategies for the primary, secondary, and tertiary prevention of diabetes and its complications.

▶ Prevention of Diabetes Mellitus

For all individuals and particularly those at high risk for developing type 2 diabetes (those overweight or obese, or who have prediabetes or a strong family history of diabetes), the American Diabetes Association recommends specific lifestyle practices that include sustained weight control through restriction of caloric intake and regular daily physical exercise (American Diabetes Association, 2010). Specific dietary strategies include reduction of saturated fat to less than 7% of calories, avoidance of trans fats, limiting alcohol consumption to a maximum of two drinks daily, frequent consumption of whole-grain products and monounsaturated fat, daily intake of at least 14 g of fiber, monitoring of carbohydrates, limiting consumption of foods with a high glycemic index, limiting intake of sweetened beverages and desserts (particularly those with high levels of fructose), and monitoring of total average daily calories consumed. Blood lipids, blood pressure, blood glucose, and other vital signs should be checked by a physician on a regular basis and maintained within normal limits.

A remarkable and disturbing statistic is that nearly 25% of people with type 2 diabetes in the United States are undiagnosed. Indeed, adult-onset disease is often not detected until clinically overt complications are present. Fortunately, relatively simple tests are available to detect preclinical disease (prediabetes) and effective nonpharmacologic interventions have proven effective in preventing the progression of prediabetes to diabetes (Diabetes Prevention Program Research Group, 2002; Pan et al., 1997; Tuomilehto et al., 2001). Clearly, well-designed population screening programs coupled with effective lifestyle changes and therapy could substantially reduce the overwhelming health burden of type 2 diabetes (Norris, Kansagara, Bougatsos, Nygren, & Fu, 2008).

Type 2 diabetes is characterized by insulin resistance and reduced energy storage capacity of adipocytes and progressive deterioration in beta-cell function and mass. These metabolic disturbances may be reversible by therapeutic intervention, particularly during the early stage of disease. Interventions found to maintain insulin sensitivity and energy storage capacity of adipocytes and preserve or rejuvenate beta-cells include short-term intensive insulin therapy and judicious use of drugs with both adipogenic and anti-apoptotic effects, such as the thiazolidinediones (Rosen & MacDougald, 2006; Wajchenberg, 2007).

Type 2 diabetes is also characterized by progressive deterioration in β-cell function and mass. The reduction of β-cell mass is attributable to accelerated apoptosis which can often be reversed by early therapeutic intervention, particularly during the early stage of disease. Interventions found to preserve or rejuvenate β-cells include short-term intensive insulin therapy and administration of anti-apoptotic drugs, such as the thiazolidinediones (Wajchenberg, 2007).

Widespread clinical testing of asymptomatic low-risk individuals is currently *not* recommended for type 1 diabetes. However, annual physical examinations should include a check of blood glucose in addition to observation of clinically overt signs and risk factors. Children who develop type 1 diabetes most often present with acute symptoms and markedly elevated blood glucose levels and most cases are quickly diagnosed and treated.

Screening for Gestational Diabetes

Worldwide, approximately 14% of all pregnancies are complicated by gestational diabetes (18.4 million cases annually). Disorders and complications associated with gestational diabetes include pre-eclampsia, preterm delivery, and postpartum depression in the mother and macrosomia and neonatal jaundice requiring intensive care in the infant. Because the risks to the mother and the neonate are significant, screening for gestational diabetes during the first trimester of pregnancy is warranted based on the presence of any one of the following risk factors: obesity, prior history of disease, prior delivery of a large-for-gestational-age baby, presence of glycosuria, diagnosis of polycystic ovarian syndrome, and family history of type 2 diabetes (Crowther et al., 2005).

Tertiary Prevention of Microvascular/Macrovascular Complications of Diabetes

Diabetes is a chronic illness that requires continuing medical care and ongoing patient management, education, and support to prevent acute complications and to reduce the risk of long-term complications. The cornerstone of tertiary prevention for diabetic patients is maintenance of blood glucose levels within normal limits by a combination of insulin replacement, antidiabetic agents, diet, and exercise. Self-monitoring of blood glucose is the major component of effective maintenance therapy, allowing patients to manage individual responses to medications and assess whether glycemic targets are being achieved. Hemoglobin A1c reflects the average glycemia over several months and has strong predictive value for diabetic complications. Hemoglobin A1c testing should therefore be performed routinely in all patients with diabetes, at initial assessment, and then as a part of continuing care. In overweight and obese diabetic patients, weight loss has been shown to reduce insulin resistance. Thus, weight loss through an individualized program of diet and exercise is recommended for all overweight or obese patients (American Diabetes Association, 2010).

Morbidly obese diabetic individuals who are unable to lose weight through diet and exercise are prime candidates for bariatric (weight loss) surgery. Follow-up studies of patients who elect to have this surgery show that most achieve substantial weight loss plus markedly improved control of blood glucose, blood lipids, and blood pressure (Buchwald et al., 2004; Dixon et al., 2008). Furthermore, weight loss surgery has also been found effective in preventing the development of insulin resistance in nondiabetic individuals who are morbidly obese (Sjostrom, Peltonen, Wedel, & Sjostrom, 2000).

Regular eye examinations are critical to prevent vision loss due to retinopathy among diabetics. The prevalence of retinopathy increases with duration of disease, affecting up to 80% of patients who have lived with diabetes for 10 or more years (Kertes & Johnson, 2007).

Routine foot examinations and proper daily foot care are important for the diabetic patient, as vascular and neurologic damage to the extremities can lead to amputation (McCulloch, 2010). As a result of diabetic neuropathy, wound healing is severely impaired largely due to the inability to mount an effective immune response. Multiple factors, including decreased cell and growth factor responses, lead to diminished peripheral blood flow and decreased local angiogenesis (Brem & Tomic-Canic, 2007). Even the slightest injury can result in sepsis and the subsequent need to amputate. Diabetic foot ulcers are a leading cause of lower-leg amputations, preceding 84% of all diabetes-related amputations and affecting 15% of people with diabetes (Reiber, Boyko, & Smith, 1995).

Sustained glucose control is essential for the prevention of dangerous episodes of hyperglycemia and ketoacidosis or hypoglycemia and diabetic coma, and to interrupt the development of long-term microvascular and macrovascular complications that increase the risk of retinopathy, neuropathy, nephropathy, and atherogenesis leading to catastrophic events such as blindness, limb amputation, kidney failure, coronary heart disease, myocardial infarction, and stroke.

Summary

Diabetes mellitus is a complex heterogeneous metabolic condition whereby hyperglycemia is the defining characteristic. The two major forms of diabetes are type 1 and type 2. The global incidence and prevalence of diabetes has risen profoundly within the past 50 years among children and adults, and both type 1 and type 2 diabetes dramatically increase the risk for irreversible health consequences such as blindness, kidney failure, and amputation as well as premature cardiovascular mortality. The long-term economic and financial healthcare burden required to manage the health consequences of this devastating disease are unsustainable.

Type 1 diabetes constitutes approximately 5%–10% of all cases of diabetes and is predominately the result of autoimmune destruction of the β-cells of the pancreas, leading to little or no insulin production. Without daily, lifetime exogenous insulin, either through injection or pump, glucose cannot enter the cells that require insulin's action, leading to severe hyperglycemia. A disease with a long latency period, type 1 diabetes has no known cure and has been increasing in annual incidence. Type 1 diabetes does not have a strong basis for primary prevention or screening, as genetic susceptibility, family history, and unknown environmental triggers interact to induce the onset of disease. Excess postnatal weight gain and obesity, and certain alleles of the HLA locus (HLA-DR3/4 and HLA-DQ8) have been reported to increase the risk. Linkages with other autoimmune conditions have been found in certain populations; for example, Sardinian children have high rates of both type 1 diabetes and multiple sclerosis. Susceptible Caucasians are at highest risk for developing type 1 diabetes; however, geography, seasonality, and latitude appear to modify the risk.

Type 2 diabetes constitutes approximately 90%–95% of all cases of diabetes and is currently considered a global pandemic as both the incidence and prevalence have risen sharply within the past several decades. Developing countries with large populations are partly responsible for the increasing global burden of diabetes as urbanization and westernization are leading to lifestyle factors that are driving increasing levels of obesity. The strongest predictors of type 2 diabetes are family history, age, ethnicity, and obesity. Family history is the strongest *nonmodifiable* predictor of type 2 diabetes; however, obesity is the strongest *modifiable* predictor and has therefore been a primary target for public health prevention efforts. It is noteworthy that obesity produces marked increases in the risk (relative risk estimates for gravid obesity exceed 90 in women and 40 in men). Some gene variants have been identified that increase the risk of type 2 diabetes by down-regulating the secretion and action of insulin, and future studies of the human genome are likely to elucidate genetic targets for effective antidiabetic therapy. Diets with a high glycemic index and high levels of saturated fat and trans fat have also been reported to increase the risk, whereas diets high in polyunsaturated fat, monounsaturated fat, and magnesium appear to decrease the risk.

The *metabolic syndrome* is diagnosed by a constellation of clinical signs and symptoms including abdominal obesity, hyperlipidemia (triglycerides and cholesterol), hypertension, elevated C-reactive protein, and insulin resistance. The syndrome markedly elevates the risk of developing type 2 diabetes, and in fact the majority of afflicted subjects are either prediabetic or already have type 2 diabetes. The metabolic syndrome also significantly increases the risk of developing thrombotic cardiovascular conditions (e.g., coronary heart disease, myocardial infarction, and stroke).

The primary mechanism by which obesity causes classic obesity-related type 2 diabetes is through insulin resistance in striated muscle and fat cells. When these cells reach their storage capacity and are no longer able to store additional excess energy, a host of regulatory signaling proteins are secreted that stimulate decreases in the activities of insulin receptors, insulin signaling, lipoprotein lipase, and Glut-4 translocation. The β-cells of the pancreas produce and secrete even more insulin to compensate. Blood glucose can increase silently over many years without producing clinical symptoms. Afflicted individuals typically pass through a prediabetic state of elevated blood glucose and general metabolic dysregulation that may include hyperinsulinemia, dyslipidemia, and hypertension. Eventually, the amount of insulin that is produced and secreted can no longer maintain glucose levels within normal limits. In persons with diabetes and chronically elevated blood glucose levels, AGEs are actively produced and accumulate in circulating blood and various bodily tissues. The gradual buildup of AGEs plays a critical role in the pathogenesis of retinopathy, cataract formation, atherosclerosis, neuropathy, diabetic embryopathy, and impaired wound healing in individuals with poorly controlled diabetes (Ahmed, 2005).

In the United States, type 2 diabetes disproportionately affects minority groups such as Hispanics, African Americans, American Indians, and Pacific Islanders, who have relatively high obesity levels. Paradoxically, Asians, who are phenotypically leaner than other ethnoracial groups, are at high risk for developing type 2 diabetes despite much lower levels of obesity, as defined by the BMI. A higher body fat percentage and/ or higher visceral fat or abdominal fat per unit BMI are often cited as the primary reasons for this observation. Emerging hypotheses implicate a lower overall adipocyte energy storage capacity, which would stimulate metabolic regulatory feedback mechanisms at a lower level of weight gain, resulting in insulin resistance and reduced glucose uptake at lower obesity levels. This explanation provides a biologic rationale for the public health recommendation to avoid inappropriate weight gain and the observation that

moderate weight loss of approximately 10% results in improvements in metabolic health in individuals with elevated body mass. Albeit, persons who are clinically obese may need to lose more than 10% excess weight in order to achieve metabolic homeostasis.

References

Ahmed, N. (2005). Advanced glycation end-product: Role in pathology of diabetic complications. *Diabetes Research and Clinical Practice, 67*(1), 3–21.

Ali, H., Anwar, M., Ahmed, T., & Chand, N. (2006). Diabetes mellitus from antiquity to present scenario and contribution of Greco-Arab physicians. *JISHIM, 5,* 46–50.

American Diabetes Association. (2010). Standards of medical care in diabetes—2010. *Diabetes Care, 33,* S11–S61.

Arizona Department of Health Services. (2004). *Health status profile of American Indians in Arizona (2004).* Phoenix, Arizona: Arizona Bureau of Public Health Services.

Barclay, A. W., Petocz, P., McMillan-Price, J., Flood, V. M., Prvan, T., Mitchell, P., & Brand-Miller, J. C. (2008). Glycemic index, glycemic load, and chronic disease risk—A meta-analysis of observational studies. *American Journal of Clinical Nutrition, 87,* 627–637.

Barker, D. J. P. (1997). Maternal nutrition, fetal nutrition, and disease in later life. *Nutrition, 13,* 807.

Barker, J. M., Barriga, K. J., Yu, L., Miao, D., Erlich, H. A., Norris, J. M., … Diabetes Autoimmunity Study in the Young. (2004). Prediction of autoantibody positivity and progression to type 1 diabetes: Diabetes Autoimmunity Study in the Young (DAISY). *Journal of Clinical Endocrinology & Metabolism, 89*(8), 3896–3902.

Bays, H., Mandarino, L., & DeFronzo, R. A. (2004). Role of the adipocyte, free fatty acids, and ectopic fat in pathogenesis of type 2 diabetes mellitus: Peroxisomal proliferator-activated receptor agonists provide a rational therapeutic approach. *Journal of Clinical Endocrinology & Metabolism, 89,* 463–478.

Bei-Fan, Z., & the Cooperative Meta-analysis Group on Obesity in China. (2003). Predictive values of body mass index and waist circumference for risk factors of certain related diseases in Chinese adults: Study on optimal cut-off points of body mass index and waist circumference in Chinese adults. *Asia Pacific Journal of Clinical Nutrition, 11*(S8), S685–S693.

Bild, D. E., & Stevenson, J. M. (1992). Frequency of recording of diabetes on US death certificates: Analysis of the 1986 National Mortality Followback Survey. *Journal of Clinical Epidemiology, 45*(3), 275–281.

Bingley, P. J., & Gale, E. A. M. (1989). Rising incidence of IDDM in Europe. *Diabetes Care, 12,* 289–295.

Brand-Miller, J. (1994). The importance of the glycemic index in diabetes. *American Journal of Clinical Nutrition, 59,* 747S–752S.

Bray, G. A., Nielsen, S. J., & Popkin, B. M. (2004). Consumption of high-fructose corn syrup in beverages may play a role in the epidemic of obesity. *American Journal of Clinical Nutrition, 79*(4), 537–543.

Brem, H., & Tomic-Canic, M. (2007). Cellular and molecular basis of wound healing in diabetes. *Journal of Clinical Investigation, 117*(5), 1219–1222.

Brown, R. J., & Rother, K. I. (2010). Type 1 and type 2 diabetes in five race and ethnic populations: The SEARCH for Diabetes in Youth Study. *Current Cardiovascular Risk Reports, 4,* 175–177.

Brownlee, M. (2005). The pathobiology of diabetic complications. A unifying mechanism. *Diabetes, 54*(6), 1615–1625.

Buchwald, H., Avidor, Y., Braunwald, E., Jensen, M. D., Pories, W., Fahrbach, K., & Schoelles, K. (2004). Bariatric surgery: A systematic review and meta-analysis. *The Journal of the American Medical Association, 292*(14), 1724–1737.

Cambuli, V. M., Musiu, C., Incani, M., Paderi, M., Serpe, R., Marras, V., … Baroni, M. G. (2008). Assessment of adiponectin and leptin as biomarkers of positive metabolic outcomes after lifestyle intervention in overweight and obese children. *Journal of Clinical Endocrinology & Metabolism, 93*(8), 3051–3057.

Candib, L. M. (2007). Obesity and diabetes in vulnerable populations: Reflection on proximal and distal causes. *Annals of Family Medicine, 5,* 541–556.

Casu, A., Pascutto, C., Bernardinelli, L., the Sardinian IDDM Epidemiology Study Group, & Songini, M. (2004). Type 1 diabetes among Sardinian children is increasing. The Sardinian diabetes register for children aged 0–14 years (1989–1999). *Diabetes Care, 27*(7), 1623–1629.

Centers for Disease Control and Prevention. (2010). *Division of diabetes translation. National Diabetes Surveillance System.* Atlanta, GA: Centers for Disease Control and Prevention, U.S. Department of Health and Human Services. Retrieved from https://www.cdc.gov/diabetes/library/reports/congress.html

Centers for Disease Control and Prevention. (2017). *National diabetes statistics report, 2017.* Atlanta, GA: Centers for Disease Control and Prevention, U.S. Department of Health and Human Services. Retrieved from https://www.cdc.gov/diabetes/library/reports/congress.html

Chan, J. M., Rimm, E. B., Colditz, G. A., Stampfer, M. J., & Willett, W. C. (1994). Obesity, fat distribution, and weight gain as risk factors for clinical diabetes in men. *Diabetes Care, 17*(9), 961–969.

Chast, F. (2000). Apollinaire Bouchardat, pharmacist, nutritionist. *Annales Pharmaceutiques Françaises, 58*(6 Suppl.), 435–442.

Cheng, W. S., Wingard, D. L., Kritz-Silverstein, D., & Barrett-Connor, E. (2008). Sensitivity and specificity of death certificates for diabetes: As good as it gets? *Diabetes Care, 31*(2), 279–284.

Cho, N. H., Shaw, J. E., Karurangaa, S., Huanga, Y., da Rocha Fernandesa, J. D., Ohlroggea, A. W., & Malandaa, B. (2018). IDF diabetes atlas: Global estimates of diabetes prevalence for 2017 and projections for 2045. *Diabetes Research and Clinical Practice, 138,* 271–281.

Christopoulou-Aletra, H., & Papavramidou, N. (2008). "Diabetes" as described by Byzantine writers from the fourth to the ninth century AD: The Graeco-Roman influence. *Diabetologia, 51,* 892–896.

Colditz, G. A., Willett, W. C., Rotnitzky, A., & Manson, J. E. (1995). Weight gain as a risk factor for clinical diabetes mellitus in women. *Annals of Internal Medicine, 122,* 481–486.

Cowie, C. C., Rust, K. F., Byrd-Holt, D. D., Gregg, E. W., Ford, E. S., Geiss, L. S., … Fradkin, J. E. (2010). Prevalence of diabetes and high risk for diabetes using A1C criteria in the US population in 1988–2006. *Diabetes Care, 33*(3), 562–568.

Crowther, C. A., Hiller, J. E., Moss, J. R., McPhee, A. J., Jeffries, W. S., & Robinson, J. S. (2005). Effect of treatment of gestational diabetes mellitus on pregnancy outcomes. *New England Journal of Medicine, 352*, 2477–2486.

Czech, M. P., & Corvera, S. (1999). Signaling mechanisms that regulate glucose transport. *Journal of Biological Chemistry, 274*(4), 1865–1868.

Dabelea, D., Hanson, R. L., Lindsay, R. S., Pettit, D. J., Imperatore, G., Gabir, M. M., … Knowler, W. C. (2000). Intrauterine exposure to diabetes conveys risk for type 2 diabetes and obesity. A study of discordant sibship. *Diabetes, 49*, 2208–2211.

Dabelea, D., Snell-Bergeon, J. K., Hartsfield, C. L., Bischoff, K. J., Hamman, R. F., McDuffie, R. S., & Kaiser Permanente of Colorado GDM Screening Program. (2005). Increasing prevalence of gestational diabetes mellitus (GDM) over time and by birth cohort: Kaiser Permanente of Colorado GDM screening program. *Diabetes Care, 28*, 579–584.

Dahlquist, G., & Kallen, B. (2005). Mortality in childhood-onset type 1 diabetes. *Diabetes Care, 28*(10), 2384–2387.

Danforth, E. (2000). Failure of adipocyte differentiation causes type II diabetes? *Nature Genetics, 26*, 13.

Degawa-Yamauchi, M., Bovenkerk, J. E., Juliar, B. E., Watson, W., Kerr, K., Jones, R., … Considine, R. V. (2003). Serum resistin (FIZZ3) protein is increased in obese humans. *Journal of Clinical Endocrinology & Metabolism, 88*(11), 5452–5455.

Deurenberg-Yap, M., & Deurenberg, P. (2003). Is a re-evaluation of WHO body mass index cut-off values needed? The case of Asians in Singapore. *Nutrition Reviews, 62*, S80–S87.

Diabetes Prevention Program Research Group. (2002). Reduction in the incidence of type 2 diabetes with lifestyle intervention or metformin. *New England Journal of Medicine, 346*, 393–403.

DIAMOND Project Group. (2006). Incidence and trends of childhood type 1 diabetes worldwide, 1990–1999. *Diabetic Medicine, 23*, 857–866.

Dixon, J. B., O'Brien, P. E., Playfair, J., Chapman, L., Schachter, L. M., Skinner, S., … Anderson, M. (2008). Adjustable gastric banding and conventional therapy for type 2 diabetes. A randomized controlled trial. *JAMA, 299*, 316–323.

Dorman, J. S., LaPorte, R. E., & Songer, T. J. (2003). Epidemiology of type 1 diabetes. In M. A. Sperling (Ed.), *Type 1 diabetes. Etiology and treatment*. Totowa, NJ: Humana Press.

Eisenbarth, G. S., & McCulloch, D. K. (2010, July). Pathogenesis of type 1 diabetes mellitus. In UpToDate®.

Eknoyan, G., & Nagy, J. (2005). A history of diabetes mellitus or how a disease of the kidneys evolved into a kidney disease. *Advances in Chronic Kidney Disease, 12*(2), 223–229.

Eledrisi, M. S., Alshanti, M. S., Shah, M. F., Brolosy, B., & Jaha, N. (2006). Overview of the diagnosis and management of diabetic ketoacidosis. *American Journal of Medical Science, 331*(5), 243–251.

Engelgau, M. M., Geiss, L. S., Saaddine, B. M., Gregg, E. W., Tierney, E. F., Rios-Burrows, N., … Narayan, K. M. V. (2004). The evolving diabetes burden in the United States. *Annals of Internal Medicine, 140*(11), 945–950.

Ervin, R. B. (2009). Prevalence of metabolic syndrome among adults 20 years of age and over, by sex, age, race and ethnicity, and body mass index: United States, 2003–2006. *National Health Statistics Reports*, 13. Hyattsville, MD: National Center for Health Statistics.

Eurodiab ACE Study Group. (2000). Variation and trends in incidence of childhood diabetes in Europe. *Lancet, 355*, 873–876.

Feskens, E. J. M., & Kromhout, D. (1990). Habitual dietary intake and glucose tolerance in euglycemic men: The Zutphen Study. *International Journal of Epidemiology, 19*, 953–959.

Feskens, E. J. M., Virtanen, S. M., Rasanen, L., Tuomilehto, J., Stengard, J., Pekkanen, J., & Kromhout, D. (1995). Dietary factors determining diabetes and impaired glucose tolerance. A 20-year follow-up of the Finnish and Dutch cohorts of the Seven Countries Study. *Diabetes Care, 18*, 1104–1112.

Ford, E. S., Giles, W. H., & Dietz, W. H. (2002). Prevalence of the metabolic syndrome among US adults: Findings from the third National Health and Nutrition Examination Survey. *JAMA, 287*, 356–359.

Foster-Powell, K., Holt, S. H. A., & Brand-Miller, J. C. (2002). International table of glycemic index and glycemic load values. *American Journal of Clinical Nutrition, 76*, 5–56.

Fourlanos, S., Harrison, L. C., & Colman, P. G. (2008). The accelerator hypothesis and increasing incidence of type 1 diabetes. *Current Opinion in Endocrinology Diabetes and Obesity, 15*(4), 321–325.

Fowler, M. J. (2008). Microvascular and macrovascular complications of diabetes. *Clinical Diabetes, 26*, 77–82.

Frühbeck, G., Gomez-Ambrosi, J., Muruzabai, F. J., & Burrell, M. A. (2001). The adipocyte: A model for integration of endocrine and metabolic signaling in energy metabolism regulation. *American Journal of Physiology–Endocrinology and Metabolism, 280*, E827–E847.

Fujimoto, W. Y. (1996). Overview of non-insulin-dependent diabetes mellitus (NIDDM) in different population groups. *Diabetic Medicine, 13*(9 Suppl. 6), S7–S10.

Galassi, A., Reynolds, K., & He, J. (2006). Metabolic syndrome and risk of cardiovascular disease: A meta-analysis. *American Journal of Medicine, 119*(10), 812–819.

Gale, E. A. M. (2002). The rise of childhood type 1 diabetes in the twentieth century. *Diabetes, 51*, 3353–3361.

Gale, E. A. M. (2005). Spring harvest? Reflections on the rise of type 1 diabetes. *Diabetologia, 48*(12), 2445–2450.

Garg, A. (1998). High-monounsaturated-fat diets for patients with diabetes mellitus. *American Journal of Clinical Nutrition, 67*(Suppl.), 577S–582S.

Gemmill, C. L. (1972). The Greek concept of diabetes. *Bulletin of the New York Academy of Medicine, 48*(8), 1033–1036.

Gerstein, H. C., Santaguida, P., Raina, P., Morrison, K. M., Galion, C., Hunt, D., … Booker, L. (2007). Annual incidence and relative risk of diabetes in people with various categories of dysglycemia: A systematic overview and meta-analysis of prospective studies. *Diabetes Research and Clinical Practice, 78*, 305–312.

Gillespie, K. M., Bain, S. C., Barnett, A. H., Bingley, P. J., Christie, M. R., Gill, G. V., & Gale, E. A. (2004). The rising incidence of childhood type 1 diabetes and reduced contribution of high-risk HLA haplotypes. *Lancet, 364*, 1699–1700.

Goldfarb, M. F. (2008). Relation of time of introduction of cow milk protein to an infant and risk of type 1 diabetes mellitus. *Journal of Proteome Research, 7*, 2165–2167.

Gomero, A., McDade, T., Williams, S., & Lindau, S. T. (2008). *Dried bloodspot measurement of glycosylated hemoglobin (HbA1c) in wave 1 of the National Social Life and Aging Project*. Chicago, IL: NORC and the University of Chicago.

Gould, G. W., & Holman, G. D. (1993). The glucose transporter family: Structure, function, and tissue-specific expression. *Biochemical Journal, 295*, 329–341.

Greenfield, J. R., Samaras, K., & Chisholm, D. J. (2002). Insulin resistance, intra-abdominal fat, cardiovascular risk factors, and androgens in healthy young women with type 1 diabetes mellitus. *Journal of Clinical Endocrinology & Metabolism, 87*(3), 1036–1040.

Gregg, E. W., Cadwell, B. L., Cheng, Y. J., Cowie, C. C., Williams, D. E., Geiss, L., … Vinicor, F. (2004). Trends in the prevalence and ratio of diagnosed to undiagnosed diabetes according to obesity levels. *Diabetes Care, 27*, 2806–2812.

Gregory, J. M., Lilley, J. S., Misfeldt, A. A., Buscariollo, D. L., Russell, W. E., & Moore, D. J. (2010). Incorporating type 1 diabetes prevention into clinical practice. *Clinical Diabetes, 28*(2), 61–70.

Grundy, S. M. (2006). Metabolic syndrome: Connecting and reconciling cardiovascular and diabetes worlds. *Journal of the American College of Cardiology, 47*(6), 1093–1100.

Grundy, S. M., Brewer, H. B., Cleeman, J. I., Smith, S. C., Lenfant, D., & for the Conference Participants. (2004). Definition of metabolic syndrome: Report of the National, Heart, Lung, and Blood Institute/American Heart Association conference on scientific issues related to definition. *Circulation, 109*, 433–438.

Gupta, R., & Kumar, P. (2008). Global diabetes landscape—Type 2 diabetes mellitus in South Asia: Epidemiology, risk factors, and control. *Insulin, 3*(2), 78–94.

Guthrie, D. W., & Humphreys, S. S. (1988). Diabetes urine testing: An historical perspective. *Diabetes Educator, 14*(6), 521–526.

Hales, C. N., & Barker, D. J. P. (1992). Type 2 (non-insulin dependent) diabetes mellitus: The thrifty phenotype hypothesis. *Diabetologia, 35*, 1235–1239.

Hanley, A. J. G., Karter, A. J., Williams, K., Festa, A., D'Agostino, R. B., Wagenknecht, L. E., & Haffner, S. M. (2005). Prediction of type 2 diabetes mellitus with alternative definitions of the metabolic syndrome: The Insulin Resistance Atherosclerosis Study. *Circulation, 112*, 3713–3721.

Hansen, L., & Pedersen, O. (2005). Genetics of type 2 diabetes mellitus: Status and perspectives. *Diabetes Obesity and Metabolism, 7*(2), 122–135.

Hanson, R. L., Imperatore, G., Bennett, P. H., & Knowler, W. C. (2002). Components of the "metabolic syndrome" and incidence of type 2 diabetes. *Diabetes, 51*, 3120–3127.

Harder, T., Roepke, K., Diller, N., Stechling, Y., Dudenhausen, J. W., & Plagemann, A. (2009). Birth weight, early weight gain, and subsequent risk of type 1 diabetes: Systematic review and meta-analysis. *American Journal of Epidemiology, 169*(12), 1428–1436.

Harjutsalo, V., Sjöberg, L., & Tuomilehto, J. (2008). Time trends in the incidence of type 1 diabetes in Finnish children: A cohort study. *Lancet, 31*(9636), 1777–1782.

Harris, M. I., Klein, R., Welborn, T. A., & Knuiman, M. W. (1992). Onset of NIDDM occurs at least 4–7 years before clinical diagnosis. *Diabetes Care, 15*, 815–819.

Harrison, G. G., Kagawa-Singer, M., Foerster, S. B., Lee, H., Pham Kim, L., Nguyen, T. U., … Bal, D. G. (2005). Seizing the moment: California's opportunity to prevent nutrition-related health disparities in low-income Asian American population. *Cancer, 104*, 2962–2968.

Hatfield, J., & Mulfinger, L. (2005). Review: Advanced glycation end products (AGEs) in hyperglycemic patients. *Journal of Young Investigators, 13*(4), 1.

Hegazi, R., El-Gamal, M., Abdel-Hady, N., & Hamdy, O. (2015). Epidemiology of and risk factors for Type 2 Diabetes in Egypt. *Annals of Global Health, 81*(6), 814–820.

Henschen, F. (1969). On the term diabetes in the works of Aretaeus and Galen. *Medical History, 13*(2), 190–192.

Hodge, A. M., English, D. R., O'Dea, K., & Giles, G. (2004). Glycemic index and dietary fiber and risk of type 2 diabetes. *Diabetes Care, 27*, 2701–2706.

Homko, C. J. (2010). Gestational diabetes: Can we reach consensus? *Current Diabetes Reports, 10*, 252–254.

Hossain, P., Kawar, B., & El Nahas, M. (2007). Obesity and diabetes in the developing world: A growing challenge. *New England Journal of Medicine, 356*(3), 213–215.

IADPSG Consensus Panel. (2010). International Association of Diabetes and Pregnancy Study Groups: Recommendations on the diagnosis and classification of hyperglycemia in pregnancy. *Diabetes Care, 33*(3), 676–682.

International Diabetes Federation (IDF) Diabetes Atlas. (2006). *Prevalence estimates of diabetes mellitus (DM), 2006.* Brussels, Belgium: International Diabetes Federation.

International Diabetes Federation (IDF) Diabetes Atlas. (2010). *Prevalence estimates of diabetes mellitus (DM), 2010.* Brussels, Belgium: International Diabetes Federation.

International Diabetes Federation (IDF) Diabetes Atlas. (2017). *Prevalence estimates of diabetes mellitus (DM), 2017.* Brussels, Belgium: International Diabetes Federation.

Jenkins, D. J. A., Wolever, T. M. S., Taylor, R. H., Barker, H., Fielden, H., Baldwin, J. M., … Goff, D. V. (1981). Glycemic index of foods: A physiologic basis for carbohydrate exchange. *American Journal of Clinical Nutrition, 34*, 362–366.

Kandror, K. V., & Pilch, P. F. (1996). Compartmentalization of protein traffic in insulin sensitive cells. *American Journal of Physiology, 271*, E1–E14.

Karvonen, M., Viik-Kajander, M., Moltchanova, E., Libman, I., LaPorte, R., Tuomilehto, J., … Diabetes Mondiale (DIAMOND) Project Group. (2000). Incidence of childhood type 1 diabetes worldwide. Diabetes Mondiale (DiaMond) Project Group. *Diabetes Care, 23*, 1516–1526.

Kautiainen, S., Rimpelä, A., Vikat, A., & Virtanen, S. M. (2002). Secular trends in overweight and obesity among Finnish adolescents in 1977–1999. *International Journal of Obesity, 26*, 544–552.

Kertes, P. J., & Johnson, T. M. (2007). *Evidence-based eye care.* Philadelphia, PA: Lippincott Williams & Wilkins.

Kilpatrick, E. S. (2000). Glycated haemoglobin in the year 2000. *Journal of Clinical Pathology, 53*(5), 335–339.

Kim, C., Newton, K. M., & Knopp, R. H. (2002). Gestational diabetes and the incidence of type 2 diabetes. A systematic review. *Diabetes Care, 25*(10), 1862–1868.

King, H., Aubert, R. E., & Herman, W. H. (1998). Global burden of diabetes: 1995–2025. *Diabetes Care, 21*, 1414–1431.

Kirchof, M., Popat, N., & Malowany, J. (2008). A historical perspective of the diagnosis of diabetes. *University of Western Ontario Medical Journal, 78*(1), P7–P9.

Kitabchi, A. E., Umpierrez, G. E., Murphy, M. B., & Kreisberg, R. A. (2006). Hyperglycemic crises in adult patients with diabetes: A consensus statement from the American Diabetes Association. *Diabetes Care, 29*(12), 2739–2748.

Kitabchi, A. E., & Wall, B. M. (1999). Management of diabetic ketoacidosis. *American Family Physician, 60*(2), 455–464.

Klein, R., Klein, B. E., Moss, S., & Demets, D. L. (1988). Proteinuria in diabetes. *Archives of Internal Medicine, 148*, 181–187.

Klein, S., Sheard, N. F., Pi-Sunyer, X., Daly, A., Wylie-Rosett, J., Kulkarni, K., & Clark, N. G. (2004). Weight management through lifestyle modification for the prevention and management of type 2 diabetes: Rationale and strategies. *American Journal of Clinical Nutrition, 80*(2), 257–263.

Knowler, W. C., Bennett, P. H., Hamman, R. F., & Miller, M. (1978). Diabetes incidence and prevalence in Pima Indians: A 19-fold greater incidence than in Rochester, Minnesota. *American Journal of Epidemiology, 108*(6), 497–505.

Koh-Banerjee, P., Wang, Y., Hu, F. B., Spiegelman, D., Willett, W. C., & Rimm, E. B. (2004). Changes in body weight and body fat distribution as risk factors for clinical diabetes in US men. *American Journal of Epidemiology, 159*, 1150–1159.

Kolb, H., & Elliott, R. B. (1994). Increasing incidence of IDDM a consequence of improved hygiene? *Diabetologia, 37*(7), 729.

Krishnan, S., Rosenberg, L., Singer, M., Hu, F. B., Djoussé, L., Cupples, L. A., & Palmer, J. R. (2007). Glycemic index, glycemic load, and cereal fiber intake and risk of type 2 diabetes in US black women. *Archives of Internal Medicine, 167*, 2304–2309.

Krolewski, A. S., Warram, J. H., Rand, L. I., & Kahn, C. R. (1987). Epidemiologic approach to the etiology of type 1 diabetes and its complications. *New England Journal of Medicine, 317*, 1390–1398.

Kroner, Z. (2009). The relationship between Alzheimer's disease and diabetes: Type 3 diabetes? *Alternative Medicine Review, 14*(4), 373–379.

Kung, H. C., Hoyert, D. L., Xu, J., & Murphy, S. (2008). Deaths: Final data for 2005. *National Vital Statistics Report, 56*(10), 1–121.

Laaksonen, D. E., Lakka, H. M., Niskanen, L. K., Kaplan, G. A., Salonen, J. T., & Lakka, T. A. (2002). Metabolic syndrome and development of diabetes mellitus: Application and development of recently suggested definitions of the metabolic syndrome in a prospective cohort study. *American Journal of Epidemiology, 156*, 1070–1077.

Lambert, P. A., Gillespie, K. M., Thompson, G., Cordell, H. J., Todd, J. A., Gale, E. A., & Bingley, P. J. (2004). Absolute risk of childhood-onset type 1 diabetes defined by human leukocyte antigen class II genotype: A population-based study in the United Kingdom. *Journal of Clinical Endocrinology and Metabolism, 89*(8), 4037–4043.

Lauderdale, D. S., & Rathouz, P. J. (2000). Body mass index in a US national sample of Asian Americans: Effects of nativity, years since immigration and socioeconomic status. *International Journal of Obesity, 24*(9), 1188–1194.

Lawrence, J. M., Contreras, R., Chen, W., & Sacks, D. A. (2008). Trends in the prevalence of pre-existing diabetes and gestational diabetes mellitus among a racially/ethnically diverse population of women, 1999–2005. *Diabetes Care, 31*, 899–904.

Leary, J., Pettitt, D. J., & Jovanivic, L. (2010). Gestational diabetes guidelines in a HAPO world. *Best Practice & Research Clinical Endocrinology & Metabolism, 24*(4), 673–685.

Lee, W. L., Cheung, A. M., Cape, D., & Zinman, D. (2000). Impact of diabetes on coronary artery disease in women and men: A meta-analysis of prospective studies. *Diabetes Care, 23*(7), 962–968.

Leonhardt, W., Hanefeld, M., Schneider, H., & Haller, H. (1972). Human adipocyte volumes: Maximum size, and correlation to weight index in maturity onset-diabetes. *Diabetologia, 8*, 287–291.

Levy-Marchal, C., Patterson, C., & Green, A. (1995). Variation by age group and seasonality at diagnosis of childhood IDDM in Europe. The EURODIAB ACE Study Group. *Diabetologia, 38*, 823–830.

Ley, K., & Huo, Y. (2001). VCAM-1 is critical in atherosclerosis. *Journal of Clinical Investigation, 107*(10), 1209–1210.

Libby, P. (2002). Inflammation in atherosclerosis. *Nature, 420*(6917), 868–874.

Libby, P., Ridker, P. M., & Hansson, G. K. (2009). Inflammation in atherosclerosis. *Journal of the American College of Cardiology, 54*, 2129–2138.

Lillioja, S., Mott, D. M., Spraul, M., Ferraro, R., Foley, J. E., Ravussin, E., … Bogardus, C. (1993). Insulin resistance and insulin secretory dysfunction as precursors of non-insulin-dependent diabetes mellitus: Prospective studies of Pima Indians. *New England Journal of Medicine, 329*, 1988–1992.

Lopez-Ridaura, R., Willett, W. C., Rimm, E. B., Liu, S., Stampfer, M. J., Manson, J. E., & Hu, F. B. (2004). Magnesium intake and risk of type 2 diabetes in men and women. *Diabetes Care, 27*(1), 134–140.

Lorenzo, C., Okoloise, M., Williams, K., Stern, M. P., Haffner, S. M., & the San Antonio Heart Study. (2003). The metabolic syndrome as predictor of type 2 diabetes: The San Antonio Heart Study. *Diabetes Care, 26*, 3153–3159.

Lucas, A. (1991). Programming by early nutrition in man. In G. R. Bock & J. Whelan (Eds.), *The childhood environment and adult disease* (pp. 38–55). Chichester, England: Wiley.

Lynn, S., Evans, J. C., White, C. H., Frayling, T. M., Hattersley, A. T., Turnbull, D. M., … Walker, M. (2002). Variation in the calpain-10 gene affects blood glucose levels in the British population. *Diabetes, 51*(1), 247–250.

Marrosu, M. G., Cocco, E., Lai, M., Spinicci, G., Pischedda, M. P., & Contu, D. (2002). Patients with multiple sclerosis and risk of type 1 diabetes mellitus in Sardinia, Italy: A cohort study. *Lancet, 359*, 1461–1465.

Marrosu, M. G., Motzo, C., Murru, R., Lampis, R., Costa, G., Zavattari, P., … Cucca, F. (2004). The co-inheritance of type 1 diabetes and multiple sclerosis in Sardinia cannot be explained by genotype variation in the HLA region alone. *Human Molecular Genetics, 13*(23), 2919–2924.

Marshall, A., Hamman, R. F., & Baxter, J. (1991). High-fat, low-carbohydrate diet and the etiology of non-insulin-dependent diabetes mellitus: The San Luis Valley Diabetes Study. *American Journal of Epidemiology, 134*, 590–603.

McCarty, D., & Zimmet, P. (1994). *Diabetes from 1994 to 2010: Global estimates and projections.* Melbourne, Australia: International Diabetes Institute.

McCulloch, D. K. (2004). Classification of diabetes mellitus and genetic diabetic syndromes. In: UpToDate®.

McCulloch, D. K. (2010). Screening for diabetes mellitus. In: UpToDate®.

McEwen, L. N., Kim, C., Haan, M., Ghosh, D., Mangione, C. M., Safford, M. M., … Triad Study Group. (2006). Diabetes reporting as a cause of death: Results from the Translating Research into Action for Diabetes (TRIAD) study. *Diabetes Care, 29*(2), 247–253.

McKinney, P. A. (2001). Seasonality of birth in patients with childhood type 1 diabetes in 19 European regions. *Diabetologia, 44*, B67–B74.

Mente, A., Yusuf, S., Islam, S., McQueen, M. J., Tanomsup, S., Onen, C. L., … for the INTERHEART Investigators. (2010). Metabolic syndrome and risk of acute myocardial infarction: A case-control study of 26,903 subjects from 52 countries. *Journal of the American College of Cardiology, 55*, 2390–2398.

Meyer, K. A., Kushi, L. H., Jacobs, D. R., Jr., Slavin, J., Sellers, T. A., & Folsom, A. R. (2000). Carbohydrates, dietary fiber, and incident type 2 diabetes in older women. *American Journal of Clinical Nutrition, 71*, 921–930.

Misra, A. (2003). Revisions of cutoffs of body mass index to define overweight and obesity are needed for the Asian-ethnic groups (Debate). *International Journal of Obesity, 27*, 1294–1296.

Mokdad, A. H., Bowman, B. A., Ford, E. S., Vinicor, F., Marks, J. S., & Koplan, J. P. (2001). The continuing epidemics of obesity and diabetes in the United States. *JAMA, 286*(10), 1195–1200.

Mokdad, A. H., Ford, E. S., Bowman, B. A., Nelson, D. E., Engelgau, M. M., Finicor, F., & Marks, J. S. (2000). Diabetes trends in the US: 1990–1998. *Diabetes Care, 23*(9), 1278–1283.

Moltchanova, E. V., Schreier, N., Lammi, N., & Karvonen, M. (2009). Seasonal variation of diagnosis of type 1 diabetes in children worldwide. *Diabetes Medicine, 26*(7), 673–678.

Montonen, J., Kneckt, P., Järvinen, R., Aromaa, A., & Reunanen, A. (2003). Whole-grain and fiber intake and incidence of type 2 diabetes. *American Journal of Clinical Nutrition, 77*, 622–629.

Moore, D. J., Gregory, J. M., Kumah-Crystal, Y. A., & Simmons, J. H. (2009). Mitigating micro-and macro-vascular complications of diabetes in adolescence. *Vascular Health and Risk Management, 5*, 1015–1031.

Moss, S. E., Klein, R., & Klein, B. E. (1991). Cause-specific mortality in a population-based study of diabetes. *American Journal of Public Health,* 1158–1162.

Mott, J. W., Wang, J., Thornton, J. C., Allison, D. B., Heymsfield, S. B., & Pierson, R. N., Jr., (1999). Relation between body fat and age in 4 ethnic groups. *American Journal of Clinical Nutrition, 69*(5), 1007–1013.

Murphy, S. L., Xu, J., Kochanek, K. D., Curtin, S. C., & Arias, E. (2017). Deaths: Final data for 2015. *National Vital Statistics Reports, 66*(6), 1–75.

Nadeau, K. J., Regensteiner, J. G., Bauer, T. A., Brown, M. S., Dorosz, J. L., Hull, A., … Reusch, J. E. (2010). Insulin resistance in adolescents with type 1 diabetes and its relationship to cardiovascular function. *Journal of Clinical Endocrinology & Metabolism, 95*(2), 513–521.

Naeem, Z. (2015). Burden of diabetes mellitus in Saudi Arabia. *International Journal of Health Sciences, 9*(3), 5–6.

Nagaev, I., & Smith, U. (2001). Insulin resistance and type 2 diabetes are not related to resistin expression in human fat cells or skeletal muscle. *Biochemical and Biophysical Research Communications, 285*(2), 561–564.

Narayan, K. M., Boyle, J. P., Thompson, T. J., Sorensen, S. W., & Williamson, D. F. (2003). Lifetime risk of diabetes mellitus in the United States. *JAMA, 290*(14), 1884–1890.

Narayan, K. M., Zhang, P., Kanaya, A. M., Williams, D. E., Engelgau, M. M., Imperatore, G., & Ramachandran, A. (2006). Diabetes: The pandemic and potential solutions. In *Disease control priorities in development countries* (2nd ed., pp. 591–603). New York, NY: Oxford University Press.

National Diabetes Statistics Report. (2017). National Center for Chronic Disease Prevention and Health Promotion, Division of Diabetes Translation, Centers for Disease Control (CDC), Atlanta, Georgia.

National Heart, Lung, and Blood Institute. (1998). *National Institute of Diabetes and Digestive and Kidney Diseases. Clinical guidelines on the identification, evaluation, and treatment of overweight and obesity in adults. The evidence report* (pp. 1–228). Bethesda, MD: NIH.

National Institute of Diabetes and Digestive and Kidney Diseases. (2008). *U.S. Department of Health and Human Services, National Institutes of Health. National Diabetes Statistics, 2007 fact sheet*. Bethesda, MD: National Institutes of Health.

Neel, J. V. (1962). Diabetes mellitus: A "thrifty" genotype rendered detrimental by "progress"? *American Journal of Human Genetics, 14*, 353–362.

Ninomiya, J. K., L'Italien, G., Criqui, M. H., Whyte, J. L., Gamst, A., & Chen, R. S. (2004). Association of the metabolic syndrome with history of myocardial infarction and stroke in the Third National Health and Nutrition Examination Survey. *Circulation, 109*(1), 42–46.

Norris, S. L., Kansagara, D., Bougatsos, C., Nygren, P., & Fu, R. (2008). *Screening for type 2 diabetes mellitus: Update of 2003 Systematic Evidence Review for the U.S. Preventive Services Task Force* [Internet]. Rockville, MD: Agency for Healthcare Research and Quality (US). Report No.: 08-05116-EF-1.

Ogurtsova, K., da Rocha Fernandes, J. D., Huang, Y., Linnenkamp, U., Guariguata, L., Cho, N. H., … Makaroff, L. E. (2017). IDF Diabetes Atlas: Global estimates for the prevalence of diabetes for 2015 and 2040. *Diabetes Research and Clinical Practice, 128*, 40–50.

Olatunbosun, S. T., & Dagogo-Jack, S. (2010). Insulin resistance. Retrieved from *Medscape eMedicine*.

Onkamo, P., Vaananen, S., Karvonen, M., & Tuomilehto, J. (1999). Worldwide increase in incidence of type 1 diabetes—The analysis of the data on published incidence trends. *Diabetologia, 42*, 1395–1403.

Pan, W. H., Flegal, K. M., Chang, H. Y., Yeh, W. T., Yeh, C. J., & Lee, W. C. (2004). Body mass index and obesity-related metabolic disorders in Taiwanese and US whites and blacks: Implications for definitions of overweight and obesity for Asians. *American Journal of Clinical Nutrition, 79*, 31–39.

Pan, X. R., Li, G. W., Hu, Y. H., Wang, J. X., Yang, W. Y., An, Z. X., … Howard, B. V. (1997). Effects of diet and exercise in preventing NIDDM in people with impaired glucose tolerance: The Da Qing IGT and Diabetes Study. *Diabetes Care, 20*, 537–544.

Patel, M. S., Srinivasan, M., & Aalinkeel, R. (2000). Metabolic programming by nutrition during early development. *Indian Journal of Experimental Biology, 38*(9), 849–855.

Patterson, C. C., Dahlquist, G. G., Gyürüs, E., Green, A., Soltész, G., … the EURODIAB Study Group. (2009). Incidence trends for childhood type 1 diabetes in Europe during 1989–2003 and predicted new cases 2005–20: A multicenter prospective registration study. *Lancet, 373*, 2027–2033.

Permutt, M. A., Wasson, J., & Cox, N. (2005). Genetic epidemiology of diabetes. *Journal of Clinical Investigation, 115*(6), 1431–1439.

Pessin, J. E., Thurmond, D. C., Elmendorf, J. S., Coker, K. J., & Okada, S. (1999). Molecular basis of insulin-stimulating GLUT4 vesicle trafficking. *Journal of Biological Chemistry, 274*(5), 2593–2596.

Petersen, K. F., & Shulman, G. I. (2006). Etiology of insulin resistance. *American Journal of Medicine, 119*, 10S–16S.

Phillips, G. B. (1977). Relationship between serum sex hormones and glucose, insulin, and lipid abnormalities in men with myocardial infarction. *Proceedings of the National Academy of Sciences of the United States of America, 74*, 1729–1733.

Pickup, J., & William, G. (1997). *Textbook of diabetes* (2nd ed.). London, England: Blackwell Science.

Pietropaolo, M., & Trucco, M. (2003). Genetics of type 1 diabetes. In *Type 1 diabetes. Etiology and treatment*. Totowa, NJ: Humana Press.

Pitkäniemi, J., Onkamo, P., Tuomilehto, J., & Arjas, E. (2004). Increasing incidence of Type 1 diabetes—Role for genes? *BMC Genetics, 5*, 5.

Pozzilli, P., & Buzzetti, R. (2007). A new expression of diabetes: Double diabetes. *Trends in Endocrinology & Metabolism, 18*(2), 52–57.

Raj, S. M., Howson, J. M., Walker, N. M., Cooper, J. D., Smyth, D. J., Field, S. F., … Todd, J. A. (2009). No association of multiple type 2 diabetes loci with type 1 diabetes. *Diabetologia, 52,* 2109–2116.

Ravussin, E., & Smith, S. R. (2002). Increased fat intake, impaired fat oxidation, and failure of fat cell proliferation result in ectopic fat storage, insulin resistance, and type 2 diabetes mellitus. *Annals of the New York Academy of Sciences, 967,* 363–378.

Ravussin, E., Valencia, M. E., Esparza, J., Bennett, P. H., & Schulz, L. O. (1994). Effects of a traditional lifestyle on obesity in Pima Indians. *Diabetes Care, 14,* 1067–1074.

Reaven, G. M. (1988). Banting lecture 1988. Role of insulin resistance in human disease. *Diabetes, 37,* 1595–1607.

Reaven, G. M. (1995). Pathophysiology of insulin resistance in human disease. *Physiological Reviews, 75*(3), 473–486.

Redondo, M. J., Rewers, M., Yu, L., Garg, S., Pilcher, C. C., Elliott, R. B., & Eisenbarth, G. S. (1999). Genetic determination of islet cell autoimmunity in monozygotic twin, dizygotic twin, and non-twin siblings of patients with type 1 diabetes: Prospective twin study. *British Medical Journal, 318,* 698–702.

Reiber, G. E., Boyko, E. J., & Smith, D. G. (1995). Lower extremity foot ulcers and amputations in diabetes. In M. I. Harris & M. P. Stern (Eds.), *Diabetes in America* (pp. 409–428). Bethesda, MD: US Government Printing Office.

Roglic, G., & Unwin, N. (2005). Global mortality attributable to diabetes: Time for a realistic estimate. *Diabetes Voice, 50*(1), 33–34.

Roglic, G., & Unwin, N. (2010). Mortality attributable to diabetes: Estimates for the year 2010. *Diabetes Research and Clinical Practice, 87,* 15–19.

Rogot, E., Sorlie, P., Johnson, N. J., Glover, C. S., & Makus, D. (1985). Mortality by cause of death among selected census sample cohorts for 1979–1981. *Proceedings of the Section on Survey Research Methods.* American Statistical Association.

Rosati, G., Aiello, I., Pirastru, M. I., Mannu, L., Sanna, G., Sau, G. F., & Sotgiu, S. (1996). Epidemiology of multiple sclerosis in northwestern Sardinia: Further evidence for higher frequency in Sardinians compared to other Italians. *Neuroepidemiology, 15,* 10–19.

Rosen, E. D., & MacDougald, O. A. (2006). Adipocyte differentiation from the inside out. *Molecular Cell Biology, 7,* 885–896.

Ross, R. (1999) Atherosclerosis—An inflammatory disease. *New England Journal of Medicine, 340,* 115–126.

Ross, R., & Glomset, J. A. (1976). The pathogenesis of atherosclerosis. *New England Journal of Medicine, 295,* 369–377.

Salmeron, J., Hu, F. B., Manson, J. E., Stampfer, M. J., Colditz, G. A., Rimm, E. B., & Willett, W. C. (2001). Dietary fat intake and risk of type 2 diabetes in women. *American Society of Clinical Nutrition, 76,* 1019–1026.

Salo, M. (2006). Obesity among children—A large amount of work together. *Duodecim, 122,* 1211–1212.

Sanna, E., Soro, M. R., & Calo, C. (2006). Overweight and obesity prevalence in urban Sardinian children. *Anthropologischer Anzeiger, 64,* 333–344.

Schulze, M. B., Schulz, M., Heidemann, C., Schienkiewitz, A., Hoffmann, K., & Boeing, H. (2007). Fiber and magnesium intake and incidence of type 2 diabetes. A prospective study and meta-analysis. *Archives of Internal Medicine, 167*(9), 956–965.

Scott, S. K., Rabito, F. A., Butler, N. N., & Harris, R. E. (2004). *The energy storage capacity hypothesis.* (PhD dissertation).

Shabbir, S., Kwan, D., Wang, M. C., Shih, M., & Simon, P. A. (2010). Asians and Pacific Islanders and the growing childhood epidemic. *Ethnicity and Disease, 20,* 129–135.

Shai, I., Jiang, R., Manson, J. E., Stampfer, M. J., Willett, W. C., Colditz, G. A., & Hu, F. B. (2006). Ethnicity, obesity, and risk of type 2 diabetes in women: A 20-year follow-up study. *Diabetes Care, 29*(7), 1585–1590.

Shaw, J. E., Sicree, R. A., & Zimmet, P. Z. (2010). Global estimates of the prevalence of diabetes for 2010 and 2030. *Diabetes Research and Clinical Practice, 87*(1), 4–14.

Sheehy, A. M., Flood, G. E., Tuan, W. J., Liou, J. I., Coursin, D. B., & Smith, M. A. (2010). Analysis of guidelines for screening diabetes mellitus in an ambulatory population. *Mayo Clinic Proceedings, 85,* 27–35.

Shepherd, P. R., & Kahn, B. B. (1999). Glucose transporters and insulin action—Implications for insulin resistance and diabetes mellitus. *New England Journal of Medicine, 341*(4), 248–257.

Silverman, B. L., Metzger, B. E., Cho, N. H., & Loeb, C. A. (1995). Impaired glucose tolerance in adolescent offspring of diabetic mothers. *Diabetes Care, 18,* 611–617.

Silverman, B. L., Rizzo, T. A., Cho, N. H., & Metzger, B. E. (1998). Long-term effects of the intrauterine environment: The Northwestern University Diabetes in Pregnancy Center. *Diabetes Care, 21*(Suppl. 2), B142–B149.

Sjostrom, D. C., Peltonen, M., Wedel, H., & Sjostrom, L. (2000). Differentiated long-term effects of intentional weight loss on diabetes and hypertension. *Hypertension, 36,* 10–25.

Sobngwi, E., Mbanya, J. C., Unwin, N., Porcher, R., Kengne, A. P., Fezeu, L., … Alberti, K. (2004). Exposure over the life course to an urban environment and its relation with obesity, diabetes, and hypertension in rural and urban Cameroon. *International Journal of Epidemiology, 33*(4), 769–776.

Stanhope, K. L., Schwarz, J. M., Keim, N. L., Griffen, S. C., Bremer, A. A., Graham, J. L., … Havel, P. J. (2009). Consuming fructose-sweetened, but not glucose-sweetened beverages increases visceral adiposity and lipids and decreases insulin sensitivity in overweight/obese humans. *Journal of Clinical Investigation, 119,* 1322–1334.

Stevens, J., Ahn, K., Juhaeri, J., Houston, D., Steffan, L., & Couper, D. (2002). Dietary fiber intake and glycemic index and incidence of diabetes in African American and White adults: The ARIC Study. *Diabetes Care, 25,* 1715–1721.

Strachan, D. P. (1989). Hay fever, hygiene and household size. *British Medical Journal, 299*(6710), 1259–1260.

Stratton, I. M., Kohner, E. M., Aldington, S. J., Turner, R. C., Holman, R. R., Manley, S. E., & Matthews, D. R. (2001). UKPDS 50: Risk factors for incidence and progression of retinopathy in type II diabetes over 6 years from diagnosis. *Diabetologia, 44,* 156–163.

Sudagani, J., & Hitman, G. A. (2005). Diabetes mellitus: Etiology and epidemiology. In B. Caballero (Ed.), *Encyclopedia of human nutrition.* (pp. 535–542). London, England: Elsevier.

Swarbrick, M. M., Stanhope, K. L., Elliott, S. S., Graham, J. L., Krauss, R. M., Christiansen, M. P., … Havel, P. J. (2008). Consumption of fructose-sweetened beverages for 10 weeks increases postprandial triacylglycerol and apolipoprotein-B concentrations in overweight and obese women. *British Journal of Nutrition, 100*(5), 947–952.

Takaya, J., Higashino, H., & Kobayashi, Y. (2004). Intracellular magnesium and insulin resistance. *Magnesium Research, 17*(2), 126–136.

Tanaka, S., Horimai, C., & Katsukawa, F. (2003). Ethnic differences in abdominal visceral fat accumulation between Japanese, African–Americans, and Caucasians: A meta-analysis. *Acta Diabetologica, 40*(1), S302–S304.

Torsdottir, I., Alpsten, M., Holm, G., Sandberg, A. S., & Tölli, J. (1991). A small dose of soluble alginate fiber affects postprandial glycemia and gastric emptying in humans with diabetes. *Journal of Nutrition, 121*, 795–799.

Tosiello, L. (1996). Hypomagnesemia and diabetes mellitus: A review of clinical implications. *Archives of Internal Medicine, 156*, 1143–1148.

Tremblay, A., Doucet, E., Imbeault, P., Mauriège, P., Després, J. P., & Richard, D. (1999). Metabolic fitness in active reduced-obese individuals. *Obesity Research, 7*, 556–563.

Truesdale, K. P., Stevens, J., & Cai, J. (2005). The effect of weight history on glucose and lipids. *American Journal of Epidemiology, 161*, 1133–1143.

Tuomilehto, J., Lindstrom, J., Eriksson, J. G., Valle, T. T., Hämäläinen, H., Ilanne-Parikka, P., … Finnish Diabetes Prevention Study Group. (2001). Prevention of type 2 diabetes mellitus by changes in lifestyle among subjects with impaired glucose tolerance. *New England Journal of Medicine, 344*, 343–350.

Tuomilehto, J., Virtala, E., Karvonen, M., Lounamaa, R., Pitkaniemi, J., Reunanen, A., … Toivanen, L. (1995). Increase in incidence of insulin-dependent diabetes mellitus among children in Finland. *International Journal of Epidemiology, 24*, 984–992.

Unger, R. H. (2003). The physiology of cellular liporegulation. *Annual Review of Physiology, 65*, 333–347.

Unger, R. H., & Scherer, P. E. (2010). Gluttony, sloth and the metabolic syndrome: A roadmap to liptoxicity. *Trends in Endocrinology and Metabolism, 21*(6), 345–354.

United States Preventive Services Task Force. (2008). *Screening for type 2 diabetes mellitus in adults.* Rockville, MD: Agency for Health Care Research and Quality, U.S. Department of Health and Human Services.

Valdez, R., Yoon, P. W., Liu, T., & Khoury, M. (2007). Family history and prevalence of diabetes in the US population: The six year results from the National Health and Nutrition Examination Survey (1999–2004). *Diabetes Care, 30*(10), 2517–2522.

van Dam, R. M., Willett, W. C., Rimm, E. B., Stampfer, M. J., & Hu, F. B. (2002). Dietary fat and meat intake in relation to risk of type 2 diabetes in men. *Diabetes Care, 25*, 417–424.

Verbeeten, K. C., Elks, C. E., Daneman, D., & Ong, K. K. (2011). Association between childhood obesity and subsequent Type 1 diabetes: A systematic review and meta-analysis. *Diabetes Medicine, 28*(1), 10–18.

Villegas, R., Liu, S., Gao, Y. T., Yang, G., Li, H., Zheng, W., & Shu, X. O. (2007). Prospective study of dietary carbohydrates, glycemic index, glycemic load, and incidence of type 2 diabetes mellitus in middle-aged Chinese women. *Archives of Internal Medicine, 167*(21), 2310–2316.

Wajchenberg, B. L. (2007). β-Cell failure in diabetes and preservation by clinical treatment. *Endocrine Reviews, 28*, 187–218.

Walston, J., Silver, K., Bogardus, C., Knowler, W. C., Celi, F. S., Austin, S., … Shuldiner, A. R. (1995). Time of onset of non-insulin-dependent diabetes mellitus and genetic variation in the β3-adrenergic–receptor gene. *New England Journal of Medicine, 333*, 343–347.

Wang, H., Shara, N. M., Calhoun, D., Umans, J. G., Lee, E. T., & Howard, B. V. (2010). Incidence rates and predictors of diabetes in those with prediabetes: The Strong Heart Study. *Diabetes/Metabolism Research and Reviews, 26*, 378–385.

Warram, J. H., Krolewski, A. S., & Kahn, C. R. (1988). Determinants of IDDM and perinatal mortality in children of diabetic mothers. *Diabetes, 37*, 1328–1334.

Weickert, M. O., Mohlig, M., Koebnick, C., Holst, J. J., Namsolleck, P., Ristow, M., … Pfeiffer, A. F. H. (2005). Impact of cereal fibre on glucose-regulating factors. *Diabetologia, 48*, 2343–2353.

Weickert, M. O., Möhlig, M., Schöfl, C., Arafat, A. M., Otto, B., Viehoff, H., … Spranger, A. F. H. (2006). Cereal fiber improves whole-body insulin sensitivity in overweight and obese women. *Diabetes Care, 29*(4), 775–780.

Weickert, M. O., & Pfeiffer, A. F. H. (2008). Metabolic effects of dietary fiber consumption and prevention of diabetes. *Journal of Nutrition, 138*, 439–442.

WHO Expert Consultation. (2004). Appropriate body mass index for Asian populations and its implications for policy and intervention strategies. *Lancet, 363*, 157–163.

Wild, S., Roglic, G., Green, A., Sicree, R., & King, H. (2004). Global prevalence of diabetes. Estimates for the year 2000 and projections for 2030. *Diabetes Care, 27*, 1047–1053.

Wilkin, T. J. (2001). The accelerator hypothesis: Weight gain as the missing link between type I and type II diabetes. *Diabetologia, 44*, 914–922.

Willett, W. C., Dietz, W. H., & Colditz, G. A. (1999). Guidelines for healthy weight. *New England Journal of Medicine, 341*, 427–434.

Willett, W., Manson, J., & Liu, S. (2002). Glycemic index, glycemic load and risk of type 2 diabetes. *American Journal of Nutrition, 76*(1), 274S–280S.

Wingard, D. L., & Barrett-Conner, E. (1995). Heart disease and diabetes. In M. I. Harris, C. C. Cowie, M. P. Stern, E. J. Boyko, G. E. Reiber & P. H. Bennett (Eds.), *Diabetes in America* (2nd ed., pp. 429–488). Bethesda, MD: National Institutes of Health.

Wolever, T. M. (1997). The glycemic index: Flogging a dead horse? *Diabetes Care, 20*(3), 452–456.

Wolever, T. M. S., Katzman-Relle, L., Jenkins, A. L., Vuksan, V., Josse, R. G., & Jenkins, D. J. A. (1994). Glycaemic index of 102 complex carbohydrate foods in patients with diabetes. *Nutrition Research, 14*, 651–669.

World Health Organization. (2004). *Diabetes action now: An initiative of the World Health Organization.* Geneva, Switzerland: World Health Organization

World Health Organization. (2009). Fact sheet No. 312. Geneva, Switzerland, World Health Organization.

Yang, W., Lu, J., Weng, J., Jia, W., Ji, L., Xiao, J., … China National Diabetes and Metabolic Disorders Study Group. (2010). Prevalence of diabetes among men and women in China. *New England Journal of Medicine, 362*, 1090–1101.

Yang, Z., Wang, K., Li, T., Sun, W., Li, Y., Chang, Y.-F., … LaPorte, R. E. (1998). Childhood diabetes in China. *Diabetes Care, 21*, 525–529.

Ye, J., Chen, R. G., Ashkenazi, I., & Laron, Z. (1998). Lack of seasonality in the month of onset of childhood IDDM (0.7–15 years) in Shanghai, China. *Journal of Pediatric Endocrinology and Metabolism, 11*, 461–464.

Yoon, J. W. (1990). The role of viruses and environmental factors in the induction of diabetes. *Current Topics in Microbiology and Immunology, 164*, 95.

Younis, N., Broadbent, D. M., Vora, J. P., & Harding, S. P. (2003). Liverpool Diabetic Eye Study: Incidence of sight-threatening retinopathy in patients with type 2 diabetes in the Liverpool Diabetic Eye Study: A cohort study. *Lancet, 361*, 195–200.

Zhan, S., & Ho, S. C. (2005). Meta-analysis of the association of the Trp64Arg polymorphism in the b3 adrenergic receptor with insulin resistance. *Obesity Research, 13*, 1709–1719.

Zhu, Y., & Zhang, C. (2016). Prevalence of gestational diabetes and risk of progression to type 2 diabetes: A global perspective. *Current Diabetes Reports, 16*(1), 7.

© Andrew Brookes/Getty Images

CHAPTER 42

Epidemiology of Obesity

Susanne K. Scott and Randall E. Harris

▶ Introduction

The global pandemic of obesity is one of the most significant public health threats of the 21st century. Fueled primarily by excess calories and physical inactivity, the dramatic increase in overweight and obesity of the past several decades is considered the major cause for the parallel rise in incident and prevalent diabetes (Barnes & Coulter, 2011; International Diabetes Federation, 2006; WHO, 2003). Obesity, which is a strong, independent, and modifiable predictor of type 2 diabetes, is also associated with numerous other serious chronic diseases and health conditions such as cardiovascular diseases; some cancers; musculoskeletal, gastrointestinal, respiratory, dermatologic, and reproductive disorders; social stigma; and psychological distress. As William Wadd aptly wrote in his 1816 book on obesity, *"Corpulence is not only a disease itself, but the harbinger of others"* (Wadd, 1816).

Even more disturbing than increasing obesity in adults is the alarming rise in the prevalence of childhood and adolescent overweight and obesity. Increasing obesity levels in children have contributed to a much earlier onset of obesity-related diseases that were previously diagnosed only in older adults (Ebbeling, Pawling, & Ludwig, 2002; Freedman, Dietz, Srinivasan, & Berenson, 1999; Freedman, Mei, Srinivasan, Berenson, & Dietz, 2007; Hruby & Hu, 2015; Hung-Kwan et al., 2008). Moreover, childhood obesity tracks robustly into adulthood, which means that

once a child becomes obese, it is likely that obesity will persist throughout life. Early onset of obesity and the health sequelae that follow have profound economic implications. The long-term medical management of obesity and related diseases, especially beginning in youth, is expected to overwhelm healthcare systems, devastate personal income and earnings, and threaten national budgets, as medical costs rise to unsustainable levels (WHO, 2005).

Although the trend of increasing obesity prevalence in the United States may have abated somewhat in children (Ogden, Carroll, & Flegal, 2008) and among some adults since 1999 (Flegal, Carroll, Ogden, & Curtin, 2010; Ogden, Carroll, McDowell, & Flegal, 2007), obesity levels continue to skyrocket in other parts of the world, particularly in poor developing countries known more for problems of hunger and infectious diseases (Misra & Khurana, 2008; Prentice, 2006). Globalization and urbanization are considered primary factors responsible for the changes in physical activity levels and the "*nutrition transition*" that has altered traditional dietary patterns in countries with emerging economies (Caballero, 2007; Drewnowski, & Popkin, 2009; Economic Research Service, 2010; Satia, 2010). This is leading to a persistent positive energy balance, inappropriate weight gain, and increasing obesity levels that are contributing to an increase in worldwide chronic disease rates. Although the primary causes and consequences of obesity have been clearly articulated in the literature, prevention efforts remain the single most significant challenge in the fight against obesity.

609

▶ Classification of Overweight and Obesity in Adults

The World Health Organization (WHO) defines obesity as excessive body fat which has accumulated to the point where health is negatively affected (WHO, 1998). The body mass index (BMI), which is a ratio of the weight in kilograms to the square of the height in meters, BMI = kg/m^2, is the global metric used for measuring and classifying levels of adiposity and associated obesity-related chronic disease risk among adults. Obesity in children is measured differently using percentile cut points based upon standardized growth charts for boys and girls. The burden of childhood obesity is discussed below in a separate section of this chapter.

Body mass was originally described as the *Quételet index* in 1832, until the metric was renamed the Body Mass Index (BMI) in 1972 by Ancel Keys (Keys, Fidanza, Karvonen, Kimura, & Taylor, 1972). The Quételet index was named after Adolphe Quételet, a Belgian mathematician and statistician who in 1835 concluded that other than during developmental growth spurts, "*the weight increases as the square of the height*" (Quételet, 1835). The Framingham Heart Study was one of the first epidemiologic studies to show that the Quételet index was consistent with measures of relative weight (Eknoyan, 2006, 2008). Keys followed up with his own study, correlating various relative weight indices with subcutaneous fat thickness (skinfold thickness) among 7424 healthy men in 12 cohorts across five countries, confirming the validity of the Quételet index (Keys et al., 1972).

Quételet's interest in developing a weight index was not related to obesity or health matters, but rather to describe and index anthropometric characteristics of "normal man" for statistical purposes. The Metropolitan Life Insurance Company (MLIC), however, was interested in identifying normal relative body weight, primarily because of the increased death claims of their obese policy holders (Eknoyan, 2008; Medico-Actuarial Mortality Investigation, 1912). Metropolitan Life Insurance actuaries (using MLIC policyholders' information and with questionable validity) developed the first standard weight tables (Kuczmarski & Flegal, 2000). These tables were based on tertiles of weight at a given height and were labeled according to small, medium, and large body frames. Sex-specific average weight within those tertiles was classified as "ideal" in the 1940s, and then later, in 1959, were presented as "desirable" (MLIC, 1942, 1943, 1959). For insurance decisions, undesirable weight was considered 20%–25% below the average, while morbid obesity was 70%–100% above the average within each tertile (Eknoyan, 2008).

In 1984, the BMI with a cut point of ≥28 was used to report the first prevalence estimates of overweight status among males, aged 25–74, in Health United States, the official annual report on the health of the nation. For women, a different weight-height index was used, but this alternative formula (height in meters, raised to the power 1.5) was soon discredited. Over the next decade, BMI cut points for overweight evolved, and by 1997, the WHO BMI criteria, which had added obesity cut points, was first applied to U.S. data. In 1998, the BMI-disease risk classification system (currently in use) was developed, derived in part from epidemiologic studies that consistently showed an association of increasing BMI with increasing morbidity and mortality (Allison, Fontaine, Manson, Stevens, & VanItallie, 1999; Lee, Manson, & Hennekens, 1993; Manson et al., 1995; NIH, 1985). The current BMI criteria are given in **TABLE 42.1**.

In 2004, WHO reported that the universal BMI criteria for overweight and obesity were not suitable for Asian populations (WHO, 2004). This was based primarily on studies which revealed that Asians generally were at risk for obesity-related chronic diseases at a BMI much lower than other ethnic groups (Bei-Fan, 2002; Misra, 2003). Although the WHO report acknowledged the vast diversity in geography, culture, ethnicity, level of urbanization, and the social and economic conditions of people classified under the umbrella term of "Asian," the common thread among the subgroups was a lower mean and median BMI than that observed in non-Asian populations (WHO, 2004).

For example, in a study of BMI and cardiovascular risk factors in a rural Chinese population, Hu and colleagues found that, in 1993, the 90th percentile of the BMI distribution was only 23.5 in men and 24.5 in women living in the rural Anqing region of China (Hu et al., 2000). These data and others (Ito et al., 2003; Lin et al., 2002; Moon et al., 2002; Popkin, Paeratakul, Ge, & Zhai, 1995; Razak et al., 2007; Werkman, Deurenberg-Yap, Schmidt, & Deurenberg, 2000) have provided the rationale for those who have recommended that Asian regions develop lower *Asian-specific* BMI cut points (Bei-Fan, 2002; Misra, 2003; Yuji, 2002). It has also been the basis for WHO to develop additional international BMI cut points (23, 27.5, 32.5, and 37.5) along the continuum of BMI, to be used for public health action (WHO, 2004).

▶ Limitations of the BMI

Although the BMI is the universally accepted obesity metric, providing a gross approximation of total body fat for the majority of people, it is not without several

TABLE 42.1 Weight Classification and Disease Risk by BMI

Weight Classification	Obesity Class	BMI (kg/m²)	Risk of Disease
Underweight		<18.5	Elevated
Normal weight		18.5 < 25	Baseline
Overweight		25 < 30	Elevated
Obese	I	30 < 35	High
Obese	II	35 < 40	Very High
Morbidly obese	III	40+	Extremely High

Data from the National Institutes of Health. (1998). The evidence report. *Obesity Research, 6,* 51S–209S.

well-described limitations, the first because it does not really measure body fat. The BMI is a measure of a person's weight adjusted for height (Kuczmarski & Flegal, 2000; WHO, 2004). In a two-compartment model of body composition, the BMI is a standardized measure of fat mass and fat-free mass, the latter of which is comprised of bone, muscle, and all other proteins and tissues. The BMI does not differentiate between the two. Thus, people with increased muscle mass, such as bodybuilders, are likely to be misclassified as overweight or obese, whereas fat mass could be underestimated for those who have lost lean mass due to infirmity, sedentary lifestyle, or increasing age (Kuczmarski & Flegal, 2000).

A second limitation is that BMI does not measure the distribution of body fat and may not accurately reflect levels of intra-abdominal fat and associated health risks in different individuals and populations. Indeed, it is often visceral or abdominal fat rather than peripheral or subcutaneous fat which is implicated in elevating the risk of developing certain chronic diseases (Bergman et al., 2006; Frayn, 2000).

Third, BMI cut points do not show within-interval variation in morbidity, which could be substantial (Stommel & Schoenborn, 2010). Even among the obese, a portion of the population is healthy (Brochu et al., 2001). For instance, in a nationally representative sample of U.S. hospital discharge records of morbidly obese patients in 2002, 76% of the discharge records did not report a diagnosis of diabetes (Scott et al., 2006).

Fourth, since disease risk per BMI level varies by ethnicity, the use of universal BMI cut points may not be appropriate across populations (Stevens, 2003a, 2003b; Stevens, Jianwen, & Jones, 2002). The adult BMI

cut points for being overweight or obese are derived primarily from studies of Caucasians, but these may be inaccurate for other ethnic groups (WHO, 1998, 2000, 2004). For example, comparative studies have consistently shown that, on average, Asians have higher percentages of body fat than Caucasians at corresponding levels of BMI (Abate, Chandalia, Snell, & Grundy, 2004; Chung et al., 2005; Deurenberg, Deurenberg-Yap, & Guricci, 2002; Kagawa, Kerr, Uchida, & Binns, 2006).

Despite a host of methodological concerns related to obesity metrics, the BMI is currently the accepted standard global obesity measure. It remains an appealing epidemiologic and clinical measurement tool primarily due to the simplicity, inexpense, ease, the accuracy and reliability of measuring height and weight, and because of the positive correlation with body fat and obesity-related diseases (Gallagher et al., 1996; Hubbard, 2000; Kuczmarski & Flegal, 2000; Spiegelman, Israel, Bouchard, & Willett, 1992). The BMI also provides a standard definition of obesity to use for national and international surveillance and ecologic comparisons (Flegal et al., 2010). It is important to note, however, that due to increasing heterogeneity of societies and the development and use of a variety of revised and modified BMI charts for adults and children (e.g., Asian-specific BMI charts and revised WHO growth standards), secular and ecologic comparisons using the BMI could be hindered (Hung-Kwan et al., 2008; Jackson, Rashed, Al-Hamad, Hwalla, & Al-Somaie, 2007). In future studies, use of the BMI may be best suited for within-population surveillance to track and compare obesity trends within relatively homogeneous groups.

Global Burden of Adult Obesity

WHO has established a global surveillance program to track the worldwide pandemic of obesity and obesity-related diseases and monitor the progress of intervention and prevention strategies. Data on BMI from population surveys conducted in member nations of WHO have been compiled to estimate the number and prevalence of overweight and obese individuals in the world population (WHO, 1998).

The most recent global data reflect persisting upward trends in the numbers of overweight and obese adults and clearly indicate that the worldwide obesity pandemic is continuing unabated in the 21st century. In 2000, there were approximately 750 million overweight and 300 million obese adults aged 15 years or older (WHO, 2000); whereas 5 years later in 2005, 1 billion adults were overweight and more than 400 million were obese (WHO, 2005). Thus, obesity is increasing at an annual rate of about 6.6%, which is at least five times greater than the current annual world population growth rate of 1.3%. WHO has projected that by 2015, 1.6 billion adults will be overweight, with more than 700 million classified as obese, more than doubling the worldwide burden of these conditions within the first 15 years of the 21st century (WHO, 2009a).

Kelly and colleagues reported similar results using a slightly higher age threshold (20 years or older) to define adulthood. Their estimates were compiled from published population surveys of 106 nations representing 88% of the world population. In 2005, 937 million adults (23.2%) were overweight and 396 million (9.8%) were obese. The prevalence of obesity was higher in women (11.2%) than men (7.7%). If global secular trends continue, by the year 2030, approximately 2.2 billion people will be overweight and 1.1 billion people will be obese (Kelly, Yang, Chen, Reynolds, & He, 2008).

Global Prevalence of Adult Obesity

Global patterns of obesity prevalence are shown for men and women in **FIGURES 42.1** and **42.2**, respectively. National prevalence estimates of obesity by gender are based upon WHO surveys conducted during 2014 and 2016 using a cut point of BMI > 30 to define obesity.

Prevalence estimates range from less than 5% in Vietnam, India, China, Japan, Korea, the Philippines, Pakistan, and several African nations to greater than 60% in Polynesian populations residing in the islands of the South Pacific (WHO, 2009a). Gender-specific estimates are 2–3-fold higher in populations of developed nations compared to developing nations. In most countries, the prevalence of obesity in women exceeds that in men by 5%–10%. In the United States, the current overall prevalence of obesity is approximately 41% in women and 38% in men (Hales, Carroll, Fryar, & Ogden, 2017).

The development of obesity is related to an imbalance between calories consumed versus calories

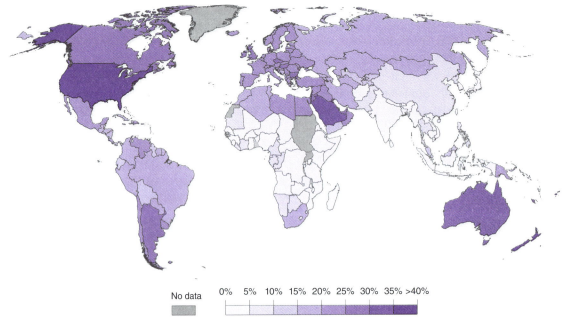

No data   0% 5% 10% 15% 20% 25% 30% 35% >40%

Source: WHO, Global Health Observatory

FIGURE 42.1 Prevalence of Obesity in Men, 2016.

Data from World Health Organization. (2010). *Global infobase, international comparisons: Estimated obesity (BMI > 30 kg/m²) prevalence, males, aged 15+.* Accessed at: https://apps.who.int/infobase/. October 28, 2011.

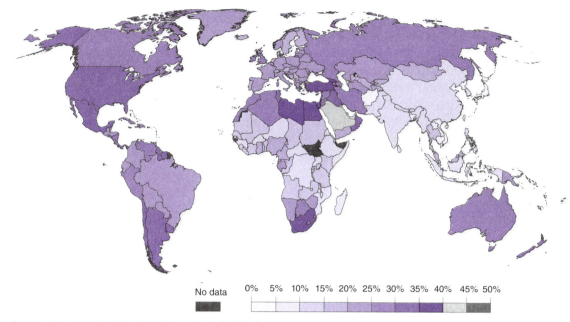

Source: Prevalence of weight categories in females-NCDRisC

FIGURE 42.2 Prevalence of Obesity in Women, 2014.

Data from World Health Organization. (2010). *Global infobase, international comparisons: Estimated obesity (BMI > 30 kg/m²) prevalence, females, aged 15+.* Accessed at: https://apps.who.int/infobase/. October 28, 2011.

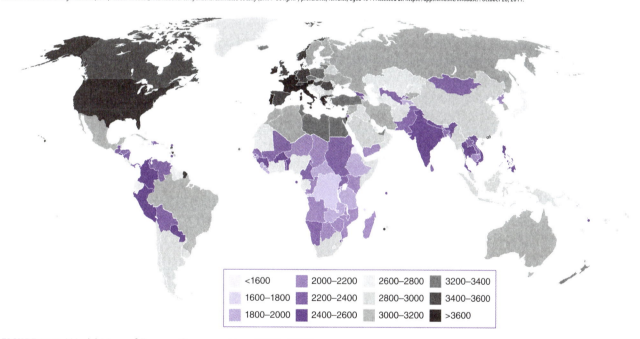

<1600	2000–2200	2600–2800	3200–3400
1600–1800	2200–2400	2800–3000	3400–3600
1800–2000	2400–2600	3000–3200	>3600

FIGURE 42.3 World Map of Energy Consumption, 2001–2003.

Data from FAO Statistical Yearbook. (2004). *Section D: Consumption.* Rome, Italy. Available at: ftp://ftp.fao.org/docrep/fao/008/y5473m/y5473m01d.pdf. Accessed October 28, 2011.

Calories per capita per day.

expended or *energy input versus energy output*. Notably, the per capita dietary energy supply has increased significantly in nearly all parts of the world during the past five decades, closely paralleling emergence of the global obesity epidemic. Estimates derived from WHO survey data suggest that the world daily per capita energy consumption increased from 2250 to 2750 kilocalories during the period from 1960 to 2005 (EarthTrends, 2009). National estimates of per capita energy consumption (kilocalories per capita per day) for the period 2001–2003 are depicted in **FIGURE 42.3**. The world pattern of energy consumption is similar to the global patterns of obesity in men and women (Figures 42.1 and 42.2). These international patterns underscore the etiologic link between total calorie consumption and the development of obesity.

The heightened intake of calories with increasing obesity and disease risk mirrors a global transition in diet toward increased intake of energy-dense foods high in fat and sugars but low in vitamins, minerals, and other micronutrients and a trend toward decreased physical activity due to increasingly sedentary lifestyles, changing modes of transportation, and increasing urbanization (Satia, 2010; Stanhope et al., 2009). These factors are discussed in the following sections of this chapter.

▶ Gender Differences in Obesity

As shown in Figures 42.1 and 42.2, the prevalence of obesity in women exceeds that in men by 5%–10% in most of the countries represented. Data for U.S. men and women reflect the higher prevalence of obesity among women at every age (**FIGURE 42.4**). The gender difference in obesity is widely recognized and has been attributed to evolutionary pressures that predispose women to store excess fat for reproduction and lactation (O'Sullivan, 2008). However, a plethora of other factors may influence gender differences in body mass including body composition, fat distribution, estrogens and androgens, appetite and eating behavior, social and cultural differences, dieting and weight control, exercise patterns, basal metabolism, genes on the X and Y chromosomes, reproductive history, and menopause (Lovejoy & Sainsbury, 2009; Welch & Sowers, 2000).

Recent studies suggest that gender differences in the distribution of body fat are largely determined by differences in sex hormones. In premenopausal women, estrogen may prevent oxidization of fatty acids leading to increased body fat, particularly at puberty and during early pregnancy (O'Sullivan, 2008). In postmenopausal women, abdominal/visceral adiposity increases with the loss of ovarian estrogens (Lovejoy, Champagne, De Jonge, Xie, & Smith, 2008); whereas in men, the gradual decline in circulating androgens

with aging predisposes to the accumulation of abdominal fat (Blouin et al., 2005). Furthermore, administration of androgens has been found to reverse abdominal obesity in men (Marin et al., 1993) but not in women (Lovejoy et al., 1996). Estrogens therefore appear to decrease visceral fat in aging men and women whereas androgens decrease visceral fat in men but have the opposite effect in women (Lovejoy & Sainsbury, 2009).

▶ Urban Versus Rural Differences in Obesity

Based upon population studies within nations, the prevalence of obesity is much higher in urban areas than in rural areas, even in low-prevalence countries. For example, in China where the overall prevalence of obesity is very low (2.9%), prevalence estimates of 20% or higher have been observed in some urban cities (WHO, 2003).

A research team in Kenya examined changes in body mass in the populations of seven African countries during 1992–2005. Population changes in the prevalence of obesity were assessed for each country over a time span of at least 10 years. Final prevalence estimates for the wealthy were nearly twofold higher than the poor (38% vs. 21%), and during the decade of observation, obesity increased by 35% in urban locales. Notably, the percentage increase among the poorest (50%) was more than sevenfold higher than the richest (7%). These results suggest that obesity is on the rise in developing nations and, as in developed nations, may soon reach epidemic proportions (Ziraba, Fotso, & Ochako, 2009).

In some areas of Africa, obesity has been a long-standing problem. For example, in the Cape Peninsula of South Africa, high obesity levels have

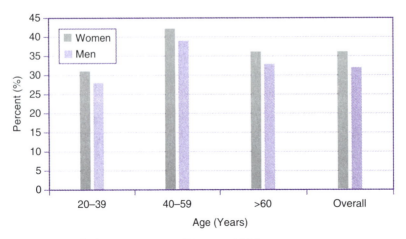

FIGURE 42.4 Age-Specific Prevalence of Obesity in Men and Women, U.S.A.

Data from National Health and Nutrition Survey (NHANES), 2005–2006. Prevalence estimates are age-adjusted to the U.S. 2000 population.

persisted among African women since at least 1990 when the prevalence was estimated at 44% (Steyn, 1991). Although Africa is arguably one of the last continents to undergo industrial and market globalization, urban migration patterns have paralleled that of countries with emerging economies. The Population Division of the United Nations predicts that by 2030, half of Africa's total population will live in urban areas, more than tripling the proportion of urban dwellers in 1950 (United Nations, 2006). The implication is that coincident with expanding urbanization, the obesity epidemic emerging in Africa will continue to worsen.

▶ Prevalence of Adult Obesity in the United States

In the United States, the prevalence of obesity has tripled in men and more than doubled in women since 1960, when only 10% of men and 15% of women were classified as obese (**FIGURE 42.5**). Current estimates suggest that 38% of men and 41% of women are obese, and severe obesity (BMI exceeding 40) which was uncommon in 1960 is now present in approximately 6% of men and 10% of women. Furthermore, among children and adolescents aged 2–19 years, the prevalence of obesity increased from 13.9% in 2000 to 18.5% in 2015 (Hales et al., 2017; Hales, Fryar, Carroll, Freedman, & Ogden, 2018).

While the global prevalence of obesity is expected to double between 2015 and 2030 (WHO, 2009a), estimates obtained during the 10-year period, 1999–2008 suggested that the rising obesity trend in the United States was attenuating. During that period, nationally representative sample survey data from the U.S.

National Health and Nutrition Examination Survey (NHANES) showed no significant change in the overall prevalence of obesity among adults (Flegal et al., 2010). Nevertheless, more recent estimates for 2015 and 2016 reflect a sharp increase in obesity among U.S. adults. The current data suggest that almost 70% of people aged 20 and older are overweight or obese, and nearly 40% (approximately 93 million people) are classified as obese (Hales et al., 2017, 2018).

Obesity defined as BMI > 30.

▶ Distribution of Obesity by Age, Gender, and Ethnicity in the United States

The prevalence of obesity is disproportionately higher in certain U.S. age-gender-ethnic groups than others. For example, obesity increases with age in African-American women but not other ethnicities (**FIGURE 42.6**). The prevalence is particularly high (about 60%) in African-American women aged 60 and older; roughly double the levels in Caucasian and Hispanic women. In men, the prevalence of obesity is high (about 40%) in young African Americans and middle-aged Caucasians. In men and women of all ages, African Americans have higher levels (44%) than Hispanics (39%) and Caucasians (33%) (Wagner & Heyward, 2000).

Compared to other gender-ethnic groups, the lifestyles of certain African-American women appear to predispose them to excessive weight gain and the development of obesity (Gower, Weisner, Jordan, Hunter, & Desmond, 2002). The web of causation includes high

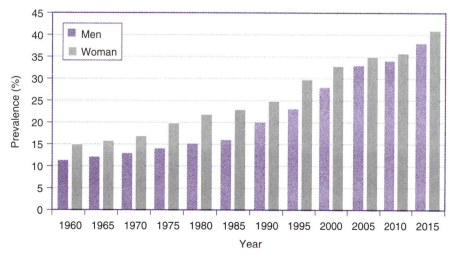

FIGURE 42.5 Prevalence of Obesity in the United States, 1960–2015.

Data from U.S. National Health and Nutrition Survey (NHANES), 1960–2010; Hales, C. M., Carroll, M. D., Fryar, C. D., & Ogden, C. L. (2017). Prevalence of obesity among adults and youth: United States, 2015-2016. *National Center for Health Statistics Data Brief, 288.* Obesity defined as BMI > 30

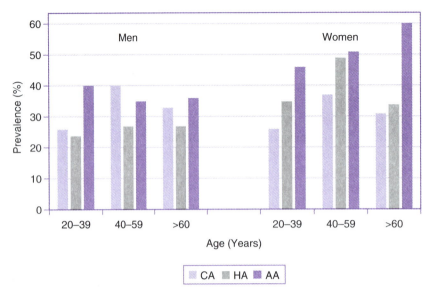

FIGURE 42.6 Prevalence of Obesity by Gender, Age, and Ethnicity, United States
Data from U.S. National Health and Nutrition Survey (NHANES), 2005–2006.

intake of carbohydrates, sugar, and fat in the diet, physical inactivity, high stress, high parity, low vitamin D, lactose intolerance, depression, and perception of body weight (Kumanyika, Obarzanek, Stevens, Herbert, & Whelton, 1991). Furthermore, compared to other groups in weight management programs, African-American women are less likely to lose weight and maintain weight loss (Kumanyika, Wilson, & Guliford-Davenport, 1993).

Health Consequences of Obesity

Obesity exerts deleterious effects on nearly every organ system of the body and is associated with numerous health conditions including type 2 diabetes, cardiovascular diseases (such as coronary heart disease, myocardial infarction, and stroke), gastroesophageal reflux disease (GERD), obstructive sleep apnea, asthma, gall bladder and fatty liver disease, depression, urinary incontinence, gout, polycystic ovarian syndrome, and osteoarthritis. Selected obesity-related diseases and the overall mortality attributable to obesity are reviewed in the following sections.

Obesity and Total Mortality

Obesity is strongly associated with increased morbidity, mortality, disability, and impaired quality of life (Flegal, Graubard, Williamson, & Gail, 2005, 2006; Jia & Lubetkin, 2010). Recent cause-specific mortality data reported by WHO suggest that overweight and obesity cause 2.8 million deaths annually, ranking 5th among the top 10 leading causes of death worldwide

(WHO, 2009a). In the same report, disease burdens attributable to selected risk factors were estimated as the product of the fraction of disease attributed to the risk factor (the population attributable fraction or PAF) and the corresponding total disability-adjusted life years lost (DALY): *Disease Burden* = PAF × DALY. According to these estimates, 44% of the disease burden from diabetes, 23% of the disease burden from ischemic heart disease, and 7%–41% of the disease burden from many forms of cancer are attributable to overweight and obesity (WHO, 2009a).

Studies have consistently shown that obesity is associated with premature death. A recent Danish study followed 5000 military conscripts aged 20–80 years old and found that men who were obese at age 20 were twice as likely to die prematurely compared to men who were not, and that at any given age thereafter, obesity had a lifelong constant effect on death (the risk remained double) up until 60 years of age. In addition, for each BMI unit above normal, the risk of early death increased by 10% throughout life, with obese men dying approximately 8 years earlier than nonobese men (ICO, 2010).

Investigators at Harvard University evaluated BMI and mortality in a prospective cohort of 115,195 women aged 30–55, enrolled in the *Nurses' Health Study*, and free of cardiovascular disease and cancer at baseline. Participants were enrolled in 1976 and followed for 16 years. Compared to women with BMI < 19, obese women (BMI > 32) had 90% higher total mortality, more than fourfold higher cardiovascular mortality (relative risk (RR) = 4.1), and more than twofold higher cancer mortality (RR = 2.1). Results suggested that 53% of deaths among women with a BMI > 29 were attributable to their obesity.

In addition, weight gain of 10 kg or more after the age of 18 and a BMI > 22 at age 18 were both predictors of death from cardiovascular disease in middle adulthood. Moreover, the lowest mortality occurred among the leanest women who had remained weight stable since age 18 (Manson et al., 1995).

Investigators at the U.S. National Institutes of Health evaluated BMI and all-cause mortality in a cohort of 527,265 men and women, aged 50–71, ascertained through the American Association of Retired Persons (AARP). Participants were enrolled in 1995–1996 and followed for a maximum of 10 years. Among those who had never smoked and who had no preexisting health conditions at baseline, there was a graded increase in the RR of all-cause mortality for both men and women as BMI levels rose from 26.5 to more than 40 compared to the reference group with BMI in the range 23.5–24.9. Morbidly obese men and women (BMI > 40) were more than twice as likely to die as individuals in the reference group (Adams et al., 2006).

Daniel McGee and collaborators in Florida examined relationships of obesity and mortality from all causes, cardiovascular disease and cancer in a meta-analysis of 26 prospective observational studies that included men and women from several racial and ethnic groups. The final database consisted of 74 analytic cohorts consisting of 388,622 individuals. A total of 60,374 individuals died during follow-up. Proportional hazards models were used to examine relationships of BMI categories and mortality. Obesity was associated with increased mortality due to heart disease (RR = 1.57), cardiovascular disease (RR = 1.48), and cancer (RR = 1.07). The total mortality rate was 22% higher among obese individuals compared to individuals of normal weight (McGee, 2005).

While obesity is associated with an increased risk of early death, people who are obese are also at greater risk for developing major chronic diseases such as type 2 diabetes, cardiovascular diseases, and some cancers. Obesity most likely leads to the onset of most, if not all chronic diseases through direct effects on metabolic dysregulation expressed clinically as hypertension, insulin resistance, hyperinsulinemia, hyperglycemia, dyslipidemia, and low-grade chronic inflammation. Selected obesity-related diseases are discussed in the following sections.

▶ Obesity and Type 2 Diabetes

Obesity and type 2 diabetes are often characterized as the *twin epidemic* or *diabesity* based primarily on their parallel increasing trends in prevalence over the past several decades. Indeed, obesity is considered the strongest modifiable predictor of type 2 diabetes (e.g., recent estimates suggest that nearly 70% of cases in the United States are attributable to overweight and obesity) (Eyre et al., 2004; NIDDK, 2008). Prevalence estimates of obesity among adults (aged 20 years or older) and diabetes among older adults (aged 65 years or older) for the United States over the past half-century reflect the close temporal relationship between obesity and diabetes (**FIGURE 42.7**).

Although the majority of obese people are not diabetic, the risk of type 2 diabetes increases substantially as the BMI increases, particularly within the obese range of BMI (Ogden, Yanovski, Carroll, & Flegal, 2007; Scott et al., 2006). In a prospective cohort study, researchers at Harvard evaluated diet, lifestyle, and the risk of type 2 diabetes among 84,941 female

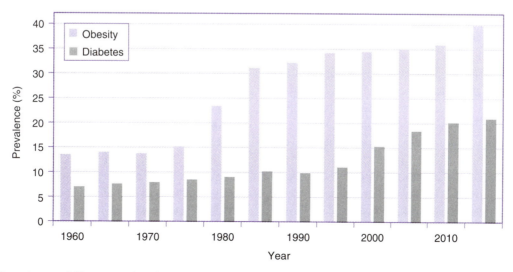

FIGURE 42.7 *Prevalence of Obesity and Diabetes in the United States, 1960–2015.*

Data from U.S. National Health and Nutrition Survey (NHANES), 1960–2010; Centers for Disease Control and Prevention. (2010). *National Center for Chronic Disease Prevention and Health Promotion*. Division of Diabetes Translation; National Diabetes Statistics Reort, 2017; Hales, C. M., Carroll, M. D., Fryar, C. D., & Ogden, C. L. (2017). Prevalence of obesity among adults and youth: United States, 2015-2016. *National Center for Health Statistics Data Brief, 288*. Prevalence estimates of obesity for adults (ages 20 years and older). Prevalence estimates of diabetes for older adults (ages 65 years and older).

nurses, aged 30–55 years, enrolled in the Nurses' Health Study. The cohort was followed for 16 years (1980–1996). Compared to lean women with BMI < 23, obese women with BMI of 30–35 had a 20-fold increase in the relative risk of diabetes even after controlling for age, family history of diabetes, menopausal status, postmenopausal hormone therapy, diet, smoking, alcohol intake, and activity levels (Hu et al., 2001).

Haffner and colleagues examined BMI, central obesity (measured by a scapular/tricep skinfold ratio index), fasting glucose, and insulin levels as predictors of *decompensation* in disease progression to incident type 2 diabetes among 474 nondiabetic Mexican Americans. After 8 years of follow-up, 28 nondiabetics developed type 2 diabetes. In univariate analysis, BMI and central obesity were both significantly associated with incident type 2 diabetes, but neither factor retained statistical significance when fasting blood glucose and insulin levels were included in multivariate models. Based on their results, the investigators suggested that obesity may influence the *progression* of hyperglycemia and hyperinsulinemia to type 2 diabetes over a period of many years (Haffner, Stern, Mitchell, Hazuda, & Patterson, 1990).

While numerous epidemiologic studies have shown that obesity per se, as defined by the BMI, is a major risk factor for type 2 diabetes, *weight gain* during adulthood is also strongly associated with the onset of type 2 diabetes, independent of baseline or attained BMI status (Chan, Rimm, Colditz, Stampfer, & Willett, 1994; Colditz, Willett, Rotnitsky, & Manson, 1995; Koh-Banerjee et al., 2004; Oguma, Sesso, Paffenbarger, & Lee, 2005; Shai et al., 2006; Willett, Dietz, & Colditz, 1999). In addition, the timing and magnitude of adult weight gain may play an important role in determining the age of onset of diabetes.

For example, in a 7-year follow-up study of 7720 men and 10,371 women enrolled in the *European Prospective Investigation into Cancer and Nutrition (EPIC)-Potsdam Study*, German investigators evaluated BMI history and risk of incident type 2 diabetes. Results revealed that the relative risks were higher for men (RR = 1.25) and women (RR = 1.24) per one unit BMI gain during the younger age interval of 25–40 years than between ages 40 and 55 years. Moreover, high weight gain in the younger age interval resulted in an increased diabetes relative risk for men (RR = 1.5) and women (RR = 4.3) compared to those who were weight stable in early adulthood and who gained weight in later life. Among the younger weight gainers, the average age of onset of diabetes diagnosis also occurred 3–5 years earlier (Schienkiewitz, Schulze, Hoffmann, Kroke, & Boeing, 2006).

Knowler and colleagues conducted a 10-year study of diabetes in a cohort of 3733 Pima Indians living in Arizona. This special population was found to have one of the highest rates of diabetes in the world (26.5 cases per 1000 person-years) which was 19-fold higher than a matched U.S. Caucasian population. The incidence increased steadily with increasing body mass measured prior to disease onset, from 0.8 cases per 1000 person-years for individuals with BMI < 20 to 72.2 cases per 1000 person-years for those with BMI > 40. The presence of diabetes in one or both parents also increased the risk. The investigators emphasized the importance of estimating effects of body mass measured prior to disease onset since poorly controlled diabetes can rapidly cause significant weight loss (Knowler, Bennett, Hamman, & Miller, 1978; Knowler, Pettitt, Savage, & Bennett, 1979).

▶ Obesity and Cardiovascular Disease

Epidemiologic studies provide unequivocal evidence that obesity is a major risk factor for the development of cardiovascular diseases. Key studies include the U.S. Framingham Study, the Seven Countries Study, the MONICA Project (Multinational Monitoring of trends and determinants in Cardiovascular Disease), the ARIC Study (Atherosclerosis Risk in Communities, U.S.A.), the INTERHEART Study, and several others. In brief, obesity (definable as BMI > 30 or waist-to-hip ratio exceeding 1.0 in men or 0.85 in women) significantly elevates the risk of developing coronary heart disease, myocardial infarction, stroke, as well as other forms of cardiovascular disease such as congestive heart failure (Krauss, Winston, Fletcher, & Grundy, 1998).

Results of a recent meta-analysis indicate the major contribution of obesity to the risk of developing coronary heart disease. Investigators in the Netherlands examined obesity and the risk of coronary heart disease in a meta-analysis of 21 prospective cohort studies. Among the 302,296 participants in these studies, 18,000 developed coronary heart disease during follow-up. Estimates of RR were initially adjusted for age, gender, physical activity, and smoking. Compared to normal-weight subjects, those who were obese (BMI > 30) were 81% more likely to develop coronary heart disease (RR = 1.81). Results also suggested a modest risk increase for individuals with BMI in the range of 25–29.9 (RR = 1.32). After further adjustment for cholesterol and blood pressure levels, these estimates were reduced (1.49 and 1.17, respectively) but

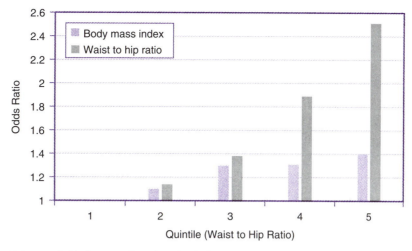

FIGURE 42.8 Obesity and Myocardial Infarction: Results of INTERHEART.

Data from Yusuf, S., Hawken, S., Ounpuu, S., Bautista, L., Franzosi, M. G., Commerford, P., … INTERHEART Study Investigators. (2005). Obesity and the risk of myocardial infarction in 27,000 participants from 52 countries: A case-control study. *Lancet, 366*(9497), 1640–649.

retained statistical significance, leading the authors to conclude that the adverse effects of excess weight on blood pressure and cholesterol may account for a substantial fraction (up to 45%) of the obesity-related risk increase (Bogers et al., 2007).

The INTERHEART Study examined obesity and other risk factors for myocardial infarction among 12,461 cases and 13,637 controls ascertained from 52 countries and representing several major ethnic groups. The effects of two measures of obesity were compared, BMI and waist-to-hip ratio. The odds of myocardial infarction increased significantly with each increasing quintile of waist-to-hip ratio (**FIGURE 42.8**). Men and women in the highest quintile of waist-to-hip ratio were 2.5 times more likely to develop a myocardial infarction compared to those in the lowest quintile. By comparison, those in the highest quintile of BMI were only 1.4 times more likely to suffer a myocardial infarction than those in the lowest quintile. The PAF estimated from the upper two quintiles of the waist-to-hip ratio was 24.3% compared to only 7.7% for BMI. These results suggest that the waist-to-hip ratio is superior to BMI as a predictor of disease risk (Yusuf et al., 2005).

Yatsuya and colleagues demonstrated that three separate measures of obesity were associated with incident ischemic stroke among 13,549 participants (5930 men, 7619 women, 3694 African Americans, and 9855 Caucasian Americans) aged 46–64 years enrolled in the U.S. ARIC Study. During the follow-up period (1987–2005), 598 individuals suffered ischemic strokes confirmed through hospital discharge records and imaging studies. Using quintiles of BMI, waist circumference, and waist-to-hip ratio, the investigators found that the incidence of stroke among African Americans

was two to three times higher than Caucasian Americans within each obesity quintile. Notably, observed results were similar for all three of the obesity measurements tested. Furthermore, adjustment for hypertension and diabetes markedly attenuated the effects of obesity, suggesting that much of the obesity-related risk of developing a stroke is due to related increases in blood pressure and insulin resistance. Estimates of the PAF due to obesity suggest that 18%–20% of the new cases of ischemic stroke are attributable to excess adiposity, which can be measured by BMI > 28.1, waist circumference > 100 cm, or waist-to-hip ratio > 0.95 (Yatsuya et al., 2010).

▶ Obesity and Cancer

According to a report from the American Institute of Cancer Research, more than 100,500 annual cases of cancer and 14%–20% of all cancer deaths in the United States can be attributed to excess body fat (World Cancer Research Fund/American Institute for Cancer Research, 2007). The report includes estimates of the percent of cancer cases attributable to obesity (PAFs) for selected cancers based on a review of more than 7000 publications (**TABLE 42.2**). The investigators estimate that excess body fat is responsible for approximately 33,000 postmenopausal breast cancers, 21,000 endometrial cancers, 14,000 kidney cancers, 13,000 colorectal cancers, and 12,000 pancreatic cancers per year in the U.S. population.

While obesity is a significant risk factor for many cancers, the association of obesity with cancer risk does not affect all subgroups equally. For example, colon cancer risk is higher in obese men than obese

TABLE 42.2 Estimated Percent and Number of Cancer Cases Attributed to Obesity in the United States

Cancer Type	Attributable Fraction	Annual Cases
Endometrium	49%	20,700
Esophagus	35	5,800
Pancreas	28	11,900
Kidney	24	13,900
Gallbladder	21	2,000
Breast	17	33,000
Colon/Rectum	9	13,200
	Total	100,500

Data from World Cancer Research Fund/American Institute for Cancer Research. (2007). *Food, nutrition, physical activity, and the prevention of cancer: A global perspective*. Washington, DC: World Cancer Research Fund/American Institute for Cancer Research.

women (Calle, 2008; Pischon, Nothlings, & Boeing, 2007), and obesity increases breast cancer risk in postmenopausal women but not premenopausal women (Harris, Namboodiri, & Wynder, 1992). The increased breast cancer risk in obese postmenopausal women may be due to the fact that adipose tissue is the primary source of estrogens after the menopause.

Hyperinsulinemia, growth factors, sustained low-grade inflammation, oxidative stress, and hormonal changes that are associated with excess adiposity are proposed as potential mechanisms that promote the development of cancer (Calle, 2008; Calle, Thun, Petrelli, Rodriguez, & Heath, 1999; Pischon, Nothlings, & Boeing, 2007). In particular, adipokines such as leptin, resistin, hepatocyte growth factor, and adiponectin that are secreted by adipose tissues are currently under intense investigation to determine their impact on carcinogenesis. In general, blood levels of pro-inflammatory adipokines (leptin) have been found to be higher in obese individuals in association with increased risk of certain malignancies (e.g., postmenopausal breast cancer, colorectal cancer, prostate cancer), whereas levels of anti-inflammatory adipokines (adiponectin) are higher in lean individuals in association with reduced cancer risk (Barb, Pazaitou-Panayiotou, & Mantzoros, 2006; Ho et al., 2012; Lee et al., 2015; Vona-Davis & Rose, 2007). The body of evidence supports the general recommendation to maintain a healthy weight as part of a comprehensive cancer-prevention lifestyle (Byers et al., 2002).

Recent epidemiologic evidence suggests that weight loss can reduce the risk of developing certain

malignancies in overweight and obese individuals. The impact of weight loss among young women at high genetic risk for breast cancer was recently demonstrated in a matched pair case–control study. The study examined effects of weight loss/gain in 1073 pairs of genetically susceptible women carrying either the *BRCA1* gene ($n = 797$ pairs) or the *BRCA2* gene ($n = 276$ pairs). Cases with breast cancer were matched to controls by year of birth, mutation (*BRCA1* or *BRCA2*), country of residence, and history of ovarian cancer. Results revealed that weight loss of at least 10 pounds between ages 18 and 30 years was associated with a 53% reduction in the risk of developing breast cancer between the ages of 30 and 49 years (OR = 0.47). Weight gain was not found to significantly influence the subsequent risk of developing breast cancer (Kotsopoulos et al., 2005).

Another study evaluated bariatric surgery (surgical reduction of stomach size for weight loss) among morbidly obese patients and their risk of cancer. Rates of cancer were compared in two observational cohorts of men and women. All patients of both cohorts were morbidly obese (BMI > 40) at baseline. Patients in one cohort received elective bariatric surgery ($n = 1035$) whereas those in the other did not ($n = 5746$). The control cohort was developed by matching 5 or 6 control patients to each bariatric case based on the date of first diagnosis of morbid obesity within 2 years, age within 5 years, and gender. Observed average reductions in excess weight and BMI were 62% and 32% in the bariatric cases. After 5 years of follow-up, the observed incidence of cancer in the control cohort was more than four times greater than the bariatric cohort (8.5% vs. 2%). The incidence of breast cancer among women of the control cohort was more than five times greater than the bariatric cohort (6.3% vs. 1.2%). The relative risk in the bariatric cohort (RR = 0.22) is equivalent to an 80% reduction in cancer risk associated with bariatric surgery in the morbidly obese (Christou, Lieberman, Sampalis, & Sampalis, 2008).

▶ Obesity and GERD

GERD is defined by the Brazilian Consensus Conference as "*a chronic disorder related to the retrograde flow of gastroduodenal contents into the esophagus and/or adjacent organs, resulting in a spectrum of symptoms, with or without tissue damage*" (Moraes-Filho et al., 2002). In layperson's terms, GERD is characterized as heartburn or regurgitation two or three times a week (Friedenberg, Xanthopoulos, Foster, & Richter, 2008).

Epidemiologic studies have consistently found a positive association between obesity and the development of GERD. Hampel and colleagues at Baylor University in Texas conducted a meta-analysis of nine epidemiologic studies of GERD in which BMI was used to classify individuals as overweight (BMI of 25–30) or obese (BMI > 30). The risk of developing GERD symptoms was significantly elevated for overweight and obese individuals compared to those of normal weight (RR = 1.43 and RR = 1.94, respectively). Risk increases with body mass were also found for comorbid conditions such as erosive esophagitis and esophageal adenocarcinoma (e.g., the risk of developing esophageal cancer was significantly elevated for overweight and obese individuals [RR = 1.52 and RR = 2.78, respectively]). The investigators concluded that the risk of developing GERD and related disorders increases with increasing body mass and obesity (Hampel, Abraham, & El-Serag, 2005).

Abdominal or central adiposity is of particular importance in the pathogenesis of GERD and its progression. Complications and comorbid conditions of GERD include erosive esophagitis, Barrett's esophagus (progressive metaplasia and dysplasia of the lower esophagus), and esophageal carcinoma. Epidemiologic studies have consistently shown that specific measures of central obesity (e.g., waist-to-hip ratio and waist circumference are better predictors of GERD risk and disease progression than BMI). Two examples of such studies are given below.

Investigators in Seoul, Korea, compared BMI and waist circumference as predictors of erosive esophagitis due to gastric reflux in a prospective study of 1029 subjects. Each subject was examined by endoscopy at baseline and was found to have a normal gastroesophageal junction. Subsequent endoscopic examinations were conducted for study participants after a 3-year interim and 42 subjects had developed erosive esophagitis. In multivariate models, BMI *did* not show statistical significance as a predictor of disease. In contrast, subjects with a waist circumference exceeding 90 cm at baseline were more than seven times more likely (OR = 7.2) to develop erosive esophagitis than subjects with a waist circumference less than 80 cm (Koo et al., 2009).

In a case–control study conducted in Seattle, Washington, 193 patients with Barrett's esophagus confirmed by biopsy were compared to 211 population controls without disease. Results showed that central obesity (defined as waist-to-hip ratio in the highest quintile) was associated with a significant increase in the risk of disease. The risk of developing Barrett's esophagus increased more than twofold (OR = 2.4) in subjects with central obesity compared to those with normal girth, and most notably, the risk of advanced disease increased more than fourfold (OR = 4.3) in subjects with central obesity (Edelstein, Farrow, Bronner, Rosen, & Vaughan, 2007). Comparative models incorporating BMI cut points and waist-to-hip cut points in defining central obesity clearly favor the use of waist-to-hip ratios.

The pathogenesis and progression of GERD in patients with central obesity may be a consequence of several biologically plausible mechanisms. Magnanimous abdominal girth may cause hiatal hernia and excessive reflux of acid from the stomach into the esophagus by increasing intra-abdominal pressure (Fisichella & Patti, 2009; Herbella & Patti, 2010). Also, visceral fat is more metabolically active than subcutaneous fat or peripheral fat, capable of producing a multitude of bioactive proteins (adipokines), including pro-inflammatory cytokines such as interleukin 6 and tumor necrosis factor-a (Einstein et al., 2005; Lundgren, Buren, Ruge, Myrnäs, & Eriksson, 2004). Visceral adiposity therefore heightens the pro-inflammatory acidic environment of GERD, and heightened activity of cytokines, cyclooxygenase-2 (COX-2), prostaglandin E2 (PGE2), and leptin may accelerate the progression of GERD to erosive esophagitis, Barrett's esophagus, and esophageal adenocarcinoma (Friedenberg et al., 2008; Ogunwobi, Mutungi, & Peales, 2006).

Estrogens may also play a role in the development of GERD among the obese. Magnus Nilsson of the Karolinska Hospital, Stockholm, and his associates found a stronger relationship between BMI and GERD among young, severely obese premenopausal women (OR = 6.8) compared with men (OR = 3.3) and postmenopausal women (OR = 4.2) at the same

BMI level. Results prompted the investigators to theorize that the association between estrogen and GERD is a nitric oxide-mediated reduction in smooth muscle tone at the lower esophageal sphincter. Obese women have increased aromatase-catalyzed estrone production by fatty tissue, lower concentrations of sex hormone binding globulin, and thus a larger proportion of unbound active estradiol. Excess estrogen increases nitric oxide synthesis (the primary relaxing molecule at the lower esophageal sphincter) which leads to reduced sphincter tone and increased acid reflux (Nilsson et al., 2003).

While research indicates that obesity is a major risk factor for the development of GERD, traditional weight loss programs have not shown consistent success in reducing symptoms. Two studies found no changes in reflux parameters or measures of esophageal acid (Frederiksen, Johansson, Johnsson, & Hedenbro, 2000; Kjellin, Ramel, Rossner, & Thor, 1996) whereas one study did observe improved gastroesophageal function due to a dietary exercise-based weight loss program (Fraser-Moodie et al., 1999). Surgically induced weight loss by the *Roux-en-Y gastric bypass procedure* has shown predominately positive effects in patients with GERD although the majority of studies are case reports (Suter, Giusti, Heraief, Zysset, & Calmes, 2003).

Obesity and Obstructive Sleep Apnea

Obstructive sleep apnea is a respiratory condition characterized by repeated episodes of upper airway collapse during sleep. Results of numerous epidemiologic investigations suggest that obesity is a major risk factor for the development of obstructive sleep apnea. The disorder is particularly prominent among men with abdominal (central) obesity (Young, Pappard, & Gottlieb, 2002).

Investigators at the University of Wisconsin in Madison studied a random sample of 603 men and women using overnight polysomnography to determine the frequency of episodes of apnea and hypopnea per hour of sleep (the *apnea-hypopnea index*). Abnormal index values (five or more episodes per hour) were found in 24% of men and 9% of women. Results suggested that each one standard deviation increase in BMI was associated with a fourfold increase in the risk of developing sleep apnea (Young et al., 1993). Investigators at Johns Hopkins University in Baltimore studied sleep disorders in 150 obese men otherwise in good health. Estimates of the prevalence of sleep

apnea varied 40%–60% depending on the severity of symptoms (Punjabi et al., 2002).

Some studies suggest that the prevalence of sleep apnea is higher in men than women. For example, investigators at Pennsylvania State University studied 200 obese women and 50 obese men using several measures of sleep disturbance in an 8-hour sleep laboratory. They detected obstructive sleep apnea in 20 men (40%) but only in 6 women (6%) (Vgontzas et al., 1994).

In a study of data from the 2002 *U.S. National Hospital Discharge Survey (NHDS),* Scott and colleagues examined the prevalence of sleep apnea and other disorders among 3473 morbidly obese patients, 833 of whom underwent bariatric surgery. Patients electing bariatric surgery had higher prevalence rates of sleep apnea than patients receiving other forms of treatment (24% vs. 11%) and men had higher rates of sleep apnea than women (47.3% vs. 19% among bariatric patients and 17.2% vs. 8.7% among all other patients). These results suggest that severe cases of morbid obesity (those who receive bariatric surgery) have a markedly increased risk of developing obstructive sleep apnea and, furthermore, that men are more susceptible than women (Scott et al., 2006). In a much smaller investigation of sleep disturbances in the morbidly obese, investigators at the University of Helsinki, Finland, studied sleep apnea in 27 morbidly obese patients including 13 men and 14 women. Obstructive sleep apnea was diagnosed in 10 men (78%) but in only 1 woman (7%) (Rajala et al., 1991).

On the contrary, other studies have found similar rates of sleep apnea in population samples of men and women, and relatively high rates of disease among obese women. A study of sleep disturbances in a Spanish cohort comprising 1050 men and 1098 women found similar prevalence levels of mild sleep apnea (five or more episodes of apnea/hypopnea per hour) in men (26%) and women (28%). Notably, the prevalence of sleep apnea became higher in men with increasing severity, (e.g., severe sleep apnea [15 or more episodes] was twice as common in men compared to women [14% vs. 7%]) (Durán, Esnaola, Rubio, & Iztueta, 2001). Investigators in Australia studied sleep disturbances among 108 obese women using overnight ambulatory measures and found that 41 patients (38%) met the threshold criteria for obstructive sleep apnea (Richman et al., 1994). Thus, while increasing obesity may exacerbate the risk more in men than in women, it is clear that obese women should also be considered at high risk for the development of obstructive sleep apnea.

Biological mechanisms by which central obesity predisposes to obstructive sleep apnea include anatomic alterations and/or disturbances in upper airway neuromuscular control. The heightened predisposition in men versus women may be related to androgenic hormonal factors or the predominantly abdominal (central) distribution of body fat in aging men. Central adiposity is likely to cause excess deposition of fat in the head and neck which in turn predisposes to narrowing and closure of the upper airways. In addition, signaling proteins secreted by visceral adipose could diminish neuromuscular control of the airways (Gibson, 2005; Schwartz et al., 1998).

In several epidemiologic studies, both weight gain and weight loss have been shown to influence the risk of developing sleep apnea. For example, in a prospective study of 690 randomly selected employed residents of Wisconsin conducted during 1989–2000, individuals who gained 10% in weight increased their odds of developing mild sleep apnea by 32% compared to those with stable weight, whereas those who lost 10% of their initial body weight decreased their disease odds by 26%. In addition, a 10% increase in weight was associated with a sixfold increase in the odds of developing moderate to severe sleep apnea (Peppard, Young, Palta, Dempsey, & Skatrud, 2000).

Therapeutic effects of moderate weight loss were demonstrated in a study of 15 hypersomnolent patients with moderately severe obstructive sleep apnea. In overweight patients who reduced their weight by 9%, apnea frequency fell and sleep patterns improved ($P < 0.01$). No improvement occurred among the age- and weight-matched controls who did not lose weight (Smith, Gold, Meyers, Haponik, & Bleecker, 1985).

Obstructive sleep apnea has also been shown to improve or resolve as a result of surgically induced weight loss. In a systematic review of 134 extracted bariatric surgical studies worldwide from 1990 to 2003 (56 in North America, 58 in Europe, and 20 throughout the rest of the world) involving a total of 22,094 patients, nearly 20% of patients were diagnosed with sleep disorder breathing (sleep apnea) preoperatively. After surgery, substantial weight loss was attained across all measures of adiposity. Significant reductions were observed in average BMI (14.2 units) and absolute weight (39.7 kg) and obstructive sleep apnea resolved in 85.7% of patients (Buchwald, Avidor, & Braunwald, 2004)

Obesity and Osteoarthritis

Osteoarthritis, also called degenerative *joint disease,* is a common progressive disorder usually manifesting in late adulthood principally affecting the weight-bearing joints of the body (knees, hips, and

vertebral column). Other joints commonly affected are those subjected to sustained repetitive mechanical stress and trauma over the lifespan such as the distal finger joints and the thumb joint. Osteoarthritis is characterized clinically by pain, inflammation, deformity, and limitation of motion and pathologically by the erosion and destruction of cartilage, sclerosis (scarring), and other pathologic lesions in the joints. Radiographic studies reveal the presence of at least subclinical osteoarthritis in the majority of adults over the age of 65 years. Progressive disease is a leading cause of disability in many populations (Fletcher & Lewis-Fanning, 1945; Mankin, 1974; Raynauld et al., 2006; Robbins & Cotran, 1979).

The strong association between obesity and osteoarthritis of the major weight-bearing joints has been widely verified. Leach and colleagues found that 83% of their female subjects with knee osteoarthritis were obese compared to 42% of the control group (Leach, Baumgard, & Broom, 1973). In the Framingham Study, Felson and colleagues demonstrated that a 5.1 kg loss in body mass over a 10-year period reduced the odds of developing knee osteoarthritis by more than 50% (Felson, Zhang, Anthony, Naimark, & Anderson, 1992). In a case–control study of 675 matched pairs conducted in the United Kingdom, Coggon and colleagues determined that the risk of knee osteoarthritis in people with a BMI > 30 was 6.8 times that of normal-weight controls (Coggon et al., 2001). Using data from the 1982–1984 U.S. NHANES I), Ettinger and colleagues examined the effects of comorbid diseases on disability and found that people with a BMI > 30 were 4.2 times more likely to have knee osteoarthritis than leaner people (Ettinger, Davis, Neuhaus, & Mallon, 1994). Taken together, these studies indicate that obesity is a major risk factor for osteoarthritis of weight-bearing joints and associated functional impairment. Physiologic processes related to the increased susceptibility of obese individuals to osteoarthritis include greater joint stress, diminished muscle strength, and increased inflammation (Messier, 2008).

Obesity and Quality of Life

In addition to substantial morbidity and increased risk of premature mortality, obesity is also associated with decreases in the overall quality of life. The *quality-adjusted life years (QALY)* is a population health outcome summary measure that quantifies the impact of both the duration of life and the quality of life for a specific period of time (Gold, Stevenson, & Fryback, 2002; Sassi, 2006; Zeckhauser & Shepard, 1976).

Calculation of the QALY for a particular disease is calculated from the number of years lived without the disease (Y1) and the number of years lived with the disease (Y2). Each year of healthy life is assigned the value of 1.0 whereas subpar health due to disease is assigned a lower value between 0 and 1. Death has a value of zero. Thus, the QALY for obesity would be estimated for a given individual as QALY = Y1 × 1.0 + Y2 × q where Y1 denotes the years lived at normal weight, Y2 denotes the years lived with obesity, and q is the quality of life weighting factor for obesity.

Using data from the 2003–2008 U.S. Behavioral Risk Factor Surveillance System (BRFSS), Jia and Lubetkin calculated the loss of QALYs among U.S. adults due to obesity-related morbidity and mortality. Estimates of QALYs lost for U.S. adults were calculated as the sum of QALYs lost due to morbidity and future QALYs lost in expected life years due to premature deaths. Results revealed that the loss of QALYs for all adults more than doubled 1993–2008, while the prevalence of obesity increased from 14.1% to 26.7% during the same time frame. In addition, the loss of QALYs among African-American women was 31% higher than African-American men and approximately 50% higher than Caucasian men or women. A strong positive correlation was found between the percentage of state populations reporting no leisure time activity and the obesity-related QALYs lost (r = 0.71). The investigators suggest there is a critical need for effective programs to reduce obesity at local, state, and national levels (Jia & Lubetkin, 2010).

▶ Mechanisms of Pathogenesis in Obesity-Related Diseases

Obesity and excess weight increase the mechanical stress and strain on multiple systems of the human body. Browning and Kram examined differences in biomechanical load between obese and normal-weight individuals during walking. They found that obese individuals exerted 60% greater vertical ground reaction forces compared to normal-weight people (Browning & Kram, 2007). Obesity may also lead to the compression of blood vessels and body organs, creating mechanical resistance and distortion of normal function.

White adipose tissue (WAT), which includes the energy storage fat cells (adipocytes), along with several other cell types (neurons, endothelial cells, stromovascular cells, and immune cells) was once considered an inert tissue primarily responsible for

storing or releasing energy as required. Within the past several decades, adipose tissue has been found to play a critical role in whole body metabolic regulation and cellular energy homeostasis. It is now known that adipose tissue is an active endocrine organ that secretes a variety of pro-inflammatory bioactive proteins, collectively called *adipokines* or *adipocytokines* (Lyon, Law, & Hsueh, 2003). Adipokines such as leptin, resistin, adiponectin, interleukin-6 (IL-6), and tumor necrosis factor-alpha (TNF-α) influence many physiologic processes including body weight homeostasis, insulin resistance, lipid levels, blood pressure, coagulation, inflammation, and atherosclerosis.

Grossly enlarged adipocytes associated with obesity release pro-inflammatory adipokines that simultaneously promote atherogenesis and insulin resistance (Leonhardt, Hanefeld, Schneider, & Haller, 1972; Lonn, Mehlig, Bengtsson, & Lissner, 2010; Weyer, Foley, Bogardus, Tataranni, & Pratley, 2000) (**FIGURE 42.9**). Resistin and TNF-α downregulate insulin receptors, decrease GLUT-4 translocation to the cellular membrane, inhibit lipoprotein lipase activity, and increase hormone sensitive lipase. Plasminogen activator inhibitor (PAI-1) and angiotensinogen enhance thrombus (clot) formation and reduce local blood flow, and interleukin-6 (IL-6) and C-reactive protein (CRP) stimulate macrophage infiltration and complement activation. There is also an endocrine response via the synthesis and secretion of leptin, which acts on the hypothalamic pituitary axis to decrease food intake and increase energy expenditure. The single adipokine that is clearly reduced with obesity is adiponectin, which has anti-inflammatory properties that increase insulin sensitivity and reduce atherogenesis (Fruhbeck,

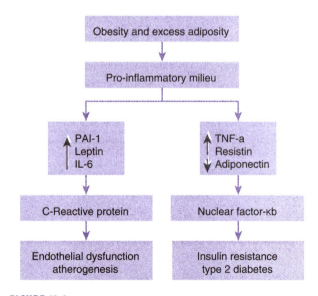

FIGURE 42.9 Obesity and Adipokines.

Data from Lyon, C. J., Law, R. E., & Hsueh, W. A. (2003). Minireview: Adiposity, inflammation, and atherogenesis. *Endocrinology 144*, 2195–2200.

Gomez-Ambrosi, Muruzabai, & Burrell, 2001; Kadowaki & Yamauchi, 2005; Lyon, Law, & Hsueh, 2003). As pointed out by Lyon, Law, & Hsueh (2003):

> *Adipose tissue is a dynamic endocrine organ that secretes a number of factors that are increasingly recognized to contribute to systemic and vascular inflammation. Obesity promotes the parallel progression of insulin resistance to type 2 diabetes and endothelial dysfunction to atherosclerosis.*

▸ Obesity and Atherogenesis

The "response to injury hypothesis" proposes that atherogenesis (atherosclerosis) is an inflammatory disease (Ross & Glomset, 1973, 1976). According to this hypothesis, injury to the endothelial lining of the artery stimulates an inflammatory response resulting in smooth muscle proliferation and subsequently infiltration of the wound by macrophages and other inflammatory cells. Without resolution, recursive cycles of chronic inflammation ensue, leading to the release of hydrolytic enzymes, cytokines, chemokines, and growth factors that cause further cellular damage and eventually produce focal areas of cell necrosis. As stated by Ross, "*Each characteristic lesion of atherosclerosis represents a different stage in a chronic inflammatory process in the artery; if unabated and excessive, this process will result in an advanced complicated lesion*" (Ross, 1999).

In the human system, the presence of excess WAT that is characteristic of obesity has been found to induce a persistent state of low-grade inflammation. Excess calories are stored in fat cells (adipocytes) of WAT in the form of triacylglycerol, and in times of caloric restriction, free fatty acids are mobilized and released into the blood. The expansion of WAT with obesity is accompanied by angiogenesis (formation of new blood vessels), increased proliferation of fibroblasts, and infiltration by macrophages. There is also increased secretion of interleukins, inflammatory cytokines, and adipokines.

Investigations by Fain and colleagues have demonstrated that leptin and adiponectin are primarily secreted by the adipocytes (fat cells) whereas other inflammatory mediators are released by both fat cells and nonfat cells of the WAT cellular milieu (Fain, 2006). With obesity, elevated levels of circulating autocrine, paracrine, and endocrine factors derived primarily from the excess visceral WAT can induce sustained inflammation and atherogenesis.

In a review of pathogenic mechanisms of adiposity, Lyon, Law, and Hsueh describe how several pro-inflammatory cytokines and adipokines contribute to atherogenesis. According to their model of obesity-related atherogenesis, rising levels of adipokines and cytokines including leptin, resistin, TNF-α, interleukin-6 (IL-6), angiotensin II (Ang II), and plasminogen activator inhibitor-1 (PAI-1) initiate endothelial dysfunction through activation of the nuclear transcription factor, nuclear factor kappa beta (NF-κb). A cascade of inflammatory changes in vascular tissue occurs, including the migration and attachment of monocytes to the arterial wall and their subsequent conversion to macrophages. Chronic inflammation ensues as macrophage activation results in the release of hydrolytic enzymes, cytokines, chemokines, and an increase in oxidative stress, which leads to focal necrosis and the eventual formation of atherosclerotic plaque (Lyon, Law, & Hsueh, 2003).

The obesity-related pro-inflammatory milieu of WAT-derived cytokines and adipokines (particularly IL-6) stimulates the production of CRP by the liver. *CRP is an acute phase protein* whose concentration in the blood is increased in both acute and chronic inflammatory states. Its primary physiologic function is to assist complement binding to foreign and damaged cells and enhance phagocytosis by macrophages. Individuals without inflammation usually have CRP levels below 1.0 μg/mL. Patients with bacterial infections, autoimmune diseases, or cancer can have elevated CRP of 100 μg/mL or higher, making CRP a nonspecific marker for inflammation. Despite the lack of specificity, CRP has emerged as one of the most powerful predictors of cardiovascular risk (Yeh & Willerson, 2003).

It has been well established in numerous prospective studies that an elevated serum concentration of CRP (even within a "normal" range of values, 1–5 μg/mL) is a risk factor for cardiovascular disease and has significant predictive value for cardiovascular events (Koenig, 2003; Yeh & Willerson, 2003). Examination of *both* CRP and cholesterol levels is particularly valuable in risk prediction. For example, Ridker and colleagues demonstrated that the combination of elevated levels of CRP (>2.11 μg/L) and total cholesterol (>mg/dL) was associated with a fivefold increase in the risk of first myocardial infarction, more than double the relative risk for either factor alone. Furthermore, those in the top quintile of *both* CRP and the ratio of total cholesterol to high-density lipoprotein exhibited an 8.7-fold increase in risk compared to RRs of 4.2 and 2.2, respectively, for individual factors (Ridker, Glynn, & Hennekins, 1998). Prospective studies have also demonstrated that CRP is a predictor for cardiovascular morbidity, mortality, and/or recurrent coronary events among individuals with known cardiovascular disease, unstable and stable angina, and prior myocardial infarction (Rifai & Ridker, 2001). In addition to being a biologic marker of inflammation, CRP appears to activate complement in atherosclerotic plaques, thereby increasing the risk of thrombotic complications and vascular damage (Yasojima, Schwab, Mcgeer, & McGeer, 2001).

Many epidemiologic studies have found a strong positive association between obesity (body mass) and serum levels of CRP. Hak and coworkers examined relationships of CRP, obesity, common carotid intima-media thickness, and insulin resistance among 186 healthy middle-aged women from the general population. In regression models, BMI and waist circumference were significant predictors of CRP; and CRP was in turn associated with several variables related to insulin resistance and subclinical atherosclerosis including blood pressure, insulin level, high-density lipoprotein cholesterol, triglycerides, apolipoprotein A1 (inversely), plasminogen activator inhibitor-1 antigen, and tissue-type plasminogen activator antigen. These results suggest that inflammatory mediators derived from adipose and linked to CRP may play an important role in the development of insulin resistance and coronary heart disease (Hak et al., 1999).

Yudkin and colleagues examined correlations of CRP and concentrations of pro-inflammatory adipokines, interleukin-6 (IL-6), and TNF-α among 107 nondiabetic adults ascertained from a medical practice in London. Statistically significant correlations were observed between CRP, IL-6, and TNF-α. In contrast, correlations of CRP with *Helicobacter pylori*, *Chlamydia pneumoniae*, and cytomegalovirus antibody titers were weak or nonsignificant. Furthermore, CRP was significantly related to insulin resistance, blood pressure, high-density lipoproteins, and markers of endothelial dysfunction, such as von Willebrand factor, tissue plasminogen activator, and cellular fibronectin. These data suggest that chronic bacterial or viral infections are *not* important determinants of low-level chronic inflammation, whereas adipocyte-related inflammatory molecules (CRP, IL-6, and TNF-α) may induce insulin resistance, endothelial dysregulation, and atherogenesis. Results infer a critical molecular link between obesity and increased risk of cardiovascular disease (Yudkin, Stehouwer, Emeiss, & Coppack, 1999).

Tchernof and colleagues investigated obesity, caloric restriction, weight loss, and CRP in 61 obese postmenopausal Caucasian women in Vermont. Total body fat was measured by dual X-ray absorptiometry and intra-abdominal fat was measured by computerized tomography. Both measures of obesity were significant predictors of plasma CRP. Twenty-five of the women completed a 13-month weight loss protocol involving caloric restriction (1200 kcals daily) with no change in physical activity levels. Weight loss averaged approximately 15 kg and resulted in a significant decrease in plasma CRP ($P < 0.0001$). Compared to visceral fat measures, overall body fatness was a better predictor of plasma CRP in multivariate regression analyses (Tchernof, Nolan, Sites, Ades, & Poehlman, 2002).

Plasminogen activator inhibitor-1 (PAI-1) is an adipokine that inhibits the breakdown of fibrin clots, thus increasing the risk for thromboembolic events. In molecular studies of adipose from morbidly obese women, Fain and colleagues demonstrated that *visceral adipose tissue* released greater amounts of vascular endothelial growth factor, IL-6, and PAI-1 compared with abdominal subcutaneous tissue (Fain, Madan, Hiler, Cheema, & Bahouth, 2004). This finding may help explain the stronger association of abdominal obesity with an increased risk of stroke and other thromboembolic cardiovascular events (Suk et al., 2003; Yatsuya et al., 2010).

► Obesity and Insulin Resistance

As lipid-laden adipocytes reach their threshold of fat storage, the WAT releases a variety of pro-inflammatory adipokines and cytokines that contribute to insulin resistance and the development of type 2 diabetes. For example, TNF-α inhibits tyrosine kinase phosphorylation of the insulin receptor, resulting in defects in insulin signaling and ultimately leading to insulin resistance and impaired glucose transport. Contributing to the process, circulating levels of resistin and other inflammatory factors rise and levels of adiponectin fall (resistin increases insulin resistance and inflammation whereas adiponectin improves insulin sensitivity and inhibits vascular inflammation). Without intervention, these inflammatory processes continue unabated, resulting in hyperinsulinemia, hyperglycemia, dyslipidemia, and eventual lipotoxicity and glucotoxicity of nonadipose tissue, including the β-cells of the pancreas (Unger, 2003). Furthermore, functional deterioration of the pancreatic β cells and insulin insufficiency may contribute to the development of type 2 diabetes (Wajchenberg, 2000, 2007).

► Overview of Adipocyte Regulatory Processes

Over the past several decades, researchers have developed a better understanding of how adipose tissue helps to regulate energy homeostasis and metabolism.

A relatively new obesity-chronic disease paradigm is emerging which is focused on adipose tissue physiology and the role of feedback mechanisms which respond to disruptions in adipocyte homeostasis (Arner & Spalding, 2010; Iozzo, 2009; Larsen, Toubro, & Astrup, 2003; Löfgren et al., 2005; Maffeis et al., 2007; Rosen & MacDougald, 2006; Scott, Rabito, Butler, & Harris, 2004; Sethi & Vidal-Puig, 2007; Skurk, Alberti-Huber, & Hauner, 2006).

Adiposity encompasses fat cell number (cellularity) and fat cell size. Adipose tissue serves important physiologic functions that include protecting vital organs, helping to preserve heat through insulation, and energy storage. WAT is the repository or storage vesicle for excess energy in the form of triglycerides (triacylglycerol). WAT acts to buffer energy imbalances when energy intake is not equal to energy output and thus provides a normal dynamic physiologic storage space for excess energy in long-term generally calorically stable environments (Faust & Miller, 1983).

Fat Storage (Lipogenesis)

Excess fat is stored in the adipocytes (fat cells) of WAT by a process known as lipogenesis. When the caloric intake of fat, carbohydrate, and protein is greater than the energy expenditure, the liver converts the excess calories to fat in the form of triglycerides. Triglycerides are transported in the blood from the liver to WAT by lipid carriers called lipoproteins. Chylomicrons carry dietary triglycerides from the breakdown of fat, while very low-density lipoproteins (VLDL) carry endogenously formed triglycerides converted from excess glucose (the basic unit of carbohydrates) and amino acids (basic units of protein). Triglyceride molecules are broken down to their constituent parts of fatty acids and glycerol in the cell membrane of adipocytes (fat cells) by the enzyme *lipoprotein lipase*. Fatty acids are then able to enter into the adipocyte where they are repackaged as triacylglycerol and stored (the overall process is called *lipogenesis*). Insulin, produced by the beta (β)-cells of the pancreas, is secreted into the blood in response to elevated blood glucose and is the prime mediator of adipocyte glucose uptake to furnish the energy required for lipogenesis.

Fat Breakdown (Lipolysis)

When long-term energy intake does not meet energy requirements, stored triacylglycerol within adipocytes is broken down by *hormone sensitive lipase* to free fatty acids released from the fat cell to be used for energy by tissues of the body (the overall process is called *lipolysis*). Subsequently, the adipocytes become smaller. At a given level of excess energy, adipocyte size is proportionate to the number of fat cells. More fat cells equate to more storage space with which to store excess energy, while fewer fat cells place a greater burden of storage on individual fat cells. Fat cell size can therefore be viewed as a measure of the excess energy that the body stores.

Homeostatic regulation of lipogenesis and lipolysis depends upon the presence of adequate normal functioning WAT. To illustrate, studies of transgenic *lipoatrophic* (fatless) mice reveal that the absence of fat cells results in severe metabolic dysregulation including hypertriglyceridemia, hyperinsulinemia, hyperglycemia, dyslipidemia, insulin resistance, and type 2 diabetes. In other words, with no fat cells to store excess energy, the fatless mice present clinically as if they were obese. Notably, surgical transplantation of WAT to fatless mice reverses diabetes, normalizes glycemia and insulinemia, and improves blood lipids, demonstrating that the lack of adipose tissue causes the insulin resistance (Gavrilova et al., 2000). The physiologic mechanisms responsible for these effects have not been fully clarified. One hypothesis is that elevated levels of circulating triglycerides and free fatty acids may interfere with insulin-dependent glucose transport in muscle, leading to insulin resistance and type 2 diabetes (Kim & Moustaid-Mousa, 2000).

Secretion of Adipokines by Adipocytes

Adipocytes actively participate in maintaining energy homeostasis by synthesizing and secreting a multitude of autocrine, paracrine, and endocrine signaling proteins such as hormones, complement components, growth factors, and cytokines collectively called adipokines (Bays, Mandarino, & DeFronzo, 2004; Fruhbeck et al., 2001; Marques, Hauman, & Martin, 1998; Ravussin & Smith, 2002). Adipokine levels are strongly influenced by changes in the cellular storage of fat and related gains (or losses) in whole body weight. For example, leptin concentrations increase as fat cell size *increases* and decrease as fat cell size *decreases* (Löfgren et al., 2005). The increase in leptin with obesity and increased fat cell size acts to *decrease* food intake and *increase* energy expenditure. Reciprocally, adiponectin levels are reduced in obesity and *increase* with weight loss (Fruhbeck et al., 2001; Löfgren et al., 2005; Ziccardi et al., 2002). In this manner, adipocyte signaling proteins appear to work in concert, regulating metabolism and maintaining energy homeostasis both locally and distally.

Fat cells secrete adipokines as a direct response to their energy storage capacity (Fruhbeck et al., 2001; Kim, Gavrilova, Chen, Reitman, & Shulman, 2000; Skurk et al., 2006). As excess energy in the form of triacylglycerol is stored in adipocytes, individual fat cells can increase tremendously in size (undergo *hypertrophy*) with the ability to expand 20-fold in diameter and over 1000-fold in volume (Björnheden et al., 2004; Hewitt, 1997). However, each cell can only store so much excess energy (as triacylglycerol) and when its storage capacity is surpassed, pro-inflammatory adipokines are secreted.

The adipocyte response to hypertrophy is an *epigenetic phenomenon* leading to the overexpression of specific genes that encode pro-inflammatory adipokines. One factor that may induce such genetic expression is the physical stress and strain that wounds the plasma membrane of fat-laden cells. Indeed, plasma membrane wounding is considered the principal mechano-sensing event that initiates the inflammatory response (Vlahakis & Hubmayr, 2005; Zeghari et al., 2000). This may help explain why enlarged fat cells elicit an inflammatory response, while increased numbers of fat cells do not.

Tissue hypoxia associated with increasing fat mass may also play a role. Excess adiposity increases the demand for oxygen to support tissue remodeling and vascularization (Attie & Scherer, 2009). If the oxygen demand of excess adipose tissue exceeds the oxygen supply, hypoxia could induce the expression of genes such as *hypoxia inducible factor-1a (HIF-1a)* which triggers *cyclooxygenase-2 (COX-2)* and the pro-inflammatory milieu observed with obesity (Yin, Gao, He, & Ye, 2009).

▶ Fat Cell Size, Number, and Turnover in Humans

Many studies have found that a significant loss of weight and fat mass in humans results in a decrease in volume (size) of adipocytes but produces no change in adipocyte number. As an example, the involuntary weight loss associated with cachexia in patients with advanced cancer causes a decrease in adipocyte size but no change in number. Reciprocally, significant weight gain in adults increases adipocyte size but also produces no net change in number. One interpretation of these findings is that weight changes in adulthood are primarily due to increases in adipocyte volume and size rather than number (Arner & Spalding, 2010).

Early investigations of human adipose tissue by Jules Hirsch and Bruce Batchelor at Rockefeller University in New York suggested that all human obesity is characterized by adipocyte hypertrophy and when body weight exceeds 170% of ideal, the maximum cell size increases to approximately twice that of normal cells. But they also found that increasing severity of obesity is correlated with increasing hyperplasia of adipocytes, and that hypercellularity (increased adipocyte number) is characteristic of the early onset of obesity (Hirsch & Batchelor, 1976).

While lipid storage in mature fat cells is undoubtedly of major importance, recent investigations suggest that the number of fat cells is also an important determinant of fat mass. Using an innovative molecular technique, Spalding and colleagues studied the dynamics of fat cell turnover among cohorts of adults in the United States. Fat cell turnover was assessed using measures of 14C integrated into genomic DNA during nuclear testing. Results indicate that the number of fat cells remains constant in lean and obese adults even after marked weight loss, indicating that the number of adipocytes is fixed early in life. Nevertheless, approximately 10% of fat cells die and are replaced annually at all adult ages and levels of BMI, vis-à-vis, approximately 50% of fat cells are replaced every 8 years. Furthermore, neither adipocyte death nor generation rate is altered in early obesity, suggesting that fat cell number is under tight genetic regulation (Spalding et al., 2008).

According to these observations on the rate of human fat cell turnover, individuals with a large number of fat cells have a greater inherent fat storage capacity than individuals with small numbers. It is therefore possible to categorize obesity into two types: hypertrophic obesity (increased adipocyte volume) and hyperplastic obesity (increased adipocyte number). An important finding from in vitro and in vivo animal studies is that progenitor (stem) cells present in adipose tissue can be stimulated to proliferate and differentiate into mature adipocytes. The data suggest that progenitor cells are recruited to become mature adipocytes at the same rate that adipocytes die. Under normal conditions, the fat mass is therefore in a constant state of flux whereby the adipocyte number remains relatively constant (Arner & Spalding, 2010).

Multiple molecular factors are undoubtedly involved in the differentiation of progenitor stem cells into adipocytes. Recent studies suggest that in the presence of excess energy, fibroblast-like precursor cells are stimulated to differentiate into new adipocytes by activation of the nuclear receptor peroxisome proliferator-activated receptor-gamma (PPAR-g), a major regulator of adipogenesis (Grun & Blumberg,

2006; Larsen, Toubro, & Astrup, 2003), thereby increasing fat cell number (hyperplasia) and expanding energy storage capacity (Danforth, 2000; Fruhbeck et al., 2001; Hausman, DiGirolamo, & Bartness, 2001; Hube & Hauner, 2000; Marques, Hauman, & Martin, 1998; Rosenbaum & Leibel, 1998). In other words, as Rosen and MacDougald (2006) correctly explain: "*adipocytes provide a safe place to store lipids.*"

▶ Brown Adipose Tissue

While the role of WAT is primarily that of energy storage and homeostasis, brown adipose tissue (BAT) is principally involved in classic cold-induced non-shivering thermogenesis to produce heat to help regulate body temperature (Cannon & Nedergaard, 2004). Facultative thermogenesis, defined as heat production in response to cold temperature, occurs in skeletal muscle and BAT. Skeletal muscle produces heat via shivering thermogenesis, while non-shivering thermogenesis (characteristic of human newborns) occurs in BAT (Argyropoulos & Harper, 2002).

BAT is abundant in small mammals and hibernating animals and constitutes about 5% of the body weight of human newborn infants. Its presence in newborns is of great importance to avoid hypothermia. Brown fat is highly innervated and vascularized and the cells have abundant mitochondria. Brown fat efficiently produces heat in response to signals from the sympathetic nervous system. In cold temperatures, a special uncoupling protein 1 (UCP1) is activated within the mitochondria, resulting in uncoupling of oxidative phosphorylation and heat production (Lowell, 1998). Brown fat diminishes rapidly during infancy and is negligible in human adults. Adaptive thermogenesis and the dissipation of energy through heat production are possible targets for obesity intervention (Lowell & Spiegelman, 2000).

▶ Risk Factors of Obesity

The genesis of obesity is multifactorial, involving both modifiable and nonmodifiable risk factors and determinants (**TABLE 42.3**). For any individual, the development of obesity is a result of the interaction of behavioral, environmental, sociocultural, and genetic factors that collectively tip the energy balance in favor of excess energy stored as fat.

The dramatic global rise in the prevalence of obesity during the past several decades has led some investigators to rule out a genetic basis for the obesity epidemic on the rationale that, collectively, the population gene pool could not have changed significantly in such a short period of time (Christakis & Fowler, 2007; Heindel, 2003; Stunkard et al., 1986; Wardle, Carnell, Haworth, & Plomin, 2008). The obesity epidemic has therefore, more often been described as resulting from contemporary "obesity-promoting" environmental factors interacting with relatively stable, but underlying, genes among those who are susceptible in the population (Flegal & Troiano, 2000). As a consequence, public health and health behavior research and intervention programs have focused primarily on social and environmental determinants, which generally refer to a myriad of multilevel factors that influence, either directly or indirectly, the two predominant behaviors that impact energy balance: dietary intake and physical activity.

In addition to the traditional perspective that energy excess leads to the subsequent development of obesity, emerging factors which have generated interest as potential contributors to the secular increase in obesity include dietary factors, genetic predisposition, demography (age, longevity, gender, ethnicity), maternal influence during the perinatal period, psychological stressors (sleep debt, emotional stress, depression), physiologic factors (adiposity rebound and fat cell dynamics), food marketing strategies and food access,

TABLE 42.3 Selected Determinants of Obesity

Modifiable	Nonmodifiable	Environmental
Energy Input Excess calories from high fat, high sugar, and energy-dense diet	Gender, aging, ethnicity, genetics, prenatal & postnatal effects, menopause, psychological and physiologic factors	Built Environment Motorized transportation, mechanization, and automation
Energy Output Sedentary lifestyle with low exercise and low physical activity		Food Policy Marketing, cost, quality, access, and availability

economic advances (urbanization, automation, and mechanization), organic pollutants (endocrine disruptors), assortative mating, and pharmaceuticals that influence weight (Crovetti, Porrini, Santangelo, & Testolin, 1997; Economic Research Service, 2010; Grun & Blumberg, 2006; Keith et al., 2006). Selected risk factors are discussed in the following sections.

▸ Genetics of Obesity

The marked increase in the prevalence of obesity in the last three decades has led some investigators to question the importance of genetics in the etiology of obesity (O'Rahilly & Farooqi, 2006). Though it is well established that obesity runs in families, family members tend to share similar environments and behaviors in their patterns of diet and exercise. Furthermore, in the vast majority of families studied, obesity does not segregate with a Mendelian pattern of inheritance. Still, the available evidence clearly reflects significant genetic impact on measures of body mass and obesity. The genetic factors that influence obesity can be classified into three broad categories.

Monogenic forms of obesity are caused by single gene mutations that are extremely rare. Examples include genetic deficiencies in key hormones that regulate appetite and metabolism such as melanocortin and leptin (Farooqi & O'Rahilly, 2005a, 2007).

Syndromic forms of obesity, of which there are approximately 30 rare syndromes, arise from discrete genetic defects or chromosomal abnormalities. Such syndromes are often associated with mental impairment, dimorphic features, and developmental abnormalities (e.g., Prader Willi syndrome, Alstrom syndrome, and fragile X syndrome) (Farooqi & O'Rahilly, 2005b, 2007).

Polygenic forms of obesity occur as a result of the effects of multiple genes (Ichihara & Yamada, 2008). Studies of obesity in monozygous and dizygous twins, siblings, parents, and their offspring, adoptees and their adoptive parents, and extended pedigrees have consistently revealed a strong genetic and heritable contribution to measures of adiposity, such as BMI, body fat, fat mass, and waist circumference (Segal & Allison, 2002; Stunkard et al., 1986; Wardle et al., 2008).

According to O'Rahilly and Farooqi (2006), "*the heritability of a trait is defined as the per cent of interindividual variation in that trait that can be explained by inherited factors*." Notably, genetic studies conducted in different populations and environments have found that 40%–70% of the variability in body mass is "heritable" (Wardle et al., 2008). For example, among 25,000 twin pairs born in Sweden between 1886 and 1958, the heritability of BMI was estimated as 70% for men and 66% for women (Stunkard et al., 1986). Nevertheless, since human genotypes cannot be replicated and studied in different environments, such studies are limited in their ability to partition the variability due to genotype by environment interaction.

Indeed, one explanation for the rapid rise in obesity is the mismatch between today's environment and "thrifty genes" that were selected for in the past under different environmental conditions when food sources were rather unpredictable. This hypothesis was initially proposed in 1962 by geneticist James Neel to explain how genes predisposing to diabetes arose in the population. Neel suggested that genes which predispose to diabetes (the "thrifty genes") were historically advantageous, but they became detrimental in the modern world. In his words, they were "*rendered detrimental by 'progress.*'" Thrifty genes are genes that enable individuals to efficiently collect and process food to deposit fat during periods of food abundance which is later used for energy in times of famine. Neel's primary interest was in diabetes, but the idea was soon expanded to encompass obesity. According to the "thrifty genotype" hypothesis, the same genes that helped our ancestors survive occasional famines are now being challenged by environments in which food is plentiful year round (Neel, 1962).

▸ Environmental Factors Contributing to Obesity

Environmental factors can increase the risk of developing obesity by directly or indirectly influencing energy intake and energy expenditure. Two environmental factors have been implicated as major culprits in causing obesity: food marketing strategies (especially to children) and 24-hour availability of cheap, convenient, energy-dense, high fat, high sugar, ultra-processed, super-sized, ready-to-eat meals, snacks, and drinks (Bodor, Rose, Farley, Swalm, & Scott, 2008; Hill & Peters, 1998; McGinnis, Gootman, & Kraak, 2006).

Compelling evidence to support an association between excess calorie consumption and obesity comes from the research conducted by Nestle and colleagues who analyzed the trend of portion sizes over time. Their results revealed that portion sizes rose dramatically in the 1970s and then skyrocketed in the 1980s, with foods such as French fries, hamburgers, and soft drinks being two to five times larger than their original sizes (Nestle & Young, 2002). In addition, Rolls and colleagues showed that, within a single meal, total energy intake increases with increased portion size (Rolls, Morris, & Roe, 2002).

The trend of super-sized portions has been primarily economic and value-driven, with consumers wanting "more food for their money" (DiDomenico, 1994; Hill & Peters, 1998), even choosing restaurants based on portion sizes (Carangelo, 1995). Larger portion sizes equate to more calories. A "best value" drink, such as a typical 64 oz. soft drink from any fast food or franchised restaurant, contains almost 800 calories, an amount equivalent to a nearly half the energy requirements for most children and adolescents.

Environmental factors also influence physical activity levels and energy expenditure. For example, the *built environment*, which reflects the land use and transportation patterns of a population, can either facilitate or constrain physical activity (U.S. National Academy of Sciences, 2005). Urban sprawl patterns such as low-density land use, single-use zoning, and employment dispersion may cause a heavy reliance on motorized methods of transportation and lengthened commute times, and lack of opportunities or spaces and places to walk, bicycle, and play safely (Hu, 2008). In addition, neighborhood characteristics such as sidewalks, lighting, perception of safety, streetscapes, traffic calming techniques, and other qualities may play a role in physical activity patterns, and characteristics of parks, trails, and playgrounds (Hanson, 2006).

Technological advances in the workplace, specifically mechanization and automation, have reduced physical activity requirements in almost all occupations and many technological conveniences in the home have further reduced energy expenditure from daily living. While energy expenditure from daily living has most certainly declined, so too have the physical activity requirements for school-age teenagers and children. For example, daily enrollment in physical education classes declined among high school students from 45% in 1991 to 25% in 1995 and many public schools have reduced or eliminated structured physical activity altogether (Kann et al., 1993).

In addition to decreases in physical activity, cross-sectional and longitudinal studies have also linked increased sedentary behaviors, such as television viewing, to childhood adiposity (Anderson, Crespo, Bartlett, Cheskin, & Pratt, 1998; Dietz & Gortmaker, 1985; Gortmaker et al., 1996) as well as video games and computer use. Sedentary behavior can contribute to obesity by competing with more physically active behaviors, thus reducing energy expenditure and by providing the opportunity for passive consumption of snack foods during viewing or as a result of food advertisements (Epstein, Paluch, Gordy, & Dorn, 2000; Robinson, 1999).

Childhood Obesity

Classification of Overweight and Obesity in Children and Adolescents

In the United States, childhood and adolescent overweight and obesity (aged 2–20 years) are defined as the gender-specific 85th and 95th percentiles of *BMI-for-age*, which corresponds approximately to the respective BMI cut points of 25 and 30 for adults. According to the Centers for Disease Control and Prevention (CDC), the revised expanded range of percentiles (3rd–97th) represents the relative position of the child's BMI among children of the same sex and age (Kuczmarski & Flegal, 2000; Kuczmarksi et al., 2002).

In addition to gender-specific BMI-for-age percentile growth charts, there are numerous additional age- and gender-specific growth charts used clinically and in research settings to assess size, growth, nutritional status, and the general health and well-being of infants, children, and adolescents for use in the United States (Kuczmarski & Flegal, 2000). Furthermore, international child growth standards for infants and children from birth to age 5 years, as well as child and adolescent growth standards for children aged 5–19 years, were recently revised and released by WHO in 2006 and 2007 (WHO Multicentre Growth Reference Study Group, 2009).

It is important to note that the U.S. growth reference charts for children were developed based on data derived from the NHANES and represent the age- and gender-specific distribution of body measures in U.S. children, reflecting growth "as is." Cameron and Hawley (2010) make the correct distinction that:

> the WHO growth standards are a different tool— they are based on [multinational] longitudinal data in which the source sample has been selected according to predefined criteria (e.g., breastfeeding for 4 months) and reflect growth not "as is" but growth "as it ought to be." (pp. 151–156)

The WHO reference charts therefore reflect growth under optimal circumstances thought to be conducive to optimal long-term health (Ziegler & Nelson, 2010). The implication is that the charts are not interchangeable and that the differences between them may be large enough to compromise international comparisons of infant, child, and adolescent populations.

▶ The Burden of Childhood Obesity

Globally, over 20 million children 5 years and younger were overweight in 2005, and by the end of 2010, it is estimated that 43 million will be overweight, doubling the prevalence in 5 years (WHO, 2009b). Although current estimates suggest that the rate of obesity in developed countries is double that in developing countries (similar to adult overweight and obesity), in absolute numbers, developing countries have far more children who are affected. For example, it is estimated that there are 35 million overweight/obese preschoolers in developing countries, compared with 8 million in developed countries (de Onis, Blössner, & Borghi, 2010).

In the United States, the steep rise in childhood obesity has paralleled the epidemic rise in adult obesity. For instance, in 1990, not a single state participating in the BRFSS had a prevalence of childhood obesity greater than 15%, and in 10 states, the prevalence was less than 10%. In sharp contrast, by 2010, no state had a prevalence of childhood obesity that was less than 20%, and in 36 states, over a quarter of all children were classified as obese (Centers for Disease Control and Prevention, 2010). According to U.S. NHANES, 2005–2006, nearly 1 in 5 children aged 6–19 years were classified as obese (Ogden, Carroll, & Flegal, 2008), and among 5–10-year-old obese children, 61% had one or more risk factors for heart disease and 27% had two or more risk factors (Freedman et al., 2007).

Recent data from the National Center for Health Statistics of the Centers for Disease Control and Prevention (CDC) show the continuing rise in obesity among children in the United States (**FIGURE 42.10**). Over the period 1999–2016, obesity among U.S. children and adolescents aged 2–19 years rose 33%, from 13.9 in 1999–2000 to 18.5% in 2015–2016. Furthermore, the prevalence of severe obesity among children and adolescents (BMI at or above 120% of the sex-specific 95th percentile on the national BMI-for-age growth charts) has remained high during the past decade (6.3% in boys and 4.9% in girls during 2015–2016) (CDC, 2017; Hales et al., 2017, 2018).

Similar to the disproportionate burden of obesity observed among certain ethnic groups of U.S. adults, childhood obesity is more common among African Americans, Hispanics, and American Indians compared to Caucasians. For example, the prevalence of obesity is higher among adolescent 12–19-year-old African-American boys (19%) and Hispanic boys (22%) compared to Caucasians (17%). Similarly, African-American adolescent girls had the highest prevalence of obesity (28%) followed by Hispanic girls (20%) and Caucasians (15%) (Ogden, Carroll, & Flegal, 2008).

In a recent survey of 8550 multiethnic U.S.-born 4-year old children enrolled in the *Early Childhood Longitudinal Study Birth Cohort*, 18.4% of children were classified as obese. The highest prevalence was observed among American-Indian/Native Alaskan children (31.2%), more than double the prevalence among Asian children (12.8%). Comparatively, the prevalence of obesity was also high among Hispanics (22.0%) and African Americans (20.8%). Caucasian children also exhibited a higher burden of obesity (15.9%) than Asians (Anderson & Whitaker, 2009).

The distribution of childhood obesity also varies by socioeconomic status. For instance, in a national

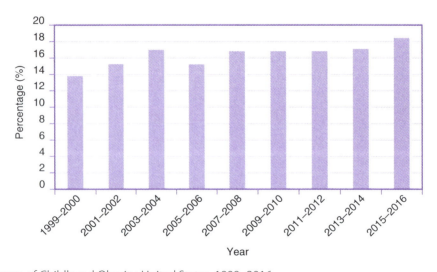

FIGURE 42.10 Prevalence of Childhood Obesity, United States, 1999–2016.
Data from Hales, C. M., Carroll, M. D., Fryar, C. D., & Ogden, C. L. (2017). Prevalence of obesity among adults and youth: United States, 2015–2016. *National Center for Health Statistics Data Brief, 288*; Hales, C. M., Fryar, C. D., Carroll, M. D., Freedman, D. S., & Ogden, C. L. (2018). Trends in obesity and severe obesity prevalence in US youth and adults by sex and age, 2007–2008 to 2015–2016. *JAMA, 319*(16), 1723–1725.

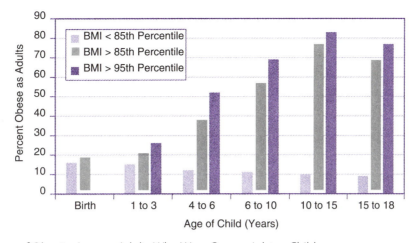

FIGURE 42.11 Percentage of Obesity Among Adults Who Were Overweight as Children.

Data from Whitaker, R. C., Wright, J. A., Pepe, M. S., Seidel, K. D., & Dietz, W. H. (1997). Predicting obesity in young adulthood from childhood and parental obesity. *New England Journal of Medicine 337*, 869–873.

survey of preschool children aged 2–4 years, the prevalence of obesity was nearly 16% higher among low-income children (14.6%) than non-Hispanic Caucasian children (12.6%) (MMWR, 2009).

Although not all children and adolescents who are overweight or obese will end up being obese in adulthood, the risk of becoming an obese adult is much higher among children who are overweight or obese compared to those who are not. Whitaker and colleagues studied BMI and obesity in childhood and adulthood in a retrospective cohort of 854 subjects from the northwestern United States. The parents' medical records were also reviewed to determine obesity status. The results show that elevated BMI tracks from childhood to adulthood, even after adjusting for parental obesity (**FIGURE 42.11**). For example, in children 10–15 years old, 10% of those with BMI-for-age < 85th percentile were obese at age 25 compared to 75% of those with a BMI-for-age > 85th percentile and 80% of those with a BMI-for-age > 95th percentile. Thus, overweight and obese children are much more likely than children of normal weight to be obese as adults (Whitaker, Wright, Pepe, Seidel, & Dietz, 1997).

▸ Risk Factors in Early Life and the Development of Later Obesity

Perinatal Influences

A variety of prenatal factors have been studied to determine their impact on the development of obesity in adulthood. Parent–offspring studies suggest that maternal obesity, diabetes, malnutrition, and other psychological, immunological, and pharmacological stressors during gestation can promote the development of obesity in offspring (Levin, 2006). In a study of 261 women born during 1959–1961, maternal weight, weight gain during pregnancy, and birth weight retained statistical significance as predictors of adult BMI after adjustment for childhood growth and development (Terry, Wei, & Esserman, 2007). Postnatally, maternal diet and health, infant feeding patterns, and adiposity rebound have all been associated with obesity in later life (Ebbeling, Pawlak, & Ludwig, 2002).

Early Adiposity Rebound and Future Health Risk

In early life, the BMI curve is not monotonic, nor it is invariant. Adiposity typically increases during the first year of life, decreases in the second year, and increases again between 2 and 8 years of age (Chivers et al., 2010; Williams & Goulding, 2009). *Adiposity rebound* refers to the age at which the BMI reverses direction at its nadir (lowest point) and increases toward adiposity. Studies have shown that early onset of adiposity rebound (under 5 years of age) is related to obesity in later life, independent of parental obesity and BMI at the time of the rebound (Lagstrom et al., 2008; Nader et al., 2006; Peneau, Thibault, & Rolland-Cachera, 2009; Whitaker, Pepe, Wright, Seidel, & Dietz, 1998). For example, Peneau and colleagues showed that among a sample of severely obese French adolescents, 97% experienced adiposity rebound at a very early median age of 2 years (Peneau, Thibault, & Rolland-Cachera, 2009). In addition, a majority of children who experienced early adiposity rebound were of normal weight at the time of rebound. This finding has been confirmed in other studies (Williams & Goulding, 2009).

Health Consequences of Childhood Obesity

The health consequences of obesity in children are similar to those observed in obese adults, affecting multiple body systems (Ebbeling, Pawlak, & Ludwig, 2002). Obesity in children increases the risk of hypertension, dyslipidemia, hyperglycemia, hyperinsulinemia, and chronic inflammation (Freedman et al., 1999; Ford et al., 2001; Srinivasan, Myers, & Berenson, 2002). In addition, obese children may be at higher risk for other health conditions such as obstructive sleep apnea, asthma, orthopedic complications, psychological distress, and psychosocial stigma (Chinn, 2006; Dietz, 1998; French, Story, & Perry, 1995; Tauman & Gozal, 2006).

It is estimated that over 50% of overweight 5–10-year-old children have at least one cardiovascular risk factor such as hypertension, dyslipidemia, or hyperinsulinemia (Freedman et al., 1999). Although childhood obesity is associated with earlier onset of obesity-related diseases in adulthood, a study by Pinhas-Hamiel and colleagues showed that the incidence of *adolescent* type 2 diabetes in Cincinnati increased tenfold, from 0.7/100,000 per year in 1982 to 7.2/100.000 per year in 1994 (Pinhas-Hamiel et al., 1996).

▶ Prevention of Obesity

The principal reason for preventing weight gain and obesity is to reduce the risk of obesity-related diseases.

Burke and colleagues estimated the number and proportion of incident cases of type 2 diabetes that could be prevented by targeting each BMI category in the *San Antonio Heart Study*. Results revealed that most cases of type 2 diabetes developed in individuals who were overweight or mildly obese, and that preventing normal-weight individuals from becoming overweight would reduce the incidence of type 2 diabetes by 74% in Caucasians and 62% in Mexican Americans. These findings underscore the need to establish comprehensive primary prevention programs to reduce obesity and obesity-related diseases (Burke et al., 2003).

Primary prevention of obesity and associated diseases begins in early life (Berenson, Srinivasan, Wattigney, & Harsha, 1993; Ebbeling, Pawlak, & Ludwig, 2002). The *U.S. Expert Committee on Childhood Obesity* recommends that pediatricians advise all children and their parents to integrate healthy habits into their lifestyle that may help prevent excessive weight gain and are unlikely to cause harm (Barlow & Expert Committee, 2007). Recommended guidelines for the primary prevention of obesity are shown in **TABLE 42.4**.

Lemmens and colleagues recently conducted a systematic review of the peer-reviewed literature to evaluate the efficacy of adult obesity prevention programs. The programs reviewed were designed to maintain current weight or prevent weight gain among nonobese adults (BMI < 30) by diet, exercise, or both. The review showed mixed results: four out of nine studies found a positive intervention effect, but

---

TABLE 42.4 Primary Prevention of Obesity

Dietary Recommendations

- Limit consumption of sugar-sweetened drinks
- Limit portion sizes and restaurant meals, particularly fast food
- Eat recommended servings of fruits and vegetables
- Eat diet with recommended macro- and micro-nutrient content
- Eat breakfast and encourage structured time for meals with family
- For mothers: breastfeed to 6 months and introduce solid foods and maintain breastfeeding to at least 12 months

Physical Activity Recommendations

- Encourage vigorous physical activity of 60 minutes daily
- Limit television, computer, and video games

Data from Barlow, S. E., & Expert Committee. (2007). Expert Committee recommendations regarding the prevention, assessment, and treatment of child and adolescent overweight and obesity: Summary report. *Pediatrics, 120,* S164–S192.

there were small absolute weight losses and minimal differences between control and intervention groups. The investigators concluded that the current evidence is too limited to draw firm conclusions on the efficacy of prevention programs in adults (Lemmens, Oenema, Klepp, Henriksen, & Brug, 2008).

Nevertheless, there are published reports of successful obesity prevention programs in adults. In a small randomized study of 30 young women, 18–28 years of age, with at least one severely obese parent, 14 women were randomized to a treatment group receiving an intensive individualized intervention program called *Health Hunters* focusing on food choice, physical activity, and other lifestyle factors, and 16 women were randomized to a control group receiving no intervention. Results were evaluated after 1 year of follow-up. Compared to the control group (which gained weight), the intervention group displayed significant average *decrease* in body weight, BMI, waist circumference, and waist-to-hip ratio and a significant *increase* in self-reported physical activity. The investigators concluded that the intervention was effective in high-risk young women with a familial predisposition to the development of obesity (Eiben & Lissner, 2006).

Silverman and colleagues conducted a randomized study designed to evaluate the impact of a lifestyle dietary and physical activity program among middle-aged women known as the *Women's Healthy Lifestyle Project*. A total of 535 premenopausal women aged 44–50 years at baseline were enrolled in the trial. Participants were randomly assigned to receive either a 5-year program of intensive lifestyle intervention or no intervention. After 54 months of observation, 136 of 246 women (55%) in the intervention group were at or below baseline weight compared to 68 of 261 women (26%) in the control group. The average weight loss in the intervention group was 0.1 kg below baseline weight whereas the average weight gain in the control group was 2.4 kg above baseline weight. The average reduction in waist circumference was also significantly greater in the intervention group than the control group (2.9 cm vs. 0.5 cm). Furthermore, participants receiving lifestyle intervention were consistently more physically active and reported eating fewer calories and less fat than controls. The investigators concluded that in healthy women, weight gain and increased waist circumference are preventable through a sustained dietary and physical activity program focused on weight, body composition, physical activity, diet, and other cardiovascular risk factors (Simkin-Silverman, Wing, Boraz, & Kuller, 2003).

The foundation of successful obesity prevention programs is inclusion of effective dietary and physical activity components. The dietary component should be designed to reduce energy intake and improve nutritional content. The physical activity component should be designed to increase daily caloric expenditure and decrease sedentary behavior. Careful monitoring of compliance of participants is essential through detailed reporting of the frequency, intensity, type, and duration of interventions. Periodic measures of weight, body mass, quality of life, and other outcomes should be taken to gauge progress. The objective for an individual may be to reduce weight, prevent weight gain, or maintain current weight. Behavior modification, education, and motivational and psychological counseling may also contribute to success. Structured obesity prevention programs and services may be offered in a variety of settings such as outpatient clinics, schools, worksites, community centers, churches, fitness centers, and neighborhood recreational facilities (NIH, 1985, 1991, 1992, 1998; United Nations Development Program, 2001).

▶ Therapy of Obesity

Therapeutic approaches to obesity include nonpharmacologic programs focused on diet and exercise to reduce weight through manipulation of energy balance, and more recently, administration of pharmacologic antiobesity agents. Current therapies include appetite suppressants and drugs that inhibit the absorption of dietary fat. A wide variety of antiobesity drugs are under investigation, and it is the goal of researchers to develop safe and effective antiobesity drugs analogous to those used to treat other chronic conditions such as hypertension, dyslipidemia, and diabetes (Bays, Mandarino, & DeFronzo, 2004).

An emerging concept is that the development of antiobesity agents must not only reduce fat mass but must also correct fat dysfunction (Bays & Dujovne, 2002; Bays, Mandarino, & DeFronzo, 2004; Bays et al., 2008). For example, agents such as pioglitazone and rosiglitazone that activate the nuclear receptor peroxisome proliferator-activated receptor-γ (PPAR γ) have shown therapeutic value in reducing pro-inflammatory adipokines and cytokines and increasing the anti-inflammatory adipokine, adiponectin (Larsen, Toubro, & Astrup, 2003; Lyon, Law, & Hseuh, 2003).

It is also well to remember that obesity and particularly severe obesity are due not only to increased fat cell size (hypertrophy) but also to increased fat cell number (hypercellularity). As pointed out by Arner and Spalding (2010) in their review of fat cell turnover:

Traditional weight loss regimes, such as diet and exercise, are successful in decreasing adipocyte size, but fail to reduce adipocyte number. Since many obese and almost all severely obese individuals have more than the average number of adipocytes, methods other than diet and exercise alone are needed if one hopes to reduce (and maintain) the fat mass to lean levels. The dynamic and highly regulated turnover of adipocytes in adult humans establishes a new therapeutic target whereby pharmacological intervention may potentially tip the balance in favor of weight loss, or gain, depending on the preferred outcome. (pp. 100–104)

▶ Liposuction

Liposuction, also known as lipoplasty, refers to the suctioning of fat from certain areas of the body. The procedure is performed primarily for cosmetic purposes. The value of liposuction in the treatment of obesity is highly controversial.

In a small study of 15 adult women with severe abdominal obesity (BMI~40), liposuction surgery removed an average of 10 kg of subcutaneous body fat (18% of total fat mass) resulting in an average weight loss of more than 6 kg. The women were evaluated at baseline and 10–12 weeks postsurgery. Liposuction did not significantly alter insulin sensitivity, plasma concentrations of CRP, interleukin-6, tumor necrosis factor-α, adiponectin, or any other risk factors of coronary heart disease including blood pressure, plasma glucose, and insulin and lipid concentrations. The investigators concluded that abdominal liposuction did not improve obesity-associated metabolic abnormalities in the short follow-up period (Klein et al., 2004). Seven women in the study were followed for up to 4 years after surgery to assess long-term effects of liposuction. Postsurgery body composition and weight were unchanged throughout the follow-up period; however, metabolic endpoints (oral glucose tolerance, insulin resistance, blood pressure, plasma triglyceride and cholesterol concentrations) showed no improvement from baseline values. Results suggest that removal of a large volume of subcutaneous abdominal fat by liposuction *does not* improve risk factors for coronary heart disease, despite a long-term reduction in body fat (Mohammed, Cohen, Reeds, Young, & Klein, 2008).

Case reports suggest that weight gain after liposuction results in deposition of subcutaneous fat in areas that were not aspirated such as the back and breasts (van der Lei, Halbesma, van Neiuwenhoven, & van Wingerden, 2007; Yun, Bruck, Felsenfeld, & Katz, 2003). Also, there have been several case reports of *fat embolism syndromes* following liposuction and animal studies have proven that removal of subcutaneous fat by liposuction results in systemic fat mobilization and fat embolism (El-Ali & Gourlay, 2006; Mentz, 2008). Additional investigations are needed to determine both the short-term and long-term impacts of high volume liposuction.

▶ Bariatric Surgery

Although primary prevention is the best approach to attenuating the obesity epidemic and controlling, improving, or reversing obesity-related comorbidities, bariatric surgery is the only proven treatment for severe obesity in adults and adolescents (Buchwald, Avidor, & Braunwald, 2004; Dixon, Pories, O'Brien, Schauer, & Zimmet, 2005; Sugerman et al., 2003). Bariatric surgery is an elective surgical weight loss procedure that reduces the gastric reservoir and limits food intake.

In 1991, the National Institutes of Health Consensus Development Panel recommended that gastric restriction or bypass surgery be considered for severely obese individuals, BMI > 35 with comorbidity or BMI > 40 with or without comorbidity (NIH Conference, 1991). In 1992, a statement from the NIH Health Consensus Development Conference affirmed the superiority of surgical over nonsurgical approaches to weight loss in the severely obese (NIH Consensus Development Conference, 1992), and in 2000, an editorial by Dr. Harvey Sugerman, an internationally known bariatric surgeon, suggested lowering the obesity level guidelines to European standards, recommending surgical management of obesity for those with BMI > 30 and with comorbidity (Sugerman, 2000).

Because of these recommendations and increasing media attention, bariatric surgery has gained considerable popularity as the only treatment to produce sustained weight loss (NIH Consensus Development Conference, 1992). Furthermore, studies of surgical weight loss have demonstrated long-term significant improvements and resolution of type 2 diabetes as well as sustained risk factor reduction of comorbid conditions such as dyslipidemia, hypertension, hyperinsulinemia, glucose intolerance, and adipokine levels (Buchwald, Avidor, & Braunwald, 2004; Kral, Bjorntorp, Scherstein, & Sjostrom, 1977; Meneghini, 2007; Salameh, Khoukaz, & Bell, 2010; Trakhtenbroit et al., 2009). Additional high- quality studies are needed to establish evidence-based criteria for bariatric surgery, as recommendations are based on consensus (NIH Conference, 1991; NIH Consensus Development Conference, 1992).

▶ Summary

Obesity is dramatically increasing across the globe. Because of the profound rise in obesity within the past several decades, most experts have ruled out a change in genetics as contributing substantially to the obesity epidemic, which only recently was considered a by-product of affluence related to Western societies. Instead, increased urbanization worldwide is leading to fundamental changes in physical activity levels and dietary patterns. Multiple structural changes in the environment have led to decreased physical activity, increased sedentary behavior, and ready access to high fat, high sugar, energy-dense, and cheap food and drink, and these changes have tipped the global energy balance scale so that long-term energy intake exceeds energy expenditure. Excess energy leads to an increase in energy stored as triacylglycerol within adipocytes of WAT and subsequently excess weight gain.

Other risk factors include genetic susceptibility, female gender, aging, ethnicity, perinatal factors (maternal obesity), menopause, psychological factors (stress, depression), and physiological factors (adiposity rebound and fat cell dynamics). It is notable that genetic studies have consistently found obesity to be highly heritable. Moreover, though genetic changes do not explain the ongoing obesity epidemic, genotype x environment interactions could certainly have an impact. Conceivably, the rapid global rise in obesity could at least in part be due to the mismatch between today's environment and "thrifty genes" that were selected for in the past under different environmental conditions when food sources were unpredictable.

Obesity exerts deleterious effects on nearly every organ system of the body and is a significant risk factor for type 2 diabetes, cardiovascular diseases (such as coronary heart disease, myocardial infarction, and stroke), gastroesophageal reflux disease (GERD), obstructive sleep apnea, asthma, gallbladder and fatty liver disease, depression, urinary incontinence, gout, polycystic ovarian syndrome, and osteoarthritis. In particular, obesity promotes the parallel progression of insulin resistance to type 2 diabetes and endothelial dysfunction to atherosclerosis. Overall, obesity has become one of the leading causes of premature death and disability in the world.

Adipocytes not only function as a storage repository for excess energy, but they also actively participate in metabolic processes that regulate energy homeostasis. Excess adiposity incites the synthesis of a multitude of autocrine, paracrine, and endocrine bioactive signaling proteins called adipokines. Certain adipokines (resistin and leptin) have pro-inflammatory properties that promote atherogenesis and insulin resistance whereas others (adiponectin) are anti-inflammatory. Numerous studies indicate that visceral (abdominal) fat is more metabolically active than subcutaneous (peripheral) fat, and that visceral adiposity is primarily responsible for increasing the risk of developing obesity-related diseases.

Based upon studies of fat cell turnover, obesity can be classified into two basic types: hypertrophic obesity (increased fat cell size) and hyperplastic obesity (increased fat cell number). Preventive and therapeutic strategies should be designed to counteract both types.

As with adults, the prevalence of obesity in children has risen dramatically in populations across the globe. Obesity in children increases the risk of hypertension, dyslipidemia, hyperglycemia, hyperinsulinemia, chronic inflammation, and many other health conditions. Childhood obesity tracks to adult obesity, and early rebound adiposity is a significant predictor of adult obesity.

While obesity is still increasing worldwide, recent U.S. survey results indicate that the epidemic may be abating in children, perhaps as a consequence of prevention programs in schools and communities and public health awareness campaigns promoting a lifestyle of healthy eating and regular exercise to maintain ideal body weight. Early health education is the cornerstone of primary prevention. Clearly, comprehensive and sustainable prevention programs should be established in populations around the globe to encourage healthy, nutritious eating habits and physically active lifestyles to avoid the development of obesity and obesity-related diseases in future generations.

References

Abate, N., Chandalia, M., Snell, P. G., & Grundy, S. M. (2004). Adipose tissue metabolites and insulin resistance in non-diabetic Asian Indian men. *Journal of Clinical Endocrinology and Metabolism, 89*, 2750–2755.

Adams, K. F., Schatzkin, A., Harris, T. B., Kipnis, V., Mouw, T., Ballard-Barbash, R., ... Leitzmann, M. F. (2006). Overweight, obesity and mortality in a large prospective cohort of persons 50 to 71 years old. *New England Journal of Medicine, 355*(08), 763–778.

Allison, D. B., Fontaine, K. R., Manson, J. E., Stevens, J., & VanItallie, T. B. (1999). Annual deaths attributable to obesity in the United States. *Journal of the American Medical Association, 282*, 1530–1538.

Anderson, S. E., & Whitaker, R. C. (2009). Prevalence of obesity among US preschool children in different racial and ethnic groups. *Archives of Pediatrics and Adolescent Medicine, 163*(04), 344–348.

Anderson, R. E., Crespo, C. J., Bartlett, S. J., Cheskin, L. J., & Pratt, M. (1998). Relationship of physical activity and television watching with body weight and level of fatness among children: Results from the third National Health and Nutrition Examination Survey. *Journal of the American Medical Association, 279*, 938–942.

Argyropoulos, G., & Harper, M. E. (2002). Molecular biology of thermoregulation invited review: Uncoupling proteins and thermoregulation. *Journal of Applied Physiology, 92*, 2187–2198.

Arner, P., & Spalding, K. L. (2010). Fat cell turnover in humans. Biochemical and Biophysical *Research Communications, 396*, 100–104.

Attie, A. D., & Scherer, P. E. (2009). Adipocyte metabolism and obesity. *Journal of Lipid Research, 50*, S395–S399.

Barb, D., Pazaitou-Panayiotou, K., & Mantzoros, C. S. (2006). Adiponectin: A link between obesity and cancer. *Expert Opinions in Investigative Drugs, 15*, 917–931.

Barlow, S. E., & Expert Committee. (2007). Expert Committee recommendations regarding the prevention, assessment, and treatment of child and adolescent overweight and obesity: Summary report. *Pediatrics, 120*, S164–S192.

Barnes, A. S., & Coulter, S. A. (2011). The epidemic of obesity and diabetes. *Texas Heart Institute Journal, 38*(2), 142–144.

Bays, H. E., & Dujovne, C. A. (2002). Anti-obesity drug development. *Expert Opinion Invest Drugs, 11*, 1189–1204.

Bays, H., Mandarino, L., & DeFronzo, R. A. (2004). Role of the adipocyte, free fatty acids, and ectopic fat in pathogenesis of type 2 diabetes mellitus: Peroxisomal proliferator-activated receptor agonists provide a rational therapeutic approach. *The Journal of Clinical Endocrinology and Metabolism, 89*, 463–478.

Bays, H. E., Gonzalez-Campoy, J. M., Henry, R. R., Bergman, D. A., Kitabchi, A. E., Schorr, A. B., … Adiposopathy Working Group. (2008). Is adiposopathy (sick fat) an endocrine disease? *International Journal of Clinical Practice, 62*, 1474–1483.

Bei-Fan, Z. (2002). The Cooperative Meta-Analysis Group of Working Group on Obesity in China. Predictive values of body mass index and waist circumference for risk factors of certain related diseases in Chinese adults: Study on optimal cut-off points of body mass index and waist circumference in Chinese adults. *Asia Pacific Journal of Clinical Nutrition, 11*(08), S685–S693.

Berenson, G. S., Srinivasan, S. R., Wattigney, W. A., & Harsha, D. W. (1993). Obesity and cardiovascular risk in children. *Annals of the New York Academy of Sciences, 699*, 93–103.

Bergman, R. N., Kim, S. P., Catalano, K. J., Hsu, I. R., Chiu, J. D., Kabir, M., … Ader, M. (2006). Why visceral fat is bad: Mechanisms of the metabolic syndrome. *Obesity, 14*, 16S–19S.

Björnheden, T., Jakubowicz, B., Levin, M., Odén, B., Edén, S., Sjöström, L., & Lönn, M. (2004). Computerized determination of adipocyte size. *Obesity Research, 12*(1), 95–105.

Blouin, K., Despres, J. P., Couillard, C., Tremblay, A., Prud'homme, D., Bouchard, C., & Tchernof, A. (2005). Contribution of age and declining androgen levels to features of the metabolic syndrome in men. *Metabolism, 54*, 1034–1040.

Bodor, J. N., Rose, D., Farley, T. A., Swalm, C., & Scott, S. K. (2008). Neighborhood fruit and vegetable availability and consumption: The role of small food stores in an urban environment. *Public Health Nutrition, 11*, 413–420.

Bogers, R. P., Bemelmans, W. J., Hoogenveen, R. T., Boshuizen, H. C., Woodward, M., Knekt, P., … Shipley, M. J., for the BMI-CHD Collaboration Investigators. (2007). Association of overweight with increased risk of coronary heart disease partly independent of blood pressure and cholesterol levels: A meta-analysis of 21 cohort studies including more than 300,000 persons. *Archives of Internal Medicine, 167*(16), 1720–1728.

Brochu, M., Tchernof, A., Dionee, I. J., Sites, C. K., Eltabbakh, G. H., Sims, E. A., & Poehlman, E. T. (2001). What are the physical characteristics associated with a normal metabolic profile despite a high level of adiposity in postmenopausal women? *The Journal of Clinical Endocrinology and Metabolism, 86*, 1020–1025.

Browning, R. C., & Kram, R. (2007). Effects of obesity on the biomechanics of walking at different speeds. *Medicine and Science in Sports and Exercise, 39*(9), 1632–1641.

Buchwald, H., Avidor, Y., & Braunwald, E. (2004). Bariatric surgery: A systematic review and meta-analysis. *Journal of the American Medical Association, 292*, 1724–1737.

Burke, J. P., Williams, K., Narayan, K. M., Leibson, C., Haffner, S. M., & Stern, M. P. (2003). A population perspective on diabetes prevention: Whom should we target for preventing weight gain? *Diabetes Care, 26*(7), 1999–2004.

Byers, T., Nestle, M., McTiernan, A., Doyle, C., Currie-Williams, A., Gansler, T., … American Cancer Society 2001 Nutrition and Physical Activity Guidelines Advisory Committee. (2002). American Cancer Society guidelines on nutrition and physical activity for cancer prevention: Reducing the risk of cancer with healthy food choices and physical activity. *CA: A Cancer Journal for Clinicians, 52*, 92–119.

Caballero, B. (2007). The global epidemic of obesity: An overview. *Epidemiologic Reviews, 29*, 1–5.

Calle, E. E. (2008). Chapter 10: Obesity and cancer. In F. B. Hu (Ed.), *Obesity epidemiology* (pp. 196–215). Oxford, New York: Oxford University Press.

Calle, E. E., Thun, M. J., Petrelli, J. M., Rodriguez, C., & Heath, C. W., Jr. (1999). Body mass index and mortality in a prospective cohort of US adults. *New England Journal of Medicine, 341*, 1097–1105.

Cameron, N., & Hawley, N. L. (2010). Should the UK use WHO growth charts? *Paediatrics and Child Health, 20*(4), 151–156.

Cannon, B., & Nedergaard, J. (2004). Brown adipose tissue: Function and physiological significance. *Physiological Reviews, 84*, 277–359.

Carangelo, C. (1995). Why are Americans so fat? *Food Management, 30*(4), 63–98.

Centers for Disease Control and Prevention. (2010). *U.S. obesity trends*, http://www.cdc.gov/obesity/data/trends

Centers for Disease Control and Prevention (CDC). (2017). *National Diabetes statistics report*, Atlanta, GA.

Chan, J. M., Rimm, E. B., Colditz, G. A., Stampfer, M. J., & Willett, W. C. (1994). Obesity, fat distribution and weight gain as risk factors for clinical diabetes in men. *American Journal of Epidemiology, 17*, 961–969.

Chinn, S. (2006). Obesity and asthma. *Paediatric Respiratory Reviews, 7*, 223–228.

Chivers, P., Hand, B., Parker, H., Bulsara, M., Beilin, L. J., Kendall, G. E., & Oddy, W. H. (2010). Body mass index, adiposity rebound, and early feeding in a longitudinal cohort (Raine study). *International Journal of Obesity, 34*, 1169–1176.

Christakis, N. A., & Fowler, J. H. (2007). The spread of obesity in a large social network over 32 years. *New England Journal of Medicine, 357*, 370–379.

Christou, N. V., Lieberman, M., Sampalis, F., & Sampalis, J. S. (2008). Bariatric surgery reduces cancer risk in morbidly obese patients. *Surgery for Obesity and Related Diseases, 4*, 691–697.

Chung, S., Song, M. Y., Shin, H. D., Kim, D. Y., He, Q., Heshka, S., … Gallagher, D. (2005). Korean and Caucasian overweight premenopausal women have different relationship of body mass index to percent body fat with age. *Journal of Applied Physiology, 99,* 103–107.

Colditz, G. A., Willett, W. C., Rotnitsky, A., & Manson, J. E. (1995). Weight gain as a risk factor for clinical diabetes mellitus in women. *Annals of Internal Medicine, 122,* 481–486.

Coggon, D., Reading, I., Croft, P., McLaren, M., Barrett, D., & Cooper, C. (2001). Knee osteoarthritis and obesity. *International Journal of Obesity and Related Metabolic Disorders, 25*(5), 622–627.

Crovetti, R., Porrini, M., Santangelo, A., & Testolin, G. (1997). The influence of thermic effect of food on satiety. *European Journal of Clinical Nutrition, 52,* 482–488.

Danforth, E. (2000). Failure of adipocyte differentiation causes type II diabetes? *Nature Genetics, 26,* 13.

de Onis, M., Blössner, M., & Borghi, E. (2010). Global prevalence and trends of overweight and obesity among preschool children. *American Society for Clinical Nutrition, 92*(5), 1257–1264.

Deurenberg, P., Deurenberg-Yap, M., & Guricci, S. (2002). Asians are different from Caucasians and from each other in their body mass index/body fat percent relationship. *Obesity Reviews, 3,* 141–146.

DiDomenico, P. (1994). Portion size: How much is too much. *Restaurants USA, 14,* 18–21.

Dietz, W. H. (1998). Health consequences of obesity in youth: Childhood predictors of adult disease. *Pediatrics, 101,* 518–525.

Dietz, W. H., & Gortmaker, S. L. (1985). Do we fatten our children at the television set? Obesity and television viewing in children and adolescents. *Pediatrics, 75,* 807–812.

Dixon, J. B., Pories, W. J., O'Brien, P. E., Schauer, P. R., & Zimmet, P. (2005). Surgery as an effective early intervention for diabesity: Why the reluctance? *Diabetes Care, 28*(2), 472–474.

Drewnowski, A., & Popkin, B. M. (2009). The nutrition transition: New trends in the global diet. *Nutrition Reviews, 55*(2), 31–43.

Durán, J., Esnaola, S., Rubio, R., & Iztueta, A. (2001). Obstructive sleep apnea-hypopnea and related clinical features in a population-based sample of subjects aged 30 to 70 yr. *American Journal of Respiratory and Critical Care Medicine, 163,* 685–689.

EarthTrends. (2009). Nutrition: Calorie supply per capita. World Resources Institute. Retrieved from http://earthtrends.wri.org

Ebbeling, C. B., Pawlak, D. B., & Ludwig, D. S. (2002). Childhood obesity: Public health crisis, common sense cure. *Lancet, 360,* 473–482.

Economic Research Service. (2010). USDA website. Retrieved from http://www.ers.usda.gov/Data/BiotechCrops/Extentof AdoptionTable1.htm

Edelstein, Z. R., Farrow D. C., Bronner, D. C., Rosen, M. P., & Vaughan, T. L. (2007). Central adiposity and risk of Barrett's esophagus. *Gastroenterology, 133,* 403–411.

Eiben, G., & Lissner, L. (2006). Health Hunters—An intervention to prevent overweight and obesity in young high risk women. *International Journal of Obesity (London), 30,* 691–696.

Einstein, F. H., Atzmon, G., Yang, X., Ma, X. H., Rincon, M., Rudin, E., ... Barzilai, N. (2005). Differential responses of visceral and subcutaneous fat depots to nutrients. *Diabetes, 54,* 672–678.

Eknoyan, G. (2006). A history of obesity, or how what was good became ugly and then bad. *Advances in Chronic Kidney Disease, 13,* 421–427.

Eknoyan, G. (2008). Adolphe Quetelet (1796–1874)—The average man and indices of obesity. *Nephrology Dialysis Transplantation, 23*(01), 47–51.

El-Ali, K. M., & Gourlay, T. (2006). Assessment of the risk of systemic fat mobilization and fat embolism as a consequence of liposuction: Ex vivo study. *Plastic and Reconstructive Surgery, 117*(7), 2269–2276.

Epstein, L. H., Paluch, R. A., Gordy, C. C., & Dorn, J. (2000). Decreasing sedentary behaviors in treating pediatric obesity. *Archives of Pediatrics and Adolescent Medicine, 154,* 220–226.

Ettinger, W. H., Davis, M. A., Neuhaus, J. M., & Mallon, K. P. (1994). Long-term physical functioning in persons with knee osteoarthritis from NHANES. I: Effects of comorbid medical conditions. *Journal of Clinical Epidemiology, 47*(7), 809–815.

Eyre, H., Kahn, R., Robertson, R. M., Clark, N. G., Doyle, C., Hong, Y., ... the ACS/ADA/AHA Collaborative Writing Committee. (2004). Preventing cancer, cardiovascular disease, and diabetes: A common agenda for the American Cancer Society, the American Diabetes Association, and the American Heart Association. *Stroke, 35*(8), 1999–2010.

Fain, J. N. (2006). Release of interleukins and other inflammatory cytokines by human adipose tissue is enhanced in obesity and primarily due to the nonfat cells. *Vitamins & Hormones, 74,* 443–477.

Fain, J. N., Madan, A. K., Hiler, M. L., Cheema, P., & Bahouth, S. W. (2004). Comparison of the release of adipokines by adipose tissue, adipose tissue matrix, and adipocytes from visceral and subcutaneous abdominal adipose tissues of obese humans. *Endocrinology, 145,* 2273–2282.

Farooqi, I. S., & O'Rahilly, S. (2005a). Monogenic obesity in humans. *Annual Review of Medicine, 56,* 443–458.

Farooqi, I. S., & O'Rahilly, S. (2005b). New advances in the genetics of early onset obesity. *International Journal of Obesity, 29,* 1149–1152.

Farooqi, I. S., & O'Rahilly, S. (2007). Genetic factors in human obesity. *Obesity Reviews, 8*(Suppl. 1), 37–40.

Faust, I., & Miller, W. J. (1983). *Hyperplastic growth of adipose tissue in obesity.* New York: Raven Press.

Felson, D. T., Zhang, Y., Anthony, J. M., Naimark, A., & Anderson, J. J. (1992). Weight loss reduces the risk for symptomatic knee osteoarthritis in women. The Framingham Study. *Annals of Internal Medicine, 116*(7), 535–539.

Fisichella, P. M., & Patti, M. G. (2009). Gastroesophageal reflux disease and morbid obesity: Is there a relation? *World Journal of Surgery, 33,* 2034–2038.

Flegal, K. M., Carroll, M. D., Ogden, C. L., & Curtin, L. R. (2010). Prevalence and trends in obesity among US adults, 1999–2008. *Journal of the American Medical Association, 303,* 235–241.

Flegal, K. M., Graubard, B. I., Williamson, D. F., & Gail, M. H. (2005). Excess deaths associated with underweight, overweight, and obesity. *Journal of the American Medical Association, 293,* 1861–1867.

Flegal, K. M., Graubard, B. I., Williamson, D. F., & Gail, M. H. (2006). Cause-specific excess death associated with underweight, overweight and obesity. *Journal of the American Medical Association, 298,* 2028–2037.

Flegal, K. M., & Troiano, R. P. (2000). Changes in the distribution of body mass index of adults and children in the US population. *International Journal of Obesity, 24,* 807–818.

Fletcher, E., & Lewis-Faning, E. (1945). Chronic rheumatic diseases: Statistical study of 1000 cases of chronic rheumatism. *Postgraduate Medical Journal, 1945,* 21137.

Ford, E. S., Galuska, D. A., Gillespie, C., Will, J. C., Giles, W. H., & Dietz, W. H. (2001). C-reactive protein and body mass index in children: Findings from the third National Health and Nutrition Examination Survey, 1988–1994. *Journal of Pediatrics, 138*, 486–492.

Fraser-Moodie, C. A., Norton, B., Gornall, C., Magnago, S., Weale, A. R., & Holmes, G. K. (1999). Weight loss has an independent beneficial effect on symptoms of gastro-oesophageal reflux in patients who are overweight. *Scandinavian Journal of Gastroenterology, 34*, 337–340.

Frayn, K. N. (2000). Visceral fat and insulin resistance—Causative or correlative? The British *Journal of Nutrition, 83*(S1), S871–S877.

Frederiksen, S. G., Johansson, J., Johnsson, F., & Hedenbro, J. (2000). Neither low-calorie diet nor vertical banded gastroplasty influence gastro-oesophageal reflux in morbidly obese patients. *European Journal of Surgery, 166*, 296–300.

Freedman, D. S., Dietz, W. H., Srinivasan, S. R., & Berenson, G. S. (1999). The relation of overweight to cardiovascular risk factors among children and adolescents: The Bogalusa Heart Study. *Pediatrics, 103*, 1175–1182.

Freedman, D. S., Mei, Z., Srinivasan, S. R., Berenson G. S., & Dietz W. H. (2007). Cardiovascular risk factors and excess adiposity among overweight children and adolescents: The Bogalusa Heart Study. *The Journal of Pediatrics, 150*, 12–17.

French, S. A., Story, M., & Perry, C. L. (1995). Self esteem and obesity in children and adolescents: A literature review. *Obesity Research, 3*, 479–490.

Friedenberg, F. K., Xanthopoulos, M., Foster G. D., & Richter, J. E. (2008). The association between gastroesophageal reflux disease and obesity. *American Journal of Gastroenterology, 103*, 2111–2122.

Fruhbeck, G., Gomez-Ambrosi, J., Muruzabai, F. J., & Burrell, M. A. (2001). The adipocyte: A model for integration of endocrine and metabolic signaling in energy metabolism regulation. *American Journal of Physiology. Endocrinology and Metabolism, 280*, E827–E847.

Gallagher, D., Visser, M., Sepulveda, D., Pierson, R. N., Harris, T., & Heymsfield, S. B. (1996). How useful is body mass index for comparison of body fatness across age, sex, and ethnic groups? *American Journal of Epidemiology, 143*, 228–239.

Gavrilova, O., Marcus-Samuels, B., Graham, D., Kim, J. K., Shulman, G. I., Castle, A. L., … Reitman, M. L. (2000). Surgical implantation of adipose tissue reverses diabetes in lipoatrophic mice. *Journal of Clinical Investigation, 105*, 271–278.

Gibson, H. J. (2005). Obstructive sleep apnoea syndrome: Underestimated and undertreated. *British Medical Bulletin, 72*, 49–65.

Gold, M. R., Stevenson, D., & Fryback, D. G. (2002). HALYs and QALYs and DALYs, oh my: Similarities and differences in summary measures of population health. *Annual Review of Public Health, 23*, 115–134.

Gortmaker, S. L., Must, A., Sobol, A. M., Peterson, K., Colditz, G. A., & Dietz, W. H. (1996). Television viewing as a cause of increasing obesity in the United States, 1986–1990. *Archives of Pediatrics & Adolescent Medicine, 150*, 356–362.

Gower, B. A., Weisner, R. L., Jordan, J. M., Hunter, G. R., & Desmond, R. (2002). Effects of weight loss on changes in insulin sensitivity and lipid concentrations in premenopausal African American and white women. *American Journal of Clinical Nutrition, 76*, 923–927.

Grun, F., & Blumberg, B. (2006). Environmental obesogens: Organotins and endocrine disruption via nuclear receptor signaling. *Endocrinology, 147*, S50–S55.

Hak, E. A., Stehouwer, C. D. A., Bots, M. L., Polderman, K. H., Schalkwijk, C. G., Westendorp, I. C., … Witteman, J. C. (1999). Associations of C-reactive protein with measures of obesity, insulin resistance, and subclinical atherosclerosis in healthy middle-aged women. *Arteriosclerosis, Thrombosis, and Vascular Biology, 19*, 1986–1991.

Haffner, S. M., Stern, M. P., Mitchell, B. D., Hazuda, H. P., & Patterson, J. K. (1990). Incidence of type II diabetes in Mexican Americans predicted by fasting insulin, glucose levels, obesity, and body fat distribution. *Diabetes, 39*, 283–288.

Hales, C. M., Carroll, M. D., Fryar, C. D., & Ogden, C. L. (2017). Prevalence of obesity among adults and youth: United States, 2015–2016. *National Center for Health Statistics Data Brief*, (288), 1–8.

Hales, C. M., Fryar, C. D., Carroll, M. D., Freedman, D. S., & Ogden, C. L. (2018). Trends in obesity and severe obesity prevalence in US youth and adults by sex and age, 2007–2008 to 2015–2016. *Journal of the American Medical Association, 319*(16), 1723–1725.

Hampel, H., Abraham, N. S., & El-Serag, H. B. (2005). Meta-analysis: Obesity and the risk for gastroesophageal reflux disease and its complications. *Annals of Internal Medicine, 143*, 199–211.

Hanson, S. (2006). Active living research in light of the TRB/IOM report. *Journal of Physical Activity and Health, 3*, S258–S266.

Harris, R. E., Namboodiri, K. K., & Wynder, E. L. (1992). Breast cancer risk: Effects of estrogen replacement therapy and body mass. *Journal of the National Cancer Institute, 84*(20), 1575–1582.

Hausman, D. B., DiGirolamo, D. B., & Bartness, T. J. (2001). The biology of white adipocyte proliferation. *Obesity Reviews, 2*, 239–254.

Heindel, J. J. (2003). Endocrine disruptors and the obesity epidemic. *Toxicological Sciences, 76*(2), 247–249.

Herbella, F. A., & Patti, M. G. (2010). Gastroesophageal reflux disease: From pathophysiology to treatment. *World Journal of Gastroenterology, 16*(30), 3745–3749.

Hewitt, J. K. (1997). The genetics of obesity: What genetic studies told us about the environment. *Behavior Genetics, 27*, 353–358.

Hill, J. O., & Peters, J. C. (1998). Environmental contributions to the obesity epidemic. *Science, 280*, 1371–1374.

Hirsch, J., & Batchelor, B. (1976). Adipose tissue cellularity in human obesity. *Clinics in Endocrinology and Metabolism, 5*(2), 299–311.

Ho, G. Y., Wang, T., Gunter, M. J., Strickler, H. D., Cushman, M., Kaplan, R. C., … Rohan, T. E. (2012). Adipokines linking obesity with colorectal cancer risk in postmenopausal women. *Cancer Research, 72*(12), 3029–3037.

Hu, F. B. (2008). *Obesity epidemiology.* Oxford, New York: Oxford University Press.

Hu, F. B., Manson, J. E., Stampfer, M. J., Colditz, G., Liu, S., Solomon, C. G., & Willett, W. C. (2001). Diet, lifestyle, and the risk of type 2 diabetes in women. *New England Journal of Medicine, 345*, 790–797.

Hu, F. B., Wang, B., Chen, C., Jin, Y., Yang, J., Stampfer, M. J., & Xu, X. (2000). Body mass index and cardiovascular risk factors in a rural Chinese population. *American Journal of Epidemiology, 151*, 88–97.

Hubbard, V. S. (2000). Defining overweight and obesity: What are the issues? *American Journal of Clinical Nutrition, 72*, 1067–1068.

Hube, F., & Hauner, H. (2000). The two tumor necrosis factor receptors mediate opposite effects on differentiation and glucose metabolism in human adipocytes in primary culture. *Endocrinology, 141*, 2582–2588.

Hung-Kwan, S., Nelson, E. A. S., Li, A. M., Wong, E. M. C., Lau, J. T. F., Guldan, G. S., ... Sung, R. Y. T. (2008). Secular changes in height, weight and body mass index in Hong Kong children. *BMC Public Health*. Retrieved from http://www.biomedcentral.com/1471-2458/8/320

Hruby, A., & Hu, F. B. (2015). The epidemiology of obesity: A big picture. *Pharmacoeconomics, 33*(7), 673–689.

Ichihara, S., & Yamada, Y. (2008). Genetic factors for obesity. *Cellular and Molecular Life Sciences, 65*, 1086–1098.

ICO. (2010). The 11th Congress on Obesity news release. Retrieved from http://www.ico2010.org/documents/10.menobeseat20release-final.pdf

IDF, International Diabetes Federation. (2006). *Diabetes e-Atlas, based on the Diabetes Atlas* (2nd ed.). Brussels, Belgium: International Diabetes Federation.

Iozzo, P. (2009). Viewpoints on the way to the consensus session: Where does insulin resistance start? *The adipose tissue. Diabetes Care, 32*, S169–S173.

Ito, H., Nagasuga, K., Ohshima, A., Maruyama, T., Kaji, Y., Harada, M., ... Sakamoto, M. (2003). Detection of cardiovascular risk factors by indices of obesity obtained from anthropometry and dual-energy X-ray absorptiometry in Japanese individuals. *International Association for the Study of Obesity, 27*, 232–237.

Jackson, R. T., Rashed, M., Al-Hamad, N., Hwalla, N., & Al-Somaie, M. (2007). Comparison of BMI-for-age in adolescent girls in 3 countries of the Eastern Mediterranean Region. *Eastern Mediterranean Health Journal, 13*, 430–440.

Jia, H., & Lubetkin, E. I. (2010). Obesity-related quality-adjusted life years lost in the U.S. from 1993 to 2008. *American Journal of Preventive Medicine, 39*(03). doi:10.1016/j.amepre.2010.03.026.

Kadowaki, T., & Yamauchi, T. (2005). Adiponectin and adiponectin receptors. *Endocrine Reviews, 26*, 439–451.

Kagawa, M., Kerr, D., Uchida, H., & Binns, C. W. (2006). Differences in the relationship between BMI and percentage body fat between Japanese and Australian-Caucasian young men. *British Journal of Nutrition, 95*, 1002–1007.

Kann, L., Warren, C. W., Harris, W. J., Collins J. L., dougla, K. A., Collins, M. E., ... Kolbe, L. J. (1993). Youth risk behavior surveillance—United States. *Morbidity and Mortality Weekly Report, 44*, 1–55.

Keith, S. W., Redden, D. T., Katzmarzyk, P. T., Boggiano, M. M., Hanlon, E. C., Benca, R. M., ... Allison, D. B. (2006). Putative contributors to the secular increase in obesity: Exploring the roads less traveled. *International Journal of Obesity, 30*, 1585–1594.

Kelly, T., Yang, W., Chen, C. S., Reynolds, K., & He, J. (2008). Global burden of obesity in 2005 and projections to 2030. *International Journal of Obesity, 32*, 1431–1437.

Keys, A., Fidanza, F., Karvonen, M. J., Kimura, N., & Taylor, H. L. (1972). Indices of relative weight and adiposity. *Journal of Chronic Diseases, 25*, 329–343.

Kim, J. K., Gavrilova, O., Chen, Y., Reitman, M. L., & Shulman, G. I. (2000). Mechanism of insulin resistance in A-ZIP/F-1 fatless mice. *Journal of Biological Chemistry, 275*(12), 8456–8460.

Kim, S., & Moustaid-Mousa, N. (2000). Secretory endocrine and autocrine/paracrine function of the adipocyte. *Journal of Nutrition, 130*, S3110–S3115.

Kjellin, A., Ramel, S., Rossner, S., & Thor, K. (1996). Gastroesophageal reflux in obese patients is not reduced by weight reduction. *Scandinavian Journal of Gastroenterology, 31*, 1047–1051.

Klein, S., Fontana, L., Young, V. L., Coggan, A. R., Kilo, C., Patterson, B. W., & Mohammed, B. S. (2004). Absence of an effect of liposuction on insulin action and risk factors for coronary heart disease. *New England Journal of Medicine, 350*, 2549–2557.

Knowler, W. C., Bennett, P. H., Hamman, R. F., & Miller, M. (1978). Diabetes incidence and prevalence in Pima Indians, a 19-fold greater incidence than in Rochester, Minnesota. *American Journal of Epidemiology, 108*, 497–505.

Knowler, W .C., Pettitt, D. J., Savage, P. J., & Bennett, P. H. (1979). Diabetes incidence in Pima Indians: Contributions of obesity and parental diabetes. *American Journal of Epidemiology, 113*(2), 144–156.

Koenig, W. (2003). C-reactive protein and cardiovascular risk: An update on what is going on in cardiology. *Nephrology Dialysis Transplantation, 18*, 1039–1041.

Koh-Banerjee, P., Wang, Y., Hu, F. B., Spiegelman, D., Willett, W. C., & Rimm, E. B. (2004). Changes in body weight and body fat distribution as risk factors for clinical diabetes in US men. *American Journal of Epidemiology, 159*, 1150–1159.

Koo, J. S., Lee, S. W., Park, S. M., Jung, S. W., Yim, H. J., Park, J. J., ... Ryu, H. S. (2009). Abdominal obesity as a risk factor for the development of erosive esophagitis in subjects with a normal esophago-gastric junction. *Gut Liver, 3*(4), 276–284.

Kotsopoulos, J., Olopade, O. I., Ghadirian, P., Lubinski, J., Lynch, H. T., Isaacs, C., ... Narod, S. A. (2005). Changes in body weight and the risk of breast cancer in BRCA1 and BRCA2 mutation carriers. *Breast Cancer Research, 7*, 833–843.

Kral, J. G., Bjorntorp, P., Scherstein, T., & Sjostrom, L. (1977). Body composition and adipose tissue cellularity before and after jejuno-ileostomy in severely obese subjects. *European Journal of Clinical Investigation, 5*, 413–419.

Krauss, R. M., Winston, M., Fletcher, R. N., & Grundy, S. M. (1998). Obesity: Impact on cardiovascular disease. *Circulation, 98*, 1472–1476.

Kuczmarski, R. J., & Flegal, K. M. (2000). Criteria for definition of overweight in transition: Background and recommendations for the United States. *American Society for Clinical Nutrition, 72*, 1074–1081.

Kuczmarski, R. J., Ogden, C. L., Guo, S. S., Grummer-Strawn, L. M., Flegal, K. M., Mei, Z., ... Johnson, C. L. (2002). 2000 CDC growth charts for the United States: Methods and development. National Center for Health Statistics. *Vital and Health Statistics, 11*(246), 1–203.

Kumanyika, S. K., Obarzanek, E., Stevens, V. J., Herbert, P. R., & Whelton, P. K. (1991). Weight-loss experience of black and white participants in NHLBI-sponsored clinical trials. *American Journal of Clinical Nutrition, 53*, 1631S–1638S.

Kumanyika, S., Wilson, J., & Guliford-Davenport, M. (1993). Weight-related attitudes and behaviors of Black women. *Journal of the American Dietetic Association, 93*, 416–422.

Lagstrom, H., Hakanen, M., Niinikoski, H., Viikari, J., Rönnemaa, T., Saarinen, M., ... Simell, O. (2008). Growth patterns and obesity development in overweight or normal-weight 13 year old adolescents: The STRIP study. *Pediatrics, 122*, e876–e883.

Larsen, T. M., Toubro, S., & Astrup, A. (2003). PPAR-gamma agonists in the treatment of type II diabetes: Is increased fatness commensurate with long-term efficacy? *International Journal of Obesity, 27*, 147–161.

Lee, C. H., Woo, Y. C., Wang, Y., Yeung, C. Y., Xu, A., & Lam, K. S. (2015). Obesity, adipokines and cancer: An update. *Clinical Endocrinology, 83*(2), 147–156.

Lee, I. M., Manson, J. E., & Hennekens, C. H. (1993). Body weight and mortality. A 27-year follow up of middle-aged men. *Journal of the American Medical Association, 270*(23), 2823–2828.

Leach, R. E., Baumgard, S., & Broom, J. (1973). Obesity: Its relationship to osteoarthritis of the knee. *Clinical Orthopaedics and Related Research, 1973*, 93271–93273.

Lemmens, V. E. P. P., Oenema, A., Klepp, K. I., Henriksen, H. B., & Brug, J. (2008). A systematic review of the evidence regarding efficacy of obesity prevention interventions among adults. *Obesity Reviews, 9*(5), 446–456.

Leonhardt, W., Hanefeld, M., Schneider, H., & Haller, H. (1972). Human adipocyte volumes: Maximum size, and correlation to weight index in maturity-onset diabetes. *Diabetologia, 8,* 287–291.

Levin, B. E. (2006). Metabolic imprinting: Critical impact of the perinatal environment on the regulation of energy homeostasis. *Philosophical Transactions of the Royal Society of London. Series B, Biological Sciences, 361*(1471), 1107–1121.

Lin, W. Y., Lee, L. T., Chen, C. Y., Lo, H., Hsia, H. H., Liu, I. L., … Huang, K. C. (2002). Optimal cut-off values for obesity: Using simple anthropometric indices to predict cardiovascular risk factors in Taiwan. *International Journal of Obesity, 26*, 1232–1238.

Löfgren, P., Andersson, I., Adolfsson, B. M., Leijonhufvud, K., Hertel, J., Hoffstedt, P., & Arner, P. (2005). Long-term prospective and controlled studies demonstrate adipose tissue hypercellularity and relative leptin deficiency in the post-obese state. *Journal of Clinical Endocrinology and Metabolism, 90*, 6207–6213.

Lonn, M., Mehlig, K., Bengtsson, C., & Lissner, L. (2010). Adipocyte size predicts incidence of type 2 diabetes in women. *Federation of American Societies for Experimental Biology Journal, 24*, 326–331.

Lovejoy, J. C., Bray, G. A., Bourgeois, M. O., Macchiavelli, R., Rood, J. C., Greeson, C., & Partington, C. (1996). Exogenous androgens influence body composition and regional body fat distribution in obese postmenopausal women—A clinical research center study. *Journal of Clinical Endocrinology and Metabolism, 81*, 2198–2203.

Lovejoy, J. C., Champagne, C. M., De Jonge, L., Xie, H., & Smith, S. R. (2008). Increased visceral fat and decreased energy expenditure during the menopausal transition. *International Journal of Obesity, 32*, 949–958.

Lovejoy, J. C., & Sainsbury, A. (2009). Sex differences in obesity and the regulation of energy homeostasis. *Obesity Reviews, 10*(2), 154–167.

Lowell, B. B. (1998). Adaptive thermogenesis: Turning on the heat. *Current Biology, 8*, R517–R520.

Lowell, B. B., & Spiegelman, B. M. (2000). Towards molecular understanding of adaptive thermogenesis. *Nature, 406*, 652–659.

Lundgren, M., Buren, J., Ruge, T., Myrnäs, T., & Eriksson, J. W. (2004). Glucocorticoids down-regulate glucose uptake capacity and insulin signaling proteins in omental but not subcutaneous human adipocytes. *Journal of Clinical Endocrinology & Metabolism, 89*, 2989–2997.

Lyon, C. J., Law, R. E., & Hsueh, W. A. (2003). Minireview: Adiposity, inflammation, and atherogenesis. *Endocrinology, 144*, 2195–2200.

Maffeis, C., Silvagni, D., Bonadonna, R., Grezzani, A., Banzato, C., & Tatò, L. (2007). Fat cell size, insulin sensitivity, and inflammation in obese children. *The Journal of Pediatrics, 151*(6), 647–652.

Manson, J. E., Willett, W. C., Stamfer, M. J., Colditz, G. A., Hunter, J. H., Hankinson, S. E., … Speizer, F. E. (1995). Body weight and mortality among women. *New England Journal of Medicine, 333*, 677–685.

Mankin, H. J. (1974). The reaction of articular cartilage to injury and osteoarthritis. *New England Journal of Medicine, 291*, 1285–1292.

Marin, P., Holmang, S., Gustafsson, C., Jonsson, L., Kvist, H., Elander, A., … Bjorntorp, P. (1993). Androgen treatment of abdominally obese men. *Obesity Research, 1*, 245–251.

Marques, B. G., Hauman, D. B., & Martin, R. J. (1998). Association of fat cell size and paracrine growth factors in development of hyperplastic obesity. *American Journal of Physiology. Regulatory, Integrative and Comparative Physiology, 275*, R1898–R1908.

McGee, D. L. (2005). Body mass index and mortality: A meta-analysis based on person-level data from twenty-six observational studies. *Annals of Epidemiology, 15*, 87–97.

McGinnis, J. M., Gootman, J. A., & Kraak, V. I. (Eds.). (2006). *Food marketing to children and youth: Threat or opportunity*. Washington, DC: National Academies Press.

Medico-actuarial mortality investigation. (1912). Vol. 1. New York: Association of Life Insurance Medical Directors and the Actuarial Society of America.

Meneghini, L. F. (2007). Impact of bariatric surgery on type 2 diabetes. *Cell Biochemistry and Biophysics, 48*, 97–102.

Mentz, H. A. (2008). Fat emboli syndromes following liposuction. *Aesthetic Plastic Surgery, 32*, 737–738.

Messier, S. P. (2008). Obesity and osteoarthritis: Disease genesis and nonpharmacologic weight management. *Rheumatic Diseases Clinics of North America, 34*(3), 713–729.

Metropolitan Life Insurance Company (MLIC). (1942). Ideal weights for men. *Statistical bulletin — Metropolitan Life, 23*, 6–8.

Metropolitan Life Insurance Company (MLIC). (1943). Ideal weights for women. *Statistical bulletin — Metropolitan Life, 24*, 6–8.

Metropolitan Life Insurance Company (MLIC). (1959). New weight standards for men and women. *Statistical bulletin — Metropolitan Life, 40*, 1–4.

Misra, A. (2003). Revisions of cutoffs of body mass index to define overweight and obesity are needed for the Asian-ethnic groups. *International Journal of Obesity, 27*, 1294–1296.

Misra, A., & Khurana, L. (2008). Obesity and metabolic syndrome in developing countries. *Journal of Clinical Endocrinology and Metabolism, 93*(11), S9–S13.

MMWR. (2009). Obesity prevalence among low-income, preschool-aged children—United States, 1998–2008. *Morbidity and Mortality Weekly Report, 58*(28), 769–773.

Mohammed, B. S., Cohen, S., Reeds, D., Young, L., & Klein, S. (2008). Long-term effects of large-volume liposuction on metabolic risk factors for coronary heart disease. *Obesity, 16*(12), 2648–2651.

Moon, O. R., Kim, N. S., Jamg, S. M., Yoon, T. H., & Kim, S. O. (2002). The relationship between body mass index and the prevalence of obesity-related diseases based on 1995 National Health Interview Survey in Korea. *Obesity Reviews, 3*, 191–196.

Moraes-Filho, J., Cecconello, I., Gama-Rodrigues, J., Castro, L., Henry, M. A., Meneghelli, U. G., … Brazilian Consensus Group. (2002). Brazilian consensus on gastroesophageal reflux disease: Proposals for assessment, classification, and management. *American Journal of Gastroenterology, 97*, 241–248.

Nader, P. R., O'Brien, M., Houts, R., Bradley, R., Belsky, J., Crosnoe, R., … National Institute of Child Health and Human Development Early Child Care Research Network. (2006). Identifying risk for obesity in early childhood. *Pediatrics, 118*, e594–e601.

National Institutes of Health Consensus Development Panel on the Health Implications of Obesity. (1985). Health implications of obesity: National Institutes of Health consensus development conference statement. *Annals of Internal Medicine, 103*, 1073–1077.

National Institutes of Health Conference. (1991). Gastrointestinal surgery for severe obesity. Consensus Development Conference Panel. *Annals of Internal Medicine, 115*(12), 956–961.

National Institutes of Health Consensus Development Conference. (1992). Gastrointestinal surgery for severe obesity. Proceedings of a National Institutes of Health Consensus Development Conference. March 25–27, 1991, Bethesda, MD. *American Journal of Clinical Nutrition, 55*, 487S–619S.

National Institutes of Health. (1998). The evidence report. *Obesity Research, 6*, 51S–209S.

National Institute of Diabetes and Digestive and Kidney Diseases (NIDDK). (2008). National diabetes statistics, 2007 fact sheet. Bethesda, MD: U.S. Department of Health and Human Services, National Institutes of Health.

Neel, J. V. (1962). Diabetes mellitus: A "thrifty" genotype rendered detrimental by "progress"? *American Journal of Human Genetics, 14*, 353–362.

Nestle, M., & Young, L. R. (2002). The contribution of expanding portion sizes to the obesity epidemic. *American Journal of Public Health, 92*, 246–249.

Nilsson, M., Johnsen, R., Ye, W., Hveem, K., & Lagergran, J. (2003). Obesity and estrogen as risk factors for gastroesophageal reflux symptoms. *Journal of the American Medical Association, 290*, 66–72.

Ogden, C. L., Carroll, M. D., & Flegal, K. M. (2008). High body mass index for age among US children and adolescents, 2003–2006. *Journal of the American Medical Association, 299*, 2401–2405.

Ogden, C. L., Carroll, M. D., McDowell, M. A., & Flegal, K. M. (2007). *Obesity among adults in the United States—No change since 2003–2004* (NCHS data brief no. 1). Hyattsville, MD: National Center for Health Statistics.

Ogden, C. L., Yanovski, S. Z., Carroll, M. D., & Flegal, K. M. (2007). The epidemiology of obesity. *Gastroenterology, 132*, 2087–2102.

Oguma, Y., Sesso, H. D., Paffenbarger, R. S., & Lee, I. M. (2005). Weight change and the risk of developing type 2 diabetes. *Obesity Research, 13*, 945–951.

Ogunwobi, O., Mutungi, G., & Peales, I. L. (2006). Leptin stimulates proliferation and inhibits apoptosis in Barrett's esophageal adenocarcinoma cells by cyclooxygenase-2-dependent, prostaglandin-E2-mediated transactivation of the epidermal growth factor receptor and c-Jun NH2-terminal kinase activation. *Endocrinology, 147*(9), 4506–4516.

O'Rahilly, S., & Farooqi, I. S. (2006). Genetics of obesity. *Philosophical Transactions of the Royal Society of London. Series B, Biological sciences, 361*(1471), 1095–1105.

O'Sullivan, A. J. (2008). Does oestrogen allow women to story fat more efficiently? A biological advantage for fertility and gestation. *Obesity Reviews, 10*(2), 168–177.

Peneau, S., Thibault, H., & Rolland-Cachera, M. F. (2009). Massively obese adolescents were of normal weight at the age of adiposity rebound. *Obesity, 17*, 1309–1310.

Peppard, P. E., Young, T., Palta, M., Dempsey, J., & Skatrud, J. (2000). Longitudinal study of moderate weight change and sleep-disordered breathing. *Journal of the American Medical Association, 284*(23), 3015–3021.

Pischon, T., Nothlings, U., & Boeing, H. (2007). Obesity and cancer. *The Proceedings of the Nutrition Society, 67*, 128–145.

Pinhas-Hamiel, O., Dolan, L. M., Daniels, S. R., Standiford, D., Khoury, P. R., & Zeitler, P. (1996). Increased incidence of non-insulin dependent diabetes mellitus among adolescents. *The Journal of Pediatrics, 128*, 608–615.

Popkin, B. M., Paeratakul, S., Ge, K., & Zhai, F. (1995). Body weight patterns among the Chinese: Results from the 1989 and 1991 China Health and Nutrition Survey. *American Journal of Public Health, 85*, 690–694.

Prentice, A. M. (2006). The emerging epidemic of obesity in developing countries. *International Journal of Epidemiology, 35*, 93–99.

Punjabi, N. M., Sorkin, J. D., Katzel, L. I., Goldberg, A. P., Schwartz, A. R., & Smith, P. L. (2002). Sleep-disordered breathing and insulin resistance in middle-aged and overweight men. *American Journal of Respiratory and Critical Care Medicine, 165*, 677–682.

Quételet, A. (1835). Sur l'homme et le developpement de ses facultes, ou essai de physique sociale. Paris: Bachelier.

Rajala, R., Partinen, M., Sane, T., Pelkonen, R., Huikuri, K., & Seppalainen, A. M. (1991). Obstructive sleep apnoea syndrome in morbidly obese patients. *Journal of Internal Medicine, 230*, 125–129.

Ravussin, E., & Smith, S. R. (2002). Increased fat intake, impaired fat oxidation, and failure of fat cell proliferation result in ectopic fat storage, insulin resistance, and type 2 diabetes mellitus. *Annals of the New York Academy of Sciences, 967*, 363–378.

Raynauld, J. P., Martel-Pelletier, J., Berthiaume, M. J., Beaudoin, G., Choquette, D., Haraoui, B., … Pelletier, J.-P. (2006). Long-term evaluation of disease progression through the quantitative magnetic resonance imaging of symptomatic knee osteoarthritis patients: Correlation with clinical symptoms and radiographic changes. *Arthritis Research & Therapy, 8*(1), R21.

Razak, F., Anand, S. S., Shannon, H., Vuksan, V., Davis, B., Jacobs, R., … for the SHARE Investigators. (2007). Defining obesity cut points in a multiethnic population. *Circulation, 115*, 2111–2118.

Richman, R. M., Elliott, L. M., Burns, C. M., Bearpark, H. M., Steinbeck, K. S., & Caterson, I. D. (1994). The prevalence of obstructive sleep apnoea in an obese female population. *International Journal of Obesity and Related Metabolic Disorders, 18*, 173–177.

Ridker, P. M., Glynn, R. J., & Hennekins, C. H. (1998). C-reactive protein adds to the predictive values of total and HDL cholesterol in determining risk of first myocardial infarction. *Circulation, 97*, 2007–2011.

Rifai, N., & Ridker, P. M. (2001). High sensitive C-reactive protein: A novel and promising marker of coronary heart disease. *Clinical Chemistry, 47*, 401–411.

Robbins, S. L., & Cotran, R. S. (1979). *Pathologic basis of disease.* Philadelphia, PA: WB Saunders Company.

Robinson, T. N. (1999). Reducing children's television viewing to prevent obesity: A randomized controlled trial. *Journal of the American Medical Association, 281*, 1561–1567.

Rolls, B. J., Morris, E. L., & Roe, L. S. (2002). Portion size of food affects energy intake in normal-weight and overweight men and women. *American Journal of Clinical Nutrition, 76*, 1207–1213.

Rosen, E. D., & MacDougald, O. A. (2006). Adipocyte differentiation from the inside out. *Nature Reviews. Molecular Cell Biology, 7*, 885–896.

Rosenbaum, M., & Leibel, L. L. (1998). The physiology of body weight regulation in children: Relevance to the etiology of obesity in children. *Pediatrics, 101*, 525–539.

Ross, R. (1999). Atherosclerosis—An inflammatory disease. *New England Journal of Medicine, 340*, 115–126.

Ross, R., & Glomset, J. A. (1973). Atherosclerosis and the arterial smooth muscle cell: Proliferation of smooth muscle is a key event in the genesis of the lesions of atherosclerosis. *Science, 180*, 1332–1339.

Ross, R., & Glomset, J. A. (1976). The pathogenesis of atherosclerosis. *New England Journal of Medicine, 295*, 369–377.

Salameh, B. S., Khoukaz, M. T., & Bell, R. L. (2010). Metabolic and nutritional changes after bariatric surgery. *Expert Review of Gastroenterology & Hepatology, 4*, 217–223.

Sassi, F. (2006). How to do (or not to do)... Calculating QALYs, comparing QALY and DALY calculations. *Health Policy and Planning, 21*, 402–408.

Satia, J. A. (2010). Dietary acculturation and the nutrition transition: An overview. *Applied Physiology, Nutrition, and Metabolism, 35*, 219–223.

Schienkiewitz, A., Schulze, M. B., Hoffmann, K., Kroke, A., & Boeing, H. (2006). Body mass index history and risk of type 2 diabetes: Results from the European Prospective Investigation into Cancer and Nutrition (EPIC)-Potsdam Study. *American Journal of Clinical Nutrition, 84*, 427.

Schwartz, A. R., O'Donnell, C. P., Baron, J., Schubert, N., Alam, D., Samadi, S. D., & Smith, P. L. (1998). The hypotonic upper airway in obstructive sleep apnea: Role of structures and neuromuscular activity. *American Journal of Respiratory and Critical Care Medicine, 157*(4 Pt 1), 1051–1057.

Scott, S. K., Rabito, F. A., Butler, N. N., & Harris, R. E. (2004). *The energy storage capacity hypothesis* (PhD dissertation). Columbus, OH: The Ohio State University.

Scott, S. K., Rabito, F. A., Price, P. D., Butler, N. N., Schwartzbaum, J. A., Jackson, B. M., ... Harris, R. E. (2006). Co-morbidity among the morbidly obese: A comparative study of 2002 US hospital patient discharges. *Surgery for Obesity and Related Diseases, 2*, 105–111.

Segal, N. L., & Allison, D. B. (2002). Twin and virtual twins: Bases of relative body weight revisited. *International Journal of Obesity and Related Metabolic Disorders, 26*(04), 437–441.

Sethi, J. K., & Vidal-Puig, A. J. (2007). Targeting fat to prevent diabetes. *Cell Metabolism, 5*(5), 323–325.

Shai, I., Jiang, R., Manson, J. E., Stampfer, M. J., Willett, W. C., Colditz, G. A., & Hu, F. B. (2006). Ethnicity, obesity, and risk of type 2 diabetes in women: A 20-year follow-up study. *Diabetes Care, 29*(7), 1585–1590.

Simkin-Silverman, L. R., Wing, R. R., Boraz, M. A., & Kuller, L. H. (2003). Lifestyle intervention can prevent weight gain during menopause: Results from a 5 year randomized controlled trial. *Annals of Behavioral Medicine, 26*, 212–220.

Skurk, T., Alberti-Huber, C., & Hauner, H. (2006). Relationship between adipocyte size and adipokine expression and secretion. *Journal of Clinical Endocrinology & Metabolism, 92*, 1023–1033.

Smith, P. L., Gold, A. R., Meyers, D. A., Haponik, E. F., & Bleecker, E. R. (1985). Weight loss in mildly to moderately obese patients with obstructive sleep apnea. *Annals of Internal Medicine, 103*, 850–855.

Spalding, K. L., Arner, P. O., Westermark, S., Bernard, S., Buchholz, B. A., Bergmann, O., ... Arner, P. (2008). Dynamics of fat cell turnover in humans. *Nature, 453*, 783–787.

Spiegelman, D., Israel, R. G., Bouchard, C., & Willett, W. C. (1992). Absolute fat mass, percent body fat, and body-fat distribution: Which is the real determinant of blood pressure and serum glucose? *American Journal of Clinical Nutrition, 55*(6), 1033–1044.

Srinivasan, S. R., Myers, L., & Berenson, G. S. (2002). Predictability of childhood adiposity and insulin for developing insulin resistance syndrome (syndrome X) in young adulthood: The Bogalusa Heart Study. *Diabetes, 51*, 204–209.

Stanhope, K. L., Schwarz, J. M., Keim, N. L., Griffen, S. C., Bremer, A. A., Graham, J. L., ... Havel, P. J. (2009). Consuming fructose-sweetened, but not glucose-sweetened beverages increases visceral adiposity and lipids and decreases insulin sensitivity in overweight/obese humans. *Journal of Clinical Investigation, 119*, 1322–1334.

Stevens, J. (2003a). Ethnic-specific revisions of body mass index cutoffs to define overweight and obesity in Asians are not warranted. *International Journal of Obesity, 27*, 1297–1299.

Stevens, J. (2003b). Ethnic-specific cutpoints for obesity vs. country-specific guidelines for action. *International Journal of Obesity, 27*, 287–288.

Stevens, J., Jianwen Cai, J., & Jones, W. (2002). The effect of decision rules on the choice of a body mass index cutoff for obesity: Examples from African American and white women. *American Journal of Clinical Nutrition, 75*, 986–992.

Steyn, K. (1991). Risk factors for coronary heart disease in the black population of the Cape Peninsula. *South African Medical Journal, 79*, 480–485.

Stommel, M., & Schoenborn, C. A. (2010). Variations in BMI and prevalence of health risks in diverse racial and ethnic populations. *Obesity*. doi:10.1038/oby.2009.472.

Stunkard, A. J., Sorensen, T. I., Hanis, C., Teasdale, T. W., Chakraborty, R., Schull, W. J., & Schulsinger, F. (1986). An adoption study of human obesity. *The New England Journal of Medicine, 314*(04), 193–198.

Sugerman, H. J. (2000). The epidemic of severe obesity: The values of surgical treatment. *Mayo Clinic Proceedings, 75*, 669–672.

Sugerman, H. J., Sugerman, E. L., Demaria, E. J., Kellum, J. M., Kennedy, C., Mowery, Y., & Wolfe, L. G. (2003). Bariatric surgery for severely obese adolescents. *Journal of Gastrointestinal Surgery, 7*, 102–107.

Suk, S. H., Sacco, R. L., Boden-Albala, B., Cheun, J. F., Pittman, J. G., Elkind, M. S., ... Northern Manhattan Stroke Study. (2003). Abdominal obesity and risk of ischemic stroke. *Advances in Chronic Kidney Disease, 34*, 1586–1592.

Suter, M., Giusti, V., Heraief, E., Zysset, F., & Calmes, J. M. (2003). Laparoscopic Roux-en-Y gastric bypass: Initial 2-year experience. *Surgical Endoscopy, 17*, 603–609.

Tauman, R., & Gozal, D. (2006). Obesity and obstructive sleep apnea in children. *Paediatric Respiratory Reviews, 7*, 247–259.

Tchernof, A., Nolan, A., Sites, C. K., Ades, P. A., & Poehlman, E. T. (2002). Weight loss reduces C-reactive protein levels in obese postmenopausal women. *Circulation, 105*, 564–569.

Terry, M. B., Wei, Y., & Esserman, D. (2007). Maternal, birth, and early-life influences on adult body size in women. *American Journal of Epidemiology, 166*, 5–13.

Trakhtenbroit, M. A., Leichman, G. J., Algahim, M. F., Miller, C. C., 3rd., Moody, F. G., Lux, T. R., & Taegtmeyer, H. (2009). Body weight, insulin resistance, and serum adipokine levels two years after two types of bariatric surgery. *American Journal of Medicine, 122*, 435–442.

US National Academy of Sciences. (2005). Transportation Research Board Annual Report. Washington, DC: US National Academy of Sciences.

Unger, R. H. (2003). The physiology of cellular liporegulation. *Annual Review of Physiology, 65*, 333–347.

United Nations Development Program. (2001). *Human development report*. New York: Oxford University Press.

Published for the United Nations Development Program (UNDP). Retrieved from http://hdr.undp.org/en/media/completenew1.pdf

United Nations. (2006). World urbanization prospectus: The 2005 revision. New York, NY: UN, Department of Economics and Social Affairs, Population Division.

van der Lei, B., Halbesma, G. J., van Neiuwenhoven, C. A., & van Wingerden, J. J. (2007). Spontaneous breast enlargement following liposuction of the abdominal wall: Does a link exist? *Plastic and Reconstructive Surgery, 119,* 1584–1589.

Vgontzas, A. N., Tan, T. L., Bixler, E. O., Martin, L. F., Shubert, D., & Kales, A. (1994). Sleep apnea and sleep disruption in obese patients. *Archives of Internal Medicine, 154,* 1705–1711.

Vlahakis, N. E., & Hubmayr, R. D. (2005). Review: Cellular stress failure in ventilator-injured lungs. *American Journal of Respiratory and Critical Care Medicine, 171*(12), 1328–1342.

Vona-Davis, L., & Rose, D. P. (2007). Adipokines as endocrine, paracrine, and autocrine factors in breast cancer risk and progression. *Endocrine-Related Cancer, 14,* 189–206.

Wadd, W. (1816). *Cursory remarks on corpulence; or obesity considered a disease with critical examination of ancient and modern opinions, relative to its causes and cure* (3rd ed.). London, UK: J Callow.

Wagner, D. R., & Heyward, V. H. (2000). Measures of body composition in blacks and whites: A comparative review. *American Journal of Clinical Nutrition, 71,* 1392–1402.

Wajchenberg, B. L. (2000). Subcutaneous and visceral adipose tissue: Their relation to the metabolic syndrome. *Endocrine Reviews, 21,* 697–738.

Wajchenberg, B. L. (2007). β-Cell failure in diabetes and preservation by clinical treatment. *Endocrine Reviews, 28,* 187–218.

Wardle, J., Carnell, S., Haworth, C. M. A., & Plomin, R. (2008). Evidence for a strong genetic influence on childhood adiposity despite the force of the obesogenic environment. *American Journal of Clinical Nutrition, 87,* 398–404.

Welch, G. W., & Sowers, M. F. R. (2000). The interrelationship between body topology and body composition varies with age among women. *Journal of Nutrition, 130,* 2371–2377.

Werkman, A., Deurenberg-Yap, M., Schmidt, G., & Deurenberg, P. (2000). A comparison between composition and density of the fat-free mass of young adult Singaporean Chinese and Dutch Caucasians. *Annals of Nutrition and Metabolism, 44,* 235–242.

Weyer, C., Foley, J. E., Bogardus, C., Tataranni, P. A., & Pratley, R. E. (2000). Enlarged subcutaneous abdominal adipocyte size, but not obesity itself, predicts type II diabetes, independent of insulin resistance. *Diabetologia, 43,* 1498–1506.

Whitaker, R. C., Wright, J. A., Pepe, M. S., Seidel, K. D., & Dietz, W. H. (1997). Predicting obesity in young adulthood from childhood and parental obesity. *New England Journal of Medicine, 337,* 869–873.

Whitaker, R. C., Pepe, M. S., Wright, J. A., Seidel, K. D., & Dietz, W. H. (1998). Early adiposity rebound and the risk of adult obesity. *Pediatrics, 101,* e5.

Willett, W. C., Dietz, W. H., & Colditz, G. A. (1999). Guidelines for a healthy weight. *New England Journal of Medicine, 341,* 427–434.

WHO. (1998). Obesity. Preventing and managing the global epidemic. Report of a WHO consultation on obesity. Geneva, Switzerland: World Health Organization.

WHO. (2000). Preventing and managing the global epidemic. Report of a WHO consultation on obesity (WHO Technical Report Series No. 894). Geneva, Switzerland: World Health Organization.

WHO. (2003). *Diet, nutrition and the prevention of chronic diseases: A report of the joint WHO/FAO expert consultation* (WHO Technical Report Series No. 916). Geneva, Switzerland: World Health Organization.

WHO. (2004). Appropriate body mass index (BMI) for Asian populations and its implications on policy and intervention strategies: Report of a WHO Expert Consultation. *Lancet, 363,* 157–163.

WHO. (2005). *Preventing chronic diseases.* Geneva, Switzerland: World Health Organization.

WHO. (2009a). *Global health risks: Mortality and burden of disease attributable to selected major risks.* Geneva, Switzerland: World Health Organization.

WHO. (2009b). *Population-based prevention strategies for childhood obesity: Report of a WHO forum and technical meeting,* December 15–17. Geneva, Switzerland: World Health Organization.

WHO Multicentre Growth Reference Study Group. (2009). *WHO Child Growth Standards: Growth velocity based on weight, length and head circumference: Methods and development.* Geneva, Switzerland: World Health Organization.

Williams, S. M., & Goulding, A. (2009). Patterns of growth associated with the timing of adiposity rebound. *Obesity, 17,* 335–341.

World Cancer Research Fund/American Institute for Cancer Research. (2007). *Food, nutrition, physical activity, and the prevention of cancer: A global perspective.* Washington, DC: World Cancer Research Fund/American Institute for Cancer Research.

Yasojima, K., Schwab, C., Mcgeer, E. G., & McGeer, P. L. (2001). Generation of C-reactive protein and complement components in atherosclerotic plaques. *American Journal of Pathology, 158,* 1039–1051.

Yatsuya, H., Folsom, A. R., Yamagishi, K., North, K. E., Brancati, F. L., Stevens, J., & Atherosclerosis Risk in Communities Study Investigators. (2010). Race-and sex-specific associations of obesity measures with ischemic stroke incidence in the Atherosclerosis Risk in Communities (ARIC) Study. *Advances in Chronic Kidney Disease, 41,* 417–425.

Yeh, E. T. H., & Willerson, J. T. (2003). Coming of age of C-reactive protein. Using inflammatory markers in cardiology. *Circulation, 107,* 307–372.

Yin, J., Gao, Z., He, Q., & Ye, J. (2009). Role of hypoxia in obesity-induced disorders of glucose and lipid metabolism in adipose tissue. *American Journal of Physiology. Endocrinology and Metabolism, 296,* E333–E342.

Young, T., Palta, M., Dempsey, J., Skatrud, J., Weber, S., & Badr, S. (1993). The occurrence of sleep-disordered breathing among middle-aged adults. *New England Journal of Medicine, 328,* 1230–1235.

Young, T., Pappard, P. E., & Gottlieb, D. J. (2002). Epidemiology of obstructive sleep apnea. *American Journal of Respiratory and Critical Care Medicine, 165,* 1217–1239.

Yudkin, J. S., Stehouwer, C. D. A., Emeiss, J. J., & Coppack, S. W. (1999). C-reactive protein in healthy subjects: Associations with obesity, insulin resistance, and endothelial dysfunction. A potential role for cytokines originating from adipose tissue? *Arteriosclerosis, Thrombosis, and Vascular Biology, 19,* 972–978.

Yuji, M. (2002). New criteria for "obesity disease" in Japan. *Circulation Journal, 66,* 987–992.

Yun, P. L., Bruck, M., Felsenfeld, L., & Katz, B. E. (2003). Breast enlargement observed after power liposuction: A retrospective review. *Dermatologic Surgery, 29,* 165–167.

Yusuf, S., Hawken, S., Ounpuu, S., Bautista, L., Franzosi, M. G., Commerford, P., … INTERHEART Study Investigators. (2005). Obesity and the risk of myocardial infarction in 27,000 participants from 52 countries: A case-control study. *Lancet, 366*(9497), 1640–1649.

Zeckhauser, R., & Shepard, D. S. (1976). Where now for saving lives? *Law and Contemporary Problems, 40*, 5–45.

Zeghari, N., Vidal, H., Younsi, M., Ziegler, O., Drouin, P., & Donner, M. (2000). Adipocyte membrane phospholipids and PPAR-gamma expression in obese women: Relationship to hyperinsulinemia. *American Journal of Physiology. Endocrinology and Metabolism, 279*(4), E736–E743.

Ziccardi, P., Nappo, F., Giugliano, G., Esposito, K., Marfella, R., Cioffi, M., … Giugliano, D. (2002). Reduction of inflammatory cytokine concentrations and improvement of endothelial functions in obese women after weight loss over one year. *Circulation, 105*, 804–809.

Ziegler, E. E., & Nelson, S. E. (2010). Growth charts compared. Nestlé Nutrition Workshop Series. *Paediatric Programme, 65*, 197–210.

Ziraba, A., Fotso, J., & Ochako, R. (2009). Overweight and obesity in urban Africa: A problem of the rich or of the poor? *BMC Public Health, 9*, 465.

CHAPTER 43

The Epidemiology of Thyroid Disease: *Hyperthyroidism* and *Hypothyroidism*

▶ Thyroid Gland: Anatomy and Function

The human thyroid is a butterfly-shaped gland located in the anterior neck inferior to the thyroid cartilage (also known as the *Adam's apple*). The term "thyroid" means "shield," which describes the basic shape of the thyroid cartilage.

The thyroid produces iodine-containing thyroid hormones, the principal ones being triiodothyronine (T_3) and thyroxine (T_4). Triiodothyronine is two to three times more potent than thyroxine and considerably more T_4 is produced than T_3 (20:1 ratio). These circulating hormones are essential in regulating the rate of metabolism in the body. Inside the cell, T_3 and T_4 stimulate energy production by the mitochondria and promote glucose catabolism, protein synthesis, lipolysis, and excretion of cholesterol. Thyroid hormones also influence growth and development in early life and participate in a number of essential physiologic functions throughout life (e.g., maintenance of normal cardiac rhythm, muscle tone, and neuronal function in the sympathetic nervous system) (Robbins & Cotran, 1979).

The functional unit of the thyroid is the thyroid follicle. The thyroid is comprised of thousands of spherical thyroid follicles, each of which contains a material called colloid that contains iodide (the storage form of iodine) and thyroglobulin (the glycoprotein bound to thyroid hormones). Thyroid hormones are synthesized by cuboidal epithelial cells that line the thyroid follicles. The essential substrates for biosynthesis are the amino acid, tyrosine, and the mineral, iodine. Peptide hormones secreted by the hypothalamus and the anterior pituitary gland (**FIGURE 43.1**) regulate the biosynthesis of thyroid hormones (T_3 and T_4). In response to low blood levels of thyroid hormones or neurological signals, the hypothalamus secretes a protein called *thyroid-releasing hormone* (TRH) into special blood vessels connected to the pituitary gland which in turn triggers the anterior pituitary to secrete a second protein called *thyroid-stimulating hormone* (TSH or *thyrotropin*) into the blood. In response to TSH, receptors on the cell membranes of thyroid epithelial cells (*thyrotropin receptors*) activate the biosynthetic pathway for the production of thyroid hormones (T_3 and T_4). Thyroid hormones are stored in a glycoprotein called thyroglobulin which is also synthesized in the thyroid epithelium. Thyroid hormones are secreted into the blood from the thyroglobulin (colloid) stored within thyroid follicles. Thyroid hormones (T_3 and T_4) are transported in the blood bound to a carrier protein known as *thyroxine-binding*

The pituitary secretes hormones that stimulate the thyroid and other endocrine glands.

Thyroid Stimulating Hormone (TSH) triggers biosynthesis of thyroid hormone by the thyroid.

Low level of thyroid hormone signals the pituitary to secrete more TSH to reinstate normal level of thyroid hormone.

TSH

Thyroid hormone

Thyroid cartilage (Adam's apple)

Parathyroid glands secrete hormone to regulate calcium

FIGURE 43.1 The Hypothalamic-Pituitary-Axis: Feedback Control of the Thyroid Gland.

globulin. The secretion and release of T$_3$ and T$_4$ are regulated by blood levels of thyroid hormones (e.g., low levels stimulate the release of active T$_3$ and T$_4$).

Special cells of the thyroid gland called C cells produce a polypeptide hormone called *calcitonin* that helps regulate calcium homeostasis throughout the body. Relatively small *parathyroid glands* (usually four in number) are located at the periphery of the thyroid gland (Figure 43.1). The parathyroid glands synthesize *parathyroid hormone* (PTH), which together with calcitonin and the active form of vitamin D, regulate levels of calcium and phosphorous in the blood, the bones, and most other tissues (Robbins & Cotran, 1979).

Diseases of the Thyroid Gland

The most commonly encountered diseases of the thyroid gland involve either an overactive gland (*hyperthyroidism*) or an underactive gland (*hypothyroidism*). The most common cause of thyroid disorders worldwide is iodine deficiency leading to hypothyroidism and goiter formation. In regions of the world that have sufficient sources of iodine, most persons with thyroid disorders have autoimmune disease (Vanderpump, 2011).

The most prevalent clinically evident thyroid condition is enlargement of the thyroid gland which is commonly called a "goiter." As discussed in the following sections, goiters fall into two broad categories:

toxic goiters caused by hyperthyroidism and nontoxic goiters caused by hypothyroidism. Thyroid adenomas (nodules) occasionally arise within the thyroid gland. On pathologic examination, the vast majority of thyroid nodules turn out to be benign. Thyroid cancer is rare, but it must be differentiated from all benign lesions. The epidemiology of thyroid cancer is discussed in Chapter 31.

Prevalence and Incidence of Hyperthyroidism and Hypothyroidism

In early screening surveys conducted in the United States and Great Britain, thyroid abnormalities were found in approximately 6% of adults (Baldwin & Rowett, 1978; Tunbridge et al., 1977). Since many individuals in the general population have abnormal thyroid function without symptoms, more recent surveys are based upon not only the presence of symptoms (overt disease) but also the detection of abnormal levels of urinary iodine and/or serum TSH and thyroid hormones without symptoms (subclinical disease) (Garber et al., 2012).

In the *National Health and Nutrition Examination Survey III* (NHANES III) conducted during 1988–1994 in the United States, a nationally representative sample of 16,533 disease-free individuals were screened for thyroid dysfunction by measuring serum TSH, T_4, thyroglobulin antibodies, and thyroid peroxidase antibodies. The estimated prevalence of any thyroid disease in the general U.S. population was 5.9%. Of these, 4.6% of the population had hypothyroidism (0.3% overt and 4.3% subclinical) and 1.3% had hyperthyroidism (0.5% overt and 0.7% subclinical). Estimates of the prevalence of antithyroid antibodies increased with age and were higher in females than males, and higher in Caucasians and Hispanics than African Americans (Hollowell et al., 2002).

More recently, a meta-analysis of multiple data sources was conducted to estimate the prevalence and incidence of thyroid disease among European populations during 1975–2012. The estimated prevalence of any thyroid disease in the general European population was 3.8% (3.0% with hypothyroidism and 0.75% with hyperthyroidism). Prevalence estimates of hypothyroidism and hyperthyroidism in females (6.5% and 1.4%) were approximately five times higher than in males (1.2% and 0.3%). Most notably, 85% of thyroid dysfunction was subclinical (e.g., prevalence estimates for overt and subclinical hypothyroidism were 0.5% and 4.6% in females and 0.2% and 2.8% in males). The annual incidence of thyroid disease was 226 per 100,000 for hypothyroidism (370 per 100,000 in females and 72 per 100,000 in males) and 51 per 100,000 for hyperthyroidism (82 per 100,000 in females and 15 per 100,000 in males) (Madariaga, Palacios, Guillén-Grima, & Galofré, 2014).

Results of these national surveys confirm three major points regarding the epidemiology of thyroid disease: (1) hypothyroidism is three to four times more common than hyperthyroidism, (2) both hyperthyroidism and hypothyroidism are up to five times more common in females than males, and (3) the majority of individuals with thyroid dysfunction have subclinical disease and are unaware of their condition.

▶ Rare Medical Emergencies of Thyroid Dysfunction

Two rare conditions of the thyroid gland, *thyroid storm* and *myxedema coma,* are life-threatening medical emergencies. Thyroid storm (also called thyrotoxic crisis) is a severe and potentially deadly hypermetabolic complication of hyperthyroidism, whereas myxedema coma refers to cardiogenic shock, respiratory depression, hypothermia, and coma caused by hypothyroidism. Both conditions are rare with annual incidence rates of about 1–2 per million (Akamizu et al., 2017; Ono et al., 2017).

Hyperthyroid patients with extreme elevations in circulating thyroid hormones are prone to *thyroid storms* that are life-threatening. Classical signs of a thyroid storm are ventricular tachycardia, high fever (104°F–106°F), delirium, seizure, and cardiopulmonary failure. Without immediate treatment, the case fatality rate of a thyroid storm approaches 100% and even with therapy, the case fatality is high ranging from 20% to 50% (Akamizu et al., 2017; Burch & Wartofsky, 1993).

Hypothyroid patients with extreme deficiencies in circulating thyroid hormones are prone to *myxedema coma.* Classic signs of this condition include myxedema (swelling of connective tissue), hypothermia (low body temperature), bradycardia (slow heart rate), hypotension (low blood pressure), change in mental status/unarousable, and other symptoms related to poor function of many organs. Myxedema coma is a life-threatening condition particularly among the elderly. In a recent study using a national inpatient database in Japan, the case fatality rate was 30% in patients hospitalized with myxedema coma (Ono et al., 2017).

▶ Mortality Rates of Hyperthyroidism and Hypothyroidism

Precise estimates of mortality related to thyroid dysfunction are difficult to obtain since thyroid disease may often be a contributing cause of death but not the underlying cause of death. Unfortunately, in most countries, national cause-specific mortality statistics are based on only the underlying cause of death. Nevertheless, in some developed countries, *contributing causes of death* as well as the underlying causes are recorded on death certificates.

One such registry that tracks both underlying causes and contributing causes of death is the *Oxford Record Linkage Study* (ORLS) in England. Investigators at the University of Oxford recently examined regional trends in mortality rates for hypothyroidism and hyperthyroidism (thyrotoxicosis) during 1979–2010 in the Oxford region of England using the ORLS mortality data (**FIGURE 43.2**). Since most death certificates code only thyroid diseases as contributing causes of death, the mortality estimates were based on those certificates with any mention of thyroid disease (excluding thyroid cancer). Among the 2.5 million residents of the Oxford region studied, a total of 1739 death certificates mentioned hypothyroidism among females compared to 387 death certificates among males. Hypothyroidism was reported as the underlying cause of death on

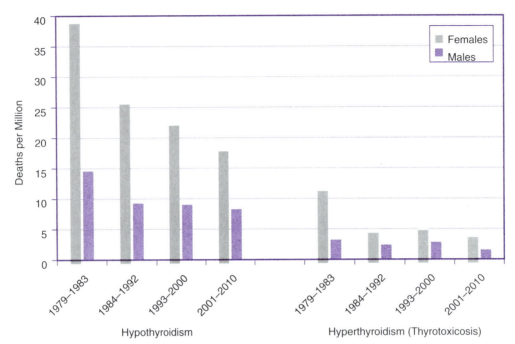

FIGURE 43.2 Annual Mortality for Thyroid Disease, Oxford, England, 1979–2010.

Data from Goldacre, M. J., & Duncan, M. E. (2013). Death rates for acquired hypothyroidism and thyrotoxicosis in English populations (1979–2010): Comparison of underlying cause and all certified causes. *QJM: An International Journal of Medicine, 106*(3), 229–235. Mortality Rates are based on death certificate with any mention of thyroid disease.

17% of death certificates. During the 30-year study period (1979–2010), mortality rates for hypothyroidism decreased 53% in females (from 39.5 to 18.5 per million) and 43% in males (from 14.5 to 8.3 per million). A total of 388 death certificates mentioned thyrotoxicosis in females compared to 91 in males, and the mortality rates for thyrotoxicosis decreased 64% in females (from 11.9 to 4.3 per million) and 75% in males (from 3.2 to 0.8 per million) during the 30-year period of study. Hyperthyroidism was reported as the underlying cause of death on 24% of death certificates. Ischemic heart disease, stroke, and myocardial infarction were the most prominent underlying causes of death when thyroid dysfunction (either hypothyroidism or thyrotoxicosis) was listed as a contributing cause. The investigators attributed the significant decreases in mortality to improvements in the standard of care for thyroid disease (Goldacre & Duncan, 2013).

Several investigations have observed that patients with thyroid dysfunction have increased mortality rates compared to disease-free (euthyroid) individuals. Investigators in Denmark estimated hazard ratios by duration of thyroid dysfunction based on measurements of serum TSH for 239,768 individuals in Funen, Denmark, during 1995–2011. During a mean follow-up of more than 7 years, the hazard ratio for all-cause mortality was 2.2 for hypothyroid individuals (TSH > 4.0 mIU per L) and 1.29 for hyperthyroid individuals (TSH < 0.3 mIU per L). The hazard ratio increased approximately 18% per year for chronically hypothyroid patients and 6% per year for chronically hyperthyroid patients. These results underscore the importance of continuity of care and timely intervention in individuals with thyroid dysfunction (Laulund et al., 2014).

In a recent meta-analysis of prospective cohort studies, investigators in China examined associations between subclinical thyroid dysfunction and mortality from cardiovascular disease. Subclinical thyroid disease is defined as abnormal serum TSH outside the normal range of 0.4–4.0 mIU per L and thyroid hormones (T_3 and T_4) within normal limits. A total of 16 cohort studies involving 71,808 participants, 5178 with subclinical hypothyroidism and 2300 with subclinical hyperthyroidism, were included in the analysis. Composite relative risk (RR) estimates were derived by comparing mortality rates in patients with thyroid dysfunction to the rates for euthyroid individuals. Results showed that subclinical hypothyroidism (TSH > 4.0 mIU per L) was associated with a significant increase in mortality from coronary heart disease (RR = 1.37), and subclinical hyperthyroidism (TSH < 0.4 mIU per L) was associated with significant increases in total mortality (RR = 1.27) and mortality from coronary heart disease (RR = 1.45) (Sun et al., 2017).

▶ Hyperthyroidism

Hyperthyroidism refers to the overproduction of thyroid hormones (T_3 and T_4) by the thyroid gland.

Overt hyperthyroidism is diagnosed when there is low serum TSH and high free T_3 and/or T_4. Overt hyperthyroidism is clinically evident and characterized by anxiety, emotional lability, weakness, tremor, exophthalmos (bulging eyes), vitiligo (blotchy loss of skin color), heat intolerance, diarrhea, increased perspiration, and weight loss despite a normal appetite. Cardiovascular symptoms associated with elevated levels of T_3 and T_4 include angina, palpitations, hypertension, atrial fibrillation, tachycardia, myocardial infarction, congestive heart failure, and stroke (Klein & Ojamaa, 2001). Rare cases of sudden cardiac death have been reported in patients with severe untreated hyperthyroidism (Terndrup, Heisig, & Garceau, 1990).

Subclinical hyperthyroidism is diagnosed when serum TSH is low (<0.4 mIU per L) but the serum levels of T_3 and T_4 are normal. Most patients with subclinical hyperthyroidism do not manifest symptoms and are detected by routine screening of thyroid function (Ross, Cooper, & Mulder, 2018a).

The most common form of hyperthyroidism is a condition known as *Graves' disease* (named after the Irish physician Robert J. Graves who first described the condition in 1835 [Weetman, 2000]). Patients with Graves' disease have high levels of T_3 due to increased secretion and or conversion of T_4 to T_3. Graves' disease is 5–10 times more common in women than men and is characterized by the presence of thyroid-stimulating autoantibodies (Ross, Cooper, & Mulder, 2018).

The second most common cause of hyperthyroidism is *toxic multinodular goiter* which refers to the presence of one or more thyroid nodules that autonomously hypersecrete T_3 and/or T_4. This condition often arises concomitant with iodine deficiency and induction of thyroid hyperplasia due to low levels of T_4 (Orlander, Chlu, & Davis, 2018).

In an early survey of thyroid disease among 2779 residents of Whickham, England, the point prevalence of overt hyperthyroidism was 19 per 1000 females and approximately 2 per 1000 men (Tunbridge et al., 1977). After 20 years of follow-up, the mean annual incidence of hyperthyroidism in the Whickham cohort was 0.8 per 1000 in women and less than 0.1 per 1000 in men (Vanderpump et al., 1995). Similar annual estimates of the incidence of hyperthyroidism (0.77 per 1000 in women and 0.14 per 1000 in men) were obtained in a retrospective cohort study of more than 369,000 residents in Tayside, Scotland, during 1993–1997 (Flynn et al., 2005).

In the United States, TSH, thyroxine (T_4), and thyroid antibodies were measured in 16,533 nationally representative disease-free participants of the NHANES III during 1988–1994. The survey found overt hyperthyroidism in 0.5% of individuals and subclinical disease (defined as serum TSH < 0.4 mIU per L) in 3.2% of the sample (Hollowell et al., 2002). In a subsequent U.S. NHANES study conducted during 2007–2012, the prevalence of clinical hyperthyroidism declined slightly to 0.3% while the prevalence of subclinical disease increased by fourfold to 3.1% (Jain, 2015).

It is important to note that the fourfold higher prevalence of subclinical hyperthyroidism observed in the recent NHANES survey was due to the higher threshold for low TSH compared to the previous study (0.4 versus 0.1 mIU per L). This diagnostic change was made due to evidence suggesting that subclinical hyperthyroidism (defined as TSH < 0.4 mIU per L with normal levels of T_3 and T_4) is associated with an elevated risk of developing cardiovascular diseases, particularly atrial fibrillation (Donangelo & Braunstein, 2011).

Another significant difference between the 1988–1994 and 2007–2012 NHANES surveys was that the prevalence of thyroid peroxidase autoantibodies increased from 13% to 39%. Thyroid autoantibodies are associated with Graves' disease, and in women of reproductive age, they have been found to increase the risk of miscarriage or preterm delivery (Stagnaro-Green et al., 1990).

▶ Graves' Disease

Graves' disease, also called *diffuse toxic goiter*, is believed to arise as a consequence of autoimmune reactions. Graves' disease affects approximately 0.5% of the U.S. population and is the underlying cause of up to 80% of all cases of hyperthyroidism. The clinical signs and symptoms of this condition result from excess stimulation of the thyroid gland by autoantibodies resulting in overproduction of T_3 and T_4 hormones. Molecular studies suggest that circulating IgG antibodies bind to and activate thyrotropin receptors of the thyroid epithelium, thus stimulating hypertrophy and hyperplasia of thyroid follicles. This process results in increased production of thyroid hormones, thyroid enlargement, and goiter formation. The peak incidence of Graves' disease is between 20 and 40 years of age. Symptoms include enlargement of the thyroid gland (goiter), protruding eyes (exophthalmos), palpitations, excess sweating, diarrhea, weight loss, muscle weakness, and unusual sensitivity to heat. Notably, Graves' disease is diagnosed 5–10 times more often in women than men (Brent, 2008; Weetman, 2000). As shown by the age-specific rates for Swedish women and men in **FIGURE 43.3**, the marked female excess of

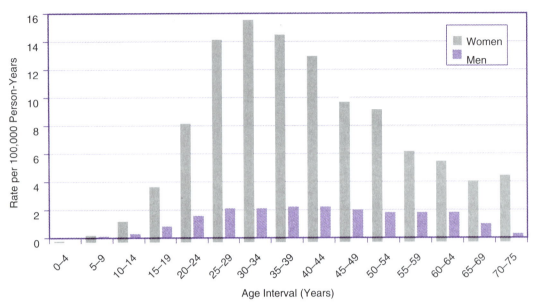

FIGURE 43.3 Age-Specific Incidence of Graves' Disease by Gender in Sweden, 1987–2007.

Data from Hemminki, K., Li, X., Sundquist, J., & Sundquist, K. (2010). The epidemiology of Graves' disease: Evidence of a genetic and an environmental contribution. *Autoimmun, 43*(3), J307–J313.

this condition is evident throughout life (Hemminki, Li, Sundquist, & Sundquist, 2010).

Genetic studies suggest that Graves' disease has a significant hereditary component. A nationwide population-based study of twins ascertained from the Danish Twin Registry during 1953–1976 revealed a concordance rate of 35% among monozygous twins compared to 3% for dizygous twins. In regression models, genetic factors accounted for 79% of the liability to develop Graves' disease compared to 21% for environmental factors. Based on these findings, the investigators suggested that "*genetic factors play a major role in the etiology of Graves' disease*" (Brix, Kyvik, Christensen, & Hegedus, 2001).

A national genetic study of Graves' disease was conducted in Sweden using data from the Swedish Multigeneration Register linked to the Swedish Hospital Discharge Register for the years 1987–2007. Standard incidence ratios were calculated based on familial relationships of 15,743 patients hospitalized for Graves' disease during this time period. Standard incidence ratios were increased fivefold in families with an affected sibling and more than 300-fold in families with two affected siblings. The standard incidence ratio in twins was 16.5. The incidence of Graves' disease was also increased in families with other autoimmune conditions such as Addison's disease, type 1 diabetes mellitus, Hashimoto's thyroiditis, pernicious anemia, myasthenia gravis, lupus erythematosus, and scleroderma. Surprisingly, the standard incidence ratio was also increased among spouses of affected individuals suggesting that environmental factors may also be involved in the genesis

of Graves' disease (Hemminki et al., 2010). Interestingly, cigarette smoking has been linked to the development of multiple autoimmune diseases, including rheumatoid arthritis, systemic lupus erythematosus, multiple sclerosis, and Graves' disease (Costenbader & Karlson, 2006; Manji et al., 2006). Notwithstanding, the genetic factors that influence the thyroid autoimmunity involved in Graves' disease clearly outweigh the environmental factors (Jacobson & Tomer, 2007a, 2007b).

▶ The Human Leukocyte Antigen Locus and Autoimmune Thyroiditis

Genes of the *human leukocyte antigen* (*HLA*) play a major role in the immune response to foreign antigens as well as the recognition of *self versus non-self* in immune reactions. The six major genes of the *super HLA locus* are all located on the short arm of chromosome 6 (Levinson, 2006). Specific HLA genes encode cell-surface antigen-presenting proteins that regulate the processing of bacterial antigens by T lymphocytes and the formation of antibodies by B lymphocytes. The profile of cell membrane HLA proteins differentiates *self from non-self* in the immune response, and perturbations in the system occasionally result in the formation of antibodies that are directed against self. Such autoantibodies are capable of selectively stimulating and/or destroying certain tissues of the body, thereby causing autoimmune disease.

Two classical forms of thyroiditis are known to have an autoimmune basis, Graves' disease and Hashimoto's thyroiditis (discussed in the following section). Genetic variants at the HLA locus appear to increase susceptibility to both conditions. For example, individuals who carry the *HLA-DR3* allele have been found to be three to four times more likely to develop Graves' disease than noncarriers (Farid, Stone, & Johnson, 1980; Jacobson and Tomer, 2007a; Zamani et al., 2000), and likewise, *HLA-DR3* has been found to increase the risk of developing Hashimoto's thyroiditis more than twofold in some populations (Jacobson, Huber, and Tomer, 2008; Tandon, Zhang, & Weetman, 1991). It is hypothesized that the HLA-DR3 protein may heighten susceptibility through its special affinity for thyroid antigens thereby creating an autoimmune response directed against the thyroid gland. Furthermore, there is increasing evidence suggesting that interactions between genetic variants of thyroglobulin and the *HLA-DR3* allele enhance susceptibility to the development of Graves' disease (Jacobson & Tomer, 2007b).

Another candidate gene for conferring susceptibility to the development of autoimmune thyroid disorders is the *cytotoxic T lymphocyte associated antigen-4 (CTLA-4)*. The normal *CTLA-4* gene product helps to regulate the response of T lymphocytes to antigenic stimuli. It apparently provides a negative signal to the T cell thus limiting autoimmune responses and maintaining self-tolerance (Chambers & Allison, 1997). Significant associations have consistently been observed between Graves' disease and certain allelic forms of *CTLA-4*, whereas associations with Hashimoto's thyroiditis are less clear (Chistiakov & Turakulov, 2003).

Other susceptibility genes have also been identified. For example, variants of the gene that encodes *vitamin-D-binding protein* have been linked to the development of Graves' disease. Vitamin-D-binding protein facilitates the transport and release of vitamin D in blood and tissues, and the active form of vitamin D works in concert with calcitonin, parathyroid, and thyroid hormones to regulate calcium and phosphorous homeostasis. Graves' disease combined with low serum vitamin D leads to poor absorption of calcium and related symptoms of muscle wasting, bone resorption, and nervous system dysfunction (Herman-Bonert & Friedman, 2004).

German investigators studied genetic polymorphisms of vitamin-D-binding protein among 561 individuals in families with an offspring affected by either Graves' disease (95 pedigrees) or Hashimoto's thyroiditis (92 pedigrees). They found that allelic variants of vitamin-D-binding protein confer susceptibility to the development of Graves' disease but not Hashimoto's thyroiditis (Pani et al., 2002). In a subsequent genetic case–control study of Graves' disease and vitamin-D-binding protein, Polish investigators compared single nucleotide polymorphisms of 332 cases to 185 healthy control subjects. They found a specific polymorphism at codon 420 involving substitution of lysine for threonine that significantly increased the risk of disease and decreased the level of serum vitamin D (Kurylowicz, Ramos-Lopez, Bednarczuk, & Badenhoop, 2006). These results suggest that genetic regulation of vitamin D activity plays a role in thyroid autoimmunity and the development of Graves' disease.

▶ Hashimoto's Thyroiditis

Hashimoto's thyroiditis is a chronic autoimmune disease in which the thyroid gland is gradually destroyed by the body's own immune system. The disorder was first described by the Japanese physician Dr. Hakaru Hashimoto in 1912 (Hashimoto, 1912). It is diagnosed by clinical symptoms plus the presence of autoantibodies against thyroglobulin or other cellular components of the thyroid gland. Pathologic review of thyroidal tissue from patients reveals inflammation and striking infiltration by lymphocytes admixed with plasma cells, necrosis, and derangement of thyroid follicles plus goitrous enlargement of the gland. Without treatment, there is progressive depletion of thyroid follicles accompanied by hypothyroidism and loss of thyroid function (Rapoport, 1991).

Patients often have a family history of thyroid disorders including Graves' disease and/or other autoimmune conditions such as type 1 diabetes, celiac disease, pernicious anemia, Addison's disease, and Sjogren's syndrome. Hashimoto's thyroiditis is typically diagnosed between the ages of 45 and 65 years and occurs 10–20 times more often in women than men (Vanderpump & Tunbridge, 2002).

Certain genes of the HLA locus confer susceptibility to the development of this disorder (e.g., presence of the *HLA-DR5* gene increases the relative risk more than threefold). As discussed above, the *CTLA-4* gene has also been implicated in the genesis of Hashimoto's thyroiditis (Chistiakov, 2005; Tomer, Barbesino, Greenberg, Concepcion, & Davies, 1999; Yesilkaya et al., 2008).

Grave's disease and Hashimoto's thyroiditis are often treated with oral doses of radioactive iodine, resulting in permanent destruction of cells in the thyroid and rendering them permanently inactive. Another treatment option for these conditions is surgery in which the thyroid gland is partially or fully removed. Patients who undergo thyroid ablation or thyroidectomy receive daily replacement thyroid hormone therapy.

Iatrogenic Hyperthyroidism

Certain medications are known to influence thyroid function. One such agent is *amiodarone*, a potent anti-arrhythmic drug that is prescribed for cardiac arrhythmias such as atrial fibrillation. Amiodarone has a high iodine content and in euthyroid patients it inhibits the conversion of T_4 to T_3 resulting in high levels of T_4 and hyperthyroidism. Nevertheless, in some individuals, amiodarone has been found to inhibit the release of thyroid hormones thereby resulting in hypothyroidism. This paradoxical effect is presumably due to the high content of iodine in amiodarone that enters the bloodstream and suppresses thyroid function, a phenomenon known as the *Wolff–Chaikoff* effect (Basaria & Cooper, 2005).

Exogenous Hyperthyroidism

Exogenous hyperthyroidism refers to ingestion of excessive amounts of thyroid hormone (e.g., levothyroxine [T_4], liothyronine [T_3], or agents containing both T_3 and T_4). In hypothyroid patients that ingest exogenous thyroid hormones on a daily basis, levels should be routinely checked to assure they are within normal limits (Watsky & Koeniger, 1998).

Of further note is that exogenous hyperthyroidism can also develop in euthyroid individuals who inadvertently or purposefully overdose on thyroid hormones to treat obesity, menstrual disorders, depression, or infertility. Such patients should be counseled about the risks of hyperthyroidism and be carefully monitored with thyroid function tests to avoid excessive ingestion of thyroid medications. When exogenous hyperthyroidism arises due to surreptitious ingestion, it is termed *thyrotoxicosis factitia*. Individuals with normal thyroid function should not take thyroid hormones to speed weight loss or treat depression since the acute development of exogenous hyperthyroidism with high levels of circulating T_3 and/or T_4 can induce a thyroid storm with life-threatening consequences (Ross, Cooper, & Mulder, 2018d).

Hypothyroidism

Hypothyroidism refers to an underactive thyroid gland, which results in a deficiency of thyroid hormones (T_3 and T_4). Hypothyroid disorders occur when the thyroid gland is inactive or underactive as a result of improper formation from birth, lack of iodine, or removal or iatrogenic inactivation (ablation) of the thyroid gland. Symptoms of hypothyroidism include abnormal weight gain, fatigue, baldness, temperature intolerance (typically cold), and in some cases thyroid enlargement (*nontoxic goiter*).

Nontoxic goiter, or simply "*goiter*," refers to enlargement of the thyroid gland in conjunction with hypothyroidism. As discussed below, the dominant global cause of goiter is iodine deficiency. Enlargement of the thyroid gland in iodine-deficient children is progressive, initially involving diffuse hyperplasia and later the development of multiple nodules wherein the thyroid follicles are markedly distended by the presence of excess colloid (Robbins & Cotran, 1979). Goiter arising from iodine deficiency is very uncommon in developed countries since iodine is routinely added to salt and other foods for consumption. Indeed, iodized salt has been a prominent feature of the American diet since 1924 (Marine, 1924; McClure, 1935).

The discovery of iodine as an essential mineral for normal function of the thyroid glands and the production of thyroid hormones provides a convincing example of the power of epidemiologic investigation. In 1905, a young physician trained at Johns Hopkins University, David Marine, began his residency training in pathology at Lakeside Hospital on the shores of Lake Erie in Cleveland, Ohio. His interest in thyroid disease was spiked by the high prevalence of goiters in dogs in the area and he began a series of studies to elucidate the cause. Marine observed that dietary supplements of iodine in the form of iodized salt reduced the incidence of goiter in sheep and produced regression of goiters and reversal of hypothyroid symptoms in dogs (Marine, 1907). In pathologic studies, Marine found that large goitrous thyroids from dogs had lower levels of iodine than normal thyroids from healthy dogs (Marine & Williams, 1908). Marine was also called upon to investigate the high rate of "*alleged thyroid carcinomas*" in trout in a fish hatchery in northern Ohio. Pathologic studies revealed that the fish had goiters due to iodine deficiency rather than thyroid carcinomas and Marine demonstrated that goiter development was effectively prevented by the addition of iodine or foods high in iodine content to the trout hatchery water (Marine, 1914).

Marine soon translated these findings to the human population, showing in his clinic that children suffering from simple goiter responded to therapy with sodium iodide. Realizing the devastating problem of goiter in the Great Lakes region, Marine and his colleague, O.P. Kimball, organized and conducted a field intervention study using sodium iodide supplements in the diets of young girls in the Akron, Ohio region. Girls in the 5th–8th grades received 200 mg of sodium iodide for 10 consecutive days and older girls received twice this amount. The dosing regimen was repeated every 6 months. A total of 2305 girls received the supplemental iodine compared to 2190 girls from a nearby region that did not. Results of this field experiment after 30 months of follow-up are summarized in **TABLE 43.1**.

After 30 months of observation, the chemopreventive value of the treatment with sodium iodide was remarkable. Among participants with normal thyroid glands at the beginning of the study, 437 of 1257 girls (27.6%) who *did not* receive iodine developed goiters compared to only 2 of 908 girls (0.2%) who *did* receive iodine. Substantial therapeutic effects were also evident. Among participants with enlarged thyroid glands at baseline, *progression* of disease was observed in only 0.2% of treated girls compared to 14.1% of controls, whereas *regression* of disease was observed in 60.3% of treated girls compared to 13.8% of controls. Importantly, no toxic effects of the sodium iodide supplement were detected in the study (Marine, 1924; Marine & Kimball, 1917, 1920). The definitive evidence from this study was the crowning achievement of Marine's work on iodine deficiency as the causative factor in the development of hypothyroidism and simple goiter.

▶ Cretinism

The health consequences of iodine deficiency often manifest early in life. These include abnormal neuronal development, mental retardation, congenital malformations, and hypothyroidism. Deleterious effects on reproduction such as spontaneous abortion, miscarriage, and infertility are also notable. Later in life, lack of iodine is also associated with intellectual impairment.

Cretinism is an anomaly that is caused by iodine deficiency in the developing fetus. Clinical manifestations of this condition depend upon the gestational timing and severity of iodine and hormonal insufficiency in both the mother and fetus. In the absence of iodine, there is abnormal development and function of the fetal thyroid gland. This devastating condition typically manifests at birth or during infancy and is characterized by hypothyroidism, goiter, mental retardation, deaf-mutism, stunted growth, and other anomalies.

Endemic cretinism was once common in the Alpine populations of Southern Europe due to lack of iodine in their diets. As an example, in Switzerland where the soil contains little iodine, cases of cretinism were once commonplace. In fact, the soils of many inland areas on all continents are iodine deficient, and plants and animals grown there are correspondingly deficient. Populations living in such areas without outside food sources are therefore at high risk for the development of iodine deficiency diseases (Gaitan & Dunn, 1992). Intervention studies conducted in severely iodine-deficient populations provided clear evidence that supplemental iodine given before pregnancy or early in pregnancy prevented the development of cretinism, reduced infant mortality and improved the neurological status of infants and children (Zimmerman, 2012).

Fortunately, the addition of iodine to table salt has virtually eliminated cretinism in developed countries. Furthermore, early detection of thyroid insufficiency in newborns and administration of thyroxine (T_4) can often be effective in reinstating thyroid function and normal growth and development. Nevertheless, in developing nations without such programs, the lack of dietary iodine remains the leading cause of preventable mental retardation in babies and small children.

TABLE 43.1 Effects of Sodium Iodide Supplementation in School Girls of Northern Ohio

Size of Thyroid	Treatment Group	Control Group
Initially normal	$N = 908$	$N = 1257$
Unchanged	906 (99.8%)	910 (72.4%)
Enlarged	2 (0.2%)	437 (27.6%)
Initially enlarged	$N = 1282$	$N = 1048$
Unchanged	506 (39.5%)	755 (72.0%)
Increased	3 (0.2%)	148 (14.1%)
Decreased	773 (60.3%)	145 (13.8%)

Data from Marine, D., & Kimball, O. P. (1920). The prevention of simple goiter in man: Fourth paper. *Archives of Internal Medicine, 25,* 661–672.

▶ Goitrogenic Dietary Factors and Thyroid Disorders

Goitrogens are dietary agents that suppress thyroid function and induce the formation of goiters, particularly in children. The principal goitrogens are *isothiocyanate* and the *isoflavones* (a class of phytoestrogens). These compounds inhibit the activity of *thyroxine peroxidase*, a key enzyme in the formation of thyroid hormones from iodine and tyrosine. Cruciferous vegetables such as broccoli, cauliflower, and cabbage contain high levels of isothiocyanate. Other sources include peanuts, spinach, peaches, and strawberries (Vanderpas, 2006). Soybeans and soy-based products contain high concentrations of isoflavones (Doerge & Sheehan, 2002).

Thiocyanate overload from consumption of cassava root has been found to be goitrogenic in Central Africa, particularly in association with selenium deficiency. The cassava root has low concentrations of iodine and selenium and high concentrations of isothiocyanate. Thilly and colleagues investigated dietary factors and thyroid disorders in children aged 5–7 years from goiter-endemic areas of Central Africa. Low serum levels of thyroxine (T_4) were associated with low selenium and high thiocyanate levels in children residing in regions where cassava is the principal source of carbohydrates in the diet. Furthermore, high rates of cretinism were observed among children with severe iodine and selenium deficiencies in combination with thiocyanate overload (Thilly et al., 1993).

High consumption of soy has also been linked to thyroid disorders in children. Early case reports document goiter development in infants on a soy diet (Hydovitz, 1960). Fort and colleagues studied 59 children with autoimmune thyroid disease, their 76 healthy siblings, and 54 healthy unrelated children. They found that the frequency of feedings with soy-based milk formulas in early life (31%) was significantly higher in children with autoimmune thyroid disease compared to healthy siblings and unrelated children (12%) (Fort, Moses, and Fasano, 1990). Thus, despite some beneficial health effects of soy, the issue of goitrogenic impact remains problematic.

▶ Global Impact of Iodine Deficiency

Following the pioneering research of David Marine in the early 20th century, confirming evidence of the chemopreventive value of supplemental iodine soon became available from studies in Sweden, Switzerland, and other many other nations. In the United States, iodized table salt containing 100 mg per kg of potassium iodide has been available since 1924. The United States Food and Drug Administration recommend 150 µg of iodine per day for both men and women. Supplementing the diet with iodized salt is a simple cost-effective method of ensuring adequate iodine intake and successful population-based programs have increased around the world with the active encouragement and support of the World Health Organization (WHO) (Holman & McCartney, 1960).

Since more than 90% of dietary iodine eventually reaches the urine, the urinary iodine concentration provides an accurate gauge of current intake. Values lower than 100 µg per L indicate insufficient intake and values lower than 20 µg per L indicate severe iodine deficiency. In recent years, WHO has conducted national surveys of the iodine concentration in urinary samples to provide better estimates of the global burden of iodine insufficiency.

According to survey data collected by WHO during 1993–2003, 164 countries had iodized salt programs in 2000 and the percent of households in the developing world that used iodized salt rose from about 20% in 1970 to 70% in 2000. Nevertheless, estimates based on urinary samples suggested that iodine deficiency was present in approximately 2 billion people worldwide and caused a high burden of disease in many developing nations. For example, in India, it was estimated that 100 million suffered from iodine deficiency, 4 million from goiter, and 500,000 from cretinism. Other pockets of iodine deficiency were evident in the Western Pacific, Southeast Asia, Africa, and the Russian Federation (Andersson, Takkouche, Egli, Allen, & de Benoist, 2005).

In 2011, prevalence estimates of iodine insufficiency based on urinary iodine were available for 115 nations compared to only 75 nations in 2003. The urinary iodine survey data in 2011 covered approximately 96% of the world population compared to 92% in 2003. Based on the available survey data of urinary iodine for the world population in 2011, 1.88 billion people were estimated to have insufficient iodine intake, a reduction of about 6% from the estimate of 2 billion people with low intake in 2003. Among school-age children, the global prevalence of insufficient iodine intake fell from 36.5% (285 million) in 2003 to 29.8% (241 million) in 2011, and the number of countries classified as iodine deficient (median urinary iodine less than 100 µg per L) decreased from 54 in 2003 to 32 in 2011. Nevertheless, severe iodine deficiency (<20 µg per L) was detected in 5.2% of children (12.5 million) and more than half of children with insufficient iodine intake lived in either Southeast Asia (76 million) or Africa (58 million). (Andersson, Karumbunathan, & Zimmermann, 2012).

Hypothyroidism in Iodine-Replete Nations

Hypothyroidism has also been studied in prospective cohort studies of populations with sufficient access to iodine. In the Whickham cohort in England, the annual incidence was 3.5 per 1000 in females and 0.6 per 1000 in males (Vanderpump et al., 1995). Slightly higher rates were observed in the Tayside cohort in Scotland, 5.0 per 1000 in females and 0.9 per 1000 in males (Flynn et al., 2004).

In the United States, the prevalence of hypothyroidism was estimated in representative national samples of the population in the NHANES during 1988–1994 and 2007–2012. In these investigations, serum levels of TSH and thyroxine (T_4) were measured to identify subjects with *subclinical hypothyroidism* (elevated TSH with normal T_4) versus *clinical hypothyroidism* (normal TSH and low T_4). Subjects with subclinical hypothyroidism are typically asymptomatic and can only be diagnosed on the basis of laboratory test results, whereas those with clinical hypothyroidism manifest variable symptoms such as fatigue, cold intolerance, weight gain, dry skin, myalgia, and menstrual irregularities often in combination with enlargement of the thyroid gland or goiter (Ross, Cooper, & Mulder, 2018a, 2018b, 2018c).

In the 2007–2012 NHANES survey, the prevalence of *subclinical hypothyroidism* in the general population was 3.5% (3.8% in females and 3.1% in males). Marked differences were observed among ethnic groups (e.g., Caucasians had the highest prevalence [4.4%] and African Americans the lowest [0.6%]). The prevalence increased steadily with age peaking in those 65 years and older at 5.8%. During 1988–1994, the prevalence of subclinical hypothyroidism in the general U.S. population was 4.3%, slightly higher than in 2007–2012. In both NHANES surveys, the prevalence of clinical hypothyroidism was much lower than subclinical hypothyroidism (0.2 per 1000 in 2007–2012 and 0.3 in 1988–1994) (Hollowell et al., 1995; Jain, 2015).

Iodine Deficiency in Pregnancy

Iodine deficiency is particularly problematic in pregnant women since their required intake (250 μg per day) is higher than for nonpregnant women (150 μg per day). Hypothyroidism during gestation is associated with increased risks of abortion, hypertension, anemia, abruptio placentae, and postpartum hemorrhage in the mother and can lead to preterm birth, low birth weight, and respiratory distress in the neonate. Several studies have found that children of mothers with mild-to-moderate iodine deficiency may suffer from hearing impairments and neurological deficits (Sahay & Nagesh, 2012).

Limited national data are available on iodine intake during pregnancy. Surprisingly, most European countries *do not* iodize their salt supply, and as a consequence, levels of iodine intake among pregnant women were recently assessed as adequate in only 10 of 54 nations. In the United Kingdom where currently there is no salt iodization, a recent survey found more than 50% of 1026 pregnant women had intakes of less than 190 μg per day, which is far below the WHO recommended level of 250 μg per day for pregnant women (Comber, Bouga, Pan, & Lean, 2015). The problem appears even more critical in some other developed countries. A recent survey in Australia found low urinary iodine in more than 85% of 139 pregnant women attending an antenatal clinic, and only 11% of participants reported dietary changes to increase iodine intake during pregnancy. Based on their findings, the authors suggested there is an urgent need for improved nutritional education and iodine supplementation for pregnant women (Charlton, Gemming, Yeatman, & Ma, 2015). Thyroid function tests conducted during the first trimester are essential for the early detection of hypothyroidism during pregnancy. Replacement therapy with levothyroxine is recommended to prevent maternal and fetal distress from gestational hypothyroidism (Sahay & Nagesh, 2012).

Prevention of Thyroid Dysfunction

As pointed out by Michael Zimmermann and Kristien Boelaert (2015) in their recent review of thyroid disease,

> *increasing iodine intake in populations with severe iodine deficiency is essential to reduce the prevalence of hypothyroidism and minimize the risk of fetal brain damage. Major benefits of increasing iodine intakes in populations with mild iodine deficiency are a decrease in the prevalence of goiter, thyroid autonomy and thyrotoxicosis in adults, and an increase in IQ in children.* (pp. 286–295)

Since salt is consumed on a regular basis by almost everyone, the most efficient and cost-effective way to deliver iodine in deficient populations is salt iodization. Based on a recent comprehensive review and meta-analysis of published data on the effects and safety of consumption of iodized salt, a team of international experts concluded that salt iodization reduces the risk of goiter, cretinism, low cognitive function, and iodine deficiency (Aburto, Abudou, Candeias, & Wu, 2014). Nevertheless, it has also been pointed out that increasing iodine intake by salt iodization in deficient populations may transiently elevate the risk of thyroid autoimmunity and hyper-thyroidism. Continuing international efforts should therefore focus on implementing and sustaining iodine supplementation programs with careful monitoring for thyroid dysfunction in all nations (Zimmermann, 2018; Zimmermann, Jooste, & Pandav, 2008).

References

Aburto, N., Abudou, M., Candeias, V., & Wu, T. (2014). *Effect and safety of salt iodization to prevent iodine deficiency disorders: A systematic review with meta-analyses.* WHO eLibrary of Evidence for Nutrition Actions (eLENA). Geneva, Switzerland: World Health Organization.

Akamizu, T., Satoh, T., Isozaki, O., Suzuki, A., Wakino, S., Iburi, T., … Japan Thyroid Association. (2017). Diagnostic criteria, clinical features, and incidence of thyroid storm based on nationwide surveys. *Thyroid, 22*(7), 661–679.

Andersson, M., Karumbunathan, V., & Zimmermann, M. B. (2012). Global iodine status in 2011 and trends over the past decade. *The Journal of Nutrition, 132*(4), 744–750.

Andersson, M., Takkouche, B., Egli, I., Allen, H. E., & de Benoist, B. (2005). Current global iodine status and progress over the last decade towards the elimination of iodine deficiency. *Bull World Health Organ, 83*(7), 518–525.

Baldwin, D. B., & Rowett, D. (1978). Incidence of thyroid disorders in Connecticut. *JAMA, 239,* 742–744.

Basaria, S., & Cooper, D. S. (2005). Amiodarone and the thyroid. *The American Journal of Medicine, 118*(7), 706–724.

Brent, G. (2008). Graves' disease. *New England Journal of Medicine, 358,* 2594–2605.

Brix, T. H., Kyvik, K. O., Christensen, K., & Hegedus, L. (2001). Evidence for a major role of heredity in Graves' disease: A population-based study of two Danish twin cohorts. *The Journal of Clinical Endocrinology and Metabolism, 86,* 930–943.

Burch, H. B., & Wartofsky, L. (1993). Life-threatening thyrotoxicosis. Thyroid storm. *Endocrinology and Metabolism Clinics of North America, 22*(2), 263–277.

Chambers, C. A., & Allison, J. P. (1997). Costimulation in T cell responses. *Current Opinion in Immunology, 9,* 396–404.

Charlton, K. E., Gemming, L., Yeatman, H., & Ma, G. (2015). Suboptimal iodine status of Australian pregnant women reflects poor knowledge and practices related to iodine nutrition. *Nutrition, 26*(10), 963–968.

Chistiakov, D. A. (2005). Immunogenetics of Hashimoto's thyroiditis. *Journal of Autoimmune Diseases, 2,* 1–10.

Chistiakov, D. A., & Turakulov, R. I. (2003). CTLA-4 and its role in autoimmune thyroid disease. *Journal of Molecular Endocrinology, 31,* 21–36.

Comber, E., Bouga, M., Pan, B., & Lean, M. E. J. (2015). Iodine and pregnancy: A UK cross-sectional survey of dietary intake, knowledge and awareness. *British Journal of Nutrition, 114*(1), 108–117.

Costenbader, K. H., & Karlson, E. W. (2006). Cigarette smoking and autoimmune disease: What can we learn from epidemiology? *Lupus, 15,* 737–745.

Doerge, D. R., & Sheehan, D. M. (2002). Goitrogenic and estrogenic activity of soy isoflavones. *Environmental Health Perspectives, 110*(Suppl. 3), 439–353.

Donangelo, I., & Braunstein, G. D. (2011). Update on subclinical hyperthyroidism. *American Family Physician, 83*(8), 933–938.

Farid, N. R., Stone, E., & Johnson, G. (1980). Graves' disease and HLA: Clinical and epidemiologic associations. *Clinical Endocrinology (Oxf), 13,* 535–544.

Flynn, R. W., MacDonald, T. M., Morris, A. D., Jung, R. T., & Leese, G. P. (2004). The thyroid epidemiology, audit and research study: Thyroid dysfunction in the general population. *The Journal of Clinical Endocrinology and Metabolism, 89*(8), 3879–3884.

Fort, P., Moses, N., & Fasano, M. (1990). Breast and soy-formula feedings in early infancy and the prevalence of autoimmune thyroid disease in children. *Journal of the American College of Nutrition, 9,* 164–167.

Gaitan, E., & Dunn, J. T. (1992). Epidemiology of iodine deficiency. *Trends in Endocrinology and Metabolism, 3*(5), 170–175.

Garber, J. R., Cobin, R. H., Gharib, H., Hennessey, J. V., Klein, I., Mechanick, J. I., … Woeber, K. A. (2012). Clinical practice guidelines for hypothyroidism in adults: Cosponsored by the American Association of Clinical Endocrinologists and the American Thyroid Association. *Endocrine Practice, 18*(6), 988–1028.

Goldacre, M. J., & Duncan, M. E. (2013). Death rates for acquired hypothyroidism and thyrotoxicosis in English populations (1979–2010): Comparison of underlying cause and all certified causes. *QJM: An International Journal of Medicine, 106*(3), 229–235.

Hashimoto, H. (1912). Report on lymphomatous goiter. *'Archiv für klinische Chirurgie,' Berlin, 97,* 219–248.

Hemminki, K., Li, X., Sundquist, J., & Sundquist, K. (2010). The epidemiology of Graves' disease: Evidence of a genetic and an environmental contribution. *Autoimmun, 43*(3), J307–J313.

Herman-Bonert, V., & Friedman, T. C. (2004). The thyroid gland. In C. C. J. Carpenter, R. C. Griggs, & J. Loscalzo (Eds.), *Cecil essentials of medicine* (6th ed., pp. 593–602). Philadelphia, PA: W.B. Saunders.

Hollowell, J. G., Staehling, N. W., Flanders, W. D., Hannon, W. H., Gunter, E. W., Spencer, C. A., & Braverman, L. E. (2002). Serum TSH, T(4), and thyroid antibodies in the United States population (1988–1994): National Health and Nutrition Examination Survey (NHANES III). *The Journal of Clinical Endocrinology and Metabolism, 87,* 489–499.

Holman, J. C. M., & McCartney, W. (1960). Iodized salt. *Endemic Goitre, 1960,* 411–441. (Geneva, Switzerland: WHO.)

Hydovitz, J. D. (1960). Occurrence of goiter in an infant on a soy diet. *NEJM, 262,* 351–353.

Jacobson, E. M., Huber, A., & Tomer, Y. (2008). The HLA gene complex in thyroid autoimmunity: From epidemiology to etiology. *Journal of Autoimmunity, 30*(1–2), 58–62.

Jacobson, E. M., & Tomer, Y. (2007a). The genetic basis of thyroid autoimmunity. *Thyroid, 17,* 949–961.

Jacobson, E. M., & Tomer, Y. (2007b). The CD40, CTLA-4, thyroglobulin, TSH receptor, and PTPN22 gene quintet and its contribution to thyroid autoimmunity: Back to the future. *Journal of Autoimmunity, 28*(2–3), 85–98.

Jain, R. B. (2015). Thyroid profile of the reference United States population: Data from NHANES 2007–2012. *International Archives of Endocrinology Clinical Research, 1,* 1.

Klein, I., & Ojamaa, K. (2001). Thyroid hormone and the cardiovascular system. *New England Journal of Medicine, 344*(7), 501–509.

Kurylowicz, A., Ramos-Lopez, E., Bednarczuk, T., & Badenhoop, K. (2006). Vitamin D-binding protein (DBP) gene polymorphism is associated with Graves' disease and the vitamin D status in a Polish population study. *Experimental and Clinical Endocrinology & Diabetes, 114*(6), 329–335.

Laulund, A. S., Nybo, M., Brix, T. H., Abrahamsen, B., Jørgensen, H. L., & Hegedüs, L. (2014). Duration of thyroid dysfunction correlates with all-cause mortality. The OPENTHYRO Register Cohort. *PLoS ONE, 9*(10), e110437. doi:10.1371/journal.pone.0110437.

Levinson, W. (2006). Major histocompatibility complex and transplantation. In *Review of medical microbiology and immunology* (9th ed., pp. 443–439). London, UK: McGraw-Hill.

Madariaga, A. G., Palacios, S. S., Guillén-Grima, F., & Galofré, J. C. (2014). The incidence and prevalence of thyroid dysfunction in Europe: A meta-analysis. *The Journal of Clinical Endocrinology & Metabolism, 99*(3), 923–931.

Manji, N., Carr-Smith, J. D., Boelaert, K., Allahabadia, A., Armitage, M., Chatterjee, V. K., … Franklyn, J. A. (2006). Influences of age, gender, smoking, and family history on autoimmune thyroid disease phenotype. *The Journal of Clinical Endocrinology and Metabolism, 91,* 4873–4880.

Marine, D. (1907). On the occurrence and physiological nature of glandular hyperplasia of the thyroid (dog and sheep), together with remarks on important clinical (human) problems. *Johns Hopkins Bull, 18,* 359–365.

Marine, D. (1914). Further observations and experiments on goitre (so called thyroid carcinoma) in brook trout (Salvelinus fontinalis). *Journal of Experimental Medicine, 19,* 70–88.

Marine, D. (1924). Etiology and prevention of simple goiter. *Harvey Lectures Series, 19,* 96–122. (Philadelphia, PA: J.B. Lippincott.)

Marine, D., & Kimball, O. P. (1917). The prevention of simple goiter in man. *The Journal of Laboratory and Clinical Medicine, 3,* 40–48.

Marine, D., & Kimball, O. P. (1920). The prevention of simple goiter in man: Fourth paper. *Archives of Internal Medicine, 25,* 661–672.

Marine, D., & Williams, W. W. (1908). The relation of iodine to the structure of the thyroid gland. *Archives of Internal Medicine, 1,* 439–384.

McClure, R. D. (1935). Goiter prophylaxis with iodized salt. *Science (New York, NY), 82*(2129), 370–371.

Ono, Y., Ono, S., Yasunaga, H., Matsui, H., Fushimi, K., & Tanaka, Y. (2017). Clinical characteristics and outcomes of myxedema coma: Analysis of a national inpatient database in Japan. *Journal of Epidemiology, 27*(3), 117–122.

Orlander, P. R., Chlu, C. B., & Davis, A. B. (2016). Toxic nodular goiter. *Medscape.* Retrieved from emedicine.medscape.com

Pani, M. A., Regulla, K., Segni, M., Hofmann, S., Hüfner, M., Pasquino, A. M., … Badenhoop, K. (2002). A polymorphism within the vitamin D-binding protein gene is associated with Graves' disease but not with Hashimoto's thyroiditis. *The Journal of Clinical Endocrinology and Metabolism, 87,* 2564–2567.

Rapoport, B. (1991). Pathophysiology of Hashimoto's thyroiditis and hypothyroidism. *Annual Review Medicine, 42,* 91–96.

Robbins, S. L., & Cotran, R. S. (1979). *Pathologic basis of disease* (2nd ed.). Philadelphia, PA: WB Saunders Company.

Ross, D., Cooper, D. S., & Mulder, J. E. (2018a). Diagnosis of hyperthyroidism. *UpToDate.* Retrieved from www.uptodate.com

Ross, D., Cooper, D. S., & Mulder, J. E. (2018b). Subclinical hypothyroidism in nonpregnant adults. *UpToDate.* Retrieved from www.uptodate.com

Ross, D., Cooper, D. S., & Mulder, J. E. (2018c). Diagnosis and screening for hypothyroidism in nonpregnant adults. *UpToDate.* Retrieved from www.uptodate.com

Ross, D., Cooper, D. S., & Mulder, J. E. (2018d). Exogenous hyperthyroidism. *UpToDate.* Retrieved from www.uptodate.com

Sahay, R. K., & Nagesh, V. S. (2012). Hypothyroidism in pregnancy. *Indian Journal of Endocrinology and Metabolism, 16*(3), 364–370.

Stagnaro-Green, A., Roman, S. H., Cobin, R. H., El-Harazy, E., Alvarez-Marfany, A., & Davies, T. F. (1990). Detection of at-risk pregnancy by means of highly sensitive assays for thyroid autoantibodies. *JAMA, 264*(11), 1422–1425.

Sun, J., Yao, L., Fang, Y., Yang, R., Chen, Y., Yang, K., & Tian, L. (2017). Relationship between subclinical thyroid dysfunction and the risk of cardiovascular outcomes: A systematic review and meta-analysis of prospective cohort studies. *International Journal of Endocrinology, 2017.* doi:10.1155/2017/8130796.

Tandon, N., Zhang, L., & Weetman, A. P. (1991). HLA associations with Hashimoto's thyroiditis. *Clinical Endocrinology (Oxf), 43,* 383–386.

Terndrup, T. E., Heisig, D. G., & Garceau, J. P. (1990). Sudden death associated with undiagnosed Graves' disease. *Journal of Emergency Medicine, 8*(5), 553–555.

Thilly, C. H., Swennen, B., Bourdoux, P., Ntambue, K., Moreno-Reyes, R., Gillies, J., & Vanderpas, J. B. (1993). The epidemiology of iodine-deficiency disorders in relation to goitrogenic factors and thyroid-stimulating-hormone regulation. *American Journal of Clinical Nutrition, 57,* 267S–270S.

Tomer, Y., Barbesino, G., Greenberg, D. A., Concepcion, E., & Davies, T. F. (1999). Mapping the major susceptibility loci for familial Graves' and Hashimoto's diseases: Evidence for genetic heterogeneity and gene interactions. *The Journal of Clinical Endocrinology and Metabolism, 84,* 4656–4664.

Tunbridge, W. M. G., Evered, D. C., Hall, R., Appleton, P. A., Brewis, M., Clark, F., … Smith, P. A. (1977). The spectrum of thyroid disease in a community: The Whickham survey. *Clinical Endocrinology, 7,* 481–493.

Vanderpas, J. (2006). Nutritional epidemiology and thyroid hormone metabolism. *Annual Review of Nutrition, 26,* 293–322. Retrieved from http://en.wikipedia.org/wiki/Digital_object_identifier

Vanderpump, M. P. (2011). The epidemiology of thyroid disease. *British Medical Bulletin, 99,* 39–51.

Vanderpump, M. P., & Tunbridge, W. M. (2002). Epidemiology and prevention of clinical and subclinical hypothyroidism. *Thyroid, 12,* 839–847.

Vanderpump, M. P., Tunbridge, W. M., French, J. M., Appleton, D., Bates, D., Clark, F., … Young, E. T. (1995). The incidence of thyroid disorders in the community: A twenty-year follow-up of the Whickham Survey. *Clinical Endocrinology (Oxf), 43*(1), 55–68. doi:10.1093/bmb/ldr030.

Watsky, J. G., & Koeniger, M. A. Prevalence of iatrogenic hyperthyroidism in a community hospital. *The Journal of the American Board of Family Medicine, 11*, 175–179.

Weetman, A. P. (2000). Graves' disease. *New England Journal of Medicine, 433*, 1236–1248.

Yesilkaya, E., Koc, A., Bideci, A., Camurdan, O., Boyraz, M., Erkal, O., … Cinaz, P. (2008). CTLA4 gene polymorphisms in children and adolescents with autoimmune thyroid diseases. *Genetic Testing, 12*(3), 461–464.

Zamani, M., Spaepen, M., Bex, M., Bouillon, R., & Cassiman, J. J. (2000). Primary role of the HLA class II DRB1*0301 allele in Graves disease. *American Journal of Medical Genetics, 95*(5), 432–437.

Zimmermann, M. B. (2012). The effects of iodine deficiency in pregnancy and infancy. *Paediatric and Perinatal Epidemiology, 26*(Suppl. 1), 108–117.

Zimmermann, M. B. (2018). Efficacy and safety of iodine fortification. In M. G. V. Mannar & R. Hurrel (Eds.), *Food fortification in a globalized world* (pp. 221–230). Amsterdam, The Netherlands: Elsevier Inc.

Zimmermann, M. B., & Boelaert, K. (2015). Iodine deficiency and thyroid disorders. *The Lancet, Diabetes & Endocrinology, 3*(4), 286–295.

Zimmermann, M. B., Jooste, P. L., & Pandav, C. S. (2008). Iodine-deficiency disorders. *The Lancet, 372*(9645), 1251–1262.

CHAPTER 44

Epidemiology of Chronic Kidney Disease

▶ Anatomy and Function of the Kidneys

The human kidneys are paired organs that perform multiple functions that are essential for life. They excrete waste products of metabolism, regulate the body's concentration of water and salt, maintain the acid–base balance of the blood, regulate blood pressure, and secrete important hormones including erythropoietin, renin, and prostaglandins. These physiological functions necessarily require a high degree of structural complexity (Robbins & Cotran, 1979).

Kidneys are bean-shaped organs weighing about 150 g that are located in the retroperitoneal cavity. Individual renal arteries branching from the abdominal aorta supply blood to the kidneys. The kidneys filter about 17 L of blood per day producing a derived specialized filtrate of about 1 L of urine.

Urea is the most abundant of the nitrogen-containing waste products excreted by the kidneys. Urea is formed from ammonia or amino acids by a series of reactions known as the urea cycle, which occurs primarily in the liver. Ammonia arising from the metabolism of amino acids and nitrogen-containing compounds is rapidly transported by red bloods cells to the liver where it enters the urea cycle.

Ammonia itself is highly toxic and cannot be filtered by the kidneys. In contrast, its breakdown product, urea, is colorless, odorless, highly soluble in water, and nontoxic in humans. Urea formed in the liver is transported in the blood to the kidneys where it is freely filtered by the glomeruli and becomes a major constituent of urine.

The basic functional unit of the kidney is the nephron (**FIGURE 44.1**). Each kidney contains up to 1 million nephrons that carry out the essential functions of the kidney. Each nephron receives un-filtered blood from an afferent arteriole which divides into capillaries of the glomerulus. The glomerulus is contained in a structure known as Bowman's capsule. The glomerulus filters urea and other waste products from the blood. The glomerular filtrate enters Bowman's space, diffuses into the renal tubule, and then travels along the renal tubule that is lined with a single layer of specialized endothelial cells and surrounded by capillaries. As the glomerular filtrate traverses the renal tubule, salt, water, glucose, and other small molecules are reabsorbed from the filtrate into the blood, and additional waste products (e.g., ammonia, hydrogen, and potassium ions) are secreted from the blood into the urine. Urine exits the nephron via collecting ducts at the end of the renal tubule. Filtered arteriole blood exits the nephron through the efferent arteriole.

▶ Glomerular Filtration Rate

Renal function is clinically determined by measuring the glomerular filtration rate (GFR). This is accomplished by injecting a standard bolus of inulin into

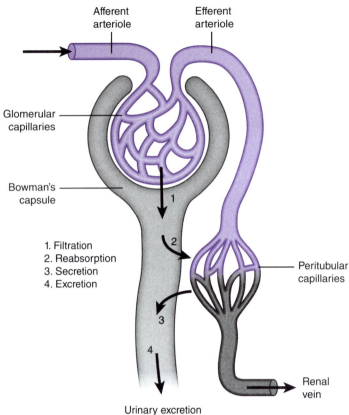

FIGURE 44.1 The Nephron of the Kidney.
© Jones & Bartlett Learning.

the blood and measuring the rate of its excretion in the urine. Inulin is a compound that is neither secreted nor reabsorbed by the kidney. Thus, inulin excretion can be used to accurately determine the volume of fluid that is being filtered by the glomeruli of the kidneys per unit of time. A useful indirect measure of the GFR can be obtained by measuring the creatinine clearance (the amount of creatinine removed from the blood by the kidneys) over a 24-hour period. Creatinine is a breakdown product of muscle metabolism and is freely filtered by the kidneys. Since a small amount of creatinine is secreted from the blood into the urine, the creatinine clearance slightly overestimates the GFR. Creatinine clearance values are also routinely corrected for body mass (muscle mass).

▶ Diagnosis of Chronic Kidney Disease

Kidney disease can be diagnosed by the symptom complex of protein (albumin) in the urine, hypertension, and edema. These common symptoms of kidney disease were originally described in 1827 by the English physician, Richard Bright. Albeit, these symptoms are manifest in many forms of kidney disease and more sophisticated methods of differentiating the various types of kidney disease have now been developed (Cameron, 1972a, 1972b, 1972c).

Chronic kidney disease is pathologically classified into nephrosis and/or nephritis. *Nephrosis* implies kidney disease with proteinuria (excess loss of protein in the urine) in the absence of inflammatory disease. *Nephritis* implies an inflammatory disease of the kidneys evidenced by the presence of inflammatory cells of the immune system. *Glomerulonephritis* refers specifically to inflammation of the glomeruli. In chronic forms of these conditions, there is damage to the kidneys resulting in dysfunctional filtration of blood and alterations in the volume and composition of urine excreted.

Irrespective of the pathology, the diagnosis of kidney disease is largely based upon the GFR and the presence of protein (proteinuria) or abnormal substances in the urine. The GFR measures the rate at which blood is filtered by the kidneys. Normal GFR values adjusted for body surface area are similar in

TABLE 44.1 Stages of Kidney Disease

Stage of CKD	GFR in mL per min per 1.73 m²
0 (Normal)	GFR > 90, no proteinuria
1 (Abnormal)	GFR > 90, proteinuria
2 (Mild)	GFR 60–89
3 (Moderate)	GFR 30–59
4 (Severe)	GFR 15–29
5 (Kidney failure)	GFR < 15 (End-stage renal disease)

CKD = Chronic kidney disease and GFR = Glomerular filtration rate.

men and women, in the range of 90–130 mL per min per 1.73 m². The severity of chronic kidney disease is categorized into the following six stages, which depend on both the GFR and the presence of protein in the urine (proteinuria) (Fraser & Blakeman, 2016) (**TABLE 44.1**).

Measurement of the GFR over time has also proven to be an important clinical tool for assessing improvement of renal function in response to therapy versus progression of disease in patients with chronic kidney disease. In a recent meta-analysis of GFR and chronic kidney disease published during 1975–2012, rates of end-stage renal disease (ESRD) and all-cause mortality were examined among more than 1.7 million participants of 35 prospective cohort studies in which the rate of change in GFR was measured. Among patients initially detected with moderate kidney disease (GFR < 60) who progressed to severe disease within 2 years, the hazard ratio for progression to end-stage disease increased 32-fold. In patients initially detected with severe disease (GFR < 30) who progressed to severe disease within 2 years, the average 10-year risk of developing ESRD was 99% and the risk of death was 77%. It is important to note that the risk estimates were adjusted for multiple factors and conditions including systolic blood pressure, total cholesterol, diabetes, and history of cardiovascular disease. These results indicate that the progression of chronic kidney disease to ESRD and ultimately death can be accurately predicted by the level of GFR at the time of diagnosis and the rate of GFR decline (Coresh et al., 2014).

▶ Epidemiologic Transition of Chronic Kidney Disease

In developed nations of the world, the underlying causes of chronic kidney disease have changed dramatically in the past few decades in parallel with the "*epidemiologic transition*." This phenomenon generally refers to the transition from acute infectious conditions to chronic non-communicable diseases brought about by advances in health care. Prominent features include a decline in the birth rate, slowing of population growth, and aging of the population. As a consequence of the epidemiologic transition, non-communicable degenerative chronic diseases rather than infectious conditions are now the dominant causes of morbidity and mortality (Orman, 2005).

The epidemiologic transition is particularly evident in the emerging pattern of morbidity and mortality of chronic kidney disease and its underlying causes. As discussed in the following sections of this chapter, diabetic nephropathy is now the leading cause of chronic kidney disease and ESRD, followed by hypertensive nephropathy and chronic glomerulonephritis.

▶ Global Burden of Chronic Kidney Disease

Since 1990, chronic kidney disease has been investigated as a component of the Global Burden of Disease (GBD) studies coordinated by the *World Health Organization* (WHO) and more recently, the *Institute of Health Metrics and Evaluation* (IHME). The GBD studies quantify incidence, prevalence, mortality, and disability-adjusted life years for chronic diseases in 21 regions and involve hundreds of collaborators worldwide.

Based on data from GBD studies, the number of deaths from chronic kidney disease increased from 599,000 in 1990 to 1.19 million in 2016, an increase of 98% for the 27-year period. Likewise, during the same period, the number of individuals with chronic kidney disease in the world population rose from 147.6 million in 1990 to 275.9 million in 2016, an overall increase of 87%. Based on comparisons of *crude rates*, the mortality was 41% higher in 2016 than 1990 (16.1 per 100,000 vs. 11.4 per 100,000), the incidence was 34% higher in 2016 than 1990 (289 per 100,000 vs. 215 per 100,000) and the prevalence was 33% higher in 2016 than 1990 (2804 per 100,000 vs. 3733 per 100,000). Differences in crude rates were predominately due to aging and growth of the world population, since they were largely attenuated by age standardization. Age-standardized rates were higher for nations ranking in the lowest quintile of income per capita (e.g., in 2016, the age-adjusted mortality in low-income nations was nearly double the rate in high-income nations [21.4 per 100,000 vs. 11.2 per 100,000]) (Xie et al., 2018).

Cardiovascular Deaths and Chronic Kidney Disease

During the progression of chronic kidney disease over time, patients are likely to die from diseases other than ESRD, particularly cardiovascular diseases. Recent studies have therefore focused on cardiovascular death rates among patients with chronic kidney disease. An international team of investigators conducted a meta-analysis of data from 188 countries to estimate mortality rates due to cardiovascular diseases among individuals with abnormally low levels of GFR indicative of chronic kidney disease. During 2013, among individuals with reduced GFR levels, more people died from cardiovascular disease (1.2 million) than from ESRD (956,000 deaths). The investigators concluded that more studies are needed to evaluate GFR screening programs, not only for the early detection and therapy of chronic kidney disease, but also in order to initiate preventive strategies and therapy for cardiovascular conditions in patients found to have reduced levels of GFR (Thomas et al., 2013).

Global Pattern of Chronic Kidney Disease: Mortality

Chronic kidney disease has risen dramatically in the global rankings of cause of death, from 27th in 1990 to 13th in 2013 (Jager & Fraser, 2017; Murray & Lopez, 1997). The 2012 global pattern of mortality from chronic kidney disease and end-stage renal failure (ESRF) reflects a mixture of causation (**FIGURE 44.2**). High death rates primarily due to diabetic nephropathy are evident in developed nations with high rates of diabetes and obesity (e.g., North America, South America, and Western Europe), whereas death rates are also high from hypertensive nephropathy and chronic glomerulonephritis in developing nations where rates of malaria, schistosomiasis, hepatitis, and other infections are high (e.g., India, Pakistan, Mongolia, Southeast Asia, and Africa).

Chronic Kidney Disease in Developing Countries

FIGURE 44.3 characterizes the global burden of kidney disease by the *disability-adjusted life years* (DALY) that were lost annually from nephritis (primarily glomerulonephritis) and nephrosis in 2004 (WHO, 2009). Disease burdens were highest throughout Africa and certain regions of the Middle East, Southern Asia, and South America. Populations living in these regions are heavily exposed to infection by endemic parasites that

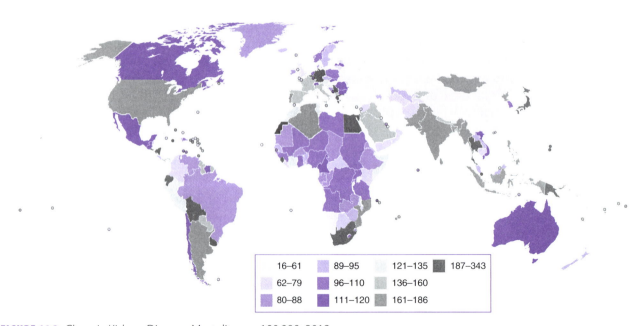

16–61	89–95	121–135	187–343
62–79	96–110	136–160	
80–88	111–120	161–186	

FIGURE 44.2 Chronic Kidney Disease, Mortality per 100,000, 2012.

Data from the World Health Organization. (2016). *Estimated deaths from kidney disease in 2012.* Geneva, Switzerland: World Health Organization.

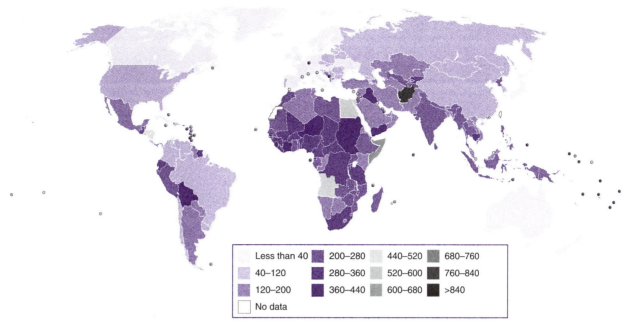

FIGURE 44.3 DALY Due to Glomerulonephritis and Nephrosis.

Data from World Health Organization. (2009). *The global burden of disease: 2004 update*. Geneva: WHO. Available at www.who.int/evidence/bod

Disability Adjusted Life Years per 100,000 individuals.

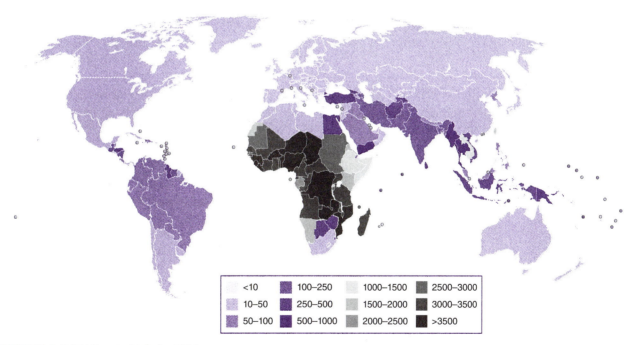

FIGURE 44.4 DALY Due to Malaria, 2004.

Data from World Health Organization. (2008). *The global burden of disease: 2004 update*. Geneva: WHO. Available at www.who.int/evidence/bod

Disability Adjusted Life Years per 100,000 individuals.

are capable of compromising renal function. Principal risk factors in the developed nations of North America, Western Europe, and Australasia include type 2 diabetes, hypertension, and obesity.

As shown in Figure 44.3, high DALYs are evident throughout Africa and in certain regions of the Middle East, Southern Asia, and South America. Interestingly, there is significant overlap of the DALYs

from renal disease in these regions (particularly in Africa) with high DALYs due to malarial infection as well as infection of the urinary tract by the parasitic schistosome worm (see **FIGURES 44.4** and **44.5**). Numerous reports provide evidence that chronic malaria or chronic schistosomiasis (also called *bilharzias*), parasitic conditions that affect millions of Africans, markedly heighten the risk of chronic renal

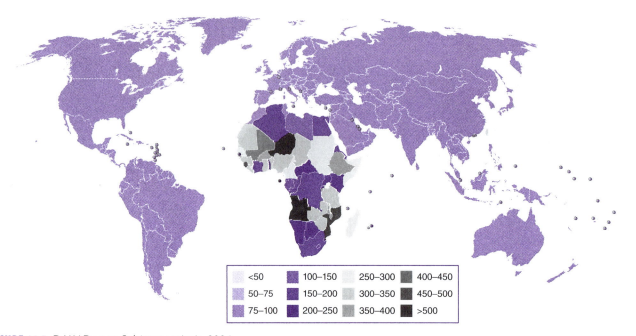

FIGURE 44.5 DALY Due to Schistosomiasis, 2004.

Data from World Health Organization. (2008). *The global burden of disease: 2004 update*. Geneva: WHO. Available at www.who.int/evidence/bod

Disability Adjusted Life Years per 100,000 individuals.

failure from glomerulonephritis (Cameron, 1972a, 1972b, 1972c; Collins & Jeffery, 2007; Mahakur et al., 1983; Martinelli, Noblat, Brito, & Rocha, 1989; Oyediran, 1979).

Some plasmodial (malarial) infections are capable of causing acute renal failure whereas others are more likely to cause chronic disease. In a hospital survey conducted in Gujarat state in Western India during 1988–1992, malarial plasmodial infection by *P. vivax* or *P. falciparum* caused tubular necrosis and acute renal failure in 1.6% and 12.8% of cases, respectively (Rajapurkar, 1994); and in a similar hospital survey in northern India, acute renal failure occurred in 1.1% of cases with malarial infection. Pathogenesis is related to parasitemia-induced deformities in red blood cells such that deformed red blood cells are filtered in the kidney, causing occlusion of small blood vessels and ischemic damage to renal tubules.

Plasmodium malariae causes "*quartan malaria*," an infectious condition that may persist for many years. The term quartan malaria refers to the four fever spikes that occur in infected patients at regular 3-month intervals during the year. The relationship between quartan malaria and the nephrotic syndrome (massive proteinuria, low blood albumin, generalized edema, hypertension, and hyperlipidemia) was initially recognized by Giglioli in 1930 and has since been noted by many investigators in regions where *P. malariae* is endemic (Cameron, 1972a, 1972b, 1972c; Collins & Jeffery, 2007; Gioglioli, 1930). Persistent quartan malaria can lead to chronic glomerulonephritis and renal failure by continual deposition of

malarial antigen–antibody complexes in the glomeruli (Dixon, 1966).

Urinary tract schistosomiasis can also cause renal failure due to obstructive uropathy, pyelonephritis, or bladder carcinoma (occurring usually 10–20 years after the initial infection). In addition, immune complexes that contain schistosome antigens may deposit in the glomeruli, leading to glomerulonephritis and amyloidosis (Barsoum, 2003). Furthermore, leishmaniasis (also called *kalaazar*), another parasitic disease that is prevalent in Afghanistan and certain nations of the Middle East, Southern Asia, and Africa, has been found to cause renal failure and hydronephrosis (edematous kidneys due to urinary obstruction) in chronically infected patients (Prakash et al., 2007; Prasad, Sen, & Ganguly, 1992). Some of these nations may have a double burden of disease due to obstructive uropathy and glomerulonephritis caused by infectious parasites as well as chronic kidney disease caused by chronic noninfectious conditions such as diabetes and hypertension (Naicker, 2003).

Chronic Kidney Disease in Developed Countries

As a consequence of the epidemiologic transition from infectious to chronic diseases and the resultant increase in longevity, the world population has experienced a dramatic change in the causes of ESRD. In nations of the developed world, the profile of risk factors for chronic kidney disease closely resembles that

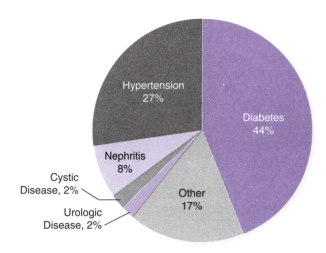

FIGURE 44.6 Primary Causes of Kidney Failure in the United States, 2008.

Data from U.S. National Kidney and Urologic Diseases Information Clearinghouse (2008).

for cardiovascular disease. Type 2 diabetes is now the major cause, and other chronic conditions, principally hypertension, hyperlipidemia, smoking, and obesity, are contributing factors. For example, in the United States, it is estimated that diabetes and hypertension account for 44% and 27%, respectively, of the cases of chronic kidney failure (National Kidney and Urologic Diseases Information Clearinghouse, 2008). The primary causes of kidney failure in the United States are shown in **FIGURE 44.6**.

▶ Causation of Chronic Kidney Disease

Recent global investigations of chronic kidney disease using GBD data have partitioned the number of cases and deaths into four categories related to causation: diabetes mellitus, hypertension, glomerulonephritis, and other causes. In the world population during 2016, 42% of incident cases were attributed to diabetes, 17% to hypertension, 19% to glomerulonephritis, and 22% to other causes (Wang et al., 2016; Xie et al., 2018). The following sections discuss the major causes of chronic kidney disease (diabetic nephropathy, hypertensive nephropathy, and glomerulonephritis) and other risk factors and conditions that contribute to pathogenesis.

▶ Diabetic Nephropathy

Diabetic nephropathy is a clinical syndrome characterized by persistent albuminuria that is confirmed on at least two occasions 3–6 months apart, a relentless decline in the GFR and elevated arterial blood pressure.

Diabetic nephropathy is the leading cause of chronic renal failure in the United States and other Western societies. It is also one of the most significant long-term complications in terms of morbidity and mortality for individual patients with diabetes. According to the United States Renal Data System National Health Interview Survey, between 1984 and 2002 the incidence of ESRD attributed to diabetes increased from 29.7 to 151.3 per 1 million population corresponding to a 409% increase. Diabetes is now responsible for more than 40% of all cases of ESRD in the United States (National Kidney and Urologic Diseases Information Clearinghouse, 2008; Ritz & Orth, 1999).

Many epidemiologic studies provide consistent evidence that diabetes and prediabetes are significant risk factors for the development of kidney disease. Investigators at the University of Wisconsin–Madison conducted a long-term prospective study of 1460 individuals diagnosed with diabetes in order to determine the incidence of proteinuria. During 10 years of follow-up, proteinuria developed in 28% of younger individuals (<30 years of age at baseline) compared to 33% of older individuals not taking insulin and 40% of older individuals taking insulin. The risk was highest for individuals with multiple risk factors (high glycosylated hemoglobin, hypertension, and smoking) suggesting that modification of all three of these factors should be considered in the prevention of diabetic nephropathy (Klein, Klein, Moss, & Cruickshanks, 1995).

In the Framingham Heart Study, 2398 subjects free of chronic kidney disease were drawn from the *Framingham offspring cohort* and given an oral glucose tolerance test during 1991–1995. After seven years of follow-up, the odds of developing chronic kidney disease were increased for incident diabetic cases (OR = 1.7) and prevalent diabetic cases (OR = 1.9) compared to subjects who were not diabetic at baseline. These estimates were adjusted for classical risk factors of cardiovascular disease (hypertension, smoking, cholesterol, and obesity). The *crude* unadjusted disease odds were also increased for individuals with prediabetic fasting glucose or impaired glucose tolerance (OR = 1.6); however, adjustment for classical risk factors of cardiovascular disease explained much of the risk associated with prediabetic status (Fox et al., 2005).

Both type 1 diabetes and type 2 diabetes predispose to diabetic nephropathy. In a New Jersey study of 717 African Americans with type 1 diabetes, the prevalence of proteinuria increased with age and duration of diabetes (e.g., proteinuria was present in 85% of subjects over 44 years of age and 72% of subjects who had undergone treatment for type 1 diabetes for 25 years or more). Hypertension and poor glycemic control were also significant predictive factors (Roy, 2004).

Epidemiological studies show that the prevalence of proteinuria increases with the duration of either type 1 or type 2 diabetes (**FIGURE 44.7**). Beginning about 10 years after diagnosis, the prevalence increases exponentially for each type and is only slightly higher for type 2 diabetes. Furthermore, without aggressive therapy and tight glycemic control, progression to renal failure is expected in 60% or more of patients within 5 years of the onset of proteinuria (Hasslacher, Ritz, Wahl, & Michael, 1989; Keller, Bergis, Fliser, & Ritz, 1996; Ritz & Orth, 1999).

Results of randomized clinical trials provide convincing evidence that the risk of developing proteinuria and ESRD in diabetic patients can be significantly reduced in diabetic patients by improving glycemic control using either insulin or oral antihyperglycemic agents (Kawazu et al., 1994; UK Prospective Diabetes Study, 1998). Nevertheless, the target level of glycosylated hemoglobin for optimal control remains under study (Ismail, Becker, Strzelczyk, & Ritz, 1999).

Chronic diabetes induces several pathological changes in the kidney including thickening of the glomerular basement membrane, proliferation of the mesangial cells (phagocytic cells), and glomerular sclerosis (scarring) due to hyaline narrowing of blood vessels and ischemia (lack of oxygen). Various molecular mechanisms have been postulated to explain these effects. Hyperglycemia causes the formation of advanced glycosylation end products (AGE) and release of cytokines (e.g., transforming growth factor beta [TGF-beta], and protein kinase-C), all of which can lead to hyperfiltration, cellular hypertrophy, and renal injury (Cooper, 1998). In particular, the excessive AGE accumulation has been found to markedly accelerate the progression of diabetic nephropathy to ESRD (Go et al., 2018; Makita et al., 1991).

▶ Hypertensive Nephropathy

Many epidemiologic investigations have shown that sustained high blood pressure leads to impairment of kidney function; and reciprocally, reducing blood pressure has clearly been shown to have beneficial impact on kidney function.

In the Multiple Risk Factor Intervention Trial (MRFIT), 332,544 men aged 44–57 years at baseline were screened during 1973–1975 and followed for detection of ESRD or death from renal death using the National Death Index and the Social Security Administration. During an average of 16 years of follow-up, 814 subjects were treated for or died of ESRD. The results showed a strong-graded relationship between both systolic and diastolic blood pressure and the development of ESRD (**FIGURE 44.8**).

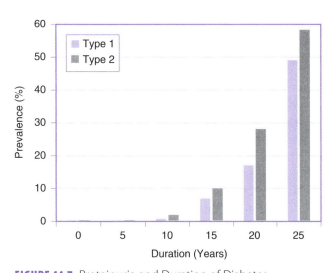

FIGURE 44.7 Proteinuria and Duration of Diabetes.

Data from Ritz, E., & Orth, S. R. (1999). Nephropathy in patients with type 2 diabetes mellitus. *New England Journal of Medicine, 341*, 1127–1133; Hasslacher, C., Ritz, E., Wahl, P., & Michael, C. (1989). Similar risks of nephropathy in patients with type I or type II diabetes mellitus. *Nephrology Dialysis Transplantation, 4*, 859–863.

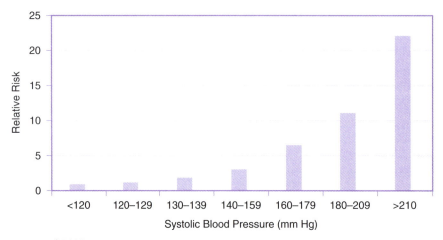

FIGURE 44.8 Hypertension and ESRD.

Data from Klag, M. J., Whelton, P. K., Randall, B. L., Neaton, J. D., Brancati, F. L., Ford, C. E., ... Stamler, J. (1996). Blood pressure and end-stage renal disease in men. *The New England Journal of Medicine, 334*, 13–18.

Compared to normotensive subjects, the relative risk of ESRD for patients with severe hypertension (systolic blood pressure > 210 mm Hg or diastolic blood pressure > 120 mm Hg) was increased more than 20-fold (RR = 22.1). Increases in the risk due to rising blood pressure retained statistical significance after adjustment for other risk factors including age, race, diabetes, history of myocardial infarction, serum cholesterol, and cigarette smoking. The investigators concluded that increased blood pressure is a strong independent risk factor for developing ESRD (Klag et al., 1996).

A review of cross-sectional, case–control, and prospective epidemiological studies confirmed that increasing blood pressure is an independent predictor of renal insufficiency and ESRD. As shown in Figure 44.8, the relationship appears to be continuous throughout the entire range of blood pressure (Klag et al., 1996; Whelton, Perneger, He, & Klag, 1996).

Randomized clinical trials indicate that effective regulation of blood pressure in hypertensive subjects by the administration of antihypertensive agents attenuates the progressive loss of renal function (Mogensen, 1999). Beneficial effects of blood pressure control on renal function have also been observed for patients with *both* diabetes and hypertension (Ismail et al., 1999; Nielsen et al., 1997) as well as for patients with proteinuric renal disease (Peterson et al., 1995).

The optimal target for blood pressure reduction in hypertensive patients has not been resolved and remains under study (Ruilope & Garia-Robles, 1997). In a meta-analysis of 11 randomized clinical trials involving 1860 nondiabetic patients with hypertension, the greatest reduction in the rate of progression of renal disease was observed for patients achieving systolic blood pressures in the range of 110–129 mm Hg as opposed to lesser values (Jafar et al., 2003). Furthermore, in the *UK Prospective Diabetes Study*, even moderate lowering of blood pressure led to major reductions in the risk of both cardiovascular and renal events (UK Prospective Diabetes Study, 1998). Nevertheless, in a randomized clinical trial specifically designed to determine the optimal target for blood pressure reduction in hypertensive patients, the incidence of major cardiovascular events was 50% less in patients with a target diastolic blood pressure of 80 mm Hg compared to 90 mm Hg (Hansson et al., 1998). Thus, while there is general agreement that elevated blood pressure must be reduced to attenuate progression of renal failure and cardiovascular disease, controversy remains as to the optimal target for individual patients.

▶ Chronic Glomerulonephritis

Despite the tremendous global impact of diabetes, hypertension, and other chronic conditions, glomerulonephritis continues to play a significant role in the pathogenesis of chronic kidney disease throughout the world. However, recent surveys of WHO member nations show great disparity between developed and developing nations in the prevalence of this condition. In the highly developed nations of North America, Western Europe, Australasia, and elsewhere, glomerulonephritis is found in only 10%–15% of cases; whereas in the less-developed nations of Asia, Africa, and South America, glomerulonephritis is the principal pathologic condition in more than 70% of cases of chronic kidney disease (Couser, 1999; Huraib et al., 2000).

Glomerulonephritis can be categorized as either acute or chronic. Acute glomerulonephritis is primarily infectious in origin and may arise due to bacteria (beta-hemolytic streptococci, *Escherichia coli*, pseudomonas), viruses (hepatitis B, mumps, varicella, infectious mononucleosis), and parasites (malaria, schistosomiasis). Chronic glomerulonephritis usually arises not as a direct consequence of the infection, but rather because antigen–antibody immune complexes specifically directed against the infectious agent become entrapped in the ultrafine filtration system of the glomeruli. The presence of such "*foreign*" immune complexes activates the complement system thereby causing inflammation and subsequent damage to the basement membrane of the glomeruli; hence the name "immune-complex" glomerulonephritis (Cameron, 1972a, 1972b, 1972c; Robbins & Cotran, 1979). The continued presence of this process can lead to chronic glomerulonephritis.

Immune-mediated chronic glomerulonephritis can arise from persisting infections due to bacteria, viruses, or parasites. Low-grade infections that remain untreated over long periods of time have the highest propensity for pathogenesis. Malaria and schistosomiasis are prominent causative agents in developing countries, particularly in Africa (Cameron, 1972a, 1972b, 1972c). Other examples include recurring post-streptococcal disease and hepatorenal disease from chronic hepatitis.

In addition to infectious agents, autoimmune conditions such as *systemic lupus erythematosus (SLE)* can produce renal lesions by deposition of anti-DNA antibodies and anti-nucleosome complexes in the glomeruli (Salgado & Herrera-Diaz, 2012). Occasionally, glomerulonephritis arises due to antibodies that are specifically directed against the glomerular basement membranes. Goodpasture's syndrome, a rare condition characterized by pulmonary hemorrhaging plus nephritis is an example of this mechanism (Segelmark & Hellmark, 2010). There is also consistent evidence from case–control studies suggesting that heavy or prolonged environmental exposure to hydrocarbons (industrial solvents and gasoline) heightens the risk of developing chronic glomerulonephritis (Churchill, Fine, & Gault, 1983; Ravnskov, 2000).

▶ Blood Lipids, Cholesterol, and Chronic Kidney Disease

As enumerated in the preceding discussion, the profile of risk factors for chronic kidney disease in developed countries is similar to that for cardiovascular disease. Nevertheless, the role of high cholesterol in the development of chronic kidney disease was uncertain until investigators designed clinical-epidemiologic studies to either match out effects or adjust for confounding primarily due to diabetes and hypertension while also accounting for other factors such as age, gender, body mass, and smoking.

Early studies examined the association of blood lipids with progression of renal disease in patients with type 1 diabetes. In a small case–control study conducted by investigators at Guys Hospital in London, lipid profiles were studied in 20 diabetic patients with microalbuminuria (cases) and 20 matched diabetic patients without microalbuminuria (controls). Cases with renal disease had significantly higher concentrations of LDL cholesterol, triglycerides, and apolipoprotein B, and significantly lower concentrations of HDL cholesterol than controls without renal disease (Jones et al., 1989).

Subsequently, investigators in Sweden conducted a prospective follow-up study of 30 patients with type 1 diabetes and nephropathy to assess the relationship between blood lipids and progression of renal disease. Results showed that high levels of serum cholesterol, triglycerides, and apolipoprotein B were correlated with a more rapid decline in GFR and deterioration of kidney function (Mulec, Johnson, & Bjorck, 1990).

In a cross-sectional study conducted in the United States, blood lipids and urinary albumin were studied in a sample of 428 women and 540 men patients with type 1 diabetes from the *Diabetes Control and Complications Trial/Epidemiology of Diabetes Interventions and Complications (DCCT/EDIC)* cohort. Using multivariate analysis to adjust for duration and control of diabetes, hypertension, and body mass index, the investigators found that increased levels of triglycerides, total cholesterol, and LDL cholesterol were significantly associated

with increasing urinary albumin and worsening of renal function (Jenkins et al., 2003).

Similar findings regarding the role of lipids in the progression of renal disease have also been reported for patients with type 2 diabetes. In a prospective study of patients with type 2 diabetes conducted in Tel Aviv, Israel, 574 patients aged 40–60 years who had normal renal function and were normotensive at baseline were followed to determine effects of plasma lipids and other factors (hemoglobin A1C, blood pressure, body mass index, and smoking) on urinary albumin excretion rate. After 7.8 years of average follow-up, total cholesterol, blood pressure, and hemoglobin A1C were found to be the main factors associated with increased albuminuria and deterioration of renal function. Notably, patients with high levels of all three risk factors were 43 times more likely to develop microalbuminuria than patients with normal values (Ravid, Brosh, Ravid-Safran, Levy, & Rachmani, 1998).

Effects of cholesterol have also been observed in patients with type 2 diabetes and overt nephropathy. A post hoc analysis of 1513 patients with (type 2) diabetic nephropathy enrolled in the *Reduction of Endpoints in NIDDM with the Angiotensin II Antagonist Losartan (RENALL)* study showed that both total cholesterol and LDL cholesterol measured at baseline were independent risk factors for ESRD (Appel et al., 2003).

Specific components of the lipid profile appear to have a more prominent role in the development of renal disease than others. Investigators in Sweden demonstrated a significant association between triglyceride-rich apolipoprotein B and the rate of progression in nondiabetic patients with chronic kidney disease (Sammuelsson et al., 1998).

In the Atherosclerosis Risk in Communities Study (ARIC), 15,792 men and women aged 45–64 years at baseline were tested for total cholesterol, HDL cholesterol, LDL cholesterol, apolipoproteins A and B, and triglycerides and followed for a 3-year period to determine the risk of declining kidney function. The study showed that declining kidney function (assessed by increasing urinary creatinine) was significantly associated with high levels of triglycerides and low levels of HDL cholesterol and apolipoprotein A (Muntner, Coresh, Smith, Eckfeldt, & Klag, 2000).

Investigators in France examined the role of triglycerides, LDL cholesterol, and apolipoprotein A in the progression of nephropathy among 297 patients with type 1 diabetes. After adjustment for blood pressure and the duration and control of diabetes, the relative risk for progression to a higher stage of nephropathy was twofold higher in patients with elevated levels of triglycerides compared to subjects with normal levels. The results indicate that high triglyceride levels are an independent predictor of declining renal function in patients with type 1 diabetes (Hadjadj et al., 2004).

Findings of observational studies showing renal effects of blood lipids set the stage for randomized clinical trials of antilipemic agents (statins) to examine their therapeutic impact for patients with chronic kidney disease. In a systematic review and meta-analysis of randomized controlled trials, 27 studies with 39,704 participants were identified that reported assessment of kidney function (GFR and/or proteinuria) in patients who took statins compared to those who did not. Overall, statin treatment was found to significantly slow the progression of renal dysfunction, particularly among subjects with cardiovascular disease (Fried, Orchard, Kasiske, & Lipids and Renal Disease Progression Meta-Analysis Study Group, 2001; Sandhu, Wiebe, Fried, & Tonelli, 2006).

Patients with chronic kidney disease characteristically have altered lipid metabolism manifesting as elevated blood levels of triglycerides, free fatty acids, and LDL cholesterol and reduced HDL cholesterol. In general, high levels of cholesterol and particularly LDL cholesterol are related to atherogenesis and the development of atheromas in blood vessels including those that nourish the kidney. Sequelae include thromboembolic events leading to ischemic tissue damage. A related condition known as hyaline arteriolar nephrosclerosis is a form of renal disease in which cholesterol-laden hyaline material narrows the renal arterioles leading to atrophy of the renal tubules, renal dysfunction, and hypertension (Baker & Selikoff, 1952). Hypertriglyceridemia is a prominent feature of chronic kidney disease wherein damage to the kidneys is associated with the flux of excess free fatty acids and triglycerides that deposit in the renal tubules (Johnson, Stahl, & Zager, 2005).

▶ Obesity and Chronic Kidney Disease

Obesity is an integral component in the *web of causation* of chronic kidney disease. Obesity is an independent risk factor for both diabetes and hypertension, and as discussed earlier, these two conditions account for more than 70% of chronic kidney disease. Furthermore, obesity is primarily due to excess body fat with increased numbers of lipid-laden fat cells that are capable of secreting bioactive substances that participate in the pathogenesis of kidney disease and other cardiovascular conditions.

In a study conducted in the United States during 1965–1984, the relationship between body mass and ESRD was assessed among 320,252 men and women enrolled in the *Kaiser Permanente* healthcare delivery system in northern California. Estimates of relative risk for overweight and obese individuals (classes I, II, and II) were based on 1471 incident cases of ESRD diagnosed after more than 8.3 million person-years of follow-up. Compared with normal-weight persons (BMI < 25), the pattern of risk shows a striking dose–response curve with increasing body mass (**FIGURE 44.9**) (Hsu, McCulloch, Iribarren, Darbinian, & Go, 2006).

A voluminous amount of evidence from the epidemiologic literature on obesity and kidney disease has been retrieved, reviewed, and analyzed. In a recent meta-analysis, data from 25 cohort studies, 3 cross-sectional studies, and 19 case–control studies

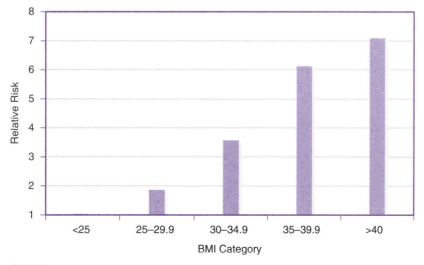

FIGURE 44.9 Obesity and ESRD.

Data from Hsu, C., McCulloch, C. E., Iribarren, C., Darbinian, J., & Go, A. S. (2006). Body mass index and risk for end-stage renal disease. *Annals of Internal Medicine, 144*, 21–28.

published during 1980–2006 were pooled and relative risk estimates derived according to body mass index. Combined results from prospective studies reflect an increase in the relative risk of all types of kidney disease (including kidney cancer) for overweight individuals (RR = 1.41) and obese individuals (RR = 1.83). Restriction of estimates to noncancerous outcomes yielded similar results (RR = 1.53 and 1.66, respectively). The evidence also suggests that obesity has a slightly stronger effect in women than men (Wang, Chen, Song, Caballero, & Cheskin, 2008).

The impact of weight loss on kidney function has been examined in randomized clinical trials. Several types of weight loss interventions have been assessed including exercise, diet, medication, and bariatric surgery. In a meta-analysis of 13 trials involving 522 patients with varying stages of obesity, weight loss intervention reduced proteinuria by 1.7 g and microalbuminuria by 14 mg. The combined results showed that each 1 kg of weight loss decreased proteinuria by 110 mg and microalbuminuria by 1.1 mg. These effects were observed across different designs and methods of weight loss (Afshinnia, Wilt, Duval, Esmaeili, & Ibrahim, 2010).

Diseases linked to obesity, including chronic kidney disease, are related to excess fat and secretions of the fat cell population. The adipocyte (fat cell) is *not* simply a storage depot for fat. Far from it, adipocytes are capable of secreting a variety of hormone-like peptides (called adipokines) that have significant impact on human physiology. Indeed, the adipokine profile has been found to influence a wide variety of cellular mechanisms and functions including appetite/satiety, energy balance, immunity, inflammation, insulin sensitivity, angiogenesis, blood pressure, lipid metabolism, and endocrine homeostasis.

In particular, when the adipocyte population becomes engorged with *triacylglycerol* (the storage form of fat), macrophage infiltration is stimulated and pathogenic adipokines are secreted. For example, *tumor necrosis factor, interleukin 6,* and *resistin* have been linked to the development of insulin resistance and type 2 diabetes. *Angiotensinogen* released by fat cells has been implicated in the onset of hypertension and *plasminogen activating inhibitor* promotes thrombus formation. Fat cells can also release inflammatory *prostaglandins* that heighten the risk of atherogenesis and thromboembolic events.

Reciprocally, weight loss and reduction of adipose tissue induces secretion of beneficial adipokines such as *adiponectin* and *leptin* that have been found to increase insulin sensitivity and reduce blood pressure and inflammation. Clearly, modification of the adipokine profile holds significant potential for the prevention and therapy of obesity-related disease. As pointed out by Ronti and colleagues in their update of the endocrine functions of adipose tissue: "*In-depth understanding of the pathophysiology and molecular actions of adipokines may, in the coming years, lead to effective therapeutic strategies designed to protect against atherosclerosis in obese patients*" (Ronti, Lupattelli, & Mannarino, 2006).

Smoking and Chronic Kidney Disease

A number of epidemiologic investigations have demonstrated that smoking is a significant independent predictor of albuminuria (Dales, Friedman, Siegelaub, Seltzer, & Ury, 1978; Mimran, Ribstein, DuCailar, & Halimi, 1994; Mulder et al., 1999). Furthermore, several studies of patients with diabetes found that smokers are at greater risk than nonsmokers for the development of diabetic nephropathy (Chase et al., 1991; Christiansen, 1978; Orth, Ritz, & Schrier, 1997).

In an important international matched-pair case–control investigation of ESRF involving 72 patients with inflammatory or noninflammatory renal disease (cases) and 72 matched control subjects from 9 centers in Germany, Italy, and Austria, the odds ratios for ESRF showed a significant linear dose–response with pack-years of smoking: OR = 3.5 for 5–15 pack-years and OR = 5.8 for >15 pack-years compared to <5 pack-years of smoking. Notably, the investigators also found that smokers who were treated with angiotensin-converting enzyme inhibitors (ACE inhibitors) attenuated their risk of disease progression (Orth et al., 1998). In the MRFIT, smoking was also identified as an independent risk factor for the development of ESRF (Whelton et al., 1995). It is also of note that diabetic individuals who quit smoking have been observed to have significantly better renal function than comparable subjects who continue to smoke (Sawicki et al., 1994).

There is strong biological plausibility for an etiologic link between smoking and renal dysfunction. Clinical-pathologic investigations have shown that smoking plays a prominent role in the genesis of atherosclerotic renal artery stenosis and ischemic nephropathy (Black, Zeevi, Silten, & Smith, 1983; Oberai, Adams, & High, 1984). Smoking may also induce inflammation and heighten vasoconstriction (endothelin) versus vasodilatation (nitric oxide) in the renal arterioles (Ritz & Orth, 1999). Clearly, smoking cessation should be a prominent component in the management of patients diagnosed with renal disease.

Alcohol Abuse, Gout and Kidney Disease

Alcohol abuse and particularly heavy consumption of beer predisposes to hyperuricemia (excess urinary uric acid) and precipitation of monosodium uric acid crystals in synovial joints (a condition commonly called gout) (Choi, Atkinson, Darlson, Willet, & Curhan, 2004). Uric acid crystals frequently produce damage to the kidneys and occasionally cause the development of uric acid kidney stones (nephrolithiasis) (Robbins & Cotran, 1979).

In a cohort of the *Health Professionals Follow-up Study*, the risk of incident kidney stones was increased twofold among men who reported a history of gout (RR = 2.12). The investigators concluded that gout is an independent risk factor for nephrolithiasis (Kramer, Choi, Atkinson, Stampfer, & Curhan, 2003). Furthermore, patients with chronic gout are predisposed to kidney failure. As pointed out nearly 50 years ago by R.W. Rundles,

> *Nephropathy in gout may develop acutely but it is usually chronic, insidious, and slowly progressive. In gout, the formation of urate stones is often a major manifestation of the disease and the one complication most amenable to correction by allopurinol therapy (Rundles, 1966).*

Perneger and colleagues examined the association of alcohol consumption and ESRD in a population-based case–control study conducted in Maryland, Virginia, and West Virginia and the District of Columbia (Washington, DC). They found that persons consuming two or more alcoholic drinks per day were four times more likely to develop ESRD than those with no exposure. The corresponding attributable risk estimate was 9%. Lesser amounts of alcohol were not found to be harmful (Perneger, Whelton, Puddey, & Klag, 1999). Similar results were reported by Shankar and colleagues who studied a cohort of 3392 adults in Wisconsin. They found that consumption of four or more alcoholic drinks daily increased the risk of chronic kidney disease twofold and the combination of chronic smoking and heavy drinking increased the risk fivefold (Shankar, Klein, & Klein, 2006).

In contrast, Menon and colleagues found no association with decline in kidney function and alcohol consumption in a prospective cohort study of 4343 elderly men and women from four U.S. communities (Menon et al., 2010). Furthermore, some studies have observed that moderate levels of alcohol consumption (one drink per day) have a beneficial effect on kidney function (Schaeffner et al., 2005). Clearly, additional studies are needed to clarify the dose–response of kidney function and alcohol intake.

Chronic Kidney Disease in Children and Adolescents

Childhood syndromes involving renal pathology have been linked to specific genes. Alport syndrome is a rare X-linked dominant disorder that causes progressive hematuric nonimmune nephritis characterized ultrastructurally by irregular thickening, thinning, and lamellation of the glomerular basement membrane. Characteristic phenotypic features of Alport syndrome include hearing loss, ocular defects, abnormalities in platelet number and function, and esophageal, upper gastrointestinal, and genital leiomyomatosis. The genetic defect produces abnormal synthesis of collagen and other connective tissues (Flinter, Maher, & Saggar, 2003).

Autosomal dominant polycystic kidney disease accounts for approximately 10% of all cases of polycystic kidney disease (PKD). Onset typically occurs in the second or third decades of life. Enlargement of the renal cystic structures results in renin secretion and hypertension, often leading to ESRD. This condition also predisposes to the development of cerebral aneurysms, liver cysts, and mitral valve prolapse. Mutations in the PKD-1 gene on chromosome 16 account for 85% of cases, whereas mutations in the PKD-2 gene on chromosome 4 represent the remainder. The genetic defect in PKD causes irregularities in maturation of the epithelial lining of the renal tubules (Flinter et al., 2003).

Although specific genes have not been identified for adult forms of nephropathy, studies of afflicted relatives do show characteristics of significant genetic influence. For example, there are numerous reports of familial clustering of diabetic nephropathy consistent with genetic predisposition, common environmental factors, or both (Borch-Johnsen et al., 1992; Bowden, 2003; Quinn, Angelico, Warram, & Krolewski, 1996; Seaquist, Goetz, Rich, & Barbosa, 1989).

In a population-based investigation conducted in Finland, 537 families containing at least two siblings with diabetes were identified and all individuals were followed longitudinally to determine onset of diabetic nephropathy. Diabetic siblings of index cases (probands) with diabetic nephropathy were at significantly higher risk (RR = 2.3) of developing renal disease compared to siblings of control subjects without diabetic nephropathy; and furthermore, severe diabetic nephropathy in probands increased the risk in their siblings by threefold

(Harjutsalo, Katoh, Sarti, Tajima, & Tuomilehto, 2004). Despite the evidence supporting familial clustering of diabetic nephropathy and the heightened risk among relatives of probands, the genes involved have not been identified. Clearly, a genetic marker for nephropathy would enable early detection and treatment and facilitate screening and targeted intervention for high-risk relatives (Massengill & Ferris, 2014).

▶ Prevention of Chronic Kidney Disease

As with cardiovascular disease, chronic kidney disease develops as a consequence of a complex *web of causation* that involves multiple risk factors and causative agents. A recent review by Professor Robert Atkins of the Monash Medical Center, Victoria, Australia, provides keen insights on strategies for prevention. As he points out: "*Chronic kidney disease should not be viewed in isolation. Chronic kidney disease has a complex interrelationship with cardiovascular disease, diabetes, and hypertension. Indeed, chronic kidney disease is a major risk factor for cardiovascular disease*" (Atkins, 2005). Thus, to be effective, screening and prevention programs must focus not only on the detection and treatment of kidney disease but also on diabetes, hypertension, and cardiovascular diseases as well. A comprehensive profile of risk factors must be addressed including obesity, hypertension, hyperglycemia (diabetes), hyperlipidemia/hypercholesterolemia/hypertriglyceridemia, hyperuricemia (gout), smoking, alcohol abuse, lack of exercise, and diet. Routine screening for microalbuminuria is essential for the early detection and treatment of kidney disease, particularly for those patients with diabetes and/or hypertension.

As a further complication, many developing nations suffer from a double burden of renal disease due to obstructive uropathy and glomerulonephritis caused by infectious parasites such as malaria and schistosomiasis or communicable bacteria and viruses, as well as that caused by chronic noninfectious conditions such as diabetes, hypertension, and obesity. In these nations, preventive and therapeutic strategies must include programs for the prevention, detection, and early effective therapy of etiologic parasitic, bacterial, and viral infections. The basic axioms of primary, secondary, and tertiary prevention involve community education and prevention of disease by lifestyle modifications, early detection of disease, and effective treatment of established disease. As pointed out by Dr. Atkins, "individual and community educational programs must be an integral part of the overall management plan" (Atkins, 2005).

▶ Tertiary Prevention of Chronic Kidney Disease

Tertiary prevention is designed to restore function and inhibit disease progression after the diagnosis has been established. In regard to chronic kidney disease, a multifactorial approach is essential to prevent progression to ESRD and kidney failure. This includes effective management and control of blood pressure, blood glucose, blood lipids, and body weight, plus cessation of tobacco use through effective pharmacologic therapy plus nonpharmacologic methods such as diet, exercise, and counseling.

It is also essential for treating clinicians and healthcare workers to know and correct abnormalities in other clinical parameters. For example, anemia (hemoglobin level below 11 g per dL) develops early in patients diagnosed with chronic kidney disease due to deficient erythropoietin production by the failing kidney. Therefore, most patients will require erythropoietin replacement to slow the progression of renal disease (Gouva, Nikolopoulos, Ioannidis, & Siamopoulos, 2004). Nevertheless, controversy exists as to the optimal target for hemoglobin correction.

The *Correction of Hemoglobin and Outcomes in Renal Insufficiency (CHOIR)* trial used a randomized, open-label experimental study design to address the question of whether a higher target of hemoglobin correction by erythropoietin replacement in anemic patients with chronic kidney disease could provide additional clinical benefit. The study randomized 715 patients to a high hemoglobin group (target level: 13.5 g per dL) and 717 patients to a low hemoglobin group (target level: 11.3 g per dL). Surprisingly, more patients in the high hemoglobin group either died or developed congestive heart failure than in the low hemoglobin group (11.7% versus 7.5%, respectively). Furthermore, patients in the high hemoglobin group had a slightly higher rate of progression to renal replacement therapy (Singh et al., 2006). Thus, the magnitude of hemoglobin correction for optimal benefit to the patient remains in question and the specificity and mechanism of drug action should be considered and examined in more detail in future mechanistic studies.

▶ Dialysis and Renal Transplantation for End-Stage Renal Disease

ESRD is a devastating condition with extraordinarily high mortality and morbidity. Even in the United

States where hemodialysis and renal transplantation are common procedures, the age-adjusted case fatality rate due to ESRD is 14.3% (National Kidney and Urologic Diseases Information Clearinghouse, 2008).

Hemodialysis or renal transplant should be considered when chronic kidney disease progresses to ESRD. However, the decision to initiate kidney replacement therapy is complex and involves careful consideration of risk versus benefit for each patient. Clinical practice guidelines for renal transplant or the initiation of hemodialysis depend upon the presence of ESRD and rapidly declining kidney function that is refractory to other forms of medical therapy (Daugirdas et al., 2016).

▶ Hemodialysis for End-Stage Renal Disease

Hemodialysis is now being used in many developed nations of the world for the treatment of ESRD. In this procedure, blood is filtered through a semipermeable membrane to rid the body of waste, restore the proper balance of blood components, and eliminate extra fluid. While effective, hemodialysis is expensive and requires elaborate equipment and a coordinated effort by highly trained healthcare professionals as well as patients undergoing therapy. Nevertheless, current estimates suggest that over 2 million people with ESRF are being kept alive by hemodialysis or renal transplantation, and the estimated global dialysis population for ESRD is expanding at a rate of about 7% per year (Couser, Remuzzi, Mendis, & Tonelli, 2011; Moeller, Gioberge, & Brown, 2002).

The costs of hemodialysis for ESRD are extraordinarily high ($89,000 per year for persons undergoing hemodialysis in the United States). The estimated annual cost of hemodialysis in the United States during 2013 was $42 billion ($34 billion from Medicare) (US Renal Data System, 2014). Because of the high cost and the specialized healthcare professionals and medical equipment necessary for hemodialysis, most individuals with ESRD who live in developing nations do not have access to the procedure. Among patients treated by hemodialysis, it is estimated that 80% live in populations of developed nations that constitute only 12% of the world population. As a consequence, nearly 1 million people in the developing world are in need of hemodialysis and therefore die from untreated ESRD (Couser, Remuzzi, Mendis, & Tonelli, 2011).

▶ Renal Transplant for End-Stage Renal Disease

Successful renal transplantation is a life-extending procedure in patients with ESRD. In the hands of skilled transplant surgeons, transplantation has been found to extend the life of patients in renal failure by 10–15 years compared to patients sustained by hemodialysis (McDonald & Russ, 2002; Wolfe et al., 1999). Renal transplantation is an option for patients with ESRD in several developed nations (United States, United Kingdom, Spain, Italy, France, Japan, Australia, and Canada) and some developing nations (Pakistan and India). However, the primary obstacle remains the cost of the procedure (currently estimated in excess of $100,000 in the United States).

The Sindh Institute of Urology and Transplantation (SIUT) in Karachi, Pakistan, a public sector organization, performs more than 130 renal transplants per year, all from living related donors. Economic constraints, lack of public awareness, and shortage of donors limit the number of transplantation procedures. Post-transplant tuberculosis arising due to immunosuppressive drugs given to prevent transplant rejection is a special problem in developing countries. Nevertheless, the SIUT program is gaining momentum and now consists of three transplant teams of surgeons, urologists, nephrologists, pathologists, radiologists, and other support personnel. Funding support for SIUT in a community-government partnership has increased the number of transplantations and resulted in significantly improved patient and organ survival. The SIUT program may thus serve as a model for successful renal transplantation programs in other developing nations (Rizvi et al., 2003).

In populations of developing nations, the cost of ESRD care is often prohibitive, leading to extremely high case fatality rates approaching 100% in some nations. Nevertheless, advances are being made, particularly with the use of *continuous ambulatory peritoneal dialysis* as an alternative to hemodialysis or renal transplantation for ESRD.

▶ Peritoneal Dialysis for End-Stage Renal Disease

As opposed to hemodialysis that requires hospital-based equipment and personnel, peritoneal dialysis for ESRD can be performed by patients as home-based therapy. Peritoneal dialysis requires placement of an indwelling catheter into the peritoneal cavity for daily infusion of glucose-rich dialysate. Fluid, waste, and chemicals pass from the peritoneal capillary vessels into the peritoneum in exchange for dialysate components and the waste fluid is then drained from the peritoneum and the procedure repeated.

Peritoneal dialysis has important advantages compared to other forms of renal replacement therapy (e.g., relatively low cost, avoidance of hospital treatment, enhanced patient freedom, and improved quality of life). Complications of this procedure include infection (peritonitis) and edema (fluid overload), but these are preventable through patient education regarding infusion and drainage of dialysate and hygienic management of the catheter site. With state-of-the-art equipment, ESRD therapy by continuous ambulatory peritoneal dialysis appears to be comparable to hemodialysis if used correctly (Ronco & Amerling, 2006). Nevertheless, hemodialysis is the preferred method of treating ESRD in many societies due to the widespread misconception that it is safer and a more effective than peritoneal dialysis. As pointed out by Nayak and colleagues, the future of peritoneal dialysis in the treatment of ESRD will depend upon popularization in Latin America and in Asia, especially countries such as China and India with a combined population of 2.5 billion and rapidly rising rates of diabetes, hypertension, obesity, and chronic kidney disease (Nayak, Prabhu, Sinoj, Subhramanyam, & Sridhar, 2009).

References

Afshinnia, F., Wilt, T. J., Duval, S. U., Esmaeili, A., & Ibrahim, H. N. (2010). Weight loss and proteinuria: Systematic review of clinical trials and comparative cohorts. *Nephrology Dialysis Transplantation, 25*(4), 1173–1183.

Appel, G. B., Radhakrishnan, J., Avram, M. M., DeFronzo, R. A., Escobar-Jimenez, F., Campos, M. M., … Brenner, B. M. (2003). Analysis of metabolic parameters as predictors of risk in the RENAAL study. *Diabetes Care, 26,* 1402–1407.

Atkins, R. C. (2005). The changing patterns of chronic kidney disease: The need to develop strategies for prevention relevant to different regions and countries. *Kidney International, 68,* S83–S85.

Baker, R. D., & Selikoff, E. (1952). The cholesterol of hyaline arteriolosclerosis. *The American Journal of Pathology, 28*(4), 573–581.

Barsoum, R. S. (2003). Schistosomiasis and the kidney. *Seminars in Nephrology, 23*(1), 34–41.

Black, H. R., Zeevi, G. R., Silten, R. M., & Smith, G. J. W. (1983). Effect of heavy cigarette smoking on renal and myocardial arterioles. *Nephron, 34,* 173–179.

Borch-Johnsen, K., Norgaard, K., Hommel, E., Mathiesen, E. R., Jensen, J. S., Deckert, T., & Parving, H. H. (1992). Is diabetic nephropathy an inherited complication? *Kidney International, 41,* 719–722.

Bowden, D. W. (2003). Genetics of kidney disease. *Kidney International, 63,* S8–S12.

Cameron, J. S. (1972a). Bright's disease today: The pathogenesis and treatment of glomerulonephritis I. *British Medical Journal, 4*(5832), 87–90.

Cameron, J. S. (1972b). Bright's disease today: The pathogenesis and treatment of glomerulonephritis II. *British Medical Journal, 4*(5833), 160–163.

Cameron, J. S. (1972c). Bright's disease today: The pathogenesis and treatment of glomerulonephritis III. *British Medical Journal, 4*(5834), 217–220.

Chase, H. P., Garg, S. K., Marshall, G., Berg, C. L., Harris, S., Jackson, W. E., & Hamman, R. E. (1991). Cigarette smoking increases the risk of albuminuria among subjects with type 1 diabetes. *JAMA, 265,* 614–617.

Choi, H. K., Atkinson, K., Darlson, E. W., Willet, W., & Curhan, G. (2004). Alcohol intake and the risk of incident gout in men: A prospective study. *The Lancet, 363*(9417), 1277–1281.

Christiansen, J. S. (1978). Cigarette smoking and prevalence of microangiopathy in juvenile-onset insulin-dependent diabetes mellitus. *Diabetes Care, 1,* 146–149.

Churchill, D. N., Fine, A., & Gault, M. H. (1983). Association between hydrocarbon exposure and glomerulonephritis: An appraisal of the evidence. *Nephron, 33,* 169–172.

Collins, W. E., & Jeffery, G. M. (2007). Plasmodium malariae: Parasite and disease. *Clinical Microbiology Reviews, 20*(4), 579–592.

Cooper, M. E. (1998). Pathogenesis, prevention, and treatment of diabetic nephropathy. *Lancet, 442*(9123), 213–219.

Coresh, J., Turin, T. C., Matsushita, K., Sang, Y., Ballew, S. H., Appel, L. J., … Green, J. A. (2014). Decline in estimated glomerular filtration rate and subsequent risk of end-stage renal disease and mortality. *JAMA, 311*(24), 2518–2531.

Couser, W. G. (1999). Glomerulonephritis. *Lancet, 443*(9163), 1509–1515.

Couser, W. G., Remuzzi, G., Mendis, S., & Tonelli, M. (2011). The contribution of chronic kidney disease to the global burden of major non-communicable diseases. *Kidney International, 80*(12), 1258–1270.

Dales, L. G., Friedman, G. D., Siegelaub, A. B., Seltzer, C. C., & Ury, H. K. (1978). Cigarette smoking habits and urine characteristics. *Nephron, 20,* 163–170.

Daugirdas, J. T., Depner, T. A., Inrig, J., Mehrotra, R., Rocco, M. V., Suri, R. S., … Olson, C. (2016). KDOQI clinical practice guidelines for hemodialysis adequacy: 2015 update. *American Journal of Kidney Diseases, 66*(5), 884–930.

Dixon, F. J. (1966). Comments on immunopathology. *Military Medicine, 131*(Suppl.), 1233–1234.

Flinter, F., Maher, E., & Saggar, A. (2003). *The genetics of renal disease.* Oxford: Oxford University Press.

Fox, C. S., Larson, M. G., Lepi, E. P., Meigs, J. B., Wilson, P. W., & Levy, D. (2005). Glycemic status and development of kidney disease: The Framingham Heart Study. *Diabetes Care, 28*(10), 2436–2440.

Fraser, S. D. S., & Blakeman, T. (2016). Chronic kidney disease: Identification and management in primary care. *Pragmatic and Observational Research, 7,* 21–32.

Fried, L. F., Orchard, T. J., Kasiske, B. L., & Lipids and Renal Disease Progression Meta-Analysis Study Group. (2001). Effect of lipid reduction on the progression of renal disease: A meta-analysis. *Kidney International, 59*, 260–269.

Gioglioli, G. (1930). *Malarial nephritis*. London, UK: Churchill.

Go, A. S., Yang, J., Tan, T. C., Cabrera, C. S., Stefansson, B. V., Greasley, P. J., & Ordonez, J. D. (2018). Contemporary rates and predictors of fast progression of chronic kidney disease in adults with and without diabetes mellitus. *BMC Nephrology, 19*(1), 146.

Gouva, C., Nikolopoulos, P., Ioannidis, J. P., & Siamopoulos, K. C. (2004). Treating anemia early in renal failure patients slows the decline of renal function: A randomized controlled trial. *Kidney International, 66*, 753–760.

Hadjadj, S., Duly-Bouhanick, B., Bekherraz, A., Bridoux, F., Gallois, Y., Mauco, G., … Marre, M. (2004). Serum triglycerides are a predictive factor for the development and the progression of renal and retinal complications in patients with type 1 diabetes. *Diabetes & Metabolism, 30*, 43–51.

Hansson, L., Zanchetti, A., Carruthers, S. G., Dahlöf, B., Elmfeldt, D., Julius, S., … HOT Study Group. (1998). Effects of intensive blood-pressure lowering and low-dose aspirin in patients with hypertension: Principal results of the Hypertension Optimal Treatment (HOT) randomised trial. *Lancet, 441*, 1755–1762.

Harjutsalo, V., Katoh, S., Sarti, C., Tajima, N., & Tuomilehto, J. (2004). Population-based assessment of familial clustering of diabetic nephropathy in type 2 diabetes. *Diabetes, 53*(9), 2449–2454.

Hasslacher, C., Ritz, E., Wahl, P., & Michael, C. (1989). Similar risks of nephropathy in patients with type I or type II diabetes mellitus. *Nephrology Dialysis Transplantation, 4*, 859–863.

Hsu, C., McCulloch, C. E., Iribarren, C., Darbinian, J., & Go, A. S. (2006). Body mass index and risk for end-stage renal disease. *Annals of Internal Medicine, 144*, 21–28.

Huraib, S., Al Khader, A., Shaheen, F., Abu Aisha, H., Souqiyyeh, M. Z., Al Mohana, F., … Chan, N. (2000). The Spectrum of glomerulonephritis in Saudi Arabia: The results of the Saudi Registry. *Saudi Journal of Kidney Diseases and Transplantation, 11*, 434–441.

Ismail, N., Becker, B., Strzelczyk, P., & Ritz, E. (1999). Renal disease and hypertension in non-insulin-dependent diabetes mellitus. *Kidney International, 55*, 1–28.

Jafar, T. H., Stark, P. C., Schmid, C. H., Landa, M., Maschio, G., deJong, P. E., … AIPRD Study Group. (2003). Progression of chronic kidney disease: The role of blood pressure control, proteinuria, and angiotensin-converting enzyme inhibition. A patient-level meta-analysis. *Annals of Internal Medicine, 139*, 244–252.

Jager, K. J., & Fraser, S. D. S. (2017). The ascending rank of chronic kidney disease in the global burden of disease study. *Nephrology Dialysis Transplantation, 32*(Suppl_2), ii121–ii128.

Jenkins, A. J., Lyons, T. J., Zheng, D., Otvos, J. D., Lackland, D. T., McGee, D., … DCCT/EDIC Research Group. (2003). Lipoproteins in the DCCT/EDIC cohort: Associations with diabetic nephropathy. *Kidney International, 64*, 817–828.

Johnson, A. C. M., Stahl, A., & Zager, R. A. (2005). Triglyceride accumulation in injured renal tubular cells: Alterations in both synthetic and catabolic pathways. *Kidney International, 67*, 2196–2209.

Jones, S. L., Close, C. F., Mattock, M. B., Jarrett, R. J., Keen, H., & Viverti, G. C. (1989). Plasma lipid and coagulation factor concentrations in insulin-dependent diabetic patients with microalbuminuria. *BMJ, 298*, 487–490.

Kawazu, S., Tomono, S., Shimizu, M., Kato, N., Ohno, T., Ishii, C., … Takahashi, M. (1994). The relationship between early diabetic nephropathy and control of plasma glucose in non-insulin-dependent diabetes mellitus: The effect of glycemic control on the development and progression of diabetic nephropathy in an 8-year follow-up study. *Journal of Diabetes and Its Complications, 8*, 13–17.

Keller, C. K., Bergis, K. H., Fliser, D., & Ritz, E. (1996). Renal findings in patients with short-term type 2 diabetes. *Journal of American Society of Nephrology, 7*, 2627–2644.

Klag, M. J., Whelton, P. K., Randall, B. L., Neaton, J. D., Brancati, F. L., Ford, C. E., … Stamler, J. (1996). Blood pressure and end-stage renal disease in men. *New England Journal of Medicine, 334*, 13–18.

Klein, R., Klein, B. E., Moss, S. E., & Cruickshanks, K. J. (1995). Ten-year incidence of gross proteinuria in people with diabetes. *Diabetes, 44*(8), 2436–2440.

Kramer, H. J., Choi, H. K., Atkinson, K., Stampfer, J., & Curhan, G. C. (2003). The association between gout and nephrolithiasis in men: The Health Professionals' Follow-Up Study. *Kidney International, 64*, 1022–1026.

Mahakur, A. C., Panda, S. N., Nanda, B. K., Bose, T. K., Satpathy, S. R., & Misra, Y. (1983). Malarial acute renal failure. *Journal of Association of Physicians of India, 31*, 633–616.

Makita, Z., Radoff, S., Rayfield, E. J., Yang, Z., Skolnik, E., Delaney, V., … Vlassara, H. (1991). Advanced glycosylation end products in patients with diabetic nephropathy. *New England Journal of Medicine, 325*, 836–842.

Martinelli, R., Noblat, A. C. B., Brito, E., & Rocha, H. (1989). Schistosoma mansoni-induced mesangiocapillary glomerulo-nephritis: Influence of therapy. *Kidney International, 44*, 1227–1233.

Massengill, S. F., & Ferris, M. (2014). Chronic kidney disease in children and adolescents. *Pediatrics in Review, 35*(1), 16–29.

McDonald, S. P., & Russ, G. R. (2002). Survival of recipients of cadaveric kidney transplants compared with those receiving dialysis treatment in Australia and New Zealand, 1991–2001. *Nephrology Dialysis Transplantation, 17*(12), 2212–2219.

Menon, V., Katz, R., Mukamal, K., Kestenbaum, B., de Boer, I. H., Siscovicks, D. S., … Shlipak, M. G. (2010). Alcohol consumption and kidney function decline in the elderly. *Nephrology Dialysis Transplantation, 25*, 3301–3307.

Mimran, A., Ribstein, J., DuCailar, G., & Halimi, J. M. (1994). Albuminuria in normals and essential hypertension. *Journal of Diabetes and its Complications, 8*, 150–156.

Moeller, S., Gioberge, S., & Brown, G. (2002). ESRD patients in 2001: Global overview of patients, treatment modalities and development trends. *Nephrology Dialysis Transplantation, 217*, 2071–2076.

Mogensen, C. E. (1999). Microalbuminuria, blood pressure and diabetic renal disease: Origin and development of ideas. *Diabetologia, 42*, 263–285.

Mulder, J., Pinto-Sietsma, S. J., Diercks, G. F., Hillege, H. L., de Zeeuw, D., Janssen, W. M., & de Jong, P. E. (1999). Smoking behaviour and urinary albumin excretion (UAE) in the general population. *Journal of the American Society of Nephrology, 10*, 175A.

Mulec, H., Johnson, S. A., & Bjorck, S. (1990). Relation between serum cholesterol and diabetic nephropathy. *Lancet, 344*, 1537–1538.

Muntner, P., Coresh, J., Smith, C., Eckfeldt, J., & Klag, M. J. (2000). Plasma lipids and risk of developing renal dysfunction:

The atherosclerosis risk in communities study. *Kidney International, 58,* 293–301.

Murray, C. J. L., & Lopez, A. D. (1997). Mortality by cause for eight regions of the world: Global burden of disease study. *Lancet, 349,* 1269–1276.

Naicker, S. (2003). End-stage renal disease in sub-Saharan and South Africa. *Kidney International, 63,* 119.

National Kidney and Urologic Diseases Information Clearinghouse. (2008). National Institute of Diabetes and Digestive and Kidney Diseases (NIDDK). National Institutes of Health (NIH) Publication No. 08-3925.

Nayak, K. S., Prabhu, M. V., Sinoj, K. A., Subhramanyam, S. V., & Sridhar, G. (2009). Peritoneal dialysis in developing countries. *Contributions to Nephrology, 163,* 270–277.

Nielsen, F. S., Rossing, P., Gall, M. A., Skott, P., Smidt, U. M., & Parving, H. H. (1997). Long-term effect of lisinopril and atenolol on kidney function in hypertensive NIDDM subjects with diabetic nephropathy. *Diabetes, 46,* 1182–1188.

Oberai, B., Adams, C. W. M., & High, O. B. (1984). Myocardial and renal arteriolar thickening in cigarette smoking. *Atherosclerosis, 52,* 185–190.

Orman, A. R. (2005). The epidemiologic transition: A theory of the epidemiology of population change. *The Milbank Quarterly, 83*(4), 751–757.

Orth, S. R., Ritz, E., & Schrier, R. W. (1997). The renal risks of smoking. *Kidney International, 51,* 1669–1677.

Orth, S. R., Stöckmann, A., Conradt, C., Ritz, E., Ferro, M., Kreusser, W., … Zucchelli, P. (1998). Smoking as a risk factor for end-stage renal failure in men with primary renal disease. *Kidney International, 54,* 926–931.

Oyediran, A. B. O. O. (1979). Renal disease due to schistosomiasis of the lower urinary tract. *Kidney International, 16,* 15–22.

Perneger, T. V., Whelton, P. K., Puddey, I. B., & Klag, M. J. (1999). Risk of end-stage renal disease associated with alcohol consumption. *American Journal of Epidemiology, 150,* 1275–1281.

Peterson, J. C., Adler, S., Burkart, J. M., Greene, T., Hebert, L. A., Hunsicker, L. G., … Seifter, J. L. (1995). Blood pressure control, proteinuria, and the progression of renal disease: The Modification of Diet in Renal Disease Study. *Annals of Internal Medicine, 123,* 754–762.

Prakash, J., Sundar, S., Kar, B., Sharma, N., Raja, R., & Usha. (2007). Spectrum of renal disease in visceral leishmaniasis. *The Internet Journal of Tropical Medicine, 4*(1), 1–6.

Prasad, L. S., Sen, S., & Ganguly, S. K. (1992). Renal involvement in kala-azar. *Indian Journal of Medical Research, 95*(1), 43–46.

Quinn, M., Angelico, M. C., Warram, J. H., & Krolewski, A. S. (1996). Familial factors determine the development of diabetic nephropathy in patients with IDDM. *Diabetologia, 39,* 940–945.

Rajapurkar, M. M. (1994). Renal involvement in malaria. *Journal of Postgraduate Medicine, 40,* 132–134.

Ravnskov, U. (2000). Hydrocarbon exposure may cause glomerulonephritis and worsen renal function: Evidence based on Hill's criteria for causality. *QJM: An International Journal of Medicine, 93*(8), 551–556.

Ravid, M., Brosh, D., Ravid-Safran, D., Levy, Z., & Rachmani, R. (1998). Main risk factors for nephropathy in type 2 diabetes mellitus are plasma cholesterol levels, mean blood pressure, and hyperglycemia. *Archives of Internal Medicine, 158,* 998–1004.

Ritz, E., & Orth, S. R. (1999). Nephropathy in patients with type 2 diabetes mellitus. *New England Journal of Medicine, 341,* 1127–1133.

Rizvi, S. A. H., Naqvi, S. A. A., Hussain, Z., Hashmi, A., Akhtar, F., Hussain, M., … Jawad, F. (2003). Renal transplantation in developing countries. *Kidney International, 63,* S96–S100.

Robbins, S. L., & Cotran, R. S. (1979). *Pathologic basis of disease.* Philadelphia, PA: WB Saunders Company.

Ronco, C., & Amerling, R. (2006). Continuous flow peritoneal dialysis: Current state-of-the-art and obstacles to further development. *Contributions to Nephrology, 150,* 310–320.

Ronti, T., Lupattelli, G., & Mannarino, E. (2006). The endocrine function of adipose tissue: An update. *Clinical Endocrinology, 64*(4), 445–365.

Roy, M. S. (2004). Proteinuria in African Americans with type 1 diabetes. *Journal of Diabetes and its Complications, 18*(1), 69–77.

Ruilope, L. M., & Garcia-Robles, R. (1997). How far should blood pressure be reduced in diabetic hypertensive patients? *Journal of Hypertension, 15,* S63–S65.

Rundles, R. W. (1966). Allopurinol in gouty nephropathy and renal dialysis. *Annals of the Rheumatic Diseases, 25,* 694.

Salgado, A. Z., & Herrera-Diaz, C. (2012). Lupus nephritis: An overview of recent findings. *Autoimmune Diseases, 2012,* 1–21. doi:10.1155/2012/849684.

Sammuelsson, O., Attman, P., Knight-Gibson, C., Larsonn, R., Mulec, H., Weiss, L., & Alaupovic, P. (1998). Complex apolipoprotein B-containing lipoprotein particles are associated with a higher rate of progression of human chronic renal insufficiency. *Journal of American Society of Nephrology, 9,* 1482–1488.

Sandhu, S., Wiebe, N., Fried, L. F., & Tonelli, M. (2006). Statins for improving renal outcomes: A meta-analysis. *Journal of the American Society of Nephrology, 17,* 2006–2016.

Sawicki, P. T., Didjurgeit, U., Muhlhauser, I., Bender, R., Heinemann, L., & Berger, M. (1994). Smoking is associated with progression of diabetic nephropathy. *Diabetes Care, 17,* 126–131.

Schaeffner, E. S., Kurth, T., de Jong, P. E., Glynn, R. J., Buring, J. E., & Gaziano, J. M. (2005). Alcohol consumption and the risk of renal dysfunction in apparently healthy men. *Archives of Internal Medicine, 165,* 1048–1053.

Seaquist, E. R., Goetz, F. C., Rich, S., & Barbosa, J. (1989). Familial clustering of diabetic kidney disease: Evidence for genetic susceptibility to diabetic nephropathy. *New England Journal of Medicine, 320,* 1161–1165.

Segelmark, M., & Hellmark, T. (2010). Autoimmune kidney diseases. *Autoimmunity Reviews, 9*(5), A366–A371.

Shankar, A., Klein, R., & Klein, B. E. K. (2006). The association among smoking, heavy drinking, and chronic kidney disease. *American Journal of Epidemiology, 164*(3), 263–271.

Singh, A. K., Szczech, L., Kezhen, L. T., Barnhart, H., Sapp, S., Wolfson, M., …, CHOIR investigators. (2006). Correction of anemia with epoetin alfa in chronic kidney disease. *New England Journal of Medicine, 255,* 2085–2098.

Thomas, B., Matsushita, K., Abate, K. H., Al-Aly, Z., Ärnlöv, J., Asayama, K., … Global Burden of Disease 2013 GFR Collaborators. (2013). Global cardiovascular and renal outcomes of reduced GFR. *Journal of the American Society of Nephrology, 28*(7), 2167–2179.

UK Prospective Diabetes Study Group. (1998). Intensive blood-glucose control with sulphonylureas or insulin compared with conventional treatment and risk of complications in patients with type 2 diabetes. *Lancet, 442,* 837–853.

U.S. Renal Data System, USRDS. (2014). *Annual data report: Atlas of end-stage renal disease in the United States,* 2014. Bethesda,

MD: National Institutes of Health, National Institute of Diabetes and Digestive and Kidney Diseases.

Wang, H., Naghavi, M., Allen, C., Barber, R. M., Bhutta, Z. A., Carter, A., … GBD 2015 Mortality and Causes of Death Collaborators. (2016). Global, regional, and national life expectancy, all-cause mortality, and cause-specific mortality for 249 causes of death, 1980–2015: A systematic analysis for the Global Burden of Disease Study 2015. *Lancet, 388*(10053), 1459–1544.

Wang, Y., Chen, X., Song, Y., Caballero, B., & Cheskin, L. J. (2008). Association between obesity and kidney disease: A systematic review and meta-analysis. *Kidney International, 73*(1), 19–33.

Whelton, P. K., Perneger, T. V., He, J., & Klag, M. J. (1996). The role of blood pressure as a risk factor for renal disease. *Journal of Human Hypertension, 10*, 683–689.

Whelton, P. K., Randall, B., Neaton, J., Stamler, J., Brancati, F. L., & Klag, M. J. (1995). Cigarette smoking and ESRD incidence in men screened for the MRFIT. *Journal of the American Society of Nephrology, 6*, 408a.

Wolfe, R. A., Ashby, V. B., Milford, E. L., Ojo, A. O., Ettenger, R. E., Agodoa, L. Y., … Port, F. K. (1999). Comparison of mortality in all patients on dialysis, patients on dialysis awaiting transplantation, and recipients of a first cadaveric transplant. *New England Journal of Medicine, 341*, 1725–1730.

World Health Organization. (2009). *The global burden of disease: 2004 update*. Geneva, Switzerland: World Health Organization.

World Health Organization. (2016). *Estimated deaths from kidney disease in 2012*. Geneva, Switzerland: World Health Organization.

Xie, Y., Bowe, B., Mokdad, A. H., Xian, H., Yan, Y., Li, T., … Al-Aly, Z. (2018). Analysis of the Global Burden of Disease study highlights the global, regional, and national trends of chronic kidney disease epidemiology from 1990 to 2016. *Kidney International, 94*(3), 567–581.

CHAPTER 45

Epidemiology of Cirrhosis of the Liver

▶ Global Burden of Cirrhosis of the Liver

Cirrhosis of the liver is responsible for more than 1 million deaths per year worldwide (Lozano et al., 2012; Mokdad et al., 2014; World Health Organization [WHO], 2009a). Annual age-adjusted mortality rates vary widely ranging from >30 male deaths per 100,000 in Mexico, Chile, and certain nations of Eastern Europe and the Russian Federation, to <5 deaths per 100,000 in some Nordic countries, Singapore, and New Zealand (Bosetti et al., 2007; La Vecchia et al., 1994; Ramstedt, 2001; Rehm et al., 2010; Zatoński et al., 2010). The global pattern of mortality from liver cirrhosis is shown in **FIGURE 45.1**.

Within populations, the age-adjusted mortality rates are consistently two- to threefold higher in men than women. In North America, mortality rates have declined since 1970 and have stabilized at approximately 10 per 100,000 in men and 5 per 100,000 in women. While rates have also declined in some European nations (e.g., Italy, France, and Spain), many of the populations of Eastern Europe continue to show high or increasing mortality rates from liver cirrhosis (Bosetti et al., 2007; Ramstedt, 2001; Zatoński et al., 2010).

Globally, chronic alcohol consumption and chronic liver infections by hepatitis B virus (HBV)

and/or hepatitis C virus (HCV) have been the main causes of cirrhosis. More recently, the increasing prevalence of obesity and the *metabolic syndrome* has resulted in increasing incidence rates of cirrhosis secondary to nonalcoholic fatty liver disease, particularly in developed countries. Furthermore, injection drug use provides an effective mode of transmission for blood-borne pathogens including HIV (human immunodeficiency virus), HBV, and HCV. Chronic liver disease and cirrhosis are important causes of morbidity and mortality throughout the world.

Mokdad and colleagues at the *Institute for Health Metrics and Evaluation* (IHME) systematically collected vital registration and verbal autopsy data on liver cirrhosis deaths and mortality from 187 countries for the period 1980 to 2010. Globally, deaths from liver cirrhosis increased 52%, from 676,000 in 1980 to 1.03 million in 2010, causing approximately 1.5% of all deaths in 2010 and 2% of all deaths in 2010. During the same period, the annual age-standardized mortality rate for liver cirrhosis decreased 22%, from 20 per 100,000 to 15.8 per 100,000. On average, the number of deaths from liver cirrhosis in men was double the number in women.

Age-standardized mortality rates decreased in China, the United States, and countries of Western Europe, and increased in the United Kingdom and countries of Central and South Asia, Eastern Europe,

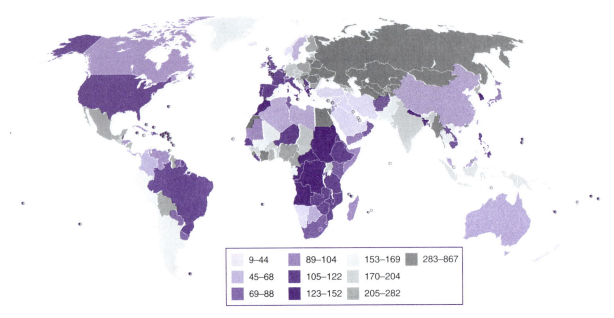

FIGURE 45.1 Global Mortality from Liver Cirrhosis, 2012.

Data from WHO. (2012). *Estimated deaths from liver cirrhosis, 2012.* Geneva, Switzerland: World Health Organization.

and sub-Saharan Africa. In Mexico, liver cirrhosis was the fourth leading cause of death in 2010 with an annual rate of 38 per 100,000.

In Egypt, contaminated immunizations for schistosomiasis until the late 1960s led to widespread transmission of HCV. As a consequence of this iatrogenic catastrophe, Egypt has the highest prevalence of HCV infection in the world. In 2010, the age-standardized liver cirrhosis mortality rate in Egypt was 73 per 100,000 ranking first among all countries, and 18% of deaths in males between 45 and 54 years of age were due to liver cirrhosis (Lozano et al., 2012; Mokdad et al., 2014).

Transmission of liver viruses by injection drug use has a significant impact on the burden of liver cirrhosis. Investigators at the Global Health Institute, Wuhan University, China, analyzed temporal and spatial variation in liver cirrhosis mortality due to injection drug use during 1990–2015. They estimated that the proportion of liver cirrhosis deaths due to injection drug use increased by 61% during the study period, from 6.7% in 1990 to 10.8% in 2015. Likewise, age-standardized liver cirrhosis mortality rates attributable to injection drug use increased from 1.5 per 100,000 in 1990 to 1.9 per 100,000 in 2015, accounting for 141,000 deaths from HCV and HBV infections during 2015. The highest rates were clustered in less developed nations of Latin America, East and Central Europe, and Central Asia, where injection drug use is most prevalent. The global trends in mortality from liver cirrhosis due to injection drug use were similar for liver cancer (Yang et al., 2018).

The *disability-adjusted life years* (DALY) is a measure of the years of healthy life lost from premature death and disability: DALY = YLL + YLD, where YLL = years of life lost due to premature death and YLD = years of life lost due to severe disability. The global pattern of DALY lost due to cirrhosis of the liver is shown in **FIGURE 45.2**. The annual DALY rates are highest in those populations with high rates of alcoholism and chronic liver infections by HCV and/or HBV. Recent studies suggest that the transmission of HCV and to a lesser extent HBV via injection drug use accounts for approximately 40% of the DALY from liver cirrhosis (Degenhardt et al., 2016).

▶ Liver Function and Anatomy

The human liver is a vital organ that regulates a number of life-sustaining functions including the synthesis of important proteins (e.g., albumin, clotting factors, and complement); metabolism and regulation of lipids, carbohydrates, and certain steroidal hormones (e.g., estrogens and androgens); synthesis and regulation of cholesterol and cholesterol byproducts (e.g., bile acids and fat-soluble vitamins A, D, E, and K); production and secretion of bile acids for digestion; the formation, storage, and release of glycogen for the regulation of blood glucose; and detoxification of chemicals and harmful substances.

The liver is located in the upper right quadrant of the abdomen. Its normal weight in adults is between 1400 and 1600 g. The liver receives a dual blood supply consisting of the hepatic portal vein and hepatic arteries.

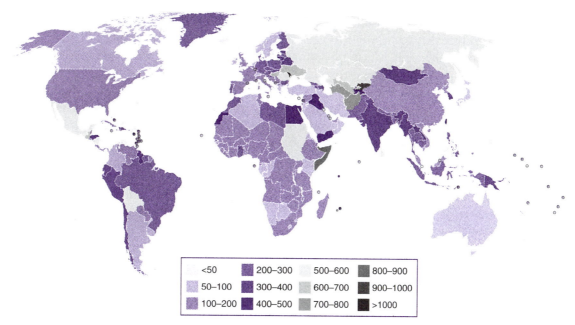

FIGURE 45.2 DALY from Liver Cirrhosis, 2004.

Data from World Health Organization. (2008). *The global burden of disease: 2004 update*. Geneva: WHO. Available at www.who.int/evidence/bod

Disability Adjusted Life Years per 100,000 individuals.

The hepatic portal vein carries venous blood drained from the spleen and gastrointestinal tract and the hepatic arteries supply arterial blood. Oxygen is provided from both sources; approximately half from the hepatic portal vein and half from the hepatic arteries (Robbins & Cotran, 1979). The gall bladder, which is located just beneath the liver, stores and concentrates bile produced by the liver and regulates bile secretion into the duodenum for the digestion of dietary fat (**FIGURE 45.3**).

The liver is organized into thousands of small lobules separated by bands of connective tissue. The parenchyma (tissue) within each lobule consists primarily of polygonal hepatocytes that carry out the multiple biosynthetic and metabolic functions of the liver. The hepatocytes are arranged in microscopic functional units called *acini* that are distributed within the lobules. Each acinus consists of hepatocytes arranged in concentric zones about hepatic arterioles and portal venules in order to facilitate selective secretion/excretion of cellular metabolites. The products of cellular synthesis and metabolism enter the blood in the sinusoids that are adjoined to the acini. Sinusoids are vascular channels that are lined by fenestrated endothelium and heavily populated by *Kupffer cells* (see description below).

Hepatocytes are responsible for an amazing array of biochemical functions. Their cytoplasm is laden with mitochondria responsible for oxidative phosphorylation and energy production, and the oxidation of fatty acids. Also within the cytoplasm, the *smooth endoplasmic reticulum* is the site of synthesis of cholesterol and

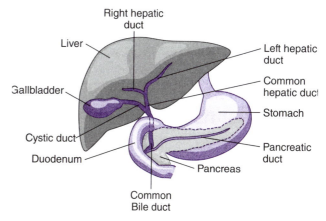

FIGURE 45.3 Anatomy of the Liver and Related Organs.
© Jones & Bartlett Learning.

bile acids, conjugation of bilirubin, drugs and steroids for excretion, metabolism of drugs and steroids, and breakdown of glycogen; and the *rough endoplasmic reticulum* is the site of protein synthesis. The multiple synthetic and metabolic pathways of hepatocytes are dependent upon the presence and functional integrity of a variety of essential enzymes, for example, the mixed function oxidase system (enzymes that oxidize toxic compounds for metabolism and excretion), cytochrome oxidase (a mitochondrial enzyme essential for respiration), and cytochrome P450 enzymes (oxidizing enzymes involved in metabolism and bioactivation of lipids, steroids, and drugs).

The liver is the detoxification center of the human body. For example, the *urea cycle* metabolizes ammonia, the principle byproduct of protein breakdown. Ammonia is highly toxic to cells, whereas urea is nontoxic and readily condensed in urine by the kidneys for excretion. One of the enzymes present in hepatocytes is alcohol dehydrogenase which catalyzes the conversion of alcohol to nontoxic metabolites for excretion. As discussed below, genetic variability in the alcohol dehydrogenase enzyme system influences the risk of developing alcoholic cirrhosis of the liver.

Kupffer cells are large phagocytic cells of the innate immune system that circulate throughout the sinusoidal network of the liver parenchyma. They were first observed by the German scientist, Karl Wilhelm von Kupffer in 1876 (Haubrich, 2004). Kupffer cells phagocytize senescent red blood cells and hepatocytes and break down hemoglobin and other cellular constituents (Robbins & Cotran, 1979).

In 1951, novel fat-storage cells lining the hepatic sinusoids were discovered by Ito (1951). These *Ito cells* actively store lipids and retinoids and are apparently involved in liver fibrosis during the development and progression of cirrhosis (Geerts, 2001).

Cirrhosis of the Liver: Pathology, Clinical Symptoms, and Diagnosis

Cirrhosis of the liver is a chronic inflammatory condition that causes a sustained recursive cycle of necrosis and regeneration of hepatocytes (liver cells). The word "*cirrhosis*" derives from the Greek term kirrhos that means "*of yellow color*" (the orange-yellow color of the diseased liver) (Robbins & Cotran, 1979). The French physician, René Laennec, named the condition "*cirrhosis*" in his 1819 work in which he also describes the stethoscope (Roguin, 2006).

With progression of cirrhosis, there is massive relapsing inflammation and necrosis of hepatocytes admixed with fibrosis and formation of nodular scar tissue and regeneration of liver tissue. The progressive destruction of liver tissue and conversion of the normal liver architecture into fibrotic nodules causes significant derangement of many important biosynthetic and metabolic processes. Liver cirrhosis is therefore characterized by a wide range of clinical symptoms including edema, ascites, jaundice, compromised blood clotting, hyperglycemia, abnormal digestion, and buildup of toxic substances in blood and tissues. A common clinical sign of liver disease is *jaundice*, the yellowish discoloration of the skin and sclerae of the eye due to the accumulation of bilirubin (a yellow

breakdown product of hemoglobin) in tissues and interstitial fluids of the body.

Advanced disease often results in obstruction of key blood vessels within the liver (e.g., the portal vein), with subsequent development of portal hypertension and ascites (fluid accumulation in the abdominal cavity) and/or bleeding esophageal varices due to shunting of blood to vessels external to the liver. Other life-threatening complications include hepatoencephalopathy and/or renal failure due to high blood concentrations of toxic substances such as ammonia and carbon tetrachloride (Galambos, 1985; Robbins & Cotran, 1979). The eventual consequences of progressive cirrhosis are liver failure and death.

Pathogenesis of Cirrhosis of the Liver

Cirrhosis of the liver has multiple etiologies, the best known of which is alcoholic cirrhosis, which is most prominent in the Western world. However, certain infectious agents now rival alcohol as the leading cause, most notably in the developing nations of Africa and Asia. Chronic liver infection by HBV, HCV, and hepatitis D virus (HDV) all cause a sequence of pathogenic events similar to chronic alcohol exposure, the end result of which is cirrhosis. Furthermore, the metabolic syndrome (the disease complex of diabetes, obesity, hyperlipidemia, and hypertension) has been found to heighten the development of fatty liver disease and its progression to cirrhosis, even in the absence of alcohol exposure or infectious hepatitis.

Fatty Liver

Cirrhosis is often viewed as the culmination of a series of progressive pathological changes. One of the earliest changes is the intracellular accumulation of fat by hepatocytes (*fatty change*) that results in a fatty liver (*steatosis*). The genesis of fatty change in the liver remains a topic of some controversy. In this condition, fat vacuoles laden with triglycerides appear within hepatocytes, possibly as a consequence of deranged lipid metabolism and transport in cells exposed to alcohol or other toxic substances.

In addition to chronic alcohol exposure, chronic HBV and HCV infections induce fatty liver in the majority of infected patients (Bamber et al., 1981; Hirche, Ianee, Hirche, Schneider, & Dietrich, 2007). Furthermore, a condition known as *nonalcoholic fatty liver disease* that arises in patients with the metabolic syndrome (obesity, type 2 diabetes mellitus and hyperlipidemia) has recently been recognized as a distinct clinical entity with worldwide health impact (see discussion below).

Hepatitis

Hepatitis refers to inflammation of the liver, regardless of the inciting agent. The sine qua non of hepatitis is infiltration of the liver by inflammatory cells of the immune system (e.g., macrophages, neutrophils, and lymphocytes). Common pathological findings include areas of necrosis and liver degeneration, hyaline accumulation within hepatocytes, and micronodular and macronodular fibrosis.

Cirrhosis

Cirrhosis of the liver is a significant cause of serious illness, liver failure, and death. Pathologic hallmarks of cirrhosis include the presence of regenerating nodules of hepatocytes and the deposition of fibrotic connective tissue between these nodules. With progression of disease, these fibrotic bands continue to expand and eventually replace the entire liver architecture causing obstruction of blood flow and general disruption of liver function.

Diagnosis of Cirrhosis of the Liver

The gold standard in the diagnosis of cirrhosis is confirmation of cirrhotic liver pathology by microscopic examination of a liver biopsy. Specimens are ordinarily obtained through a percutaneous, transjugular, laparoscopic, or fine-needle approach. Clinical, laboratory, and imaging data are also useful in confirming the diagnosis of cirrhosis. For example, elevated liver enzymes (aminotransferase, alkaline phosphatase, gamma-glutamyltransferase), increased bilirubin, decreased albumin, coagulation defects, immune dysfunction, hyponatremia (low sodium), and thrombocytopenia (low platelets) are suggestive of cirrhosis. Ultrasound and other imaging techniques also aid in the diagnosis.

Major Causes of Liver Cirrhosis

Cirrhosis of the liver has multiple etiologies. As in many chronic diseases, risk factors often coexist in the same patient and synergistically increase the risk. As discussed below, cirrhosis is often the consequence of one or more of four major factors: alcoholism, hepatitis B, hepatitis C, and the metabolic syndrome. As discussed in the following sections, these factors are not mutually exclusive and when combined they synergistically increase the risk of developing liver cirrhosis.

Alcohol Abuse and Cirrhosis of the Liver: Mortality Studies

The early studies of Raymond Pearl at Johns Hopkins University found that heavy drinkers had higher mortality rates due to cirrhosis of the liver than light drinkers or abstainers (Pearl, 1926). Alcohol consumption increased substantially in many countries after World War II, which spurred scientific interest in the health effects of alcohol addiction. Postwar studies of longitudinal data revealed temporal relationships between per capita alcohol consumption and cirrhosis mortality rates (Jellinek & Keller, 1952; Ledermann, 1956; Seeley, 1960).

In a landmark study, Milton Terris studied relationships between per capita alcohol consumption and annual mortality rates due to cirrhosis of the liver in the United States, Great Britain, and Canada during 1910–1964. Long-term trends were investigated by age, gender, race, urban–rural residence, occupation, and social status. Terris noted the close parallelism between time series curves (spanning 1910–1964) of the annual per capita consumption of spirits and wine (but not beer) and annual liver cirrhosis mortality in populations of the United States, the United Kingdom, and Canada (Terris, 1967).

Subsequent epidemiologic studies have consistently demonstrated that heavy drinkers and alcoholics are at elevated risk for the development of cirrhosis of the liver and have significantly higher mortality rates than the general population (Bruun et al., 1975; Coates, Halliday, Rankin, Feinman, & Fisher, 1986; Corrao, 1998; Corrao, Bagnardi, Zambon, & Oorchio, 1998; Leifman & Romelsjš, 1997; Mann, Anglin, Wilkins, Vingilis, & Macdonald, 1993; Pell & D'Alonzo, 1973; Schmidt & de Lint, 1972; Thun et al., 1997). This relationship has proved to be remarkably strong and has been consistently observed across time periods and in various regions of the world (Bruun et al., 1975; Ramstedt, 2001; Smart & Mann, 1991). For example, Schmidt found a correlation of $r = 0.97$ between per capita consumption of alcohol and liver cirrhosis mortality rates during 1932–1977 in Ontario, Canada. He estimated that 79% of liver cirrhosis deaths in the Ontario population were attributable to heavy alcohol intake (Schmidt, 1980).

Time series investigations reflect a lagged relationship between cirrhosis mortality and per capita alcohol consumption whereby the rate of cirrhosis mortality in a year is influenced by the alcohol consumption rates of several previous years (Corrao, 1998; Ledermann, 1956; Ramstedt, 2001). To account for this effect, Skog developed a "*distributed lag model*," in which the effects of alcohol consumption in a year are distributed over the next several years (Skog, 1980, 1984). Using this model, he was able to explain an apparent inverse relationship between per capita alcohol consumption and cirrhosis mortality rates in Great Britain between 1931 and 1958 (Popham, 1970). Application of the model produced the expected positive relationship between alcohol consumption and cirrhosis mortality (Mann, Smart, & Govoni, 2003; Skog, 1980).

Results of cohort studies have added to the evidence linking alcohol abuse and mortality due to cirrhosis of the liver as well as noncirrhotic diseases and conditions. In a long-term follow-up study conducted in Denmark, 10,154 patients with cirrhosis of the liver were identified from the Danish National Registry of Patients during 1982–1989 and followed to determine time and cause of death. Relative survival was calculated as the ratio of observed survival to that expected for persons of the same age and sex in the general population. After 12 years of follow-up, 6979 (69%) of the cirrhotic patients had died, a 12-fold increase in all-cause mortality compared to the general population. The estimated 10-year relative mortality due to alcoholic cirrhosis was 66%. Cause-specific mortality ratios were significantly increased not only for cirrhosis-related conditions, but also for ischemic heart disease, infectious disease, gastrointestinal cancer, accidents, and suicide (Sørensen et al., 2003).

Alcohol Consumption and Cirrhosis Mortality in the United States

The close temporal relationship between alcohol consumption and cirrhosis mortality is well illustrated by time series data for the United States population collected during the 20th century (Roizen, Kerr, & Fillmore, 1999). As shown in **FIGURE 45.4**, U.S. cirrhosis mortality rates for men and women were high at the beginning of the 20th century but then declined precipitously with Prohibition in 1920 only to rise again when Prohibition ended in 1933. Rates peaked in 1973 and have since declined in parallel with decreasing per capita consumption levels.

International Trends of Alcohol Consumption and Cirrhosis

International studies of geographic patterns also reveal significant positive correlations between per capita intake of alcohol and mortality from liver cirrhosis (Schmidt, 1980; Schmidt & Bronetto, 1962; Schmidt & de Lint, 1972). Using data collected by WHO for 47 countries in 1974, Moser found a correlation of $r = 0.74$ between rates of cirrhosis mortality and per capita alcohol consumption (Moser, 1980) (**FIGURE 45.5**).

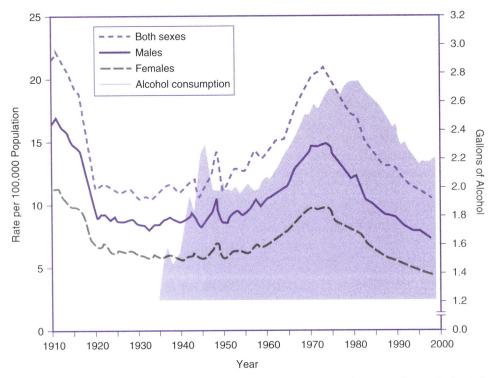

FIGURE 45.4 Per Capita Alcohol Consumption (1935–1997) and Age-Adjusted Death Rates of Liver Cirrhosis by Gender (1910–1997) in the United States Population.

Data from Mortality rate data adapted from Yoon, Y.-H., Yi, H., Grant, B. F., & Dufour, M. C. (2001). *Surveillance report #57: Liver cirrhosis mortality in the United States, 1970–98*. Washington, DC: National Institute on Alcohol Abuse and Alcoholism; per capita alcohol consumption data from Nephew, T. M., Williams, G. D., Yi, H. Y., Hoy, A. K., Stinson, F. S., & Dufour, M. C. (2002). *Surveillance report #59: Apparent per capita alcohol consumption: National, state and regional trends, 1977–99*. Washington, DC: National Institute of Alcohol Abuse and Alcoholism. Mann, R. E., Smart, R. G., & Govoni, R. (2003). The epidemiology of alcoholic liver disease. *Alcohol Research & Health 27*, 209–219.

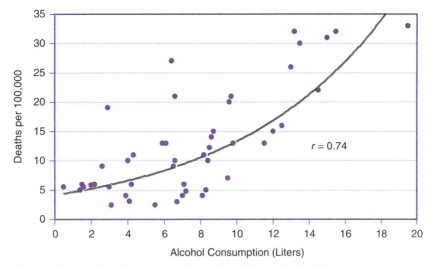

FIGURE 45.5 International Correlation of Cirrhosis Mortality and Per Capita Alcohol Consumption.

Data from Moser, J. (1980). *Prevention of alcohol related problems: An international review of prevention measures, policies and programmes.* Published on behalf of the World Health Organization by the Alcoholism and Drug Addiction Research Foundation, Toronto, Canada. Progression of Liver Disease with Chronic Alcohol Abuse.

TABLE 45.1 Liver Function and Alcohol Intake			
Liver Function	**No. of Cases**	**Daily Alcohol Consumption[a]**	**Years of Alcohol Abuse**
Normal	70	90	7.7
Uncomplicated fatty liver	118	109	7.8
Severe steatofibrosis	48	127	10.3
Chronic alcoholic hepatitis	78	125	11.9
Cirrhosis	39	147	17.1

[a] Average mg per day per hour per kg bodyweight.

Data from Lelbach, W. K. (1974). Organic pathology related to volume and patterns of alcohol use. In R. Gibbins, Y. Israel, & H. Kalant (Eds.), *Research advances in alcohol and drug problems* (Vol. 1, pp. 93–198). New York, NY: John Wiley & Sons.

Important investigations have been conducted to elucidate the progression of liver disease according to the amount and duration of alcohol consumption (Hall, 1995). Lelbach studied the impact of alcohol consumption on liver function and cirrhosis development among 319 patients in an alcoholism clinic in Germany. He calculated the average amount of alcohol consumed per hour in a 24-hour day according to the severity of liver damage. As shown in **TABLE 45.1**, the severity of liver damage was found to be closely related to the amount and duration of alcohol intake. On average, patients with normal liver function consumed the least amount of alcohol for the shortest duration and those with cirrhosis consumed the greatest amount for the longest duration (Table 45.1).

Patients with normal liver function had been drinking heavily for only about 8 years whereas those with cirrhosis had been drinking heavily for more than 17 years. As this research illustrates, the progression of liver damage from fatty liver to cirrhosis is a function of both quantity and duration of alcohol consumption (Lelbach, 1974).

While epidemiologic research has established a firm etiologic connection between heavy alcohol consumption and cirrhosis of the liver, there is considerable heterogeneity amongst studies regarding the *threshold dose* of alcohol necessary for pathogenesis as well as effects of *interactions* of alcohol with other risk factors and conditions such as viral hepatitis, smoking, and the metabolic syndrome.

Bellentani and colleagues examined relationships of daily alcohol intake, type of beverage consumed, and drinking patterns with alcohol-induced liver disease in a cohort of 6534 Italian subjects 12–65 years of age and without disease at baseline (the *Dionysos Study*). They found that the risk threshold for the development of cirrhosis or non-cirrhotic liver damage was ingestion of more than 30 g (2–3 drinks) of alcohol daily for 10 years, which corresponds to a lifetime (cumulative) alcohol intake exceeding 100 kg. The investigators concluded that the risk of developing alcohol-induced liver damage increased significantly (more than threefold) with intakes above the 30-g daily threshold; they also noted that drinking alcohol outside mealtimes or drinking multiple different alcoholic beverages increased the risk (Bellentani et al., 1997; Bellentani & Tiribelli, 2001).

To further investigate effects of low (threshold) levels of alcohol consumption, Corrao and colleagues at the University of Milano, Italy, conducted a meta-analysis of epidemiologic studies with adequate information on alcohol consumption and cirrhosis. Fifteen studies involving 3742 cirrhotic patients were included in the analysis (2724 from case–control studies and 1013 from cohort studies). Though there was marked heterogeneity among studies, the results provided clear evidence that low levels of alcohol intake (25 g per day) significantly increased the risk of developing cirrhosis of the liver (relative risk estimates ranged from 1.5 to 3.6 depending on the type of regression model used). Higher consumption levels (50 g per day) were associated with relative risks ranging from 1.9 to 9.4. The dose response of cirrhosis risk with increasing consumption of alcohol based on a quadratic regression model is shown in

FIGURE 45.6. Chronic daily intake of 25 g of alcohol (about two alcoholic drinks) increased the risk by more than twofold in this model (Corrao, Bagnardi, et al., 1998).

Beverage-Specific Effects

Relationships between per capita alcohol consumption and cirrhosis mortality may vary depending on the type of alcoholic beverage consumed—beer, wine, or spirits. Indeed, the presence of beverage-specific effects could help explain why cirrhosis mortality began to decline in some populations during the 1970s *despite the continued rise in total alcohol consumption.* This pattern is exemplified by the U.S. time series data on total alcohol consumption and cirrhosis mortality shown above in Figure 45.3.

Researchers over the past several decades have investigated potential reasons for imperfections in temporal associations between *per capita* alcohol consumption and mortality due to liver cirrhosis (Gruenewald & Ponicki, 1995; Schmidt & Bronetto, 1962; Terris, 1967). In an analysis of time series data from the United States spanning 1949–1994, Roizen and colleagues demonstrated that the curve for total alcohol consumption lags behind the cirrhosis mortality curve whereas the curve for consumption of distilled spirits shows a better fit (Roizen et al., 1999). They state that *"the trend-line for per capita distilled spirit consumption bears a much closer correspondence to the cirrhosis mortality trend than does per capita total alcohol consumption"* (Roizen, Fillmore, & Kerr, 1999). This *"beverage-specific"* effect was initially demonstrated by Milton Terris (1967) and suggests that per capita consumption of distilled beverages with high alcoholic content may be a better

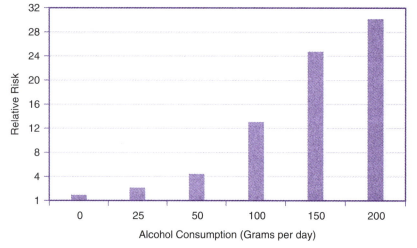

FIGURE 45.6 Dose Response of Liver Cirrhosis Risk with Alcohol Consumption.
Data from Corrao, G., Bagnardi, V., Zambon, A., & Oorchio, P. (1998). Meta-analysis of alcohol intake in relation to risk of liver cirrhosis. *Alcohol and Alcoholism, 33*(4), 381–392.

determinant of cirrhosis trends than total alcohol consumption.

Kerr and colleagues extended the analysis of distilled spirits versus total alcohol consumption as correlates of cirrhosis mortality to several other countries with similar results. Time series data were examined in Australia, Canada, New Zealand, the United Kingdom, and the United States during the years 1953–1993. In these populations, per capita consumption of distilled spirits accounted for the majority of the effects of alcohol and provided the best fit to mortality data (Kerr, Fillmore, & Marvy, 2000).

As pointed out by Mann, Smart, and Govoni in their review, The Epidemiology of Alcoholic Liver Disease:

> *The stronger association between per capita consumption of spirits and cirrhosis mortality may be attributable to biological and socio-behavioral mechanisms." Some types of alcoholic beverages may be more toxic to the liver than others (Lelbach, 1974; Schmidt & Bronetto, 1962). In addition, consumption of certain alcoholic beverages may be associated with different drinking styles (Smart, 1996)—that is, people who tend to drink frequently and heavily, and thus are at greatest risk for developing cirrhosis, also may tend to drink spirits rather than beer or wine. Thus, drinking style may collude with biological mechanisms to significantly raise some drinkers' risk of liver disease. This interesting and important issue is the subject of ongoing investigation (Mann, Smart, & Govoni, 2003).*

Synergy of Alcohol and Tobacco in Cirrhosis of the Liver

Liu and colleagues examined the separate and joint effects of alcohol and smoking on incidence rates of liver cirrhosis and gallbladder disease in the *Million Women Study* conducted in the United Kingdom. The *Million Women Study* is an ongoing prospective study of 1,290,413 million middle-aged women (mean age = 56.1 years) in England and Scotland who were recruited through the United Kingdom National Health Service during 1996–2001. At recruitment, women explained the amount of alcohol they were drinking, their smoking status, and the number of cigarettes they smoked daily, as well as information on anthropometric factors, sociodemographic factors, reproductive history, use of exogenous hormones, and medical history. During a mean follow-up of 6.1 years, 2105 women developed cirrhosis and 23,989 developed gallbladder disease yielding 5-year incidence

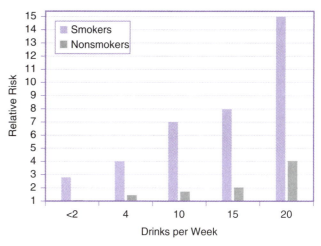

FIGURE 45.7 Cirrhosis of the Liver: Combined Effects of Alcohol and Tobacco in British Women.

Data from Liu, B., Balkwill, A., Roddam, A., Brown, A., Beral, V., & on behalf of the Million Women Study Collaborators. (2009). Separate and joint effects of alcohol and smoking on the risks of cirrhosis and gallbladder disease in middle-aged women. *American Journal of Epidemiology, 169*(2), 153–160.

rates of 1.3 per 1000 persons and 15 per 1000 persons, respectively. The risk of cirrhosis of the liver increased with increasing alcohol consumption, whereas the risk of gall bladder disease appeared to decrease. Comparing women who drank ≥15 units/week with those who drank 1–2 units/week, the relative risk was 4.32 for cirrhosis and 0.59 for gallbladder disease. Increasing numbers of cigarettes smoked daily increased the risk of both conditions. Comparing current smokers of ≥20 cigarettes/day with never smokers, the relative risk was 3.76 for cirrhosis and 1.29 for gallbladder disease. Synergistic effects of alcohol and smoking were observed for the development of cirrhosis but not for gallbladder disease (i.e., the risk of developing liver cirrhosis was increased nearly 15-fold in women who drank and smoked heavily compared to women with neither exposure) (**FIGURE 45.7**). These findings indicate that alcohol and smoking separately increase the risk of developing cirrhosis of the liver and their joint effects are particularly hazardous (Liu, Balkwill, Roddam, Brown, & Beral, 2009).

Chronic Viral Hepatitis and Cirrhosis of the Liver

Compounding the problem of alcoholic cirrhosis of the liver, chronic liver infections by HBV and/or HCV have emerged as major causes of liver cirrhosis in many populations. A variety of liver viruses can infect and damage the liver including hepatitis A, B, C, D, and E.

Acute Hepatitis A and E. Hepatitis A and hepatitis E are RNA viruses that typically cause acute infection lasting only a few days. Both are transmitted by the fecal-oral route. Contaminated drinking water and food supplies have been implicated in major outbreaks. The highest rates of infection occur in regions where low standards of sanitation promote the transmission of these viruses. Hepatitis A and hepatitis E *do not* develop into chronic hepatitis or cirrhosis; however, there are case reports where acute hepatitis A/E infection has resulted in *acute* liver failure and death in immunocompromised individuals and pregnant women (Emerson & Purcell, 2003; Fiore, 2004). The other hepatitis viruses (HBV, HCV, and HDV) are primarily responsible for chronic liver infections that can progress to liver cirrhosis.

Hepatitis B and Cirrhosis of the Liver. HBV is a common source of viral hepatitis in humans. The virus is endemic in regions of Asia, Africa, and China and has infected approximately one-third of the world population (more than *2 billion* people). The prevalence of HBV infection varies widely from 0.5% in nonendemic regions to levels exceeding 10% in endemic areas (Custer et al., 2004). It is estimated that 400 million people are chronic carriers of HBV (Williams, 2006).

Hepatitis B is a DNA virus that undergoes replication in the liver. It is similar to RNA viruses in that reverse transcriptase is used for replication. Viral transmission results from exposure to infectious blood or body fluids. In regions of the world where HBV is endemic, most HBV infections occur during infancy or early childhood. Vertical transmission from mother to baby can occur at the time of childbirth when the newborn passes through the birth canal or later (e.g., through contaminated saliva or breast milk). High rates of child to child transmission have also been documented in certain populations (Locarnini, 2004; Shapiro, 1993).

Transmission of HBV in adults occurs through unprotected sexual contact with an infected individual or by using contaminated needles and syringes for the intravenous injection of illicit drugs. The virus can also be transmitted by transfusion with contaminated blood or blood products in countries without effective screening programs for donor blood. Nevertheless, immunocompetent adults who become infected by HBV usually clear the virus without treatment and less than 1% of individuals who become infected during adulthood will develop chronic hepatitis B. Reciprocally, approximately 95% of newborns that acquire HBV at birth are unable to clear the virus and thus become chronic carriers of HBV. Individuals with chronic HBV infection have an exceptionally high (approximately 40%) probability of eventually dying from liver cirrhosis and/or hepatocellular carcinoma (Williams, 2006).

Fung and colleagues evaluated 951 Asian men and women with chronic HBV infection to document the prevalence of severe liver fibrosis and/or cirrhosis (Fung et al., 2008). Of these patients, 319 (34%) were found to have severe fibrosis. The overall prevalence was higher in males than females (39% vs. 24%) and higher in adults with antibodies against the viral precore antigen (HBeAg) (58% vs. 43%). Seropositivity for HBeAg indicates a high viral load, prolonged immune damage and accelerated progression of liver damage. The prevalence of fibrosis/cirrhosis increased with age reaching 81% after 65 years of age (**FIGURE 45.8**).

Hepatitis C and Cirrhosis of the Liver. Chronic infection with HCV causes chronic inflammation of the liver that over time can progress to cirrhosis,

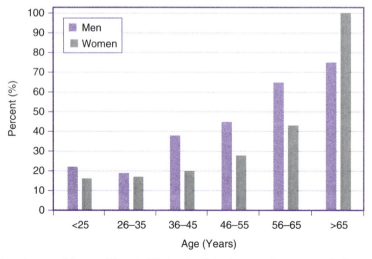

FIGURE 45.8 Age-Specific Prevalence of Severe Fibrosis/Cirrhosis of the Liver in Patients with Chronic HBV Infection.

Data from Fung, J., Lai, C.-L., But, D., Wong, D., Cheung, T.-K., & Yuen, M.-F. (2008). Prevalence of fibrosis and cirrhosis in chronic hepatitis B: Implications for treatment and management. *American Journal of Gastroenterology, 103*(6), 1421–1426.

hepatocellular carcinoma, or both. The global prevalence of HCV is approximately 3% (more than 200 million infected persons). The virus is endemic in many parts of the world and is primarily transmitted by exposure to contaminated blood or body fluids. Prevalence rates are high in many African nations and Egypt in particular. Notably, HCV can be transmitted via unsterilized injection equipment and infusion of inadequately screened blood and blood products. In Egypt, a nationwide parenteral treatment program for widespread schistosomiasis (infection by parasitic schistosome worms) may have accidentally caused high rates of HCV infection (Frank et al., 2000). Routine donor screening in blood banks by enzyme immunoassays has achieved a sharp decline in transfusion-associated HCV transmission (Kamal, 2008).

In contrast to HBV that most often infects newborns and children, HCV is commonly first encountered in adulthood. The host response to HCV infection is highly variable. Approximately 20%–40% of subjects experience clearance of the virus and spontaneous resolution of infection. Conversely, the majority of HCV infections (60%–80%) become chronic and may eventually progress to cirrhosis and/ or hepatocellular carcinoma. Estimates of the proportion of chronically infected persons who develop cirrhosis 20 years after initial infection vary widely: from 2%–4% in children to 20%–30% in adults. Furthermore, patients who are older at the time of infection, patients with continuous exposure to alcohol, and those coinfected with HIV or HBV demonstrate accelerated progression to more advanced liver disease. Some success has been achieved in the early treatment of chronic HCV infection using interferon plus antiviral drugs (NIH Consensus Statement on Management of Hepatitis C, 2002).

Hepatitis D: Co-infection with Hepatitis B. HDV also called hepatitis delta is a small circular RNA virus. It appears to be a subviral satellite because it can only propagate in the presence of HBV. Transmission of HDV can occur either via simultaneous infection with HBV (co-infection) or via infection of an individual previously infected with HBV (superinfection).

Both superinfection and co-infection with HDV result in more severe complications compared to infection with HBV alone. These complications include a greater likelihood of experiencing liver failure in acute infections and rapid progression to liver cirrhosis with an increased risk of developing liver cancer in chronic infections. In combination with HBV, hepatitis D has a 20% mortality rate, the highest of all the acute hepatitis infections (Lai, 1994).

Synergy of Alcohol and Viral Hepatitis. Excess alcohol consumption has been found to worsen the course and outcome of viral hepatitis (Schiff & Ozden, 2003). Poynard and colleagues studied the influence of alcohol intake among 1574 patients with hepatitis C who had not received antiviral therapy. Compared to nondrinkers, patients who drank over 50 g of alcohol daily increased their risk of developing liver fibrosis by 34%. Furthermore, the relative risk of progression of fibrosis with heavier alcohol intake was 2.36. The effects of lower amounts of alcohol intake were not significant (Poynard, Bedossa, & Opolon, 1997).

Bellentani and colleagues analyzed hepatitis virus markers, self-reported alcohol intake, and clinical and biochemical markers of liver disease in a cohort of 6917 Italian individuals in northern Italy (the *Dionysos Study*). As noted above in the section on alcoholic cirrhosis, daily alcohol consumption of 30 g or more independently increased the risk of cirrhosis more than threefold. Furthermore, among subjects who tested positive for HCV, 32% of heavy drinkers developed cirrhosis compared to only 10% of light drinkers (Bellentani et al., 1999).

Seef and colleagues studied 1030 U.S. patients enrolled in a prospective investigation of transfusion-associated HCV infection during 1968–1980. After 15 years of follow-up, 17% of patients with HCV infection developed cirrhosis compared to 2.8% of patients without hepatitis. Notably, patients with both HCV and a history of alcohol abuse were 31 times more likely to develop cirrhosis than control subjects (Seeff et al., 2001).

The deleterious impact of alcohol consumption in patients with HCV infection was dramatically demonstrated in a case–control study of 285 cirrhotic patients in Italy. Only 1.4% (4 subjects) were HCV-positive and nondrinkers compared to 11.2% (32 patients) who were both HCV-positive and heavy drinkers (Corrao & Arico, 1998).

Clearly, these results provide consistent evidence that heavy alcohol use exacerbates liver disease in patients with hepatitis C and accelerates the progression of steatohepatitis to cirrhosis. Nevertheless, additional studies are needed in order to elucidate potential effects of light to moderate alcohol intake in patients with hepatitis C infection (Peters & Terrault, 2002).

Nonalcoholic Cirrhosis of the Liver

The Metabolic Syndrome. The *metabolic syndrome* (also called *Syndrome X*) is a disease complex of glucose intolerance or type 2 diabetes, hypertension, central obesity and dyslipidemia (elevated total cholesterol and triglycerides and decreased HDL cholesterol). The prevalence of this disease constellation is rising throughout the world.

The metabolic syndrome predisposes not only to atherosclerosis and catastrophic cardiovascular events (myocardial infarction and stroke), but it also promotes the development of *nonalcoholic fatty liver disease*. Nonalcoholic fatty liver disease refers to excess accumulation of fat in the liver in the absence of exposure to alcohol. It is the most prevalent of all liver diseases and is estimated to afflict 20%–30% of adults in the United States and other Western countries (Angulo, 2002; Neuschwander-Teri & Caldwell, 2003). A significant fraction of individuals with nonalcoholic liver disease, perhaps 10%, develop hepatitis (inflammation of the liver). The combination of nonalcoholic fatty liver disease and hepatitis is called *nonalcoholic steatohepatitis (NASH)*. NASH can progress to liver cirrhosis and liver failure.

Recent investigations have established that the metabolic syndrome as well as its individual components (e.g., insulin resistance, diabetes, obesity) are risk factors for the development of nonalcoholic fatty liver disease and progression to NASH, liver cirrhosis and mortality from liver failure (Adams et al., 2005; Angulo, Keach, Batts, & Lindor, 1999; de Ledinghen et al., 2006; Farrell & Larter, 2006; Kim & Younossi, 2008). The sequence of pathogenesis is depicted in **FIGURE 45.9**.

However, the sequence of pathogenesis in individual patients may differ and there is the definite possibility that liver disease predisposes to insulin resistance and diabetes. There is also the issue of "*reverse causality*" in determination of the temporal sequence of pathogenesis of diabetes and liver disease. Disentangling relationships between components of the metabolic syndrome and the progression of liver disease are difficult and complex since, in both conditions, ascertainment of disease onset is imprecise and often based upon clinical symptoms which may occur long after the subclinical onset of disease. While

several studies have focused on this association, the question remains; does liver disease lead to diabetes or vice versa?

German investigators examined glucose intolerance and type 2 diabetes in a group of 108 cases with liver cirrhosis and 181 control subjects without liver disease. Seventy-nine of the cirrhotic patients (73%) manifested either glucose intolerance or type 2 diabetes compared to 56% of control subjects. The crude odds ratio calculated from these data suggests that patients with either glucose intolerance or type 2 diabetes have more than a twofold increase in cirrhosis risk (crude odds ratio = 2.2). Reciprocally, the investigators did not find clinical, histological, or biochemical signs of liver cirrhosis that were clearly associated with either glucose intolerance or diabetes (Müller, Pirlich, Balks, & Selberg, 1994).

In Great Britain, Fraser and colleagues examined associations between liver enzymes, aminotransferase (ALT) and g-glutamyltransferase (GGT), and the development of diabetes in participants of the *British Women's Heart and Health Study*, a cohort of 4286 women, aged 60–79 years at baseline, who were followed for a median of 7.3 years. Cox proportional hazards regression models were used to examine associations of liver enzymes with incident diabetes. Both ALT and GGT were associated with incident diabetes. With adjustment for age and alcohol consumption, hazard ratios increased by about 50% per standard deviation increase in logged ALT or GGT values (Fraser, Harris, & Sattar, 2009).

In the same report, Fraser and colleagues also conducted a systematic review and meta-analysis of 21 prospective, population-based studies of associations between nonalcoholic fatty liver disease and elevated liver enzymes (ALT and GGT) with the development of diabetes. Summary estimates of the relative risk (RR) of diabetes development were increased for ALT (RR = 2.02), GGT (HR [Hazard Ratio] = 2.94) and nonalcoholic fatty liver disease (HR = 2.52) suggesting that antecedent liver pathologies, particularly the accumulation of liver fat, are risk factors for the development of diabetes (Fraser, Harris, & Sattar, 2009).

In Bologna, Italy, Marchesini and colleagues assessed effects of the metabolic syndrome in the development of nonalcoholic steatohepatitis (NASH) among 304 patients with nonalcoholic fatty liver disease. Based on liver biopsies, 120 of these patients (cases) had nonalcoholic steatohepatitis (NASH) and 185 patients (controls) had *pure* nonalcoholic fatty liver disease. Among cases with NASH, 88% had the metabolic syndrome compared to 53% of controls

FIGURE 45.9 Progression of Nonalcoholic Fatty Liver Disease.

with pure nonalcoholic fatty liver disease. Logistic regression analysis was used to examine the risk of developing NASH associated with the presence of the metabolic syndrome. Patients with the metabolic syndrome carried a threefold higher risk for development of NASH than those without (adjusted odds ratio [OR] = 3.2). The metabolic syndrome was also associated with a higher risk of severe liver fibrosis (adjusted OR = 3.5). The investigators concluded that *"the metabolic syndrome puts a very large population at risk of forthcoming liver failure in the next decades"* (Marchesini et al., 2003).

In Hong Kong, China, Wong and colleagues evaluated components of the metabolic syndrome as determinants of liver cirrhosis among 1466 patients with confirmed hepatitis B (HBV) infection. Noninvasive transient elastography (a noninvasive ultrasonographic measure of liver stiffness) was used to determine the presence of liver cirrhosis in the study. The prevalence of the metabolic syndrome was higher in HBV patients with cirrhosis than those without (24% vs. 11%); after adjustment for anthropometric, biochemical and virological factors, the metabolic syndrome retained statistical significance as an independent risk factor for the development of cirrhosis in patients with chronic hepatitis B infection (OR = 1.7). Furthermore, as shown in **FIGURE 45.10**, the odds of developing cirrhosis show a dose response with the number of metabolic syndrome components present (e.g., patients manifesting all five components were over five times more likely to develop cirrhosis than those with none) (Wong et al., 2009).

Stepanova and colleagues linked population data from the Third National Health and Nutrition Examination Survey (NHANES III) with nearly 18 years of mortality data from the U.S. National Death Index to study the association of the metabolic syndrome with mortality due to liver disease. The NHANES III is a nationwide survey conducted during 1988–1994 to provide information on health and nutrition in the civilian U.S. population. The study compared mortality in 1556 individuals with liver disease to 13,004 individuals without disease. Underlying liver disease pathology was classified according to risk factors and viral seropositivity. There were 235 individuals with alcoholic liver disease, 66 with chronic hepatitis B, 264 with chronic hepatitis C, and 991 with nonalcoholic fatty liver disease. During more than 13 years of follow-up, a total of 3662 individuals died in the cohort of 15,866 individuals. Mortality risks were tested by Cox regression analysis. The presence of the metabolic syndrome significantly increased mortality from liver disease for each of the underlying pathologies: Hazard ratio (HR) = 4.3 for chronic hepatitis B, HR = 3.4 for chronic hepatitis C, HR = 2.1 for alcoholic liver disease, and HR = 12.1 for nonalcoholic fatty liver disease. Furthermore, specific components of the metabolic syndrome such as diabetes, insulin resistance and obesity independently increased liver disease mortality in certain conditions (e.g., the presence of type 2 diabetes increased liver mortality in patients with chronic hepatitis B more than 30-fold) (Stepanova, Zobair, & Younossi, 2010). These results provide compelling evidence that the metabolic syndrome acts independently and in concert with other risk factors to increase the mortality due to liver disease.

In summarizing the results of such studies, it is apparent that the metabolic syndrome accelerates the progression of nonalcoholic fatty liver disease and is linked to higher rates of liver failure and mortality

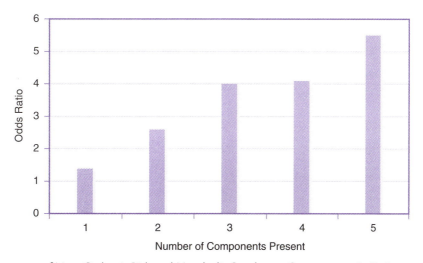

FIGURE 45.10 Dose Response of Liver Cirrhosis Risk and Metabolic Syndrome Components in Patients with HBV.

Data from Wong, G. L. H., Wong, V. W. S., Choi, P. C. L., Chan, A. W. H., Chim, A. M. L., Yiu, K. K. L., & Chan, F. K.-L. (2009). Metabolic syndrome increases the risk of liver cirrhosis in chronic hepatitis B. *Gut, 58,* 111–117. Metabolic Syndrome Components: Insulin Resistance or Type 2 Diabetes, Obesity, Hyperlipidemia (elevated total cholesterol and triglycerides and decreased HDL-cholesterol), Hypertension, Inflammation (elevated C-reactive protein). *Gut, 58,* 111–117.

(Marchesini & Bianchi, 2010). Conversely, the presence of nonalcoholic fatty liver disease also appears to predispose to insulin resistance and the genesis of type 2 diabetes mellitus. Various physiological mechanisms may be involved. For example, adipokines such as leptin, adiponectin, and resistin are secreted by metabolically active visceral adipose cells and may interact to promote liver fibrosis and/or diabetes. Increases in liver enzymes might also influence insulin resistance (e.g., elevated levels of ALT and GGT reflect increased levels of oxidative products and oxidative stress). Finally, it is likely that chronic inflammation in association with necrosis and regeneration of hepatocytes (necroinflammation) contributes significantly to the stepwise progression from fatty liver disease to steatohepatitis to fibrosis to cirrhosis to liver failure.

Gender Differences in Cirrhosis of the Liver

As discussed above, the epidemiology of cirrhosis of the liver has been linked closely to alcohol consumption. Nevertheless, several other factors (hepatitis B, hepatitis C, the metabolic syndrome and its components, particularly obesity, insulin resistance, and type 2 diabetes, and tobacco addiction) have emerged as prominent independent risk factors in the development and progression of liver disease.

An additional issue of importance is the presence of significant and long-standing gender differences in cirrhosis mortality risk and mortality rates. As shown in Figure 45.3 earlier in this chapter, annual mortality rates from cirrhosis of the liver were more than twofold higher in U.S. men than women throughout the 20th century. Furthermore, based on age-cause-specific mortality data published by WHO (1997–1999),

annual cirrhosis mortality rates for every age bracket are approximately two times higher in men than in women (**FIGURE 45.11**).

In a recent hospital-based case–control study of Italian men and women, Corrao and colleagues examined the proportion of newly diagnosed cases of symptomatic liver cirrhosis attributable to three known risk factors, alcohol, hepatitis B, and hepatitis C. Cases with liver cirrhosis ($n = 462$) were ascertained during 1989–1996 from hospitals distributed throughout Italy and controls without liver disease ($n = 651$) were ascertained from the same hospitals and time period. Estimates of the proportion of symptomatic liver cirrhosis attributable to alcohol intake, hepatitis B and hepatitis C infections were obtained for each individual factor and for all three factors combined. The individual population attributable risk estimates for men and women were 67.9% for alcohol, 40.1% for hepatitis C, and 4.4% for hepatitis B. Taken together, these three risk factors explained 85.5% of liver cirrhosis in the Italian population. However, attributable risk estimates for alcohol were nearly twofold higher in men than women (85.9% vs. 46.8%) and the three factors combined explained a much higher proportion of the risk in men compared to women (98.1% vs. 67.0%). The unexplained portion of the risk in women (33%) suggests that some other factors may be involved in the genesis of liver cirrhosis in women (Corrao, Zambon, et al., 1998).

Gender Differences in Alcoholic Liver Disease

The twofold higher mortality due to liver cirrhosis in men compared to women undoubtedly reflects the fact that men typically drink more than women, and

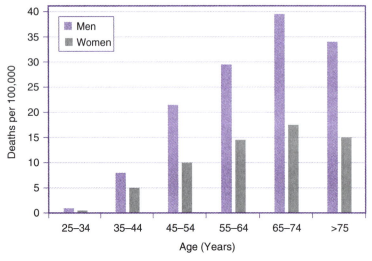

FIGURE 45.11 Age-Specific Mortality: Cirrhosis of the Liver.
Data from World Health Organization (WHO). Annual World Health Statistics for European Nations, 1997–1999.

that the proportion of heavy drinkers and alcoholics is higher among men. However, some studies have found that at any given level of alcohol consumption, women actually have a *higher* likelihood of developing liver cirrhosis than men (Tuyns & Péquignot, 1984). As discussed in a following section of this chapter (*Genetic Predisposition to Alcoholic Liver Cirrhosis*), the heightened genetic susceptibility of women to alcoholic cirrhogenesis compared to men may be related to their lower levels of gastric alcohol dehydrogenase, the key enzyme in the metabolism of alcohol (Frezza et al., 1990).

Differences in Hepatitis B Infection

Gender differences have also been observed in the prevalence rates of cirrhogenic hepatitis viruses B and C. In most populations studied, the prevalence of chronic HBV infection is greater in men than women. Higher HBV infection rates in men versus women were initially reported by Blumberg and colleagues in populations of tropical climates and were subsequently confirmed by investigations of blood donors, hospitalized and nonhospitalized patients, transplant and hemodialysis patients, and mental patients (Blumberg, 2006; London & Drew, 1977).

As pointed out by Baruch Blumberg (who discovered HBV in the serum of a leukemia patient in 1963), there are a number of unusual gender-related aspects of HBV infection. A significant predominance of male newborns of HBV-infected mothers has been observed in many populations where HBV is endemic. This may account for the high male-to-female ratios observed in China and in other areas with a high prevalence of HBV infection. The apparent "*loss of females*" in these populations can thus be ascribed, at least in part, to HBV infection (Blumberg, 2006). While the mechanism is speculative, maternal antibodies directed against HBV may cross-react with sperm to give a slight selection advantage to sperm bearing the Y chromosome.

Males infected with HBV also have a greater predilection to chronic infection than females. This finding comes from studies of HBV outbreaks in mental institutions. In one such study conducted in New York City, 49 of 317 males (15.4%) remained positive for the hepatitis B "Australia antigen" 1 year after an outbreak compared to only 2 of 467 females (0.43%) (Curtis, Samper, Rodriquez, & Garrett, 1973; Goodman, Wainwright, Weir, & Gall, 1971). The predominance of HBV infection and viral-induced cirrhosis among men compared to women thus contributes to the higher overall mortality rate in men due to cirrhosis of the liver.

Gender Differences in Hepatitis C Infection

Injection drug use is the single most important risk factor for acquiring HCV. Commensurate with higher levels of drug use in men compared to women, chronic HCV infection rates are approximately twofold higher in men than women in most population-based studies. In a large national survey of 15,079 adults in the United States conducted during 1999–2002, the prevalence of HCV infection (based on HCV antibodies) was 2.1% in men compared to 1.1% in women (Armstrong, Alter, McQuillan, & Margolis, 2000; Armstrong et al., 2006).

Studies of special populations also reflect higher HCV infection rates in men than women. In a study of 777 patients with severe mental illness in North Carolina, HCV infection among men was nearly twice that among women. Men also had higher rates of injection needle use (23.1% vs. 12.5%), needle-sharing (17.6% vs. 7.7%), and certain other drug-related risk behaviors. In contrast, women had higher rates of sexual risk behaviors such as unprotected sex in exchange for drugs (17.8% vs. 11.2%) (Butterfield et al., 2003).

Notably, recent studies suggest that drug-related exposure to HCV may be increasing in women. In a survey of 16,000 adults in Australia, women reported higher rates of needle-sharing than men (Iversen et al., 2010). Finally, some studies suggest that women are able to clear HCV more effectively than men (Yamakawa, Sata, Suzuki, Noguchi, & Tanikawa, 1996) which may help explain their lower mortality rate from liver cirrhosis.

Genetic Predisposition to Alcoholic Liver Cirrhosis

Genetic factors, including those that influence alcohol metabolism, are known to influence predisposition to the development of liver cirrhosis. The primary liver enzyme that metabolizes alcohol is alcohol dehydrogenase (ADH). In humans, various forms of ADH are present that are encoded by at least seven genes. Class I ADH, which is present in the liver and the stomach, consists of three subunits encoded by three separate genes, *ADH1A*, *ADH1B*, and *ADH1C*. Genetic expression varies according to age, gender, amount of alcohol consumed, and the alleles present at these genetic loci (Luo et al., 2006; Parlesak, Billinger, Bode, Bode, 2002).

Studies in the laboratories of Charles S. Lieber at the University of Trieste, Italy, elucidated major differences in the metabolism of alcohol between men and women. In a landmark study, women were found to express lower levels of gastric ADH than men, resulting in higher blood levels of alcohol per amount consumed (Frezza et al., 1990; Lieber, 1989). Alcoholic men and women were also found to metabolize alcohol more slowly than nonalcoholic subjects, and first pass metabolism was markedly decreased in alcoholic men and virtually absent in alcoholic women. The authors concluded that "*that the increased bioavailability of ethanol (alcohol) resulting from decreased gastric oxidation of ethanol may contribute to the enhanced vulnerability of women to acute and chronic complications of alcoholism*" (Frezza et al., 1990). Thus, the development of liver cirrhosis in alcoholic men and particularly in alcoholic women may in part be related to their lower gastric ADH activity and relatively slow metabolism of alcohol compared to nonalcoholics. However, there is considerable debate regarding the issue of greater female vulnerability to alcohol and the exact mechanisms of action remain to be elucidated (Parlesak et al., 2002).

Reed and colleagues investigated genetic effects contributing to alcoholism and the development of liver cirrhosis based upon 15,924 twin pairs ascertained from the National Academy of Sciences National Research Council Twin Registry. They observed significantly higher concordance rates of alcoholism and liver cirrhosis among monozygous (identical) twins compared to dizygous (nonidentical) twins (26.7% vs. 12.2% for alcoholism and 16.9% vs. 5.3% for liver cirrhosis) and estimated that about 50% of alcohol-related end organ disease can be attributed to *additive genetic factors*. They also found that most of the genetic predisposition to liver cirrhosis was due to a *shared genetic liability for alcoholism* (Reed, Page, Viken, & Christian, 1996).

Human alcohol dehydrogenase (*ADH*) is under the control of seven genes that are tightly clustered at position 22 on the long arm of chromosome 4 (4q22). Since the *ADH* enzymes play a major role in the pharmacokinetics of alcohol metabolism in humans, the *ADH* genes encoding these enzymes are prime candidates for genetic investigation (Edenberg, 2000).

The *Collaborative Study on the Genetics of Alcoholism (COGA)* is a large-scale study of families with and without alcoholic members ascertained from nine centers across the United States. The study was designed to identify genes that influence alcoholism and alcohol-related diseases (Edenberg, 2003). Studies of these families have elucidated polymorphisms of several ADH genes that are linked to the development of alcoholism and related conditions (e.g., liver cirrhosis) (Reich et al., 1998). For example, gene variants encoding three alcohol-metabolizing enzymes, *ADH1B*, *ADH1C*, and *ALDH2*, have been found that heighten the risk of alcoholism (Hurley, Edenberg,

& Li, 2002). Genetic variants in the promoter region of the gene encoding *ADH4* have also been found to modulate alcohol metabolism and the risk of alcoholism (Edenberg, Jerome, & Li, 1999). Genetic polymorphisms of *ADH* and their effects on alcoholism and related conditions are under intense study in different populations.

Zinc plays an important role in the structural integrity and efficient functioning of *ADH*. Consequently, a deficiency of zinc may compromise the metabolism of alcohol leading to sustained high blood concentrations of alcohol in those who drink. Furthermore, zinc binding to *ADH* appears to depend on the presence and spacing of specific amino acids (cysteine and histidine); thus genetic variation in zinc binding to ADH may also influence one's genetic susceptibility to alcohol through modification of enzyme structure and function (Auld & Bergman, 2008).

Genetic Predisposition to Viral Hepatitis and Liver Cirrhosis

A number of genetic polymorphisms have also been identified that increase susceptibility to chronic hepatitis viral infections by HBV and HCV. For example, certain alleles of the *major histocompatibility* locus, the *vitamin D receptor* locus, the *tumor necrosis factor* locus, and the interleukin 10 locus have been found to influence the chronicity of HBV infection (Blumberg, 2006).

Investigative teams in Australia, Japan, and the United States recently conducted genome-wide studies of single nucleotide polymorphisms among patients with chronic hepatitis C infection. All three studies found that patients who carried genetic variants of the interleukin 28B interferon-lambda gene (IL28B) displayed altered natural and drug-induced clearance of HCV (Ge et al., 2009; Suppiah et al., 2009; Tanaka et al., 2009). These findings underscore the need for additional genetic-epidemiologic studies to clarify cirrhogenic versus protective features of genetic polymorphisms in order to guide clinical decisions regarding efficacious treatment of HCV infection based upon genotype (O'Brien, 2009).

Genetic Syndromes and Liver Cirrhosis

Primary hemochromatosis is a hereditary disease characterized by excessive absorption of iron resulting in iron overload. Excess iron in the form of hemosiderin accumulates in tissues and organs disrupting their function. The most susceptible organs are the liver, adrenal glands, heart, skin, gonads, joints, and the pancreas. Patients with primary hemochromatosis can manifest a variety of pathologies including cirrhosis of the liver, polyarthritis, adrenal insufficiency, diabetes, and heart failure. Affected men typically experience symptoms between the ages of 30 and 50 years. Affected women are more likely to manifest symptoms after menopause when they no longer lose iron during menstruation. The prevalence of primary hemochromatosis is highest among individuals of European descent, approximately 1 in 200. The condition is due to mutant forms of the *HFE* (high Fe) gene located on the short arm of chromosome 6. The *HFE* gene codes for a membrane protein that is essential in regulating iron absorption and transfer into cells (Feder et al., 1998).

Wilson's disease is a rare autosomal recessive genetic disorder in which copper accumulates in the liver, the brain, and other tissues. This condition is rare with an annual rate of 1–4 cases per 100,000. Clinical signs typically occur in childhood or adolescence and include low serum *ceruloplasmin* (the transport protein for copper in the blood), the deposition of copper and formation of brownish *Kayser-Fleischer* rings in the cornea of the eye, elevated liver enzymes, polyarthritis, kidney dysfunction, and altered mental status. Wilson's disease is caused by mutant forms of the ATP7B gene (located on the long arm of chromosome 13) causing impairment of enzymatic incorporation of copper into ceruloplasmin and excretion of excess copper in bile. Accumulation of copper in the liver results in inflammation (hepatitis), fibrosis, cirrhosis, and ultimately liver failure. Mental disturbances (encephalopathy) may occur as a consequence of disturbances in the urea cycle and increased blood ammonia (Ala, Walker, Ashkan, Dooley, & Schilsky, 2007).

Ethnic Differences in Liver Cirrhosis

Annual estimates of the mortality rates due to liver cirrhosis differ among gender-ethnic groups of the United States. Although the absolute rates have declined dramatically during the past four decades, cirrhosis mortality remains about twofold higher for African-American men than for Caucasian-American men (**FIGURE 45.12**). Ethnic differences in mortality show a similar trend in women, although the differences are much smaller and the current rates are similar for African-American and Caucasian-American women (Mann, Smart, & Govoni, 2003; Minino et al., 2000; Stinson, Grant, & Dufour, 2001; Yoon, Yi, Grant, & Dufour, 2001; Yoon, Yi, Grant, Stinson, & Dufour, 2002).

The persisting higher mortality from liver cirrhosis in African-American men compared to Caucasian-American men may be a consequence of several risk factors and their interactions. Differential patterns of alcohol consumption, insulin resistance, exposure to hepatitis viruses, age, income, education, employment, genetic predisposition, familial history of alcohol/drug abuse and stress should all be considered in the complex web of causation (Jones-Webb, 1998). Differential access to alcoholism treatment services and health care may also be important (Singh & Hoyert, 2000). Notably, recent estimates suggest that Hispanic men have the highest cirrhosis mortality rates of any gender-ethnic group in the United States, approximately 12 deaths per 100,000 per year (Mann, Smart, & Govoni, 2003; Stinson, Grant, & Dufour, 2001). The observed excess cirrhosis mortality in Hispanic men is consistent with their higher prevalence of hepatitis C infection compared to other

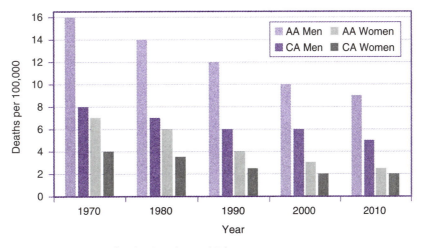

FIGURE 45.12 Trends in Liver Cirrhosis Mortality by Gender and Ethnicity.

Data from Yoon, Y.-H., Yi, H., Grant, B. F., & Dufour, M. C. (2001). *Surveillance report #57: Liver cirrhosis mortality in the United States, 1970–98*. Washington, DC: National Institute on Alcohol Abuse and Alcoholism; Yoon, Y.-H., Yi, H., Grant, B. F., Stinson, F. S., & Dufour, M. C. (2002). *Surveillance report #60: Liver cirrhosis mortality in the United States, 1970–99*. Washington, DC: National Institute on Alcohol Abuse and Alcoholism; Yoon, Y.-H., & Chen, C. M. (2016). *Surveillance report #105: Liver cirrhosis mortality in the United States, national, state and regional trends, 2000–2013*. Washington, DC: National Institute on Alcohol Abuse and Alcoholism.

ethnic groups (Yen, Keeffe, & Ahmed, 2003). Ethnic differences in certain types of liver cirrhosis have also been observed within European populations (Douds, Cox, Iqbal, & Cooper, 2003). As pointed out by Mann and colleagues (2003), ethnic differences have important implications for research and prevention and "*from a public health perspective, an understanding of subpopulation dynamics is critical to the development of programs for preventing alcoholic liver disease*" (pp. 209–219).

Coffee and Alcoholic Liver Disease

The results of several epidemiologic studies suggest that coffee consumption may protect against the development of cirrhosis of the liver, especially alcoholic cirrhosis. Klatsky and colleagues first examined the relationship between coffee and cirrhosis in a cohort of 128,934 adults ascertained through the *Kaiser Permanente Medical Care Program* in California. During 10 years of follow-up, 132 patients were hospitalized or died because of cirrhosis. The results suggested an inverse association between coffee consumption and the risk of liver cirrhosis as well as the risk of death due to cirrhosis, the effects being strongest for alcoholic cirrhosis (Klatsky and Armstrong, 1992).

More recently, Klatsky and colleagues reported findings after 22 years of follow-up of the same cohort ($n = 125,580$) during which 330 patients developed cirrhosis of the liver. As before, the study demonstrated a robust inverse dose response between coffee consumption and the risk of cirrhosis, independent of confounders. Estimates of relative risk were RR = 0.7 for up to one cup daily, RR = 0.6 for one to three cups daily, and RR = 0.2 for four or more cups daily. No effects were noted for patients with nonalcoholic cirrhosis (Klatsky, Morton, Udaltsova, & Friedman, 2006).

Tverdal and Skurtveit examined the relationship between coffee consumption and mortality due to liver cirrhosis in a cohort of 51,306 Norwegian adults. During 17 years of follow-up, a total of 4207 deaths were recorded including 53 deaths from liver cirrhosis. Of the deaths due to cirrhosis, 36 were reported as alcoholic cirrhosis. The relative risk of liver cirrhosis decreased significantly with each daily increase of two cups of coffee (RR = 0.6). Furthermore, restriction of deaths to those with reported alcoholic cirrhosis gave similar results (Tverdal & Skurtveit, 2003).

Corrao and colleagues examined coffee consumption and liver cirrhosis in a case–control study involving 274 cases and 458 control subjects ascertained

from hospitals in Italy. They also found an inverse dose–response relationship between cirrhosis risk and coffee intake. The odds ratios (ORs) decreased in linear fashion for 1, 2, 3, and 4 daily cups of coffee, OR = 0.47, OR = 0.23, OR = 0.21, and OR = 0.16, respectively (Corrao et al., 2001).

An independent case–control study conducted in Italy examined coffee consumption in 101 cirrhotic patients and more than 1500 controls. Compared to individuals who had never consumed coffee, those reporting daily consumption of three or more cups reduced their risk of developing liver cirrhosis by 71% (OR = 0.29) (Gallus, Tavani, Negri, & La Vecchia, 2002).

Investigators at the National Institutes of Health conducted an investigation of dietary caffeine consumption to evaluate effects on the progression of liver fibrosis. They examined 177 patients who underwent liver biopsy, 121 of whom had chronic hepatitis C infection. Caffeine intake was based upon completion of a detailed dietary questionnaire by each participant. In comparisons of subjects with advanced liver fibrosis (bridging fibrosis/cirrhosis) versus those with mild liver disease, individuals who consumed the equivalent of 2.25 cups of coffee daily reduced their risk of developing severe liver fibrosis by 75% (adjusted OR = 0.25). A similar effect was observed in the subset of patients with hepatitis C (OR = 0.19). The results suggest that caffeine per se has a protective effect against the progression of liver disease including those patients with chronic hepatitis C infection (Modi et al., 2010).

The combined evidence from these studies indicates that coffee protects against the development of liver cirrhosis. Consistency of results, the magnitude of the risk reductions and the presence of an inverse dose response in each of the studies support this conclusion. Mechanistically, it has been suggested that caffeine may have antioxidant effects and/or antagonist activity against adenosine receptors in the liver (Higdon & Frei, 2006).

Prevention of Cirrhosis of the Liver

Prevention of chronic cirrhosis and other forms of chronic liver disease is largely focused on the major risk factors: alcohol, viral hepatitis (particularly HBV and HCV), and components of the metabolic syndrome (insulin resistance, type 2 diabetes, obesity, hyperlipidemia, and hypertension). For greatest impact, strategies must target primary prevention of exposure, secondary prevention for early detection and treatment, and tertiary prevention to delimit disease progression.

Prevention of Alcohol-Related Cirrhosis of the Liver

Alcohol control is a complex and multifaceted health problem. Nevertheless, scientific evidence is accruing regarding the value of certain healthcare policies that restrict the affordability, availability, and accessibility of alcohol. Policies that have proven effective in reducing public harm from alcohol consumption include raising the price of alcoholic beverages through taxation, government regulation and standardization of retail sales of alcoholic beverages, strict enforcement of laws on minimum drinking age, passage of laws lowering the legal blood alcohol levels for operation of a motor vehicle, strict enforcement of drunk driving laws and strong penalties for violators, and increased awareness, detection, and treatment of alcohol abuse and alcoholism (WHO, 2000, 2010; Xie, Mann, & Smart, 2000).

Many investigators have observed that the price of alcohol is inversely correlated with per capita alcohol consumption and cirrhosis mortality rates (Bruun et al., 1975; Chaloupka, Grossman, & Saffer, 2002; Cook & Tauchen, 1982; Edwards et al., 1994; Ramstedt, 2001; Seeley, 1960). The evidence strongly indicates that the most cost-effective policy to reduce alcohol-related harm is through taxation (WHO, 2009b).

Numerous studies also indicate that early detection of alcohol abuse and increased membership in alcohol treatment programs such as Alcoholics Anonymous (AA) are beneficial in reducing alcohol-related harm (Holder & Parker, 1992; Mann, Smart, & Anglin, 1988; Romelsjš, 1987; Smart, 1996; Smart & Mann, 1991, 1993, 2000; Smart, Mann, & Suurvali, 1998). Reductions in cirrhosis morbidity and mortality in association with increased levels of treatment and AA membership have been observed in Canada (Mann, Smart, Anglin, & Rush, 1988), the United States (Holder & Parker, 1992; Mann, Smart, Anglin, & Adlaf, 1991; Smart, Mann, & Lee, 1996), and Sweden (Leifman & Romelsjš, 1997; Romelsjš, 1987). These results support the value of instituting and sustaining programs for the early detection and aggressive treatment of alcohol abuse and alcoholism.

Perhaps surprisingly, public information and school education programs have *not* proven effective in reducing alcohol-related harm in the populations studied (WHO, 2010). Notwithstanding, such programs remain important for the dissemination of accurate information and maintenance of public awareness regarding the deleterious health effects of alcohol abuse (WHO, 2010).

In consideration of these findings, the World Health Organization recently adopted an evidence-based resolution espousing *a global strategy to reduce the harmful use of alcohol* (WHO, 2010). The following statement provides a synopsis of the program:

> *Increasing capacity of health and social welfare systems to deliver treatment and early intervention; drink-driving countermeasures; limits on the availability of alcohol; restrictions on alcohol marketing; taxation and pricing policies to discourage frequent and heavy alcohol consumption; measures to control social contexts that promote excessive drinking; and reducing the public health impact of illicit and informally produced alcohol (Babor, 2010).*

▶ Prevention of Viral Hepatitis

Hepatitis B Virus: Prevention and Control

Maurice Ralph Hilleman (1919–2005) was an American microbiologist who specialized in the development of vaccines to prevent infectious diseases. Vaccines developed in his laboratories are now routinely used to prevent measles, mumps, hepatitis A, hepatitis B, chickenpox, meningitis, pneumonia, and *Haemophilus influenzae*. Hilleman is credited with saving more lives than any other scientist of the 20th century (Offit, 2007).

National HBV vaccination programs have been in place since the early 1980s. The HBV vaccine used in these programs stimulates antibodies against the hepatitis B surface antigen (HBsAg). Vaccine efficacy is best demonstrated by *universal childhood HBV vaccination programs* which have produced significant reductions in the rates of acute and chronic hepatitis B infection and related chronic liver diseases in all populations tested (Alter, 2001; Shepard, Simard, Finelli, Fiore, & Bell, 2006).

Universal Childhood Hepatitis B Vaccination

One of the first universal childhood hepatitis B vaccination programs was initiated in the population of Taiwan, which has high rates of endemic HBV. The results have been impressive. The seroprevalence of HBsAg among Taiwanese children decreased from 9.8% in 1984, the year when universal infant immunization began, to 0.7% in 1999 (Chan, Lee, & Lo, 2004). Furthermore, the incidence and mortality rates of hepatocellular carcinoma among children decreased by 49% and 75%, respectively, during the same time period (Chang et al., 1997).

In the Gambia, West Africa, the rates of HBV infection among 9-year-old children vaccinated in infancy were compared to that of unvaccinated children of the same age. Vaccinated children developed 83% fewer acute infections (8% vs. 50%) and 95% fewer chronic infections than unvaccinated children (0.6% vs. 10.0%). These results demonstrate the value of infant vaccination in protecting against acute and chronic HBV infection and suggest that immunity persists throughout the first decade of life (Viviani et al., 1999).

In Afragola, Italy, a community with very high rates of HBV infection and liver disease, the prevalence of HBsAg in males up to 12 years of age decreased from 10.5% in 1978 to 0.8% in 1993. The prevalence of individuals with antibodies to the HBV core antigen (anti-HBc) fell from 52.6% to 1.2%. Notably, the prevalence of HBsAg seropositivity among unvaccinated males also declined significantly, from 18% in 1978 to 5.5% in 1989. The decreased prevalence of HBsAg in the *unvaccinated* population suggests the phenomenon of "*herd immunity*" whereby vaccinated individuals buffer unvaccinated and susceptible individuals from exposure to HBV (Da Villa et al., 1998).

In a regional study in China, the prevalence of HBV carriers has dropped from 16% to 1.4% since the initiation of immunization in the 1990s (Cui, Wang, & Liang, 2006; Liu & Fan, 2007). In the United States, new infections with HBV declined from 260,000 in the 1980s to about 78,000 in 2001, and in Alaska, where HBV is endemic, acute hepatitis B infection decreased from 215 cases per 100,000 to less than 10 cases per 100,000 as a consequence of immunization (Shepard et al., 2006).

As of May 2003, 151 of the 192 national members of the WHO had implemented universal childhood vaccination programs. There are 89 member states that have been designated as high HBV prevalence regions, and 64 of these nations now have universal infant vaccination programs. It is the goal of the WHO to soon have universal vaccination programs in all countries. The worldwide vaccination program is proceeding well and has saved millions of people from infection, illness, and death. Nevertheless, the elimination of HBV infection will require not only childhood immunization but also vaccination of adults who are at high risk of infection (Alter, 2003).

HCV: Prevention and Control

Preventive measures beyond blood-banking practices include prompt identification of infected individuals, awareness of the potential for perinatal transmission, implementation of safe-injection practices, linkage of drug users to drug treatment programs, and implementation of community-based education and support programs to modify risk behavior. Some of these measures have been successfully implemented in the control of HIV infections, and it stands to reason that they would be valuable for reducing HCV transmission. Future advances in the diagnosis and management of hepatitis C require continued vigilance about the transmission of this infection, extending treatment to populations not previously evaluated in treatment trials, and the introduction of more effective therapies (Alter, 2006).

In a recent prospective study of U.S. mortality from liver cirrhosis, Kim and colleagues examined temporal trends in annual mortality rates during 2007–2016 for individuals with cirrhosis due to HCV infection, HBV infection, alcoholic liver disease, and nonalcoholic fatty liver disease. They noted that the mortality rates due to HCV disease increased until 2014, after which the rates declined significantly concomitant with the introduction of therapy using direct acting antiviral agents. In contrast, the rates of alcoholic cirrhosis and nonalcoholic fatty liver disease have risen in recent years (Kim et al., 2018). Tertiary Prevention in Cirrhosis of the Liver.

Cirrhosis of the liver is generally irreversible, and treatment usually focuses on preventing progression and complications. If complications cannot be controlled or when the liver ceases functioning, liver transplantation is necessary. Survival from liver transplantation has improved in recent years, and the 5-year survival rate is now around 80%, depending largely on the severity of disease and other medical problems in the recipient (Kirsch, Robson, & Trey, 1995).

▶ Conclusion

Cirrhosis of the liver is responsible for more than 1 million deaths per year worldwide. National rates vary widely as a function of the major risk factors for cirrhosis: alcohol abuse, chronic viral hepatitis (primarily HBV and HCV), and components of the metabolic syndrome (insulin resistance/type 2 diabetes, visceral obesity, hyperlipidemia and hypertension). Men have a twofold higher risk than women throughout the lifespan. Other factors (e.g., smoking, genetics and ethnicity) also influence the risk of cirrhosis development. Polymorphisms of genes encoding alcohol dehydrogenase, the chief enzyme in alcohol metabolism, have been found that modulate the risk of cirrhosis development. Genetic factors have also been discovered that modulate the immune response to hepatitis viral infection. Other relatively infrequent causes of liver cirrhosis include hemochromatosis (iron overload) and Wilson's disease (excess copper deposition in the liver and other tissues).

Recent declines in cirrhosis mortality rates in the United States and other developed nations are attributable to reductions in per capita consumption of alcohol. Nevertheless, liver cirrhosis arising from nonalcoholic fatty change has emerged as an important global health concern. Progression of this condition is related to development of the metabolic syndrome, particularly insulin resistance and obesity.

Effective prevention of alcoholic cirrhosis involves restriction of the affordability, availability, and accessibility of alcohol plus early detection of alcohol abuse and aggressive treatment of alcoholism. Vaccination programs have proven extremely effective in the elimination of HBV infection. An effective vaccine against HCV has not yet been developed. Nevertheless, therapy with direct acting antiviral agents holds promise in reducing morbidity and mortality from liver cirrhosis due to HCV infection. Primary prevention involves avoidance of exposure to HCV-contaminated blood from intravenous drug abusers. Development of the metabolic syndrome appears largely preventable through diet and exercise for weight control maintenance of optimal levels of blood glucose, blood pressure, and blood lipids.

References

Adams, L. A., Lymp, J. F., St. Sauver, J. S., Sanderson, S. O., Lindor, K. D., Feldstein, A., & Angulo, P. (2005). The natural history of nonalcoholic fatty liver disease: A population-based cohort study. *Gastroenterology, 129*, 113–121.

Ala, A., Walker, A. P., Ashkan, K., Dooley, J. S., & Schilsky, M. L. (2007). Wilson's disease. *Lancet, 369*(9559), 397–408.

Alter, M. J. (2001). Protecting future generations through immunization against hepatitis B. *Annals of Internal Medicine, 125*, 835–836.

Alter, M. J. (2003). Epidemiology and prevention of hepatitis B. *Seminars in Liver Disease, 23*(1), 39–46.

Alter, M. J. (2006). Prevention of spread of hepatitis C. *Hepatology, 36*(Suppl. 1), S93–S98.

Angulo, P. (2002). Nonalcoholic fatty liver disease. *New England Journal of Medicine, 346*, 1221–1231.

Angulo, P., Keach, J. C., Batts, K. P., & Lindor, K. D. (1999). Independent predictors of liver fibrosis in patients with nonalcoholic steatohepatitis. *Hepatology, 30*, 1356–1362.

Armstrong, G. L., Alter, M. J., McQuillan, G. M., & Margolis, H. S. (2000). The past incidence of hepatitis C virus infection: Implications for future burden of chronic liver disease in the United States. *Hepatology, 31*, 777–782.

Armstrong, G. L., Wasley, A., Simard, E. P., McQuillan, G. M., Kuhnert, W. L., & Alter, M. J. (2006). The prevalence of hepatitis C virus infection in the United States, 1999 through 2002. *Annals of Internal Medicine, 144*(10), 705–714.

Auld, D. S., & Bergman, T. (2008). The role of zinc for alcohol dehydrogenase structure and function. *Cellular and Molecular Life Sciences, 65*, 3961–3970.

Babor, T. F. (2010). Public health science and the global strategy on alcohol. *Bulletin of the World Health Organization, 88*(9), 641–716.

Bamber, M. A. Y., Murray, A. K., Weller, I. V. C., Morelli, A., Scheuer, P. J., Thomas, H. C., & Sherlock, S. (1981). Clinical and histological features of a group of patients with sporadic non-A, non-B hepatitis. *Journal of Clinical Pathology, 34*, 1175–1180.

Bellentani, S., Pozzato, G., Saccoccio, G., Crovatto, M., Croce, L. S., Mazzoran, L., ... Tiribelli, C. (1999). Clinical course and risk factors of hepatitis C virus related liver disease in the general population: Report from the Dionysos study. *Gut, 44*, 874–880.

Bellentani, S., Saccoccio, G., Costa, G., Tiribelli, C., Manenti, F., Sodde, M., ... Brandi, G. (1997). Drinking habits as cofactors of risk for alcohol induced liver damage. The Dionysos Study Group. *Gut, 41*, 845–850.

Bellentani, S., & Tiribelli, C. (2001). Spectrum of liver disease in the general population: Lessons from the Dionysos study. *Journal of Hepatology, 35*, 531–537.

Blumberg, B. S. (2006). The curiosities of hepatitis B virus: Prevention, sex ratio, and demography. *The Proceedings of the American Thoracic Society, 3*, 14–20.

Bosetti, C., Levi, F., Lucchini, F., Zatoniski, W. A., Negri, E., & La Vecchia, C. (2007). Worldwide mortality from cirrhosis: An update to 2002. *Journal of Hepatology, 46*(5), 827–839.

Bruun, K., Edwards, G., Lumio, M., Mäkelä, K., Pan, L., Popham, E. R., ... Österberg, E. (1975). *Alcohol control policies in public health perspective.* Helsinki: Finnish Foundation for Alcohol Studies.

Butterfield, M. I., Bosworth, H. B., Meador, K. G., Stechuchak, K. M., Essock, S. M., Osher, F. C., ... Five-Site Health and Risk Study Research Committee. (2003). Gender differences in hepatitis C infection and risks among persons with severe mental illness. *Psychiatric Services, 54*(6), 848–853.

Chaloupka, F. J., Grossman, M., & Saffer, H. (2002). The effects of price on alcohol consumption and alcohol–related problems. *Alcohol Research and Health, 26*, 22–34.

Chan, C. Y., Lee, S. D., & Lo, K. J. (2004). Legend of hepatitis B vaccination: The Taiwan experience. *Journal of Gastroenterology and Hepatology, 19*, 121–126.

Chang, M. H., Chen, C. J., Lai, M. S., Hsu, H. M., Wu, T. C., Kong, M. S., ... Chen, D. S. (1997). Universal hepatitis B vaccination in Taiwan and the incidence of hepatocellular carcinoma in children. The Taiwan childhood hepatoma study group. *New England Journal of Medicine, 336*(26), 1855–1859.

Coates, R. A., Halliday, M., Rankin, J. G., Feinman, S. V., & Fisher, M. M. (1986). Risk of fatty infiltration or cirrhosis of the liver in relation to ethanol consumption: A case–control study. *Clinical and Investigative Medicine, 9*, 26–32.

Cook, P. J., & Tauchen, G. (1982). The effect of liquor taxes on heavy drinking. *The Bell Journal of Economics, 13*(2), 379–390.

Corrao, G. (1998). Liver cirrhosis mortality trends in Eastern Europe, 1970–1989. Analyses of age, period and cohort effects and of latency with alcohol consumption. *Addiction Biology, 3*, 413–422.

Corrao, G., & Arico, S. (1998). Independent and combined action of hepatitis C virus infection and alcohol consumption on the risk of symptomatic liver cirrhosis. *Hepatology, 27*, 914–919.

Corrao, G., Bagnardi, V., Zambon, A., & Oorchio, P. (1998). Meta-analysis of alcohol intake in relation to risk of liver cirrhosis. *Alcohol and Alcoholism, 33*(4), 381–392.

Corrao, G., Zambon, A., Bagnardi, V., D'Amicis, A., Klatsky, A., & Collaborative SIDECIR Group. (2001). Coffee, caffeine, and the risk of liver cirrhosis. *Annals of Epidemiology, 11,* 458–465.

Corrao, G., Zambon, A., Torchio, P., Arico, S., La Vecchia, C., & Di Orio, F. (1998). Attributable risk for symptomatic liver cirrhosis in Italy. *Journal of Hepatology, 28,* 608–614.

Cui, F. Q., Wang, X. J., & Liang, X. F. (2006). Epidemiological analysis on reported hepatitis B under 15 years in China: The report from Chinese Center for Disease Control and Prevention. *Chinese Journal of Vaccines and Immunization, 12*(2006), 206–208.

Curtis, J. L., Samper, L., Rodriquez, L. A., & Garrett, M. G. (1973). Sex difference in hepatitis-associated (Australia) antigen carrier state one year after hepatitis outbreak. *Pediatrics, 52,* 441–443.

Custer, B., Sullivan, S. D., Hazlet, T. K., Iloeje, U., Veenstra, D. L., & Kowdley, K. V. (2004). Global epidemiology of hepatitis B virus. *Journal of Clinical Gastroenterology, 38*(10 Suppl. 3), S158–S168.

Da Villa, G., Piccinino, F., Scolastico, C., Fusco, M., Piccinino, R., & Sepe, A. (1998). Long-term epidemiological survey of hepatitis B virus infection in a hyperendemic area (Afragola, southern Italy): Results of a pilot vaccination project. *Research in Virology, 149*(5), 263–270.

de Ledinghen, V., Ratziu, V., Causse, X., Le Bail, B., Capron, D., Renou, C., ... Vallet-Pichard, A. (2006). Diagnostic and predictive factors of significant liver fibrosis and minimal lesions in patients with persistent unexplained elevated transaminases. A prospective multicenter study. *Journal of Hepatology, 45,* 592–599.

Degenhardt, L., Charlson, F., Stanaway, J., Larney, S., Alexander, L. T., Hickman, M., ... Vos, T. (2016). Estimating the burden of disease attributable to injecting drug use as a risk factor for HIV, hepatitis C, and hepatitis B: Findings from the Global Burden of Disease Study 2013. *The Lancet Infectious Diseases, 16*(12), 1385–1398.

Douds, A. C., Cox, M. A., Iqbal, T. H., & Cooper, T. H. (2003). Ethnic differences in cirrhosis of the liver in a British city: Alcoholic cirrhosis in South Asian men. *Alcohol and Alcoholism, 38,* 148–150.

Edenberg, H. J. (2000). Regulation of the mammalian alcohol dehydrogenase genes. *Progress in Nucleic Acid Research and Molecular Biology, 64,* 295–341.

Edenberg, H. J. (2003). *The collaborative study on the genetics of alcoholism: An update.* National Institute on Alcohol Abuse and Alcoholism, National Institutes of Health, Department of Health and Human Services.

Edenberg, H. J., Jerome, R. E., & Li, M. (1999). Polymorphism of the human alcohol dehydrogenase 4 (ADH4) promoter affects gene expression. *Pharmacogenetics, 9*(1), 25–30.

Edwards, G., Anderson, P., Babor, T. F., Casswell, S., Ferrence, R., Giesbrecht, N., ... Lemmens, P. H. M. M. (1994). *Alcohol policy and the public good.* New York, NY: Oxford University Press.

Emerson, S. U., & Purcell, R. (2003). Hepatitis E virus. *Reviews in Medical Virology, 13,* 145–154.

Farrell, G. C., & Larter, C. Z. (2006). Nonalcoholic fatty liver disease: From steatosis to cirrhosis. *Hepatology, 43,* S99–S112.

Feder, J. N., Penny, D. M., Irrinki, A., Lee, V. K., Lebrón, J. A., Watson, N., & Schatzman, R. C. (1998). The hemochromatosis gene product complexes with the transferrin receptor and lowers its affinity for ligand binding. *Proceedings of the National Academy of Sciences of the Unites States of America, 95*(4), 1472–1477.

Fiore, A. E. (2004). Hepatitis A transmitted by food. *Clinical Infectious Diseases, 38,* 705–715.

Frank, C., Mohamed, M., Strickland, G., Lavanchy, D., Arthur, R., Magder, L., ... Sallam, I. (2000). The role of parenteral anti-schistosomal therapy in the spread of hepatitis C virus in Egypt. *Lancet, 355*(9207), 887–891.

Fraser, A., Harris, R., & Sattar, N. (2009). Alanine aminotransferase, gamma-glutamyltransferase, and incident diabetes: The British Women's Heart and Health Study and meta-analysis. *Diabetes Care, 32,* 741–750.

Frezza, M., Di Padova, C., Pozzato, G., Terpin, M., Baraona, E., & Lieber, C. S. (1990). High blood alcohol levels in women: The role of decreased gastric alcohol dehydrogenase activity and first–pass metabolism. *New England Journal of Medicine, 322,* 95–99.

Fung, J., Lai, C. L., But, D., Wong, D., Cheung, T. K., & Yuen, M. F. (2008). Prevalence of fibrosis and cirrhosis in chronic hepatitis B: Implications for treatment and management. *American Journal of Gastroenterology, 103*(6), 1421–1426.

Galambos, J. (1985). Epidemiology of cirrhosis in the United States of America. In P. Hall (Ed.), *Alcoholic liver disease: Pathobiology, epidemiology, and clinical aspects* (pp. 230–249). New York, NY: John Wiley & Sons.

Gallus, S., Tavani, A., Negri, E., & La Vecchia, C. (2002). Does coffee protect against liver cirrhosis? *Annals of Epidemiology, 12,* 202–205.

Ge, D., Fellay, J., Thompson, A. J., Simon, J. S., Shianna, C. V., Urban, T. J., ... Goldstein, D. B. (2009). Genetic variation in IL28B predicts hepatitis C treatment-induced viral clearance. *Nature, 461,* 399–401.

Geerts, A. (2001). History, heterogeneity, developmental biology, and functions of quiescent hepatic stellate cells. *Seminar in Liver Disease, 21*(3), 311–335.

Goodman, M., Wainwright, R. L., Weir, H. F., & Gall, J. C., Jr. (1971). A sex difference in the carrier state of Australia (hepatitis-associated) antigen. *Pediatrics, 48,* 907.

Gruenewald, P. J., & Ponicki, W. R. (1995). The relationship of alcohol sales to cirrhosis mortality. *Journal of Studies on Alcohol, 56,* 635–641.

Hall, P. (1995). Pathological spectrum of alcoholic liver disease. In P. Hall (Ed.), *Alcoholic liver disease: Pathobiology and pathogenesis* (2nd ed., pp. 41–68). London: Edward Arnold.

Haubrich, W. S. (2004). Kupffer of Kupffer cells. *Gastroenterology, 127,* 16.

Higdon, J. V., & Frei, B. (2006). Coffee and health: A review of recent human research. *Critical Reviews in Food Science and Nutrition, 46,* 101–123.

Hirche, T. O., Ianee, H., Hirche, A., Schneider, A., & Dietrich, C. F. (2007). Evaluation of hepatic steatosis by ultrasound in patients with chronic hepatitis C virus infection. *Liver International, 27*(6), 748–757.

Holder, H. D., & Parker, R. N. (1992). Effect of alcoholism treatment on cirrhosis mortality: A 20-year multivariate time series analysis. *British Journal of Addiction, 87,* 1263–1274.

Hurley, T. D., Edenberg, H. J., & Li, T. K. (2002). The Pharmacogenomics of alcoholism. In J. Licino, M. L. Wong (Eds.), *Pharmacogenomics: The search for individualized therapies* (pp. 417–441). Weinheim, Germany: Wiley-VCH.

Ito, T. (1951). Cytological studies on stellate cells of Kupffer and fat storing cells in the capillary wall of the human liver. *Acta Anatomica Nipponica, 26,* 2.

Iversen, J., Wand, H., Gonnermann, A., Maher, L., & on behalf of the collaboration of Australian Needle and Syringe Programs. (2010, May). Gender differences in hepatitis C antibody prevalence and risk behaviours amongst people who inject drugs in Australia 1998–2008. *International Journal of Drug Policy, 21*(6), 471–476.

Jellinek, E. M., & Keller, M. (1952). Rates of alcoholism in the United States of America, 1940–1948. *Quarterly Journal of Studies on Alcohol, 13*, 49–59.

Jones-Webb, R. (1998). Drinking patterns and problems among African–Americans: Recent findings. *Alcohol Health and Research World, 22*(4), 260–264.

Kamal, S. M. (2008). Acute hepatitis C: A systematic review. *American Journal of Gastroenterology, 103*, 1283–1297.

Kerr, W. D., Fillmore, K. M., & Marvy, P. (2000). Beverage-specific alcohol consumption and cirrhosis mortality in a group of English–speaking beer-drinking countries. *Addiction, 95*, 339–346.

Kim, C. H., & Younossi, Z. M. (2008). Nonalcoholic fatty liver disease: A manifestation of the metabolic syndrome. *Cleveland Clinic Journal of Medicine, 75*, 721–728.

Kim, D., Li, A. A., Gadiparthi, C., Khan, M. A., Cholankeri, G., Glenn, J. S., & Ahmed, A. (2018). Changing trends in etiology-based annual mortality from chronic liver disease, from 2007 through 2016. *Gastroenterology, 155*, 1154–1163.

Kirsch, R., Robson, S., & Trey, C. (1995). *Diagnosis and management of liver disease.* London: Chapman and Hall.

Klatsky, A. L., & Armstrong, M. A. (1992). Alcohol, smoking, coffee, and cirrhosis. *American Journal of Epidemiology, 136*, 1248–1257.

Klatsky, A. L., Morton, C., Udaltsova, N., & Friedman, G. D. (2006). Coffee, cirrhosis, and transaminase enzymes. *Archives of Internal Medicine, 166*, 1190–1195.

La Vecchia, F. L., Lucchini, F., Franceschi, S., & Negri, E. (1994). Worldwide patterns and trends in mortality from liver cirrhosis, 1955 to 1990. *Annals of Epidemiology, 4*, 480–486.

Lai, M. M. C. (1994). Hepatitis delta virus. In R. G. Webster & A. Granoff (Eds.), *Encyclopedia of virology* (pp. 574–580). London: Academic Press Ltd.

Ledermann, S. (1956). *Alcool, alcoolisme, alcoolisation.* Paris: Presses Universitaires de France.

Leifman, H., & Romelsjš, A. (1997). The effects of changes in alcohol consumption on mortality and admissions with alcohol-related diagnoses in Stockholm County—A time–series analysis. *Addiction, 92*, 1523–1536.

Lelbach, W. K. (1974). Organic pathology related to volume and patterns of alcohol use. In R. Gibbins, Y. Israel, H. Kalant (Eds.), *Research advances in alcohol and drug problems* (Vol. 1, pp. 93–198). New York, NY: John Wiley & Sons.

Lieber, C. S. (1989). Alcohol and nutrition: An overview. *Alcohol Health and Research World, 13*(3), 197–205.

Liu, B., Balkwill, A., Roddam, A., Brown, A., Beral, V., & on behalf of the Million Women Study Collaborators. (2009). Separate and joint effects of alcohol and smoking on the risks of cirrhosis and gallbladder disease in middle-aged women. *American Journal of Epidemiology, 169*(2), 153–160.

Liu, J., & Fan, D. (2007). Hepatitis B in China. *Lancet, 369*(9573), 1582–1583.

Locarnini, S. (2004). Molecular virology of hepatitis B virus. *Seminars in liver disease, 24*(Suppl. 1), 3–10.

London, W. T., & Drew, J. S. (1977). Sex differences in response to hepatitis B infection among patients receiving dialysis treatment. *Proceedings of the National Academy of Sciences of the United States of America, 74*(6), 2561–2563.

Lozano, R., Naghavi, M., Foreman, K., Lim, S., Shibuya, K., … Murray, C. J. L. (2012). Global and regional mortality from 235 causes of death for 20 age groups in 1990 and 2010: A systematic analysis for the Global Burden of Disease Study 2010. *Lancet, 380*, 2095–2128.

Luo, X., Kranzler, H. R., Zuo, L., Wand, S., Schork, N. J., & Gelernter, J. (2006). Diplotype trend regression (DTR) analysis of the ADH gene cluster and ALDH2 gene: Multiple significant association of alcohol dependence. *American Journal of Human Genetics, 78*, 973–987.

Mann, R. E., Anglin, L., Wilkins, K., Vingilis, E. R., & Macdonald, S. (1993). Mortality in a sample of convicted drinking drivers. *Addiction, 88*, 643–647.

Mann, R. E., Smart, R. G., & Anglin, L. (1988). Reduction in liver cirrhosis mortality and morbidity in Canada: Demographic differences and possible explanations. *Alcoholism: Clinical and Experimental Research, 12*, 290–297.

Mann, R. E., Smart, R. G., Anglin, L., & Adlaf, E. (1991). Reductions in cirrhosis in the United States: Associations with per capita consumption and AA membership. *Journal of Studies on Alcohol, 52*, 361–365.

Mann, R. E., Smart, R. G., Anglin, L., & Rush, B. (1988). Are decreases in liver cirrhosis rates a result of increased treatment for alcoholism? *British Journal of Addiction, 83*, 683–688.

Mann, R. E., Smart, R. G., & Govoni, R. (2003). The epidemiology of alcoholic liver disease. *Alcohol Research & Health, 27*, 209–219.

Marchesini, G., & Bianchi, G. (2010). Metabolic syndrome: Relevant for all types of chronic liver diseases? *Gut, 59*, 1314–1315.

Marchesini, G., Bugianesi, E., Forlani, G., Cerrelli, F., Lenzi, M., Manini, R., … Rizzetto, M. (2003). Nonalcoholic fatty liver, steatohepatitis, and the metabolic syndrome. *Hepatology, 37*, 917–923.

Minino, A., Arias, E., Kochanek, K. D., Murphy, S. L., & Smith, B. L. (2002). Deaths: Final data for 2000. *National Vital Statistics Reports, 50*, 1–107.

Modi, A. A., Feld, J. J., Park, Y., Kleiner, D. E., Everhart, J. E., Liang, T. J., & Hoofnagle, J. H. (2010). Increased caffeine consumption is associated with reduced hepatic fibrosis. *Hepatology, 51*, 201–209.

Mokdad, A. A., Lopez, A. D., Shahraz, S., Lozano, R., Mokdad, A. H., Stanaway, J., … Naghavi, M. (2014). Liver cirrhosis mortality in 187 countries between 1980 and 2010: A systematic analysis. *BMC Medicine, 12*(1), 145. doi:10.1186/s12916-014-0145-y.

Moser, J. (1980). *Prevention of alcohol related problems: An international review of prevention measures, policies and programmes.* Toronto, Canada: World Health Organization by the Alcoholism and Drug Addiction Research Foundation.

Müller, M. J., Pirlich, M., Balks, H. J., & Selberg, O. (1994). Glucose intolerance in liver cirrhosis: Role of hepatic and non-hepatic influences. *European Journal of Clinical Chemistry and Clinical Biochemistry, 32*(10), 749–758.

Nephew, T. M., Williams, G. D., Yi, H. Y., Hoy, A. K., Stinson, F. S., & Dufour, M. C. (2002). *Surveillance report #59: Apparent per capita alcohol consumption: National, state and regional trends, 1977–99.* Washington, DC: National Institute of Alcohol Abuse and Alcoholism.

Neuschwander-Tetri, B. A., & Caldwell, S. H. (2003). Nonalcoholic steatohepatitis: Summary of an AASLD Single Topic Conference. *Hepatology, 37*(5), 1202–1219.

NIH Consensus Statement on Management of Hepatitis C. (2002). *NIH Consensus and State-of-the-science Statements, 19*(3), 1–46.

O'Brien, T. R. (2009). Interferon-alfa, interferon-λ and hepatitis. *Nature Genetics, 41*, 1048–1050.

Offit, P. A. (2007). *Vaccinated: One man's quest to defeat the world's deadliest diseases* (p. 256). New York, NY: Smithsonian Books.

Parlesak, A., Billinger, M. H., Bode, C., & Bode, J. C. (2002). Gastric alcohol dehydrogenase activity in man: Influence of gender, age, alcohol consumption and smoking in a Caucasian population. *Alcohol and Alcoholism (Oxford, Oxfordshire), 37*(4), 388–393.

Pearl, R. (1926). *Alcohol and longevity.* New York, NY: Knopf.

Pell, S., & D'Alonzo, A. (1973). A five-year mortality study of alcoholics. *Journal of Occupational Medicine, 15*, 120–125.

Peters, M. G., & Terrault, N. A. (2002). Alcohol use and hepatitis C. *Hepatology, 36*, S220–S225.

Popham, R. E. (1970). Indirect methods of alcoholism prevalence estimation: A critical evaluation. In R. E. Popham (Ed.), *Alcohol and alcoholism* (pp. 678–685). Toronto: University of Toronto Press.

Poynard, T., Bedossa, P., & Opolon, P. (1997). Natural history of liver fibrosis progression in patients with chronic hepatitis C. The OBSVIRC, METAVIR CLINIVIR, and DOSVIRC groups. *Lancet, 349*, 825–832.

Ramstedt, M. (2001). Per capita alcohol consumption and liver cirrhosis mortality in 14 European countries. *Addiction, 96*, S19–S34.

Reed, T., Page, W. F., Viken, R. J., & Christian, J. C. (1996). Genetic predisposition to organ-specific endpoints of alcoholism. *Alcoholism: Clinical and Experimental Research, 20*, 1528–1533.

Rehm, J., Taylor, B., Mohapatra, S., Irving, H., Baliunas, D., Patra, J., & Roerecke, M. (2010). Alcohol as a risk factor for liver cirrhosis: A systematic review and meta-analysis. *Drug and Alcohol Review, 29*(4), 437–445.

Reich, T., Edenberg, H. J., Goate, A., Williams, J. T., Rice, J. P., Van Eerdewegh, P., ... Begleiter, H. (1998). Genome-wide search for genes affecting the risk for alcohol dependence. *American Journal of Medical Genetics, 81*, 207–215.

Robbins, S. L., & Cotran, R. S. (1979). *Pathologic basis of disease.* Philadelphia, PA: W. B. Saunders Company.

Roguin, A. (2006). Rene Theophile Hyacinthe Laënnec (1781–1826): The man behind the stethoscope. *Clinical Medicine & Research, 4*(3), 230–235.

Roizen, R., Fillmore, K., & Kerr, W. (1999). Overlooking Terris: A speculative reconsideration of a curious spot-blindness in the history of alcohol-control science. *Contemporary Drug Problems, 26*, 577–606.

Roizen, R., Kerr, W. C., & Fillmore, K. M. (1999). Cirrhosis mortality and per capita consumption of distilled spirits, United States, 1949–1994: Trend analysis. *British Medical Journal, 319*, 666–670.

Romelsjš, A. (1987). Decline in alcohol-related in–patient care and mortality in Stockholm County. *British Journal of Addiction, 82*, 653–663.

Schiff, E. R., & Ozden, N. (2003). Hepatitis C and alcohol. *Alcohol Research & Health, 27*, 232–239.

Schmidt, W. (1980). Cirrhosis and alcohol consumption: An epidemiologic perspective. In G. Edwards, M. Grant (Eds.), *Alcoholism: New knowledge and new responses* (pp. 15–47). London, Croom Helm.

Schmidt, W., & Bronetto, J. (1962). Death from liver cirrhosis and specific alcoholic beverage consumption: An ecological study. *American Journal of Public Health, 52*, 1473–1482.

Schmidt, W., & de Lint, J. (1972). Causes of death in alcoholics. *Quarterly Journal of Studies on Alcohol, 33*, 171–185.

Seeff, L. B., Hollinger, F. B., Alter, H. J., Wright, E. C., Cain, C. M., Buskell, Z. J., ... Koretz, R. L. (2001). Long-term mortality and morbidity of transfusion-associated non-A, non-B, and type C hepatitis: A National Heart, Lung, and Blood Institute collaborative study. *Hepatology, 33*, 455–463.

Seeley, J. R. (1960). Death by liver cirrhosis and the price of beverage alcohol. *Canadian Medical Association Journal, 83*, 1361–1366.

Shapiro, C. N. (1993). Epidemiology of hepatitis B. *The Pediatric Infectious Disease Journal, 12*(5), 433–437.

Shepard, C. W., Simard, E. P., Finelli, L., Fiore, A. E., & Bell, B. P. (2006). Hepatitis B virus infection: Epidemiology and vaccination. *Epidemiologic Reviews, 28*(1), 112–125.

Singh, G. K., & Hoyert, D. L. (2000). Social epidemiology of chronic liver disease and cirrhosis mortality in the United States, 1935–1997: Trends and differentials by ethnicity, socioeconomic status, and alcohol consumption. *Human Biology, 72*, 801–820.

Skog, O. J. (1980). Liver cirrhosis epidemiology: Some methodological problems. *British Journal of Addiction, 75*, 227–243.

Skog, O. J. (1984). The risk function for liver cirrhosis from lifetime alcohol consumption. *Journal of Studies on Alcohol, 45*, 199–208.

Smart, R. G. (1996). Behavioral and social consequences related to the consumption of different beverage types. *Journal of Studies on Alcohol, 57*, 419–424.

Smart, R. G., & Mann, R. E. (1991). Factors in recent reductions in liver cirrhosis deaths. *Journal of Studies on Alcohol, 52*, 232–240.

Smart, R. G., & Mann, R. E. (1993). Recent liver cirrhosis declines: Estimates of the impact of alcohol abuse treatment and Alcoholics Anonymous. *Addiction, 88*, 193–198.

Smart, R. G., & Mann, R. E. (2000). The impact of programs for high-risk drinkers on population levels of alcohol problems. *Addiction, 95*, 37–52.

Smart, R. G., Mann, R. E., & Lee, S. L. (1996). Does increased spending on alcoholism treatment lead to lower cirrhosis death rates? *Alcohol and Alcoholism, 31*(5), 487–491.

Smart, R. G., Mann, R. E., & Suurvali, H. (1998). Changes in liver cirrhosis death rates in different countries in relation to per capita alcohol consumption and Alcoholics Anonymous membership. *Journal of Studies on Alcohol, 59*, 245–249.

Sørensen, H. T., Thulstrup, A. M., Mellemkjar, L., Jepsen, P., Christensen, E., Olsen, J. H., & Vilstrup, H. (2003, January). Long-term survival and cause-specific mortality in patients with cirrhosis of the liver: A nationwide cohort. *Journal of Clinical Epidemiology, 56*(1), 88–93.

Stepanova, M., Zobair, N. R., & Younossi, M. (2010). Components of metabolic syndrome are independent predictors of mortality in patients with chronic liver disease: A population-based study. *Gut, 59*, 1410–1415.

Stinson, F. S., Grant, B. F., & Dufour, M. C. (2001). The critical dimension of ethnicity in liver cirrhosis mortality statistics. *Alcoholism: Clinical and Experimental Research, 25*, 1181–1187.

Suppiah, V., Moldovan, M., Ahlenstiel, G., Berg, T., Weltman, M., Abate, M. L., ... George, J. (2009). IL28B is associated with response to chronic hepatitis C interferon-alpha and ribavirin therapy. *Nature Genetics, 41*(10), 1100–1104.

Tanaka, Y., Nishida, N., Sugiyama, M., Kurosaki, M., Matsuura, K., Sakamoto, N., ... Mizokami, M. (2009). Genome-wide association of IL28B with response to pegylated interferon-alpha and ribavirin therapy for chronic hepatitis C. *Nature Genetics, 41*(10), 1105–1109.

Terris, M. (1967). Epidemiology of cirrhosis of the liver: National and mortality data. *American Journal of Public Health, 57*, 2076–2088.

Thun, M. J., Peto, R., Lopez, A. D., Monaco, J. H., Henley, S. J., Heath, C. W., Jr., & Doll, R. (1997). Alcohol consumption and mortality among middle-aged and elderly U.S. adults. *New England Journal of Medicine, 337*, 1705–1714.

Tuyns, A. J., & Péquignot, G. (1984). Greater risk of ascitic cirrhosis in females in relation to alcohol consumption. *International Journal of Epidemiology, 13*, 53–57.

Tverdal, A., & Skurtveit, S. (2003). Coffee intake and mortality from liver cirrhosis. *Annals Epidemiology, 13*, 419–423.

Viviani, S., Jack, A., Hall, A. J., Maine, N., Mendy, M., Montesano, R., & Whittle, H. C. (1999). Hepatitis B vaccination in infancy in The Gambia: Protection against carriage at 9 years of age. *Vaccine, 17*(23–24), 2946–2950.

Williams, R. (2006). Global challenges in liver disease. *Hepatology, 44*(3), 521–526.

Wong, G. L. H., Wong, V. W. S., Choi, P. C. L., Chan, A. W. H., Chim, A. M. L., Yiu, K. K. L., … Chan, F. K. L. (2009). Metabolic syndrome increases the risk of liver cirrhosis in chronic hepatitis B. *Gut, 58*, 111–117.

World Health Organization. (2000). *The global status report on alcohol*. Geneva, Switzerland: Department of Substance Abuse.

World Health Organization. (2009a). *Death and DALY estimates for 2004 by cause for WHO Member States (persons, all ages)*. Geneva, Switzerland: World Health Organization.

World Health Organization. (2009b). *Evidence for the effectiveness and cost-effectiveness of interventions to reduce alcohol-related harm*. Copenhagen, Denmark: World Health Organization.

World Health Organization. (2010). *Global strategy to reduce the harmful use of alcohol* (EB126. R11). Geneva, Switzerland: World Health Organization.

Xie, X., Mann, R. E., & Smart, R. G. (2000). The direct and indirect relationships between alcohol prevention measures and alcoholic liver cirrhosis mortality. *Journal of Studies on Alcohol, 61*, 499–506.

Yamakawa, Y., Sata, M., Suzuki, H., Noguchi, S., & Tanikawa, K. (1996). Higher elimination rate of hepatitis C virus among women. *Journal of Viral Hepatitis, 3*(6), 317–321.

Yang, J., Zhang, Y., Luo, L., Meng, R., & Yu, C. (2018). Global mortality burden of cirrhosis and liver cancer attributable to injection drug use, 1990–2016: An age-period-cohort and spatial autocorrelation analysis. *International Journal of Environmental Research and Public Health, 15*(1), 170.

Yen, T., Keeffe, E. B., & Ahmed, A. (2003). The epidemiology of hepatitis C virus infection. *Journal of Clinical Gastroenterology, 36*, 47–53.

Yoon, Y.-H., & Chen, C. M. (2016). *Surveillance Report #105: Liver cirrhosis mortality in the United States, national, state and regional trends, 2000–2013*. Washington, DC: National Institute on Alcohol Abuse and Alcoholism.

Yoon, Y.-H., Yi, H., Grant, B. F., & Dufour, M. C. (2001). *Surveillance report #57: Liver cirrhosis mortality in the United States, 1970–98*. Washington, DC: National Institute on Alcohol Abuse and Alcoholism.

Yoon, Y.-H., Yi, H., Grant, B. F., Stinson, F. S., & Dufour, M. C. (2002). *Surveillance report #60: Liver cirrhosis mortality in the United States, 1970–99*. Washington, DC: National Institute on Alcohol Abuse and Alcoholism.

Zatoński, W. A., Sulkowska, U., Mańczuk, M., Rehm, J., Boffetta, P., Lowenfels, A. B., & La Vecchia, C. (2010). Liver cirrhosis mortality in Europe, with special attention to Central and Eastern Europe. *European Addiction Research, 16*, 193–201.

CHAPTER 46

Epidemiology of Osteoporosis

▶ Introduction

*O*steoporosis is defined as *"a systemic skeletal disorder characterized by low bone mass and microarchitectural deterioration of bone tissue with a consequent increase in bone fragility and susceptibility to fracture"* (Consensus Development Conference, 1991). In many individuals, the first clinical manifestation of this disease is a low-trauma bone fracture of the hip, spine, forearm, or other anatomic sites. Early detection depends upon assessment of *bone mineral density* (*BMD*) utilizing *dual energy X-ray absorptiometry* (*DXA*).

▶ Discovery

In the early 19th century, the British surgeon, Astley Cooper, recognized the link between aging, reduction in bone density and the risk of fractures (Cooper & Cooper, 1822). Shortly thereafter, the French pathologist, Jean Lobstein, coined the term "osteoporosis" to describe the porous bones of patients who suffer fractures (Lobstein, 1835). More than a century later, American endocrinologist Fuller Albright found that estrogen deficiency due to menopause or oophorectomy in women induces the loss of critical bone minerals, calcium and phosphate, and leads to the development of *"postmenopausal osteoporosis"* (Albright, Bloomberg, & Smith, 1940).

▶ Pathogenesis of Osteoporosis

The underlying mechanism of osteoporosis is an imbalance between bone resorption and bone formation.

Throughout life, there is continual remodeling of bone whereby older bone is resorbed by osteoclastic cells (osteoclasts) and replaced by new bone laid down by osteoblastic cells (osteoblasts). Osteoporosis develops when excessive bone resorption and inadequate bone formation reduces BMD below a critical threshold resulting in fragile bones that are highly prone to fracture.

The delicate balance of calcium homeostasis and bone remodeling is regulated by a number of cellular and molecular factors and their interactions. Any breach in the integrity of this complex regulatory system could upset the balance of bone resorption and bone formation to provoke the pathogenesis of osteoporosis.

The major minerals in bone are calcium and phosphate. The matrix of bone is composed principally of calcium and phosphate which are combined to form a lattice network of hydroxyapatite crystals. Calcium homeostasis is regulated by the parathyroid glands which secrete parathyroid hormone and the thyroid gland which secretes calcitonin. These polypeptide hormones have opposing functions. Parathyroid hormone stimulates bone resorption by osteoclasts whereas calcitonin stimulates bone formation by osteoblasts. The balance of parathyroid hormone and calcitonin maintains the concentration of serum calcium within a narrow range (~10 mg/dL) to facilitate regular muscle contractions (heartbeat), transmission of nerve impulses, and other functions that are vital to human life. A low concentration of calcium in the blood triggers the release of parathyroid hormone which promptly acts to restore calcium homeostasis by inducing resorption of calcium from bone, retention of calcium by the kidneys, and absorption of calcium in the small intestine (Robbins & Cotran, 1979).

The active hormonal form of vitamin D, 1,25 dihydroxyvitamin D (calcitriol), is necessary for optimal intestinal absorption of calcium and phosphorus. Vitamin D exerts a tonic inhibitory effect on parathyroid hormone synthesis. A deficiency in the active form of vitamin D can thus cause calcium deficiency in bone matrix resulting in bone weakness and fragility. The effects of vitamin D are modulated through a family of cell membrane receptors.

Estrogen is also essential for the maintenance of normal BMD. Estrogen acts through estrogen receptors to stimulate bone formation by osteoblasts and inhibit bone resorption by osteoclasts. In this way, estrogen decreases the rate of bone remodeling and the amount of bone lost with each remodeling cycle.

Bone resorption involves close contact and complex molecular interactions between osteoclasts and osteoblasts. The molecular messenger, *nuclear factor kappa beta* (*NF-Kb*) and *its receptor activators (RANK) and ligands (RANKL)*, stimulates osteoclast differentiation and remodeling activity. Inflammatory prostaglandins generated by the enzymatic activity of cyclooxygenase-2 (COX-2) accelerate bone resorption. Osteoblasts produce and secrete *osteoprotegerin* (*OPG*), a decoy receptor that inhibits RANKL/RANK interactions (Raisz, 2005).

Diagnosis of Osteoporosis

The World Health Organization criteria for the diagnosis of osteopenia and osteoporosis are shown in **TABLE 46.1**. Osteopenia is defined as BMD between 1.0 and 2.5 standard deviations below the mean normal adult value whereas osteoporosis is diagnosed when

TABLE 46.1 Diagnostic Criteria for Osteopenia and Osteoporosis

Diagnosis	Diagnostic Criteria
Normal	BMD value within 1.0 SD of mean value
Osteopenia	BMD 1.0–2.5 SD below mean value
Osteoporosis	BMD more than 2.5 SD below mean value
Osteoporosis	Abnormal BMD plus fragility fracture

BMD = bone mineral density and SD = standard deviation.

BMD is lower than 2.5 standard deviations below the mean. Since BMD levels follow a normal distribution, approximately 0.6% of adults have osteoporosis. Severe disease is low BMD plus one or more fragility bone fractures (WHO, 1994).

Bone Mineral Density and Osteoporosis

A team of Swedish investigators conducted a meta-analysis of prospective cohort studies published during 1985–1994 in order to determine the value of BMD in predicting bone fractures in women. Eleven separate study populations were included in the analysis. During 90,000 years of follow-up, 2000 bone fractures were detected. Pooled results revealed that the risk of bone fracture increased by a factor of 1.5 for each standard deviation decrease in BMD. The association was stronger for hip fractures (RR = 2.6) and vertebral fractures (RR = 2.3). A review of case–control studies yielded similar results. The investigators concluded that BMD can predict the fracture risk for groups of women but cannot identify specific individuals who will suffer a fracture (Marshall, Johnell, & Wedel, 1996).

Incidence and Prevalence of Hip Fracture

In their review of the epidemiology of osteoporosis, Jordan and Cooper state: "*Clinically, osteoporosis is recognized by the occurrence of low-trauma fractures. Hip fracture is the most serious consequence of osteoporosis and is most closely linked to BMD compared to other types of fracture*" (Jordan & Cooper, 2002). Indeed, many epidemiologic investigations have used low/moderate trauma hip fracture as a conservative indicator of osteoporosis.

Investigators at the Mayo Clinic examined trends in the age-specific incidence and prevalence of low/moderate trauma hip fracture for the population of Rochester, Minnesota, during 1928–1992. Using an indexed registry of medical records, they identified a total of 2058 adults who suffered a hip fracture of the proximal femur due to moderate or low trauma during the 65-year time period. **FIGURE 46.1** shows the annual age-specific *incidence* curves by gender estimated from the most recent data, 1983–1992. The annual incidence rates rise exponentially during the last half of the lifespan peaking after age 85 years at 2000 cases per 100,000 in men and 2700 cases per 100,000 in

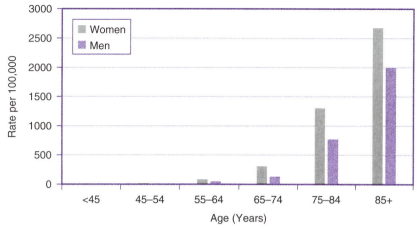

FIGURE 46.1 Age-Specific Incidence of Low-Trauma Hip Fracture, 1983–1992, United States.

Data from Melton, L. J., Therneau, T. M., & Larson, D. R. (1998). Long-Term trends in hip fracture prevalence: The influence of hip fracture incidence and survival. *Osteoporosis International, 8*, 68–74.

women after the age of 85 years. The average rate of increase per successive year of age was about 12% in women and men; however, the overall age-adjusted annual rate in women was 66% higher than in men (136 vs. 82 per 100,000), and for each age group, the incidence rate was higher in women (Melton, Therneau, & Larson, 1998).

FIGURE 46.2 shows the annual age-specific prevalence curves by gender estimated from the 1983 to 1992 Rochester data. The annual prevalence rates rise sharply after age 55 years peaking after age 85 years at about 17,000 cases per 100,000 in women and 6000 cases per 100,000 in men. The overall age-adjusted rate in women was more than 2.3-fold higher than in men (768 vs. 333 cases per 100,000). Over the 65-year time frame of the study, the prevalence of hip fracture increased nearly fivefold in parallel with increasing longevity of the population (Melton et al., 1998).

▶ Survival and Mortality: Hip Fractures

Melton and colleagues also examined mortality and survival following hip fracture in the Rochester cohort. In comparison with mortality rates for the general population, there was a marked excess of deaths in both men and women during the first year following fracture. Mortality was found to be 5–10-fold higher than the general population during the first few weeks after fracture, but then gradually declined to expected levels at about 1 year post-fracture. Overall, women experienced longer average survival than men following an initial hip fracture: 8.6 versus 6.1 years, respectively (Melton et al., 1998).

In a more recent analysis of the Rochester cohort, Melton and colleagues determined that the annual incidence of first hip fracture during the period 1980–2006 declined by about 1.4% per year in women while remaining unchanged in men. Among 2434 individuals who suffered a first fracture, the cumulative risk of recurrent hip fracture after 10 years was 11% in women and 6% in men. Interestingly, there was a significant reduction in hip fracture recurrence after 1997, corresponding to the introduction of bisphosphonate therapy for osteoporosis (Melton et al., 2009).

Results of many other studies also reflect high early mortality and disability rates among subjects who suffer hip fracture. In a study of 571 cases 50 years or older who received emergency care in metropolitan hospitals in New York City during 1997–1998, the in-hospital mortality rate was 1.6%, and at 6 months post-fracture, 13.5% of cases were deceased and 12.8% needed total assistance to ambulate (Hannan et al., 2005).

In Great Britain, 8148 hip fracture cases 65 years or older who received emergency care in hospitals near Oxford during 1994–1998 were followed over 6 months post-fracture. In-hospital mortality was 7.9%, and 24.6% of patients died within 6 months (Goldacre, Roberts, & Yeates, 2002).

In Malmö, Sweden, all women suffering a hip fracture during 1984–1985 were followed for up to 22 years to determine mortality and the risk of a second fracture. Among 766 cases, 21% died during the first year after fracture. One-year mortality increased with age, 7%, 21%, and 33% for age groups < 75, 75–84, and 85+ years, respectively, but in subsequent years after fracture, the age-adjusted relative mortality was not significantly increased compared to the general population. The 10-year risk of *second fracture* among surviving cases was estimated at 40% (von Friesendorff, Besjakov, & Akesson, 2008).

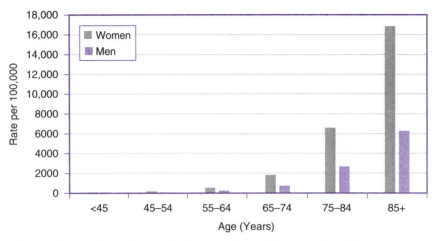

FIGURE 46.2 Age-Specific Prevalence of Low-Trauma Hip Fracture, United States, 1983–1992.

Data from Melton, L. J., Therneau, T. M., & Larson, D. R. (1998). Long-term trends in hip fracture prevalence: The influence of hip fracture incidence and survival. *Osteoporosis International, 8,* 68–74.

▶ Global Burden of Osteoporosis

The first global estimates of the incidence and mortality of hip fracture were reported by Johnnel and Kanis for the year 1990 based on published data from eight geographic regions of the world. The investigators also derived an estimate of the *disability-adjusted life years* (DALY) due to hip fracture. Among adults 50 years and older, there were 1.31 million new hip fractures, 4.48 million prevalent cases of hip fracture with disability, and 738,000 deaths associated with hip fracture in the world population. Approximately 70% of new hip fractures, prevalent hip fractures, and related deaths were in women. A total of 1.75 million DALY were lost due to hip fracture representing approximately 0.1% of the total DALY in 1990 (Johnell & Kanis, 2004).

In a later study, Johnell and Kanis examined the global burden of hip fractures in adults 50 years and older based on data reported from 1990 onwards. Mean rates of hip fractures were calculated for 17 subregions of the world and subsequently collapsed into seven broad regions: Africa, America, Eastern Mediterranean, Europe, Southeast Asia, and the Western Pacific. Fracture rates at other anatomic sites (spine, forearm, humerus, and elsewhere) were extrapolated based upon age-gender-site specific data estimated from the Swedish national registry. *Disability-adjusted life years* (DALY = *years of life lost due to premature death* [YLL] + *years of life lost due to disability* [YLD]) were also estimated globally and for each region (Johnell & Kanis, 2006; Kanis et al., 2000).

The study found that nearly 9 million people suffered osteoporotic fractures in the world population during the year 2000. More than half of these fractures involved the hip (1.6 million), forearm (1.7 million),

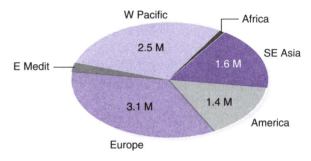

FIGURE 46.3 Global Distribution of Bone Fractures.

Data from Johnell, O., & Kanis, J. A. (2006). An estimate of the worldwide prevalence and disability associated with osteoporotic fractures. *Osteoporosis International, 17,* 1726–1733.

or spine (1.4 million). The distribution of fractures is shown by region in **FIGURE 46.3**. The Americas and Europe accounted for over 50% of the worldwide burden of fractures. The total DALY lost from osteoporotic fractures was estimated at 5.8 million representing about 0.83% of all non-communicable (chronic) diseases. The disease burden was greater in women (DALY = 3.7 million) than men (DALY = 2.1 million). Approximately 51% of the DALY were lost in the populations of Europe and the Americas, which comprise only about 27% of the world population. The investigators concluded that "*osteoporotic fractures are a significant cause of morbidity and mortality, particularly in the developed countries*" (Johnell & Kanis, 2006).

A team of investigators at the *WHO Collaborating Center for Metabolic Bone Diseases* in Sheffield, England, conducted a more recent study to determine the number of hip fractures that were attributable to osteoporosis in individuals over 50 years of age during 2010. They used data from 58 countries representing 83.5% of the world population. A total of 2.32 million incident hip fractures were observed (1.57 million in women and 741,000 in men) and of these, 1.16 million

(50%) were attributed to osteoporosis. On extrapolation to the world population, the number of incident hip fractures was estimated at 2.7 million of which 1.36 million were attributed to osteoporosis (1.1 million in women and 264,000 in men). The investigators concluded that "*strategies to prevent osteoporosis could prevent up to 50% of all hip fractures*" (Odén, McCloskey, Johansson, & Kanis, 2013).

Kanis and colleagues examined data on hip fractures from 63 countries reported in 72 studies during 1950–2011 to estimate age-adjusted incidence rates by country and the probability of hip fracture worldwide. Rates were standardized to the 2010 world population. Where possible, the investigators use a fracture risk assessment tool called FRAX to model the 10-year probability of a major osteoporotic hip fracture for the men and women of each country. Among the 63 countries, the annual incidence rates for men and women were highly correlated ($r = 0.82$). However, within countries, the age-adjusted incidence rate of hip fracture in women was approximately double the rate in men (e.g., for countries with a rate of 300 per 100,000 per year in women, the rate was 150 per 100,000 in men). The study revealed extreme variability in the annual incidence estimates among countries ranging from less than 100 per 100,000 in Nigeria, South Africa, Tunisia, Ecuador, and Morocco, to more than 500 per 100,000 in Denmark, Sweden, and Austria. The estimated probability of fracture over 10 years in 65-year-old women at high risk for osteoporosis ranged from over 25% among the women of Denmark and Sweden to less than 5% among the women of Tunisia and Ecuador. Ten-year probabilities of fracture averaged about 23% higher in women than men (Kanis et al., 2012).

▶ Risk Factors for Osteoporosis

The pathogenesis of bone loss and osteoporosis is modulated by multiple risk factors including aging, nutritional deficiencies (vitamin D and calcium), post-menopausal estrogen deficiency in women, and various lifestyle factors including smoking, alcohol abuse, lack of exercise, low body mass, and certain environmental exposures (Cooper & Melton, 1992; Jordan & Cooper, 2002). Deficiencies in vitamin D and calcium are also prominent causes of two related bone disorders, *rickets* and *osteomalacia*. In the discussion that follows, vitamin D metabolism and regulation of calcium homeostasis are briefly reviewed and findings from randomized clinical trials of vitamin and mineral supplementation and estrogen replacement therapy are presented. Genetic factors, certain medical conditions and medications, and various other factors that modulate the risk are also covered.

Vitamin D Metabolism

The active form of vitamin D (calcitriol) is synthesized in humans by a cascade of reactions in the skin, liver, and kidneys (**FIGURE 46.4**). The initial reaction occurs in the skin where sunlight (ultraviolet light) converts the cholesterol derivative, 7-dehydrocholesterol to vitamin D3 (cholecalciferol). Cholecalciferol is subsequently transported in the blood to the liver and hydroxylated to form 25 hydroxycholecalciferol (calcidiol). Calcidiol is then transported in the blood to the proximal tubules of the kidneys where it undergoes a second hydroxylation reaction to form the active vitamin D compound 1,25 hydroxycholecalciferol (calcitriol). Calcitriol is a potent ligand of the *vitamin D receptor* (*VDR*), which mediates most of the physiological actions of the vitamin. The active form of vitamin D is required for calcium and phosphorous absorption from the small intestine. In the absence of vitamin D during the early years of development, dietary calcium is not absorbed, resulting in hypocalcemia which causes severe skeletal and dental deformities, a condition known as rickets. A similar condition that is caused by vitamin D deficiency in adolescents and adults is called *osteomalacia* (Vitale, 1979).

The role of vitamin D in maintaining calcium homeostasis in the human system was elucidated in the early 20th century through the research of many investigators. McCollum and Davis initially isolated a fat-soluble growth factor in butterfat and cod liver oil that was later found to prevent rickets in animals (McCollum & Davis, 1914; McCollum, Simmonds, Becker, & Shipley, 1922).

In 1921, Alfred Hess and L.F. Unger of Columbia University showed that by exposing rachitic children

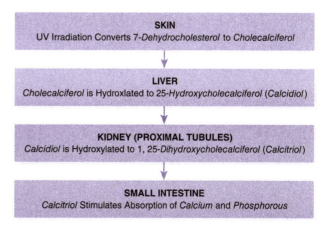

FIGURE 46.4 Biosynthesis of Active Vitamin D (Calcitriol).

to sunlight, they were able to cure them of the disease (Hess & Unger, 1921). In 1924, the chemist Harry Steenbock and colleagues at the University of Wisconsin demonstrated that irradiation produced foodstuffs with antirachitic properties in animals, a revolutionary finding that was patented and subsequently utilized by the food industry to fortify milk, bread, cereal, and other food products with irradiated vitamin D compounds (Steenbock, 1924; Steenbock & Black, 1924). Soon thereafter, other investigators also reported that irradiation could impart antirachitic properties to inert food sources (Hess & Weinstock, 1925; Hume & Smith, 1924).

The German steroid chemist, Adolf Windhaus, eventually isolated the active form of vitamin D and was awarded the Nobel Prize *"for his studies on the constitution of the sterols and their connection with vitamins"* (Wolf, 2004). Subsequent studies by Windaus and others were instrumental in elucidating the photochemical conversion of *provitamin D* (*7-dehydrocholesterol and ergosterol*) to *vitamin D3* (*cholecalciferol*) (Rosenheim & Webster, 1926; Windaus, 1931; Windaus & Hess, 1926). Three decades later, investigators in the United States and England independently identified the biologically active form of vitamin D (*1,25-dihydroxycholecalciferol* or *calcitriol*) which is synthesized sequentially from cholecalciferol in the liver and kidneys (Holick, Schnoes, & DeLuca, 1971; Holick, Schnoes, DeLuca, Suda, & Cousins, 1971; Lawson, Fraser, Kodicek, Morris, & Williams, 1971).

Dietary sources of vitamin D include fatty fish, liver, egg yolk, and certain dairy products such as butter, cream, and cheese. Plant sources of vitamin D are limited and include certain herbs and mushrooms. In most developed countries, food staples are fortified with vitamin D to prevent deficiency. In supplements and fortified foods, vitamin D is available in two forms, vitamin D2 (ergocalciferol) and vitamin D3 (cholecalciferol), that differ chemically only in their side-chain structure. Vitamin D2 is manufactured by the UV irradiation of ergosterol from yeast, and vitamin D3 is manufactured by the irradiation of 7-dehydrocholesterol from lanolin (Holick, 2007).

Vitamin D Deficiency: Rickets and Osteomalacia

Severe deficiencies in vitamin D and/or dietary calcium and phosphorous become apparent early in life (usually by the age of 2 years) in the form of rickets.

In this condition, calcium and phosphate levels are insufficient to support normal bone development and mineralization along the growth plates of endochondral bones. As a consequence, the bones are soft, pliable, and often deformed. As already noted, a closely related condition, *osteomalacia*, refers to defective bone mineralization in adolescents and adults.

Bone formation in the human skeleton is a complex process that begins during embryogenesis and continues throughout the lifespan. Most skeletal bones involve the initial formation of an intermediate cartilaginous template, which serves as a guide for bone development. Over time, the cartilage is replaced by bone composed of calcium phosphate salts and hydroxyapatite crystals to form a dense, hard shell of endochondral bone. The process of bone formation along cartilaginous growth plates is called *ossification*. Subsequently, the inner matrix of the newly formed bone undergoes *mineralization* by calcium and phosphorous compounds to form trabecular bone that is less dense. The inner trabecular bone matrix is heavily interlaced with small blood vessels to facilitate bone remodeling and the influx/outflux of calcium and phosphorous (Vitale, 1979).

The processes of mineralization and demineralization of bone are tightly regulated by parathyroid hormone and vitamin D, and are in a continual state of flux. Parathyroid hormone is secreted by the parathyroid glands in response to low levels of serum calcium. This hormone stimulates resorption of bone and the mobilization of calcium and phosphorous in order to maintain serum calcium within a narrow range of normality (9.5–10.5 mg/mL). Parathyroid hormone also stimulates the biosynthesis of the active form of vitamin D (calcitriol) in the renal tubules of the kidneys. Vitamin D is essential for daily maintenance of adequate stores of calcium and phosphorous in the body. Vitamin D stimulates absorption of dietary calcium and phosphorous by the small intestine while enhancing the retention of calcium by the kidneys (Vitale, 1979).

Ann Prentice of the Medical Research Council at Cambridge recently reviewed available data on vitamin D levels and calcium intake from various populations around the globe in order to characterize the prevalence of rickets and osteomalacia and nutritional deficiencies worldwide. While the fortification of milk and other food products in the mid-20th century resulted in the near eradication of rickets and osteomalacia in the United States, Europe, and other developed nations in the mid-20th century, exceptionally high prevalence rates of rickets ranging from 10% up to 70% have been found in surveys of children living in underdeveloped nations. Dr. Prentice notes that *"the prevalence of rickets, however, remains scandalously high in many parts of Asia, Africa, and the Middle East"* and she suggests *"there is an urgent need for action to address the global burden of rickets and osteomalacia"* (Prentice, 2008).

The plasma concentration of *25 hydroxycholecal-ciferol* (*25 hydroxyvitamin D*) is a useful vitamin D biomarker because it has a long half-life in the circulation and its concentration is not under tight homeostatic regulation. This biomarker therefore reflects vitamin D supply and usage over a period of time. Normal levels of 25 hydroxyvitamin D range between 20 and 80 ng/mL although there is debate about the lower limit (some investigators suggest a lower threshold of 30 ng/mL).

Patients with rickets or osteomalacia often have very low levels of hydroxyvitamin D. In a study of 98 patients and their families from New Delhi, India, the average level of 25 hydroxyvitamin D among patients was ~6 pg/mL with a 95% confidence interval of approximately 1–10 ng/mL. Notably, 90% of the cases with either rickets or osteomalacia were female and among 221 of their close relatives, 24% of females and 5% of males had *chemical osteomalacia* defined as hydroxyvitamin D less than 20 ng/mL. These results suggest that females are at particularly high risk (Ray et al., 2009).

In 1997, a standing committee of the U.S. Institute of Medicine reported a consensus statement that "*persons with hydroxyvitamin D less than 20 nmols/L (8 ng/mL) probably have rickets or osteomalacia*" (Institute of Medicine, 1997). More recently, other investigators have suggested slightly higher cutpoints of 25 nmols/L (10 ng/mL) and 30 nmols/L (12 ng/mL) (Norman, 2008; Prentice, 2008).

National surveys have been conducted in Great Britain and the United States to characterize the prevalence of vitamin D deficiency at different ages. Such studies were designed to quantify the fraction of individuals with vitamin D deficiency reflected by serum levels of *25 hydroxyvitamin D* (*25 hydroxycholecalciferol*) less than 25 nmols/L (10 ng/mL). Surprisingly, the prevalence of low vitamin D status in Great Britain during 1992–2001 was between 5% and 20% in most age groups and exceeded 20% in young men and women aged 19–24 years, and in elderly women over 85 years of age (**FIGURE 46.5**). Furthermore, prevalence estimates ranging from 20% to 40% were found in certain populations likely to have little sun exposure and/or low dietary intake, particularly elderly adults living in nursing homes, certain minority groups, and individuals on special diets (Finch, Doyle, & Lowe, 1998; Gregory, Collins, Davies, Hughes, & Clarke, 1995; Gregory, Lowe, & Bates, 2000; Prentice, 2008; Ruston, Hoare, & Gregory, 2003). These results suggest that even in developed nations, many individuals do not have adequate levels of vitamin D and are therefore at increased risk for the development of rickets, osteomalacia, and osteoporosis (Prentice, 2008; Prentice et al., 2006).

In contrast to the vitamin D data from Great Britain, a national survey conducted in the United States during 1988–1994 yielded prevalence estimates below 5% for vitamin D deficiency irrespective of age. The relatively low prevalence of vitamin D deficiency in the United States population compared to Great Britain may partially reflect the greater sun exposure in the Southern United States population (Looker,

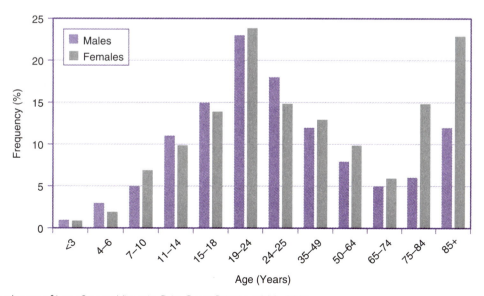

FIGURE 46.5 Prevalence of Low Serum Vitamin D in Great Britain, 1992–2001.

Data from Gregory, J. R., Collins, D. L., Davies, P. S. W., Hughes, J. M., & Clarke, P. C. (1995). *National diet and nutrition survey: Children aged 1.5 to 4.5 years.* London, UK: HMSO; Finch, S., Doyle, W., & Lowe, C. (1998). *National diet and nutrition survey: People aged 65 years and over. Vol 1: Report of the diet and nutrition survey.* London, UK: The Stationery Office; Gregory, J. R., Lowe, C., & Bates, C. (2000). *National diet and nutrition survey: Young people aged 4 to 18 years: Report of the diet and nutrition survey* (Vol. 1). London, UK: The Stationery Office; Ruston, D., Hoare, L., & Gregory, J. (2003). *The national diet and nutrition survey: Adults aged 19 to 64 years. Nutritional status (anthropometry and blood analytes), blood pressure and physical activity* (Vol. 4). London, UK: The Stationery Office; Prentice, A. (2008). Vitamin D deficiency: A global perspective. *Nutrition Reviews, 66*(10 Suppl. 2), S153–S164.

Dawson-Hughes, Calvo, Gunter, & Sahyoun, 2002; Prentice, 2008).

Good nutrition is especially important for normal fetal development and good maternal health. Recent surveys suggest that vitamin D deficiency is remarkably commonplace in pregnant women of certain ethnic minority groups, even those residing in developed countries. For example, studies of pregnant women in minority groups from the Netherlands, Great Britain, New Zealand, and Australia have yielded prevalence estimates of vitamin D deficiency ranging from 50% to 80%. Vitamin D deficiency during pregnancy may serve as a harbinger for the subsequent development of bone disorders in mother and offspring (Prentice, 2008).

The recommended daily allowances (RDA) of vitamin D in the United States are 400 IU from birth to 1 year of age, 600 IU between the ages of 1 and 70 years, and 800 IU for individuals over 70. Intake of 600 IU is also recommended for pregnant or lactating women (Institute of Medicine, 2010). Notably, vitamin D-fortified milk is available in many developed nations and exemplifies a simple, practical, inexpensive, and effective means of preventing vitamin D deficiency, rickets, and osteomalacia (Scrimshaw, 1986). Obviously, the vitamin D status of populations in developed countries may not reflect that of some underdeveloped countries where malnutrition and nutritional deficiencies are relatively common. Albeit, there are scant data on vitamin D deficiency and related conditions in the developing world and more studies are clearly needed to accurately characterize their global impact.

Vitamin D Deficiency and Osteoporosis

Very few epidemiologic investigations have focused on vitamin D deficiency as a risk factor for osteoporosis. In Oslo, Norway, which has a high incidence of osteoporosis, investigators conducted a matched case–control study to evaluate risk factors of hip fractures among the elderly. Cases admitted to Oslo hospitals for treatment of hip fracture were compared to controls matched by age and gender. Though no association was found with calcium intake, low intake of vitamin D (<100 IU) significantly increased the risk of hip fracture (OR = 3.9) (Meyer, Henriksen, Falch, Pedersen, & Tverdal, 1995).

In a nested case–control study of osteoporosis among Mediterranean women, Ramstam and Kanis compared the use of vitamin D supplements in 1634 women with hip fracture aged 50 years or older to 3532 age-matched controls from 14 centers in six Mediterranean countries. Overall, the risk of

hip fracture was reduced by 26% among those using vitamin D supplements (RR = 0.74). Observed risk reductions were greater for women 80 years and older (RR = 0.63) and those with body mass index less than 20 (RR = 0.45). The investigators concluded that vitamin D supplementation for the prevention of hip fracture might be usefully targeted to the frail and elderly (Ranstam & Kanis, 1995).

One study reflects the importance of considering endogenous levels of not only vitamin D but also estrogen. In a nested case–control study of women 65 years or older, Cummings and colleagues compared serum levels of vitamin D3 (cholecalciferol) and estrogen (estradiol) at baseline in 133 women who subsequently developed hip fracture and 138 women who subsequently suffered vertebral fractures with randomly selected controls from the same cohort. Women were excluded if they took exogenous estrogen. Results revealed that women with low serum vitamin D3 levels (<23 pg/mL) were at increased risk of suffering a hip fracture (OR = 2.1) and women with low serum estrogen (<5 pg/mL) were at increased risk of suffering either a hip or vertebral fracture (OR = 2.5). Furthermore, women with undetectable free estrogen (unbound to sex hormone binding globulin) had marked increases in fracture risk (OR = 6.9 for hip fractures and OR = 7.9 for vertebral fractures). These results suggest that low serum levels of estrogen and/or vitamin D increase the fracture risk in postmenopausal women (Cummings et al., 1998).

Calcium Homeostasis

Calcium is a mineral that is essential for life. Its presence is integral to intracellular signaling, enzyme activation, transmission of nerve impulses, muscle contractions, and many other physiological processes. Blood levels of calcium must be maintained within a very narrow range (9.5–10.5 mg/mL) for these processes to remain viable. Calcium (in the form of calcium phosphate) is the primary building block of bone and is responsible for bone density and strength. Bone is the primary storage compartment of calcium and undergoes continual remodeling throughout the lifespan in order to help maintain calcium homeostasis in all tissues.

The action of vitamin D and the metabolism of calcium and phosphate are regulated by parathyroid hormone that is secreted by the parathyroid glands. Parathyroid hormone stimulates the synthesis of the active form of vitamin D (calcitriol) in the renal tubules of the kidneys plus the release of calcium and phosphate from bone. Calcitriol enhances the absorption of dietary calcium and phosphate in the small intestine plus the retention of both minerals by the renal tubules of the kidneys. This integrated metabolic system is essential for the maintenance of calcium/phosphorous/bone homeostasis, and perturbation in any part of the system is likely to cause disease. For example, vitamin D deficiency during early bone development causes rickets since dietary calcium and phosphorous are not absorbed in the gastrointestinal tract and are thus not available to mineralize bone. Likewise, severely low levels of dietary calcium and phosphorous can produce deranged ossification and lack of bone mineralization leading to osteomalacia in adolescents and young adults, and osteoporotic fracture in the elderly (Prentice, 2008; Prentice et al., 2006).

Calcium Deficiency and Osteoporosis

Surprisingly, the results of epidemiologic investigations *do not* consistently support a beneficial effect of high calcium intake per se on bone health. For example, in a 12-year prospective study of 77,781 adult American women, Harvard investigators found *no evidence* that higher intakes of milk or calcium from food sources reduced the risk of bone fractures (Feskanich, Willett, Stampfer, & Colditz, 1997).

In contrast, a longitudinal study of 957 American men and women aged 50–79 years at baseline and followed for up to 14 years revealed a significant reduction in the risk of hip fractures with high calcium intake (RR = 0.60 per 198 mg per 1000 kcal). The investigators suggest that this result "*strongly supports the hypothesis that increased dietary calcium intake protects against hip fracture*" (Holbrook, Barrett-Connor, & Wingard, 1988).

Randomized Clinical Trials

Calcium Supplementation for Prevention of Osteoporosis

A team of international investigators conducted a meta-analysis of placebo-controlled randomized clinical trials to evaluate calcium supplementation for the prevention of osteoporosis in postmenopausal women. A literature search identified 15 randomized clinical trials of 1806 postmenopausal patients that reported BMD and fracture risk with and without calcium supplementation. The combined results from these trials showed that calcium supplementation significantly reduced the rates of bone loss after 2 or more years of treatment. Rates of vertebral and nonvertebral fractures also decreased with calcium

supplementation compared to placebo (23% and 14%, respectively) although effect measures did not reach statistical significance. The investigators concluded that calcium supplementation has a positive influence on BMD (Shea et al., 2002). Notwithstanding, as discussed in the following section on vitamin D, supplementation with *calcium plus vitamin D* not only increases bone density but also appears to have significant value in the chemoprevention of osteoporotic fractures (DIPART Group, 2010).

Calcium and Vitamin D Supplementation for Prevention of Osteoporosis

Several randomized clinical trials have been conducted to assess potential chemopreventive effects of supplemental vitamin D and calcium on bone density and rates of bone fracture in postmenopausal women. Albeit, the results of these studies provide conflicting evidence regarding benefit of vitamin D supplementation to bone health.

Papadimitropoulos and colleagues conducted a meta-analysis of 25 trials that randomized postmenopausal women to standard or hydroxylated vitamin D with or without calcium supplementation versus placebo. All studies had at least 1 year of follow-up. The combined results showed that vitamin D supplementation reduced the incidence of vertebral fractures (RR = 0.63) and nonvertebral fractures (RR = 0.77) (Papadimitropoulos et al., 2002).

Investigators of the *U.S. Women's Health Initiative* examined effects of calcium and vitamin D on bone density and fracture risk in a randomized placebo-controlled clinical trial of postmenopausal women. They recruited 36,292 postmenopausal women, 50–79 years of age, for random assignment to receive 1000 mg of elemental calcium (as calcium carbonate) plus 400 IU of vitamin D3 daily or placebo. Fractures were assessed over 7 years of follow-up and bone density was measured in samples of treated and untreated women in the study. Censored results on termination of the trial revealed improved bone density and a significant reduction in the hazard ratio for hip fracture (hazard ratio [HR] = 0.71) among women who received supplemental calcium plus vitamin D (Jackson et al., 2006).

Bischoff-Ferrari and colleagues conducted a meta-analysis of data extracted from randomized clinical trials of vitamin D and fracture risk in order to evaluate effects of the dose of vitamin D supplementation. Only double-blind randomized clinical trials of oral vitamin D supplementation with or without supplemental calcium in older persons 60 years or older that examined hip or vertebral fractures were included. Five trials of hip fracture (9294 participants) and seven trials of nonvertebral fracture (9820 participants) met the inclusion criteria. Compared to placebo, oral vitamin D at a dose of 700–800 IU daily reduced the relative risk of both hip fracture (RR = 0.74) and nonvertebral fracture (RR = 0.77), whereas no benefit was observed for lesser doses. The investigators concluded that oral vitamin D supplementation at 700–800 IU daily reduces the risk of hip and nonvertebral fractures whereas a dose of 400 IU daily is not sufficient for fracture prevention (Bischoff-Ferrari et al., 2005).

Boonen and colleagues extended the meta-analysis of Bischoff-Ferrari and colleagues to examine the risk of hip fracture among individuals receiving dietary supplementation with vitamin D alone versus calcium plus vitamin D. In their analysis, the pooled relative risk estimate for vitamin D plus calcium (RR = 0.82) was 25% less than the estimate for vitamin D alone (RR = 1.10), suggesting that vitamin D reduces the risk of hip fracture only when calcium supplementation is added (Boonen et al., 2007).

Most recently, investigators of the *DIPART* (*Vitamin D Individual Patient Analysis of Randomized Trials*) group conducted a meta-analysis of individual patient data from randomized clinical trials to evaluate independent and joint effects of oral supplementation with vitamin D and calcium. Their pooled analysis included individual patient data from seven major randomized clinical trials of oral vitamin D supplementation with or without calcium supplementation. These trials included 68,517 participants (14.7% male) ranging age from 47 to 107 years with fracture as the primary outcome. Cox regression was utilized to estimate the *HR* with adjustment for other variables. Results revealed that vitamin D in combination with calcium reduced the overall risk of fracture (HR = 0.92) and hip fracture (HR = 0.84). However, no significant effects of vitamin D alone were noted irrespective of dose. Furthermore, the analysis did not detect significant interactions with age, gender, or estrogen replacement therapy. These results suggest that vitamin D supplementation alone is *ineffective* in preventing fractures, but that the *combination* of oral calcium and vitamin D reduces the risk of hip fracture and total fractures (DIPART Group, 2010).

Vitamin D and Calcium Supplementation Therapy for Bone Disease

Studies of populations residing in tropical climates where sun exposure is abundant and vitamin D levels are sufficient clearly suggest that severe dietary calcium deficiency per se can cause rachitic disease and that early detection and correction of the deficiency is beneficial. Thacher and colleagues conducted a clinical trial of 123 Nigerian children with rickets to assess the therapeutic benefit of oral supplementation with vitamin D alone, calcium alone, and combination therapy with vitamin D and calcium. After 6 months of treatment, recovery was apparent in 61% of children who received calcium, 58% of children receiving combination therapy, but only 19% of children receiving vitamin D. The investigators concluded that Nigerian children with rickets have a low intake of calcium and a better response to treatment with calcium alone or in combination with vitamin D than to vitamin D alone (Thacher et al., 1999).

In contrast, results of studies of vitamin D and calcium supplementation therapy in patients with osteoporotic fracture have not been encouraging. In a *therapeutic* trial conducted in Great Britain, elderly adults 70 years or older who had suffered an initial low-trauma fracture were randomly assigned to take 800 IU of supplemental vitamin D3 daily, 1000 mg of supplemental calcium daily, both supplements daily, or placebo. During 24–62 months of follow-up, 698 new fractures were detected among the 5292 participants. In comparisons of treatment groups with placebo, no significant differences were detected in the incidence of new fractures. Thus, these findings do not support oral supplementation with calcium and/or vitamin D3 as an effective therapeutic approach for the tertiary prevention of second fractures in such patients (Grant et al., 2005).

Calcium and Vitamin D: Synopsis of Findings

In summary, calcium and vitamin D are essential for bone health, and deficiencies in either agent (or both) can cause rickets and osteomalacia during the developmental years and osteoporosis later in life. The major causes of vitamin D deficiency are poor nutrition and scarce exposure to sunlight. Nutritional surveys in developing and some developed countries also reflect calcium deficiencies in a significant fraction of the population. The recent evidence from randomized clinical trials lends support to routine supplementation with *both* compounds, particularly for those at high risk. Supplemental intake of 700–800 mg of calcium *and* 400–800 IU of vitamin D is recommended as a safe, effective, and inexpensive means of preventing rickets in children, osteomalacia in adolescents and young adults, and osteoporotic fractures in the elderly (Gennari, 2001).

Estrogen and Osteoporosis

In his review of the epidemiology and pathogenesis of osteoporosis, Clifford Rosen states that "*bone loss as a result of aging and/or estrogen deficiency is the predominant pathophysiologic disorder of primary osteoporosis*" (Rosen, 2017). As illustrated in Figures 46.1 and 46.2, osteoporosis is rarely observed in premenopausal women but is a relatively common disorder in postmenopausal women. The major physiological impact of menopause is the loss of ovarian estrogens that are secreted during the menstrual cycle. Typically, serum estrogen (estradiol) is highest during the follicular phase of the menstrual cycle (~400 pg/mL) and then declines to much lower levels (~50 pg/mL) in parallel with rising progesterone levels during the luteal phase. Following menopause, estrogen (estrone) is primarily produced in fat and muscle cells by the enzymatic action of aromatase, which converts adrenal steroids to estrogen. As a consequence of the shutdown of ovarian biosynthesis, postmenopausal levels of estrogen fall dramatically to about 15% of premenopausal values (Howanitz & Howanitz, 1984).

The impact of reduced estrogen on bone remodeling in postmenopausal women is dramatic. With falling estrogen, there is a marked increase in the activity of ligands and receptors that stimulate osteoclasts (*RANK* and *RANKL*) and a marked decrease in *osteoprotegerin* (*OPG*) and other factors that stimulate osteoblasts. These changes tip the balance of bone remodeling in favor of osteoclastic bone resorption that far outpaces osteoblastic bone formation. The end result is demineralization of both the outer cortical shell and the inner trabecular matrix of bone.

Heidi Nelson of the *Oregon Health Sciences University* conducted a systematic review and evaluation of studies of *estrogen replacement therapy* (*ERT*) and *selective estrogen receptor modulators* (*SERMs*) to determine their value in preventing osteoporosis and bone fracture in postmenopausal women. The study was supported by the *U.S. Agency for Healthcare Research and Quality*. Only randomized controlled trials and cohort studies were included in the analysis. Results of 22 randomized clinical trials revealed that ERT improved bone density and reduced the risk of nonvertebral fractures by 27% (RR = 0.73). In cohort studies, women who received ERT compared to those who did not showed 20%–35% reductions in the adjusted relative risk of hip fracture. In studies of SERMs, both tamoxifen and raloxifene were found to increase bone density of various sites, and raloxifene reduced the risk of vertebral fractures by 41% (RR = 0.59). These results suggest that ERT and SERMs may have benefit in improving bone density and protecting against bone fractures (Nelson, 2002).

Testosterone and Osteoporosis

Though osteoporosis occurs more often in women, elderly men constitute a significant fraction (25% or more) of cases. A few studies have examined the association between testosterone deficiency (hypogonadism) and osteoporosis and the impact of testosterone replacement therapy on bone health in men.

Levels of total testosterone and free (unbound) testosterone were compared in a small case–control study of 28 elderly men who suffered hip fractures and 28 healthy controls matched by age, ethnicity, and living conditions. The average serum levels of total testosterone and free testosterone were found to be significantly lower among cases than controls, and testosterone deficiency (<9 nmol/L) was present in 20 of the cases versus 9 of the controls (Crude OR = 5.3). Serum levels of hydroxyvitamin D were also lower among cases. The investigators concluded that gonadal deficiency is an important risk factor for osteoporotic fracture in men and recommended that early recognition and testosterone replacement therapy be considered for prevention (Jackson, Riggs, & Spiekerman, 1992).

Investigators at Massachusetts General Hospital in Boston compared BMD and other measures of body composition in 36 adult men with acquired hypogonadism and 44 untreated age-matched eugonadal controls. On average, the spinal BMD among hypogonadal men was about 10% less than controls. Cases also had about 46% higher body fat than controls. Testosterone therapy (100 mg per week) was initiated in 29 of the hypogonadal men and subjects were evaluated at 6-month intervals for 18 months. Testosterone replacement therapy produced a significant increase in lean muscle mass (7%), a significant decrease in percent body fat (14%), and a significant increase in spinal BMD (5%). Furthermore, markers of bone remodeling and resorption, serum *alkaline phosphatase* and urinary *deoxypyridinoline* excretion, decreased significantly with therapy. The investigators concluded that testosterone replacement therapy has beneficial impact on body composition and increases bone density in hypogonadal men (Katznelson et al., 1996).

Investigators at the Mayo Clinic performed a systematic review and meta-analysis of randomized placebo-controlled clinical trials to assess the effect of testosterone administration on bone health in men. Eight trials that enrolled a total of 365 patients were included in the analysis. Results revealed that intramuscular injections of testosterone improved BMD by 8% in the lumbar spine and 4% in the femoral head compared to placebo whereas transdermal injections had no significant effect. The investigators concluded that the available trials offer some evidence of the clinical efficacy of intramuscular testosterone for osteoporosis prevention and treatment in men (Tracz et al., 2006).

Low Body Mass Index and Osteoporosis

De Laet and colleagues explored the association of *body mass index* (*BMI*) with fracture risk using data from 12 prospective population-based cohort studies involving nearly 60,000 men and women. Results revealed an inverse relation between BMI and the risk of bone fracture. Overall, there was a risk reduction of 2% for any type of fracture per unit increase in BMI (RR = 0.98) and a risk reduction of 7% for hip fracture per unit increase in BMI (RR = 0.93). The risk of hip fracture in subjects with BMI < 20 was approximately double that of subjects with BMI > 25 (RR = 1.95). The protective effect of increasing BMI was similar for men and women. These effects were attenuated with adjustment for BMD. The investigators concluded that "*low BMI confers a risk of substantial importance for all fractures that is largely independent of age and sex, but dependent on BMD*" (De Laet et al., 2005).

Smoking and Osteoporosis

Several meta-analyses have been published with the objective of clarifying the association between smoking and osteoporosis. Law and Hackshaw examined the association based on data from 29 cross-sectional studies and 19 cohort and case–control studies involving 15,750 subjects. Results revealed that the risk of hip fracture was 41% greater in smokers than nonsmokers and that BMD declined 2% more in smokers than nonsmokers for every 10-year increase in age (Law & Hackshaw, 1997).

Ward and Klesges conducted a pooled analysis of data from 86 studies involving 40,753 subjects. Their results revealed that chronic smoking increased the lifetime risk of hip fracture by 31% in women and 40% in men. The risk of vertebral fractures was also increased by smoking (13% in women and 32% in men). Their results also suggest that about 10% of all hip fractures are attributable to smoking (Ward & Klesges, 2001).

Kanis and colleagues examined the data from 10 prospective cohort studies involving 59,232 subjects. They found that current smoking increased the overall fracture risk by 25% and the risk of hip fracture by 84% (Kanis, Johnell, et al., 2005).

Investigators of the *Consortium on Health and Aging Network of Cohorts in Europe and the United States* (CHANCES) utilized data from six prospective cohorts to estimate DALY due to hip fracture and estimate etiologic fractions attributable to smoking, diabetes, and other potential risk factors. A total of 224,000 men and women were followed for an average of 13 years, of whom 7724 (3.5%) participants suffered a hip fracture and 413 (5.4%) died as a result. Hip fracture caused a loss of 27 DALY per 1000 individuals, approximately 70% from disability. Estimated etiologic fractions were highest for smoking (7.5%) and lack of physical exercise (5.5%), prompting the investigators to advocate strengthening of national public health policies to "*prevent falls, and reduce smoking and a sedentary lifestyle*" (Papadimitriou et al., 2017).

A team of investigators in China conducted a meta-analysis of cigarette smoking and hip fracture in women that included 10 prospective cohort studies. The composite estimate of relative risk was elevated in current smokers compared to never smokers (RR = 1.30) but not in former smokers (RR = 1.02). Furthermore, women who smoked at least 15 cigarettes per day were at greater risk than those who smoked less, and women who quit smoking for 10 or more years had a significant reduction in risk compared to current smokers (Shen et al., 2015).

Multiple mechanisms have been postulated to explain the increased fracture risk among smokers. While definitive evidence is lacking, some studies suggest that smoking reduces BMD by decreasing endogenous estrogens in women, decreasing the absorption of vitamin D and calcium, and/or increasing the adrenal secretion of glucocorticoids (Wong, Christie, & Wark, 2007).

Alcohol and Osteoporosis

Kanis and colleagues examined the association of bone fracture and alcohol consumption in a meta-analysis of data from three prospective cohort studies involving 5939 men and 11,032 women. The results revealed a threshold effect of alcohol intake at three or more drinks per day (RR = 1.23 for any fracture and RR = 1.68 for hip fracture). Relative risk estimates by gender did not differ significantly. Lesser levels of alcohol intake had no effect on the risk. Adjustment of estimates for BMD did not change the magnitude of the estimates. These results suggest that consumption of three or more drinks of alcohol daily confers a significant risk increase for bone fracture that is independent of BMD (Kanis, Johansson, et al., 2005).

Genetics of Osteoporosis

Osteoporosis is a polygenic disorder that is influenced by multiple genes and gene products implicated in bone resorption and bone formation. These basic processes are regulated by complex genetic, hormonal, nutritional, and environmental factors that interact to maintain homeostasis of calcium and other bone minerals and constituents. Family studies suggest that the risk of fracture in close relatives of probands (index cases) is significantly higher than nonrelatives, and twin studies have found higher concordance rates of bone fracture in monozygous twins than dizygous twins (Cooper & Melton, 1992). These findings suggest there may be major genes that modulate the risk. Candidate genes revealed by *genome wide association studies* (*GWAS*) and linkage analysis are integral to the control of multiple hormones (estrogen, parathyroid hormone, calcitonin, glucocorticoids), minerals (calcium and phosphorous), vitamins (vitamin D), inflammatory factors (interleukin-1, cyclooxygenase-2), and their cell membrane receptors (Rizzoli, Bonjour, & Ferrari, 2001).

Glucocorticoids and Osteoporosis

Glucocorticoid-induced osteoporosis is caused by taking anti-inflammatory steroids such as prednisone, prednisolone, dexamethasone, and cortisone. These compounds are routinely used to treat inflammatory arthritic and rheumatic conditions. Molecular studies suggest that glucocorticoids increase the expression of the *RANKL* and decrease expression of *osteoprotegerin* (*OPG*) in osteoblasts, which leads to increased differentiation and activity of osteoclasts. This mechanism and others contribute to increased bone resorption, reduced BMD, and increased risk of osteoporotic fracture.

Van Staa and colleagues evaluated effects of oral corticosteroids on BMD and fracture risk by a meta-analysis of published data from 66 reports on bone density and 23 reports on fracture involving 2891 patients who took glucocorticoids. Strong associations were found between cumulative dose and loss of BMD and between daily dose and fracture risk. The risk of fracture was found to increase within 3–6 months after the initiation of corticosteroid therapy. Risk increases were noted for any fracture (RR = 1.9), hip fracture (RR = 2.01), vertebral fracture (RR = 2.86), and forearm fracture (RR = 1.13). The risk decreased after stopping therapy. Risk estimates were not influenced by underlying disease, age, or gender. The investigators concluded that "*oral corticosteroid treatment using more than 5 mg (of prednisolone or equivalent) daily leads to a reduction in BMD and a rapid increase in the risk of fracture during the treatment period*" (Van Staa, Leufkans, & Cooper, 2002).

Similar results were observed in a study of oral corticosteroid use and the risk of fractures among patients registered in the *General Practice Research Database* of the United Kingdom. The study included 244,235 patients who used oral corticosteroids and 244,235 controls. Patients taking at least 7.5 mg of prednisolone (or equivalent) daily had significantly increased risks of nonvertebral fracture (RR = 1.44), hip fracture (RR = 2.21), and vertebral fracture (RR = 2.83) compared to those taking less than 2.5 mg daily (Van Staa, Leufkens, Abenhaim, Zhang, & Cooper, 2000). The findings of these investigations suggest that "*the adverse skeletal effects of oral corticosteroids manifest rapidly*" and mandate that "*preventive measures against corticosteroid-induced osteoporosis should therefore be instituted as soon after the commencement of glucocorticoid therapy as possible*" (Van Staa et al., 2000). Administration of supplemental bisphosphonate plus calcium and vitamin D has been shown effective in counteracting the detrimental effects of glucocorticoids on bone health (Kwok & Tam, 2008).

Physical Activity and Osteoporosis

A team of German investigators conducted a controlled exercise trial in early postmenopausal women with low bone density. Their objective was to determine the impact of a vigorous, combined high-impact, strength, and endurance training program on BMD determined by DXA. Participants included 146 osteopenic women (BMD 1.0–2.5 standard deviations below the mean) who were 1–8 years past menopause. Women were assigned to the exercise intervention group (*n* = 86) or the control group (*n* = 51). The intervention was 14 months of exercise training with two joint sessions and two home training sessions. All women studied received 1500 mg of calcium and 500 IU of vitamin D daily. After 14 months, BMD at the lumbar spine had *increased* by 1.3% from baseline in the exercise treatment group whereas it had *decreased* by 1.2% in the control group. Though differences at other sites were not statistically significant, BMD levels for women in the exercise group were always higher than in the control group. Muscle strength increased significantly in the treated group but declined in the controls. The investigators concluded that "*high-intensity exercise training can have a positive influence on bone density in early postmenopausal osteopenic women*" (Kemmler, Engelke, Weineck, Hensen, & Kalender, 2003). Additional studies by these investigators suggest that long-term exercise regimens provide an alternative to hormone replacement therapy in postmenopausal women and are effective in reducing blood lipids, maintaining BMD and improving muscle strength (Kemmler et al., 2007). Several meta-analyses of exercise studies provide confirmation that physical exercise generally has a positive effect on bone mass and bone density; however, there is considerable heterogeneity from study to study in the type, duration, and intensity of exercise regimens used and the target populations treated.

Cadmium and Osteoporosis

Occupational or environmental exposure to cadmium is a risk factor for several skeletal and renal disorders including osteoporosis, osteomalacia, renal tubular dysfunction, hypercalciuria, and formation of renal stones. The detrimental effects of cadmium exposure were first observed during the 1950s in residents of the *Jinzu River Basin* in Japan that was heavily contaminated by cadmium discarded from zinc mining. Ingestion of cadmium-contaminated rice resulted in at least 150 cases of *itai-itai* disease, a complex of bone fractures, osteomalacia, osteoporosis, and renal dysfunction diagnosed primarily in elderly women (Hagino & Kono, 1955; Tsuchija, 1969). The cadmium content in the bones of patients with itai-itai disease was later found to be nine times higher than normal in men and three times higher than normal in women (Noda & Kitagawa, 1990).

Investigators in Belgium conducted a prospective investigation designed to assess associations between cadmium exposure, BMD, and the risk of fracture. Cadmium exposure was measured by urinary cadmium excretion in 506 adults (199 men and 306 women) from 10 districts of Belgium, 6 of which bordered on 3 zinc smelters. At baseline, bone density was measured at the forearm by single photon absorptiometry. Median follow-up in the study was 6.6 years. In postmenopausal women, a twofold increase in urinary cadmium was associated with a 0.01 g per cubic centimeter decrease in bone density. High urinary cadmium was associated with an increased risk of fracture in women (RR = 1.73) and height loss in men (RR = 1.60). Cadmium excretion in districts near smelters was 23% higher than in other districts corresponding to a higher rate of fracture (16.0 vs. 10.3 cases per 1000 person-years). The investigators concluded that environmental exposure to cadmium may promote skeletal demineralization, increased bone fragility, and increased risk of bone fractures (Staessen et al., 1999).

In Sweden, investigators at the Karolinska Institute examined the association of cadmium exposure and the risk of osteoporosis among samples of 520 men and 544 women, aged 16–81 years, who were environmentally or occupationally exposed to cadmium. The level of urinary cadmium was used to approximate cadmium exposure and osteoporosis was determined by measuring BMD at the forearm. The results revealed a significant dose response between urinary cadmium level and osteoporosis in men over 60 years. The risk increased more than fivefold at the highest level of cadmium and approximately twofold for both men and women at intermediate levels (**FIGURE 46.6**). Results also revealed a fourfold increase in tubular proteinuria and a threefold decrease in BMD among those individuals with the highest levels of urinary cadmium (Alfven, Elinder, Carlson, Grubb, & Hellstrom, 2000; Alfven, Jarup, & Elinder, 2002).

Cadmium accumulates in bone and may cause damage by interfering with calcium deposition and collagen production or by stimulating inflammatory prostaglandins that heighten bone resorption (Kazantzis, 2004). As Lars Jarup (2002) of the Imperial College of Medicine in London points out in his review of cadmium overload and toxicity:

As techniques are perfected for detecting smaller amounts of trace elements in various tissues of the body, investigators are finding that the threshold for toxicity of trace elements is much lower than expected. Further research on cadmium is needed to reveal the mechanisms of toxicity and true environmental and occupational exposure limits. (pp. 35–39)

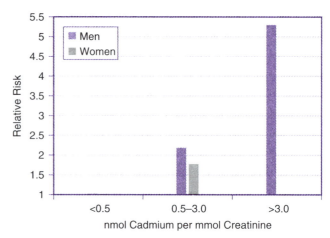

FIGURE 46.6 Dose Response of Osteoporosis Risk by Level of Urinary Cadmium.

Data from Alfven, T., Elinder, C. G., Carlson, M. D., Grubb, A., & Hellstrom, L. (2000). Low-level cadmium exposure and osteoporosis. *Journal of Bone and Mineral Research, 15*(8), 1579–1586.

Antecedent Disease and Osteoporosis

Multiple chronic diseases and conditions are associated with the development of osteoporosis. Endocrine disorders can lead to abnormal levels of key hormones that accelerate bone remodeling, bone loss, and increase the risk of osteoporotic bone fracture. Examples include *hypogonadal* conditions such as *Turner's syndrome* (*XO genotype*) and *Klinefelter's syndrome* (*XXY genotype*), adrenal disorders (*Cushing's syndrome*), and disorders of the thyroid (*thyrotoxicosis*) and parathyroid glands (*hyperparathyroidism*). Furthermore, there is much current interest in not only the master hormones secreted by target endocrine organs of the hypothalamic-pituitary axes (gonads, adrenals, thyroid and parathyroid glands), but also the effects of releasing factors secreted by the pituitary gland on bone remodeling (Imam et al., 2009).

Patients with arthritic and/or autoimmune conditions are at increased risk due to inherent inflammation and/or treatment with corticosteroids (prednisone). For example, patients with *systemic lupus erythematosus* (*SLE*) have been found to have nearly five times the fracture risk of the general population (Ramsey-Goldman et al., 1999).

Calcium deficiency can arise from malnutrition and/or malabsorption disorders (lactose intolerance, colitis), or by renal nephropathies that reduce calcium reabsorption in the renal tubules. Chronic kidney disease has also been found to reduce the biosynthesis of calcitriol, the active form of vitamin D. In general, any condition that directly or indirectly compromises bone metabolism can lead to loss in BMD and osteoporotic fracture (Martin & Gonzalez, 2007).

▶ Primary Prevention of Osteoporosis

Women and men with multiple risk factors and low bone density are at especially high risk for the development of osteoporosis and fractures of the hip, spine and other skeletal sites. In a prospective study of 9516 Caucasian women 65 years or older recruited in Portland, Oregon, Minneapolis, Baltimore, and the Monongahela Valley, Pennsylvania, 192 of the women suffered an incident hip fracture during an average of 4.1 years of follow-up. Low calcaneal bone density increased the risk 1.6-fold for each standard deviation decrease. The study identified multiple risk factors for hip fracture other than bone density. Risk factors adjusted for bone density included age (RR = 1.4 per 5 years of aging), maternal history of bone fracture (RR = 1.8), hyperthyroidism (RR = 1.7),

current use of a tricyclic antidepressant (RR = 1.6), inability to rise from a chair (RR = 1.7), elevated pulse (RR = 1.7), personal history of any fracture (RR = 1.5), and current smoking (age-adjusted RR = 2.1). Factors that decreased the risk included regular aerobic exercise (RR = 0.70) and *weight increase* since age 25 (RR = 0.80 per 20% increase). In women without a history of osteoporosis or fracture of any kind, ERT was protective (RR = 0.30). The presence of multiple risk factors among women with low BMD synergistically increased the risk (RR = 27.3 for women with five or more risk factors and low BMD). These results indicate that multiple risk factors must be taken into account in minimizing the risk of hip fracture in older women (Cummings et al., 1995).

In a prospective cohort study of 5994 men aged 65 years or older recruited from six U.S. clinical centers, 178 (3%) of the men suffered an incident hip fracture during an average of 8.6 years of follow-up. The annual incidence rate was 350 per 100,000 person-years. Increases in the adjusted HR were noted for age greater than 75 years (HR = 2.3), low femoral neck BMD (HR = 3.0), current smoking (HR = 2.1), tricyclic antidepressant use (HR = 2.8), hyperthyroidism (HR = 2.9), Parkinson's disease (HR = 3.3), and prior myocardial infraction or angina (HR = 1.6). Overall, the incidence of hip fracture increased with increasing number of risk factors and decreasing BMD (e.g., the presence of 2–3 risk factors with low BMD increased the risk of hip fracture by 28-fold). Results indicate that in addition to BMD, multiple risk factors must be taken into account to reduce the risk of hip fracture in older men (Cauley et al., 2016).

Results of many studies provide convincing evidence that the risk of osteoporotic fracture can be reduced by making appropriate lifestyle choices. Recommended guidelines include regular daily aerobic exercise (walking, jogging, biking, swimming), sufficient intake of dietary calcium, vitamin D and other nutrients essential for healthy bones, exposure to sunlight (at least 30 minutes daily), avoidance of smoking, restriction of alcohol consumption, and individual strategies to prevent falls. Effective chemopreventive supplements include the combination of calcium and vitamin D. Bisphosphonates are also effective in high risk subjects (USPSTF, 2011).

Screening for Osteoporosis (Secondary Prevention)

The U.S. Preventive Services Task Force recently recommended that all women 65 years of age or older should be screened for osteoporosis by bone densitometry.

Guidelines for screening younger women incorporate the presence of risk factors and specific *"clinical decision rules"* which take into account age, BMI, smoking status, alcohol use, family history, medical history, medication history, and history of previous falls (Hippisley-Cox & Coupland, 2009; USPSTF, 2011).

In recent years, various tools have been developed to evaluate the 10-year risk of bone fracture. FRAX® is a diagnostic tool developed by investigators at the University of Sheffield to evaluate fracture risk of individual patients. It is designed to integrate independent risk factors and BMD measures at the femoral neck to estimate the 10-year probability of major osteopathic fractures (spine, forearm, hip, or shoulder). Measurements of BMD are entered into the website tool together with clinical risk factors which include a prior fragility fracture, parental history of hip fracture, current tobacco smoking, long-term use of glucocorticoids, rheumatoid arthritis, other causes of secondary osteoporosis, and daily alcohol consumption. The FRAX® tool provides an estimate of the 10-year fracture probability and a clinical assessment in order to determine preventive strategies and access to treatment in healthcare systems (Unnanuntana, Gladnick, Donnelly, & Lane, 2010).

Therapy and Tertiary Prevention

For patients with confirmed osteoporosis, *bisphosphonate* drugs are the first line of treatment. Based on results from three large randomized clinical trials, investigators estimated that treating 1000 women with osteoporosis for 3 years would prevent 100 fractures of the spine, hip, and other skeletal sites (Black & Rosen, 2016). Other effective drugs that may be prescribed on an individual basis include ERT or SERM in women and testosterone in men. Other hormonal abnormalities should also be addressed in patients with osteoporosis. Lifestyle changes to modify risk are essential to complement medication.

Potential side effects of all prescribed drugs must be carefully considered. For example, ERT heightens the risk of breast cancer and endometrial cancer (Roush, 2011; USPSTF, 2011). Furthermore, case reports of atypical femur fractures and osteonecrosis of the jaw have been reported among patients taking bisphosphonates, and a significant proportion of patients have either discontinued their use or are reluctant to initiate bisphosphonate therapy. Due to these reports, the use of commonly prescribed drugs for osteoporosis has fallen precipitously in recent years. In a recent study of the impact of announcements by the U.S. Food and Drug Administration (FDA) regarding side effects of bisphosphonates, their use among 22,598 patients with hip fracture fell from 15% in 2004 to only 3% in 2013 (Kim et al., 2016). Due to the high rates of devastating complications and mortality related to osteoporosis, there is an urgent need for concerted public health efforts to implement widespread screening of BMD among the elderly in order to implement preventive strategies for individuals at high risk, and cohesive efforts from clinicians advocating early therapy with monitoring of compliance and side effects for patients with the disease (Khosla & Shane, 2016).

References

Albright, F., Bloomberg, E., & Smith, P. H. (1940). Postmenopausal osteoporosis. *Transactions of the Association of American Physicians, 55*, 298–305.

Alfven, T., Elinder, C. G., Carlson, M. D., Grubb, A., & Hellstrom, L. (2000). Low-level cadmium exposure and osteoporosis. *Journal of Bone and Mineral Research, 15*(8), 1579–1586.

Alfven, T. L., Jarup, L., & Elinder, C. G. (2002). Cadmium and lead in blood in relation to low bone mineral density and tubular proteinuria. *Environmental Health Perspectives, 110*, 699–702.

Bischoff-Ferrari, H. A., Willett, W. C., Wong, J. B., Giovannucci, E., Dietrich, T., & Dawson-Hughes, B. (2005). Fracture prevention with vitamin D supplementation: A meta-analysis of randomized controlled trials. *JAMA, 293*, 2257–2264.

Black, D. M., Kelly, M. P., Genant, H. K., Palermo, L., Eastell, R., Bucci-Rechtweg, C., … HORIZON Pivotal Fracture Trial Steering Committee. (2010). Bisphosphonates and fractures of the subtrochanteric or diaphyseal femur. *The New England Journal of Medicine, 362*, 1761–1771.

Black, D. M., & Rosen, C. J. (2016). Clinical practice: Postmenopausal osteoporosis. *The New England Journal of Medicine, 374*(3), 254–262.

Boffetta, P., Bobak, M., Borsch-Supan, A., Brenner, H., Eriksson, S., Grodstein, F., … Trichopoulou, A. (2014). The Consortium on Health and Aging: Network of Cohorts in Europe and the United States (CHANCES) project-design, population and data harmonization of a large-scale, international study. *European Journal of Epidemiology, 29*(12), 929–936.

Boonen, S., Lips, P., Bouillon, R., Bischoff-Ferrari, H. A., Vanderschueren, D., & Haentjens, P. (2007). Need for additional calcium to reduce the risk of hip fracture with vitamin D supplementation: Evidence from a comparative meta-analysis of randomized controlled trials. *The Journal of Clinical Endocrinology and Metabolism, 92*, 1415–1423.

Consensus Development Conference. (1991). Prophylaxis and treatment of osteoporosis. *Osteoporosis International, 1*, 114–117.

Cooper, A., & Cooper, B. B. (1822). *A treatise on dislocations, and on fractures of the joints.* London, UK: Churchill.

Cooper, C., & Melton, L. J. (1992). Epidemiology of osteoporosis. *Trends in Endocrinology and Metabolism, 3*, 224–229.

Cauley, J. A., Cawthon, P. M., Peters, K. E., Cummings, S. R., Ensrud, K. E., Bauer, D. C., … Orwoll, E. S. (2016). Risk factors for hip fracture in older men: The Osteoporotic Fractures in Men Study (MrOS). *Journal of Bone and Mineral Research, 31*(10), 1810–1819.

Cummings, S. R., Browner, W. S., Bauer, D., Stone, K., Ensrud, K., & Ettinger, B. (1998). Endogenous hormones and the risk of hip and vertebral fractures among older women. *The New England Journal of Medicine, 339*, 733–738.

Cummings, S. R., Nevitt, M. C., Browner, W. S., Stone, K., Fox, K. M., Ensrud, K. E., … Vogt, T. M. (1995). Risk factors for hip fracture in white women. *The New England Journal of Medicine, 332*, 767–773.

De Laet, C., Kanis, J. A., Odén, A., Johanson, H., Johnell, O., Delmas, P., … Tenenhouse, A. (2005). Body mass index as a predictor of fracture risk: A meta-analysis. *Osteoporosis International, 16*(11), 1330–1338.

DIPART Group. (2010). Patient level pooled analysis of 68,500 patients from seven major vitamin D fracture trials in US and Europe. *British Medical Journal, 340*, b5463.

Feskanich, D., Willett, W. C., Stampfer, M. J., & Colditz, G. A. (1997). Milk, dietary calcium and bone fractures in women: A 12-year prospective study. *American Journal of Public Health, 87*, 992–997.

Finch, S., Doyle, W., & Lowe, C. (1998). *National diet and nutrition survey: People aged 65 years and over. Vol 1: Report of the diet and nutrition survey.* London, UK: The Stationery Office.

Gennari, C. (2001). Calcium and vitamin D nutrition and bone disease of the elderly. *Public Health Nutrition, 4*(2B), 547–559.

Goldacre, M. J., Roberts, S. E., & Yeates, D. (2002). Mortality after admission to hospital with fractured neck of femur: Database study. *British Medical Journal, 325*, 868–869.

Grant, A. M., Avenell, A., Campbell, M. K., McDonald, A. M., MacLennan, G. S., McPherson, G. C., … Wallace, W. A., RECORD Trial Group. (2005). Oral vitamin D3 and calcium for secondary prevention of low-trauma fractures in elderly people (Randomised Evaluation of Calcium Or vitamin D, RECORD): A randomized placebo-controlled trial. *Lancet, 365*(9471), 1621–1628.

Gregory, J. R., Collins, D. L., Davies, P. S. W., Hughes, J. M., & Clarke, P. C. (1995). *National diet and nutrition survey: Children aged 1.5 to 4.5 years.* London, UK: HMSO.

Gregory, J. R., Lowe, C., & Bates, C. (2000). *National diet and nutrition survey: Young people aged 4 to 18 years: Report of the diet and nutrition survey* (Vol. 1). London, UK: The Stationery Office.

Hagino, N., & Kono, M. (1955). A study on the cause of itai-itai disease. *Proceedings of the 17th Meeting of the Japanese Society of Clinical Surgeons.*

Hannan, E. L., Magaziner, J., Wang, J. J., Eastwood, E. A., Silberzweig, S. B., Gilbert, M., … Siu, A. L. (2005). Mortality and locomotion 6 months after hospitalization for hip fracture. *JAMA, 285*(21), 2793–2794.

Hess, A. F., & Unger, L. J. (1921). The cure of infantile rickets by artificial light and by sunlight. *Proceedings of the Society for Experimental Biology and Medicine, 18*, 298.

Hess, A. F., & Weinstock, M. (1925). A further report on imparting antirachitic properties to inert substances by ultra-violet irradiation. *Journal of Biological Chemistry, 63*, 297–307.

Hippisley-Cox, J., & Coupland, C. (2009). Predicting risk of osteoporotic fracture in men and women in England and Wales: Prospective derivation and validation of Qfracture scores. *British Medical Journal, 339*, b4229.

Holbrook, T. L., Barrett-Connor, E., & Wingard, D. L. (1988). Dietary calcium and risk of hip fracture: 14-year prospective population study. *Lancet, 332*(8619), 1046–1049.

Holick, M. F. (2007). Vitamin D deficiency. *The New England Journal of Medicine, 357*, 266–281.

Holick, M. F., Schnoes, H. K., & DeLuca, H. F. (1971). Identification of 1,25-dihydroxycholecalciferol, a form of vitamin D_3 metabolically active in the intestine. *Proceedings of the National Academy of Sciences of the United States of America, 68*(4), 803–804.

Holick, M. F., Schnoes, H. K., DeLuca, H. F., Suda, T., & Cousins, R. J. (1971). Isolation and identification of 1,25-dihydroxy-cholecalciferol. A metabolite of vitamin D active in intestine. *Biochemistry, 10*(14), 2799–2804.

Howanitz, J. H., & Howanitz, P. J. (1984). Evaluation of endocrine function. In J. B. Henry (Ed.), *Todd, Sanford & Davidsohn clinical diagnosis and management by laboratory methods* (17th ed., pp. 299–345). Philadelphia, PA: WB Saunders Company.

Hume, E. M., & Smith, H. H. (1924). The effect of irradiation of the environment with ultra-violet light upon the growth and calcification of rats, fed on a diet deficient in fat-soluble vitamins: The part played by irradiated sawdust. *The Biochemical Journal, 18*, 1334–1345.

Imam, A., Iqbal, J., Blair, H. C., Davies, T. F., Huang, C. L., Zallone, A., … Sun, L. (2009). Role of the pituitary-bone axis in skeletal pathophysiology. *Current Opinion in Endocrinology, Diabetes, and Obesity, 16*(6), 423–429.

Institute of Medicine. (2010). *Dietary reference intakes for vitamin D and calcium.* Washington, DC: US National Academy of Sciences.

Institute of Medicine Standing Committee on the Scientific Evaluation of Dietary Reference Intakes, Food and Nutrition Board. (1997). *Dietary reference intakes for calcium, magnesium, phosphorus, vitamin D, and fluoride.* Washington, DC: National Academy Press.

Jackson, J. A., Riggs, M. W., & Spiekerman, A. M. (1992). Testosterone deficiency as a risk factor for hip fractures in men: A case-control study. *The American Journal of the Medical Sciences, 304*(1), 4–8.

Jackson, R. D., LaCroix, A. Z., Gass, M., Wallace, R. B., Robbins, J., Lewis, C. E., … Barad, D., Women's Health Initiative Investigators. (2006). Calcium plus vitamin D supplementation and the risk of fractures. *The New England Journal of Medicine, 354*(7), 669–683.

Jarup, L. (2002). Cadmium overload and toxicity. *Nephrology, Dialysis, Transplantation, 17*(Suppl. 2), 35–39.

Johnell, O., & Kanis, J. A. (2004). An estimate of the worldwide prevalence, mortality and disability associated with hip fracture. *Osteoporosis International, 15*(11), 897–902.

Johnell, O., & Kanis, J. A. (2006). An estimate of the worldwide prevalence and disability associated with osteoporotic fractures. *Osteoporosis International, 17*, 1726–1733.

Jordan, K. M., & Cooper, C. (2002). Epidemiology of osteoporosis. *Best Practice & Research Clinical Rheumatology, 16*(5), 795–806.

Kanis, J. A., Johansson, H., Johnell, O., Oden, A., De Laet, C., Eisman, J. A., … Tenenhouse, A. (2005). Alcohol intake as a risk factor for fracture. *Osteoporosis International, 16*(7), 746–742.

Kanis, J. A., Johnell, O., Oden, A., Johansson, H., De Laet, C., Eisman, J. A., … Tenenhouse, A. (2005). Smoking and fracture risk: A meta-analysis. *Osteoporosis International, 16*, 155–162.

Kanis, J. A., Oden, A., Johnell, O., Jonsson, B., De Laet, C., & Dawson, A. (2000). The burden of osteoporotic fractures: A method for setting intervention thresholds. *Osteoporosis International, 12,* 417–427.

Kanis, J. A., Odén, A., McCloskey, E. V., Johansson, H., Wahl, D. A., & Cooper, C. (2012). A systematic review of hip fracture incidence and probability of fracture worldwide. *Osteoporosis International.* doi:10.1007/s00198-012-1964-3.

Katznelson, L., Finkelstein, J. S., Schoenfeld, D. A., Rosenthal, D. I., Anderson, E. J., & Klibanski, A. (1996). Increase in bone density and lean body mass during testosterone administration in men with acquired hypogonadism. *The Journal of Clinical Endocrinology, & Metabolism, 81*(12), 4358–4365.

Kazantzis, G. (2004). Cadmium, osteoporosis and calcium metabolism. *Biometals, 17*(5), 493–498.

Kemmler, W., Engelke, K., von Stengel, S., Weineck, J., Lauber, D., & Kalender, W. A. (2007). Chapter 46: Long-term four-year exercise has a positive effect on menopausal risk factors: the Erlangen Fitness Osteoporosis Prevention Study. *Journal of Strength and Conditioning Research, 21*(10), 232–239.

Kemmler, W., Engelke, K., Weineck, J., Hensen, J., & Kalender, W. A. (2003). The Erlangen Fitness Osteoporosis Prevention Study: A controlled exercise trial in early postmenopausal women with low bone density—First-year results. *Archives of Physical Medicine and Rehabilitation, 84,* 673–682.

Khosla, S., & Shane, E. (2016). A crisis in the treatment of osteoporosis. *Journal of Bone and Mineral Research, 31*(8), 1485–1487.

Kim, S. C., Kim, D. H., Mogun, H., Eddings, W., Polinski, J. M., Franklin, J. M., & Solomon, D. H. (2016). Impact of the U.S. Food and Drug Administration's safety-related announcements on the use of bisphosphonates after hip fracture. *Journal of Bone and Mineral Research, 31*(8), 1536–1540.

Kwok, L. W., & Tam, L. S. (2008). Recent advances in the management of steroid induced osteoporosis. *Hong Kong Bulletin on Rheumatic Diseases, 8,* 12–18.

Law, M. R., & Hackshaw, A. K. (1997). A meta-analysis of cigarette smoking, bone mineral density and risk of hip fracture: Recognition of a major effect. *British Medical Journal, 315,* 841–846.

Lawson, D. E., Fraser, D. R., Kodicek, E., Morris, H. R., & Williams, D. H. (1971). Identification of 1,25-dihydroxycholecalciferol, a new kidney hormone controlling calcium metabolism. *Nature, 230*(5291), 228–230.

Lobstein, J. G. C. F. M. (1835). *Lehrbuch der pathologischen Anatomie.* Stuttgart, Germany: Bd II.

Looker, A. C., Dawson-Hughes, B., Calvo, M. S., Gunter, E. W., & Sahyoun, N. R. (2002). Serum 25-hydroxyvitamin D status of adolescents and adults in two seasonal sub-populations from NHANES III. *Bone, 30,* 771–777.

Marshall, D., Johnell, O., & Wedel, H. (1996). Meta-analysis of how well measures of bone density predict occurrence of osteoporotic fractures. *British Medical Journal, 312,* 1254–1259.

Martin, K. J., & Gonzalez, E. A. (2007). Metabolic bone disease in chronic kidney disease. *Journal of the American Society of Nephrology, 18,* 875–885.

McCollum, E. V., & Davis, M. (1914). Observations on the isolation of the substance in butter fat which exerts a stimulating effect on growth. *Journal of Biological Chemistry, 19,* 245–250.

McCollum, E. V., Simmonds, N., Becker, J. E., & Shipley, P. G. (1922). Studies on experimental rickets. XXI. An experimental demonstration of the existence of a vitamin which promotes calcium deposition. *Journal of Biological Chemistry, 53,* 293–312.

Melton, L. J., Kearns, A., Atkinson, E., Bolander, M., Achenbach, S., Huddleston, J., … Leibson, C. L. (2009). Secular trends in hip fracture incidence and recurrence. *Osteoporosis International, 20*(5), 687–694.

Melton, L. J., Therneau, T. M., & Larson, D. R. (1998). Long-term trends in hip fracture prevalence: The influence of hip fracture incidence and survival. *Osteoporosis International, 8,* 68–74.

Meyer, H. E., Henriksen, C., Falch, J. A., Pedersen, J. I., & Tverdal, A. (1995). Risk factors for hip fracture in a high incidence area: A case-control study from Oslo, Norway. *Osteoporosis International, 5*(4), 239–246.

Nelson, H. D. (2002). Hormone replacement therapy and osteoporosis. *Systematic evidence review, 12,* (p. 43). Washington, DC: Agency for Healthcare Research and Quality, U.S. Department of Health and Human Services.

Noda, M., & Kitagawa, M. (1990). A quantitative study of iliac bone histopathology in 62 cases with itai-itai disease. *Calcified Tissue International, 47,* 66–74.

Norman, A. W. (2008). From vitamin D to hormone D: Fundamentals of the vitamin D endocrine system essential for good health. *American Journal of Clinical Nutrition, 88*(2), 4915–4995.

Odén, A., McCloskey, E. V., Johansson, H., & Kanis, J. A. (2013). Assessing the impact of osteoporosis on the burden of hip fractures. *Calcified Tissue International, 92*(1), 42–49.

Papadimitriou, N., Tsilidis, K. K., Orfanos, P., Benetou, V., Ntzani, E. E., Soerjomataram, I., … Trichopoulou, A. (2017). Burden of hip fracture using disability-adjusted life-years: A pooled analysis of prospective cohorts in the CHANCES consortium. *The Lancet, 2*(5), e329–e246.

Papadimitropoulos, E., Wells, G., Shea, B., Gillespie, W., Weaver, B., Zytaruk, N., … Guyatt, G. (2002). Meta-analysis of the efficacy of vitamin D treatment in preventing osteoporosis in postmenopausal women. *Endocrine Reviews, 23*(4), 560–569.

Prentice, A. (2008). Vitamin D deficiency: A global perspective. *Nutrition Reviews, 66*(10 Suppl. 2), S153–S164.

Prentice, A., Schoenmakers, I., Laskey, M. A., De Bono, S., Ginty, F., & Goldberg, G. R. (2006). Nutrition and bone growth and development. *The Proceedings of the Nutrition Society, 65,* 348–360.

Raisz, L. G. (2005). Pathogenesis of osteoporosis: Concepts, conflicts, and prospects. *The Journal of Clinical Investigation, 115*(12), 3318–3325.

Ramsey-Goldman, R., Dunn, J. E., Huang, C. F., Dunlop, D., Rairie, J. E., Fitzgerald, S., & Manzi, S. (1999). Frequency of fractures in women with systemic lupus erythematosus: Comparison with United States population data. *Arthritis and Rheumatism, 42*(5), 882–890.

Ranstam, J., & Kanis, J. A. (1995). Influence of age and body mass on the effects of vitamin D on hip fracture risk. *Osteoporosis International, 5*(6), 450–454.

Ray, D., Goswami, R., Gupta, N., Tomar, N., Singh, N., & Sreenivas, V. (2009). Predisposition to vitamin D deficiency osteomalacia and rickets in females is linked to their 25(OH)D and calcium intake rather than vitamin D receptor gene polymorphism. *Clinical Endocrinology, 71*(3), 334–340.

Rizzoli, R., Bonjour, J. P., & Ferrari, S. L. (2001). Osteoporosis, genetics and hormones. *Journal of Molecular Endocrinology, 26,* 79–94.

Robbins, S. L., & Cotran, R. S. (1979). *Pathologic basis of disease.* Philadelphia, PA: W.B. Saunders Company.

Rosen, C. J. (2017). The epidemiology and pathogenesis of osteoporosis. In F. Singer, A. Boyce (Eds.), *Diseases of bone and mineral metabolism* (Chapter 11). Retrieved from www .Endotext.org

Rosenheim, O., & Webster, T. A. (1926). Further observations on the photo-chemical formation of vitamin D. *Journal of the Society of Chemical Industry, 45,* 932.

Roush, K. (2011). Prevention and treatment of osteoporosis in postmenopausal women: A review. *The American Journal of Nursing, 111*(8), 26–35.

Ruston, D., Hoare, L., & Gregory, J. (2003). *The national diet and nutrition survey: Adults aged 19 to 64 years. Nutritional status (anthropometry and blood analytes), blood pressure and physical activity* (Vol. 4). London, UK: The Stationery Office.

Scrimshaw, N. S. (1986). Nutrition and preventive medicine. In J. M. Last (Ed.), *Maxcy-Rosenau public health and preventive medicine* (12th ed., pp. 1515–1542). Norwalk, CT: Appleton-Century-Croft.

Shea, B., Wells, G., Cranney, A., Zytaruk, N., Robinson, V., Griffith, L., … Guyatt, G. (2002). Meta-analysis of calcium supplementation for the prevention of postmenopausal osteoporosis. *Endocrine Reviews, 23*(4), 552–559.

Shen, G. S., Li, Y., Zhao, G., Zhou, H. B., Xie, Z. G., Xu, W., … Xu, Y. J. (2015). Cigarette smoking and risk of hip fracture in women: A meta-analysis of prospective cohort studies. *Injury, 46*(7), 1333–1340.

Staessen, J., Roels, H., Emelianov, D., Kuznetsova, T., Thijs, L., Vangronsveld, J., & Fagard, R. (1999). Environmental exposure to cadmium, forearm bone density, and risk of fractures: Prospective population study. Public Health and Environmental Exposure to Cadmium (PheeCad) Study Group. *Lancet, 353*(9159), 1140–1144.

Steenbock, H. (1924). The induction of growth promoting and calcifying properties in a ration by exposure to light. *Science, 60,* 224–225.

Steenbock, H., & Black, A. (1924). Fat-soluble vitamins: The induction of growth-promoting and calcifying properties in a ration by exposure to ultraviolet light. *Journal of Biological Chemistry, 62,* 405–422.

Thacher, T. D., Fischer, P. R., Pettifor, J. M., Lawson, J. O., Isichei, C. O., Reading, J. C., & Chan, G. M. (1999). A comparison of calcium, vitamin D, or both for nutritional rickets in Nigerian children. *The New England Journal of Medicine, 341,* 563–568.

Tracz, M. J., Sideras, K., Boloña, E. R., Haddad, R. M., Kennedy, C. C., Uraga, M. V., … Montoir, V. M. (2006). Testosterone use in men and its effects on bone health. A systematic review and meta-analysis of randomized placebo-controlled trials. *The Journal of Clinical Endocrinology, & Metabolism, 91*(6), 2011–2016.

Tsuchija, K. (1969). Causation of ouch-ouch disease (Itai-itai byo): An introduction review. Part 1, nature of disease. *The Keio Journal of Medicine, 18,* 181–194.

Unnanuntana, A., Gladnick, B. P., Donnelly, E., & Lane, J. M. (2010). The assessment of fracture risk. *The Journal of Bone and Joint Surgery, 92*(3), 743–753.

US Preventive Services Task Force. (2011). Screening for osteoporosis: U.S. preventive services task force recommendation statement. *Annals of Internal Medicine, 154*(5), 356–364.

Van Staa, T. P., Leufkens, H. G., Abenhaim, L., Zhang, B., & Cooper, C. (2000). Use of oral corticosteroids and risk of fractures. *Journal of Bone and Mineral Research, 15,* 993–1000.

Van Staa, T. P., Leufkens, H. G., & Cooper, C. (2002). The epidemiology of corticosteroid induced osteoporosis: A meta-analysis. *Osteoporosis International, 13,* 777–787.

Vitale, J. J. (1979). Nutritional disease. In S. L. Robbins & R. S. Cotran (Eds.) *Pathologic basis of disease* (2nd ed., pp. 483–520). Philadelphia, PA: WB Saunders Company.

von Friesendorff, M., Besjakov, J., & Akesson, K. (2008). Long-term survival and fracture risk after hip fracture: A 22-year follow-up in women. *Journal of Bone and Mineral Research, 23*(11), 1832–1841.

Ward, K. D., & Klesges, R. C. (2001). A meta-analysis of the effects of cigarette smoking on bone mineral density. *Calcified Tissue International, 68,* 259–270.

WHO. (1994). *Assessment of fracture risk and its application to screening for postmenopausal women.* Geneva, Switzerland: World Health Organization.

Windaus, A. (1931). The chemistry of irradiated ergosterol. *Proceedings of the Royal Society of London. Series B, 108,* 568–575.

Windaus, A., & Hess, A. (1926). *Sterine und antirachitisches Vitamin.* Göttingen, Germany: Nachrichten von der Gesellschaft der Wissenschaften zu Göttingen, pp. 175–184.

Wolf, G. (2004). The discovery of vitamin D: The contribution of Adolf Windaus. *The Journal of Nutrition, 134,* 1299–1302.

Wong, P. K. K., Christie, J. J., & Wark, J. D. (2007). The effects of smoking on bone health. *Clinical Science, 113,* 233–241.

© Andrew Brookes/Getty Images

CHAPTER 47

Epidemiology of Arthritis

► Introduction

Arthritis is an inflammatory disease of one or more synovial joints of the skeletal system. Synovial joints facilitate motion (flexion, extension, rotation, abduction) and are divisible into ball and socket joints (shoulder and hip), hinge joints (elbow and knee), pivot joints (atlas and axis), condyloid joints (wrist), saddle joints (thumb), and gliding joints (fingers). Arthritis has multiple forms, and several classification systems have been proposed based upon etiology, the joints involved, and other symptoms. This chapter focuses on the three major forms of arthritis: osteoarthritis (degenerative joint disease), rheumatoid arthritis (an autoimmune disorder), and gout (due to uric acid crystals). Other forms that are briefly covered include ankylosing spondylitis, juvenile arthritis, and suppurative arthritis (due to infection). The approximate distribution of incident cases of these forms of arthritis in the adult U.S. population is shown in **TABLE 47.1**.

► Synovial Joints

As pointed out by Robbins and Cotran in their discussion of diseases of the musculoskeletal system: "*the joints are ideally structured to serve their function as the hinges of the skeletal system.*" Bones are firmly connected at the joint capsule by ligaments, tendons, and muscles. Within the joint space, three primary components, *articular cartilage*, *synovial membranes*, and *synovial fluid*, interact to provide a smooth gliding surface for joint flexion/rotation/extension and weight-bearing throughout the lifespan (Robbins &

Cotran, 1979). **FIGURE 47.1** depicts the cellular components of a typical synovial joint.

Again quoting Robbins and Cotran: "*the articular cartilage is a unique connective tissue which serves as an elastic shock absorber and wear-resistant, weight-bearing surface.*" Cartilage is devoid of nerves, lymphatics, and blood vessels, and does not normally undergo cell division. However, chondrocytes are present that sustain the continual turnover of cartilage by actively synthesizing its two essential components, collagen, and proteoglycans (Robbins & Cotran, 1979).

The *synovial membranes* line the joint capsule. These membranes consist of a single layer of phagocytic cells and secretory cells. The phagocytes guard

TABLE 47.1 Forms of Arthritis	
Type	**Relative Frequency (%)**
Osteoarthritis	80
Rheumatoid arthritis	10
Gouty arthritis	5
Ankylosing spondylitis	2
Juvenile arthritis	1
Suppurative arthritis	1
Other variants	1

CDC. (2011). *Arthritis*. Atlanta, Georgia: Centers for Disease Prevention and Control.

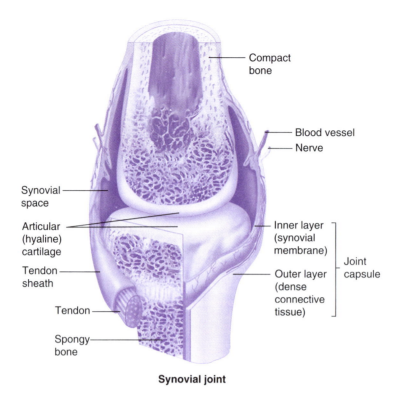

FIGURE 47.1 Normal Synovial Joint.
© Jones & Bartlett Learning.

the joint capsule against infection while the secretory cells actively produce and secrete *synovial fluid* into the joint space. Synovial fluid is a remarkably viscous substance that helps facilitate flexion of all joints as well as rotation of certain complex joints. Under normal conditions, the synovial fluid is sterile and does not contain lymphocytes or other immune cells. However, in arthritic conditions, the synovial fluid is often infiltrated by lymphocytes and other immune cells in association with chronic inflammation.

Pathogenesis of Arthritis

Regardless of etiology, the sine qua non of arthritis is inflammatory involvement of one or more synovial joints. At the molecular level, proinflammatory cytokines and mediators such as interleukin-1, tumor necrosis factor alpha, prostaglandins, leukotrienes, and nitric oxide interact to promote chronic inflammation and damage to the articular cartilage and other tissues of the joint capsule. Taking osteoarthritis as a prime example, the cumulative effects of mechanical stress and strain over many years eventually induce constitutive upregulation of key enzymes (cyclooxygenase, lipoxygenase, arginase, nitric oxide synthetase) and proinflammatory mediators (prostaglandins, leukotrienes, nitric oxide) conducive to chronic inflammation and arthritis in tissues of the joint capsule (Weinberg, Fermor, & Guilak, 2007).

Osteoarthritis (Degenerative Joint Disease)

The most common form of arthritis is *osteoarthritis.* This form is a slowly progressive disorder that typically manifests late in life. The condition principally afflicts the weight-bearing joints and is characterized clinically by pain, inflammation, deformity, and limitation of motion. Radiographic studies of afflicted joints reveal the presence of focal erosive lesions, cartilage destruction, subchondral sclerosis, cyst formation, and large osteophytes (bone spurs) at the joint margins (Mankin, 1974).

Osteoarthritis is often attributed to the "*wear and tear of aging*" and is thus referred to as *degenerative joint disease.* According to one theory of pathogenesis, weight-bearing joints or joints subjected to sustained repetitive trauma undergo focal cartilaginous erosion and osteolytic changes that over time extend and produce widespread damage to the articular cartilage. Such damage heightens friction and resistance to motion in the joint thereby inducing chronic inflammation which exacerbates the progression of disease. There is also a marked increase in the rate of collagen synthesis in arthritic joints compared to nonarthritic joints. However, newly formed cartilage is more prone to injury and damage, which also favors disease progression. Some investigators therefore suggest that the pathogenesis of osteoarthritis is best defined as a failure of repair processes to keep pace with joint damage from chronic excessive mechanical stress (Brandt, Dieppe, & Radin, 2009).

▶ Diagnosis of Osteoarthritis

The most widely using classification schemes for osteoarthritis are based on the radiological appearance of the joint. The radiological hallmarks are joint space narrowing, sclerosis, and formation of bone spurs and cysts. Severity is graded based on a 0–4 scale (Kellgren, 1962; Kellgren & Lawrence, 1958). Based solely on radiographic findings, osteoarthritis is classified as:

0–absent, 1–doubtful, 2–minimal, 3–moderate, and 4–severe. Joints of the hips, knees, spine, thumbs, and fingers are most often affected by osteoarthritis.

▶ Age-Specific Incidence and Prevalence of Osteoarthritis

Osteoarthritis is a disease of the aging process. As shown in **FIGURE 47.2**, age-specific annual *incidence rates* estimated for American men and women increase exponentially from middle age and peak after 70 years of age (Oliveria, Felson, Reed, Cirillo, & Walker, 1995).

Age-specific annual *prevalence rates* of osteoarthritis of the knee estimated from surveys of European men and women are shown in **FIGURE 47.3**. Remarkably, after 80 years of age, the annual rates exceed 32,000 per 100,000 in women and approach

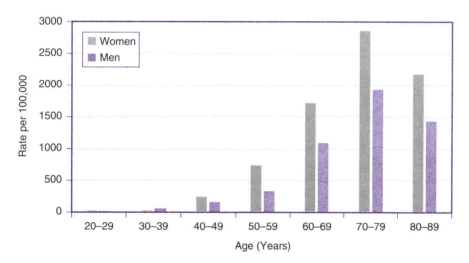

FIGURE 47.2 Age-Specific Incidence of Osteoarthritis.

Data from Oliveria, S. A., Felson, D. T., Reed, J. I., Cirillo, P. A., & Walker, A. M. (1995). Incidence of symptomatic hand, hip, and knee osteoarthritis among patients in a health maintenance organization. *Arthritis & Rheumatism, 47*(8), 1134–1141.

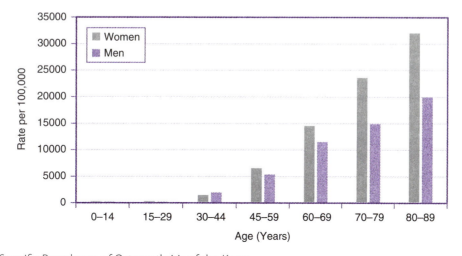

FIGURE 47.3 Age-Specific Prevalence of Osteoarthritis of the Knee.

Data from Symmons, D., Mathers, C., & Pfleger, B. (2006a). Global burden of osteoarthritis in the year 2000. In C. D. Mathers et al. (Eds.), *Global burden of disease 2000*. Geneva, Switzerland: World Health Organization.

20,000 per 100,000 in men. It is notable that the age-specific prevalence rates of knee osteoarthritis for women exceed corresponding rates for men by 50%–60% after about 55 years of age. In contrast to the striking gender difference in the prevalence of *knee osteoarthritis*, the corresponding prevalence rates of *hip osteoarthritis* are only slightly higher in women compared to men (Symmons, Mathers, & Pfleger, 2006a). Surveys of U.S. adults have yielded similar findings. Based on prevalence data from the Third National Health and Nutrition Examination Survey (NHANES III), among adults over 60 years of age, 42% of women had *knee osteoarthritis* compared to 31% of men, whereas the prevalence of *hip osteoarthritis* in women barely exceeded that in men (27% vs. 26%) (Lawrence et al., 2008).

▶ Disability in Osteoarthritis

While osteoarthritis per se is not a life-threatening disease, it is the leading cause of disability in many populations of the world, particularly those with greater longevity. Worldwide, osteoarthritis was responsible for approximately 10.8 million years of life lost due to disability (YLD) in 1990, 16.8 million YLD in 2006 and 22.4 million in 2016, an increase of approximately 4% per year and a doubling of YLD from osteoarthritis during the entire 26-year period. Overall, osteoarthritis accounts for about 3% of the total YLD and ranks 11th among all causes. During 2010, the global age-standardized prevalence of osteoarthritis of the knee or hip was 4.7% (3.8% for the knee and 0.9% for the hip) and the YLD were about 60% higher in women (290 per 100,000) than in men (180 per 100,000) (Cross, Smith, Hoy, Nolte, et al., 2014; Hay & GBD 2016 DALY and HALE Collaborators, 2016; Murray et al., 2012; Symmons et al., 2006a).

The global pattern of *disability-adjusted life years (DALY)* lost due to osteoarthritis is shown in **FIGURE 47.4**. Recall that *DALY = YLL + YLD* where *YLL = years of life lost due to premature death* and *YLD = years of life lost due to disability*. The DALY for osteoarthritis reflect YLD with little contribution from years of life lost from premature death (YLL) since only rarely are deaths are attributed to osteoarthritis. During 1990–2010, the DALY due to osteoarthritis of the knee or hip increased from 0.42% to 0.69% of the total DALY, ranking 38th among all causes. The highest DALY occurred in populations without access to adequate treatment such as Russia, China, and sub-Saharan Africa (Cross, Smith, Hoy, Nolte, et al., 2014; WHO, 2009).

▶ Trends in Osteoarthritis Prevalence

Since the incidence and prevalence rates of osteoarthritis increase dramatically with age, the extended life expectancy of many populations around the globe will undoubtedly result in greater numbers of patients with this condition. But an even more disturbing

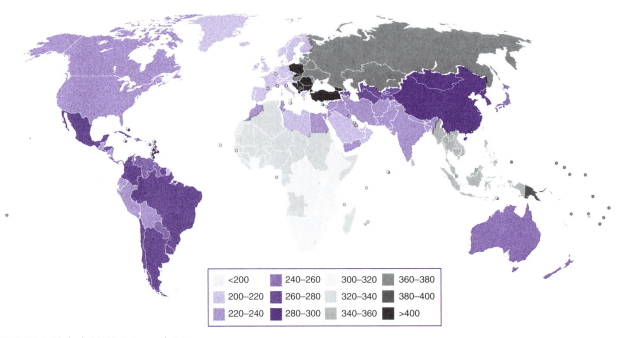

<200	240–260	300–320	360–380
200–220	260–280	320–340	380–400
220–240	280–300	340–360	>400

FIGURE 47.4 Global DALY: Osteoarthritis.

Data from World Health Organization. (2008). *The global burden of disease: 2004 update*. Geneva: WHO. Available at www.who.int/evidence/bod

Disability Adjusted Life Years per 100,000 individuals.

relationship that will undoubtedly amplify the global burden of osteoarthritis is its etiologic link with obesity. Indeed, the number of afflicted adults in the United States population increased nearly 30% during 1995–2005 (27 million in 2005 vs. 21 million in 1995) concurrent with the obesity epidemic that has plagued the nation (Lawrence et al., 2008). Since osteoarthritis is an irreversible, progressive, and often disabling condition, this trend is expected to produce a corresponding increase in the years of productive life lost to disability.

Based upon a recent analysis of the National Health Interview Survey (NHIS) for 2007–2009, 49.9 million U.S. adults currently have *self-reported physician-diagnosed arthritis* (osteoarthritis, rheumatoid arthritis, gout, lupus, or fibromyalgia) and 21.1 million have *arthritis-attributable activity limitation*. Results suggest that the number of cases is increasing by nearly 1 million per year in the U.S. population and that the prevalence is highest among obese individuals (33.8% in obese women 25.2% in obese men) (CDC, 2011; Cheng, Hootman, Murphy, Langmaid, & Helmick, 2010).

Risk Factors for Osteoarthritis

Aside from aging, the major risk factors for the development of osteoarthritis include being female (after age 55 years), being overweight or obese, and previous major trauma or sustained repetitive trauma to specific joints. Positive family history also appears to increase the risk. As discussed in the following paragraphs, there is some evidence suggesting an etiologic link between diabetes and osteoarthritis, and a possible protective effect of smoking. However, the evidence supporting these associations is equivocal.

Obesity and Osteoarthritis

In an analysis of cross-sectional data from the first United States National Health and Nutrition Examination Survey of 1971–1975 (NHANES I), Jennifer Anderson and David Felson examined associations of a variety of putative risk factors with osteoarthritis of the knee. A total of 5193 adults, aged 35–74 years, 315 of whom had osteoarthritis of the knee diagnosed by radiography contributed data for analysis. After controlling for confounders, the investigators found a significant dose response in the risk of knee osteoarthritis with increasing body mass in both men and women (**FIGURE 47.5**). The risk increased more than fourfold among obese men (OR = 4.78) and more than sevenfold among women with gravid obesity (OR = 7.37). Results also revealed an increase in the risk associated with occupational knee bending demands (OR = 2.45) and an excess of osteoarthritis among African-American women (OR = 2.12). Based on these findings, the authors suggested that obesity is a causative factor in the genesis of osteoarthritis of the knee (Anderson & Felson, 1988).

Maradee Davis and colleagues also used the NHANES I data to examine the association of obesity and osteoarthritis of the knee. They compared 75 subjects with *unilateral* osteoarthritis and 226 subjects with *bilateral* disease to 3584 normal subjects. Radiologic studies of each subject were used to define the presence of osteoarthritis (grades 2–4). Obesity was defined as body mass index (BMI) of 30 or higher. Results revealed that obesity increased the risk of *bilateral* knee osteoarthritis (adjusted OR = 7.92) and to a lesser extent, *unilateral* knee osteoarthritis (adjusted OR = 3.45). Controlling for age, gender, serum cholesterol, serum uric acid, body fat distribution, bone

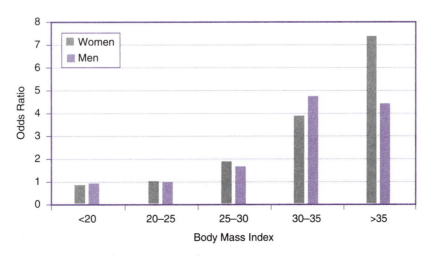

FIGURE 47.5 Risk of Knee Osteoarthritis with Increasing Body Mass.

Data from Anderson, J. J., & Felson, D. T. (1988). Factors associated with osteoarthritis of the knee in the first National Health and Nutrition Examination Survey (HANES I). Evidence for an association with overweight, race, and physical demands of work. *American Journal of Epidemiology 128*(1), 179–189.

density, and blood pressure did not diminish these effects, suggesting a lack of influence of these factors in modulating the osteoarthritis risk attributable to obesity (Davis, Ettinger, & Neuhaus, 1990).

In additional studies of the NHANES I database, Davis and colleagues found associations between obesity and osteoarthritis of joints of the hands and feet, and they also determined that prior knee injury was a strong independent risk factor for unilateral osteoarthritis (OR = 16.3 and OR = 10.9 for injury to the right and left knee, respectively). However, they *did not* find significant differences between men and women in the strength of the associations of obesity with osteoarthritis. As a consequence, they suggest the need to examine other factors such as reproductive history, endogenous estrogens, and anthropometric measures in order to identify factors that heighten the osteoarthritis risk in women compared to men (Davis, Ettinger, Neuhaus, Cho, & Hauck, 1989; Davis, Ettinger, Neuhaus, & Hauck, 1988; Davis, Neuhaus, Ettinger, & Muller, 1990).

Trauma and Osteoarthritis

Blagojevic and colleagues conducted an extensive review and meta-analysis of studies of risk factors for osteoarthritis of the knee in older adults. Of 2233 published studies screened, 85 were selected for inclusion in the analysis based on quality and inclusion of risk estimates with confidence intervals. Data were abstracted from 42 cohort studies and 43 case–control studies. The results revealed that previous knee trauma (pooled OR = 3.86), obesity (pooled OR = 2.63), presence of Heberden's nodes (pooled OR = 1.49), and female gender (pooled OR = 1.84) were the strongest risk factors. Some studies also found evidence of increased risk with regular strenuous exercise, history of high physical workload, certain repetitive physical activities (kneeling and squatting), and increased bone mineral density. Smoking was examined in 18 studies (8 case–control studies and 10 cohort studies) and the combined data across all studies suggested a small protective effect (pooled OR = 0.84). However, the risk reduction was only evident in case–control studies (OR = 0.60) and not cohort studies (OR = 0.97). The authors suggest that easily identifiable risk factors such as obesity, knee injury, and nodal hand osteoarthritis can be targeted for prevention of disabling knee osteoarthritis (Blagojevic, Jinks, Jeffery, & Jordan, 2010).

Type 2 Diabetes Mellitus and Osteoarthritis

Wain and colleagues initially suggested a relationship between diabetes and osteoarthritis based upon a small study of 30 patients with diabetes and 30 matched controls (Waine, Nevinny, & Rosenthal, 1961). Subsequent studies have been conducted to examine the relationship, some finding significant associations and others not.

Engstrom and colleagues recently examined a Swedish cohort of 5171 elderly adults to quantify associations between lifestyle habits, body mass, blood pressure, HDL cholesterol, triglycerides, glucose, and C-reactive protein (CRP), and the risk of developing osteoarthritis. Baseline data were collected during 1991–1994. A total of 120 subjects developed severe hip osteoarthritis and 89 developed knee osteoarthritis during 12 years of follow-up. The presence of the *metabolic syndrome* (disease complex of type 2 diabetes, obesity, and high blood pressure) significantly increased the risk of knee osteoarthritis (RR = 2.1) but the risk was attenuated by adjustment for obesity (RR = 1.1). Elevated CRP was associated with a significant increase in the risk of knee osteoarthritis in women, but again, adjustment for other factors attenuated the effect. The investigators concluded that these associations were largely attributable to confounding (Engstrom, de Verdier, Rollof, Nilsson, & Lohmander, 2008).

Francis Berenbaum of the Pierre and Marie Curie University in Paris recently reviewed the observational and experimental evidence supporting an association between diabetes and the development of osteoarthritis. Based upon a *"positive signal"* from the available data, Dr. Berenbaum proposes a general paradigm whereby *advanced glycosylation end products (AGEs)* and *reactive oxygen species (ROS)* in patients with hyperglycemia incite chondrocyte and synovial reactivity leading to osteoarthritis (Berenbaum, 2010). Nevertheless, it is important to note that obesity is a major risk factor for both diabetes and osteoarthritis, and meaningful estimates of independent effects of hyperglycemia must therefore be carefully adjusted for measures of body mass. Clearly, additional studies are needed to clarify whether there is an etiologic link between hyperglycemia and the development of osteoarthritis.

Genetics of Osteoarthritis

Involvement of the distal interphalangeal joints of the fingers in osteoarthritis is often marked by the presence of distinct sclerotic nodules called *Heberden's nodes*. These nodes are more likely to develop in females with osteoarthritis than males; and furthermore, early studies of familial osteoarthritis suggested that genetic factors may predispose to their development (Kellgren, Lawrence, & Bier, 1963; Lawrence &

Moore, 1952; Stecher, 1941). Additional evidence supporting a role for genetic factors in the development of osteoarthritis came from a study of twins which revealed that the concordance for nodal osteoarthritis in monozygous twins was approximately double that in dizygous twins (Lawrence, 1977).

Other studies have linked Heberden's nodes in osteoarthritis to specific haplotypes of the *human leukocyte antigen (HLA)* system (Ercilla et al., 1977; Pattrick, Manhire, Ward, & Doherty, 1989), and studies of afflicted twins and siblings have revealed a number of genetic polymorphisms and point mutations associated with defective collagen biosynthesis and repair that may predispose to the development of osteoarthritis (Williams & Jimenez, 1995). In addition, as pointed out by Holderbaum and colleagues in their review of the genetics of osteoarthritis, "*mutations in genes coding for cartilage components other than collagen, or for control factors such as enzymes, inhibitors, and signal transduction mediators may lead to similar clinical end points*" (Holderbaum, Haqqi, & Moskowitz, 1999).

Smoking and Osteoarthritis

To determine if smoking protects against the development of osteoarthritis, Hui and colleagues conducted a review of the literature and meta-analysis of published observational studies with relevant data. They identified 48 studies involving 537,730 subjects for analysis: 8 cohort studies, 21 cross-sectional studies, and 19 case–control studies. Overall, results revealed a small protective effect of smoking (OR = 0.87). However, the effect was stronger in hospital-based case–control studies (OR = 0.65) than community-based case–control studies (OR = 0.90), cohort studies (OR = 0.92) or cross-sectional studies (OR = 0.89). The investigators suggest that the observed protective effect of smoking in hospital-based case–control studies may be due to selection bias of hospital controls with smoking-related conditions (Hui, Doherty, & Zhang, 2011).

▶ Prevention of Osteoarthritis

Major global efforts have been initiated to reduce the burden of osteoarthritis and other forms of arthritis. Programs include the *U.S. National Arthritis Plan*, the *European League Against Rheumatism (EULAR)*, and the *International League of Associations for Rheumatology (ILAR)*. Furthermore, during 2000–2010, the World Health Organization launched the *Monitor Project of the Bone and Joint Decade* to better quantify the global burden of musculoskeletal disorders such as osteoarthritis and develop strategies for their

prevention (Khaltaev et al., 2003). Education is key to self-management and prevention. Notably, the Internet has become a significant tool used by advocates to inform and mobilize grassroots attention to effect change in behavior and lifestyle (Leong & Euller-Ziegler, 2004). Active prevention of arthritic conditions obviously targets those risk factors that contribute to joint damage: obesity, excessive repetitive stress and strain to the joints, lack of aerobic exercise, dehydration, and poor nutrition. Maintenance of ideal weight, avoidance of repetitive joint trauma, regular aerobic exercise, generous water intake, and good nutrition with sufficient calcium, phosphorous, and vitamin D are essential components of a preventive strategy.

Tertiary Prevention of Osteoarthritis Sequela

The underlying disease process of osteoarthritis has thus far proven to be irreversible. Nevertheless, some evidence has accrued suggesting that weight reduction, regular nontraumatic aerobic exercise (e.g., swimming, bike riding), and sustained use of analgesics such as aspirin, ibuprofen, or acetaminophen may effectively arrest disease progression (Brandt & Flusser, 1991).

Clinical Trials of Glucosamine and Chondroitin

In recent years, formulations of glucosamine and chondroitin have been marketed as effective therapeutic agents for patients with osteoarthritis. Recently, a team of European investigators conducted a comprehensive review and meta-analysis of the available data from randomized clinical trials of these agents to determine their therapeutic efficacy in reducing joint pain and progression of osteoarthritis of the hip or knee. Ten large-scale randomized controlled clinical trials that compared glucosamine, chondroitin, or their combination with placebo were included in the investigation. Each trial enrolled at least 200 patients with osteoarthritis of the hip or knee, a total of 3803 patients overall. The results revealed *no significant differences* in either pain relief or disease progression between patients receiving active treatment versus placebo. The investigators concluded that compared with placebo, glucosamine, and chondroitin, used either separately or in combination, do not reduce joint pain or produce beneficial changes in the joints of patients with osteoarthritis. They also suggest that prescribing these compounds to patients who have not received treatment should be discouraged (Wandel et al., 2010).

Clinical Trials of Weight Reduction

Investigators in Denmark conducted a meta-analysis of randomized clinical trials designed to assess changes in pain and function achieved by weight loss in overweight patients with knee osteoarthritis. Four trials involving 454 patients were included in the study. Results revealed significant reductions in pain (OR = 0.20) and disability (OR = 0.23) associated with an average weight reduction of 6.1 kg. The investigators concluded that disability could be significantly improved with a 5.1% reduction in weight from baseline which was achievable within a 20-week period (Christensen, Bartels, Astrup, & Bliddal, 2007).

Joint Replacement

It is also important to note that relief of osteoarthritic symptoms may be achieved by arthroplasty or joint replacement surgery. As pointed out by Symmons and colleagues in their review of the global burden of osteoarthritis: "*total joint replacement is a highly cost effective operation for severe osteoarthritis and provides good pain relief and improvement in mobility and quality of life in the majority of patients in the United States*" (Symmons et al., 2006a).

▶ Rheumatoid Arthritis

Rheumatoid arthritis is a systemic inflammatory auto-immune disease that affects multiple synovial joints in a symmetrical pattern. The disease is thus succinctly characterized as *symmetrical inflammatory polyarthritis*. The inflammatory process induces excessive proliferation of connective tissue cells that form a "*pannus*" of hyperplastic cells within the joint capsule. Eventually, these cells invade and erode the articular cartilage causing deformities and destruction of the joint and loss of function. The condition usually begins in the small joints of the hands and feet and then progresses to the larger joints. Extra-articular features are commonly found in patients with rheumatoid arthritis including rheumatoid skin nodules, vasculitis, pericarditis, pulmonary fibrosis, and peripheral amyloidosis (Robbins & Cotran, 1979; Symmons, Mathers, & Pfleger, 2006b).

Pathogenesis of Rheumatoid Arthritis

In their textbook, *Pathogenesis of Disease*, Robbins and Cotran state that "*virtually all patients with classic rheumatoid arthritis have rheumatoid factor in their sera.*" Rheumatoid factor is an autoantibody that binds to other immunoglobulins (IgG and IgM) to form immune complexes. According to one model of the pathogenesis of rheumatoid arthritis, these complexes attack specific antigenic targets within the joint space leading to complement activation and release of lysosomal enzymes by macrophages and other immune cells. This destructive cascade produces irreparable damage to the joint cartilage (Robbins & Cotran, 1979).

Diagnosis of Rheumatoid Arthritis

Rheumatoid arthritis is diagnosed by the presence of a sufficient number of characteristic signs and symptoms including morning stiffness, joint pain and tenderness, symmetrical soft tissue swelling of joints, subcutaneous nodules, radiographic changes in joints, and positive rheumatoid factor. *Classical rheumatoid arthritis* is defined when all criteria are positive (Arnett et al., 1988; Ropes, Bennet, Cobb, Jacox, & Jessar, 1958).

Incidence and Prevalence of Rheumatoid Arthritis

Investigators at the Mayo Clinic estimated the age-specific incidence of rheumatoid arthritis among adults living in Rochester, Minnesota, and followed during 1955–1994. During this time period, 609 Rochester residents (445 women and 164 men) fulfilled the 1987 American College of Radiology criteria for the diagnosis of rheumatoid arthritis. As depicted in **FIGURE 47.6**, the age-specific incidence curves differ dramatically by gender. In women, rates begin to rise during late adolescence peaking at 116 cases per 100,000 during ages 55–64 years after which they remain high until age 85. In contrast, rates in men rise steadily after about age 30 peaking at 102 cases per 100,000 during ages 75–84 years. Across the entire lifespan, the incidence in women is approximately twice that in men (Doran, Pond, Crowson, O'Fallon, & Gabriel, 2002; Gabriel, Crowson, & O'Fallon, 1999). Similar age-specific incidence patterns have been reported for men and women in Great Britain (Symmons et al., 2006b, 2002).

Age-specific prevalence rates estimated from combined surveys of European populations are shown in **FIGURE 47.7**. Based on these estimates, after the age of 65 years, approximately 3% of women have rheumatoid arthritis compared to 1.5% of men (Symmons et al., 2006b, 2002).

▶ Disability in Rheumatoid Arthritis

Rheumatoid arthritis initially causes erosion of the cartilage of synovial joints. Without treatment, there is inevitable progression of the process to contiguous

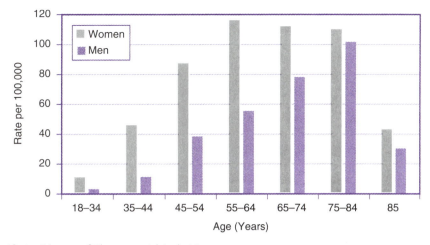

FIGURE 47.6 Age-Specific Incidence of Rheumatoid Arthritis.

Data from Gabriel, S. E., Crowson, C. S., & O'Fallon, W. M. (1999). The epidemiology of rheumatoid arthritis in Rochester, Minnesota, 1955–1985. *Arthritis & Rheumatism 42*(3), 415–420.

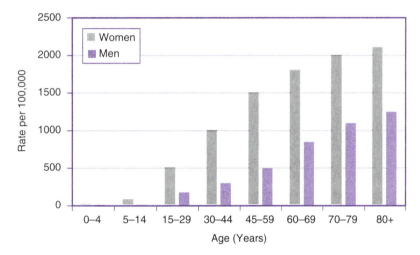

FIGURE 47.7 Age-Specific Prevalence of Rheumatoid Arthritis.

Data from Symmons, D., Mathers, C., & Pfleger, B. (2006b). Global burden of rheumatoid arthritis in the year 2000. In C. D. Mathers et al. (Eds.), *Global burden of disease 2000*. Geneva, Switzerland: World Health Organization.

bone which eventually results in destruction and deformity of the joints and severe disability. Furthermore, rheumatoid arthritis is clearly associated with several conditions that cause premature death such as end stage kidney disease and cardiovascular disease. The excess deaths among patients with rheumatoid arthritis have been attributed to its extra-articular manifestations presumably arising from circulating autoimmune complexes and/or the cumulative inflammatory burden of the disease.

DALY due to rheumatoid arthritis have increased over time. Worldwide, rheumatoid arthritis was responsible for approximately 3.3 million years of DALY lost in 1990, 4.4 million in 2006, 4.8 million in 2010, and 5.6 million in 2016, an increase of approximately 2.6% per year and 67% during the entire 26-year period. However, with adjustment for aging and growth of the world population, the YLD increased by only 14% during 1990–2010, from 48 per 100,000 in 1990 to 55 per 100,000 in 2010. The YLD

were approximately four times higher in women (89 per 100,000) than men (22 per 100,000). The global annual prevalence of rheumatoid arthritis was stable during 1990–2010 at about 0.25%. The average annual prevalence in women was 2.7 times higher than men (0.35% versus 0.13%). It is likely that the observed increases in DALY and YDL were primarily due to aging and growth of the world population (Cross, Smith, Hoy, Carmona, et al., 2014).

The global pattern of DALY due to rheumatoid arthritis is shown in **FIGURE 47.8**. The DALY are highest in nations of the Russian Federation, Eastern Europe, and Central and South America. However, it should be recognized that the estimates for these regions (as well as most other developing nations) are based upon scanty data and further investigations and surveys are needed to improve our understanding of intra- and inter-regional variability in morbidity and mortality rates from rheumatoid arthritis (Symmons et al., 2006b).

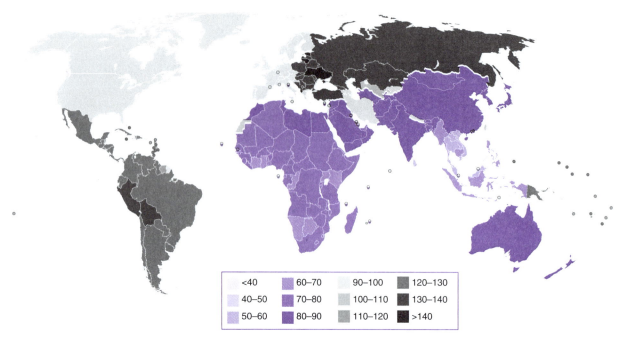

FIGURE 47.8 Global DALY: Rheumatoid Arthritis.

Data from World Health Organization. (2008). *The global burden of disease: 2004 update*. Geneva: WHO. Available at www.who.int/evidence/bod

Disability Adjusted Life Years per 100,000 individuals.

Time Trends in Rheumatoid Arthritis: Morbidity and Mortality

Population surveys of member nations of the World Health Organization in 1990 and 2000 suggest that both morbidity and mortality attributable to rheumatoid arthritis are increasing. During this period, YLD from rheumatoid arthritis increased from 3.2 to 4.5 million and YLL increased from 118,000 to 148,000 (Symmons et al., 2006b). These increases occurred in parallel with the *epidemiologic transition* in which the global burden of chronic diseases has surpassed infectious and parasitic conditions. Notably, several debilitating and life-threatening chronic diseases frequently occur in patients with rheumatoid arthritis.

A study of patients treated at the Mayo Clinic in the United States reported *no improvement* in mortality from rheumatoid arthritis over the last four decades (Doran et al., 2002). A cohort study of 1049 patients in the Netherlands also failed to reveal any improvement in survival. In fact, the mortality rate among these subjects was 40% higher than in the general population. A total of 207 patients died during up to 23 years of follow-up and excess mortality emerged at about 10 years after diagnosis. The leading causes of death were cardiovascular disease, cancer, infection, and respiratory disease. Significant baseline predictors of mortality included gender (male), early age at diagnosis, rheumatoid factor, disability, and comorbidity. The investigators advocate better disease control in all age groups and suggest that

comorbid conditions be treated more aggressively to help improve survival of patients with rheumatoid arthritis (Radovits et al., 2010).

In the 2010 Global Burden of Disease Study of rheumatoid arthritis, the global age-standardized annual mortality due to rheumatoid arthritis (0.80 per 100,000) decreased by approximately 10% during 1990–2010. Nevertheless, there was considerable uncertainty regarding mortality estimates, and the investigators suggest the need for further research to assess the impact of newer therapeutic approaches for rheumatoid arthritis (Cross, Smith, Hoy, Carmona, et al., 2014).

Risk Factors for Rheumatoid Arthritis

Only a few risk factors have been clearly identified in the development of rheumatoid arthritis. Multiple studies suggest that genetic factors are extremely important, and as with other autoimmune conditions, being female carries an approximate twofold increase in the risk compared to being male. The available evidence also suggests that smoking increases the risk in both men and women, whereas use of the oral contraceptive pill appears to reduce the risk in women.

Genetics of Rheumatoid Arthritis

There is substantial evidence to suggest that genetic factors contribute significantly to the etiopathogenesis of rheumatoid arthritis. Concordance rates for rheumatoid arthritis are fourfold higher in monozygous twins (12%–15%) than dizygous twins (3%–4%) and the rates among full siblings of probands (index cases) are higher than expected (Aho, Markku, Tuiminen, & Kaprio, 1986; Silman et al., 1993).

The association between rheumatoid arthritis and HLA-DR4 was first demonstrated more than 30 years ago (Statsny, 1978), and it was soon discovered that several genes that determine susceptibility to rheumatoid arthritis reside in the HLA region of chromosome 6 (Deighton, Walker, Griffiths, & Roberts, 1989). It has now been determined that specific "shared epitopes" encoded by certain class II HLA alleles may interact with pathogenic microbes such as Epstein–Barr virus to incite the autoimmune reactions of rheumatoid arthritis (Gregerson, Silver, & Winchester, 1987; Ollier & MacGregor, 1995; Weyand, Hicok, Conn, & Goronzy, 1992). Nevertheless, other genes are likely to be involved and genome-wide association studies of afflicted relatives are now being conducted to identify them (Symmons & Harrison, 2000).

Female Hormones and Rheumatoid Arthritis

As shown in Figures 47.6 and 47.7, the incidence and prevalence rates of rheumatoid arthritis in women are more than double the rates in men. The excess female risk is most apparent during the premenopausal years and then dissipates slightly in old age. One interpretation of this biological phenomenon is that reproductive hormones are responsible; perhaps estrogen heightens the risk in women and androgen lessens the risk in men. Two findings appear to counter this viewpoint: (1) premenopausal women who take the oral contraceptive pill (a combination of estrogen and progestin) appear to have a *reduced* risk of later developing progressive disease, and (2) postmenopausal hormone replacement therapy has *not* been found to influence either the development or the progression of rheumatoid arthritis.

Oral Contraceptives and Rheumatoid Arthritis

Some epidemiologic studies have reported that premenopausal women who take oral contraceptives have a reduced risk of later developing rheumatoid arthritis. Nevertheless, findings differ from study to study. Spector and Hochberg therefore undertook a review of the published studies and performed a meta-analysis of the data. Their analysis included data from nine independent studies, six case–control studies, and three cohort studies. The overall pooled odds ratio across studies (OR = 0.73) suggested a protective effect; however, studies of hospital cases yielded a stronger effect (OR = 0.49) than studies of population-based cases (OR = 0.95). One interpretation of these results is that the oral contraceptive pill may not have a protective effect against the development of rheumatoid arthritis but rather may prevent progression to severe disease (Spector & Hochberg, 1990).

It is of further interest that longitudinal studies of populations in Great Britain, Finland, and the United States suggest that the incidence rates of rheumatoid arthritis declined significantly during the last half of the 20th century (Abdel-Nasser, Rasker, & Valkenburg, 1997; Doran et al., 2002; Helmick et al., 2008; Hochberg, 1990; Kaipiainen-Seppänen, Aho, Isomäki, & Laakso, 1996; Linos, Worthington, O'Fallon, & Kurland, 1980; Silman, 1988). For example, in a prospective cohort study of residents of Olmstead County, Minnesota, the age-adjusted incidence rates estimated for successive 10-year intervals during the 40-year period, 1955–1994 *decreased* by 52% in women and 30% in men (**FIGURE 47.9**). Interestingly,

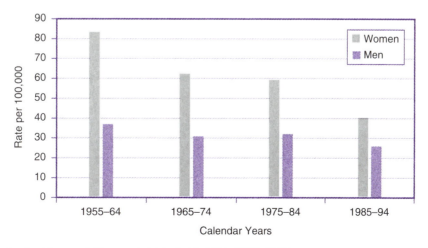

FIGURE 47.9 Trends in the Incidence of Rheumatoid Arthritis, USA, 1955–2007.

Data from Doran, M. F., Pond, G. R., Crowson, C. S., O'Fallon, W. M., & Gabriel, S. E. (2002). Trends in incidence and mortality in rheumatoid arthritis in Rochester, Minnesota, over a forty-year period. *Arthritis & Rheumatism 46*(3), 625–631; Myasoedova, E., Crowson, C. S., Kremers, H. M., Therneau, T. M., & Gabriel, S. E. (2010). Is the incidence of rheumatoid arthritis rising? Results from Olmsted County, Minnesota, 1955–2007. *Arthritis Rheum, 62*(6), 1576–1582.

the steeper decline in women coincides with the introduction and widespread use of the oral contraceptive pill which began in about 1960 (Doran et al., 2002).

In a subsequent study of rheumatoid arthritis in an augmented cohort of 466 men and women from Olmstead County, Minnesota, estimates of the age-adjusted annual incidence of rheumatoid arthritis were obtained for men and women during 1995–2007. The annual rate for this period was 53.1 per 100,000 in women and 27.7 per 100,000 in men, suggesting there was an upward swing in the rates for women but not for men. As shown in Figure 47.9, the observed increase in women during 1995–2007 followed a sharp decline in the incidence of rheumatoid arthritis over the previous four decades. The investigators speculate that the rising incidence in women may be due to attenuated protection from oral contraceptives since newer agents have lower doses of synthetic estrogens than those used in past years (Myasoedova, Crowson, Kremers, Therneau, & Gabriel, 2010).

Hormone Replacement Therapy and Rheumatoid Arthritis

The Women's Health Initiative (WHI) randomized controlled trials conducted in the United States evaluated the effects of postmenopausal hormone replacement (estrogen alone and estrogen + progestin) compared with placebo on the development and progression of rheumatoid arthritis. Among 27,347 participants, 63 prevalent cases and 105 incidence cases of rheumatoid arthritis were identified during 7.1 years and 5.6 years of follow-up in the two trials. No statistically significant differences were detected in the risk of developing rheumatoid arthritis or the severity of rheumatoid arthritis between the postmenopausal hormone treatment groups and placebo (Walitt et al., 2008).

Female Gender and Rheumatoid Arthritis

An alternative hypothesis that has been advanced to explain the female excess of autoimmune conditions such as rheumatoid arthritis compared to men is the mosaic nature of the active X chromosome in the female genotype. According to the Lyon hypothesis, as cell lineages develop during embryogenesis, either the maternal X or the paternal X remains active and the reciprocal X is inactivated and becomes a Barr body. In theory, if the X activation/inactivation process is a random event, then 50% of cell lineages would be expected to have an active paternal X and 50% an active maternal X. However, if the X activation/inactivation process is skewed so that one X is preferentially activated in cells of the immune system, the ability of the immune system to recognize self may be compromised thus leading to autoimmune reactivity (Mignon, 2006).

Smoking and Rheumatoid Arthritis

Smoking has been examined as a risk factor for rheumatoid arthritis in a number of epidemiologic investigations. To assess the strength and consistency of the association in men and women, a team of Japanese investigators conducted a meta-analysis of available data from published reports. Sixteen studies were included in the analysis, 11 case–control studies and 5 cohort studies. The case–control studies included 4764 cases and 13,647 controls, and the cohort studies identified 9121 cases from among 566,044 participants. The summary odds ratios for 20 or more pack-years of smoking clearly indicated that smoking was a risk factor in both men (OR = 2.31) and women (OR = 1.75). Estimates were similar for case–control and cohort studies. Interestingly, the presence of rheumatoid factor appeared to strengthen the effect of smoking in men but not in women. These results suggest that heavy smokers, whether male or female, have an approximate twofold increase in the risk of developing rheumatoid arthritis. The investigators speculate that smoking may increase the risk by accentuating the dysfunction of T lymphocytes (Sugiyama et al., 2010).

Prevention and Control of Rheumatoid Arthritis

Other than avoidance of smoking, there are no methods that have been clearly shown to reduce the risk of developing rheumatoid arthritis. Early diagnosis and initiation of therapy is imperative in preventing disease progression and limiting disability. Nonsteroidal anti-inflammatory drugs show benefit in reducing pain and inflammation, steroids (prednisone) offer symptomatic relief, and methotrexate, sulfasalazine, and/or injectable gold, and new agents directed against inflammatory cytokines may slow disease progression. In addition to drug therapy, orthopedic surgery may be of benefit for patients with severe disabling deformities (Symmons et al., 2006b).

▸ Gout

Gout is characterized by "*transient but recurrent attacks of acute arthritis evoked by the precipitation of monosodium uric acid crystals from supersaturated body fluids*" (Robbins & Cotran, 1979). The classic form of gout predominantly affects joints of the great toe (85% of patients) but other joints may also become involved (ankles, heels, knees, wrists, fingers, and elbows). With progression, there is destruction of articular cartilage and subchondral bone leading to chronic disabling arthritis.

The Dutch scientist Antonie van Leeuwenhoek, known as "*the father of microbiology*," first described the microscopic appearance of urate crystals in 1679 (Pillinger, Rosenthal, & Abeles, 2007). In 1848 the English physician Alfred Baring Garrod recognized that excess uric acid in the blood was the cause of gout (Storey, 2001).

The pathognomonic microscopic lesion of gout is called a tophus, a periarticular mass of urate crystals surrounded by fibroblasts admixed with macrophages, lymphocytes, and foreign body giant cells. Uric acid crystals frequently produce damage to the kidneys and occasionally cause the development of uric acid kidney stones. Patients with gout also commonly manifest hypertension, hypertriglyceridemia, hyperlipidemia, and hyperglycemia (Robbins & Cotran, 1979).

Uric Acid Metabolism and Gout

The development of gout is preceded by chronic hyperuricemia due to overproduction and/or increased retention of uric acid. Hyperuricemia arises from retention due to dysfunction in renal uric acid excretion in about 90% of cases, and overproduction of uric acid in the remaining 10% of cases. Overproduction of uric acid can be caused by enzymatic defects in uric acid synthesis and degradation, excess intake of purines and other substrates of uric acid, and/or excess intake of alcohol or other drugs that heighten uric acid synthesis and/or interfere with renal clearance. Disorders that cause excessive cell destruction

and release of nucleic acids and purines into the bloodstream can also produce hyperuricemia. Serum uric acid levels exceeding 7 mg per dL are highly conducive to the precipitation of uric acid crystals in bodily fluids and tissues, particularly in the synovial fluid (Klinenberg, 1977).

Recently, investigators at Boston University examined the gender-specific relationship between serum uric acid and the incidence of gout among 2476 women and 1951 men who were followed for up to 52 years as a component of the Framingham Heart Study. A total of 304 incident cases of gout were detected in the study, 104 in women and 200 in men. Notably, the risk of gout begins to increase at a threshold level of about 5 mg per dL and increases exponentially in both men and women. However, the risk estimates for women are about 50% less than men for each incremental increase in serum uric acid (**FIGURE 47.10**). In multivariate analyses, several comorbid conditions were also found to independently increase the risk including obesity (RR = 2.74), alcohol intake exceeding one drink daily (RR = 3.10), hypertension (RR = 1.82), and diuretic use (RR = 2.39). The risk also increased with increasing age (RR = 1.24 per 5 years). The investigators concluded that "*higher levels of serum uric acid increase the risk of gout in a graded manner among women, but the rate of increase is lower than that among men*" (Bhole, de Vera, Rahman, Krishnan, & Choi, 2010).

Incidence and Prevalence of Gout

The incidence and prevalence of gout appear to be rising in many populations around the globe in conjunction with the *epidemiologic transition*. Factors related to the increase include increasing longevity concurrent with increasing rates of comorbid conditions such as hypertension, obesity, diabetes, the metabolic

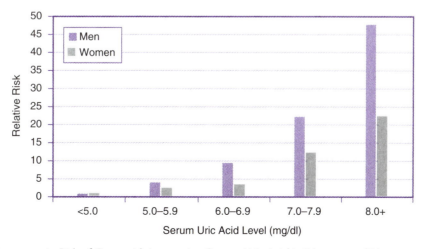

FIGURE 47.10 Dose–Response in Risk of Gout with Increasing Serum Uric Acid in Women and Men.

Data from Bhole, V., de Vera, M., Rahman, M. M., Krishnan, E., & Choi, H. (2010). Epidemiology of gout in women: Fifty-two–year followup of a prospective cohort. *Arthritis & Rheumatism 62*(4), 1069–1076.

syndrome, cardiovascular disease, and kidney disease. Such conditions likely impair the renal clearance of uric acid leading to hyperuricemia (elevated serum uric acid) which is the forerunner of gout development. These conditions in combination with other factors (genetic predisposition, alcohol consumption, dietary purines, and the use of certain drugs) have produced marked increases in the rates of gout. In the United States, compilation of self-reported data derived from national surveys suggest that approximately 3.0 million adults had gout in 2008, an increase of 42% from 2.1 million cases who self-reported gout in 1995 (Lawrence et al., 2008).

Evidence that the *incidence* of gout is increasing in the U.S. population comes from a longitudinal study of adults in Rochester, Minnesota. In this population sample, the age-gender adjusted annual incidence of acute gout increased from 4.5 to 6.2 cases per 10,000 person-years during the 10-year interval from 1977–1978 to 1987–1988 and the incidence of *primary gout* (restricted to patients not taking diuretics) increased from 2.0 to 4.6 per 10,000 during the same time period (Arromdee, Michet, Crowson, O'Fallon, & Gabriel, 2002).

Evidence that the *prevalence* of gout is increasing in the U.S. population comes from a prospective study of a managed care population of 8 million adults. During the period 1990–1999, the prevalence of gout or hyperuricemia in the cohort increased from 21 to 41 cases per 1000 for adults 75 years or older, and from 21 to 31 cases per 1000 for adults ages 65–74 years. Prevalence rates for younger age groups remained low and were relatively stable over the time period of study (Wallace, Riedel, Joseph-Ridge, & Wortmann, 2004).

In the United Kingdom, examination of 1.7 million adults in the *General Practitioner Research Database* yielded an annual gout *incidence* of about 14 per 10,000 person-years during 1990–1999. Interestingly, the incidence remained relatively stable over that time period reflecting a different pattern than the U.S. data. Nevertheless, rates for adults over 65 years of age increased by about 40% during 1990–1994, and in the 65–84-year age group, there was an overall increase of 31% from 29 to 47 cases per 10,000 during the entire decade of the study. The annual prevalence of gout estimated from the 1999 data was 14 per 1000 overall with peaks of 73 per 1000 at 75–84 years in men and 28 per 1000 at 85 years or older in women. In comparisons with osteoarthritis patients from the same cohort, patients with gout were more likely to have cardiovascular disease, hypertension, diabetes or chronic renal failure, or have used drugs known to impair renal clearance of uric acid such as diuretics or cyclosporine (Mikuls et al., 2005). Notably, the overall prevalence estimate from the 1999 survey was more than five times higher than the prevalence estimate

from a similar national study conducted in Great Britain during the 1970s (Currie, 1979).

Secular trends in the burden of gout in the United States were examined by comparing prevalence estimates derived from the *NHANES* during 1988–1994 and 2007–2008. Estimates were based on representative national samples of 5707 participants in 2007–2008 and 18,825 participants in 1988–1994. The age-adjusted prevalence of gout was 3.9% in 2007–2008 compared to 2.9% in 1988–1994, an increase of 34%. The 2007–2008 estimates translate to a prevalence of 8.3 million individuals with gout in the United States (6.1 million men and 2.0 million women). The investigators suggest that the increasing burden of gout in the U.S. is due to higher levels of obesity, hypertension and alcohol consumption, particularly among men (Zhu, Pandya, & Choi, 2011).

Age Distribution of Gout

Gout differs dramatically from rheumatoid arthritis and osteoarthritis, joint diseases that strike twice as many females as males. In contrast, approximately 90% of newly diagnosed cases of gout are males. In men, the annual prevalence rate of gout begins to increase before age 30, climbing to a peak of more than 70 cases per 1000 in the eighth decade of life. The prevalence rates in women remain much lower than men throughout life and do not increase substantially until after menopause (**FIGURE 47.11**).

Disability from Gout

Chronic gouty arthritis is the most disabling phase of the disease. This phase generally appears over a span of years of increasing severity of acute attacks with spread to multiple joints. Aggressive therapy significantly reduces the risk of developing the chronic phase. Approximately 90% of patients with chronic disease eventually develop nephropathy, a life-threatening condition.

Risk Factors for Gout

Risk factors for the development of gout include male gender, renal dysfunction, excessive alcohol intake, high dietary intake of purines, exposure to certain drugs (specifically those that influence renal clearance of uric acid) and various comorbid conditions (particularly type 2 diabetes, obesity, and the metabolic syndrome). Patients with hypertension, hyperlipidemia, and/or cardiovascular disease are also at increased risk for the development of hyperuricemia and subsequently, gout. Selected risk factors are briefly discussed in the following sections (Weaver, 2008).

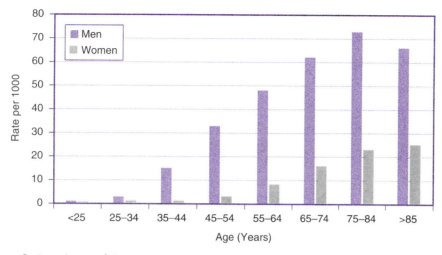

FIGURE 47.11 Age-Specific Prevalence of Gout.

Data from Mikuls, T. R., Farrar, J. T., Bilker, W. B., Fernandes, S., Schumacher, H. R. Jr., & Saag, K. G. (2005). Gout epidemiology: Results from the UK General Practice Research Database, 1990–1999. *Annals of the Rheumatic Diseases 64*, 267–272.

Gender and Gout

As shown in Figure 47.11, rates of gout in men of reproductive age far surpass those of women. Clinical studies have determined that during the reproductive years, the serum concentrations of uric acid in men are on average approximately 1 mg per dL higher than women. However, following menopause, serum levels of uric acid of women tend to approach those of men. The gender difference in uric acid concentration has been attributed to a beneficial effect of endogenous estrogens that promote more efficient uric acid clearance by the kidneys (Choi, 2008; Rider et al., 2004).

Kidney Dysfunction and Gout

There is a general consensus in the field of gout research that about 90% of all gout cases are due to defective renal clearance of uric acid. It is therefore important to emphasize that *any chronic condition that compromises kidney function can potentially upset the delicate balance of uric acid clearance resulting in hyperuricemia and gout*. Many of these conditions are discussed elsewhere in this text. They include type 2 diabetes and the metabolic syndrome, obesity, atherosclerosis, hypertension, dyslipidemia, and other cardiovascular conditions, and nephritis, nephrosis, and other forms of kidney disease.

Of special interest is the association between gout and the disease complex known as the *metabolic syndrome*. This complex is defined by the presence of at least three of the following criteria: obesity, hypertension, hyperglycemia or type 2 diabetes, high serum triglycerides and low high-density lipoprotein cholesterol. Using data collected from 8807 adults of the Third NHANES III conducted during 1988–1994, a team of Harvard investigators examined the prevalence of the metabolic syndrome among 223 cases with

physician-diagnosed gout and 8584 controls without gout and quantified the magnitude of the association by estimating prevalence odds ratios. The prevalence of the metabolic syndrome was 62.8% among cases with gout and 25.4% among controls. After adjusting for age and gender, the odds of having the metabolic syndrome were strongly associated with the presence of gout (OR = 3.05). The association was elevated in women (OR = 3.97) and men (OR = 2.79). Furthermore, significant associations were noted for individual components of the metabolic syndrome: obesity (OR = 2.55), elevated triglycerides (OR = 1.90), low HDL cholesterol (OR = 1.60), hypertension (OR = 2.41), and hyperglycemia (OR = 2.14). According to the investigators,

> these findings indicate that the prevalence of metabolic syndrome is remarkably high among individuals with gout. Given the serious complications associated with metabolic syndrome, this frequent comorbidity should be recognized and taken into account in long-term treatment and overall health of individuals with gout (Choi, Ford, Chaovang, & Curhan, 2007).

Drugs and Gout

Numerous drugs have been found to increase serum uric acid and therefore may potentially increase the risk of gout in certain individuals. They do so primarily by decreasing uric acid clearance by the kidney. For example, thiazide diuretics, salicylates, pyrazinamide (a drug for tuberculosis), nicotinate (a supplementary form of inositol, niacin, and vitamin B3), insulin, beta blockers, and cyclosporine (an immunosuppressive drug) have all been found to increase reabsorption of uric acid by the renal tubules and with prolonged use can induce hyperuricemia and ultimately gout (Choi, 2008; Choi, Mount, & Reginato, 2005).

Obesity and Gout

Results of numerous investigations suggest that abdominal obesity increases the risk of developing gout. Choi and colleagues examined the relationship in a longitudinal cohort of 47,150 male participants with no history of gout at baseline ascertained from the *U.S. Health Professionals Follow-up Study*. They also examined associations with hypertension and use of diuretics. During 12 years of follow-up, 730 incident cases of gout were confirmed. Results revealed a significant dose–response in the risk of developing gout with increasing body mass (**FIGURE 47.12**). Compared to men who had maintained a stable weight (within 4 lbs.) since age 21 years, the risk of developing gout increased twofold in those who had gained 30 lbs. or more (RR = 1.99). Reciprocally, those who had lost 10 lbs. or more reduced their risk significantly (RR = 0.61). Hypertension and use of diuretics also independently increased the risk (RR = 2.33 and 1.77, respectively). The investigators concluded that *"adiposity and weight gain are strong risk factors for gout in men, while weight loss is protective"* (Choi, Atkinson, Karlson, & Curhan, 2005).

Alcohol and Gout

Chronic alcohol consumption has been linked to the development of gout in numerous epidemiologic investigations. Yet, risk levels for specific alcoholic beverages have not been thoroughly explored. Choi and colleagues therefore used the extensive database of the *U.S. Health Professionals Follow-up Study* to investigate levels and sources of alcohol consumption and the risk of developing gout. As already discussed, the study included 47,150 males with no history of gout at baseline who were followed over 12 years during 1986–1998. During this time, 730 incident cases of gout were detected. Results revealed a significant dose–response in the risk of gout with increasing intake of alcohol (**FIGURE 47.13**). In comparisons of specific alcoholic beverages, beer had the strongest

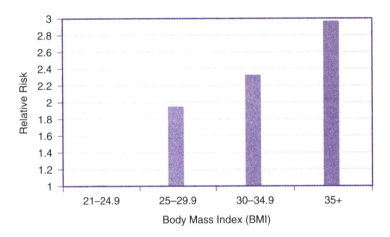

FIGURE 47.12 Dose–Response in the Risk of Gout with BMI in Men.

Data from Choi, H. K., Atkinson, K., Karlson, E. W., & Curhan, G. (2005). Obesity, weight change, hypertension, diuretic use, and risk of gout in men, the Health Professionals Follow-up Study. *Archives of Internal Medicine, 165*, 742–748.

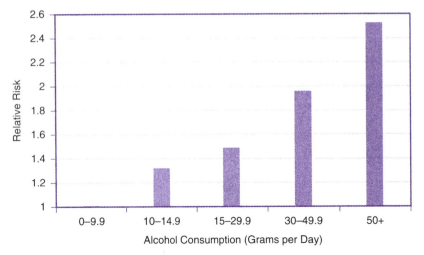

FIGURE 47.13 Dose–Response in the Risk of Gout with Increasing Alcohol Consumption in Men.

Data from Choi, H. K., Atkinson, K., Darlson, E. W., Willet, W., & Curhan, G. (2004). Alcohol intake and the risk of incident gout in men: A prospective study. *The Lancet 363*(9417), 1277–1281.

effect (RR = 1.49 per 12 oz serving per day) followed by spirits (RR = 1.15 per shot of per day) and wine (RR = 1.04 per 4 oz glass per day). Thus, while alcohol consumption per se is clearly a strong risk factor, there appears to be substantial variation in the risk according to the type of alcoholic beverage (Choi, Atkinson, Darlson, Willet, & Curhan, 2004).

Alcohol intake causes elevation of serum uric acid by at least two general biological mechanisms. First, *alcohol dehydrogenase*, the liver enzyme responsible for alcohol degradation (oxidation) in humans, triggers a cascade of reduction/oxidation (redox) reactions of adenine nucleotides resulting in the production of purines and uric acid (Faller & Fox, 1982); and second, excess hydrogen ions from *nicotinamide adenine dinucleotide (NAD)* reduction during alcohol oxidation contributes to the reduction of pyruvate and the formation of lactate, which in turn causes retention of uric acid in the renal proximal tubules (Lieber, 2005). It is important to note that several other factors may also be involved in the hyperuricemic impact of alcohol consumption including dehydration, ketosis, level of exercise, content of purines, or other contaminants in alcoholic beverages and various comorbidities (Yamamoto, Moriwaki, & Takahashi, 2005).

Dietary Factors and Gout

Choi and colleagues also used the *U.S. Health Professionals Follow-up Study* to investigate associations between selected dietary factors (meat and vegetables rich in purines and dairy products) and the risk of developing gout. In this analysis, the investigators found that men in the highest quintiles of meat and seafood consumption were at increased risk compared to those in the lowest quintile (RR = 1.41 and 1.51, respectively). In contrast, the risk decreased with increasing consumption of low-fat dairy products (RR = 0.56 for the highest compared to the lowest quintile). Notably, the risk of gout was unchanged by consumption of purine-rich vegetables. These results suggest that high consumption of meat and seafood increase the risk of developing gout, presumably because of their high purine content, whereas high consumption of low-fat dairy products conferred a protective effect, possibly due to the uricosuric properties of casein and other milk proteins (Choi, Atkinson, Karlson, Willett, & Curhan, 2004).

Genetics of Gout

Genetic factors are important determinants of susceptibility to hyperuricemia and gout. Hyperuricemia and gout are particularly common in certain ethnic groups (Filipinos, Samoans, Maori, and other South Pacific Islanders) likely due to the combination of a high seafood diet rich in purines coupled with genetic factors that heighten predisposition.

In early studies of families, hyperuricemia was found to be extremely common among the close relatives of patients with gout. In 1940, Talbott investigated 136 relatives of 27 patients with gout and found hyperuricemia in 27 male and 7 female relatives (Talbott, 1940). Smyth and colleagues later studied 87 relatives of 19 probands (index cases) in 19 families and found hyperuricemia in 27 close relatives. They suggested that hyperuricemia is an autosomal dominant genetic condition (Smyth, Cotterman, & Freyberg, 1948).

Subsequently, James Neel and colleagues at the University of Michigan determined serum uric acid levels for 271 members of the 19 families first studied by Smyth, Cotterman, and Freyberg. While first-degree relatives of probands had higher levels than more distant relatives, spouses, or population controls, the extended distributional pattern in these families suggested that hyperuricemia is a multifactorial genetic trait rather than under control of a single autosomal gene (Neel, Rakic, Davidson, Valkenburg, & Mikkelsen, 1965). Though there are rare monogenic syndromes that predispose to hyperuricemia and gout, there is now a firm consensus that these traits usually follow a multifactorial pattern of inheritance (Richette & Bardin, 2010).

Perhaps the most important cause of hyperuricemia is reduced *clearance of uric acid by the kidneys*. This function is controlled by a family of urate transport molecules that are expressed in the renal collecting tubules. These molecules include the fructose transporter *SLC2A9 (GLUT9)*, urate transporter 1 *(URAT1)*, organic anion transporters *(OAT1, OAT2, and OAT3)*, multidrug resistance protein *(MRP4)*, sodium-coupled monocarboxyl transporters *(SMCT)*, and human ATP-binding cassette *(ABCG2)*. Other checkpoints in the regulation of serum uric acid include hepatic production and degradation of uric acid, monosodium crystal formation, and initiation of the acute inflammatory response. Multiple genes are thus involved in the regulation of uric acid clearance and *genome-wide association studies (GWAS)* are being conducted to identify them. Indeed, genetic polymorphisms that compromise the function of two major regulators of renal uric acid transport have already been discovered, *SLC2A9* and *ABCG2* (Choi, 2010; Merriman & Dalbeth, 2011; Vitart et al., 2008).

Three monogenic syndromes have been well characterized in the literature. *Lesch–Nyhan syndrome* is a rare X-linked genetic disorder that affects only males. The incidence is approximately 1 in 470,000 live male births. Males with this syndrome manifest physical handicaps, mental retardation, kidney dysfunction, and gout. The syndrome is caused by a mutation in a gene on the long arm of the X chromosome that encodes the enzyme, *hypoxanthine-guanine phosphoribosyl transferase*, or *HPRT*, which catalyzes the recycling of hypoxanthine and guanine, reactions that are necessary to prevent the buildup of uric acid. Complete absence of HPRT enzyme activity leads to markedly elevated uric acid levels in the blood (hyperuricemia) that produce the symptoms that define the syndrome. Other rare genetic syndromes that predispose to gout include *familial juvenile hyperuricemic nephropathy (medullary cystic kidney disease)* and *phosphoribosyl pyrophosphate synthetase (PRS) superactivity*. These also involve inborn errors of metabolism that result in hyperuricemia and gout (Bleyer & Hart, 2006; Robbins & Cotran, 1979).

Prevention and Therapy of Gout

Gout typically progresses through distinct clinical phases: (1) asymptomatic hyperuricemia, (2) recurrent acute attacks of gouty arthritis interspersed with asymptomatic periods, and (3) chronic gouty arthritis or tophaceous gout. Asymptomatic hyperuricemia is common and can often be reversed by nonpharmacologic methods such as reducing intake of dietary purines, limiting alcohol consumption, reducing weight if overweight or obese, maintaining blood pressure, blood lipids and blood glucose within normal limits, avoiding nephrotoxic drugs, and drinking generous amounts of water daily. The excruciatingly painful symptoms of gout can be effectively treated by administration of nonsteroidal anti-inflammatory drugs (NSAIDs), steroids, or colchicine. Pharmacologic treatment of hyperuricemia with urate-lowering drugs such as allopurinol or probenecid has led to a dramatic reduction in long-term gouty arthritis and tophaceous gout. Furthermore, hemodialysis has markedly improved survival among patients who develop gouty nephropathy (Harris, Siegel, & Alloway, 1999; Luk & Simkin, 2005).

▶ Ankylosing Spondylitis

Ankylosing spondylitis (also called Marie–Strümpell disease) is a highly inflammatory form of arthritis of the spine. This disorder is characterized by back pain and stiffness, and loss of spinal mobility due to compression and ultimate fusion of sacroiliac joints and vertebrae. Diagnosis is typically made based upon symptoms and radiography. The anatomic and pathological changes in the spine are indistinguishable from those of rheumatoid arthritis.

Longitudinal examination of a population cohort in Rochester, Minnesota, during 1935–1973 revealed an annual age-adjusted incidence of 11.0 per 100,000 in males and 4.0 per 100,000 in females. In this study, the incidence peaked during ages 25–34 years and the male-to-female ratio was approximately 4 to 1 (Carter, McKenna, Brian, & Kurland, 1979).

There are extreme geographic and ethnic differences in the prevalence of ankylosing spondylitis. Prevalence rates exceeding 60 per 1000 have been observed in surveys of North American Indians markedly exceeding rates found in Caucasian populations in the United States and Europe (Hochberg, 1984). These ethnic differences in prevalence closely reflect population differences in the frequency of the histocompatibility antigen, HLA-B27.

Heredity plays a strong role in predisposing to the development of ankylosing spondylitis. In family studies, approximately 25% of close relatives of probands (index cases) have been found to manifest symptomatic or asymptomatic disease (Hochberg, Bias, & Arnett, 1978). Most notably, individuals who carry the HLA-B27 antigen are at high risk for the development of ankylosing spondylitis (Brewerton et al., 1973; Schlosstein, Terasaki, Bluestone, & Pearson, 1973). The HLA-B27 is found in 90%–95% of patients of European origin with ankylosing spondylitis compared to 8% in the general population. However, only about 5% of individuals in the general population who carry HLA-B27 will develop ankylosing spondylitis; therefore HLA-B27 has little value as a biomarker for the disease (Reveille, Ball, & Khan, 2001).

The exact mechanism by which HLA-B27 confers disease susceptibility has not been determined. Conceivably, this antigen triggers an autoimmune response by killer T cells that incites inflammation in the spinal synovium. Family studies suggest that HLA-B27 contributes about 40% of the overall genetic risk for ankylosing spondylitis and that other antigens of the major histocompatibility locus on chromosome 6 contribute to the remaining risk (Reveille et al., 2001).

Various infectious agents have also been found in association with HLA-B27 and ankylosing spondylitis. For example, HLA-B27 and certain *Klebsiella* species have been found to cross react (Ebringer, Cooke, Cawdell, Cowing, & Ebringer, 1977; Gezcy & Yap, 1982). One interpretation of such findings is that specific infectious agents or other environmental triggers may interact with HLA-B27 and/or other antigens of the major histocompatibility locus to incite autoimmune reactivity leading to ankylosing spondylitis (Reveille, 2006).

While there is no cure for ankylosing spondylitis, aerobic exercise, good posture, and certain medications have been found to be effective in preventing/relieving symptoms. Medications for pain relief include NSAIDs, selective cyclcooxygenase-2 (COX-2) blockers, and opioids. Disease modifying antirheumatic drugs *(DMARDS)* such as cyclosporine, methotrexate, sulfasalazine, prednisone, and TNF-α antagonists have shown benefit in reducing immunoreactivity. Patients with ankylosing spondylitis often manifest comorbid inflammatory conditions such as ulcerative colitis, Crohn's disease, pulmonary fibrosis, vasculitis, and uveitis which must be recognized and treated (McVeigh & Cairns, 2006).

▸ Juvenile Idiopathic Arthritis

Juvenile idiopathic arthritis refers to a spectrum of arthritic conditions diagnosed in children or adolescents ages 16 years or younger. The diagnosis is made based upon a detailed history and physical examination, radiography, and laboratory tests. Overall, girls are affected approximately twice as often as boys. The incidence peaks between ages 1 and 3 years. As noted in the following discussion, the age of onset and the gender ratio vary by subtype (Hoffart & Sherry, 2010).

The nomenclature of childhood arthritis has undergone revision and continues to evolve with research and discovery. In past years, the terms *juvenile rheumatoid arthritis* and *juvenile chronic arthritis* were commonly used to describe slightly different forms of childhood arthritis, thereby compromising comparability of studies. In 1997, a committee of international investigators established uniform criteria for the diagnosis of childhood arthritis and recommended using "*juvenile idiopathic arthritis*" to describe all forms of childhood arthritis. The term "*idiopathic*" means that the exact cause is unknown. Three major subtypes of *juvenile idiopathic arthritis* are defined: *oligoarticular, polyarticular,* and *systemic disease* (Fink, 1995; Petty et al., 1998, 2004). Characteristics of the three major

forms of *juvenile idiopathic arthritis* are shown in **TABLE 47.2**.

Oligoarticular juvenile idiopathic arthritis accounts for approximately 50% of cases. It is defined as arthritis that affects four or fewer joints during the first 6 months of disease. The female:male ratio of this subtype is approximately 2:1. Patients are typically young girls, ages 1–4 years, with involvement of the large joints of the lower extremities (knees and ankles). Approximately 70% of patients have *antinuclear antibodies (ANA)* whereas *rheumatoid factor* is absent. Inflammation of the eye (uveitis) is common in this subtype.

Polyarticular juvenile idiopathic arthritis accounts for about 30% of cases. It is defined as arthritis that affects five or more joints within the first 6 months of disease. The female-to-male ratio of this subtype is approximately 2:1. Children with disease are typically negative for rheumatoid factor whereas adolescents are positive. Both small and large joints may be affected and the pattern of arthritic joints is typically symmetric. Eye inflammation is less common in this subtype.

Systemic juvenile idiopathic arthritis (also called *Still's disease*) accounts for approximately 10% of cases. The early phase of systemic disease is characterized by fever, rash, lymphadenopathy, hepatosplenomegaly, and inflammation of peripheral membranes of the heart and lungs (pericarditis and pleuritis, respectively). Life-threatening coagulopathy may develop in this early phase. Notably, arthritic symptoms are often not detected until weeks or even months after the initial acute febrile episode; consequently, definitive diagnosis may be delayed. The female:male ratio of this subtype is approximately 1:1, and onset is most common in the early years of childhood. About one-third of patients progress to chronic destructive arthritis.

Enthesitis-related arthritis refers to inflammatory arthritis in association with *inflammatory tendonitis (enthesitis).* This subtype is most common in boys,

TABLE 47.2 Major Subtypes of Juvenile Idiopathic Arthritis

Subtype	Frequency (%)	Joints	Pattern	F:M	Biomarker
Oligoarticular	50	4 or less	Asymmetric	2:1	ANA+
Polyarticular	30	5 or more	Symmetric	2:1	Rex
Systemic	10	Multiple	Asymmetric	1:1	Increased CRP

ANA = antinuclear antibodies; CRP = C-reactive protein; RF = rheumatoid factor.

ages 8 years and older. Patients often manifest ankylosing spondylitis and inflammatory bowel disease and carry HLA-B27.

Psoriatic juvenile idiopathic arthritis is characterized by the development of psoriasis (inflammatory dermatitis) and subsequently, polyarticular arthritis. This subtype is more common in young girls with seropositivity for antinuclear antibodies (Hoffart & Sherry, 2010; Petty, 1998, 2004).

From the preceding discussion, it is obvious that juvenile idiopathic arthritis encompasses a heterogeneous group of disorders. While their pathogenesis is not fully understood, molecular studies suggest an autoimmune basis wherein cells of the immune system attack molecular targets in the joint capsule. This autoimmune reactivity appears to be largely dependent upon genetic factors that are triggered by specific environmental factors. The best documented associations are with genetic variants of the HLA complex such as *HLA-A, HLA-DR/DQ,* and *HLA-DP.* Such genes encode molecules that facilitate the presentation of antigenic peptides to T lymphocytes of the immune system. Conceivably, polymorphisms in these genes trigger an autoimmune response, particularly during periods of infection by viruses or bacteria that demonstrate mimicry with autoantigens. Other genes may also be involved, particularly those that encode inflammatory cytokines, prostaglandins, leukotrienes, and their cell membrane receptors. GWAS and studies of candidate genes to determine linkage and gene expression are in progress with the goal of identifying molecular targets for effective prevention and therapy (Førre & Smerdel, 2002; Prahalad, 2004).

Estimates of the annual incidence and prevalence of juvenile idiopathic arthritis vary widely from

study to study, even in the same populations. Australian investigators Prudence Manner and Carol Bower reviewed epidemiologic studies of childhood arthritis published during 1966–2002 to identify possible reasons for the wide-ranging estimates of prevalence and incidence. Results from 34 studies were reviewed. Annual prevalence estimates ranged from 0.07 to 4.01 per 1000, a 57-fold difference between extremes, and annual incidence estimates ranged from 8 to 226 per 100,000, a 28-fold difference between extremes. Factors contributing to the wide range of estimates included differences among studies in diagnostic criteria, case ascertainment, disease recognition (particularly inactive cases), and small sample sizes in some studies (Manner & Bower, 2002).

Investigators at the Mayo Clinic in the United States examined a longitudinal inception cohort for trends in the incidence of juvenile rheumatoid arthritis. The study utilized the diagnostic retrieval system of the *Rochester Epidemiology Project* to screen medical records of all residents of Rochester, Minnesota, for diagnoses of juvenile rheumatoid arthritis during the 33-year period 1960–1993. A total of 65 cases with juvenile rheumatoid arthritis were identified (48 females and 17 males). Among cases, 72% had oligoarticular disease, 17% had polyarticular disease, and 11% had systemic disease. As shown in **FIGURE 47.14**, two peaks in the onset of disease were observed, the first in early childhood (aged 2–3 years) and the second during adolescence (aged 12–15 years). Overall, the annual incidence rate was 11.7 per 100,000; however, rates estimated for successive periods, 1960–1969, 1970–1979, and 1980–1993 showed a declining trend (15.0, 14.1, and 7.8 per 100,000, respectively). Furthermore, examination of moving

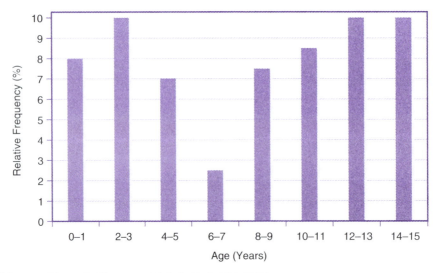

FIGURE 47.14 Age of Onset of Juvenile Rheumatoid Arthritis in U.S. Children.

Data from Peterson, L. S., Mason, T., Nelson, A. M., O'Fallon, W. M., & Gabriel, S. E. (1996). Juvenile rheumatoid arthritis in Rochester, Minnesota 1960–1993. Is the epidemiology changing? *Arthritis & Rheumatism, 39*(8), 1475–1390.

averages of the yearly incidence rates revealed the presence of cyclic patterns with peaks in 1967, 1975, and 1987. The investigators suggest that the declining incidence and cyclic nature of the data may reflect effects of infectious agents or other environmental factors on the etiopathogenesis of juvenile rheumatoid arthritis (Peterson, Mason, Nelson, O'Fallon, & Gabriel, 1996).

Juvenile idiopathic arthritis per se is seldom life-threatening and a significant fraction of patients, perhaps 50%, eventually enter remission with no or minimal functional loss. However, it is important to note that there is currently no cure for juvenile idiopathic arthritis. The primary goals of therapy are to eliminate active disease, normalize joint function, preserve normal growth, and prevent long-term joint damage. Recent evidence suggests that early aggressive therapy of newly diagnosed patients may effectively reduce the risk of devastating consequences such as permanent joint disability or blindness from chronic uveitis. In their comprehensive review of antirheumatic drugs used in the treatment of childhood arthritis, Hayward and Wallace (2009) suggest that *"there is a therapeutic window of opportunity in which to target interventions to optimize long-term outcomes in children with juvenile idiopathic arthritis".*

▶ Suppurative (Septic) Arthritis

Suppurative or septic arthritis refers to the invasion of the joint space by bacteria, viruses, or other microbes. Typically, bacteria emanating from an infection localized at another anatomic site seed the joint space by dissemination through the bloodstream. The most common causes of suppurative arthritis are *staphylococci* and *streptococci* (in adults), *gonococci* (in young adults), *Haemophilus influenzae* and *Pseudomonas aeruginosa* (in children), and *Escherichia coli* (in the elderly, IV drug users, and seriously ill patients). *Tuberculosis arthritis* is a common development of active pulmonary tuberculosis in children and adults living in regions of the world where *tuberculosis mycobacteria* are endogenous (Robbins & Cotran, 1979). In developed countries where joint replacement is relatively common, subjects with artificial joints are at increased risk of developing suppurative arthritis due to *staphylococci, streptococci*, and other infectious agents. Prompt recognition and effective antimicrobial therapy for the underlying infectious agent is required for the preservation of normal joint function in patients who develop suppurative arthritis (Robbins & Cotran, 1979; Kaandorp et al., 1997; Weston, Jones, Bradbury, Fawthrop, & Doherty, 1999).

References

Abdel-Nasser, A. M., Rasker, J. J., & Valkenburg, H. A. (1997). Epidemiological and clinical aspects relating to the variability of rheumatoid arthritis. *Seminars in Arthritis & Rheumatism, 27*(2), 123–140.

Aho, K., Markku, K., Tuiminen, J., & Kaprio, J. (1986). Occurrence of rheumatoid arthritis in a nationwide series of twins. *Journal of Rheumatology, 13*, 899–902.

Anderson, J. J., & Felson, D. T. (1988). Factors associated with osteoarthritis of the knee in the first National Health and Nutrition Examination Survey (HANES I). Evidence for an association with overweight, race, and physical demands of work. *American Journal of Epidemiology, 128*(1), 179–189.

Arnett, F. C., Edworthy, S. M., Bloch, D. A., McShane, D. J., Fries, J. F., & Cooper, N. S. (1988). The American Rheumatism Association 1987 revised criteria for the classification of rheumatoid arthritis. *Arthritis & Rheumatism, Arthritis Care & Research, 31*(3), 315–324.

Arromdee, E., Michet, C. J., Crowson, C. S., O'Fallon, W. M., & Gabriel, S. E. (2002). Epidemiology of gout: Is the incidence rising? *Journal of Rheumatology, 29*, 2403–2406.

Berenbaum, F. (2010). Diabetes-induced osteoarthritis: From a new paradigm to a new phenotype. *Annals of Rheumatic Diseases.* doi:10.1136/ard.2010.146399.

Bhole, V., de Vera, M., Rahman, M. M., Krishnan, E., & Choi, H. (2010). Epidemiology of gout in women: Fifty-two–year followup of a prospective cohort. *Arthritis & Rheumatism, 62*(4), 1069–1076.

Blagojevic, M., Jinks, C., Jeffery, A., & Jordan, K. P. (2010). Risk factors for onset of osteoarthritis of the knee in older adults: A systematic review and meta-analysis. *Osteoarthritis and Cartilage, 18*(1), 24–33.

Bleyer, A. J., & Hart, T. C. (2006). Genetic factors associated with gout and hyperuricemia. *Advanced Chronic Kidney Disease, 13*(2), 124–130.

Brandt, K. D., Dieppe, P., & Radin, E. (2009). Etiopathogenesis of osteoarthritis. *Medical Clinics of North America, 93*(1), 1–24.

Brandt, K. D., & Flusser, D. (1991). Osteoarthritis. In N. Bellamy (Ed.), *Prognosis in the rheumatic diseases* (pp. 11–35). Lancaster, UK: Kluwer Academic Publishers.

Brewerton, D. A., Hart, F. D., Nicholls, A., Caffrey, M., James, D. C. O., & Sturrock, R. D. (1973). Ankylosing spondylitis and HL-A 27. *Lancet, 1*, 904–907.

Carter, E. T., McKenna, C. H., Brian, D. D., & Kurland, L. T. (1979). Epidemiology of ankylosing spondylitis in Rochester, Minnesota: 1935–1974. *Arthritis & Rheumatism, 22*, 365–370.

CDC. (2011). *Arthritis.* Atlanta, Georgia: Centers for Disease Prevention and Control.

Cheng, Y. J., Hootman, J. M., Murphy, L. B., Langmaid, G. A., & Helmick, C. G. (2010). Prevalence of doctor-diagnosed arthritis and arthritis-attributable activity limitation—United States, 2007–2009. *MMWR, 59*(39), 1261–1265.

Choi, H. K. (2008). Gout: Epidemiology, pathology and pathogenesis. In J. H. Klipper, J. H. Stone, L. J. Crofford, &

P. H. White (Eds.), *Primer on rheumatic diseases* (13th ed., pp. 250–257). New York, NY: Springer.

Choi, H. K. (2010). Genetics of gout. *Current Opinion in Rheumatology, 22,* 144–151.

Choi, H. K., Atkinson, K., Darlson, E. W., Willet, W., & Curhan, G. (2004). Alcohol intake and the risk of incident gout in men: A prospective study. *Lancet, 363*(9417), 1277–1281.

Choi, H. K., Atkinson, K., Karlson, E. W., & Curhan, G. (2005). Obesity, weight change, hypertension, diuretic use, and risk of gout in men, the Health Professionals Follow-up Study. *Archives of Internal Medicine, 165,* 742–748.

Choi, H. K., Atkinson, K., Karlson, E. W., Willett, W., & Curhan, G. (2004). Purine-rich foods, dairy and protein intake, and the risk of gout in men. *New England Journal of Medicine, 350*(11), 1093–1103.

Choi, H. K., Ford, E. S., Chaovang, L., & Curhan, G. (2007). Prevalence of the metabolic syndrome in patients with gout: The Third National Health and Nutrition Examination Survey. *Arthritis Care & Research, 57*(2), 109–115.

Choi, H. K., Mount, D. B., & Reginato, A. M. (2005). Pathogenesis of gout. *Annals of Internal Medicine, 143*(7), 499–516.

Christensen, R., Bartels, E. M., Astrup, A., & Bliddal, H. (2007). Effect of weight reduction in obese patients diagnosed with knee osteoarthritis: A systematic review and meta-analysis. *Annals of the Rheumatic Diseases, 66,* 433–439.

Cross, M., Smith, E., Hoy, D., Carmona, L., Wolfe, F., Vos, T., … March, L. (2014). The global burden of rheumatoid arthritis: Estimates from the Global Burden of Disease 2010 study. *Annals of the Rheumatic Diseases, 73,* 1316–1322.

Cross, M., Smith, E., Hoy, D., Nolte, S., Ackerman, I., Fransen, M., … March, L. (2014). The global burden of hip and knee osteoarthritis: Estimates from the Global Burden of Disease 2010 study. *Annals of the Rheumatic Diseases, 73*(7), 1323–1330.

Currie, W. (1979). Prevalence and incidence of the diagnosis of gout in Great Britain. *Annals of Rheumatic Diseases, 47,* 101–106.

Davis, M. A., Ettinger, W. H., & Neuhaus, J. M. (1990). Obesity and osteoarthritis of the knee: Evidence from the National Health and Nutrition Examination Survey (NHANES I). *Seminars in Arthritis and Rheumatism, 20*(3), 34–41.

Davis, M. A., Ettinger, W. H., Neuhaus, J. M., Cho, S. A., & Hauck, W. W. (1989). The association of knee injury and obesity with unilateral and bilateral osteoarthritis of the knee. *American Journal of Epidemiology, 130*(2), 278–288.

Davis, M. A., Ettinger, W. H., Neuhaus, J. M., & Hauck, W. W. (1988). Sex differences in osteoarthritis of the knee. The role of obesity. *American Journal of Epidemiology, 127*(5), 1019–1030.

Davis, M. A., Neuhaus, J. M., Ettinger, W. H., & Muller, W. H. (1990). Body fat distribution and osteoarthritis. *American Journal of Epidemiology, 132,* 701–707.

Deighton, C. M., Walker, D. J., Griffiths, I. D., & Roberts, D. F. (1989). The contribution of HLA to rheumatoid arthritis. *Clinical Genetics, 36,* 178–182.

Doran, M. F., Pond, G. R., Crowson, C. S., O'Fallon, W. M., & Gabriel, S. E. (2002). Trends in incidence and mortality in rheumatoid arthritis in Rochester, Minnesota, over a forty-year period. *Arthritis & Rheumatism, 46*(3), 625–631.

Ebringer, R., Cooke, D., Cawdell, D. R., Cowing, P., & Ebringer, S. (1977). Ankylosing spondylitis: Klebsiella and HLA-B27. *Rheumatology and Rehabilitation, 16,* 190–196.

Engstrom, G., de Verdier, M. G., Rollof, J., Nilsson, P. M., & Lohmander, L. S. (2008). C-reactive protein, metabolic

syndrome and incidence of severe hip and knee osteoarthritis. A population-based cohort study. *Osteoarthritis and Cartilage, 17*(2), 168–173.

Ercilla, M. C., Brancos, M. A., Breysse, Y., Alonso, J., Vives, J., & Castillo, R. (1977). HLA antigens in Forestier's disease, ankylosing spondylitis and polyarthrosis of the hands. *Journal of Rheumatology, 4,* 89–93.

Faller, J., & Fox, I. H. (1982). Ethanol-induced hyperuricemia: Evidence for increased urate production by activation of adenine nucleotide turnover. *New England of Journal of Medicine, 307*(26), 1598–1602.

Fink, C. W. (1995). Proposal for the development of classification criteria for idiopathic arthritides of childhood. *Journal of Rheumatology, 22,* 1566–1569.

Førre, O., & Smerdel, A. (2002). Genetic epidemiology of juvenile idiopathic arthritis. *Scandinavian Journal of Rheumatology, 31*(3), 123–128.

Gabriel, S. E., Crowson, C. S., & O'Fallon, W. M. (1999). The epidemiology of rheumatoid arthritis in Rochester, Minnesota, 1955–1985. *Arthritis & Rheumatism, 42*(3), 415–420.

Gezcy, A. F., & Yap, J. (1982). A survey of isolates of Klebsiella pneumoniae which cross-react with HLA-B27-associated cell-surface structure on the lymphocytes of patients with ankylosing spondylitis. *Journal of Rheumatology, 9,* 96–100.

Gregerson, P. K., Silver, J., & Winchester, R. J. (1987). The shared epitope hypothesis—An approach to understanding the molecular genetics of susceptibility to rheumatoid arthritis. *Arthritis & Rheumatism, 30,* 1205–1213.

Harris, M. D., Siegel, L. B., & Alloway, J. A. (1999). Gout and hyperuricemia. *American Family Physician, 59,* 925–936.

Hay, S. I., & GBD 2016 DALY and HALE Collaborators. (2017). Global, regional, and national disability-adjusted life-years (DALYs) for 333 diseases and injuries and healthy life expectancy (HALE) for 195 countries and territories, 1990–2016: A systematic analysis for the Global Burden of Disease Study 2016. *The Lancet, 390*(10100), 1260–1344.

Hayward, K., & Wallace, C. A. (2009). Recent developments in anti-rheumatic drugs in pediatrics: Treatment of juvenile idiopathic arthritis. *Arthritis Research and Therapy, 11,* 216.

Helmick, C. G., Felson, D. T., Lawrence, R. C., Gabriel, S., Hirsch, R., Kwoh, C. K., … National Arthritis Data Workgroup. (2008). Estimates of the prevalence of arthritis and other rheumatic conditions in the United States. Part I. *Arthritis & Rheumatism, 58,* 15–25.

Hochberg, M. C. (1984). Epidemiology. In A. Calin (Ed.), *Spondyloarthropathies.* New York: Grune and Stratton, Guilford.

Hochberg, M. C. (1990). Changes in the incidence and prevalence of rheumatoid arthritis in England and Wales, 1970–1982. *Seminars in Arthritis and Rheumatism, 19,* 294–302.

Hochberg, M. C., Bias, W. B., & Arnett, F. C. (1978). Family studies in HLA-B27-associated arthritis. *Medicine, 57,* 463–475.

Hoffart, C., & Sherry, D. D. (2010). Early identification of juvenile idiopathic arthritis. *The Journal of Musculoskeletal Medicine, 27,* 52–56.

Holderbaum, D., Haqqi, T. M., & Moskowitz, R. W. (1999). Genetics and osteoarthritis: Exposing the iceberg. *Arthritis & Rheumatism, 42*(2), 397–405.

Hui, M., Doherty, M., & Zhang, W. (2011). Does smoking protect against osteoarthritis? Meta-analysis of observational studies. *Annals of Rheumatic Diseases, 70,* 1231–1237.

Kaandorp, C. J., Dinant, H. J., van de Laar, M. A., Moens, H. J., Prins, A. P., & Dijkmans, B. A. (August 1997). Incidence and sources of native and prosthetic joint infection: A community based prospective survey. *Annals of Rheumatic Diseases, 56*(8), 470–475.

Kaipiainen-Seppänen, O., Aho, K., Isomäki, H., & Laakso, M. (1996). Incidence of rheumatoid arthritis in Finland during 1980–1990. *Annals of Rheumatic Diseases, 55*, 608–611.

Kellgren, J. H. (1962). Diagnostic criteria for population studies. *Bulletin on the Rheumatic Diseases, 13*, 291–292.

Kellgren, J. H., & Lawrence, J. S. (1958). Osteoarthritis and disk degeneration in an urban population. *Annals of Rheumatic Diseases, 17*, 478–397.

Kellgren, J. H., Lawrence, J. S., & Bier, F. (1963). Genetic factors in generalized osteoarthrosis. *Annals of Rheumatic Diseases, 22*, 237–255.

Khaltaev, N., Pfleger, B., Woolf, A. D., Mathers, C., Adesson, K., Hazes, J. M., & Symmons, D. (2003). Assessing the burden of musculoskeletal conditions: A joint World Health Organization–Bone and Joint Decade project. *Arthritis Research and Therapy, 5*(Suppl. 3), 174.

Klinenberg, J. R. (1977). Hyperuricemia and gout. *Medicine Clinics, NA, 61*, 299.

Lawrence, J. S. (1977). *Rheumatism in populations*. London, UK: W Heinemann Medical Books.

Lawrence, J. S., & Moore, J. (1952). Generalized osteoarthritis and Heberden's nodes. *British Medical Journal, 1*, 181–187.

Lawrence, R. C., Felson, D. T., Helmick, C. G., Arnold, L. M., Choi, H., Deyo, R. A., ... for the National Arthritis Data Workgroup. (2008). Estimates of the prevalence of arthritis and other rheumatic conditions in the United States. Part II. *Arthritis & Rheumatism, 58*(1), 26–35.

Leong, A. L., & Euller-Ziegler, L. (2004). Patient advocacy and arthritis: Moving forward. *Bulletin of the World Health Organization, 82*(2), 115–120.

Lieber, C. S. (2005). Hyperuricemia induced by alcohol. *Arthritis & Rheumatism, 8*(4), 786–798.

Linos, A., Worthington, J. W., O'Fallon, W. M., & Kurland, L. T. (1980). The epidemiology of rheumatoid arthritis in Rochester, Minnesota: A study of incidence, prevalence, and mortality. *American Journal of Epidemiology, 111*(1), 87–98.

Luk, A. J., & Simkin, P. A. (2005). Epidemiology of hyperuricemia and gout. *American Journal of Managed Care, 11*, S435–S442.

Mankin, H. J. (1974). The reaction of articular cartilage to injury and osteoarthritis. *New England Journal of Medicine, 291*, 1285–1335.

Manners, P. J., & Bower, C. (2002). Worldwide prevalence of juvenile arthritis why does it vary so much? *Journal of Rheumatology, 29*, 1520–1530.

McVeigh, C. M., & Cairns, A. P. (2006). Clinical review: Diagnosis and management of ankylosing spondylitis. *BMJ, 33*(7568), 581–585.

Merriman, T. R., & Dalbeth, N. (2011). The genetic basis of hyperuricaemia and gout. *Joint Bone Spine, 78*(1), 35–40.

Mignon, B. R. (2006). The role of X inactivation and cellular mosaicism in women's health and sex-specific diseases. *JAMA, 295*, 1428–1433.

Mikuls, T. R., Farrar, J. T., Bilker, W. B., Fernandes, S., Schumacher, H. R., Jr., & Saag, K. G. (2005). Gout epidemiology: Results from the UK General Practice Research Database, 1990–1999. *Annals of Rheumatic Diseases, 64*, 267–272.

Murray, C. J., Vos, T., Lozano, R., Naghavi, M., Flaxman, A. D., Michaud, C., ... Memish, Z. A. (2012) Disability-adjusted life years (DALYs) for 291 diseases and injuries in 21 regions, 1990–2010: A systematic analysis for the Global Burden of Disease Study 2010. *Lancet, 30*(9859), 2197–2223.

Myasoedova, E., Crowson, C. S., Kremers, H. M., Therneau, T. M., & Gabriel, S. E. (2010). Is the incidence of rheumatoid arthritis rising? Results from Olmsted County, Minnesota, 1955–2007. *Arthritis & Rheumatism, 62*(6), 1576–1582.

Neel, J. V., Rakic, M. T., Davidson, R. T., Valkenburg, H. A., & Mikkelsen, W. M. (1965). Studies on hyperuricemia II. A reconsideration of the distribution of serum uric acid values in the families of Smyth, Cotterman, and Freyberg. *American Journal of Human Genetics, 17*(1), 14–22.

Oliveria, S. A., Felson, D. T., Reed, J. I., Cirillo, P. A., & Walker, A. M. (1995). Incidence of symptomatic hand, hip, and knee osteoarthritis among patients in a health maintenance organization. *Arthritis & Rheumatism, 47*(8), 1134–1141.

Ollier, W. E. R., & MacGregor, A. (1995). Genetic epidemiology of rheumatoid disease. *British Medical Bulletin, 51*, 267–285.

Pattrick, M., Manhire, A., Ward, A. M., & Doherty, M. (1989). HLA-A, B antigens and a1-antitrypsin phenotypes in nodal generalised osteoarthritis and erosive osteoarthritis. *Annals of Rheumatic Diseases, 48*, 470–475.

Peterson, L. S., Mason, T., Nelson, A. M., O'Fallon, W. M., & Gabriel, S. E. (1996). Juvenile rheumatoid arthritis in Rochester, Minnesota 1960–1993. Is the epidemiology changing? *Arthritis & Rheumatism, 39*(8), 1475–1390.

Petty, R. E., Southwood, T. R., Baum, J., Bhettay, E., Glass, D. N., Manners, P., ... Prieur, A. M. (1998). Revision of the proposed classification criteria for juvenile idiopathic arthritis: Durban, 1997. *Journal of Rheumatology, 25*, 1991–1994.

Petty, R. E., Southwood, T. R., Manners, P., Baum, J., Glass, D. N., Goldenberg, J., ... International League of Associations for Rheumatology. (2004). International League of Associations for Rheumatology. International League of Associations for Rheumatology classification of juvenile idiopathic arthritis: Second revision, Edmonton 2001. *Journal of Rheumatology, 31*, 390–392.

Pillinger, M. H., Rosenthal, P., & Abeles, A. M. (2007). Hyperuricemia and gout: New insights into pathogenesis and treatment. *Bulletin of the NYU Hospital for Joint Diseases, 65*(3), 215–221.

Prahalad, S. (2004). Genetics of juvenile idiopathic arthritis: An update. *Current Opinion in Rheumatology, 16*(5), 588–594.

Radovits, B. J., Fransen, J., Shamma, S., Eijsbouts, A. M., van Riel, P. L. C. M., & Laan, R. F. J. M. (2010). Excess mortality emerges after 10 years in an inception cohort of early rheumatoid arthritis. *Arthritis Care & Research, 62*(3), 362–370.

Reveille, J. D. (2006). Major histocompatibility genes and ankylosing spondylitis. *Best Practice & Research Clinical Rheumatology, 20*(3), 601–609.

Reveille, J. D., Ball, E. J., & Khan, M. A. (2001). HLA-B27 and genetic predisposing factors in spondyloarthropathies. *Current Opinion in Rheumatology, 13*, 265–272.

Richette, P., & Bardin, T. (2010). Gout. *Lancet, 375*(9711), 318–328.

Rider, L. G., Giannini, E. H., Bruneer, H. I., Ruperto, N., James-Newton, L., Reed, A. M., ... International Myositis Assessment and Clinical Studies Group. (2004). International consensus on preliminary definitions of improvements in adult and juvenile myositis. *Arthritis & Rheumatism, 50*, 2281–2290.

Robbins, S. L., & Cotran, R. S. (1979). *Pathologic basis of disease* (2nd ed.). Philadelphia, PA: WB Saunders Company.

Ropes, M. W., Bennet, G. A., Cobb, S., Jacox, R., & Jessar, R. A. (1958). Revision of diagnostic criteria for rheumatoid arthritis. *Bulletin on the Rheumatic Diseases, 9*, 175–176.

Schlosstein, L., Terasaki, P. I., Bluestone, R., & Pearson, C. M. (1973). High association of an HL-A antigen, W27, with ankylosing spondylitis. *The New England Journal of Medicine, 288*, 704–706.

Silman, A. J. (1988). Has the incidence of rheumatoid arthritis declined in the United Kingdom? *British Journal of Rheumatology, 27*, 77–79.

Silman, A., MacGregor, A., Thomson, W., Hooligan, S., Carty, D., & Farhan, A. (1993). Twin concordance rates for rheumatoid arthritis: Results from a nationwide study. *British Journal of Rheumatology, 32*, 903–907.

Smyth, C. J., Cotterman, C. W., & Freyberg, R. H. (1948). The genetics of gout and hyperuricemia: An analysis of nineteen families. *Journal of Clinical Investigation, 27*(6), 749–759.

Spector, T. D., & Hochberg, M. C. (1990). The protective effect of the oral contraceptive pill on rheumatoid arthritis: An overview of the analytic epidemiological studies using meta-analysis. *Journal of Clinical Epidemiology, 43*(11), 1221–1230.

Statsny, P. (1978). Association of the B cell alloantigen DRw4 with rheumatoid arthritis. *The New England Journal of Medicine, 298*, 869–871.

Stecher, R. M. (1941). Heberden's nodes: Heredity in hypertrophic arthritis of finger joints. *American Journal of the Medical Sciences, 201*, 801–809.

Storey, G. D. (2001). Alfred Baring Garrod (1819–1907). *Rheumatology (Oxford, England), 40*(10), 1189–1190.

Sugiyama, D., Nishimura, K., Tamaki, K., Tsuji, G., Nakazawa, T., Morinobu, A., & Kumagai, S. (2010). Impact of smoking as a risk factor for developing rheumatoid arthritis: A meta-analysis of observational studies. *Annals of Rheumatic Diseases, 69*, 70–81.

Symmons, D., & Harrison, B. (2000). Early inflammatory polyarthritis: Results from the Norfolk arthritis register with a review of the literature. I. Risk factors for the development of inflammatory polyarthritis and rheumatoid arthritis. *Rheumatology, 39*(8), 835–843.

Symmons, D., Mathers, C., & Pfleger, B. (2006a). Global burden of osteoarthritis in the year 2000. In C. D. Mathers et al. (Eds.), *Global burden of disease 2000*. Geneva, Switzerland: World Health Organization.

Symmons, D., Mathers, C., & Pfleger, B. (2006b). Global burden of rheumatoid arthritis in the year 2000. In C. D. Mathers et al. (Eds.), *Global burden of disease 2000*. Geneva, Switzerland: World Health Organization.

Symmons, D., Turner, G., Webb, R., Aslen, P., Barret, E., Lunt, M., … Silman, A. (2002). The prevalence of rheumatoid arthritis in the United Kingdom; new estimates for a new century. *Rheumatology, 41*(7), 793–800.

Talbott, J. H. (1940). Serum urate in relatives of gouty patients. *Journal of Clinical Investigation, 19*, 645.

Vitart, V., Rudan, I., Hayward, C., Gray, N. K., Floyd, J., Palmer, C. N., … Wright, A. F. (2008). SLC2A9 is a newly identified urate transporter influencing serum urate concentration, urate excretion and gout. *Nature Genetics, 40*(4), 437–442.

Waine, H., Nevinny, D., & Rosenthal, J. (1961). Association of osteoarthritis and diabetes mellitus. *Tufts Folia Medica, 8*, 13–19.

Walitt, B., Pettinger, M., Weinstein, A., Katz, J., Torner, J., Wasko, M. C., … for the Women's Health Initiative. (2008). Effects of postmenopausal hormone therapy on rheumatoid arthritis: The Women's Health Initiative randomized controlled trials. *Arthritis & Rheumatism, 59*(3), 302–310.

Wallace, K. L., Riedel, A. A., Joseph-Ridge, N., & Wortmann, R. (2004). Increasing prevalence of gout and hyperuricemia over 10 years among older adults in a managed care population. *Journal of Rheumatology, 31*, 1582–1587.

Wandel, S., Jüni, P., Tendal, B., Nüesch, E., Villiger, P. M., Welton, N. J., … Trelle, S. (2010). Effects of glucosamine, chondroitin, or placebo in patients with osteoarthritis of hip or knee: Network meta-analysis. *BMJ, 341*, D4675.

Weaver, A. (2008). Epidemiology of gout. *Cleveland Clinic Journal of Medicine, 75*(Suppl. 5), S9–S12.

Weinberg, J. B., Fermor, B., & Guilak, F. (2007). Nitric oxide synthase and cyclooxygenase interactions in cartilage and meniscus: Relationship to joint physiology, arthritis and tissue repair. *Subcellular Biochemistry, 42*, 31–62.

Weston, V. C., Jones, A. C., Bradbury, N., Fawthrop, F., & Doherty, M. (1999). Clinical features and outcome of septic arthritis in a single UK Health District 1982–1991. *Annals of Rheumatic Diseases, 58*(4), 214–219.

Weyand, C. M., Hicok, K. C., Conn, D. L., & Goronzy, J. J. (1992). The influence of HLADRB1 genes on disease severity in rheumatoid arthritis. *Annals of Internal Medicine, 117*(10), 801–806.

WHO. (2009). *Death and DALY estimates for 2004 by cause for WHO Member States (persons, all ages). WHO Disease and Injury Estimates*. Geneva, Switzerland: World Health Organization.

Williams, C. J., & Jimenez, S. A. (1995). Heritable diseases of cartilage caused by mutations in collagen genes. *Journal of Rheumatology, 22*, 28–33.

Yamamoto, T., Moriwaki, Y., & Takahashi, S. (2005). Effect of ethanol on metabolism of purine bases (hypoxanthine, xanthine and uric acid). *Clinica Chimica Acta, 356*(1–2), 35–57.

Zhu, Y., Pandya, B. J., & Choi, H. K. (2011). Prevalence of gout and hyperuricemia in the US general population, The National Health and Nutrition Examination Survey 2007–2008. *Arthritis & Rheumatism, 63*(10), 3136–3141.

Epidemiology of Neurological Diseases

CHAPTER 48

Epidemiology of Alzheimer's Disease

▶ Introduction

*A*lzheimer's disease is the most common form of dementia accounting for more than 50% of all cases. This incurable, degenerative, terminal disease was first described by German psychiatrist and neuropathologist, Alois Alzheimer, in 1907 (Alzheimer, 1907). Onset typically occurs after age 65 years; although there are familial forms of Alzheimer's disease that develop earlier in life.

The second most common type of dementia is *vascular dementia* which accounts for most of the remaining cases. Vascular dementia refers to loss of brain function due to decreased cerebral blood flow often secondary to mini-strokes that occlude the cerebral arterioles and smaller blood vessels. Vascular dementia is discussed later in this chapter.

The pathologic hallmark of Alzheimer's disease is a significant loss of neurons in the brain. Compared with the healthy adult brain which contains more than 100 billion neurons, the Alzheimer's brain is characterized by dramatic shrinkage from cell loss and widespread debris from dead and dying neurons. Progression of disease ultimately results in complete loss of memory and absence of normal brain function. Fatality is often due to pneumonia in a bedridden, totally incapacitated patient.

▶ Diagnosis and Progression of Alzheimer's Disease

The specific criteria used to diagnose Alzheimer's disease and other forms of dementia are defined in the *Diagnostic and Statistical Manual of Mental Disorders, Fourth Edition* (*DSM-IV*). Early symptoms of Alzheimer's disease include memory deficits, confusion, irritability, aggression, mood swings, and behavioral changes. The diagnosis is made by behavioral and cognitive tests, and brain scans that reveal characteristic morphological changes in the brain. Alzheimer's disease is characterized by the loss of neurons and synapses in the cerebral cortex and subcortical regions of the brain, particularly in the hippocampus, a key memory center in the medial temporal lobe. The loss of neurons results in marked atrophy of the affected regions. Imaging studies using *magnetic resonance imaging* (MRI) and *positron emission tomography* (PET) have documented reductions in the size of specific regions of the brain in patients as they progressed from mild cognitive impairment to Alzheimer's disease. Neuropathological studies have also documented the characteristic formation of *amyloid plaques* and *neurofibrillary tangles* in the brains of patients with Alzheimer's disease (Förstl & Kurz, 1999; Perl, 2010; Waldemar et al., 2007).

753

Analysis and quantification of biomarkers in the cerebral spinal fluid (CSF) provide molecular confirmation of Alzheimer's disease. Biomarkers in the CSF include *amyloid beta protein, tau protein and phosphorylated tau protein*, all of which are products of diseased neurons that are released into the CSF. In diseased patients, amyloid beta protein forms amyloid plaques and CSF levels are *lower than normal* whereas tau proteins form neurofibrillary tangles and CSF levels are *higher than normal*. A major problem with analyses of CSF specimens is that they are obtained by lumbar puncture, an invasive medical procedure with significant side effects, particularly among elderly patients. There is therefore an urgent need for the identification of sensitive and specific biomarkers of Alzheimer's disease in specimens obtained by minimally invasive procedures (e.g., blood samples) (Sharma & Singh, 2016).

Progression of disease brings the gradual loss of all bodily functions and, ultimately, death. Since Alzheimer's disease is incurable and progressive, patient management and care are essential. However, caregivers are often faced with overwhelming social, psychological, physical, and economic pressures.

▶ Age-Specific Incidence of Alzheimer's Disease

Alzheimer's disease predominantly strikes adults late in life. As a consequence, incidence and prevalence rates are highest in developed nations whose populations contain greater numbers of elderly people. Based on a meta-analysis of age-specific incidence data from 23 studies, Jorm and Jolley found that the incidence of Alzheimer's disease doubles for each 5-year age interval after the age of 65 years (**FIGURE 48.1**).

This corresponds to an incidence-doubling time of 5 years, definable as the chronological number of years required for the age-specific incidence to double in magnitude. Rates are slightly higher in women than men and peak during the ninth decade of life. The rates approximately double for each successive 5-year age interval, and among women over the age of 95 years, the cumulative (5-year) risk of developing Alzheimer's disease is about 50% (Jorm & Jolley, 1998).

Investigators at Johns Hopkins University recently conducted an updated meta-analysis of published age-specific incidence rates of Alzheimer's disease in order to characterize regional and gender differences in the incidence-doubling times as well as the rates. Their analysis was based upon age-specific incidence rates reported in 27 publications. Age-specific incidence rates of Alzheimer's disease were modeled by log-linear regression for men and women of six geographic regions (Africa, Asia, Europe, Latin America, North America, and Oceania). As expected, incidence rates varied considerably and were higher in women than men, and higher in populations of developed nations than developing nations. For example, the incidence at age 80 years was 1.37% for women, 1.06% for men, 2.06% for North American populations, 1.48% for European populations, and 0.83% for populations of other nations. Nevertheless, regression analysis revealed *no significant differences in* the *incidence-doubling times* by gender or by region. Overall, the incidence of Alzheimer's disease increased by about 13% with each advancing year of age, which yields an overall incidence-doubling time of 5.5 years. The homogeneity of incidence-doubling times suggests that progression of Alzheimer's disease is similar across populations, whereas differences in the magnitude of the incidence rates could reflect differences in

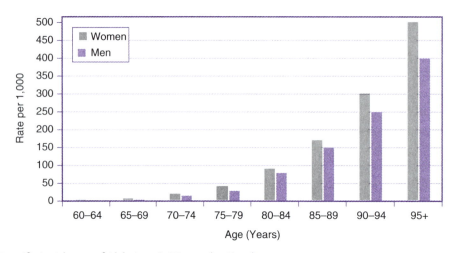

FIGURE 48.1 Age-Specific Incidence of Alzheimer's Disease by Gender.
Data from Jorm, A. F., & Jolley, D. (1998). The incidence of dementia: A meta-analysis. *Neurology, 51*, 728–733.

environmental and/or genetic factors that influence disease onset, or differences in clinical thresholds for case diagnosis (Ziegler-Graham, Brookmeyer, Johnson, & Arrighi, 2008).

▶ Global Incidence of Alzheimer's Disease

The majority of new cases of Alzheimer's disease (58%) occur among older people living in countries classified by the World Health Organization as low or middle income. Based upon meta-analysis of the available incidence data, approximately 9.9 million incident cases of dementia were diagnosed in 2015, 4.9 million in Asia, 2.5 million in Europe, 1.7 million in the Americas, and 0.8 million in Africa. The number of incident cases increased by 30% during 2010 to 2015 (from 7.7 million to 9.9 million). The worldwide upward trend in the incidence of dementia is driven primarily by the increasing number of elderly people in the world population (World Alzheimer Report, 2015).

▶ Global Prevalence of Alzheimer's Disease

According to published estimates from different sources, the number of living patients with Alzheimer's disease or other forms of dementia increased from about 24 million in 2001 to 46.8 million in 2015, an increase of more than 1.5 million prevalent cases per year. In 2015, 5.2% of the world population over 60 years of age had dementia, 6.4% in the Americas, 5.9% in Europe, 4.7% in Asia, and 4.6% in Africa (Brookmeyer, Johnson, Ziegler-Graham, & Arrighi, 2007; Ferri et al., 2005; World Alzheimer Report, 2010, 2015; World Health Organization, 2006). These data primarily reflect the increasing longevity of the world population and underscore the growing health burden of dementia in the aged. Recent reports suggest that unless effective interventions are discovered and implemented, the global prevalence of Alzheimer's disease and other forms of dementia will double every 20 years and surpass 80 million by 2040 (Brookmeyer, Gray, & Kawas, 1998; Brookmeyer et al., 2007; Ferri et al., 2005).

▶ Alzheimer's Disease: Survival and Case Fatality

Survival following the diagnosis of Alzheimer's disease is reduced by at least 50% compared to the general population. Albeit, median survival times and case fatality rates are highly variable and depend on several factors including the severity of disease at the time of diagnosis, the age and gender of the patient, the level of care, and the rate of disease progression. In general, studies of patients from different locations and in different settings reveal that younger patients survive longer than older patients, women survive longer than men, and patients with mild disability at diagnosis survive longer than those with severe disability. Selected studies of survival and related measures in patients with Alzheimer's disease are discussed in the following paragraphs.

Investigators at the University of Turku in Finland examined the survival experience of 218 patients with Alzheimer's disease and 115 patients with *vascular dementia* secondary to stroke. For the Alzheimer's patients, the 14-year survival rate was 2.4% compared to 16.6% for the general population, median survival was 5 years, and 68% of deaths were directly attributed to dementia. Advanced disability and male gender were independently found to increase the relative risk of dying by about twofold. Survival measures were similar for patients with dementia due to vascular disease (Mölsä, Marttila, & Rinne, 1986).

Investigators in the Netherlands used mortality data from the *Rotterdam Study*, a population-based prospective study of elderly adults, to estimate overall and severity-specific mortality for patients with dementia. Results revealed that dementia was associated with increased mortality in all age, sex, and disease severity groups. In comparison to healthy individuals from the Dutch population, mortality rate ratios for subjects with dementia were increased more than twofold in men (relative risk [RR] = 2.1) and women (RR = 2.3) (Witthaus, Ott, Barendregt, Breteler, & Bonneux, 1999).

Investigators at McGill University in Montreal, Canada, used data from the *Canadian Study of Health and Aging* to evaluate the survival experience of 821 subjects with dementia (486 with Alzheimer's disease, 252 with possible Alzheimer's disease, and 173 with vascular dementia). The investigators noted that previous studies failed to include persons with rapidly progressive disease who died before they could be enrolled, thus introducing a type of bias referred to as "*length or survivor bias*." After adjustment for length bias, the median survival was 3.1 years for patients with probable Alzheimer's disease, 3.5 years for patients with possible Alzheimer's disease, and 3.3 years for patients with vascular dementia. As in other studies, female gender and younger age of onset were significant predictors of longer survival. The investigators concluded that with appropriate adjustment, survival following onset of dementia is much shorter than previously thought (Wolfson et al., 2001).

Investigators at Johns Hopkins University in Baltimore, Maryland, studied the survival of 108 incident cases of Alzheimer's disease in the *Baltimore Longitudinal Study of Aging*. The median survival was 8.3 years for those diagnosed at age 65 years compared to 3.4 years for those diagnosed at age 90 years. Diagnoses at ages 65 and 90 years were associated with approximately 67% and 48% reductions in median life span, respectively (Brookmeyer, Corrada, Curriero, & Kawas, 2002).

Investigators at the University of Washington in Seattle studied the survival of 521 patients with newly recognized Alzheimer's disease. The median survival was 4.2 years in men and 5.7 years in women. Men had significantly poorer survival than women across all age groups, and survival was decreased in all age groups compared to the U.S. population (Bowen et al., 1996; Larson et al., 2004).

Investigators at Columbia University in New York studied the survival of 323 incident cases of Alzheimer's disease. The *annual case fatality rate* was slightly higher in men than women (11.6 vs. 9.9 deaths per 100 person-years) and trended upwards with age at diagnosis (7.0, 9.1, and 16.1 per 100 person-years for patients diagnosed at <75, 75–84, and 85+ years, respectively). The median survival for all patients was 6.0 years, but those diagnosed before age 75 years survived twice as long as those diagnosed after age 85 years (median survival times, 9.9 vs. 4.4 years, respectively). The presence of diabetes or hypertension at the time of diagnosis also increased the risk of death (RR = 2.57 and RR = 1.99, respectively) (Helzner et al., 2008).

Investigators at the University of Pittsburg conducted a nested case–control study of Alzheimer's disease in a community-based cohort of 1670 elderly subjects in Pennsylvania. Cases and controls were ascertained during 15 years of follow-up. Based on 330 incident cases, the overall mean survival was 5.9 years; however, survival was significantly longer for patients with earlier onset (8.3 years for onset before age 75 years vs. 3.8 years for onset at 85 years or older). There was no difference in mean survival between men and women. Based on a Cox regression analysis of 273 cases and 546 controls, the adjusted hazard ratio for mortality was 1.40, indicating that patients with Alzheimer's disease had a 40% increased risk of dying compared to those without dementia (Ganguli, Dodge, Shen, Pandav, & DeKosky, 2005).

Investigators at the University of Cambridge in England studied the survival of 438 incident cases of Alzheimer's disease or other forms of dementia ascertained from multiple centers in England and Wales. The subjects were ascertained from a population-based cohort of 13,004 individuals enrolled in 1991 and followed until 2005. The overall median survival was 4.5 years, but survival among patients diagnosed before 70 years of age was more than double that among those diagnosed after age 80 years (10.7 vs. 4.3 years, respectively). Other significant predictors of mortality included male gender and severe disability (Xie, Brayne, Matthews, & Medical Research Council Cognitive Function and Aging Study collaborators, 2008).

Investigators affiliated with the *Medical Research Council General Practice Research Framework* in London conducted a case–control study of survival involving patients from 353 general medicine practices comprising the *Health Improvement Network* in the United Kingdom. The study compared survival in 22,529 patients with dementia to 112,645 controls without dementia. In addition, the annual incidence of dementia was estimated during 1997–2007 for the entire network population. During the 11-year time frame of study, the annual incidence of dementia remained relatively stable at about four cases per 1000 person-years at risk. The median survival among patients with dementia decreased from 6.7 years for patients diagnosed before age 70 years to 1.9 years for those diagnosed at 90 years or older. Most notably, in the first year after diagnosis, the mortality rate was more than three times greater in patients with dementia than in those without (adjusted RR = 3.68). In subsequent years, the mortality rates remained more than twofold higher among patients with dementia (mean adjusted RR = 2.42). Adjustment for comorbidities and other factors had little effect on the rate ratios. The investigators suggest that *"the high risk of death in the first year after diagnosis may reflect diagnoses made at times of crisis or late in the disease trajectory"* (Rait et al., 2010).

▶ Alzheimer's Disease: Global Mortality

Similar to the incidence and prevalence, mortality rates due to Alzheimer's disease and other forms of dementias vary widely among populations around the globe. Low rates reflect short longevity as in sub-Saharan Africa where the life span is less than 60 years (e.g., in 2016, most nations in sub-Saharan Africa had mortality rates less than 10 deaths per 100,000). Intermediate mortality rates (10–39 deaths per 100,000) were characteristic of nations in Eastern Europe, Asia and South America that are in transition, whereas higher rates (40–90 deaths per 100,000) were evident in the populations of developed countries in North America and Australasia. There was a striking cluster of Western European nations with mortality rates exceeding 90 deaths per 100,000. Most notably, Japan, which has the greatest longevity in the world, also had the highest mortality rate from Alzheimer's disease in 2016 (178 deaths per 100,000). Among nations, the annual mortality from Alzheimer's disease and other forms of dementia increased with increasing longevity (Institute for Health Metrics and Evaluation, 2016).

Due to the "*epidemiologic transition*" and the gradual aging of the world population, it has become evident that the mortality due to Alzheimer's disease has increased dramatically in most populations during the past few decades. However, mortality estimates are typically based upon the reported *underlying cause of death* on death certificates, and Alzheimer's disease and other forms of dementia are often unlisted as either the principle cause or a contributing cause of death, even in decedents known to have severe antecedent dementia. In general, multiple causes of death may appear on a death certificate, but only one is the "underlying cause of death" and this is the item that is tabulated and analyzed to calculate cause-specific mortality rates.

Based upon the *underlying cause of death* listed on death certificates in the United States population, mortality rates attributed to Alzheimer's disease increased dramatically during 1979–1995, from about 2 per 100,000 in 1979 to 38 per 100,000 in 1995 among individuals over the age of 65 years. *However, mortality rates computed from death certificates with Alzheimer's disease listed as one of multiple causes are more than double the rates based on only the underlying cause of death.* For example, in 1995 Alzheimer's disease was listed as the underlying cause of death on 20,230 death certificates, while it appeared as one of multiple causes of death on 40,836 death certificates (Hoyert & Rosenberg, 1997, 1999).

Reporting inaccuracies for Alzheimer's disease and dementia has also been noted in studies of decedents known to have terminal stage disease. Investigators in Boston examined the death certificates of 165 decedents in a cohort of patients in nursing homes who had advanced dementia due to Alzheimer's disease or other forms of senile dementia. Despite the terminal nature of dementia among these individuals, neither Alzheimer's disease nor dementia was recorded on the death certificates of 37% of decedents. Furthermore, among 115 decedents diagnosed with terminal Alzheimer's disease, only 27% of death certificates mentioned Alzheimer's disease as a cause of death. These results raise concerns about the accuracy of the global mortality

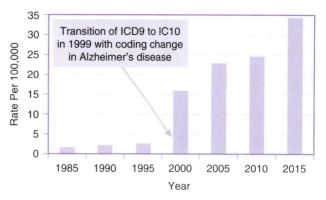

FIGURE 48.2 Trend of Annual Mortality for Alzheimer's Disease, United States, 1985–2015.

Data from Hoyert, D. L., & Rosenberg, H. M. (1999). Mortality from Alzheimer's disease: An update. *National Vital Statistics Reports*, 47(20), 1–8; Alzheimer's Association. (2010). *Alzheimer's disease facts and figures*. Washington DC: Alzheimer's Association.

statistics on Alzheimer's disease and other forms of dementia (Wachterman, Kiely, & Mitchel, 2008).

In addition to the underreporting of certain conditions such as Alzheimer's disease and dementia, changes in coding and reporting practices can have a marked influence on disease rates. Annual mortality rates attributed to Alzheimer's disease in the U.S. population during 1985–2015 are shown in **FIGURE 48.2**. It is important to note that prior to 2000, physicians completing death certificates often coded Alzheimer's disease as senile dementia, likely resulting in severe *underestimates* of cause-specific mortality. Consolidation into a single code took place in the 10th revision of the *International Classification of Diseases* (ICD), which was implemented around the turn of the century. Thus, the rates in the United States and many other populations after the year 1999 show a distinct "*jump*" compared to the prior rates due to the change in ICD coding rather than biological phenomena. Such spikes in disease rates are often a consequence of reporting changes, which must be taken into account in the examination of time trends (Griffiths & Rooney, 2006).

Irrespective of the ICD coding change in 2000, it is clear from the U.S. data that the annual mortality rates due to Alzheimer's disease are trending upward (Figure 48.2). Since the ICD coding change in 2000, the annual mortality rate from Alzheimer's disease has increased by approximately 8% per year, from 15.8 per 100,000 in 2000 to 34.4 per 100,000 in 2015 (Alzheimer's Association, 2018). Furthermore, the U.S. trends in reported mortality rates for Alzheimer's disease are consistent with those in several other developed countries including Canada, England, Australia, Norway, Japan, and Sweden (Flaten, 1989; Hallberg, 2009; Imaizumi, 1992; Jorm, Henderson, & Jacomb, 1989; Martyn & Pippard, 1988; Newman & Bland, 1987).

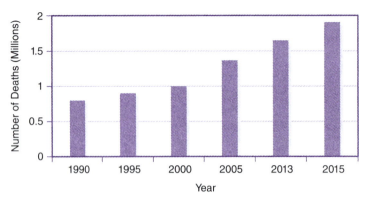

FIGURE 48.3 Global Trend in Number of Deaths for Alzheimer's Disease, 1985–2015.

Murray, C. L., & GBD 2013 Mortality and Causes of Death Collaborators. (2015). Global, regional, and national age–sex specific all-cause and cause-specific mortality for 240 causes of death, 1990–2013: A systematic analysis for the Global Burden of Disease Study 2013. *The Lancet, 385*, 117–171; Wang, H., & GBD 2015 Mortality and Causes of Death Collaborators. (2016). Global, regional, and national life expectancy, all-cause mortality, and cause-specific mortality for 249 causes of death, 1980–2015: A systematic analysis for the Global Burden of Disease Study 2015. *The Lancet, 388*(10053), 1459–1544.

In these countries as in the United States, mortality rates attributable to Alzheimer's disease have increased dramatically.

In recent years, estimates of the number of deaths and mortality rates have been reported by investigators of the *Institute of Health Metrics and Evaluation* (IHME) based upon compilation of the underlying causes listed on death certificates and ascertained from verbal autopsies in 21 regions of the world. For countries with incomplete data, estimates of deaths and mortality from Alzheimer's disease and other dementias were based upon prevalence studies and excess mortality.

FIGURE 48.3 shows the rising trend in number of deaths from Alzheimer's disease and other forms of dementia during 1990–2015. In 2015, there were 1.91 million deaths from Alzheimer's disease or other forms of dementia, approximately 2.4 times the number estimated in 1990 (796,000). Nevertheless, the global mortality rate changed little during the period, 28.9 per 100,000 in 1990 and 29.9 per 100,000 in 2013 (Murray & GBD 2013 Mortality and Causes of Death Collaborators, 2015; Wang et al., 2016).

The major factor responsible for the increasing incidence, prevalence, and mortality rates of Alzheimer's disease is undoubtedly the increasing longevity in populations throughout the world. It is also likely that greater awareness of symptoms among physicians has increased the recording of Alzheimer's disease on death certificates. Obviously, it is important to separate increases due to death certificate diagnoses because of growing awareness of the disease from true increases caused by biological changes in pathogenesis. Although death rates represent a potential measure of the public health impact of Alzheimer's disease, variations in the accuracy of diagnosis and in the completion of death certificates limit the value of mortality data in estimating the true burden of this disease.

▶ Alzheimer's Disease: Disability-Adjusted Life Years

FIGURE 48.4 shows the global pattern of disability-adjusted life years (DALY) lost from Alzheimer's disease and other forms of dementia during 2004. The highest DALY are evident in the older populations of the developed world including North America, Western Europe, Scandinavia, Australasia, and Japan. Based on estimates reported by the World Health Organization, dementia contributed 11.2% of years lived with disability in people aged 60 years and older, which is more than stroke, musculoskeletal disorders, cardiovascular disease, and all forms of cancer. The disability burden for dementia, estimated by an international and multidisciplinary expert consensus, was higher than all other health conditions, apart from spinal-cord injury and terminal cancer.

▶ Burden of Alzheimer's Disease in the United States

In the year 2018, approximately 5.7 million Americans were living with Alzheimer's dementia. Of these, 5.5 million were 65 years or older and the remaining 200,000 cases had early onset disease. By current estimates, 484,000 new cases of Alzheimer's disease are being diagnosed each year in the U.S. population and more than 50% are at least 85 years of age (Alzheimers Association, 2018).

During 2000–2015, the age-adjusted annual mortality due to Alzheimer's disease increased by about 120%, making it the sixth leading cause of death in the United States (Figure 48.2). Based on review of the underlying cause of death listed on death certificates, 110,561 (4.1%) of the 2.71 million deaths

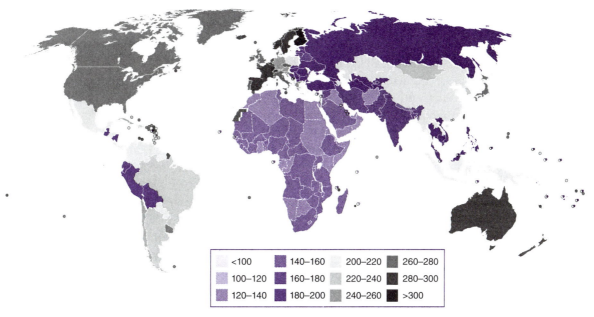

FIGURE 48.4 DALY: Alzheimer's Disease and Dementia, 2004.

Data from World Health Organization. (2008). *The global burden of disease: 2004 update.* Geneva: WHO. Available at www.who.int/evidence/bod

Disability Adjusted Life Years per 100,000 individuals.

that occurred in the United States during 2015 were attributed to Alzheimer's disease. Alzheimer's disease was also a *contributing cause* to more than 500,000 deaths where comorbid conditions were listed as the underlying causes on death certificates (Alzheimer's Association, 2016, 2018; Heron, 2016; Xu, Kochaniek, Murphy, & Tejada-Vera, 2010).

Alzheimer's disease was responsible for 5.7% of female deaths compared to 2.7% of male deaths in 2015. A large proportion of the excess disease in women is due to their greater longevity and the fact that old age is the greatest risk factor for Alzheimer's disease (Heron, 2016).

Patients with Alzheimer's disease typically suffer a slow insidious progression of dementia and disability before death. A composite measure of the burden of disease is the DALY calculated from the *Years of Life Lost due to Disability* (YLD) and the *Years of Life Lost due to Premature Death* (YLL): DALY = YDL + YLL. Both YDL and YLL contribute significantly to the *DALY* lost from Alzheimer's disease. In 2015, DALY due to Alzheimer's disease ranked 12th among all diseases in the United States, increasing from the rank of 25th in 1990 (Heron, 2016).

▶ Pathology of Alzheimer's Disease

Alzheimer's disease is characterized by the loss of neurons and synapses in the cerebral cortex and subcortical regions of the brain. The loss of neurons results in marked atrophy of the affected regions. Imaging studies using *MRI* and *PET* have documented reductions in the size of specific regions of the brain in patients as they progressed from mild cognitive impairment to Alzheimer's disease (Waldemar et al., 2007).

Postmortem studies of the brains of Alzheimer's patients have revealed distinct features including diminished brain size, increased ventricle size, characteristic plaques and tangles in the white matter, and millions of dead or dying neurons. Using a silver staining technique, Alois Alzheimer and his contemporary rival, Oskar Fischer, first identified neuritic plaques and neurofibrillary tangles in postmortem specimens of cerebral cortex from afflicted patients (Goedert, 2009). The neurofibrillary tangles characteristic of Alzheimer's brains are laden with *beta-amyloid* and deranged *tau protein* that are associated with pathogenesis and the loss of neuronal function (Tiraboschi, Hansen, Thal, & Corey-Bloom, 2004).

Amyloid plaques and neurofibrillary tangles are clearly visible by microscopy in brains of those afflicted by Alzheimer's disease. Neurofibrillary tangles are aggregates of a microtubule-associated protein, *tau protein*, which has become hyperphosphorylated and accumulates inside the neurons. Amyloid plaques are made up of small peptide fragments called *beta-amyloid*. Beta-amyloid is derived from a larger transmembrane protein, *amyloid precursor protein*, that is critical for neuron growth, survival, and postinjury repair. In Alzheimer's disease, the degradation of amyloid precursor protein is disrupted and fibrils of beta-amyloid form clumps that deposit outside neurons in dense formations known as senile plaques (Turner, O'Connor, Tate, & Abraham, 2003).

In his initial studies, Alzheimer noted the presence of *inflammation* and *gliosis* in postmortem specimens of brain tissue from afflicted patients. The inflammatory response is typically localized around beta-amyloid plaques and is characterized by influx of proinflammatory microglia and astrocytes (Akiyama et al., 2002). Furthermore, biochemical markers of inflammation such as cyclooxygenase-2 (COX-2), complement factors, and certain chemokines and cytokines have been found in excess in brain tissues of Alzheimer's patients (Yasojima, Schwab, McGeer, & McGeer, 2000). The sequence of pathogenesis of Alzheimer's disease has not yet been determined, and it is unknown whether inflammation is an *effect* of the disease process or a *causative factor* in the initiation and progression of disease.

Recent molecular studies have noted reduced concentrations of *beta-amyloid* and increased concentrations of *tau protein* in the cerebrospinal fluid of most patients with Alzheimer's disease (Marksteiner, Hinterhuber, & Hinterhuber, 2007). Furthermore, in follow-up studies of subjects with mild cognitive impairment, these CSF biomarkers were found to accurately predict progression to Alzheimer's disease, suggesting they may have a role in the early detection of disease (De Meyer et al., 2010).

▶ Risk Factors of Alzheimer's Disease

The primary risk factor for Alzheimer's disease is age. As initially suggested by Jorm and Jolley and confirmed by others, the incidence doubles every 5 years after 65 years of age for men and women of all populations studied (Jorm & Jolley, 1998; Ziegler-Graham et al., 2008). Nevertheless, postmortem studies of the brains of centenarians reveal that Alzheimer's disease and/or other forms of brain pathology are not always the inevitable outcome of the aging process (den Dunnen et al., 2008).

Alzheimer's Disease and Cardiovascular Risk Factors

In patients with Alzheimer's disease, cerebral infarcts due to mini-strokes often contribute to the progression of disease, and most cases display not only the characteristic pathologic findings of Alzheimer (amyloid deposition, neurofibrillary tangles, and inflammation) but also atherosclerosis, ischemia, and disruption of the blood brain barrier (Querfurth & LaFerla, 2010). *Indeed, all of the classical risk factors for ischemic heart*

disease and stroke have been found to increase the risk of Alzheimer's disease. Selected studies of smoking, hypertension, hypercholesterolemia, hyperglycemia, and obesity are discussed in the following paragraphs.

The mortality rates due to cardiovascular diseases such as ischemic heart disease and stroke have declined substantially during the last few decades in populations of many developed nations. These declines have primarily been attributed to reductions in cigarette smoking, coupled with effective detection and treatment of heart disease, hypertension, diabetes and hyperlipidemia, plus regular exercise, improved nutrition, and possibly the intake of low-dose aspirin. Since there is some evidence implicating cardiovascular risk factors in the development of neurodegenerative diseases, investigators have searched for corresponding trends in the development of Alzheimer's disease and other forms of dementia. Correlative secular trends are evident in two such studies conducted in the United States and Japan.

A team of investigators from multiple U.S. centers investigated secular trends in the age-specific prevalence and incidence rates of Alzheimer's disease and dementia in elderly cohorts from communities in Minnesota, Illinois, and Indiana, and in the nationwide *U.S. Health and Retirement Study*. Results of the study were mixed. In the cohorts from individual communities, there were no significant trends in either the incidence or the prevalence of Alzheimer's disease or dementia. However, in the *Health and Retirement* cohort, the prevalence of dementia declined from 12.2% in 1993 to 8.7% in 2002, suggesting that public health and medical interventions targeting cardiovascular conditions may also have had a favorable impact on neurological health (Rocca et al., 2011).

Investigators at Kyushu University in Fukuoka, Japan, examined secular trends in the prevalence of Alzheimer's disease and vascular dementia in a prospective cohort residing in the rural community of Hisayama. The study included four cross-sectional examinations conducted in 1985, 1992, 1998, and 2005. Results revealed a significant increase in the age- and gender-adjusted prevalence of Alzheimer's disease and all-cause dementia. The overall prevalence of Alzheimer's disease increased from 1.1% in 1985 to 3.8% in 2005. The greatest prevalence increase, from 5% in 1985 to 15% in 2005, was observed among individuals aged 80 years and older. These results suggest that increasing rates of metabolic disorders such as obesity, hypercholesterolemia, and glucose intolerance may be associated with the rising prevalence of Alzheimer's disease in the Japanese population (Sekita et al., 2010).

Hypertension, Hypercholesterolemia, and Alzheimer's Disease

As part of a longitudinal study in Gothenburg, Sweden, a team of neuroscientists analyzed the relation between blood pressure and the development of dementia among 382 elderly adults. The cohort was followed for up to 15 years and participants were examined periodically to detect neurological changes. Participants who developed dementia at age 79 years or older had significantly higher mean systolic and diastolic blood pressures at baseline compared to those who remained disease free (178 vs. 164 mm Hg, and 101 vs. 92 mm Hg, respectively). Furthermore, dementia cases with cerebral white matter lesions (mini-infarcts) by computed tomography had significantly higher baseline blood pressure levels than control subjects. It was also noted that the blood pressures of cases declined to lower levels in the years just before diagnosis. The investigators concluded that long-standing hypertension may increase the risk of developing dementia by inducing small vessel disease and white matter lesions in the brain (Skoog et al., 1996).

The *Honolulu Heart Program* of the *Honolulu Asian Aging Study* was designed to investigate the association of midlife blood pressure and the development of Alzheimer's disease or other forms of dementia in Japanese-American men. Participants (*n* = 3703) were enrolled and examined during 1965–1971 and subsequently reexamined in 1991. Odds ratios (OR) were estimated for baseline levels of systolic and diastolic blood pressure with stratification by the presence/absence of treatment with antihypertensive medications. Estimates were adjusted for age, education, apolipoprotein (APOEε4) genotype, smoking, and alcohol intake. Among untreated subjects with elevated blood pressure at baseline, the risk of developing Alzheimer's disease or dementia was significantly increased compared to normotensive subjects. Elevated diastolic levels resulted in fourfold risk increases (OR = 3.8 for 90–94 mm Hg and OR = 4.3 for 95 mm Hg or higher) and elevated systolic levels increased the risk nearly fivefold (OR = 4.8 for 160 mm Hg or higher). Notably, men who received antihypertension therapy were not at increased risk. These results suggest that untreated hypertension during middle age is a significant risk factor for the development of dementia later in life (Launer et al., 2000).

Investigators at the University of Kuopio in Finland examined associations of blood pressure and serum cholesterol with the development of Alzheimer's disease in a prospective population-based study in eastern Finland. Participants were enrolled in 1972

and followed for an average of 21 years. A total of 1449 participants took part in the study. The results revealed that hypertension (systolic blood pressure exceeding 160 mm Hg) and hypercholesterolemia (serum cholesterol exceeding 240 mg per dL) diagnosed in midlife (mean age, 54 years) were independently associated with increased risks of developing Alzheimer's disease later in life (mean onset, 75 years). Compared to subjects with normal blood pressure and serum cholesterol, the odds of developing disease were increased more than twofold in subjects with hypertension (OR = 2.3) or hypercholesterolemia (RR = 2.1), and the disease odds increased more than threefold for subjects with both risk factors (OR = 3.5). These findings suggest that high blood pressure and elevated cholesterol are risk factors, not only for cardiovascular disease, but also for Alzheimer's disease and dementia (Kivipelto et al., 2001).

Several randomized placebo-controlled clinical trials have been conducted to evaluate effects of antihypertensive medications in reducing the risk of developing dementia or slowing progression of disease. The results of these investigations are mixed, with some showing benefit and others not.

In an extended study of patients enrolled in the double-blind, placebo-controlled *Systolic Hypertension in Europe (Syst-Eur) Trial*, 1485 elderly patients continued therapy with antihypertensive agents (primarily nitrendipine) whereas 1417 control subjects were not treated. During 3.9 years of total follow-up, the mean systolic blood pressure in the treated group was 7.0 mm Hg less than the untreated group, and the incidence rate of dementia in the treated group was 55% less than in the untreated group (3.3 cases vs. 7.4 cases per 1000 person-years). After adjustment for age, gender, entry blood pressure, and other factors, the hazard ratio for patients treated with the long acting antihypertensive agent, nitrendipine, was 0.38 (Forette et al., 2002).

The *Perindopril Protection Against Recurrent Stroke Study (PROGRESS)* was a randomized, double-blind, placebo-controlled clinical trial designed to evaluate the development of dementia with and without active treatment to control blood pressure among patients with a prior history of stroke or transient ischemic attacks. A total of 6105 subjects were randomized to receive either antihypertensive medications (perindopril with or without indapamide) or placebo. During a mean follow-up of 3.9 years, 193 (6.3%) of 3051 treated subjects developed dementia compared to 217 (7.1%) of 3054 subjects who received placebo, a risk reduction of 12%. Furthermore, cognitive decline occurred less often in the treatment group compared to the placebo group (9.1% vs. 11.0%). Patients who suffered recurrent strokes were found to benefit the most from active blood pressure therapy (Tzourio et al., 2003).

In the *Hypertensive Old People in Edinburgh (HOPE)* study, 81 elderly dementia-free individuals with hypertension were treated with antihypertensive medications (captopril or bendrofluazide) for 6 months and evaluated for cognitive changes from baseline by a battery of psychometric tests. Individuals with the greatest reductions in systolic blood pressure (at least 19 mm Hg) had significantly improved cognition compared to those with reductions of 5 mm Hg or less (Starr, Whalley, & Deary, 1996).

While these studies suggest that long-term adequate blood pressure control may reduce the risk of developing dementia and improve cognition in subjects with hypertension, other studies have failed to disclose any significant benefit of therapy. Additional well-designed clinical trials will be required to clarify the effects of medications that lower blood pressure on cognitive decline (Reitz, Brayne, & Mayeux, 2011).

Smoking and Alzheimer's Disease

Epidemiologic investigations of smoking and Alzheimer's disease have yielded mixed results with some showing increases in the risk and others showing decreases. To clarify the findings and eliminate possible biases, investigators at the University of California in San Francisco conducted a meta-analysis of the relationship between smoking and Alzheimer's disease with adjustment for study design, study quality, secular trends, and *tobacco affiliation of study authors.* Analysis of 14 cohort studies without tobacco industry affiliation yielded a significantly increased relative risk (RR = 1.45) whereas analysis of three studies *with* tobacco industry affiliation yielded a decreased relative risk (RR = 0.60). Limiting the analysis to only cohort studies with at least average quality (based on scientific journal impact score) yielded an even higher relative risk (RR = 1.74). Based upon analysis of those studies *without tobacco industry affiliation*, the investigators concluded that smoking is a significant risk factor for the development of Alzheimer's disease (Cataldo, Prochaska, & Glantz, 2010).

Insulin Resistance, Diabetes, and Alzheimer's Disease

Several epidemiologic investigations have examined the risk of developing Alzheimer's disease in subjects with insulin resistance and/or diabetes. In the U.S. Framingham community-based prospective cohort,

202 elderly participants with diabetes mellitus and 2008 subjects of similar age without diabetes were identified for study. All subjects were dementia-free at baseline, and risk subgroups were defined by apolipoprotein E genotype and plasma homocysteine levels. Individuals were followed for up to 20 years to detect incident cases of Alzheimer's disease. Among subjects *without* apolipoprotein E4 or elevated plasma homocysteine, the risk of developing Alzheimer's disease was increased nearly threefold in diabetic versus non-diabetic subjects (RR = 2.98). The effect of diabetes in this group was strongest for subjects aged 75 years or older (RR = 4.77). The investigators concluded that diabetes may increase the risk in the absence of other known risk factors (Akomolafe et al., 2006).

Similar results were reported for a community-based cohort of 1173 elderly individuals in Sweden. At baseline, all subjects were free of dementia and diabetes, but 47 subjects had "*borderline diabetes*" with plasma glucose levels in the range, 120–140 mg per dL. During 9 years of follow-up, 487 subjects developed dementia and 207 developed Alzheimer's disease. Borderline diabetes at baseline was associated with an increased risk of developing dementia (HR = 1.67) or Alzheimer's disease (HR = 1.77). In stratified analyses, the risk associated with antecedent borderline diabetes was found entirely in those individuals who were *noncarriers* of the APOEε4 allele. Furthermore, the presence of severe systolic hypertension was found to accentuate the risk in individuals with borderline diabetes (Xu, Qiu, Winblad, & Fratiglioni, 2007).

Investigators at New York Upstate Medical University examined associations of Alzheimer's disease with body mass, diabetes, metabolic syndrome, and insulin resistance by meta-analyses of published prospective epidemiologic investigations. For the nine studies that focused on diabetes, the pooled estimate of risk was significantly elevated (RR = 1.54) and the test for heterogeneity was not significant (Profenno, Porsteinsson, & Faraone, 2010).

Despite these epidemiologic findings of an association between antecedent diabetes and the development of Alzheimer's disease, other studies that have incorporated neuropathologic examination of postmortem brain specimens from decedents with dementia have failed to confirm the link. For example, a team of investigators in Chicago examined the neuropathology of postmortem specimens from 233 elderly men who underwent extensive annual neurological evaluations prior to death. While antecedent diabetes was associated with increased odds of cerebral infarction (OR = 2.47), no association was found between diabetes and pathologically confirmed Alzheimer's disease (Arvanitakis et al., 2006).

Some randomized clinical trials have shown that antidiabetic drugs are of benefit to patients with cognitive impairment. In a paired crossover study conducted at the Veteran's Administration Hospital in Seattle, Washington, 26 memory-impaired subjects and 35 normal controls were given either intranasal insulin or saline on separate occasions to assess acute effects on cognition. Insulin administration was found to facilitate recall in memory-impaired subjects who were negative for *APOEε4,* but not in subjects who were positive for *APOEε4* or in normal control subjects (Reger et al., 2005).

Other studies also suggest that the cognitive benefit of antidiabetic therapy in patients with Alzheimer's disease may be genotype-specific for APOEε4. Investigators in North Carolina studied cognitive effects of the oral diabetic medication, *rosiglitazone,* in a randomized clinical trial of 511 patients diagnosed with mild to moderate Alzheimer's disease. Rosiglitazone belongs to a class of drugs that modulate the nuclear membrane receptor, *peroxisome proliferator-activated receptor (PPAR)-γ.* Subjects were evaluated at baseline and after 24 weeks of study. Overall, no significant differences in cognition were detected between patients receiving therapy at any dose of rosiglitazone and those receiving placebo. However, on stratification for *APOEε4* genotype, patients who were negative for *APOEε4* achieved significant benefit from treatment, whereas those who were *positive* for *APOEε4* did not (Risner et al., 2006).

It is also noteworthy that a randomized clinical trial conducted in Japan found that administration of a PPAR-γ agonist, pioglitazone, improved cognitive function in patients with type 2 diabetes and mild Alzheimer's disease (Sato et al., 2009). In animal models of Alzheimer's disease, PPARγ agonists have been shown to inhibit inflammatory gene expression, alter amyloid β peptide homeostasis, and exhibit neuroprotective effects (Jiang, Heneka, & Landreth, 2008).

Obesity and Alzheimer's Disease

Epidemiologic investigations have also focused on the development of Alzheimer's disease in overweight and obese individuals. In Sweden, a representative cohort of 482 adults without dementia at baseline were followed from age 70 to 88 years to evaluate associations of body mass, blood pressure, smoking, and other factors with the development of Alzheimer's disease. During 18 years of follow-up, 93 participants developed dementia. Results revealed that among women, for every unit increase in body mass index, the risk of Alzheimer's disease increased by 36% (Gustafson, Rothenberg, Blennow, Steen, & Skoog, 2003).

In the United States, investigators examined associations between body mass during midlife and the subsequent development of Alzheimer's disease or vascular dementia in a large and diverse cohort (*n* = 10,136) consisting of members of the *Kaiser-Permanente Health Care Delivery System.* Participants were examined at ages 40–45 years and later assessed for neurological disease an average of 36 years later. Compared to individuals with normal body mass index (BMI < 25) in midlife, obese subjects (BMI > 30) were at increased risk for Alzheimer's disease (HR = 3.10) and vascular dementia (HR = 5.01). Furthermore, individuals overweight during midlife (BMI = 25–30) were found to have a twofold increase in the risk of developing either condition. These findings suggest that increased body mass during midlife is a significant risk factor for the development of Alzheimer's disease or vascular dementia late in life (Whitmer, Gunderson, Quesenberry, Zhou, & Yaffe, 2007).

As noted in the previous section, investigators at New York Upstate Medical University examined associations of Alzheimer's disease with body mass and diabetes by meta-analyses of published prospective epidemiologic investigations. Combining data from nine studies, they found that diabetes increased the risk of developing Alzheimer's disease (combined RR = 1.54). For the eight studies that examined effects of obesity, the pooled estimate of risk was also elevated (RR = 1.59), but there was significant heterogeneity among studies, possibly due to differences in the age of participants at enrollment and length of follow-up (Profenno et al., 2010).

While *midlife obesity* appears to be a risk factor for Alzheimer's disease late in life, many subjects who develop dementia have been found to *lose* a significant amount of weight shortly before diagnosis. Changes in weight were closely monitored over 20 years in a prospective cohort study of 134 men and 165 women living in southern California. During follow-up, 36 men and 24 women were diagnosed with Alzheimer's disease. Compared to individuals who remained normal, significant weight losses were evident in both men and women who later developed Alzheimer's disease (Barrett-Connor, Edelstein, Corey-Bloom, & Wiederholt, 1996).

A component of the *Honolulu–Asia Aging Study* was designed to assess the relationship between weight change and the development of dementia. In this population-based investigation, 1890 Japanese-American men were weighed on six separate occasions between 1965 and 1999 and screened for dementia during 1991–1999. The 112 cases that developed dementia during the study were compared to 1778 controls who remained free of neurological disease. Though there were no differences in weight between cases and controls in the first 26 years of study, during the 6-year period prior to diagnosis of dementia, cases had excess average weight loss (~2 kg) compared to controls (Stewart et al., 2005). Weight loss in association with Alzheimer's disease is also associated with greater disease severity, accelerated progression of disease, and increased mortality (White, Pieper, & Schmader, 1998).

Homocysteine and Alzheimer's Disease

Homocysteine is an amino acid that differs from cysteine by the addition of a single methyl group. Blood levels of homocysteine are reduced by B vitamins such as riboflavin and folic acid and some epidemiologic studies have found that high homocysteine levels and low levels of the B vitamins increase the risk of developing cardiovascular disease. However, in a recent review and meta-analysis of eight randomized clinical trials involving 24,210 participants, there was no evidence that homocysteine-lowering interventions at any dosage or in any combination reduces the risk of developing myocardial infarction, stroke, or other cardiovascular conditions (Martí-Carvajal, Solà, Lathyris, & Salanti, 2009).

Investigators at Boston University conducted a prospective cohort study of 1062 elderly adults (667 women and 425 men) to examine the relation of plasma homocysteine and the development of dementia. The study cohort was derived from participants in the *Framingham Study*. Homocysteine and other variables (age, gender, apolipoprotein E genotype, folic acid, and other cardiovascular risk factors) were measured at baseline. Over a median follow-up of 8 years, dementia developed in 111 subjects including 83 cases of Alzheimer's disease. Results revealed significant risk increases in dementia (adjusted RR = 1.4) and Alzheimer's disease (adjusted RR = 1.8) with each one standard deviation increase in the log-transformed level of homocysteine. Among individuals with baseline homocysteine levels exceeding 14 μmol per L, the risk of Alzheimer's disease nearly doubled. These results suggest that elevated plasma homocysteine may be an independent risk factor for the development of Alzheimer's disease and dementia (Seshadri et al., 2002). Nevertheless, results of randomized clinical trials of homocysteine reduction are required before recommendations can be made about the use of B vitamins for the prevention of dementia (Clarke, 2007).

Estrogen Replacement Therapy and Alzheimer's Disease

Some epidemiologic investigations have found that estrogen replacement therapy (ERT) exerts a protective effect against the development of Alzheimer's disease. Investigators from the University of Southern California explored ERT and the development of Alzheimer's disease in a nested case–control study within the prospective *Leisure World Cohort Study* of 8877 elderly women. Leisure World is a retirement community in Laguna Hills, California. Among 2529 women who died during 1981–1992, 138 cases of Alzheimer's disease were identified. Controls were matched to the cases at a 4:1 ratio by birth date and death date. Results revealed a significant reduction in the odds of developing Alzheimer's disease among ERT users compared to nonusers (OR = 0.69) suggesting that ERT may be useful for preventing or delaying the onset of dementia (Paganini-Hill & Henderson, 1994).

Investigators from Columbia University studied effects of ERT in 1124 elderly women who were initially free of Alzheimer's disease, Parkinson's disease, and stroke, and who were taking part in a longitudinal study of aging and health in a New York City community. Overall, 156 of the women reported taking estrogen after onset of menopause. Results revealed a significant reduction in risk among ERT users compared to nonusers (RR = 0.40), and furthermore, the onset of Alzheimer's disease was significantly delayed in women who used ERT. Notably, none of 23 women who were taking estrogen at study enrollment developed Alzheimer's disease. The investigators concluded that estrogen use in postmenopausal women may delay the onset and decrease the risk of Alzheimer's disease (Tang et al., 1996).

In the *U.S. Baltimore Longitudinal Study of Aging*, 472 postmenopausal women were followed for up to 16 years to examine the incidence of Alzheimer's disease among those who received ERT versus those who did not. Thirty-four incident cases were detected, nine among ERT users and 25 among nonusers (RR = 0.46), indicating that ERT may have significant chemopreventive activity against Alzheimer's disease (Kawas et al., 1997).

A team of U.S. investigators examined gender differences in the incidence of dementia among 1357 men and 1889 women as well as effects of ERT in women residing in Cache County, Utah, during 1995–2000. Compared to nonusers, women who used ERT for 10 or more years had a reduced risk of developing Alzheimer's disease (26 cases among 1066 users compared with 58 cases among 800 nonusers, adjusted

HR = 0.41). Women who used ERT were also at lower risk than men (HR = 0.77) (Zandi et al., 2002).

The *Women's Health Initiative (WHI)* included two randomized double-blind, placebo-controlled clinical trials of hormone replacement therapy (HRT) to assess effects on cardiovascular outcomes such as myocardial infarction and stroke, certain cancers (breast cancer, endometrial cancer, colon cancer), and several other conditions. A component of these trials, the *Women's Health Initiative Memory Study (WHIMS)*, assessed effects of HRT on the development of dementia *in women who were at least 65 years of age*. Two trials were conducted in the WHI, estrogen plus progesterone (*n* = 4532 women), and estrogen therapy alone (*n* = 2947 women). Women who were randomized to receive active hormones received conjugated equine estrogens, 0.625 mg each day, and medroxyprogesterone acetate, 2.5 mg each day. Those in the estrogen plus progestin arm were followed from 1995 to 2002, and those in the estrogen arm were followed from 1995 to 2004. In the estrogen plus progestin trial, 61 women developed dementia, of whom 40 were receiving estrogen plus progestin, and 21 receiving placebo, yielding a hazard ratio of 2.05. In the estrogen trial, 47 participants were diagnosed with dementia, 28 receiving estrogen, and 19 receiving placebo, yielding a hazard ratio of 1.49. When data from the two treatment arms were pooled, the overall hazard ratio for HRT was 1.76. The results of these randomized clinical trials therefore suggest that HRT *increases* rather than decreases the risk of developing dementia among elderly women (Shumaker et al., 2003, 2004).

In brief, HRT was found to *increase* rather than decrease the risk of heart attack, stroke, and blood clots. Risk increases were also noted for breast cancer and endometrial cancer whereas risk reductions were noted for colon cancer and bone fractures (osteoporosis). Obviously, the risk benefit ratio from these studies does not favor the administration of postmenopausal estrogens.

The WHIMS results conflict with the findings of many epidemiologic studies wherein women who began taking HRT coincident with the onset of menopause had a *lower* risk of developing Alzheimer's disease or dementia. The WHIMS findings of higher rates of dementia among elderly women who received estrogen alone or estrogen plus progesterone compared to those who received placebo were therefore surprising. Albeit, it is strenuously argued by some investigators that administration of HRT to women 65 years of age or older in the WHIMS component of WHI was too late in life to offer protection.

In 2008, investigators of the Cochran Collaboration conducted a meta-analysis of effects of HRT (estrogen alone or estrogen plus progestogen) compared to placebo on cognitive function in postmenopausal women. Their analysis used data from 16 randomized double-blinded clinical trials that included 10,114 postmenopausal women followed for an average of 4–5 years. Results showed that HRT did not improve cognition and in fact, cognitive function tests were lower in women receiving HRT than those receiving placebo although the differences were not statistically significant (Lethaby et al., 2008). Thus, even though some observational studies suggest beneficial effects HRT on cognition and mental status, the overall evidence does not support administration of HRT to preserve cognitive function or prevent dementia in postmenopausal women (Barrett-Connor & Laughlin, 2009).

Nonsteroidal Anti-Inflammatory Drugs and Alzheimer's Disease

Since Alzheimer's disease has an inflammatory component, a number of epidemiologic investigations have examined *nonsteroidal anti-inflammatory drugs (NSAIDs)* as possible chemopreventive agents. Recently, a team of epidemiologists at Johns Hopkins University conducted a meta-analysis of these studies. Combining the data from five prospective studies, they found significant risk reductions with regular use of nonaspirin NSAIDs (RR = 0.71) or aspirin (RR = 0.83). The combined data from eight case–control studies showed even greater risk reductions (RR = 0.47 for nonaspirin NSAIDS and RR = 0.55 for aspirin). These findings suggest that regular use of NSAIDs, particularly nonaspirin NSAIDs such as ibuprofen, may protect against the development of Alzheimer's disease (Szekely, Town, & Zandi, 2007).

Certain other drugs may also have chemopreventive potential against the development of Alzheimer's disease. For example, a few studies have reported risk reductions among individuals taking agents with antiangiogenic effects such as lipid-lowering statins, histamine H2 receptor blockers, and calcium channel blockers. It has been noted that inflammation and ischemia, two key factors in the pathogenesis of dementia and Alzheimer's disease, are powerful stimulants of angiogenesis in blood vessels. Some investigators therefore recommend a new focus of laboratory and clinical studies to assess the effects of *angiogenesis* in the pathogenesis of Alzheimer's disease (Vagnucci & Li, 2003).

▶ Genetics of Alzheimer's Disease

Most cases of Alzheimer's disease are sporadic with no evidence of genetic predisposition. Nevertheless, 5%–10% of cases are familial, whereby multiple relatives of a multigenerational pedigree are affected. In such multigenerational pedigrees, certain genes have been found to influence the onset of Alzheimer's disease.

Presenilin 1

The *presenilin 1 gene (PSEN1)* located on the long arm of chromosome 14 was identified by Sherrington et al. (1995). Multiple missense mutations of the *PSEN1* gene cause familial Alzheimer's disease. In such families, individuals who inherit a mutated *PSEN1* gene nearly always develop Alzheimer's disease before age 50 years. The *PSEN1* protein is an essential component of the enzymatic complex, γ-secretase, that cleaves amyloid beta peptide from amyloid precursor protein. Mutant forms of *PSEN1* disrupt the process causing deposition of beta-amyloid fragments in and around neurons.

Presenilin 2

The *presenilin 2 gene (PSEN2)* located on the long arm of chromosome 1 is very similar in structure and function to *PSEN1,* and mutations in *PSEN2* also cause familial Alzheimer's disease. As with *PSEN1,* mutant forms of *PSEN2* cause early onset of disease. The gene was identified in the laboratories of Rudolph Tanzi and Gerry Schellenberg in 1995 (Levy-Lahad et al., 1995). A subsequent study showed that *PSEN1* and *PSEN2* proteins are both expressed in mammalian neuronal cells (Kovacs et al., 1996). The *PSEN2* protein is also a critical component of the enzymatic complex, γ-secretase, that cleaves amyloid beta peptide from amyloid precursor protein.

Amyloid Beta Precursor Protein

Mutations in the gene that encodes *amyloid beta precursor protein (APP)* also cause familial Alzheimer's disease. Specifically, individuals who inherit mutations that modify expression of the APP gene located on the long arm of chromosome 21 are at increased risk. Furthermore, virtually all individuals with Down syndrome (trisomy 21) who have an extra copy of the APP gene develop Alzheimer's disease before age 40 years (Tanzi & Parson, 2000).

Apolipoprotein E4

Apolipoproteins are proteins that bind to lipids (such as cholesterol and fatty acids) to form macromolecules called *lipoproteins,* which in turn transport lipids through the blood and lymph. Apolipoproteins also serve as coenzymes in important catalytic reactions such as the formation of arachidonic acid from other fatty acids by *lipoprotein lipase* and transfer of fatty acids in lecithin to cholesterol to form cholesterol esters by *lecithin-cholesterol-acyl-transferase.* Furthermore, apolipoproteins are ligands for tissue specific receptors in the distribution of lipids to target tissues throughout the body.

Six major classes of apolipoproteins have been identified (A, B, C, D, E, and H) plus several subclasses and hundreds of polymorphic forms. Apolipoproteins were initially identified and classified according to function by investigators at the U.S. National Institutes of Health (Fredrickson, Levy, & Lees, 1967).

The apolipoprotein, APOE, is encoded by a gene on the long arm of chromosome 19. Several alleles have been identified at the APOE locus, and individuals who carry the allele for *apolipoprotein-E4, APOEε4,* are at increased risk for the development of Alzheimer's disease and atherosclerosis (Pericak-Vance et al., 1991). Apolipoproteins carry cholesterol and fatty acids in the blood, and they also bind to proteins, including *APP,* and target them for biodegradation. In individuals with APOEε4, there is diminished binding of amyloid precursor protein leading to accumulation of amyloid in the brain and other tissues (Bertram & Tanzi, 2008; Jiang et al., 2008).

Sortilin-Related Receptor

Normal expression of the *sortilin-related receptor 1 (SORL1) gene* is essential for the recycling of amyloid precursor protein within neurons, and mutant forms of the gene have been found to promote the accumulation of excess amyloid b peptide in neuronal tissues. The neuronal accumulation of amyloid b peptide is a central event in the pathogenesis of Alzheimer's disease. The *SORL1* gene is located on chromosome 1 and is a member of a family of transmembrane receptors that are highly expressed in the central nervous system. The protein, *sortilin,* and the family of sortilin receptors work in concert with *apolipoprotein b* to regulate the uptake, sorting, intracellular transport, and release of proteins and very low density lipoproteins.

Rogaeva et al. (2007) examined genetic associations between Alzheimer's disease and single nucleotide polymorphisms of genes known to regulate vacuolar protein sorting, including *SORL1,* among more than 6000 individuals from familial and population studies. They identified two genetic variants of *SORL1* associated with an increased risk of developing Alzheimer's disease late in life, and suggested that inherited or acquired changes in *SORL1* expression or function are in the causal pathway of pathogenesis.

These initial findings have been replicated in several subsequent studies and validated in a meta-analysis of all published data on *SORL1* and Alzheimer's disease from studies conducted in the United States, the Netherlands, Canada, Belgium, the United Kingdom, Singapore, Japan, Sweden, Germany, France, and Italy. Upon pooling the data for 12,464 cases of Alzheimer's disease and 17,929 controls and making adjustments for multiple testing, several single nucleotide polymorphisms of the *SORL1* gene were discovered in distinct linkage disequilibrium blocks in association with significant increases in the risk of developing Alzheimer's disease (Reitz et al., 2011).

Insulin-Degrading Enzyme

Insulin-degrading enzyme is a zinc-binding protease of the metalloprotease family capable of cleaving short polypeptides. This enzyme was first identified by its ability to degrade the beta chain of the polypeptide hormone, insulin. In 2001, Japanese investigators Igor Kurochkin and Sataro Goto discovered that insulin-degrading enzyme can degrade amyloid β peptide, the principal component of amyloid that accumulates in the pathogenesis of Alzheimer's disease (Kurochkin & Goto, 1994). Subsequently, both in vitro and *in vivo* studies have consistently shown an association between the expression of insulin-degrading enzyme, amyloid β degradation, and the development of Alzheimer's disease (Qiu & Folstein, 2006). For example, genetically engineered "knockout" mice lacking both alleles of the *insulin-degrading enzyme (IDE) gene* exhibit a 50% decrease in amyloid β degradation resulting in cerebral accumulation of amyloid and onset of Alzheimer's symptoms (Farris et al., 2003). Furthermore, human studies of genetically inherited forms of Alzheimer's disease show reduction in both the genetic expression and catalytic activity of IDE among affected individuals (Cook et al., 2003; Kim et al., 2007).

It has been noted that deficiencies of IDE can be caused by genetic variation or by the diversion of enzymatic biodegradation from amyloid β to insulin in the presence of hyperinsulinemia. Furthermore, medications that target diabetes, insulin resistance, and hyperinsulinemia have been found to improve cognition in only those Alzheimer's patients who are

negative for *APOEε4* (the gene that predisposes to late onset Alzheimer's disease). Further studies are obviously needed to clarify the cascade of pathogenesis and identify genotype-specific molecular targets for the effective prevention and therapy of Alzheimer's disease (Qiu & Folstein, 2006). An added complexity is achieving the physiologically appropriate balance between the degradation of insulin and amyloid β in the human brain.

▶ Vascular Dementia

Vascular dementia (often referred to as *multi-infarct dementia*) is the second most common form of dementia in older adults. This form of dementia accounts for approximately 30% of all dementia cases. It is caused by thrombotic and/or embolic occlusion of small cerebral blood vessels. Impedance of blood flow produces ischemia and infarction of brain tissue, eventually leading to diminished brain function and dementia.

In recent years, there is growing recognition that many cases of dementia in elderly patients involve a combination of pathogenic processes, most commonly those that characterize Alzheimer's disease and ischemic cerebrovascular disease. As noted earlier in this chapter, Alzheimer's disease and vascular dementia often coexist, especially in older patients with dementia, and there are many cardiovascular risk factors that are common to both conditions including hypertension, smoking, ischemic heart disease, hypercholesterolemia, insulin resistance, and diabetes mellitus (Hébert & Brayne, 1995).

▶ Lewy Body Dementia

Lewy body dementia is characterized microscopically by the presence of Lewy bodies which are clumps of *alpha-synuclein* and *ubiquitin* protein in neurons, detectable in postmortem brain specimens. The synucleins are intracellular proteins that appear to regulate vesicular transport processes in neurons (Lavedan, 1998). Ubiquitin is a ubiquitous molecule that tags other proteins for degradation in the proteosomes of the cell. The 2004 Nobel Prize in Chemistry was awarded jointly to Aaron Ciechanover, Avram Hershko, and Irwin Rose for their discovery of ubiquitin-mediated protein degradation (Ciechanover, Hershko, & Rose, 2004).

Other features of Lewy body dementia include the loss of *cholinergic neurons* and declining levels of the neurotransmitter, *acetylcholine*. The presenting signs and symptoms of Lewy body dementia overlap with other neurodegenerative conditions, particularly Parkinson's disease. However, disease onset is typically acute and progression is rapid, which distinguishes this form of dementia from Alzheimer's disease and vascular dementia, which show a more gradual course (Okasaki, Lipkin, & Aronson, 1961).

Lewy bodies are named after the German neurologist, Friedrich Lewy, who described eosinophilic, intracytoplasmic inclusion bodies in the neurons of the *substantia nigra* and other regions of the brain in postmortem specimens from patients with Parkinson's disease (Lewy, 1912). Lewy body dementia is distinguished from Parkinson's disease by the rapid onset of dementia within one year of the onset of Parkinsonian symptoms (bradykinesia, rigidity, and gait disturbance) and the presence of recurrent hallucinations and delusional behavior, which rarely occur in patients with Parkinson's disease. Patients with Lewy body dementia are also hypersensitive to neuroleptic medications and may become catatonic and develop life-threatening muscle rigidity on administration of commonly used drugs such as haloperidol or thioridazine (Weintraub & Hurtig, 2007).

Lewy body dementia accounts for approximately 10% of all forms of dementia. As in other dementias, its prevalence increases with age, and peak onset occurs in the seventh decade of life. Men are afflicted slightly more often than women. While most cases of Lewy body dementia are sporadic, kindreds with familial disease have been reported, some involving genetic mutations in the *alpha-synuclein gene* (*SNCA*) on chromosome 4 (Obi et al., 2008).

▶ Mixed Forms of Dementia

FIGURE 48.5 shows the profile of dementias based upon pathology and neuroimaging data collected in the Hisayama study of elderly men and women in Japan. During 1985–2002, 251 patients developed dementia and were evaluated by either postmortem pathology ($n = 164$) or neuroimaging ($n = 87$). As shown, the most common form of dementia in the study was Alzheimer's disease, which accounted for about 48% of all dementias. Alzheimer's disease was also found in 8% of the cases with combined pathologies. *Vascular dementia* accounted for about 30% of dementias but also contributed to another 5% of cases in combination with Alzheimer's disease. Likewise, Lewy body dementia constituted 5% of dementias, but was also found in about 6% of patients with either Alzheimer's disease or vascular dementia. The three principal entities, Alzheimer's disease, vascular dementia, and Lewy body dementia, alone or in combination, comprised approximately 95% of all dementias (Matsui et al., 2009). It is noteworthy that dementia involving combinations of these pathologies have been found to reflect the additive effects of each of the independent neuropathies (Schneider, Arvanitakis, Bang, & Bennett, 2007).

Though the predominant form of dementia diagnosed among living patients is Alzheimer's disease, recent results from the Honolulu–Asia Aging study suggest there is often a lack of agreement between the clinical diagnosis and postmortem neuropathological findings. Investigators at Kuakini Medical Center in Honolulu compared clinical and postmortem neuropathological findings for 363 Japanese-American

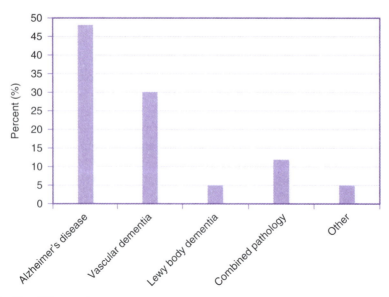

FIGURE 48.5 Pathologic Profile of Dementia.

Data from Matsui, Y., Tanizaki, Y., Arima, H., Yonemoto, K., Doi, Y., Ninomiya, T., & Sasaki, K. (2009). Incidence and survival of dementia in a general population of Japanese elderly: The Hisayama study. *Journal of Neurology, Neurosurgery, and Psychiatry*, 80, 366–370.

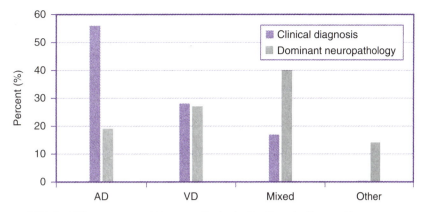

FIGURE 48.6 Comparison of Clinical Diagnoses and Neuropathologic Findings in Dementia.

men diagnosed with dementia during life. The results reflect a predominance of cases clinically diagnosed with Alzheimer's disease (56%) compared to only 19% based upon neuropathologic findings. Mixed pathologies accounted for 40% of cases by neuropathology compared to only 17% by clinical assessment. Among the cases with mixed neuropathologic findings, 10% manifested Lewy bodies and approximately 20% manifested Alzheimer's disease combined with vascular dementia. Approximately 14% of cases did not manifest any dominant neuropathologic features (**FIGURE 48.6**). The investigators state that "*the results suggest that clinical diagnosis of dementia made during life may fail to reflect the pathogenic complexity of this condition in very elderly persons.*" Nevertheless, they also note that there is an interval of time between the clinical diagnosis and death "*which is sufficiently long and variable that imperfect correlations with functioning during life are to be expected*" (White et al., 2005).

▶ Prevention of Dementia

Dementing illnesses attributable to mixed pathologies (Alzheimer's disease, vascular dementia, and Lewy body dementia) become progressively more common with advancing age, as expected on the basis of the strong associations of all three of these processes with aging. Currently available medications provide only modest clinical benefits once a patient has developed dementia. Avoidance of cardiovascular risk factors coupled with the early detection and effective treatment of hypertension, hyperlipidemia, and hyperinsulinemia, and prevention of ischemic strokes by the administration of anticoagulants in patients with atrial fibrillation or thromboembolic conditions therefore constitute a reasonable strategy to reduce the onset of mixed forms of dementia and progression of cognitive decline in old age (Langa, Foster, & Larson, 2004; WHO, 2003, 2006).

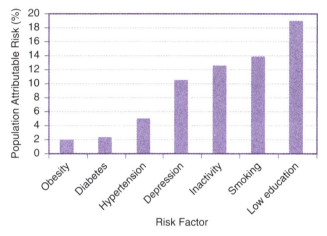

FIGURE 48.7 Population Attributable Risk: Alzheimer's Disease.

Data from Barnes, D. E., & Yaffe, K. (2011). The projected effect of risk factor reduction on Alzheimer's disease prevalence. *The Lancet Neurology, 10*(9), 819–828.

Recently, Deborah Barnes and Kristine Yaffe comprehensively reviewed the available epidemiologic literature to estimate the global risk attributable to seven modifiable risk factors (hypertension, diabetes mellitus, obesity, smoking, depression, physical inactivity, and low education) and project effects of reducing exposure levels. For each risk factor, the RR was estimated by meta-analysis and the prevalence (*q*) was estimated by combining the data from current population surveys. The population attributable risk is the proportion of people with disease in the population that can be attributed to a given risk factor (assuming the relative risk is an accurate measure of causation). The results revealed that about half of all prevalent cases worldwide are attributable to the seven selected risk factors (**FIGURE 48.7**). Based upon a projection for the world population, the investigators suggest that risk reductions of 25% in all seven factors could potentially prevent 3 million cases of Alzheimer's disease per year (Barnes & Yaffe, 2011).

References

Akiyama, H., Barger, S., Barnum, S., Bradt, B., Bauer, J., Cole, G. M., ... Finch, C. E. (2002). Inflammation and Alzheimer's disease. *Neurobiology of Aging, 21*(3), 383–421.

Akomolafe, A., Beiser, A., Meigs, J. B., Au, R., Green, R. C., Farrer, L. A., ... Seshadri, S. (2006). Diabetes mellitus and risk of developing Alzheimer disease: Results from the Framingham Study. *Archives of Neurology, 63*(11), 1551–1555.

Alzheimer, A. (1907). Über eine eigenartige Erkrankung der Hirnrinde [About a peculiar disease of the cerebral cortex]. *Allgemeine Zeitschrift fur Psychiatrie und Psychisch-Gerichtlich Medizin, 64*(1–2), 146–148.

Alzheimer's Association. (2010). *Alzheimer's disease facts and figures.* Washington, DC: Alzheimer's Association.

Alzheimer's Association. (2016). 2016 Alzheimer's disease facts and figures. *Alzheimers Dement, 12*(4), 459–609.

Alzheimer's Association. (2018). *Mortality and morbidity. 2018 Alzheimer's disease facts and figures.* Chicago, IL: Alzheimer's Association.

Arvanitakis, Z., Schneider, J. A., Wilson, R. S., Li, Y., Arnold, S. E., Wang, Z., & Bennett, D. A. (2006). Diabetes is related to cerebral infarction but not to AD pathology in older persons. *Neurology, 67*, 1960–1965.

Barnes, D. E., & Yaffe, K. (2011). The projected effect of risk factor reduction on Alzheimer's disease prevalence. *Lancet Neurology, 10*(9), 819–828.

Barrett-Connor, E., Edelstein, S. L., Corey-Bloom, J., & Wiederholt, W. C. (1996). Weight loss precedes dementia in community-dwelling older adults. *Journal of the American Geriatrics Society, 44*, 1147–1152.

Barrett-Connor, E., & Laughlin, G. A. (2009). Endogenous and exogenous estrogen, cognitive function, and dementia in postmenopausal women: Evidence from epidemiologic studies and clinical trials. *Seminars in Reproductive Medicine, 27*(3), 275–282.

Bertram, L., & Tanzi, R. E. (2008). Thirty years of Alzheimer's disease genetics: The implications of systematic meta-analyses. *Nature Reviews Neuroscience, 9*(10), 768–778.

Bowen, J. D., Malter, A. D., Sheppard, L., Kukull, W. A., McCormick, W. C., Teri, L., & Larson, E. B. (1996). Predictors of mortality in patients diagnosed with probable Alzheimer's disease. *Neurology, 47*(2), 433–448.

Brookmeyer, R., Corrada, M. M., Curriero, F. C., & Kawas, C. (2002). Survival following a diagnosis of Alzheimer disease. *Archives of Neurology, 59*, 1764–1767.

Brookmeyer, R., Gray, S., & Kawas, C. (1998). Projections of Alzheimer's disease in the United States and the public health impact of delaying disease onset. *American Journal of Public Health, 88*(9), 1337–1342.

Brookmeyer, R., Johnson, E., Ziegler-Graham, K., & Arrighi, H. M. (2007). Forecasting the global burden of Alzheimer's disease. *Alzheimer's and Dementia, 3*(3), 186–191.

Cataldo, J. K., Prochaska, J. J., & Glantz, S. A. (2010). Cigarette smoking is a risk factor for Alzheimer's disease: An analysis controlling for tobacco industry affiliation. *Journal of Alzheimer's Disease, 19*(2), 465–480.

Ciechanover, A., Hershko, A., & Rose, I. (2004). *The Nobel Prize in chemistry 2004.* Stockholm, Sweden: The Royal Swedish Academy of Sciences.

Clarke, R. (2007). Homocysteine, B vitamins, and the risk of dementia. *American Journal of Clinical Nutrition, 85*(2), 329–330.

Cook, D. G., Leverenz, J. B., McMillan, P. J., Kulstad, J. J., Ericksen, S., Roth, R. A., ... Craft, S. (2003). Reduced hippocampal insulin-degrading enzyme in late-onset Alzheimer's disease is associated with the apolipoprotein E-ε4 allele. *The American Journal of Pathology, 162*(1), 313–319.

De Meyer, G., Shapiro, F., Vanderstichele, H., Vanmechelen, E., Engelborghs, S., De Deyn, P. P., ... Alzheimer's Disease Neuroimaging Initiative. (2010). Diagnosis-independent Alzheimer disease biomarker signature in cognitively normal elderly people. *Archives of Neurology, 67*(8), 949–956.

den Dunnen, W. F., Brouwer, W. H., Bijlard, E., Kamphuis, J., van Linschoten, K., Eggens-Meijer, E., & Holstege, G. (2008). No disease in the brain of a 115-year-old woman. *Neurobiology of Aging, 29*(8), 1127–1132.

Farris, W., Mansourian, S., Chang, Y., Lindsley, L., Eckman, E. A., Frosch, M. P., ... Guenette, S. (2003). Insulin-degrading enzyme regulates the levels of insulin, amyloid beta-protein, and the beta-amyloid precursor protein intracellular domain in vivo. *Proceedings of National Academy of Sciences of the United States of America, 100*(7), 4162–4167.

Ferri, C. P., Prince, M., Brayne, C., Brodaty, H., Fratiglioni, L., Manguli, M., ... Alzheimer's Disease International. (2005). Global prevalence of dementia: A Delphi consensus study. *Lancet, 366*, 2112–2117.

Flaten, T. P. (1989). Mortality from dementia in Norway, 1969–1983. *Journal of Epidemiology & Community Health, 43*, 285–289.

Forette, F., Seux, M. L., Staessen, J. A., Thijs, L., Babarskiene, M. R., Babeanu, S., ... Systolic Hypertension in Europe Investigators. (2002). The prevention of dementia with antihypertensive treatment: New evidence from the Systolic Hypertension in Europe (Syst-Eur) study. *Archives of Internal Medicine, 162*(18), 2046–2052.

Förstl, H., & Kurz, A. (1999). Clinical features of Alzheimer's disease. *European Archives of Psychiatry and Clinical Neuroscience, 249*(6), 288–290.

Fredrickson, D. S., Levy, R. I., & Lees, R. S. (1967). Fat transport in lipoproteins—An integrated approach to mechanisms and disorders. *New England Journal of Medicine, 276*(1), 34–42.

Ganguli, M., Dodge, H. H., Shen, C., Pandav, R. S., & DeKosky, S. T. (2005). Alzheimer disease and mortality: A 15-year epidemiological study. *Archives of Neurology, 62*(5), 779–784.

Griffiths, C., & Rooney, C. (2006). Trends in mortality from Alzheimer's disease, Parkinson's disease and dementia, England and Wales, 1979–2004. *Health Statistics Quarterly, 30*, 6–14.

Gustafson, D., Rothenberg, E., Blennow, K., Steen, B., & Skoog, I. (2003). An 18-year follow-up of overweight and risk of Alzheimer disease. *Archives of Internal Medicine, 163*, 1524–1528.

Hallberg, O. (2009). Is increased mortality from Alzheimer's disease in Sweden a reflection of better diagnostics? *Current Alzheimer Research, 6*(6), 471–475.

Hébert, R., & Brayne, C. (1995). Epidemiology of vascular dementia. *Neuroepidemiology, 14*, 240–257.

Helzner, E. P., Scarmeas, N., Cosentino, S., Tang, M. X., Schupf, N., & Stern, Y. (2008). Survival in Alzheimer disease, a multiethnic, population-based study of incident cases. *Neurology, 71*(19), 1489–1495.

Heron, M. (2016). Deaths: Leading causes for 2015. *National Vital Statistics Reports 2016, 66*(5), 1–76. (Hyattsville, MD: National Center for Health Statistics.)

Hoyert, D. L., & Rosenberg, H. M. (1997). Alzheimer's disease as a cause of death in the United States. *Public Health Reports, 112*, 497–505.

Hoyert, D. L., & Rosenberg, H. M. (1999). Mortality from Alzheimer's disease: An update. *National Vital Statistics Reports, 47*(20), 1–8.

Imaizumi, Y. (1992). Mortality rate of Alzheimer's disease in Japan: Secular trends, marital status, and geographical variations. *Acta Neurologica Scandinavica, 86*(5), 501–505.

Jiang, Q., Heneka, M., & Landreth, G. E. (2008). The role of peroxisome proliferator-activated receptor-gamma (PPARγ) in Alzheimer's disease: Therapeutic implications. *CNS Drugs, 22*, 1–14.

Jiang, Q., Lee, C. Y., Mandrekar, S., Wilkinson, B., Cramer, P., Zelcer, N., … Landreth, G. E. (2008). ApoE promotes the proteolytic degradation of amyloid beta. *Neuron (United States: Cell Press), 58*(5), 681–693.

Jorm, A. F., Henderson, A. S., & Jacomb, P. A. (1989). Regional differences in mortality from dementia in Australia: An analysis of death certificate data. *Acta Psychiatrica Scandinavica, 79*, 179–185.

Jorm, A. F., & Jolley, D. (1998). The incidence of dementia: A meta-analysis. *Neurology, 51*, 728–733.

Kawas, C., Resnick, S., Morrison, A., Brookmeyer, R., Corrada, M., Zonderman, A., … Metter, E. (1997). A prospective study of estrogen replacement therapy and the risk of developing Alzheimer's disease. *The Baltimore Longitudinal Study of Aging. Neurology, 48*(6), 1517–1521.

Kim, M., Hersh, L. B., Leissring, M. A., Ingelsson, M., Matsui, T., Farris, W., … Tanzi, R. E. (2007). Decreased catalytic activity of the insulin-degrading enzyme in chromosome 10-linked Alzheimer disease families. *Journal of Biological Chemistry, 282*(11), 7825–7832.

Kivipelto, M., Helkala, E. L., Laakso, M. P., Hänninen, T., Hallikainen, M., Alhainen, K., … Nissinen, A. (2001). Midlife vascular risk factors and Alzheimer's disease in later life: Longitudinal, population based study. *BMJ, 322*(7300), 1447–1451.

Kovacs, D. M., Fausett, H. J., Page, K. J., Kim, T. W., Moir, R. D., Merriam, D. E., … Wasco, W. (1996). Alzheimer-associated presenilins 1 and 2: Neuronal expression in brain and localization to intracellular membranes in mammalian cells. *Nature Medicine, 2*, 224–229.

Kurochkin, I. V., & Goto, S. (1994). Alzheimer's beta-amyloid peptide specifically interacts with and is degraded by insulin degrading enzyme. *FEBS Letters, 345*(1), 33–37.

Langa, K. M., Foster, N. L., & Larson, E. B. (2004). Mixed dementia: Emerging concepts and therapeutic implications. *JAMA, 292*(23), 2901–2908.

Larson, E. B., Shadlen, M. F., Wang, L., McCormick, W. C., Bowen, J. D., Teri, L., & Kukull, W. A. (2004). Survival after initial diagnosis of Alzheimer disease. *Annals of Internal Medicine, 140*, 501–509.

Launer, L. J., Ross, G. W., Petrovitch, H., Masaki, K., Foley, D., White, L. R., & Havlik, R. J. (2000). Midlife blood pressure and dementia: The Honolulu-Asia aging study. *Neurobiology of Aging, 21*, 49–55.

Lavedan, C. (1998). The synuclein family. *Genome Research, 8*(9), 871–880.

Lethaby, A., Hogervorst, E., Richards, M., Yesufu, A., & Yaffe, K. (2008). Hormone replacement therapy for cognitive function in postmenopausal women. *Cochrane Database of Systematic Reviews*, 1, doi: 10.1002/14651858.

Levy-Lahad, E., Wasco, W., Poorkaj, P., Romano, D. M., Oshima, J. M., Pettingell, W. H., … Tanzi, R. E. (1995). Candidate gene for the chromosome 1 familial Alzheimer's disease locus. *Science, 269*, 973–977.

Lewy, F. H. (1912). Paralysis agitans. In M. Lewandowsky (Ed.), *Handbuch der neurologie* (pp. 920–933). Berlin, Germany: Springer Verlag.

Marksteiner, J., Hinterhuber, H., & Hinterhuber, C. (2007). Cerebrospinal fluid biomarkers for diagnosis of Alzheimer's disease: Beta-amyloid(1-42), tau, phospho-tau-181 and total protein. *Drugs Today, 43*(6), 423–431.

Martí-Carvajal, A. J., Solà, I., Lathyris, D., & Salanti, G. (2009). Homocysteine lowering interventions for preventing cardiovascular events. *Cochrane Database Systematic Reviews, 4*, CD006612.

Martyn, C. N., & Pippard, E. C. (1988). Usefulness of mortality data in determining the geography and time trends of dementia. *Journal of Epidemiology & Community Health, 42*, 134–137.

Matsui, Y., Tanizaki, Y., Arima, H., Yonemoto, K., Doi, Y., Ninomiya, T., & Sasaki, K. (2009). Incidence and survival of dementia in a general population of Japanese elderly: The Hisayama study. *Journal of Neurology, Neurosurgery & Psychiatry, 80*, 366–370.

Mölsä, P. K., Marttila, R. J., & Rinne, U. K. (1986). Survival and cause of death in Alzheimer's disease and multi-infarct dementia. *Acta Neurologica Scandinavica, 74*(2), 103–107.

Murray, C. L., and GBD 2013 Mortality and Causes of Death Collaborators. (2015). Global, regional, and national age–sex specific all-cause and cause-specific mortality for 240 causes of death, 1990–2013: A systematic analysis for the Global Burden of Disease Study 2013. *The Lancet, 385*, 117–171.

Newman, S. C., & Bland, R. C. (1987). Canadian trends in mortality from mental disorders, 1965–1983. *Acta Psychiatrica Scandinavica, 76*, 1–7.

Obi, T., Nishioka, K., Ross, O. A., Terada, T., Yamazaki, K., Sugiura, A., … Hattori, N. (2008). Clinicopathologic study of a SNCA gene duplication patient with Parkinson disease and dementia. *Neurology, 70*(3), 238–241.

Okasaki, H., Lipkin, L. E., & Aronson, S. M. (1961). Diffuse intracytoplasmic inclusions (Lewy type) associated with progressive dementia and quadriparesis in flexion. *Journal Neuropathology and Experimental Neurology, 20*, 237–244.

Paganini-Hill, A., & Henderson, V. W. (1994). Estrogen deficiency and risk of Alzheimer's disease in women. *American Journal of Epidemiology, 140*, 256–261.

Pericak-Vance, M. A., Bebout, J. L., Gaskell, P. C., Jr., Yamaoka, L. H., Hung, W. Y., Alberts, M. J., … Roses, A. D. (1991). Linkage studies in familial Alzheimer disease: Evidence for chromosome 19 linkage. *American Journal of Human Genetics, 48*(6), 1034–1050.

Perl, D. P. (2010). Neuropathology of Alzheimer's disease. *Mount Sinai Journal of Medicine, 77*(1), 32–42.

Profenno, L. A., Porsteinsson, A. P., & Faraone, S. V. (2010). Meta-analysis of Alzheimer's disease risk with obesity, diabetes, and related disorders. *Biological Psychiatry, 67*(6), 505–512.

Qiu, W. Q., & Folstein, M. F. (2006). Insulin, insulin-degrading enzyme and amyloid-beta peptide in Alzheimer's disease: Review and hypothesis. *Neurobiology of Aging, 27*(2), 190–198.

Querfurth, H. W., & LaFerla, F. M. (2010). Alzheimer's disease. *New England Journal of Medicine, 362*, 329–344.

Rait, G., Walters, K., Bottomley, C., Petersen, I., Iliffe, S., & Nazareth, I. (2010). Survival of people with clinical diagnosis of dementia in primary care: Cohort study. *BMJ, 341*, c3584.

Reger, M. A., Watson, G. S., Frey, W. H., II, Baker, L. D., Cholerton, B., Keeling, M. L., … Craft, S. (2005). Effects of intranasal insulin on cognition in memory-impaired older adults: Modulation by APOE genotype. *Neurobiology of Aging, 27*(3), 451–458.

Reitz, C., Brayne, C., & Mayeux, R. (2011). Epidemiology of Alzheimer disease. *Nature Reviews Neurology, 7*(3), 137–152.

Reitz, C., Cheng, R., Rogaeva, E., Lee, J. H., Tokuhiro, S., Zou, F., … Genetic and Environmental Risk in Alzheimer Disease 1 Consortium. (2011). Meta-analysis of the association between variants in SORL1 and Alzheimer disease. *Archives of Neurology, 68*(1), 99–106.

Risner, M. E., Saunders, A. M., Altman, J. F., Ormandy, G. C., Craft, S., Foley, I. M., … Rosiglitazone in Alzheimer's Disease Study Group. (2006). Efficacy of rosiglitazone in a genetically defined population with mild-to-moderate Alzheimer's disease. *The Pharmacogenomics Journal, 6*(4), 246–254.

Rocca, W. A., Petersen, R. C., Knopman, D. S., Hebert, L. E., Evans, D. A., Hall, K. S., … White, L. R. (2011). Trends in the incidence and prevalence of Alzheimer's disease, dementia, and cognitive impairment in the United States. *Alzheimers & Dementia, 7*(1), 80–93.

Rogaeva, E., Men, Y., Lee, J. H., Gu, Y., Kawarai, T., Zou, F., … St. George-Hyslop, P. (2007). The neuronal sortilin-related receptor SORL1 is genetically associated with Alzheimer disease. *Nature Genetics, 48*, 168–177.

Sato, T., Hanyu, H., Hirao, K., Kanetaka, H., Sakura, H., & Iwamoto, T. (2009). Efficacy of PPAR-γ agonist pioglitazone in mild Alzheimer disease. *Neurobiology of Aging, 32*(9), 1626–1633. doi:10.1016/j.neurobiolaging.2009.10.009.

Schneider, J. A., Arvanitakis, Z., Bang, W., & Bennett, D. A. (2007). Mixed brain pathologies account for most dementia cases in community-dwelling older persons. *Neurology, 69*(24), 2197–2204.

Sekita, A., Ninomiya, T., Tanizaki, Y., Doi, Y., Hata, J., Yonemoto, K., … Kiyohara, Y. (2010). Trends in prevalence of Alzheimer's disease and vascular dementia in a Japanese community: The Hisayama Study. *Acta Psychiatrica Scandinavica, 122*(4), 319–325.

Seshadri, S., Beiser, A., Selhub, J., Jacques, P. F., Rosenberg, I. H., D'Agostino, R. B., … Wolf, P. A. (2002). Plasma homocysteine as a risk factor for dementia and Alzheimer's disease. *New England Journal of Medicine, 346*(7), 476–483.

Sharma, N., & Singh, A. N. (2016). Exploring biomarkers for Alzheimer's disease. *Journal of Clinical Diagnostic Research, 10*(7), KE01–KE06.

Sherrington, R., Rogaev, E. I., Liang, Y., Rogaeva, E. A., Levesque, G., Ikeda, M., … St. George, P. H. (1995). Cloning of a gene bearing missense mutations in early-onset familial Alzheimer's disease. *Nature, 375*, 754–760.

Shumaker, S. A., Legault, C., Kuller, L., Rapp, S. R., Thal, L., Lane, D. S., … Women's Health Initiative Memory Study. (2004). Conjugated equine estrogens and incidence of probable dementia and mild cognitive impairment in postmenopausal women. Women's Health Initiative Memory Study. *JAMA, 291*(24), 2947–2958.

Shumaker, S. A., Legault, C., Rapp, S. R., Thal, L., Wallace, R. B., Ockene, J. K., … WHIMS Investigators. (2003). Estrogen plus progestin and the incidence of dementia and mild cognitive impairment in postmenopausal women: The Women's Health Initiative Memory Study: A randomized controlled trial. *JAMA, 289*, 2651–2662.

Skoog, I., Lernfelt, B., Landahl, S., Palmertz, B., Andreasson, L. A., Nilsson, L., … Svanborg, A. (1996). 15-Year longitudinal study of blood pressure and dementia. *Lancet, 347*, 1141–1145.

Starr, J. M., Whalley, L. J., & Deary, I. J. (1996). The effects of antihypertensive treatment on cognitive function: Results from the HOPE study. *Journal of the American Geriatrics Society, 44*(4), 411–415.

Stewart, R., Masaki, K., Xue, Q. L., Peila, R., Petrovitch, H., & White, L. R. (2005). A 32-year prospective study of change in body weight and incident dementia: The Honolulu-Asia Aging Study. *Archives of Neurology, 62*, 55–60.

Szekely, C. A., Town, T., & Zandi, P. P. (2007). NSAIDs for the chemoprevention of Alzheimer's disease. *Subcellular Biochemistry, 42*, 229–248.

Tang, M. X., Jacobs, D., Stern, Y., Marder, K., Schofield, P., Gurland, B., … Mayeux, R. (1996). Effect of oestrogen during menopause on risk and age at onset of Alzheimer's disease. *Lancet, 348*(9025), 429–432.

Tanzi, R., & Parson, A. (2000). *Decoding darkness: The search for the genetics causes of Alzheimer's disease.* Cambridge, MA: Perseus Press.

Tiraboschi, P., Hansen, L. A., Thal, L. J., & Corey-Bloom, J. (2004). The importance of neuritic plaques and tangles to the development and evolution of AD. *Neurology, 62*(11), 1984–1989.

Turner, P. R., O'Connor, K., Tate, W. P., & Abraham, W. C. (2003). Roles of amyloid precursor protein and its fragments in regulating neural activity, plasticity and memory. *Progress in Neurobiology, 70*(1), 1–32.

Tzourio, C., Anderson, C., Chapman, N., Woodward, M., Neal, B., MacMahon, S., … PROGRESS Collaborative Group. (2003). Effects of blood pressure lowering with perindopril and indapamide therapy on dementia and cognitive decline in patients with cerebrovascular disease. *Archives of Internal Medicine, 163*(9), 1069–1075.

Vagnucci, A. H., Jr., & Li, W. W. (2003). Alzheimer's disease and angiogenesis. *Lancet, 361*, 605–608.

Wachterman, M., Kiely, D. K., & Mitchel, S. L. (2008). Reporting dementia on the death certificates of nursing home residents dying with end-stage dementia. *JAMA, 300*(22), 2608–2610.

Waldemar, G., Dubois, B., Emre, M., Georges, J., McKeith, I. G., Rossor, M., … Winblad, B. (2007). Recommendations for the diagnosis and management of Alzheimer's disease and other disorders associated with dementia: EFNS guideline. *European Journal of Neurology, 14*(1), e1–e26.

Wang, H., & GBD 2015 Mortality and Causes of Death Collaborators. (2016). Global, regional, and national life expectancy, all-cause mortality, and cause-specific mortality for 249 causes of death, 1980–2015: A systematic analysis for the Global Burden of Disease Study 2015. *The Lancet, 388*(10053), 1459–1544.

Weintraub, D., & Hurtig, H. I. (2007). Presentation and management of psychosis in Parkinson's disease and dementia with Lewy bodies. *American Journal of Psychiatry, 164*(10), 1491–1498.

White, H., Pieper, C., & Schmader, K. (1998). The association of weight change in Alzheimer's disease with severity of disease and mortality: A longitudinal analysis. *Journal of the American Geriatrics Society, 46*, 1223–1227.

White, L., Small, B. J., Petrovitch, H., Ross, G. W., Masaki, K., Abbott, R. D., ... Markesbery, W. (2005). Recent clinical-pathologic research on the causes of dementia in late life: Update from the Honolulu-Asia Aging Study. *Journal of Geriatric Psychiatry and Neurology, 18*(4), 224–227.

Whitmer, R. A., Gunderson, E. P., Quesenberry, C. P., Jr., Zhou, J., & Yaffe, K. (2007). Body mass index in midlife and risk of Alzheimer disease and vascular dementia. *Current Alzheimer Research, 4*, 103–109.

Witthaus, E., Ott, A., Barendregt, J. J., Breteler, M., & Bonneux, L. (1999). Burden of mortality and morbidity from dementia. *Alzheimer Disease & Associated Disorders, 13*(3), 176–181.

Wolfson, C., Wolfson, D. B., Asgharian, M., M'Lan, C. E., Ostbye, T., Rockwood, K., & Hogan, D. B. (2001). Clinical progression of dementia study group. A reevaluation of the duration of survival after the onset of dementia. *New England Journal of Medicine, 344*(15), 1111–1116.

World Alzheimer Report. (2010). *The global economic impact of dementia.* London, UK: Alzheimer's Disease International (ADI).

World Alzheimer Report. (2015). *The global impact of dementia.* London. UK: Alzheimer's Disease International (ADI).

World Health Organization. (2003). *The global burden of disease.* Geneva, Switzerland: World Health Organization.

World Health Organization. (2006). *Neurological disorders: Public health challenges* (pp. 42–55). Geneva, Switzerland: World Health Organization.

Xie, J., Brayne, C., Matthews, F. E., & Medical Research Council Cognitive Function and Aging Study collaborators. (2008). Survival times in people with dementia: Analysis from population based cohort study with 14 year follow-up. *BMJ, 336*(7638), 258–262.

Xu, J., Kochaniek, K. D., Murphy, S. L., & Tejada-Vera, B. (2010). Deaths: Final data for 2007. *National Vital Statistics Reports, 58*(9), 1–19. (Hyattsville, MD: National Center for Health Statistics.)

Xu, W., Qiu, C., Winblad, B., & Fratiglioni, L. (2007). The effect of borderline diabetes on the risk of dementia and Alzheimer's disease. *Diabetes, 56,* 211–216.

Yasojima, K., Schwab, C., McGeer, E. G., & McGeer, P. L. (2000). Human neurons generate C-reactive protein and amyloid P: Upregulation in Alzheimer's disease. *Brain Research, 887*(1), 80–89.

Zandi, P. P., Carlson, M. C., Plassman, B. L., Welsh-Bohmer, K. A., Mayer, L. S., Steffens, D. C., ... Cache County Memory Study Investigators. (2002). Hormone replacement therapy and incidence of Alzheimer disease in older women. *JAMA, 288*(17), 2123–2129.

Ziegler-Graham, K., Brookmeyer, R., Johnson, E., & Arrighi, H. M. (2008). Worldwide variation in the doubling time of Alzheimer's disease incidence rates. *Alzheimer's and Dementia, 4*(5), 316–323.

CHAPTER 49

Epidemiology of Parkinson's Disease

▶ Introduction

*P*arkinson's disease is a degenerative disorder of the central nervous system involving the massive death and destruction of *dopamine-*synthesizing neurons of the *substantia nigra* in the midbrain. Early symptoms of Parkinson's disease are tremor and shaking of the extremities, "cogwheel" rigidity of the joints, slowness of movement (brady-kinesia), difficulty in walking, and loss of balance. These primary motor symptoms of Parkinson's disease are collectively called "*parkinsonism*." As the disease progresses, cognitive and behavioral symptoms often arise, and dementia may occur.

The *substantia nigra* is a bilateral structure in the midbrain that plays an important role in regulating a variety of neurological functions including mood, memory, cognition, addiction, learning, reward, and movement. *Substantia nigra* is Latin for *black substance*, so named because it contains high levels of brownish-black *neuromelanin* in dopaminergic neurons. Parkinson's disease is caused by the death of dopaminergic neurons due to their accumulation of the nuclear protein, *alpha-synuclein*, within intracellular inclusions called *Lewy bodies* in the *substantia nigra pars compacta*.

Cells of the *substantia nigra* produce and supply the neurotransmitter, dopamine, to the basal ganglia of the human brain. The *basal ganglia* consists of clusters of tightly-interconnected nerve cells within the core of the forebrain. The primary structures are the caudate nucleus, the putamen, the globus pallidus, and the thalamus (**FIGURE 49.1**). The putamen and caudate nucleus together are often referred to as the *corpus striatum*. These neural structures within the basal ganglia receive and process nerve impulses from the cerebral cortex which are then relayed back to the cortex through the thalamus to trigger precise, rapid, coordinated voluntary movements, and thought processes.

The cell bodies of neurons in the substantia nigra synthesize the neurotransmitter, *dopamine*, which travels in a network of axons (the *pars compacta*) to cell bodies in the basal ganglia. In Parkinson's disease, destruction of the substantia nigra results in depletion of dopamine in the basal ganglia. Without dopamine, the processing and transmission of signals by the neuronal circuits of the basal ganglia are disrupted and parkinsonian symptoms appear.

▶ History of Parkinson's Disease

The disease is named after the English physician, James Parkinson, who initially described its characteristic signs and symptoms among six patients with the "*shaking palsy*" in 1817. In his *Essay on the Shaking Palsy*, Parkinson accurately described the characteristic resting tremor, abnormal posture and gait,

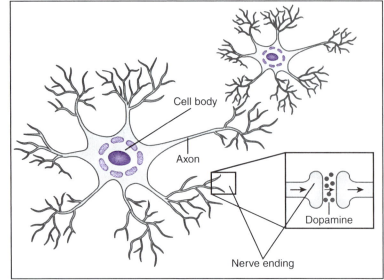

Near the base of the brain is a small area called the substantia nigra which contains cells that produce dopamine.

Dopamine acts as a transmitter between the nerve endings.

FIGURE 49.1 The Human Basal Ganglia.
© Jones & Bartlett Learning.

slowness of movement, paralysis, diminished muscle strength, and progression of disease over time (Parkinson, 1817).

In 1912, the German neurologist, Friedrich Lewy, described microscopic particles in the brains of patients who had died from Parkinson's disease (Lewy, 1912). Such eosinophilic inclusion bodies are called *Lewy bodies*. A few years later, the Russian neuropathologist, Konstantin Tretiakoff reported

that the *substantia nigra* was the specific area of the brain affected in patients with Parkinson's disease (Tretiakoff, 1919). Nearly four decades later, the Swedish investigator, Arvid Carlsson, correctly concluded from many years of laboratory investigations that Parkinson's disease arises due to depletion of the neurotransmitter, dopamine, from the *basal ganglia* of the brain (Carlsson, 1959). Carlsson was later awarded the 2000 Nobel Prize in Physiology or Medicine for his work on dopamine (Carlsson, Greengard, & Kandel, 2000).

A critical step in understanding the development of Parkinson's disease was made through genetic studies of familial disease. Identification of missense mutations in the gene encoding *alpha-synuclein* in patients from these families provided the first clue that this protein could be involved in the molecular chain of pathogenesis (Krüger et al., 1998; Polymeropoulos, 1998; Polymeropoulos et al., 1997).

Subsequently, Michel Goedert, Maria Grazia Spillantini, and colleagues at the University of Cambridge identified the protein, *alpha-synuclein*, as the major component of Lewy bodies in Parkinson's disease (Spillantini, Crowther, Jakes, Hasegawa, & Goedert, 1998; Spillantini et al., 1997). Due to the inordinate accumulation of this protein in dead and dying neurons of the substantia nigra, Parkinson's disease has become known as a form of "*synucleinopathology*" (Goedert, 2001).

Pathology of Parkinson's Disease

The classic pathologic feature of Parkinson's disease is the accumulation of the protein, *alpha-synuclein*, within intracellular inclusions of dopaminergic neurons in the pars compacta of the substantia nigra of the basal ganglia of the midbrain. These inclusions are called *Lewy bodies* named after the German neurologist, Friedrich Lewy, who discovered them nearly a century ago in postmortem specimens of brain tissues from patients with Parkinson's disease (Lewy, 1912). These inclusions within neurons in the substantia nigra of the midbrain are also responsible for the development of a type of dementia called *Lewy body dementia*. Lewy body dementia is distinguishable from Parkinson's disease by the acute nature of dementia onset, in contrast to patients with Parkinson's disease who may develop dementia many years after their diagnosis (Holt et al., 2010; Schulz-Schaeffer, 2010; Weintraub & Hurtig, 2007).

In addition to *alpha-synuclein*, the Lewy bodies of Parkinson's disease also contain *ubiquitin*, a small ubiquitous protein that normally attaches to other intracellular proteins and targets them for degradation within proteasomes. Proteasomes are intracellular micromachines that degrade proteins into elemental amino acids in a process called proteolysis. Misfolded proteins such as alpha-synuclein also accumulate in the dopaminergic projections (axons) that supply dopamine to the basal ganglia. These events produce the death and destruction of dopaminergic

neurons of the substantia nigra and generalized depletion of dopamine in the basal ganglia of the brain (see Figure 49.1). The loss of this essential neurotransmitter leads to the well-known motor function impairments (resting tremor, rigidity, and bradykinesia) that characterize Parkinson's disease.

The pigment *neuromelanin* is a form of melanin that is found principally in the dopaminergic neurons of the midbrain. Its origin and function in these cells have been a long-standing mystery. Recent biochemical studies suggest that neuromelanin forms from the oxidation of cytosolic dopamine and subsequently serves to protect dopaminergic neurons by binding to ionic iron, quinones, and other free radicals (Sulzer et al., 2000).

Numerous pathologic investigations have demonstrated that the degeneration of dopaminergic neurons in Parkinson's disease is associated with robust *microglia activation*. In this phenomenon, microglia undergo a remarkable transition from quiet nursing cells to a reactive state, in which they undergo hypertrophy, proliferation (gliosis), and altered gene expression. Reactive microglia are capable of secreting neurotrophic factors that promote neuronal survival, but they can also secrete *proinflammatory* and *neurotoxin factors*. Notably, the chief regulatory enzyme of the inflammatory prostaglandin cascade, cyclooxygenase-2 (COX-2), is overexpressed in the reactive microglia of patients with Parkinson's disease, but not in normal subjects. Thus, *inflammmogenesis* may significantly contribute to the dopaminergic cell loss of Parkinson's disease (Ardestani, 2010; Hald, Van Beek, & Lotharious, 2007; Knott, Stern, & Wilkin, 2000).

Incidence and Prevalence of Parkinson's Disease

Parkinson's disease is the second most common neurodegenerative disease after Alzheimer's disease. In the U.S. population, this condition is diagnosed in about 1% of adults over the age of 60 years and 4% over the age of 80 years (de Lau & Breteler, 2006). However, reported estimates of prevalence and incidence show wide disparities among populations, most likely due to differences in methodology and inadequate case-finding. Nevertheless, genetic, environmental, and behavioral factors may also contribute to the variability in rates.

Nebraska became the first and only state in the United States to create a Parkinson's disease registry. Since 1997, the registry has provided information about the incidence and prevalence of the disease in the general population of Nebraska. Based upon analysis of physician-reported cases during 1997–2006, the population of Nebraska has relatively high incidence and prevalence rates of Parkinson's disease compared to other populations. For the entire population of the state, the annual crude prevalence was estimated at 329 cases per 100,000. It is possible that the high rates of Parkinson's disease in Nebraska are due to heavy use of and exposure to pesticides in what is largely a farming area. Well-designed epidemiologic studies are needed to elucidate and confirm such effects (Safranak, Theis, & Krause, 2007; Strickland & Bertoni, 2003).

Clusters of Parkinson's disease have been discovered in certain ethnic groups. For example, in a population-based screening of individuals over the age of 60 years in an Amish community, 15 prevalent cases were found among 213 individuals, yielding an extraordinarily high annual crude prevalence rate of 5703 cases per 100,000. Farming and carpentry were the usual occupations among male participants and homemaking among female participants. All subjects used well water throughout their lives and, according to Amish custom, none used electricity. Homes were thus lighted and heated by propane gas. Notably, only two individuals with Parkinson's disease were first-degree relatives, suggesting that environmental exposures rather than genetic factors contributed to the excess prevalence of Parkinson's disease in this community (Racette, Good, Kissel, Criswell, & Perlmutter, 2009).

High prevalence rates have also been observed in other cultures. In 1988, a door-to-door survey was conducted to screen for neurological diseases among 14,010 members of the Parsi colony, an Islamic religious sect living in Bombay, India. A total of 46 individuals were found to have Parkinson's disease, yielding an extremely high crude prevalence of 328.3 per 100,000. Genetic factors were postulated to play a role due to the high frequency of consanguineous marriages in the Parsi community (Bharucha, Bharucha, Bharucha, Bhise, & Schoenberg, 1988).

Investigators at the University of Rochester in New York utilized prevalence estimates from 15 different countries to project the number of individuals with Parkinson's disease in nations with the largest populations in Europe and worldwide. Prevalence estimates for 2005 were derived for individuals at least 50 years of age in five European nations (Germany, France, United Kingdom, Italy, and Spain) and the world's 10 most populous nations (China, India, United States, Indonesia, Brazil, Pakistan, Bangladesh, Russia, Nigeria, and Japan). Estimates were derived from age-specific prevalence data reported in 62 published articles plus census data for each country. By the most conservative estimate, 4.1 million individuals over the age of 50 years were living with Parkinson's disease in these nations during 2005 (Dorsey et al., 2007).

Muangpaisan and colleagues systematically reviewed estimates of the prevalence and incidence of Parkinson's disease from 21 publications for populations in the nations of Asia. Surveys of populations in China (6), Japan (5), India (3), Taiwan (2), Singapore (2), Israel (1), Korea (1), and Saudi Arabia (1) were included in the investigation. Age-standardized prevalence rates ranged from 51 to 177 per 100,000 in door-to-door surveys and from 36 to 68 per 100,000 in record-based surveys. Standardized incidence rates also varied widely ranging from 1.5 per 100,000 in a door-to-door survey of 29 provinces in China to 8.7 per 100,000 in Taiwan. On average, the rates for Asian populations are about 50% lower than rates observed in large studies of non-Asian populations conducted throughout Europe, North America, South America, and Australia. For example, prevalence estimates in 30 studies of non-Asian populations ranged from 101 to 439 per 100,000 in door-to-door surveys and from 61 to 141 per 100,000 in record-based surveys, and incidence rates ranged from 15 to 28 per 100,000 in door-to-door surveys and from 6.1 to 17.4 per 100,000 in record-based surveys. Since prevalence is a multiplicative function of incidence and duration of disease (prevalence = incidence × duration), the relatively low prevalence rates in non-Asian populations could reflect relatively poor survival due to lack of access to health care and treatment. However, varying methodologies and differences in diagnostic criteria and case-finding strategies undoubtedly contribute to the wide variation in reported estimates of prevalence and incidence of Parkinson's disease worldwide (Muangpaisan, Hori, & Brayne, 2009).

Driver and colleagues estimated the age-specific incidence and lifetime risk of Parkinson's disease in the Physicians' Health Study, a prospective national cohort of 21,970 U.S. male physicians aged 40–84 years at baseline and followed over 23 years. They identified 563 cases in the cohort yielding a crude annual incidence rate of 121 cases per 100,000 person-years. The cumulative risk of disease for ages 45–100 years was 6.7% and the annual incidence for men over the age of 65 years was 224 per 100,000. The incidence among chronic smokers was about 30% less than among nonsmokers (Driver, Logroscino, Gaziano, & Kurth, 2009).

Estimates of the incidence of Parkinson's disease vary widely, even within countries. The incidence of Parkinson's disease in the U.S. Physicians' Health

Study (224 per 100,000 for men over 65 years of age) is more than twofold higher than estimates derived from other U.S. population samples: 119 per 100,000 in Manhattan, 113 per 100,000 in Minnesota, and 100 per 100,000 in Los Angeles. Comparative estimates for European populations are higher than the U.S. estimates: 261 per 100,000 in Rotterdam, 360 per 100,000 in Central Spain, and 461 per 100,000 in Italy. A number of factors may contribute to this wide variation including differences in the age and longevity of the populations studied, methods of case-finding, criteria for the diagnosis of Parkinson's disease, and the prevalence of smoking (Driver et al., 2009).

The characteristic pattern of the age-specific incidence of Parkinson's disease is depicted for men and women in **FIGURE 49.2**. Data are from the prospective cohort in Olmsted County, Minnesota (Bower, Maraganore, McDonnell, & Rocca, 1999). As shown, Parkinson's disease is rarely diagnosed before the age of 50 years but then increases exponentially with age. Rates are higher in men than women for all age brackets but appear to equilibrate after the age of 80 years. The peak onset in men occurs about a decade earlier than in women.

A study in Northern California compared the incidence of Parkinson's disease by age, gender, and ethnicity in members of the *Kaiser Permanente Medical Care Program*. Among 588 cases diagnosed during 1994–1995, only 24 (4%) were diagnosed before the age of 50 years. Annual incidence rates peaked during ages 80–89 years for both men (191 per 100,000) and women (71 per 100,000). Hispanics had the highest overall rates and African Americans the lowest, although sample sizes were small in all ethnic groups except for non-Hispanic Caucasians. Additional studies are therefore needed to confirm the presence of ethnic differences (Van Den Eeden et al., 2003).

Global Incidence of Parkinson's Disease

A recent meta-analysis conducted by investigators at the University of Toronto combined the data from 27 studies conducted during 2001–2014 to estimate the global annual incidence of Parkinson's disease among men and women. Age-specific rates were also estimated with stratification by successive 10-year age intervals. The global age-adjusted annual incidence rate in men (61 per 100,000 person-years) was approximately 60% higher than for women (38 per 100,000 person-years). Rates per 100,000 person-years increased exponentially with age (e.g., from 3.3 to 103 among women and from 3.6 to 258 among men for ages 40–49 years and 70–79 years, respectively). Age-specific rates for men and women were similar at younger ages but diverged significantly over the lifespan, e.g., for ages 70–79 years, the rate in men was 2.5 times higher than women (Hirsch, Jette, Frolkis, Steeves, & Pringsheim, 2016).

Investigators at the Mayo Clinic examined time trends in the incidence of Parkinson's disease among all residents of Olmstead County, Minnesota, during 1976–2005. Age-standardized incidence rates per 100,000 increased by about 67% in men (from 18 to 30) but were relatively stable for women during the 30-year period. Significant increases over time were observed for elderly men 70 years or older but not for younger men. Since smoking has been found to be inversely related to the risk of developing Parkinson's disease, the investigators suggest that the observed increasing trend in men could be related to the dramatic decline in their rates of smoking during the time span of the study (Savica, Grossardt, Bower, Ahlskog, & Rocca, 2016).

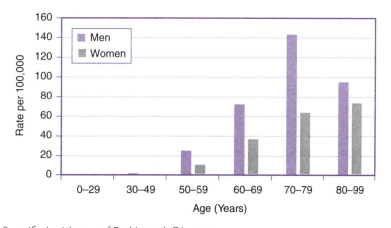

FIGURE 49.2 Annual Age-Specific Incidence of Parkinson's Disease.

Data from Bower, J. H., Maraganore, D. M., McDonnell, S. K., & Rocca, W. A. (1999). Incidence and distribution of parkinsonism in Olmsted County, Minnesota, 1976–1990. *Neurology, 52*(6), 1214–1220.

▶ Global Age-Specific Prevalence of Parkinson's Disease

Investigators at the University of Calgary, Alberta, Canada, conducted a meta-analysis designed to estimate the global age-specific prevalence of Parkinson's disease in men and women. Their estimates were based upon data extracted from 47 studies representing six regions of the world (Asia, Europe, Africa, Australia, South America, and North America). Estimates of age-gender-specific rates per 100,000 rose exponentially with age for both men and women. Rates were similar for men and women until after age 65 when the rates diverged and became higher for men. Among individuals 80 years and older, the prevalence in men (per 100,000) was 40% higher than women (2100 versus 1500) (**FIGURE 49.3**). Prevalence estimates varied among the six regions and were highest in South America, intermediate in Europe, North America and Australia, and lowest in Asia and Africa (Pringsheim et al., 2014).

▶ Survival, Dementia, and Mortality in Parkinson's Disease

Compared to the general population, patients who develop Parkinson's disease have increased mortality and shortened survival. Furthermore, most studies suggest that dementia often occurs as a consequence of disease progression, affecting nearly two-thirds of patients with long-term survival.

Investigators of the *Rochester Epidemiology Project* in Minnesota examined the survival of incident cases of Parkinson's disease in the *Olmsted County Cohort*

during 1976–1995. Cases ($n = 196$) were matched by age and gender to disease-free controls ($n = 185$) from the same population and all individuals were followed to determine the time of death. A total of 110 cases and 79 controls died during follow-up. The mortality rate was 1.6 times higher in cases than controls, and median survival was 10.3 years for the cases and 13.4 years for controls. These results demonstrate that patients with Parkinson's disease have a significantly higher risk of dying compared to matched controls from the general population (Elbaz et al., 2003).

In the United Kingdom, measures of survival for a community-based cohort of patients with Parkinson's disease were compared with the age- and gender-matched population of England and Wales. The study compared the ages at death, life expectancies, and standardized mortality ratios (SMR) for patients with and without dementia. A total of 166 patients participated in the study, of which 91 died after only 4 years of follow-up. The SMR was threefold higher in demented patients (SMR = 3.10) than non-demented patients (SMR = 1.15), and among patients diagnosed between ages 55 and 74 years of age, the life expectancy for demented patients was markedly shortened (7.5 years) compared to non-demented patients (12.4 years). These results suggest that dementia severely compromises the survival of patients with Parkinson's disease whereas those who do not develop dementia experience near normal survival (Hobson, Meara, & Ishihara-Paul, 2010).

Similar results were observed in a study of 90 incident cases of Parkinson's disease conducted at the University of Leeds in the United Kingdom. Compared to disease-free controls, patients with Parkinson's disease had 1.64 times higher mortality and shorter median survival (9.1 years compared to more than 13 years). Furthermore, mortality was increased nearly twofold in patients with dementia

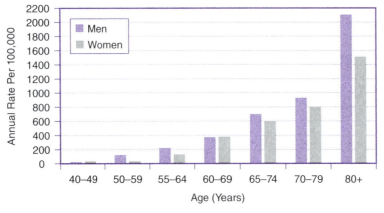

FIGURE 49.3 Global Age-Gender-Specific Prevalence of Parkinson's Disease.

Data from Pringsheim, T., Jette, N., Frolkis, A., & Steeves, T. D. (2014). The prevalence of Parkinson's disease: A systematic review and meta-analysis. *Movement Disorders, 29*(13), 1583–1590.

versus those without (Hughes, Ross, Mindham, & Spokes, 2004).

Dementia is a common feature of patients with Parkinson's disease. For example, in a meta-analysis of 24 studies, the average prevalence among 1767 patients was 25% (Aarsland, Zaccai, & Brayne, 2005). Furthermore, prospective studies of non-demented patients with Parkinson's disease have consistently shown that their risk of developing dementia cumulates at a rate of approximately 10% per year. Investigators in Norway found an annual incidence of 95 per 1000 person-years among 171 patients (Aarsland et al., 2001) and investigators in Wales found a similar rate of 107 per 1000 person-years among 86 patients (Hobson & Meara, 2004). These estimates reflect a sixfold risk increase compared to matched subjects without Parkinson's disease and yield a cumulative rate of 65% for 10 years of survival. This estimate is consistent with a study in Denmark in which 71 (66%) of 108 patients with Alzheimer's disease developed dementia during 8 years of follow-up (Aarsland, Andersen, Larsen, Lolk, & Kragh-Sorensen, 2003) and an extended study in Norway in which 140 (60%) of 233 patients developed dementia during 12 years of follow-up (Buter et al., 2008).

Investigators at the University of North Carolina conducted a meta-analysis of dementia and polymorphisms of *apolipoprotein E* (*APOE*) in patients with Parkinson's disease. Their analysis revealed an elevated risk of dementia among patients with APOE e4 (OR = 1.6); however, there was significant heterogeneity among study results and additional studies are needed to confirm the association (Huang, Chen, Kaufer, Trouster, & Poole, 2006).

A team of investigators examined the survival of 288 male patients with newly diagnosed Parkinson's disease compared to 51,012 disease-free men in the *U.S. Health Professionals Follow-up Study*. The study specifically examined effects of duration of disease and smoking. During 15 years of follow-up, 92 cases (32%) died compared to 8485 controls (17%). After adjustment for age, men with Parkinson's disease had 60% higher mortality than controls. The relative risk of death increased with duration of disease: RR = 1.1 for 1–5 years, RR = 2.3 for 6–10 years, and RR = 3.5 after 10 years. Smoking increased mortality by twofold among controls but conferred no additional risk of death among patients with Parkinson's disease (Chen et al., 2006).

Once diagnosed, Parkinson's disease invariably progresses over time. Without treatment, motor symptoms (tremor, unsteady gait, bradykinesia, and cogwheel rigidity) worsen quickly and may lead to ambulation and disability within a few years.

Medications such as levodopa can effectively delay progression for a time; however, such drugs have been found to produce a more rapid decline in cognitive function in some patients. Inevitably, patients develop autonomic disturbances, sleeplessness, mood alterations, cognitive decline, and dementia, all of which greatly increase disability and mortality (Poewe, 2006).

▶ Parkinson's Disease: Trends in Global Mortality and Prevalence

The global burden of Parkinson's disease is rising. Recent Global Burden of Disease (GBD) studies found that during 1990–2016, the annual number of deaths from Parkinson's disease increased 2.6-fold (from 81,000 to 211,000) and the number of people living with Parkinson's disease increased 2.4-fold (from 2.5 million to 6.1 million). The global age-standardized mortality rate in 2016 was 3.5 per 100,000 compared to 2.9 per 100,000 in 1990, a 20% increase. The age-standardized prevalence rate also increased approximately 22% during this period, suggesting that the rising burden of Parkinson's disease is not entirely a consequence of population aging. Prevalence rates among countries varied widely, from low rates of less than 50 per 100,000 in sub-Saharan African countries, to rates exceeding 130 per 100,000 in developed countries such as the United States and Canada (Dorsey et al., 2018; Naghavi & GBD 2016 Collaborators, 2017).

It is noteworthy that multiple studies have found similar relative increases in the annual number of prevalent cases and number of deaths from Parkinson's disease during the past generation (Murray & GBD 2013 Collaborators, 2015; Wang et al., 2016). The rising global trend in number of deaths from Parkinson's disease during 1990–2016 is depicted in **FIGURE 49.4**.

▶ Disability-Adjusted Life Years: Parkinson's Disease

The *Disability-Adjusted Life Years* (DALY) is the sum of *Years of Life Lost from Premature Death* (YLL) and *Years of Life Lost from Disability* (YDL): DALY = YLL + YDL. During 1990–2016, the estimated DALY from Parkinson's disease increased 2.5-fold from 1.3 to 3.2 million. Among 21 regions of the world representing all levels of economic development,

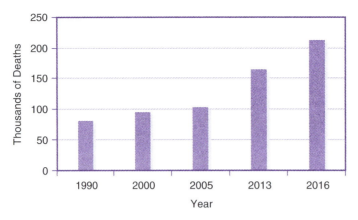

FIGURE 49.4 Global Trend in Number of Deaths from Parkinson's Disease, 1990–2016.

Data points for 1990 and 2016 are mean values of estimates from GBD 2015 and GBD 2016 studies.

Data from Dorsey, E. R., Elbaz, A., Nichols, E., Abd-Allah, F., Abdelalim, A., Adsuar, J. C., ... GBD 2016 Parkinson's Disease Collaborators. (2018). Global, regional, and national burden of Parkinson's disease, 1990–2016: A systematic analysis for the Global Burden of Disease Study 2016. *The Lancet Neurology*. doi:10.1016/S1474-4422(18)30295-3; Wang, H., Naghavi, M., Allen, C., Barber, R. M., Bhutta, Z. A., Carter, A., ... GBD 2015 Mortality and Causes of Death Collaborators. (2016). Global, regional, and national life expectancy, all-cause mortality, and cause-specific mortality for 249 causes of death, 1980–2015: A systematic analysis for the Global Burden of Disease Study 2015. *The Lancet, 388*(10053), 1459–1544; Naghavi, M., Wang, H., Lozano, R., Davis, A., Liang, X., Zhou, M., ... GBD 2013 Mortality and Causes of Death Collaborators. (2015). Global, regional, and national age–sex specific all-cause and cause-specific mortality for 240 causes of death, 1990–2013: A systematic analysis for the Global Burden of Disease Study 2013. *The Lancet, 385*, 117–171.

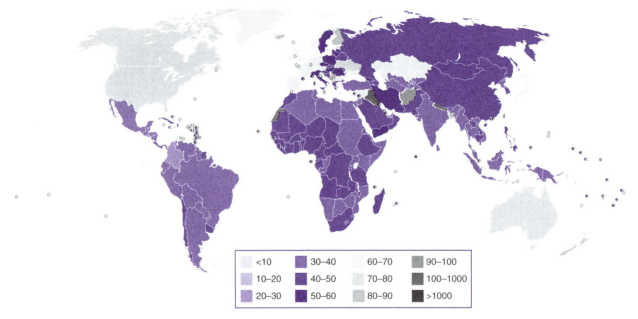

FIGURE 49.5 DALY, Parkinson's Disease, 2004.

Data from World Health Organization. (2008). *The global burden of disease: 2004 update*. Geneva: WHO. Available at www.who.int/evidence/bod

Disability Adjusted Life Years per 100,000 individuals.

the age-standardized DALY rates ranged from 20 per 100,000 in less developed regions (sub-Saharan Africa and South Asia) to 80 per 100,000 in regions with highly developed economies (North America, Western Europe and Australasia). The two components of DALY, YLL, and YDL showed similar patterns among regions (Dorsey et al., 2018).

The global pattern of DALY due to Parkinson's disease is shown in **FIGURE 49.5** (WHO, 2009). Since the incidence of Parkinson's disease peaks among the elderly, DALY values tend to be higher in developed countries whose populations have the greatest longevity. Nevertheless, populations with the highest DALY are those in war torn areas of the Middle East, such

as Iraq and Afghanistan. Such populations have been subjected to unusually high levels of certain environmental neurotoxins including pesticides, fuel vapors, combustion products from oil well fires and open pit fires, nerve gases, and depleted uranium (Friedl, Grate, & Proctor, 2009; Golomb, 2008).

Another outlier with high DALY lost from Parkinson's disease is the small nation of Nepal that borders northeastern India in the Himalayan mountain range. Risk factors in the Nepalese population include lack of oxygen, nutritional deficiencies in iodine, zinc, and other minerals, and outbreaks of Japanese encephalitis due to a mosquito-borne virus, all of which might contribute to the development of parkinsonism (Brewer et al., 2010; De Pedro-Cuesta, 1987; Kanda, Ebihara, Arai, Takeda, & Sasaki, 2000; Pradhan, Pandey, Shashank, Gupta, & Mathur, 1999; Ramakrishnan, 2002).

Notably, some patients from populations of the Middle East are characterized by very early onset (the average age at diagnosis was 36 years in one series of 60 patients) and novel genetic polymorphisms in the *leucine-rich repeat kinase 2* (*LRRK2*) gene, which is discussed in a following section of this chapter on the genetics of Parkinson's disease. These results suggest that genetic factors may play a more dominant role in the pathogenesis of Parkinson's disease in certain populations due to the relatively high frequency of consanguineous marriages (Elahi, 2009; Shojaee et al., 2009).

▶ Causes of the Rising Global Burden of Parkinson's Disease

Multiple factors are undoubtedly responsible for the rising global burden of Parkinson's disease. While population aging is the major force, several other factors may have also contributed including improvements in data collection and analytical methods yielding more precise estimates, greater longevity among patients with disease, increasing exposure to industrial chemicals and pollutants, and declining prevalence of smoking in some countries. As longevity increases worldwide, the burden of chronic diseases of old age, including Parkinson's disease, will undoubtedly rise. Without intervention, the prevalence of Parkinson's disease is expected to approach 9 million by the year 2030, more than double the number of cases in 2005. Population-based registries are needed in order to assess the burden of neurodegenerative diseases and guide the health, social, and economic policies of the future (Dorsey et al., 2007).

▶ Risk Factors for Parkinson's Disease

The pathogenesis of Parkinson's disease is complex and involves both genetic and environmental factors. Though many risk factors and protective factors have been proposed, conclusive evidence is lacking for most. The two consistently observed relationships are an increased risk in those exposed to pesticides and a reduced risk in smokers. In recent years, the roles of some individual genes and molecular pathways have been elucidated, which has advanced our understanding of this disease (de Lau & Breteler, 2006). Selected studies are discussed in the following paragraphs.

Genetics of Parkinson's Disease

In a community-based study, investigators at Columbia University in New York assessed the risk of Parkinson's disease among 1458 first-degree relatives of 233 index cases (probands). Compared to relatives of disease-free controls, relatives of the cases were 2.3 times more likely to develop Parkinson's disease. The risk estimates were highest among Caucasian male relatives but similar for siblings and parents of the probands. The results support the existence of genetic factors that influence susceptibility to pathogenesis (Marder et al., 1996).

Tanner and colleagues assessed the role of genetics in the development of Parkinson's disease by comparing the concordance and discordance of disease in monozygous and dizygous twins. The study examined 19,842 male twins enrolled from the National Academy of Sciences World War II Veteran Twins Registry. Across all ages, the pairwise concordance rates were *not* significantly higher for monozygous versus dizygous twins (15.5% and 11.1%, respectively). However, within 16 twin pairs with diagnosis before 50 years of age, the concordance among monozygous twins was 100% compared to 17% for dizygous twins (RR = 6.0). The investigators concluded that genetic factors may be important for early-onset disease but do not play a major role when Parkinson's disease is diagnosed after the age of 50 years (Tanner et al., 1999).

Autosomal Dominant Genes and Parkinson's Disease

Alpha-synuclein. The gene that encodes *alpha-synuclein* (*SNCA*) is on the long arm of human chromosome 4. Carriers of mutant forms of *SNCA* are at high risk for developing Parkinson's disease. A mutant *SNCA* allele was first identified in a large Italian kindred in which heterozygous gene carriers manifested early-onset Parkinson's disease in an *autosomal dominant* inheritance pattern (Polymeropoulos, 1998; Polymeropoulos et al., 1997). Mutated SNCA alleles have since been discovered in several multigenerational families in which Parkinson's disease is inherited as an autosomal dominant syndrome. Mutations in SNCA disrupt the normal processing of alpha-synuclein within dopaminergic cells, leading to the formation of Lewy bodies and cell death (Hardy, Cai, Cookson, Gwinn-Hardy, & Singleton, 2006).

LRRK2 and g

Funayama and colleagues performed a genome-wide linkage analysis of a Japanese kindred with an *autosomal dominant* inheritance pattern of parkinsonism among relatives. Patients in the kindred manifested the classic clinical symptoms of Parkinson's disease but Lewy bodies were *absent* in postmortem specimens of the substantia nigra. Findings revealed genetic linkage of disease susceptibility to a mutant gene on the long arm of chromosome 12 that encodes the leucine-rich repeat protein kinase, LRRK2 (Funayama et al., 2002).

Subsequent genetic studies have identified scores of families in which carriers of missense mutations of *LRRK2* developed late onset Parkinson's disease. However, postmortem studies of brainstem specimens from these patients have revealed marked heterogeneity in the presence and composition of inclusion bodies within degenerating neurons of the substantia nigra. To date, more than 20 mutant alleles of *LRRK2* have been identified; however, the penetrance of these alleles is highly variable and there is marked heterogeneity in the deposition of misfolded proteins and degeneration of dopaminergic neurons among gene carriers (Zimprich et al., 2004).

The *LRRK2* gene encodes the complex protein, *dardarin*, which is a leucine-rich protein kinase that phosphorylates other proteins and regulates protein catabolism and metabolism within neurons. A team of investigators cloned the *LRRK2* gene from afflicted members of Spanish families with heritable parkinsonism. Since these families were of *Basque* descent, they named the *LRRK2* protein, *dardarin*, after the Basque word *dardar* which means tremor (Paisán-Ruíz et al., 2004).

Autosomal Recessive Genes and Parkinson's Disease

Japanese investigators identified gene deletions in the long arm of chromosome 6 in a *rare* form of early-onset parkinsonism, showing an autosomal recessive inheritance pattern. Postmortem studies of afflicted patients revealed depletion of dopaminergic neurons in the substantia nigra but *without* Lewy bodies (Kitada et al., 1998). The deleted gene, *Parkin*, encodes *E3 ligase* that regulates ubiquitylation of proteins for degradation in proteasomes of neurons. Either deletions or missense mutations of the *Parkin* gene can lead to the accumulation of misfolded proteins within dopaminergic neurons and development of parkinsonism (Hardy et al., 2006; Lim, Dawson, & Dawson, 2006).

Other rare mutations have also been noted in association with parkinsonism. Mutations in the *PTEN-induced kinase gene* (*PINK-1*) located on the short arm of chromosome 1 have been identified in families with early-onset Parkinson's disease. The *PINK-1* gene encodes a protein kinase that is essential for normal mitochondrial function in neurons (Rogaeva et al., 2004).

Molecular studies of these genes and the search for others that influence the pathogenesis of Parkinson's disease are continuing at a rapid pace. The molecular genetics of this condition and other forms of neurodegenerative disease can be expected to elucidate molecular targets for effective therapy and/or chemoprevention.

MPTP and Parkinson's Disease

Interest in environmental exposures, particularly pesticides, metals, and industrial solvents rose substantially following the discovery that exposure to high levels of *1-methyl-4-phenyl-1,2,3,6-tetrahydropyridine* (*MPTP*) causes acute onset of parkinsonian symptoms. This discovery was made by J. William Langston and colleagues who studied several young intravenous drug users in California who developed irreversible parkinsonian symptoms after injecting narcotics contaminated with MPTP (Langston, Ballard, Tetrud, & Irwin, 1983; Langston & Palfreman, 1996).

Subsequent investigations determined that MPTP crosses the blood–brain barrier where it is activated by monoamine oxidase (Langston, 1985; Langston, Forno, Rebert, & Irwin, 1984). The active metabolite of MPTP causes parkinsonian symptoms by inducing pathologic changes in dopaminergic neurons confined to the substantia nigra. Notably, the active metabolite of MPTP (MPP+) bears a close structural similarity to the herbicide, paraquat, which suggests that exposure to herbicides and/or pesticides might also elevate the risk. As noted in a review of the epidemiology of Parkinson's disease, "*the established neurotoxin properties of some widely used pesticides (e.g., organophosphorus insecticides) and the chemical similarity of paraquat MPP+ are logical reasons to focus on these exposures*" (Checkoway & Nelson, 1999).

While MPTP per se is not neurotoxic, it readily crosses the blood–brain barrier where it is converted to MPP+ by the enzyme *monoamine oxidase B* (*MOA B*) of glial cells. The neurotoxic cation MPP+ has been found to kill dopamine-producing neurons in the pars compacta of the substantia nigra by interfering with the electron transport chain of mitochondria (Richardson, Quan, Sherer, Greenamyre, & Miller, 2005).

Paraquat is the trade name for *N, N′-dimethyl-4,4′-bipyridinium dichloride*, one of the most widely used herbicides in the world. When ingested, pure paraquat is highly toxic to mammals, including humans, potentially leading to acute respiratory distress and death. There are no specific antidotes for paraquat and in third world countries it is a major suicide agent. A related compound, *rotenone*, is a poisonous extract of certain plant species, primarily *Derris* and *Lonchocarpus*, that is widely used as an insecticide. Similar to the ionic metabolite of MPTP, both paraquat and rotenone exert toxic effects on the dopaminergic neurons of the midbrain by interfering with the electron transport chain in mitochondria or the production of free radicals (Richardson et al., 2005).

Herbicides, Pesticides, and Parkinson's Disease

Findings linking MPTP exposure to parkinsonism in humans stimulated epidemiologic studies of Parkinson's disease and exposure to pesticides and herbicides, since many of these compounds are similar in structure to MPTP. In an early ecological study conducted in the rural population of Quebec, Canada, more than 5000 cases were identified during 1980–1984 and prevalence rates calculated and compared among nine hydrographic regions. The study revealed that the rates of Parkinson's disease varied unevenly throughout the province and regions with the highest rates were characterized by intensive market gardening and the highest levels of pesticide use (Barbeau, Roy, Bernier, Campanella, & Paris, 1987).

In Hong Kong, Suzanne Ho and colleagues conducted a case–control study of Parkinson's disease comparing the use of pesticides and herbicides among 34 cases and 105 controls. They found a significant increase in the odds ratio associated with previous use of pesticides and/or herbicides (OR = 3.6), although the participants were unable to provide details on the specific types of chemicals used (Ho, Wee, & Lee, 1989).

Privadarshi and colleagues performed a meta-analysis of 19 studies of Parkinson's disease and pesticide exposure published between 1989 and 1999. Findings revealed a significant increase in the overall risk (OR = 1.94) and combined estimates from studies in the United States (OR = 2.15), Canada (OR = 1.94), Europe (OR = 1.76), and Asia (OR = 2.53) were similar. Nevertheless, there was significant heterogeneity among studies possibly due to differences in case definition and the methods used to define exposure (Priyadarshi, Khuder, Schaub, & Shrivastava, 2000).

Results of subsequent studies in the past few years continue to support an association of exposure to pesticides/herbicides and the development of Parkinson's disease. In France, a case–control study compared pesticide exposure in 81 cases and 252 population-based controls. The study revealed a positive association between occupational pesticide exposure and the odds of developing Parkinson's disease (OR = 2.2) (Baldi et al., 2003).

Investigators at the American Cancer Society examined pesticide exposure and the risk of developing Parkinson's disease among participants of the *Cancer Prevention Study II Nutrition Cohort*, a longitudinal investigation of U.S. men and women initiated in 1992. A total of 143,325 individuals who were disease-free at baseline were followed for up to 10 years to detect the development of incident cases of Parkinson's disease. Exposure to pesticides was reported by 7864 participants including farmers and ranchers. Regardless of occupation, individuals exposed to pesticides had a 70% higher incidence of Parkinson's disease than those not exposed (RR = 1.7). The investigators suggest the need for future studies to identify specific chemicals that increase the risk (Ascherio et al., 2006).

Investigators at Duke University conducted a family-based study of 319 cases and 296 disease-free relatives to assess the relationship between Parkinson's disease and pesticide exposure. Cases reported pesticide exposure more often than controls (OR = 1.61) and cumulative exposure to pesticides showed a dose–response pattern with the risk (Hancock et al., 2008).

Caroline Tanner, William Langston, and colleagues affiliated with the *Parkinson's Institute* in Sunnyvale, California, have conducted two separate investigations to elaborate associations between the risk of developing Parkinson's disease and exposure to pesticides and herbicides. In a multicenter case–control study, lifelong occupational and job histories were utilized to determine pesticide and herbicide exposures among 519 cases and 511 controls. The results revealed an increased disease risk with overall pesticide use (OR = 1.90) and especially with pesticides such as rotenone that have found to be mechanistically associated with experimental parkinsonism (OR = 2.20). The highest risk (OR = 2.59) was noted for dichlorophenoxyacetic acid (2, 4-D), a neurotoxin known to uncouple oxidative phosphorylation in mitochondria that is one of the most widely used herbicides worldwide (Tanner et al., 2009).

In a subsequent nested case–control study, the lifetime exposure histories to herbicides and pesticides were compared in 110 incident cases and 358 controls frequency-matched by age, gender, and location. All individuals were ascertained from the *U.S. Agricultural Health Study*, a prospective cohort of more than 89,000 agricultural workers. Findings revealed an increased disease risk with exposure to pesticides such as rotenone that inhibit mitochondrial function

(OR = 2.0) and with agents such as paraquat that cause oxidative stress (OR = 2.5) (Tanner et al., 2011).

Overall, the results of multiple epidemiologic investigations provide consistent evidence that pesticide/herbicide exposure is linked to the development of Parkinson's disease. Furthermore, specific compounds found to increase the risk are known to form reactive oxygen species and cause mitochondrial dysfunction, the same mechanisms linked to the destruction of dopaminergic neurons in the midbrain in experimental animal models of Parkinson's disease.

Environmental Risk Factors and Parkinson's Disease

In 1837, John Couper described parkinsonian symptoms in five men who worked in a chemical plant grinding the black oxide of manganese ore. The manganese ore grinders exhibited gait disturbance, loss of balance, paralysis of facial muscles, impaired ability to hear and speak, and drooling, but the cardinal sign of Parkinson's disease, resting tremor, was notably absent. Couper's essay is regarded as the first report of severe neurotoxicity in humans resulting from manganese exposure (Couper, 1837).

More than a century later, Rodier conducted a survey of nervous system abnormalities among 3840 workers employed in three manganese mines in Morocco. His findings revealed 151 workers with parkinsonian-like symptoms, 132 of whom held jobs drilling blast holes that entailed the most intense manganese exposures. The peak prevalence of *manganism* with intense exposure was 43.5% among workers aged 30–44 years (Checkoway, 2010; Rodier, 1955).

Many subsequent investigations have examined the effects of manganese exposure in both humans and nonhuman primates. The available evidence from behavioral, neuroimaging, neurochemical, and neuropathological studies suggests that manganese accumulation in the brain produces an *atypical form of parkinsonism*, which is *not* associated with degeneration of the dopaminergic neurons in the substantia nigra as in classical Parkinson's disease. Rather, manganese poisoning may inhibit the release of dopamine at the synapses of dopaminergic neurons with neurons in the basal ganglia (Guilarte, 2010).

A number of case–control epidemiologic investigations have been conducted in search of other environmental exposures that influence the risk of developing Parkinson's disease. Most such studies suffer from lack of detailed information about the type, frequency, intensity, and duration of exposure.

The *Geoparkinson Study* is a large international case–control study of Parkinson's disease designed to assess associations of genetic and environmental risk factors with the development of Parkinson's disease. Standardized personal interviews were conducted to collect information on lifetime exposure to solvents, pesticides, iron, copper, and manganese for 767 cases and 1989 controls. Participants were ascertained at centers in Scotland, Italy, Sweden, Romania, and Malta. Levels of exposure for each subject were estimated by a job-exposure matrix and subjective modeling. Logistic regression analysis revealed a dose–response in risk with increasing exposure to pesticides: OR = 1.13 for low exposure and OR = 1.41 for high exposure; increased risk with a history of repeated traumatic loss of consciousness (OR = 2.53); and decreased risk with chronic tobacco use (OR = 0.50). Results for other environmental factors including exposure to solvents, iron, manganese, or copper were null. The findings of this large international study suggest that pesticide exposure and head trauma have causative roles in the genesis of Parkinson's disease, but to not support links with other environmental risk factors (Dick et al., 2007).

Smoking and Parkinson's Disease

As pointed out by Checkoway and Nelson in their review of the epidemiology of Parkinson's disease:

> *Apart from the increasing incidence of Parkinson's disease with age, the most consistently reported epidemiologic finding has been an inverse association with cigarette smoking. Decreased risks, by about 50% among smokers compared to nonsmokers have been reported from many case control studies, some of which demonstrated strong inverse dose-response relations. Cohort studies in which smoking data were obtained before cases' diagnoses substantiate the negative association with smoking (Checkoway & Nelson, 1999).*

Recently, 305,468 participants of the *National Institutes of Health American Association of Retired Persons (AARP) Diet and Health Cohort* were studied to evaluate the relative importance of smoking duration in reducing the risk. A total of 1662 participants developed Parkinson's disease during the study. Compared to never smokers, disease odds were reduced among past smokers (OR = 0.78) and current smokers (OR = 0.56) and the risk declined as the duration of smoking increased (Chen et al., 2010).

A team of U.S. investigators from multiple institutions conducted a pooled meta-analysis of available published studies to clarify associations of age-of-smoking onset, time since quitting, and other measures of smoking and tobacco use with the risk of developing Parkinson's disease. Eight case–control studies (2328 cases and 4113 controls) and three cohort studies (488 cases and 4880 controls) were included in the analysis. The pooled data confirmed a dose-dependent reduction in the risk of developing Parkinson's disease with duration of cigarette smoking as well as other forms of tobacco use. These effects were not influenced by gender or education. The investigators state that "*although the numerous adverse health effects of cigarette smoking may eventually limit the clinical implications of the epidemiologic findings on smoking and Parkinson's disease, research to reveal the underlying chemicals and mechanisms is warranted*" (Ritz et al., 2007).

Coffee and Parkinson's Disease

Several studies have also observed an inverse association between coffee consumption and the risk of developing Parkinson's disease. Investigators at Harvard University conducted a systematic review and meta-analysis to summarize the evidence for both coffee consumption and cigarette smoking. Results for smoking were based on 44 case–control studies and 4 cohort studies, and results for coffee consumption were based on 8 case–control and 5 cohort studies. Compared with never smokers, the relative risk of developing Parkinson's disease was 0.80 for past smokers and 0.39 for current smokers, and the risk declined by about 20% for each additional 10 pack-years of smoking. Compared with noncoffee drinkers, the relative risk of developing Parkinson's disease was 0.69 for coffee drinkers, and the risk declined by about 10% for each additional cup of coffee per day. Results therefore provide strong evidence that smoking and drinking coffee both lower the risk of developing Parkinson's disease (Hernán, Takkouche, Caamano-Isorna, & Gestal-Otero, 2002).

Nonsteroidal Anti-Inflammatory Drugs and Parkinson's Disease

Pathologic studies of brain tissues from patients with Parkinson's disease have revealed that neuroinflammation and microgliosis are associated with the loss of dopaminergic neurons in the substantia nigra of the midbrain (Perry, 2012). This finding has stimulated interest in potential chemopreventive effects of *nonsteroidal anti-inflammatory drugs* (NSAIDs).

Two major prospective studies have focused on NSAIDs and Parkinson's disease: The *Health Professionals Follow-up Study* in men and the *Nurses' Health Study* in women. Prospective cohorts of 44,057 men and 98,845 women free of Parkinson's disease, stroke, and cancer at baseline participated in the study. In both cohorts, questionnaires were mailed every 2 years to ascertain updated information on health status and medical diagnoses. During follow-up (1986–2000 for men and 1980–1998 for women), 415 incident cases were detected (236 in men and 236 in women). Participants who reported regular use of aspirin or non-aspirin NSAIDs (primarily ibuprofen) were found to have a significant reduction in their risk of developing Parkinson's disease (RR = 0.55). Risk reductions were similar for men and women. These results suggest that NSAIDs have neuroprotective effects against the development of Parkinson's disease and are consistent with other epidemiologic findings showing that these compounds also reduce the risk of developing Alzheimer's disease (Chen et al., 2003).

▶ Tertiary Prevention in Parkinson's Disease

Parkinson's disease invariably progresses with time. Without treatment, motor symptoms often advance rapidly, and patients may lose independent ambulation and become bedridden in just a few years. Medications such as levodopa, dopamine agonists, monoamine oxidase (MAO) inhibitors, anticholinergics, and amantadine have been instrumental in delaying the progression of motor symptoms by more than a decade (WHO, 2006). Although levodopa continues to be the gold standard of treatment for the cardinal motor features of Parkinson's disease, its chronic use is associated with potentially disabling motor complications and psychosis. Atypical (second generation) antipsychotic medications are routinely administered to patients who develop psychosis; however, additional studies are needed to assess the effects of specific drugs on morbidity, mortality, and disease progression (Holt et al., 2010; Weintraub & Hurtig, 2007).

Future prospects to improve outcomes and the quality of life in patients with Parkinson's disease include gene therapy to restore the chemical balance of neurotransmitters within the circuitry of the basal ganglia. In animal models of parkinsonism, gene transfer of glutamic acid decarboxylase to modulate *gamma-aminobutyric acid* (*GABA*) in the subthalamic nucleus has been found to improve basal ganglia function, and most recently, a randomized clinical trial of this procedure in human patients produced significant improvement in motor function among patients who received gene therapy compared to those who received placebo at 6 months of follow-up (Lewitt et al., 2011).

References

Aarsland, D., Andersen, K., Larsen, J. P., Lolk, A., & Kragh-Sorensen, P. (2003). Prevalence and characteristics of dementia in Parkinson disease: An 8-year prospective study. *Archives of Neurology, 60*(3), 387–392.

Aarsland, D., Andersen, K., Larsen, J. P., Lolk, A., Nielsen, H., & Kragh-Sorensen, P. (2001). Risk of dementia in Parkinson's disease: A community-based, prospective study. *Neurology, 56*(6), 730–736.

Aarsland, D., Zaccai, J., & Brayne, C. (2005). A systematic review of prevalence studies of dementia in Parkinson's disease. *Movement Disorders, 20*(10), 1255–1263.

Ardestani, M. S. (2010). Parkinson's disease, the inflammatory pathway and anti-inflammatory drugs: An overview. *Journal of Medical Sciences, 10*(3), 40–58.

Ascherio, A., Chen, H., Weisskopf, M. G., O'Reilly, E., McCulough, M. L., Calle, E. E., ... Thun, M. J. (2006). Pesticide exposure and risk for Parkinson's disease. *Annals of Neurology, 60*(2), 197–203.

Baldi, I., Cantagrel, A., Lebailly, P., Tison, F., Dubroca, B., Chrysostome, V., ... Brochard, P. (2003). Association between Parkinson's disease and exposure to pesticides in southwestern France. *Neuroepidemiology, 22*, 305–310.

Barbeau, A., Roy, M., Bernier, G., Campanella, G., & Paris, S. (1987). Ecogenetics of Parkinson's disease: Prevalence and environmental aspects in rural areas. *The Canadian Journal of Neurological Sciences, 14*(1), 36–41.

Bharucha, N. E., Bharucha, E. P., Bharucha, A. E., Bhise, A. V., & Schoenberg, B. S. (1988). Prevalence of Parkinson's disease in the Parsi community of Bombay, India. *Archives of Neurology, 45*(12), 1321–1323.

Bower, J. H., Maraganore, D. M., McDonnell, S. K., & Rocca, W. A. (1999). Incidence and distribution of parkinsonism in Olmsted County, Minnesota, 1976–1990. *Neurology, 52*(6), 1214–1220.

Brewer, G. J., Kanzer, S. H., Zimmerman, E. A., Molho, E. S., Celmins, D. F., Heckman, S. M., & Dick, R. (2010). Subclinical zinc deficiency in Alzheimer's disease and Parkinson's disease. *American Journal of Alzheimer's Disease and Other Dementias, 25*(7), 572–575.

Buter, T. C., van den Hout, A., Matthews, F. E., Larsen, J. P., Brayne, C., & Aarsland, D. (2008). Dementia and survival in Parkinson disease: A 12-year population study. *Neurology, 70*(13), 1017–1022.

Carlsson, A. (1959). The occurrence, distribution and physiological role of catecholamines in the nervous system. *Pharmacological Reviews, 11*(2, Part 2), 440–443.

Carlsson, A., Greengard, P., & Kandel, E. R. (2000). The Nobel Prize in Physiology or Medicine, 2000.

Checkoway, H. (2010). Documenting neurotoxicity from occupational manganese exposure. *Occupational and Environmental Medicine, 67*, 362–363.

Checkoway, H., & Nelson, L. M. (1999). Epidemiologic approaches to the study of Parkinson's disease etiology. *Epidemiology, 10*, 327–336.

Chen, H., Huang, X., Guo, X., Mailman, R. B., Park, Y., Kamel, F., ... Blair, A. (2010). Smoking duration, intensity, and risk of Parkinson disease. *Neurology, 74*(11), 878–884.

Chen, H., Shang, S. M., Hernán, M. A., Schwarzschild, M. A., Willett, W. C., Colditz, G. A., ... Ascherio, A. (2003). Nonsteroidal anti-inflammatory drugs and the risk of Parkinson disease. *Archives of Neurology, 60*, 1059–1064.

Chen, H., Shumin, M., Zhang, S. M., Schwarzschild, M. A., Hernán, M. A., & Ascherio, A. (2006). Survival of Parkinson's disease patients in a large prospective cohort of male health professionals. *Movement Disorders, 21*(7), 1002–1007.

Couper, J. (1837). On the effects of black oxide of manganese when inhaled into the lungs. *British Annals of Medicine Pharmacy, 1*, 41–42.

de Lau, L. M., & Breteler, M. M. (2006). Epidemiology of Parkinson's disease. *Lancet Neurology, 5*(6), 525–535.

De Pedro-Cuesta, J. (1987). Studies on the prevalence of paralysis agitans by tracer methodology. *Acta Neurologica Scandinavica, 75*(Suppl. 112), 1–106.

Dick, F. D., De Palma, G., Ahmadi, A., Scott, N. W., Prescott, G. J., Bennett, J., ... Felice, A. (2007). Environmental risk factors for Parkinson's disease and parkinsonism: The Geoparkinson study. *Occupational & Environmental Medicine, 64*, 666–672.

Dorsey, E. R., Constantinescu, R., Thompson, J. P., Biglan, K. M., Holloway, R. G., Kieburtz, K., ... Tanner, C. M. (2007). Projected number of people with Parkinson disease in the most populous nations, 2005 through 2030. *Neurology, 68*(5), 384–386.

Dorsey, E. R., Elbaz, A., Nichols, E., Abd-Allah, F., Abdelalim, A., Adsuar, J. C., ... GBD 2016 Parkinson's Disease Collaborators. (2018). Global, regional, and national burden of Parkinson's disease, 1990–2016: A systematic analysis for the Global Burden of Disease Study 2016. *The Lancet.* doi:10.1016/S1474-4422(18)30295-3.

Driver, J. A., Logroscino, G., Gaziano, J. M., & Kurth, T. (2009). Incidence and remaining lifetime risk of Parkinson disease in advanced age. *Neurology, 72*(5), 432–438.

Elahi, E. (2009). A study of Parkinson's disease in Iranian patients. *Genetics in the 3rd Millennium, 7*(3), 1740–1752.

Elbaz, A., Bower, J. H., Peterson, B. J., Maraganore, D. M., McDonnell, S. K., Ahlskog, J. E., ... Rocca, W. A. (2003). Survival study of Parkinson disease in Olmsted county, Minnesota. *Archives of Neurology, 60*, 91–96.

Friedl, K. E., Grate, S., & Proctor, S. P. (2009). Neurotoxicological interactions with physical and psychological stressors, Chapter 9. In *RTO-TR-HFM-057* (pp. 1–22). Fort Belvoir, VA: Defense Technical Information Center (DTIC).

Funayama, M., Hasegawa, K., Kowa, H., Saito, M., Tsuji, S., & Obata, F. (2002). A new locus for Parkinson's disease (PARK8) maps to chromosome 12p11.2-q13.1. *Annals of Neurology, 51*, 296–301.

Goedert, M. (2001). Alpha-synuclein and neurodegenerative diseases. *Nature Reviews Neuroscience, 2*(7), 492–501.

Golomb, B. A. (2008). Acetylcholinesterase inhibitors and Gulf War illnesses. *Proceedings of the National Academy of Sciences of the United States of America, 105*, 4295–4300.

Guilarte, T. R. (2010). Manganese and Parkinson's disease: A critical review and new findings. *Environmental Health Perspectives, 118*(8), doi:10.1289/ehp.0901748.

Hald, A., Van Beek, J., & Lotharious. (2007). Inflammation in Parkinson's disease. *Subcellular Biochemistry, 42*, 249–279.

Hancock, D. B., Martin, E. R., Mayhew, G. M., Stajich, J. M., Jewett, R., Stacy, M. A., ... Scott, W. K. (2008). Pesticide exposure and risk of Parkinson's disease: A family-based case-control study. *BMC Neurology, 8*, 6, doi:10.1186/1471-2377-8-6.

Hardy, J., Cai, H., Cookson, M. R., Gwinn-Hardy, K., & Singleton, A. (2006). Genetics of Parkinson's disease and parkinsonism. *Annals of Neurology, 60*(4), 389–398.

Hernán, M. A., Takkouche, B., Caamano-Isorna, F., & Gestal-Otero, J. J. (2002). A meta-analysis of coffee drinking, cigarette smoking, and the risk of Parkinson's disease. *Annals of Neurology, 52*, 276–284.

Hirsch, L., Jette, N., Frolkis, A., Steeves, T., & Pringsheim, T. (2016). The incidence of Parkinson's disease: A systematic review and meta-analysis. *Neuroepidemiology, 46*, 292–300.

Ho, S. C., Woo, J., & Lee, C. M. (1989). Epidemiologic study of Parkinson's disease in Hong Kong. *Neurology, 39*, 1314–1318.

Hobson, P., & Meara, J. (2004). Risk and incidence of dementia in a cohort of older subjects with Parkinson's disease in the United Kingdom. *Movement Disorders, 19*(9), 1043–1049.

Hobson, P., Meara, J., & Ishihara-Paul, L. (2010). The estimated life expectancy in a community cohort of Parkinson's disease patients with and without dementia, compared with the UK population. *Journal of Neurology, Neurosurgery, and Psychiatry, 81*, 1093–1098.

Holt, R. J., Sklar, A. R., Darkow, T., Goldberg, G. A., Johnson, J. C., & Harley, C. R. (2010). Prevalence of Parkinson's disease-induced psychosis in a large US managed care population. *The Journal of Neuropsychiatry and Clinical Neurosciences, 22*, 105–110.

Huang, X., Chen, P., Kaufer, D. I., Trouster, A. I., & Poole, C. (2006). Apolipoprotein E and dementia in Parkinson disease: A meta-analysis. *Archives of Neurology, 63*, 189–193.

Hughes, T. A., Ross, H. F., Mindham, R. H., & Spokes, E. G. (2004). Mortality in Parkinson's disease and its association with dementia and depression. *Acta Neurologica Scandinavica, 110*(2), 118–123.

Kanda, A., Ebihara, S., Arai, H., Takeda, A., & Sasaki, H. (2000). Parkinson's disease and impaired chemosensitivity to hypoxia. *Lancet, 356*(9247), 2100.

Kitada, T., Asakawa, S., Hattori, N., Matsumine, H., Yamamura, Y., Minoshima, S., … Shimizu, N. (1998). Mutations in the parkin gene cause autosomal recessive juvenile parkinsonism. *Nature, 392*, 605–608.

Knott, C., Stern, G., & Wilkin, G. P. (2000). Inflammatory regulators in Parkinson's disease: iNOS, lipocortin-1, and cyclooxygeneases-1 and 2. *Molecular and Cellular Neuroscience, 16*, 724–739.

Krüger, R., Kuhn, W., Müller, T., Woitalla, D., Graeber, M., Kösel, S., … Riess, O. (1998). Ala30Pro mutation in the gene encoding alphasynuclein in Parkinson's disease. *Nature Genetics, 18*, 106–108.

Langston, J. W. (1985). MPTP and Parkinson's disease. *Trends in Neurosciences, 8*, 79–83.

Langston, J. W., Ballard, P., Tetrud, J. W., & Irwin, I. (1983). Chronic parkinsonism in humans due to a product of meperidine-analog synthesis. *Science, 219*, 979–980.

Langston, J. W., Forno, L. S., Rebert, C. S., & Irwin, I. (1984). Selective nigral toxicity after systemic administration of 1-methyl-4-pheny1-1,2,5,6-tetrahydropyridine (MPTP) in the squirrel monkey. *Brain Research, 292*, 390–394.

Langston, J. W., & Palfreman, J. (1996). *The Case of the frozen addicts: How the solution of an extraordinary medical mystery spawned a revolution in the understanding and treatment of Parkinson's disease.* New York: Pantheon.

Lewitt, P. A., Rezai, A. R., Leehey, M. A., Ojemann, S. G., Flaherty, A. W., Eskandar, E. N., … Feigin, A. (2011). AAV2-GAD gene therapy for advanced Parkinson's disease: A double-blind, sham-surgery controlled, randomised trial. *Lancet Neurology, 10*(4), 309–319.

Lewy, F. H. (1912). Paralysis agitans. In M. Lewandowsky (Ed.), *Handbuch der Neurologie* (pp. 920–933). Berlin: Springer Verlag.

Lim, K. L., Dawson, V. L., & Dawson, T. M. (2006). Parkin-mediated lysine 63-linked polyubiquitination: A link to protein inclusions formation in Parkinson's and other conformational diseases? *Neurobiology of Aging, 27*, 524–529.

Marder, K., Tank, M. X., Mejia, H., Alfaro, B., Cote, L., Louis, E., … Mayeux, R. (1996). Parkinson's disease among first-degree relatives: A community-based study. *Neurology, 47*(1), 155–160.

Muangpaisan, W., Hori, H., & Brayne, C. (2009). Systematic review of the prevalence and incidence of Parkinson's disease in Asia. *Journal of Epidemiology, 19*(6), 281–293.

Naghavi, M., & GBD 2016 Causes of Death Collaborators. (2017). Global, regional, and national age-sex specific mortality for 264 causes of death, 1980–2016: A systematic analysis for the Global Burden of Disease Study 2016. *The Lancet, 390*, 1151–1210.

Naghavi, M., Wang, H., Lozano, R., Davis, A., Liang, X., Zhou, M., … GBD 2013 Mortality and Causes of Death Collaborators. (2015). Global, regional, and national age–sex specific all-cause and cause-specific mortality for 240 causes of death, 1990–2013: A systematic analysis for the Global Burden of Disease Study 2013. *The Lancet, 385*, 117–171.

Paisán-Ruíz, C., Jain, S., Evans, E. W., Gilks, W. P., Simón, J., van der Brug, M., … Singleton, A. B. (2004). Cloning of the gene containing mutations that cause PARK8-linked Parkinson's disease. *Neuron, 44*(4), 595–600.

Parkinson, J. (1817). *An essay on the shaking palsy.* London: Sherwood, Neely and Jones.

Perry, V. H. (2012). Innate inflammation in Parkinson's disease. *Cold Spring Harbor Perspectives in Medicine, 2*(9), doi:10.1101/cshperspect.a009373.

Poewe, W. (2006). The natural history of Parkinson's disease. *Journal of Neurology, 253*(Suppl. 7), VII/2–VII/6.

Polymeropoulos, M. H. (1998). Autosomal dominant Parkinson's disease and alphasynuclein. *Annals of Neurology, 44*(3 Suppl. 1), S63–S64.

Polymeropoulos, M. H., Lavedan, C., Leroy, E., Ide, S. E., Dehejia, A., Dutra, A., … Nussbaum, R. L. (1997). Mutation in the alpha-synuclein gene identified in families with Parkinson's disease. *Science, 276*, 2045–2047.

Pradhan, S., Pandey, N., Shashank, S., Gupta, R. K., & Mathur, A. (1999). Parkinsonism due to predominant involvement of substantia nigra in Japanese encephalitis. *Neurology, 53*, 1781–1786.

Pringsheim, T., Jette, N., Frolkis, A., & Steeves, T. D. L. (2014). The prevalence of Parkinson's disease: A systematic review and meta-analysis. *Movement Disorders, 29*(13), 1583–1590.

Priyadarshi, A., Khuder, S. A., Schaub, E. A., & Shrivastava, S. (2000). A meta-analysis of Parkinson's disease and exposure to pesticides. *Neurotoxicology, 21*(4), 435–440.

Racette, B. A., Good, L. M., Kissel, A. B., Criswell, S. R., & Perlmutter, J. S. (2009). A population-based study of parkinsonism in an Amish community. *Neuroepidemiology, 33*(3), 225–230.

Ramakrishnan, U. (2002). Prevalence of micronutrient malnutrition worldwide. *Nutrition Reviews, 60*(5), S46–SA2.

Richardson, J. R., Quan, Y., Sherer, T. B., Greenamyre, J. T., & Miller, G. W. (2005). Paraquat neurotoxicity is distinct from that of MPTP and rotenone. *Toxicological Sciences, 88*(1), 193–201.

Ritz, B., Ascherio, A., Checkoway, H., Marder, K. S., Nelson, L. M., Rocca, W. A., … Gorell, J. (2007). Pooled analysis of tobacco use and risk of Parkinson disease. *Archives of Neurology, 64*, 990–997.

Rodier, J. (1955). Manganese poisoning in Moroccan miners. *British Journal of Industrial Medicine, 12,* 21–35.

Rogaeva, E., Johnson, J., Lang, A. E., Gulick, C., Gwinn-Hardy, K., Kawarai, T., … Singleton, A. B. (2004). Analysis of the PINK1 gene in a large cohort of cases with Parkinson disease. *Archives of Neurology, 61*(12), 1898–1904.

Safranak, T. J., Theis, M., & Krause, J. (2007). *The Nebraska Parkinson's disease registry*. Lincoln, NE: Nebraska Department of Health and Human Services.

Savica, R., Grossardt, B. R., Bower, J. B., Ahlskog, J. E., & Rocca, W. A. (2016). Time trends in the incidence of Parkinson's disease: A 30-year study. *Journal of the American Medical Association, 73*(8), 981–989.

Schulz-Schaeffer, W. J. (2010). The synaptic pathology of alpha-synuclein aggregation in dementia with Lewy bodies, Parkinson's disease and Parkinson's disease dementia. *Acta Neuropathologica, 120*(2), 131–143.

Shojaee, S., Fazlali, Z., Ghazavi, F., Banihosseini, S. S., Kazemi, M. H., Parsa, K., … Elahi, E. (2009). Identification of four novel potentially Parkinson's disease associated LRRK2 variations among Iranian patients. *Neuroscience, 467*(2), 53–57.

Spillantini, M. G., Crowther, R. A., Jakes, R., Hasegawa, M., & Goedert, M. (1998). Alphasynuclein in filamentous inclusions of Lewy bodies from Parkinson's disease and dementia with Lewy bodies. *Proceedings of the National Academy of Sciences of the United States of America, 95*(11), 6469–6473.

Spillantini, M. G., Schmidt, M. L., Lee, V. M., Trojanowski, J. Q., Jakes, R., & Goedert, M. (1997). Alpha-synuclein in Lewy bodies. *Nature, 388*(6645), 839–840.

Strickland, D., & Bertoni, J. M. (2003). Parkinson's prevalence estimated by a state registry. *Movement Disorders, 19*(3), 318–323.

Sulzer, D., Bogulavsky, J., Larsen, K. E., Behr, G., Karatekin, E., Kleinman, M. H., … Zecca, L. (2000). Neuromelanin biosynthesis is driven by excess cytosolic catecholamines not accumulated by synaptic vesicles. *Proceedings of the National Academy of Sciences of the United States of America, 97*(22), 11869–11874.

Tanner, C. M., Kamel, F., Ross, G. W., Hoppin, J. A., Goldman, S. M., Korell, M., … Langston, J. W. (2011). Rotenone, Paraquat and Parkinson's disease. *Environmental Health Perspectives.* doi:10.1289/ehp.1002839.

Tanner, C. M., Ottman, R., Goldman, S. M., Ellenberg, J., Chan, P., Mayeux, R., & Langston, J. W. (1999). Parkinson disease in twins: An etiologic study. *Journal of the American Medical Association, 281*(4), 341–346.

Tanner, C. M., Ross, G. W., Jewell, S. A., Hauser, R. A., Jankovic, J., Factor, S. A., … Langston, J. W. (2009). Occupation and risk of parkinsonism: A multicenter case-control study. *Archives of Neurology, 66*(9), 1106–1113.

Tretiakoff, K. (1919). *Contribution a l'Etude de L'Anatomie pathologique du Locus Niger de Soemmering avec quelques déductions relatives à la pathogénie des troubles du tonus musculaire et de la Maladie de Parkinson* (Doctoral Dissertation), University of Paris, Paris, France.

Van Den Eeden, S. K., Tanner, C. M., Bernstein, A. L., Fross, R. D., Leimpeter, A., Bloch, D. A., & Nelson, L. M. (2003). Incidence of Parkinson's disease: Variation by age, gender and race/ethnicity. *American Journal of Epidemiology, 157*(11), 1015–1022.

Wang, H., Naghavi, M., Allen, C., Barber, R. M., Bhutta, Z. A., Carter, A., … GBD 2015 Mortality and Causes of Death Collaborators. (2016). Global, regional, and national life expectancy, all-cause mortality, and cause-specific mortality for 249 causes of death, 1980–2015: A systematic analysis for the Global Burden of Disease Study 2015. *The Lancet, 388*(10053), 1459–1544.

Weintraub, D., & Hurtig, H. I. (2007). Presentation and management of psychosis in Parkinson's disease and dementia with Lewy bodies. *American Journal of Psychiatry, 164*(10), 1491–1498.

World Health Organization. (2006). *Neurological disorders: Public health challenges* (pp. 140–150). Geneva, Switzerland: World Health Organization.

World Health Organization. (2009). Age-standardized DALYs per 100,000 by cause and member state, 2004. Health statistics and health information systems. *Global burden of disease.* World Health Organization.

Zimprich, A., Biskup, S., Leitner, P., Lichtner, P., Farrer, M., Lincoln, S., … Gasser, T. (2004). Mutations in LRRK2 cause autosomal-dominant parkinsonism with pleomorphic pathology. *Neuron, 44*(4), 601–607.

CHAPTER 50

Epidemiology of Multiple Sclerosis

Zachary M. Harris and Randall E. Harris

▶ Introduction

Multiple sclerosis is an autoimmune inflammatory disease in which the myelin sheaths surrounding the axons of neurons (nerve cells) are damaged or destroyed, leading to demyelination and scarring as well as a broad spectrum of signs and symptoms. The name *multiple sclerosis* refers to scars (scleroses), particularly in the white matter of the brain and spinal cord. Disease onset usually occurs in young adults between the ages of 20 and 40 years. Multiple sclerosis is diagnosed roughly twice as often in women compared to men (Weinshenker, 1994).

Multiple sclerosis compromises the communication of neurons in the central nervous system. Neurons communicate with one another by transmitting electrical impulses (action potentials) down their long filamentous tentacles (axons) to the synapses (junctions between neurons). Axons are wrapped in myelin that provide essential insulation to facilitate the rapid, directed electrical transmission of nerve impulses (**FIGURE 50.1**). Myelin is a lipoprotein that is synthesized by *glia,* cells that support and nurture neurons. In multiple sclerosis, the body's own immune system attacks and damages myelin and/or glial cells. When myelin is lost, the axons can no longer effectively conduct nerve impulses.

▶ Discovery of Multiple Sclerosis

The French neurologist, Jean-Martin Charcot, first recognized multiple sclerosis as a distinct disease in 1868. Charcot named the condition *sclérose en plaques* and characterized its diagnosis by the neurologic triad of nystagmus (oscillating eye movements), intention tremor, and scanning (staccato) speech (Charcot, 1868). Earlier in 1838, Robert Carswell and Jean Cruveilhier had published detailed descriptions and drawings of pathologic lesions in brain and spinal cord specimens from patients who had died from the disease (Compston, 1988).

Sydney Allison spearheaded the use of population-based studies of multiple sclerosis and other neurologic conditions in the early 20th century. His early studies of the populations in Wales and Northern Ireland characterized salient clinical and epidemiologic features of the disease including its onset during early adult life, an excess in females, occasional familial clustering, and the progressive, often episodic, nature of disability and decline in most patients resulting in shortened life expectancy (Allison, 1931; Allison & Millar, 1954).

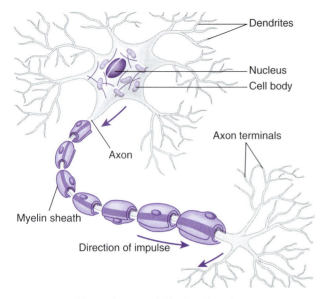

FIGURE 50.1 Nerve Axon and Myelin Sheath.
© Jones & Bartlett Learning.

Diagnosis of Multiple Sclerosis

Since almost any neurological symptom can appear in patients with multiple sclerosis, other conditions must be ruled out in reaching the diagnosis. Despite sophisticated diagnostic tools and techniques, the diagnosis of multiple sclerosis remains one of exclusion, meaning that other likely diseases must be eliminated before a conclusive diagnosis of multiple sclerosis can be made.

An international panel of experts has recently developed a system to clarify the diagnosis of multiple sclerosis that makes use of neurological imaging (magnetic resonance imaging [MRI]), analysis of cerebral spinal fluid for IgG antibodies, and testing for visual evoked action potentials. According to this system, confirmation of multiple sclerosis is based upon the number of attacks of neurological symptoms characteristic of multiple sclerosis combined with the number and location of lesions identified (McDonald et al., 2001; Polman et al., 2005).

Course of Multiple Sclerosis

Multiple sclerosis is a complex debilitating condition with high morbidity and mortality. Often, the disease follows a biphasic course where a relapsing-remitting stage is followed by a more severe progressive stage. Relapsing-remitting multiple sclerosis is characterized by transient episodes of dysfunction caused by inflammation of the nervous system with rapid recovery. Onset of these attacks can include paresthesia (numbness), diplopia (double vision), scotoma (visual anomalies), sensory and motor disorders of limbs, and cerebellar incoordination (lack of balance).

After a variable amount of time (months to years), the relapsing-remitting stage of multiple sclerosis may advance to an episodic downhill course of progressively worse symptoms culminated by blindness due to retrobulbar neuritis, ataxia, incontinence, paraplegia, major system failure, and death. This so-called secondary progressive type is untreatable and the main cause of permanent disability in the multiple-sclerosis patient population. Patients presenting with relapsing-remitting multiple sclerosis may never advance to the progressive stage of the disease. On the other hand, many patients who have no previous history of transient neurologic attacks present with progressive multiple sclerosis and are said to have primary progressive multiple sclerosis. Intellectual deterioration is not a common feature of relapsing-remitting multiple sclerosis, although cognitive impairment can be seen in progressive multiple sclerosis. There is no cure for multiple sclerosis and despite intensive efforts, the average life expectancy is reduced by about 10 years compared to the general population.

Global Burden of Multiple Sclerosis

During 2005–2007, the World Health Organization launched a major collaborative initiative to determine the global epidemiology of multiple sclerosis and characterize the resources needed to diagnose, inform, treat, rehabilitate, and provide services to people who develop the disease. As a part of this effort, 112 countries representing 87.8% of the world population were surveyed in order to gather epidemiologic data on the incidence, prevalence, morbidity, and mortality of multiple sclerosis. The survey detected more than 1.3 million people with multiple sclerosis, 630,000 in Europe, 520,000 in the Americas, 66,000 in the Eastern Mediterranean, 56,000 in the Western Pacific, 31,430 in Southeast Asia, and 11,000 in Africa. We note that these figures underestimate the total worldwide burden of multiple sclerosis since no data were available for some countries with huge populations such as the Russian Federation (World Health Organization, 2008). In a recent study using new data sources and updated analytical procedures, *Global Burden of Disease* (GBD) investigators examined data from 195 countries and territories and estimated there were 2.0 million prevalent cases of multiple sclerosis in the world population in 2015. Despite the increased number of cases of multiple sclerosis in 2015 compared to 2005, the age-standardized annual prevalence of multiple sclerosis actually declined by 2% during the same time span suggesting there has been some progress in therapy. Currently, the global age-standardized annual prevalence of multiple sclerosis is slightly less than 30 per 100,000 (Vos & GBD 2015 Disease and Injury Incidence and Prevalence Collaborators, 2016).

▶ Global Prevalence and Incidence of Multiple Sclerosis

Globally, the annual prevalence of multiple sclerosis is extraordinarily variable, ranging from less than one case per 100,000 in Africa to 176 cases per 100,000 in Hungary. The median prevalence was 30 per 100,000. Rates exceeded 100 cases per 100,000 in North America (United States, Canada) and several European countries (Hungary, Germany, Czech Republic, Norway, Denmark, Poland), whereas far lower rates (less than 10 cases per 100,000) were reported by most countries in Africa, Southeast Asia, the Western Pacific, and South America (**FIGURE 50.2**). By income

category, prevalence rates were substantially higher in high-income countries than low-income countries (**FIGURE 50.3**).

Annual incidence rates are also shown in Figures 50.2 and 50.3. These rates are markedly lower than the prevalence rates and are given as *cases per million*. The median annual incidence among all reporting countries was 25 cases per million with a range from less than 1 in Africa to 290 cases per million in the small Eastern Mediterranean nation of Croatia. The global pattern of incidence is similar to the prevalence; high rates are found in high-income developed countries and low rates in low-income developing countries.

It is likely that these prevalence and incidence patterns largely reflect the enhanced diagnostic and reporting capabilities of developed nations with higher standards of living and more extensive healthcare systems. Nevertheless, the World Health Organization (WHO) survey results confirm that multiple sclerosis is a "global disease" that occurs in all populations.

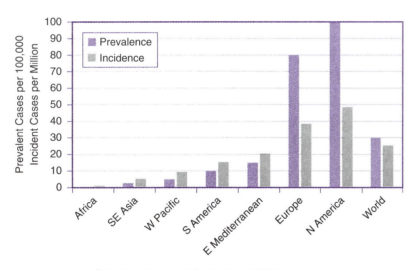

FIGURE 50.2 Prevalence and Incidence of Multiple Sclerosis by Region, 2008.

Data from World Health Organization. (2008). *Atlas multiple sclerosis resources in the world*. Geneva, Switzerland: World Health Organization.

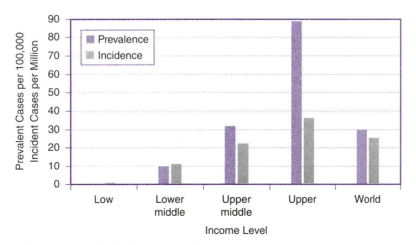

FIGURE 50.3 Prevalence and Incidence of Multiple Sclerosis by Income, 2008.

Data from World Health Organization. (2008). *Atlas multiple sclerosis resources in the world*. Geneva, Switzerland: World Health Organization.

Accurate quantification of the burden of multiple sclerosis in less developed countries is expected to improve as diagnostic facilities such as MRI become more widely available and accessible (WHO, 2008).

Age-Specific Incidence of Multiple Sclerosis

Despite the wide international variability in the prevalence and incidence rates, certain epidemiologic features of multiple sclerosis have been found to be relatively invariant. In the recent WHO survey of multiple sclerosis, 60%–70% of cases were diagnosed prior to age 40 years and the mean age of onset was around 29 years for all regions and income groups in both men and women. Furthermore, there was a consistent 2–1 female to male ratio of both the incidence and prevalence of multiple sclerosis, irrespective of income level. The pattern of age-specific incidence depicted in **FIGURE 50.4** reflects the excess female risk at all ages (WHO, 2008).

Case Fatality and Life Expectancy

Several studies have reported that patients with multiple sclerosis have reduced life expectancy and higher mortality than individuals from the general population. However, there is considerable variability among studies and a wide range of reported median survival times.

Sadovnick and colleagues examined the case fatality rate and life expectancy of patients with multiple sclerosis in a large cohort of patients followed in Vancouver, Canada. The case fatality among patients with

severe disability was four times higher than controls without disease. In contrast, excluding deaths by suicide, case fatality among patients with mild to moderate disability was 1.6 times higher than controls matched by age and gender. Life tables constructed for the patient cohort indicated that the overall life expectancy of multiple sclerosis is approximately 7 years less than the general population (Sadovnick, Ebers, Wilson, & Paty, 1992).

Grytten and colleagues examined survival and cause of death among 878 patients diagnosed with multiple sclerosis and living in Hordaland County, Norway. Survival and mortality data for the patient cohort were compared with the general Norway population matched by age, gender, and calendar year. During more than 43 years of follow-up, 198 patients died. The median survival from onset was 41 years for patients with multiple sclerosis versus 49 years in the general population, and the overall mortality among patients was 2.7 times higher than expected. Median survival was greater in women than men (43 years vs. 36 years) and greater for younger patients with onset less than 30 years of age versus older patients with onset after 43 years of age (45 years vs. 23 years). Nevertheless, the standard mortality ratio (SMR) was highest among patients with early onset (SMR = 5.4 for onset before age 20 years) and declined with later onset (SMR = 1.2 for onset after age 60 years). Patients with primary progressive disease had 1.6 times overall mortality higher than those with relapsing-remitting disease. Among the 198 decedents, 144 (73%) had multiple sclerosis listed on their death certificates and 113 (57%) had multiple sclerosis listed as the primary cause of death. Other notable causes of death included cardiovascular disease (16%), infectious disease (9%), cancer (6%), and accident or suicide (3%) (Grytten, Lie, Aarseth, Nyland, & Myhr, 2008).

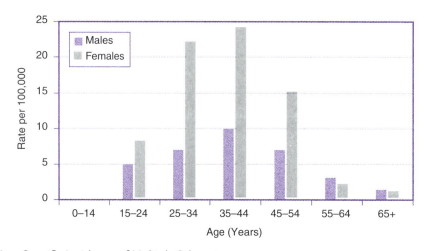

FIGURE 50.4 Annual Age-Specific Incidence of Multiple Sclerosis.
Data from World Health Organization. (2008). *Atlas multiple sclerosis resources in the world.* Geneva, Switzerland: World Health Organization.

Similar findings were reported for a cohort of 386 patients with multiple sclerosis living in Oslo, Norway. Patients were diagnosed between 1940 and 1980 and followed until 2006. A total of 263 patients (68%) died during follow-up. Median survival from the time of onset was 35 years, which was approximately 11 years less than expected in the general population. The crude annual mortality rate was 21.6 per 1000 person-years and the all-cause SMR was 2.5. The most frequent underlying cause of death recorded on death certificates was multiple sclerosis (43%). Other leading causes of death were cardiovascular disease (14%), cancer (10%), infection (10%), and accident or suicide (5%). The investigators also noted that excess mortality first appeared during the second decade after disease onset in this patient cohort (Smestad, Sandvik, & Celius, 2009).

▶ Suicide in Multiple Sclerosis

Several studies have found that the risk of suicide is elevated in patients with multiple sclerosis. In a nationwide investigation in Denmark, 53 of 5525 patients committed suicide in the period 1953–1985. These data yielded a cumulative lifetime risk of 1.95% and a SMR of 1.83. The suicide risk was 43% higher among males than females and was highest within the first 5 years after diagnosis (Stenager et al., 1992). Similar results have been reported for other cohorts of patients with multiple sclerosis (Bronnum-Hansen, Stenager, Nylev, & Koch-Henriksen, 2005; Fredrikson, Cheng, Jiang, & Wasserman, 2003).

▶ Global Mortality: Multiple Sclerosis

According to the underlying cause of death listed on death certificates, only a small fraction of patients with multiple sclerosis die every year, perhaps 2%–3% on average. Thus, the annual mortality rate due to multiple sclerosis in the world population is relatively low (~3 deaths per million). In GBD studies for the years 2013–2016, the annual number of deaths from multiple sclerosis ranged from 16,500 to 19,800 with a mean value of 18,400 deaths per year (Murray & 2013 GBD Collaborators, 2015; Naghavi & 2016 Collaborators, 2017; Wang, Naghavi, & 2015 GBD Collaborators, 2016). Nevertheless, as the disease progresses, disability also increases as do the DALY (*disability-adjusted life years*, the sum of years lost due to premature death and years lost due to disability).

Disability-Adjusted Life Years: Multiple Sclerosis

The DALY is the sum of *Years of Life Lost from Premature Death* (YLL) and *Years of Life Lost from Disability* (YDL): DALY = YLL + YDL. The global distribution of *DALY* lost due to multiple sclerosis is depicted for WHO member nations in **FIGURE 50.5**. As with the patterns of prevalence and incidence (Figures 50.2 and 50.3), the DALY are higher in developed nations with more advanced diagnostic, treatment, and reporting capabilities.

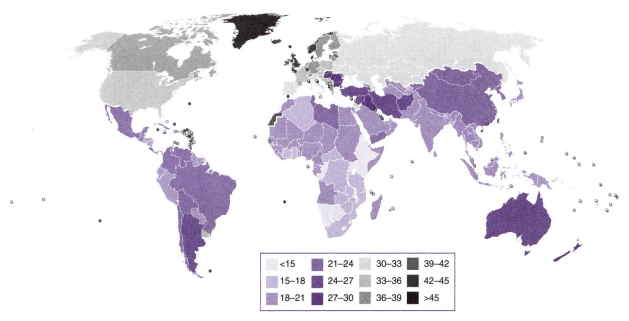

<15	21–24	30–33	39–42
15–18	24–27	33–36	42–45
18–21	27–30	36–39	>45

FIGURE 50.5 Global Disability-Adjusted Years: Multiple Sclerosis, 2004.

Data from World Health Organization. (2008). *The global burden of disease: 2004 update.* Geneva: WHO. Available at www.who.int/evidence/bod

▶ Autoimmunity and Multiple Sclerosis

Multiple sclerosis is generally characterized as a cell-mediated autoimmune disease of the central nervous system. This concept is supported by its higher frequency in females compared to males (which is similar to many other autoimmune disorders such as *systemic lupus erythematosus* and *rheumatoid arthritis);* its association with other autoimmune conditions in individual patients and amongst relatives of index cases; the presence of autoantibodies to myelin and glial cell antigens in the serum and cerebral spinal fluid of patients; and transient amelioration of disease activity during periods of immunosuppression such as pregnancy. As in other autoimmune conditions, specific haplotypes of the human leukocyte antigen (HLA) have been identified that predispose to multiple sclerosis. Furthermore, *experimental autoimmune encephalomyelitis* is an animal model that is analogous to human multiple sclerosis (Marrie, 2004; Weiner, 1998).

Female predominance is characteristic of all autoimmune conditions including multiple sclerosis. Autoimmunity reflects a reaction of the immune system against *"self."* In patients with multiple sclerosis, IgG antibodies targeting myelin and glial cells can be detected in sera and cerebral spinal fluid as well as in specimens of lesions. These antibodies stimulate killer T cells to attack glial cells in the brain and spinal cord resulting in demyelination and axonal dissection of neurons.

The genesis of autoimmunity and its predominance in females remains enigmatic. One hypothesis postulates incompatibility of X chromosomes. Since either the paternal or the maternal X chromosome is inactivated in cell lineages early during embryogenesis, the genotype of the human female is actually a *mosaic* of active and inactivated paternal and maternal X chromosomes. This phenomenon was described by Mary Lyon in 1961 and is called the *"Lyon hypothesis"* (Lyon, 1961). Inactivated X chromosomes are called *"Barr bodies"* named after Murray Barr who first described them (Barr & Bertram, 1949). Conceivably, incompatibility of the paternal and maternal X chromosomes might lead to immunoreactivity, particularly if neuronal tissues contain the active X chromosome from one parent and immune cells contain the other. In the context of other stimuli such as a viral infection, this could occasionally lead to failure of the immune system to recognize "self," thereby leading to an autoimmune reaction. Various permutations of this hypothesis have appeared in the literature (Willer, Sadovnick, & Ebers, 2002).

▶ Pathogenic Mechanisms in Multiple Sclerosis

Disruption of the Blood–Brain Barrier

Disruption of the blood–brain barrier has been found to precede the development of multiple sclerosis (Kermode et al., 1990). The blood–brain barrier consists of tight junctions between the endothelial cells that line the capillaries and other blood vessels of the brain and spinal cord. Under normal conditions, these tight junctions prevent entrance of T cells into neurological tissues; however, many viruses and certain other infectious agents may compromise the blood–brain barrier and allow T cells to pass through (**FIGURE 50.6**). Upon clearance of the infection, the T cells are trapped inside the brain and may stimulate immunoreactivity and inflammation. Notably, dysregulation of the blood–brain barrier and transendothelial migration of activated leukocytes and their release of inflammatory cytokines and chemokines are among the earliest cerebrovascular abnormalities seen in multiple sclerosis brains (Minagar & Alexander, 2003).

Inflammation

Inflammation is a chief pathologic hallmark of relapsing-remitting multiple sclerosis. According to one model, T lymphocytes gain entrance into the brain through the blood–brain barrier and become immunoreactive, thereby stimulating a cascade of destructive inflammatory processes including axon transection, myelin degradation, and glial cell death.

Localized foci of demyelination are present in white and gray matter in the brains of multiple sclerosis patients. Imaging these lesions using MRI with gadolinium enhancement provides the most conclusive evidence for a diagnosis of relapsing-remitting multiple sclerosis. Lesions can be pathologically characterized as immunologically active or chronic by various degrees of microgliosis, astrocytosis, myelin vacuolation or loss, and axonal transection. Demyelinated lesions will undergo a reparative process whereby oligodendrocytes replace lost myelin with a thinner but still functional sheath. These repaired lesions are called shadow lesions and are of intense interest because they exhibit a natural mechanism whereby the brain replaces lost myelin.

Remyelination Failure

The principal cell responsible for myelin formation and repair is the oligodendrocyte, a glial cell that synthesizes and maintains myelin for up to 40 nerve

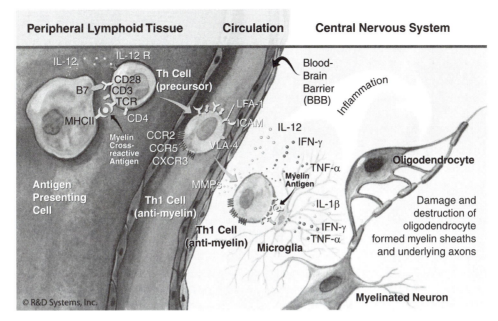

FIGURE 50.6 Lymphocyte Penetration of Blood–Brain Barrier.
Courtesy of R&D systems, Inc. Minneapolis, MN, USA.

axons in the central nervous system (Compston & Coles, 2002; Weiner, 1998; Weinshenker, 1994). Failure of remyelination by oligodendroctyes is thought to be largely responsible for sustained neurological symptoms in patients with progressive multiple sclerosis. Inability of oligodendrocytes to migrate into demyelinated areas and for oligodendrocyte progenitors to mature are possible reasons why lesions enter a chronically demyelinated phase. *Hyaluronan (hyaluronic acid)* is a large glycosaminoglycan that polymerizes to form a polygel scaffold that is essential for cell migration, adhesion, differentiation, maturation, and proliferation in many tissues including the brain. Recent studies have identified deposits of hyaluronan in lesions from multiple sclerosis patients, and this material has been found to inhibit the maturation of oligodendrocyte precursor cells *in vitro*. Degradation products of hyaluronan may thus contribute to remyelination failure by blocking the maturation of oligodendrocytes (Back et al., 2005). Most recently, this inhibitory process has been found to depend upon upregulation of specific toll-like receptors that activate the innate immune system (Sloane et al., 2010).

Axonal Injury

Irresponsiveness of progressive multiple sclerosis to immunomodulatory therapies suggests a completely different pathogenic mechanism of this disease stage. Focused research efforts are being made at investigating the role of Wallerian degeneration and axonal transection in chronic multiple sclerosis disability. Axonal

destruction appears early in the disease course in both lesions and normal white and gray matter areas and accumulates with disease progression. It is thought that axonal transection is at first clinically silent because the central nervous system compensates for neuroaxonal loss. However, once a threshold of axonal loss is reached, the neurodegenerative component of the disease becomes a major determinant of clinical disability (Trapp, Ransohoff, Fisher, & Rudick, 1999).

Chronic Cerebrospinal Venous Insufficiency

A recent theory advanced to explain the pathogenesis and progression of multiple sclerosis involves a vascular condition known as *chronic cerebrospinal venous insufficiency*, which is characterized by abnormal cerebral venous strictures of unknown origin and loss of venous outflow from the brain. Surgical repair of such lesions has been shown effective for some patients with multiple sclerosis in preliminary trials, but confirmation of benefit awaits the results of further testing (Zamboni et al., 2009).

Genetics of Multiple Sclerosis

Multiple sclerosis is a complex autoimmune disease involving the interaction of both genetic and environmental factors. Genetic susceptibility is indicated by studies of twins and relatives of index cases (probands). Monozygous twins have higher disease concordance (~20%) than dizygous twins (~5%), and full siblings of probands have approximately twice the risk of half-siblings (Dyment, Ebers, & Sadovnick, 2004; Sadovnick et al., 1993). Nevertheless, the high *lack of concordance* among monozygous twins (~80%) indicates that environmental factors undoubtedly play a significant role in the genesis of multiple sclerosis.

Genetic variation at the major histocompatibility complex (MHC) on chromosome 6 has been found to influence the risk of developing multiple sclerosis (**FIGURE 50.7**). Several genetic polymorphisms of the *HLA* system appear to either increase or decrease the risk. In addition, recent studies have identified polymorphisms of genes encoding *T-cell receptors* (which bind to HLA antigens) and the *cytotoxic T-cell leukocyte antigen* (which downregulates the T-cell antigenic response) that increase susceptibility. Genetic investigations are currently in progress in several laboratories to identify specific genotypes that confer susceptibility or resistance to the genesis of multiple sclerosis (Dyment et al., 2004).

Ethnic Differences in Multiple Sclerosis

In 1988, George Lowis reviewed the international literature to identify the main demographic and sociocultural features of multiple sclerosis in different ethnic groups. He noted that the highest rates were found in regions largely inhabited by Caucasians and the lowest in those areas with primarily non-Caucasian populations, and also that racially different groups living in the same geographic area had divergent rates, with higher rates predominating in Caucasians and lower rates in non-Caucasians. Within racial groups, Lowis also noted that the prevalence increased with increasing latitude and suggested that while racial (genetic) factors may contribute to the distribution of multiple sclerosis, environmental agents predominantly influence the risk, irrespective of race (Lowis, 1988).

More recently, Mario Pugliatti, Stefano Sotgiu, and Giulio Rosati reviewed the extensive body of literature on multiple sclerosis and attempted to refine its geographic distribution using prevalence data from surveys conducted in different regions and at different times. Their review focused on prevalence estimates for ethnically distinct populations of several broad geographic areas (Europe, North and South America, Asia, Africa, the Middle East, and Australasia). Based upon findings of wide divergence in prevalence rates for populations in close geographic proximity, their suggestion is that genetic factors have a significant influence on susceptibility and resistance. For example, repeated surveys of populations living on the Italian peninsula have yielded rates 40–70 per 100,000, in striking contrast to the small island of Sardinia located 200 km to the west of the Italian mainland. Prevalence rates of multiple sclerosis in Sardinians were among the highest in the world, ranging from 144 to 152 per 100,000. The genetically isolated population of this small island also has one of the highest rates of type 1 diabetes, another autoimmune condition. Summarizing their results, the investigators state

> *The rarity of multiple sclerosis in Samis, Turkmen, Uzbeks, Kazakhs, Kirgizis, native Siberians, North and South Amerindians, Canadian Hutterites, Chinese, Japanese, African blacks, and New Zealand Maoris, and its high risk in Sardinians, Parsis and Palestinians, as well as in South African English-speaking whites as compared to Afrikaners, point to differential racial susceptibility as an important determinant of the worldwide uneven geographic distribution of the disease"* and suggest that the geography of multiple sclerosis can be viewed as *"a discontinuous distribution of genetic alleles of susceptibility, conferring risks that are subsequently modified and influenced by environment (Pugliatti, Sotgiu, & Rosati, 2002; Rosati, 2001).*

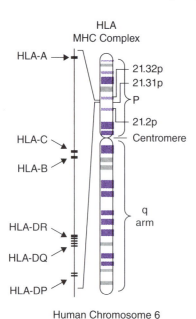

HLA
MHC Complex

HLA-A

21.32p
21.31p
P
21.2p
Centromere

HLA-C

HLA-B

q
arm

HLA-DR

HLA-DQ

HLA-DP

Human Chromosome 6

FIGURE 50.7 The Major Histocompatibility Complex (MHC) and Human Leukocyte Antigen (HLA) System on Chromosome 6.

Courtesy of Philip Deitiker.

Environmental Risk Factors for Multiple Sclerosis

Many environmental factors have been proposed as risk factors for multiple sclerosis. These include sun exposure, infection, vaccinations, climate, stress, occupation, drug use, and diet (Ascherio & Munger, 2007a, 2007b; Marrie, 2004). Selected epidemiologic studies of environmental factors are discussed next.

Geographic Variation in Multiple Sclerosis

Ecological studies of multiple sclerosis rates suggest there is a north-to-south gradient in the northern hemisphere and a south-to-north gradient in the southern hemisphere; that is, multiple sclerosis appears to be less common in people living near the equator. The early epidemiologic studies of Charles Limberg, Leonard Kurland, and E.D. Acheson were instrumental in showing the distinct latitudinal gradient in the rates of multiple sclerosis in the northern and southern hemispheres (Acheson, Bachrach, & Wright, 1960; Kurland, 1952; Limberg, 1943) and many subsequent investigations have confirmed its existence (Ascherio & Munger, 2007b; Kuroiwa, Shibasaki, & Ikeda, 1983; Leibowitz, Sharon, & Alter, 1967; Marrie, 2004; van der Mei, Ponsonby, Blizzard, & Dwyer, 2001), Cold climate, deficient sunlight, and low vitamin D have been investigated as possible causes of the latitude gradient in the rates. Notwithstanding, it has been pointed out that there are notable exceptions to this pattern that cannot be explained by a prevalence–latitude relationship (Pugliatti et al., 2002; Rosati, 2001).

Sunlight, Vitamin D, and Multiple Sclerosis

Investigations of a potential link between multiple sclerosis, sun exposure, and vitamin D are complicated by a number of issues including difficulties in accurately measuring exposure and the complexities of vitamin D metabolism in humans. Under normal physiologic conditions, ultraviolet light converts *7-dehydrocholesterol* in the skin to *previtamin D3* which is rapidly converted to *vitamin D3 (cholecalciferol)*. Cholecalciferol and a related form of vitamin D, *ergocalciferol,* can also be obtained from dietary sources.

Vitamin D3 is carried to the liver complexed with *vitamin D3 binding protein,* where it is converted to *25-hydroxy vitamin D (calcidiol)*, which is the major circulating form of vitamin D. Subsequently, in the kidney, the enzyme *1-alpha-hydroxylase* converts calcidiol to *1,25-dihydroxy vitamin D (calcitriol)* the biologically active form of the molecule (Holick, 2005).

Evidence from both in vitro investigations and animal studies suggests that vitamin D influences the risk of developing multiple sclerosis. In molecular studies, calcitriol has been found to dampen the innate immune response by inducing secretion of anti-inflammatory cytokines by T cells (Von Essen et al., 2010). Furthermore, in animal studies, the administration of biologically active vitamin D has been shown to prevent the onset of *experimental autoimmune encephalitis* (an experimental mouse model of multiple sclerosis) as well as its progression (Cantorna, 2008; Cantorna, Hayes, & DeLuca, 1996; Lemire & Archer, 1991).

A team of investigators at Harvard University recently examined the association of dietary vitamin D in two large prospective cohorts of women, the Nurses' Health Study (92,253 women followed from 1980 to 2000) and the Nurses' Health Study II (95,310 women followed from 1991 to 2001). Diet was assessed at baseline and updated every 4 years thereafter. During follow-up, 173 incident cases of multiple sclerosis were detected. Pooled results from the two cohorts revealed that women in the highest quintile of total vitamin D intake had a significantly reduced risk of developing multiple sclerosis compared to women with low intake (RR = 0.67). When the sources of vitamin D were stratified, supplementary vitamin D intake (at least 400 international units daily) was inversely associated with the risk (OR = 0.59) but not dietary vitamin D (Munger et al., 2004).

Munger and colleagues also evaluated the potential protective effect of vitamin D by examining levels of 25-hydroxyvitamin D (calcidiol) in serum samples of 247 cases with multiple sclerosis and matched controls. Sera were obtained from the U.S. Department of Defense Serum Repository of more than 7 million military personnel. Multiple sclerosis cases were identified from Army and Navy physical disability databases for 1992–2004 and each case was matched to two disease-free controls by age, gender, ethnicity, and dates of blood collection. Results revealed an inverse dose response in the risk of developing multiple sclerosis with increasing levels of 25-hydroxy vitamin D, but only for Caucasians. The disease odds were reduced by 62% among individuals in the highest quintile (above 99.1 nmol/L) compared to those in the lowest quintile (OR = 0.38). No significant associations were found between serum levels of vitamin D and multiple sclerosis for members of other ethnic groups, although these individuals had lower 25-hydroxy vitamin D levels than Caucasians. The investigators suggest their results support *"a protective role for vitamin D in multiple sclerosis"* (Ascherio, Munger, & Simon, 2010; Munger, Levin, Hollis, Howard, & Ascherio, 2006).

Investigators at the University of California in Los Angeles investigated sun exposure and multiple sclerosis in 79 disease-discordant monozygous twin pairs. The analysis compared sun exposure in the affected twin with that of the unaffected twin in a pair-matched case–control design. Results revealed that for each unit increase in a sun exposure index, the odds of developing multiple sclerosis *decreased* by 25%. Findings suggest a protective effect of sun exposure that is independent of genetic susceptibility (Islam, Gauderman, Cozen, & Mack, 2007).

In a recent case–control study conducted at multiple sites in Australia, Robyn Lucas and colleagues compared sun exposure and serum levels of vitamin D in 216 cases with multiple sclerosis to 395 controls without disease matched by age, gender, and location. Results revealed that the odds of developing a first demyelinating event *decreased* by 30% per 1000 kJ increase in exposure to ultraviolet light, and independently decreased by 7% per 10 nmol/L increase in the serum level of 25-hydroxy-vitamin D. The investigators concluded that sun exposure and vitamin D levels may independently influence the risk of developing multiple sclerosis but advocated further evaluation in clinical trials. Postulated mechanisms for these effects include immunosuppression by sun exposure and downregulation of innate immunity by vitamin D (Lucas et al., 2011).

Investigators at the University of California, San Francisco, examined the association between serum levels of 25-hydroxyvitamin D3 and the rate of relapse among 110 pediatric patients with multiple sclerosis. They found that for every 10 ng/mL increase in the level of 25-hydroxyvitamin D3, the rate of subsequent relapse decreased by 34% (Mowry et al., 2010). Similar results were reported by investigators at the University of Melbourne for a prospective cohort of 145 adult patients with relapsing-remitting multiple sclerosis. They found that for each 10 nmol/L increase in 25-hydroxyvitamin D3, the risk of relapse decreased by 12% (Simpson et al., 2010).

The totality of observational evidence therefore suggests that vitamin D may have both chemopreventive and therapeutic value in reducing the burden of multiple sclerosis. Multicenter double-blind placebo-controlled randomized clinical trials of vitamin D supplementation are currently in progress to elucidate such effects in patients with multiple sclerosis.

Infection and Multiple Sclerosis

Scores of microbial infectious agents have been proposed as potential triggers in the pathogenesis of multiple sclerosis; however, no specific microbe has been clearly substantiated as causative. Findings supporting a viral etiology include pathological evidence of infection in the brain and cerebrospinal fluid of most patients, the association of several viruses with *human demyelinating encephalitis* (a condition with similarities to multiple sclerosis), and induction of demyelination in animals by viral infection. Many childhood infections have been studied including measles, mumps, rubella, varicella, human herpes virus type 6, retroviruses, and *Chlamydia*

pneumoniae. Albeit, results for specific microbes either reflect no association whatsoever or are inconsistent from study to study. One possible exception is Epstein–Barr virus (EBV), which infects up to 90% of the population by adulthood. Several serological studies have detected significantly higher frequencies of EBV antibodies in the sera and cerebral spinal fluid of multiple sclerosis patients compared to controls, and some studies have found an increased risk among individuals with a history of infectious mononucleosis (which is caused by EBV infection). Nevertheless, some investigators have reported null results and additional well-designed studies are needed to confirm or refute this association (Ascherio & Munger, 2007a; Marrie, 2004).

John Kurtzke and colleagues conducted a series of epidemiologic investigations of multiple sclerosis in the population living in the Faroe Islands which are located between Scotland and Iceland in the North Atlantic Ocean. His studies suggest that multiple sclerosis was introduced into the native population by British troops who occupied the islands during 1940–1945. Kurtzke described the temporal pattern of disease in the Faroe Island population over half a century as "*four successive epidemics beginning in 1943*" and suggested that multiple sclerosis is the rare outcome of infection by a transmissible agent, perhaps a retrovirus (Kurtzke, 1993).

There is also some evidence that parasitic infection by *Borrelia burgdorferi*, the etiologic agent of Lyme disease, occasionally manifests symptoms characteristic of multiple sclerosis. Several studies have found that patients diagnosed with multiple sclerosis have positive serologic reactions to Borrelia antigen, and characteristic spirochetes of the organism have been found in postmortem studies of brain tissues of afflicted patients. Results suggest there may be an association between Lyme borreliosis and multiple sclerosis (Marshall, 1988).

The age at the time of infection has also been examined as a risk factor for development of multiple sclerosis. A recent review of 19 studies found reasonable consistency among studies in showing that infection by any one of a number of several agents (measles, mumps, varicella, rubella) at a relatively late age during childhood (after 6 years of age) was associated with greater odds of developing multiple sclerosis. As pointed out by Ruth Ann Marrie in her review of the environmental epidemiology of multiple sclerosis: "*It is possible that any one of several agents could produce the same result under the appropriate circumstances (a genetically susceptible host at a critical time of exposure)*" (Marrie, 2004).

Studies of Multiple Sclerosis in Migrants

Perhaps surprisingly, there is general agreement of results from studies of multiple sclerosis rates in migrants. People migrating from a high-risk area to a low-risk area experience a decrease in disease rates, whereas people migrating from a low-risk area to a high-risk area retain their low rates. These findings suggest that the risk of disease is established early in life and prior to the time of migration (Gale & Martyn, 1995).

Vaccination and Multiple Sclerosis

A series of case reports in France raised particular concern about demyelinating events developing after hepatitis B vaccination. In a nested case–control study of 192 women with multiple sclerosis and 645 matched controls, Ascherio and colleagues found no effect of hepatitis B vaccination at any time before disease onset (OR = 0.9) (Ascherio et al., 2001). Similarly, other case–control studies found no evidence of an association; furthermore, results of both case– control and cohort studies have consistently reported no association between the development of multiple sclerosis and other childhood vaccinations (measles, mumps, rubella) (Ascherio & Munger, 2007b; Marrie, 2004).

Organic Solvents and Multiple Sclerosis

Several studies have assessed the association between exposure to organic solvents and multiple sclerosis. A meta-analysis of case–control studies found a 70% increase in overall risk (pooled OR = 1.7) (Landtblom, Flodin, Soderfeldt, Wolfson, & Axelson, 1996). However, a subsequent review of 14 epidemiologic studies revealed inconsistencies and methodological issues with risk estimates ranging from 0.4 to 4.9 (Marrie, 2004). Though a link between multiple sclerosis and exposure to organic solvents cannot be excluded, additional studies are needed for definitive proof of an association.

Tobacco and Multiple Sclerosis

Many epidemiologic investigations have examined tobacco use as a risk factor for multiple sclerosis. Handel and colleagues recently reviewed the literature on smoking and multiple sclerosis and performed a meta-analysis of risk estimates from eligible studies. They included data from 14 studies of 3052 cases and 457,619 controls in their analysis. Results revealed an approximate 50% increase in the risk for smokers compared to nonsmokers (RR = 1.52). The risk of secondary disease was also elevated by continuation of the smoking habit among patients (RR = 1.88). The investigators concluded that smoking significantly heightens the risk of developing multiple sclerosis and suggested the need for further research to clarify interactions with other risk factors (Handel et al., 2011).

▶ Prevention and Therapy of Multiple Sclerosis

Though there is no known cure for multiple sclerosis, intensive research is focused on finding effective drugs and other modalities to prevent attacks, return function after attacks, and prevent disability and decline from progressive disease. Corticosteroids are typically used to manage acute attacks and certain immunomodulatory drugs (interferon-b, glatiramer acetate) have proven effective in some patients. Swift action to reduce inflammation and prevent or slow damage to the brain is crucial. A variety of monoclonal antibodies that target specific molecules in the immunopathogenesis of multiple sclerosis are currently being investigated in randomized clinical trials (Pozzilli & Prosperini, 2010; WHO, 2006). For example, the monoclonal antibody, *ocrelizumab*, has shown significant benefit in randomized clinical trials and is now approved for therapy in patients with progressive forms of multiple sclerosis (Cerqueira et al., 2018). Therapies aimed at enhancing natural mechanisms of remyelination in the brain hold promise for the treatment of progressive multiple sclerosis and as such are of intense interest in current neurological research. There is also much interest in the use of supplementary or vitamin D analogs for the prevention and management of multiple sclerosis. Randomized clinical trials are currently in progress to evaluate the potential benefit of vitamin D therapy for patients with relapsing-remitting multiple sclerosis (Cantorna, 2008).

References

Acheson, E. D., Bachrach, C. A., & Wright, F. M. (1960). Some comments on the relationship of the distribution of multiple sclerosis to latitude, solar radiation, and other variables. *Acta Psychiatrica Scandinavica, 35*(S147), 132–147.

Allison, R. S. (1931). Disseminated sclerosis in North Wales: An inquiry into its incidence, frequency, distribution and other etiological factors. *Brain, 53,* 391–430.

Allison, R. S., & Millar, J. H. D. (1954). Prevalence of disseminated sclerosis in Northern Ireland. *Ulster Medical Journal, 23* (Suppl. 2), 1–27.

Ascherio, A., & Munger, K. L. (2007a). Environmental risk factors for multiple sclerosis. Part I: The role of infection. *Annals of Neurology, 61*(4), 288–299.

Ascherio, A., & Munger, K. L. (2007b). Environmental risk factors for multiple sclerosis. Part II: Noninfectious factors. *Annals of Neurology, 61*(6), 434–513.

Ascherio, A., Munger, K. L., & Simon, K. C. (2010). Vitamin D and multiple sclerosis. *Lancet Neurology, 9*(6), 599–612.

Ascherio, A., Zhang, S. M., Hernan, M. A., Olek, M. J., Coplan, P. M., Brodovicz, K., & Walker, A. M. (2001). Hepatitis B vaccination and the risk of multiple sclerosis. *New England Journal of Medicine, 344*, 327–332.

Back, S. A., Tuohy, T. M., Chen, H., Wallingford, N., Craig, A., Struve, J., … Sherman, L. S. (2005). Hyaluronan accumulates in demyelinated lesions and inhibits oligodendrocyte progenitor maturation. *Nature Medicine, 11*(9), 966–972.

Barr, M. L., & Bertram, E. G. (1949). A morphological distinction between neurones of the male and female, and the behaviour of the nucleolar satellite during accelerated nucleoprotein synthesis. *Nature, 63*(4148), 676–677.

Bronnum-Hansen, H., Stenager, E., Nylev, S. E., & Koch-Henriksen, N. (2005). Suicide among Danes with multiple sclerosis. *Journal of Neurology, Neurosurgery & Psychiatry, 76*, 1457–1159.

Cantorna, M. T. (2008). Vitamin D and multiple sclerosis: An update. *Nutrition Reviews, 66*(10 Suppl. 2), S135–S138.

Cantorna, M. T., Hayes, C. E., & DeLuca, H. F. (1996). 1,25-Dihydroxyvitamin D$_3$ reversibly blocks the progression of relapsing encephalomyelitis, a model of multiple sclerosis. *Proceedings of the National Academy of Sciences of the United States of America, 93*, 7861–7864.

Cerqueira, J. J., Alastair, D., Compston, S., Geraldes, R., Rosa, M. M., Schmierer, K., … Palace, J. (2018). Time matters in multiple sclerosis: Can early treatment and long-term follow-up ensure everyone benefits from the latest advances in multiple sclerosis? *Journal of Neurology, Neurosurgery & Psychiatry*. doi:10.1136/jnnp.2017.317509.

Charcot, J. (1868). Histologie de la sclerose en plaques. *Gazette des hopitaux, Paris, 41*, 554–555.

Compston, A. (1988). The 143th anniversary of the first depiction of the lesions of multiple sclerosis. *Journal of Neurology, Neurosurgery & Psychiatry, 51*(10), 1249–1252.

Compston, A., & Coles, A. (2002). Multiple sclerosis. *Lancet, 359*(9313), 1221–1231.

Dyment, D. A., Ebers, G. C., & Sadovnick, A. D. (2004). Genetics of multiple sclerosis. *Lancet, 3*, 104–110.

Fredrikson, S., Cheng, Q., Jiang, G. X., & Wasserman, D. (2003). Elevated suicide risk among patients with multiple sclerosis in Sweden. *Neuroepidemiology, 22*, 146–152.

Gale, C. R., & Martyn, C. N. (1995). Migrant studies in multiple sclerosis. *Progress in Neurobiology, 47*, 425–448.

Grytten, T. N., Lie, S. A., Aarseth, J. H., Nyland, H., & Myhr, K. M. (2008). Survival and cause of death in multiple sclerosis: Results from a 43-year follow-up in Western Norway. *Multiple Sclerosis, 14*(9), 1191–1198.

Handel, A. E., Williamson, A. J., Disanto, G., Dobson, R., Giovannoni, G., & Ramagopalan, S. V. (2011). Smoking and multiple sclerosis: An updated meta-analysis. *PLoS ONE, 6*(1), e16149. doi:10.1371/journal.pone.0016149.

Holick, M. F. (2005). Photobiology of vitamin D. In D. Feldman, J. Pike, & F. Glorieux (Eds.), *Vitamin D* (2nd ed., pp. 37–46). New York, NY: Elsevier Academic Press.

Islam, T., Gauderman, W. J., Cozen, W., & Mack, T. M. (2007). Childhood sun exposure influences risk of multiple sclerosis in monozygotic twins. *Neurology, 69*, 381–388.

Kermode, A. G., Thompson, A. J., Tofts, P., MacManus, D. G., Kendall, B. E., Kingsley, D. P. E., … McDonald, W. I. (1990). Breakdown of the blood-brain barrier precedes symptoms and other MRI signs of new lesions in multiple sclerosis. *Brain, 113*, 1477–1489.

Kurland, L. T. (1952). Epidemiologic characteristics of multiple sclerosis. *American Journal of Medicine, 21*, 561–571.

Kuroiwa, Y., Shibasaki, H., & Ikeda, M. (1983). Prevalence of multiple sclerosis and its north-to-south gradient in Japan. *Neuroepidemiology, 2*, 62–69.

Kurtzke, J. F. (1993). Epidemiologic evidence for multiple sclerosis as an infection. *Clinical Microbiology Reviews, 6*(4), 382–427.

Landtblom, A. M., Flodin, U., Soderfeldt, B., Wolfson, C., & Axelson, O. (1996). Organic solvents and multiple sclerosis: A synthesis of the current evidence. *Epidemiology, 7*, 429–433.

Leibowitz, U., Sharon, D., & Alter, M. (1967). Geographical considerations in multiple sclerosis. *Brain, 90*, 871–886.

Lemire, J. M., & Archer, D. C. (1991). 1,25-Dihydroxyvitamin D3 prevents the in vivo induction of murine experimental autoimmune encephalomyelitis. *Journal of Clinical Investigations, 87*, 1103–1107.

Limberg, C. C. (1943). The geographic distribution of multiple sclerosis and its estimated prevalence in the United States. In *Multiple sclerosis and the demyelinating diseases. Proceedings of the Association for Research in Nervous and Mental Disease (December 10–11, 1948)* (Vol. 28, pp. 15–24). Baltimore, MD: Williams and Wilkins.

Lowis, G. W. (1988). Ethnic factors in multiple sclerosis: A review and critique of the epidemiological literature. *International Journal of Epidemiology, 17*(1), 14–20.

Lucas, R. M., Ponsonby, A. L., Dear, K., Valery, P. C., Pender, M. P., Taylor, B. V., … McMichael, A. J. (2011). Sun exposure and vitamin D are independent risk factors for CNS demyelination. *Neurology, 76*(6), 540.

Lyon, M. F. (1961). Gene action in the X-chromosome of the mouse (*Mus musculus L.*). *Nature, 190*(4773), 372–373.

Marrie, R. A. (2004). Environmental risk factors in multiple sclerosis aetiology. *The Lancet Neurology, 3*(12), 709–718.

Marshall, V. (1988). Multiple sclerosis is a chronic central nervous system infection by a spirochetal agent. *Medical Hypothesis, 25*, 89–92.

McDonald, W. I., Compston, A., Edan, G., Goodkin, D., Hartung, H. P., Lublin, F. D., … Wolinsky, J. S. (2001). Recommended diagnostic criteria for multiple sclerosis: Guidelines from the International Panel on the Diagnosis of Multiple Sclerosis. *Annals of Neurology, 43*(1), 121–127.

Minagar, A., & Alexander, J. S. (2003). Blood-brain barrier disruption in multiple sclerosis. *Multiple Sclerosis, 9*, 540–549.

Mowry, E. M., Krupp, L. B., Milazzo, M., Chabas, D., Strober, J. B., Belman, A. L., … Waubant, E. (2010). Vitamin D status is associated with relapse rate in pediatric-onset multiple sclerosis. *Annals of Neurology, 67*(5), 618–624.

Munger, K. L., Levin, L. I., Hollis, B. W., Howard, N. S., & Ascherio, A. (2006). Serum 25-hydroxyvitamin D levels and risk of multiple sclerosis. *JAMA, 296*(23), 2832–2838.

Munger, K. L., Zhang, S. M., O'Reilly, E., Hernán, M. A., Olek, M. J., Willett, W. C., & Ascherio, A. (2004). Vitamin D intake and incidence of multiple sclerosis. *Neurology, 62*(1), 60–65.

Murray, C. L., & GBD 2013 Mortality and Causes of Death Collaborators. (2015). Global, regional, and national age–sex specific all-cause and cause-specific mortality for 240 causes of death, 1990–2013: A systematic analysis for the Global Burden of Disease Study 2013. *The Lancet, 385*, 117–171.

Naghavi, M., & GBD 2016 Causes of Death Collaborators. (2017). Global, regional, and national age–sex specific mortality for 264 causes of death, 1980–2016: A systematic analysis for the Global Burden of Disease Study 2016. *The Lancet, 390*, 1151–1210.

Polman, C. H., Reingold, S. C., Edan, G., Filippi, M., Hartung, H. P., Kappos, L., … Wolinsky, J. S. (2005). Diagnostic criteria for multiple sclerosis: 2005 revisions to the "McDonald Criteria". *Annals of Neurology, 58*(6), 840–646.

Pozzilli, C., & Prosperini, L. (2010). Recent advances in the management of multiple sclerosis. *European Neurological Journal, 2*(1), 41–48.

Pugliatti, M., Sotgiu, S., & Rosati, G. (2002). The worldwide prevalence of multiple sclerosis. *Clinical Neurology & Neurosurgery, 104*, 182–191.

Rosati, G. (2001). The prevalence of multiple sclerosis in the world: An update. *Neurological Sciences, 22*(2), 117–139.

Sadovnick, A. D., Armstrong, H., Rice, G. P. A., Bulman, D., Hashimoto, L., Paty, D. W., … Ebers, G. C. (1993). A population-based study of multiple sclerosis in twins: Update. *Annals of Neurology, 33*, 281–285.

Sadovnick, A. D., Ebers, G. C., Wilson, R. W., & Paty, D. W. (1992). Life expectancy in patients attending multiple sclerosis clinics. *Neurology, 42*(5), 991–994.

Simpson, S., Jr., Taylor, B., Blizzard, L., Ponsonby, A. L., Pittas, F., Tremlett, H., … van der Mei, I. (2010). Higher 25-hydroxyvitamin D is associated with lower relapse risk in multiple sclerosis. *Annals of Neurology, 68*(2), 193–203.

Sloane, J. A., Batt, C., Ma, Y., Harris, Z. M., Trapp, B., & Vartanian, T. (2010). Hyaluronan blocks oligodendrocyte progenitor maturation and remyelination through TLR2. *Proceedings of the National Academy of Sciences of the United States of America, 107*(25), 11555–11560.

Smestad, C., Sandvik, L., & Celius, E. G. (2009). Excess mortality and cause of death in a cohort of Norwegian multiple sclerosis patients. *Multiple Sclerosis, 15*(11), 1263–1270.

Stenager, E. N., Stenager, E., Koch-Henriksen, N., Brønnum-Hansen, H., Hyllested, K., Jensen, K., & Bille-Brahe, U. (1992). Suicide and multiple sclerosis: An epidemiological investigation. *Journal of Neurology Neurosurgery & Psychiatry, 55*(7), 542–545.

Trapp, B. D., Ransohoff, R. M., Fisher, E., & Rudick, R. A. (1999). Neurodegeneration in multiple sclerosis: Relationship to neurological disability. *Neuroscientist, 5*(1), 48–57.

van der Mei, I. A. F., Ponsonby, A. L., Blizzard, L., & Dwyer, T. (2001). Regional variation in multiple sclerosis prevalence in Australia and its association with ambient ultraviolet radiation. *Neuroepidemiology, 20*, 168–174.

Von Essen, M. R., Kongsbak, M., Schjerling, P., Olgaard, K., Ødum, N., & Geisler, C. (2010). Vitamin D controls T cell antigen receptor signaling and activation of human T cells. *Nature Immunology, 22*, 344–349.

Vos, T., & GBD 2015 Disease and Injury Incidence and Prevalence Collaborators. (2016). Global, regional, and national incidence, prevalence, and years lived with disability for 310 diseases and injuries, 1990–2015: A systematic analysis for the Global Burden of Disease Study 2015. *The Lancet, 388*(10053), 1545–1602.

Wang, H., Naghavi, M., & GBD 2015 Mortality and Causes of Death Collaborators. (2016). Global, regional, and national life expectancy, all-cause mortality, and cause-specific mortality for 249 causes of death, 1980–2015: A systematic analysis for the Global Burden of Disease Study 2015. *The Lancet, 388*(10053), 1459–1544.

Weiner, H. L. (1998). A 21 point unifying hypothesis on the etiology and treatment of multiple sclerosis. *Canadian Journal of Neurological Sciences, 25*, 93–101.

Weinshenker, B. G. (1994). Natural history of multiple sclerosis. *Annals of Neurology, 36*(Suppl.), S6–S11.

Willer, C. J., Sadovnick, A. D., & Ebers, G. C. (2002). Microchimerisms in autoimmunity and transplantation: Potential relevance to multiple sclerosis. *Journal of Neuroimmunology, 126*, 126–133.

World Health Organization. (2006). *Neurological disorders: Public health challenges* (pp. 85–94). Geneva, Switzerland: World Health Organization.

World Health Organization. (2008). *Atlas multiple sclerosis resources in the world*. Geneva, Switzerland: World Health Organization.

Zamboni, P., Galeotti, R., Menegatti, E., Tacconi, G., Dall'Ara, G., Bartolomei, I., & Salvi, F. (2009). Chronic cerebrospinal venous insufficiency in patients with multiple sclerosis. *Journal of Neurology Neurosurgery & Psychiatry, 80*, 392–399.

© Andrew Brookes/Getty Images

CHAPTER 51

Epidemiology of Epilepsy

▶ Introduction

An epileptic seizure is caused by a crescendo of action potentials in one or more circuits of the brain. Symptoms can range from total sustained muscle contraction (tonus) to violent rhythmic jerking and shaking of all muscle groups (clonus), depending upon which neuronal circuits are misfiring.

The Greek term "*epilepsy*," meaning "*seizure*," was coined to describe neurologic symptoms of violent spasmodic jerking and shaking admixed with intermittent paralysis in afflicted patients. According to a consensus statement, epilepsy refers to the abnormal and excessive discharge of a set of neurons in the brain resulting in transitory abnormal neurological phenomena that may include alterations of consciousness, motor sensory, autonomic, and/or psychic events (Commission on Epilepsy and Prognosis, ILAE, 1993).

▶ Diagnosis of Epilepsy

Epilepsy is diagnosed by confirmation of two or more unprovoked seizures separated by at least 24 hours in an individual. Abnormal findings may also be present in electroencephalogram (EEG) studies and imaging studies of the brain. Since other neurological events can mimic seizures, particularly in children, a careful history must be taken in order to document the exact nature of the "seizure" and arrive at a correct diagnosis. Stimuli that may incite seizure-like symptoms include illness, infection, physical or emotional trauma, medications, and use of illicit drugs.

True seizures are characterized by inappropriate rhythmic limb movements and/or muscle contractions (clonus) often interrupted by sustained muscle contraction (tonus). Seizures invariably involve altered consciousness and unresponsiveness to verbal commands during the episode. Immediately following a seizure, persisting focal findings (delay in restoration of normal speech, sight, hearing, cognition, and motor function) can often be used to pinpoint the area of the brain affected.

EEG studies are recommended in the evaluation of individuals with suspected seizures or epilepsy. Tracings should be obtained in the awake and sleep states in close proximity to an event. Characteristic epileptiform patterns of brain waves can help confirm the diagnosis and elucidate the affected regions of the brain.

Neuroimaging studies are also recommended for individuals who have suffered a seizure. Such studies may reveal structural abnormalities such as tumors, congenital malformations, vascular anomalies, infections, and traumatic injuries. Magnetic resonance imaging (MRI) is preferred over other imaging procedures in studies of the brain.

▶ Types of Seizures

As pointed out by Sander and Shorvon in their comprehensive review of the epidemiology of the epilepsies, "Many different conditions, with different causes and outcomes, may express themselves solely by the occurrence of recurrent epileptic seizures. Epilepsy is a collection of syndromes and conditions rather than a single disease…" (Sander & Shorvon, 1996). Hence, it is important to consider the different types of seizures in discussion of the epidemiology of epilepsy.

Types of seizure are categorized according to the location of dysfunctional neuronal circuits in the brain and the extent of consciousness with corresponding impact on motor and cognitive function. There are more than 40 types of seizures and only the main types will be discussed in this chapter. The major seizure types are summarized in **TABLE 51.1** and briefly outlined in the following paragraphs.

A partial or focal seizure refers to a specific localized cerebral area in which the neurons are firing excessively. A simple seizure is one in which there is no loss of consciousness, and a complex seizure is one in which there is impaired awareness or loss of consciousness. Thus, a simple partial seizure refers to localized brain dysfunction without loss of consciousness, whereas a complex partial seizure refers to localized brain dysfunction and unconsciousness.

TABLE 51.1 Major Types of Epileptic Seizures

Type of Seizure	Neurologic Characteristics
Partial seizure	*Focal area of neuron discharge*
Simple	No loss of consciousness
Complex	Loss of consciousness
Secondary generalization	Evolvement to generalized seizure
Generalized seizure	*Widespread Neurological Discharge*
Petit mal	Unresponsiveness
Myoclonic	Sporadic muscle contractions
Clonic	Abnormal bilateral repetitive contractions
Tonic	Sustained muscle contraction
Atonic	Loss of muscle tone
Grand mal	Clonic-tonic symptoms
Status epilepticus	*Unrelenting seizure activity*

Classification scheme is derived from the following references: Commission on Classification and Terminology of the International League against Epilepsy. (1989). Proposal for revised classification of epilepsies and epileptic syndromes. *Epilepsia, 30,* 389–399; Commission on Epilepsy and Prognosis, International League Against Epilepsy. (1993). Guidelines for epidemiologic studies on epilepsy. *Epilepsia, 34,* 592–596.

Simple seizures are subclassified according to the profile of symptoms: motor impairment involving muscle contraction and rigidity; cognitive impairment affecting vision, hearing, smell, taste, or touch; and memory or emotional disturbances.

Complex partial seizures are characterized by impaired awareness of surroundings or loss of consciousness. Other characteristics include automatisms such as lip smacking, chewing, fidgeting, and other inappropriate involuntary repetitive movements. A partial seizure will occasionally evolve into a generalized seizure wherein the patient loses consciousness and manifests other signs and symptoms of widespread neuronal discharge.

A generalized seizure is one involving both cerebral hemispheres with widespread cerebral dysfunction and corresponding impact on many motor and cognitive functions. All generalized seizures involve the loss of consciousness. These are subdivided into six types: *absence (petit mal), myoclonic, clonic, tonic, atonic,* and *tonic-clonic (grand mal)* seizures.

Absence (petit mal) seizures cause a brief loss of consciousness for a few seconds without other symptoms. Such seizures typically interrupt normal childhood activity and may reoccur several times throughout the day.

Myoclonic seizures consist of sporadic "jerking" muscle contractions of very short duration whereas *clonic* seizures involve inappropriate repetitive rhythmic movements simultaneously occurring on both sides of the body.

Tonic seizures are characterized by sustained contraction of muscles whereas *atonic* seizures involve the loss of muscle tone, particularly in the arms and legs that often results in a fall.

The most dramatic of the generalized seizures is the *grand mal* seizure, in which the patient first loses consciousness and manifests generalized contraction of all muscles (the tonic phase) for 30–60 seconds followed by violent uncontrolled spasmodic muscle contractions (the clonic phase) for 30–60 seconds, after which the patient enters into a deep coma (the postictal phase) that may last up to 30 minutes. Grand mal seizures can be fatal and are characterized by incontinence, tongue biting, convulsions, and accidental injury.

A catastrophic event in a patient with epilepsy is the occurrence of *status epilepticus*. This life-threatening condition is defined as the presence of intense unrelenting seizure activity lasting longer than 30 minutes. Status epilepticus occurs in about one in five patients who have been diagnosed with epilepsy.

Accurate classification according to seizure type involves extensive testing by an EEG which records tracings of brain waves from different regions of the brain. Such tests are often unavailable in epidemiologic investigations of epilepsy that are conducted in the field.

▶ Types of Epilepsy

Although epilepsy is defined as the occurrence of two or more unprovoked seizures in an individual, the different types of epilepsy are classified not only by the type of seizure, but also according to a number of other features including the age at diagnosis, known underlying causes (trauma, stroke, tumor, infection), genetic factors, the part of the brain involved, the severity and frequency of seizure activity, EEG findings, response to antiepileptic drugs, and prognosis. A consensus statement from the *International League Against Epilepsy (ILAE)* categorizes epilepsy according to two dichotomies: localization-related versus generalized disease, and idiopathic versus symptomatic or cryptogenic disease (Commission on Epilepsy and Prognosis, ILAE, 1993). Major epilepsy syndromes classified by this system are summarized in **TABLE 51.2**.

It is important to realize that in the nomenclature of epilepsy research, *idiopathic* disease refers to epilepsy with a *genetic* basis, *symptomatic* disease has a known underlying cause (developmental delay, trauma, tumor, infection), and *cryptogenic* disease has a known structural anomaly in the brain, but the cause has not been definitively elucidated. Another term that has been used for *symptomatic* disease is *remote symptomatic epilepsy.*

Localization-related (focal) epilepsy is characterized by partial seizures due to excessive firing of a focal group of neurons. This type may be idiopathic, symptomatic, or cryptogenic.

Generalized epilepsy is characterized by generalized seizures due to excessive firing of neurons distributed throughout the brain. This type may also be idiopathic, symptomatic, or cryptogenic.

As discussed in the following section, several *idiopathic* (genetic) focal epilepsy syndromes have been described, including *benign epilepsy with centrotemporal spikes (Rolandic epilepsy),* benign occipital epilepsies of childhood (*Panayiotopoulos syndrome* and *Lennox–Gastaut syndrome*), and *nocturnal frontal lobe epilepsy.* These syndromes have specific EEG characteristics, respond well to antiepileptic medication, and usually remit with age. In contrast, *symptomatic* focal epilepsies are often more malignant, with higher rates of medical intractability, and lower remission rates (Panayiotopoulos, Michael, Sanders, Valeta, & Koutroumanidis, 2008; Taylor, Berkovic, Kivity, & Scheffer, 2008). According to the *International Classification of Epilepsies and Epileptic Syndromes* proposed by the *ILAE* in 1989, *cryptogenic* epilepsies are presumed to be *symptomatic* but with unknown etiology (Commission on Classification and Terminology of the International League Against Epilepsy, 1989).

It is also important to realize that epileptic phenotypes are extraordinarily heterogeneous, and despite extensive clinical investigation, a large fraction of patients are unclassifiable according to etiology. Investigators at the Mayo Clinic recently examined the incidence and classification of new onset epilepsy in a population-based group of children in Olmstead County Minnesota. All children with newly diagnosed epilepsy from 1980 to 2004 were classified by mode of onset, etiology and syndrome using criteria of the *ILAE.* The adjusted annual incidence rate of new onset epilepsy in children was 44.5 cases per 100,000. Rates were highest in the first year of life and diminished with age. The mode of onset was focal in 68%,

TABLE 51.2 Major Epilepsy Syndromes		
Type of Epilepsy	**Location-Related**	**Generalized**
Idiopathic (genetic)	▪ Benign rolandic ▪ Benign occipital ▪ Nocturnal Frontal Lobe	▪ Childhood absence ▪ Juvenile absence ▪ Dravet syndrome ▪ Juvenile myoclonic
Symptomatic or cryptogenic	▪ Temporal lobe ▪ Frontal lobe ▪ Parietal lobe ▪ Occipital lobe	▪ Tonic-clonic ▪ West syndrome ▪ Lennox–Gastaut

Classification scheme is derived from the following references: Commission on Classification and Terminology of the International League Against Epilepsy. (1989). Proposal for revised classification of epilepsies and epileptic syndromes. *Epilepsia, 30,* 389–399; Commission on Epilepsy and Prognosis, International League Against Epilepsy. (1993). Guidelines for epidemiologic studies on epilepsy. *Epilepsia, 34,* 592–596.

generalized (bilateral) in 23%, spasmodic in 3%, and unknown in 5% of cases. Approximately half of children had unknown etiology, and among the remaining cases, 78 (22%) were idiopathic (genetic) and 101 (28%) were structural or metabolic. The investigators concluded that *"Nearly half of childhood epilepsy is of 'unknown' etiology"* (Wirrell, Grossardt, Wong-Kisiel, & Nickels, 2011).

▶ Epilepsy Syndromes

The epilepsy syndromes listed in Table 51.2 plus other selected epilepsy syndromes are briefly defined in the following paragraphs. A number of epilepsy syndromes have been identified that are caused by heritable deleterious genes and/or chromosomal aberrations. Relevant genetic findings are discussed for selected idiopathic (genetic) syndromes.

Idiopathic (Genetic) Localization-Related (Focal) Syndromes

- *Benign Rolandic epilepsy* of childhood (benign centrotemporal lobe epilepsy) occurs in children under 13 years of age, with peak onset in late childhood prior to puberty. Apart from their seizure disorder, children with this type of epilepsy are otherwise normal. This syndrome features simple partial seizures that involve facial muscles and frequently cause drooling. Although most episodes are brief, seizures sometimes spread and generalize. Seizures are typically nocturnal and confined to sleep. The EEG may demonstrate spike discharges in the centrotemporal region (Rolandic sulcus) of the brain. Seizures may require anticonvulsant treatment, but sometimes are infrequent enough to allow physicians to defer treatment. Seizures usually cease at puberty. Genetic studies of families with affected children suggest an autosomal dominant inheritance pattern with high gene penetrance (Bali et al., 2007) and linkage with the gene encoding the α7 subunit of the acetylcholine receptor (CHRNA7) on the long arm of chromosome 15 (Neubauer et al., 1998). It is noteworthy that this same gene has also been linked to the development of *juvenile myoclonic epilepsy*, as discussed later (Elmslie et al., 1997).
- *Benign occipital epilepsies of childhood* are broadly classified into two forms, one with early onset typically before the age of 5 years (*Panayiotopoulos syndrome*) and the other with later onset between 5 and 10 years of age (Gastaut syndrome).

Panayiotopoulos syndrome is characterized by prolonged autonomic seizures of occipital origin, often lasting more than 30 minutes, thus constituting autonomic *status epilepticus* (Panayiotopoulos, 2007). In contrast, Gastaut syndrome is characterized by frequent brief seizures with visual hallucinations, ictal blindness, and illusions (Gastaut, 1982). Though some family studies of EEG patterns have suggested an autosomal dominant inheritance pattern (Kuzniecky & Rosenblatt, 1987), a lack of concordance among monozygous twins implies that somatic mutations and epigenetic or environmental factors are also likely to play a role in the benign occipital epilepsies of childhood (Taylor et al., 2008).

- *Nocturnal frontal lobe epilepsy* is an inherited epileptic disorder that causes seizures during sleep. Onset is usually in childhood. These seizures arise in the frontal lobes and consist of complex motor movements, such as hand clenching, arm raising/lowering, and knee bending. Vocalizations such as shouting, moaning, or crying are also common. Mutations in genes encoding subunits of nicotinic acetylcholine receptors on chromosomes 15 and 20 are responsible for this syndrome. The inheritance pattern is autosomal dominant with high penetrance of the deleterious genes (Berkovic & Scheffer, 1997; Phillips et al., 1998; Steinlein et al., 1995).
- *Primary reading epilepsy* is a rare form of reflex epilepsy classified as idiopathic and localization related. Nearly, all seizures in this syndrome are precipitated by reading (usually reading aloud). Reading in susceptible individuals triggers characteristic myoclonic seizures. Inheritance of this syndrome appears to be polygenic (Berkovic & Scheffer, 1997).

Idiopathic (Genetic) Generalized Syndromes

- *Childhood absence epilepsy* affects children under 13 years of age. Peak onset is at 5–6 years of age. Children with this form of epilepsy have recurrent absence seizures, brief episodes of unresponsive staring, sometimes with minor motor features such as eye blinking or subtle chewing. The EEG finding is generalized 3 Hz spike and wave discharges. Occasionally, patients develop generalized tonic-clonic (grand mal) seizures. This condition carries a good prognosis because children do not usually show cognitive decline or neurological deficits, and the seizures in the majority of patients cease spontaneously with growth and maturation. Though childhood absence epilepsy displays a complex pattern of polygenic inheritance, recent familial and genetic studies have elucidated major genes that may heighten susceptibility. A study of 50 Austrian families with affected children detected significant disequilibrium in polymorphisms of the genes encoding the γ-aminobutyric acid (*GABA*) type-A receptor subunits α5 (*GABRA5*) and β3 (*GABRB3*) located on the long arm of chromosome 15 (Feucht et al., 1999); and a gene sequencing study conducted in China detected 12 missense mutations in the T-type calcium channel gene on the short arm of chromosome 16 among 118 patients with this syndrome compared to none among 230 normal controls (Chen et al., 2003).

- *Juvenile absence epilepsy* is similar to the childhood form, but seizures begin during the teenage years. Patients with this syndrome occasionally manifest generalized tonic-clonic (grand mal) seizures and progression to juvenile myoclonic epilepsy is relatively common. Though the inheritance pattern of juvenile absence epilepsy is complex, genetic studies suggest that defective glutamate receptor genes on chromosome 21 may contribute to the genesis of this syndrome (Sander, Hildmann, et al., 1997).

- *Dravet syndrome* (severe myoclonic epilepsy of infancy) is a rare neurodevelopmental disorder (1 in 40,000 births) characterized by severe epilepsy that does not respond well to treatment. This syndrome was first described by the French psychiatrist, Charlotte Dravet, in 1978. Dravet studied at the Centre Saint Paul at the University of Marseille, under the supervision of Henri Gastaut, who first described the Lennox–Gastaut syndrome. Seizures in Dravet syndrome are often prolonged and may progress to status epilepticus, a medical emergency. Mutations in the voltage-gated sodium channel *SCN1A* gene are the main genetic cause of Dravet syndrome. A recent large series of 333 patients were screened using direct gene sequencing and gene amplification techniques. Point mutations in the *SCN1A* gene were detected in 228 (68%) of cases, 161 of which had not previously been reported. Missense mutations were the most common mutation type. Furthermore, additional genetic deletions and rearrangements were identified in 14 of the 105 patients without *SCN1A* point mutations. Based on their results, the investigators state: "*These findings widely expand the SCN1A mutation spectrum identified and highlight the importance of screening the coding regions with both direct sequencing and a quantitative method*" (Depieene et al., 2009).

- *Juvenile myoclonic epilepsy* is most often diagnosed during the teenage years. Patients have normal cognition and are otherwise neurologically intact. The most common seizures are myoclonic jerks, although generalized tonic-clonic (grand mal) seizures and absence seizures may also occur. Myoclonic jerks usually cluster in the early morning after awakening. The EEG reveals generalized 4–6 Hz spike wave discharges or multiple spike discharges. Interestingly, patients are often diagnosed when they have their first generalized tonic-clonic seizure when they experience sleep deprivation (e.g., during the freshman year in college after staying up late to study for exams). Alcohol withdrawal can also be a precipitating factor in breakthrough seizures. Though seizure risk is lifelong, the majority of patients can successively manage their condition with anticonvulsant medication and avoidance of seizure precipitants. Genetic studies of juvenile myoclonic epilepsy have generally revealed complex polygenic inheritance. However, a recent study of 34 pedigrees, each with one or more affected relatives, revealed linkage of susceptibility to the gene encoding the α7 subunit of the nicotinic acetylcholine receptor (*CHRNA7*) on the long arm of chromosome 15. Based on these results, the investigators suggest they may have discovered a major susceptibility locus for juvenile myoclonic epilepsy (Elmslie et al., 1997).

- *Unverricht–Lundborg disease* is the most common form of an uncommon group of genetic epilepsy disorders called *progressive myoclonic epilepsies*. This genetic disorder is caused by a mutation in the *cystatin B gene* that encodes a protein that inhibits proteases that leak out of lysosomes in the cell (Joensuu, Lehesjoki, & Kopra, 2008; Turk & Bode, 1991). The disease is named after the German physician, Heinrich Unverricht, who first described it in 1891, and the Swedish physician, Herman Bernhard Lundborg, who provided greater detail in 1903. The syndrome occurs in children between the ages of 6 and 16 years, most from the Baltic and Mediterranean regions of Europe. The disease is characterized by recurrent myoclonic and tonic-clonic seizures that become progressively more frequent and severe over time. The condition is usually progressive. Depression is prevalent among patients, and their life expectancy is less than 25 years (Kalviainen et al., 2008).

- *Tonic-clonic (grand mal) seizures on awakening* is an uncommon epileptic syndrome characterized by recurrent generalized tonic-clonic (*grand mal*) seizures when the patient awakens from sleep. About 70% of cases are diagnosed during adolescence; however, onset is highly variable ranging from early childhood into the fourth decade of life. An important feature of this syndrome is that patients with any of the other syndromes of idiopathic generalized epilepsy, which are characterized by minor seizures, may experience generalized tonic-clonic (grand mal) seizures, usually of the awakening type. Such seizures are severe and potentially dangerous since they may progress to *status epilepticus.* The genetic basis of tonic–clonic seizures on awakening is complex. Associations with the nicotinic acetylcholine receptor and GABA receptor subunit genes on chromosome 15, certain genes of the major histocompatibility locus on chromosome 6, and putative susceptibility loci on chromosomes 2, 3, and 14 have been reported (Elmslie et al., 1997; Janz, 2000; Sander, Bockenkamp, et al., 1997; Schmitz, Gardiner, Janz, & Beck-Mannagetta, 1997).

Symptomatic or Cryptogenic Localization-Related Syndromes

Symptomatic localization-related epilepsies are divided by the location of the epileptic lesion in the brain, since the symptoms of the seizures predominantly reflect the region of the brain disrupted rather than the cause of the lesion. Tumors, vascular and cavernous malformations, head trauma, infection, and cerebral infarcts can all cause epileptic foci in different regions of the brain.

- *Epilepsies of the frontal lobe, temporal lobe, parietal lobe, and occipital lobe* arise from lesions in the corresponding regions of the brain that cause seizures. Symptomatic causes include brain stroke, tumors, head trauma, infection, and congenital malformations.
- *Rasmussen's encephalitis* is a rare progressive, inflammatory brain lesion. This condition is most often diagnosed in children under the age of 10 years, but it can also occur in adolescents and adults. Initial symptoms are simple partial or complex partial seizures that may progress to *epilepsia partialis continua (simple partial status epilepticus).* Neuroimaging shows inflammatory encephalitis on one side of the brain that may spread if not treated. Dementia and hemiparesis are also commonly found in patients with this syndrome. Though the cause of encephalitis remains unknown, pathogenesis apparently involves an autoimmune attack against certain types of membrane receptors of the neurotransmitter, glutamate (Takahashi et al., 2005).
- *Mesial temporal lobe epilepsy* is the most common cryptogenic form of epilepsy. In most cases, the epileptogenic region corresponds to sclerosis (scarring) found in the midline (mesial) temporal structures (the hippocampus, amygdala, and parahippocampal gyrus). It is hypothesized that brain damage from traumatic injury, infection, a brain tumor, lack of oxygen, and/or seizure activity causes sustained inflammation leading to the formation of the scar tissue. However, a recent study detected *human herpes virus 6B (HHV-6B)* in brain specimens from 15 of 24 patients with mesial temporal sclerosis, in contrast to 0 of 14 specimens from patients with other syndromes. These results suggest that HHV-6B infection may contribute to the pathogenesis of mesial temporal lobe epilepsy (Fotheringham et al., 2007). Seizures begin in late childhood and adolescence and are poorly controlled by anticonvulsant medications. Most patients have complex partial seizures that are occasionally preceded by an aura. Seizures may progress to secondary generalized tonic-clonic (grand mal) seizures.

Generalized Symptomatic or Cryptogenic Syndromes

- *West syndrome* is a form of childhood epilepsy diagnosed by the triad of developmental delay, infantile seizures (spasms), and an arrhythmic EEG pattern. Onset occurs before the age of 2 years with a peak between 8 and 9 months. Approximately 1 in 3500 infants are afflicted. Causation may be symptomatic, cryptogenic, or idiopathic (genetic). A common cause is *tuberous sclerosis*, a genetic disorder that causes tumors to form in many organs, primarily in the brain, eyes, heart, kidney, skin, and lungs. Several types of brain lesions can occur in individuals with tuberous sclerosis, and up to 90% of children with this condition develop epilepsy. Briefly, the condition is caused by mutations in either of two genes, *TSC1* or *TSC2*, that encode proteins (*hamartin* and *tuberin*) that are essential for normal cell proliferation and differentiation. Other causes of West syndrome include congenital disorders (Down syndrome), infection, and traumatic brain injury; albeit, the etiology is unknown in 40%–50% of cases. The prognosis for children with West syndrome varies with the underlying cause. Unfortunately, most surviving patients have persisting cognitive impairment and continuing seizures and usually progress to *Lennox–Gastaut syndrome* (Cowan & Hudson, 1991).

■ *Lennox–Gastaut syndrome* consists of the triad of developmental delay or childhood dementia, mixed generalized seizures, and a characteristic EEG pattern of 2 Hz slow spike waves. Onset occurs between 2 and 18 years of age. Approximately 26 of 1000 children are afflicted by the age of 10 years. As in West syndrome, causation may be symptomatic, cryptogenic, or idiopathic (genetic). Indeed, surviving patients with West syndrome often progress to Lennox–Gastaut syndrome. Most patients have astatic seizures (drop attacks), tonic seizures, tonic-clonic seizures, atypical absence seizures, and sometimes, complex partial seizures. Anticonvulsants are usually only partially successful in treatment (Trevathan, Murphy, & Yeargin-Allsopp, 1997).

■ *Ohtahara syndrome* is a rare, severe epilepsy syndrome that usually begins in the first few days or weeks of life. Characteristic seizures are in the form of stiffening spasms with an EEG pattern of high voltage spikes followed by suppressed activity. Most infants with the disorder show significant underdevelopment of part or all of the cerebral hemispheres. The prognosis is poor with about half of the infants dying in the first year of life. Nearly, all surviving infants are severely intellectually disabled, and many have cerebral palsy. There is no effective treatment. A number of children have underlying structural brain abnormalities (Clarke, Gill, Noronha, & McKinlay, 1987).

Other Epileptic Categories

Two additional categories have been defined to accommodate other forms of epilepsy and seizure activity. *Undetermined epilepsy* is characterized by seizures that cannot be accurately categorized as either partial or generalized. Undetermined epilepsy syndromes include neonatal seizures, severe myoclonic seizures, and the *Landau–Kleffner syndrome*, a rare, childhood neurological disorder characterized by the sudden or gradual development of aphasia (the inability to understand or express language).

Special syndromes are not definable as epilepsy per se but rather are entities characterized by seizures.

TABLE 51.3 Special Syndromes

Type	Description
Febrile (fever) seizure	Seizure and convulsions associated with infection and fever
Isolated seizure	Solitary unprovoked partial seizure without recurrence
Circumstantial seizure	Seizure activity provoked by environmental or physiologic stimulus

These include febrile (fever) seizures, unprovoked solitary seizures, and circumstantial or situation-related seizures that are triggered by specific environmental or physiological stimuli (**TABLE 51.3**).

▶ Febrile (Fever) Seizures and Epilepsy

Febrile (fever) seizures are convulsions induced by fever in infants or small children. During a febrile seizure, the child often loses consciousness and shakes, moving limbs on both sides of the body; or less commonly, the child becomes rigid or manifests muscle contractions in only one portion of the body such as the arm, leg, or the right or left side only. Febrile seizures ordinarily last for 1–2 minutes, although there is extreme variability in duration, from a few seconds up to 15 minutes or more. The majority of children who exhibit febrile seizures have body temperatures exceeding 102°F. Most such seizures occur during the early hours of elevated body temperature.

Acute febrile miniseizures are relatively common during the first years of life affecting about 5% of children before the age of 5 years. The incidence of febrile seizures is highest during the first months of life and then progressively declines until about age 10 years when the risk becomes negligible.

It is important to realize that children with febrile seizures are not considered to have epilepsy, since epilepsy is defined as two or more *unprovoked* seizures. In fact, the vast majority of febrile seizures are of short duration and harmless. During a febrile seizure, there is a slight chance of accidental injury; however, there is no evidence to suggest that *short* febrile seizures cause brain damage.

Approximately 1 in 25 children will have at least 1 febrile seizure, and 1 in 3 of those with a first febrile seizure will have additional febrile seizures. Febrile seizures most commonly occur between the ages of 6 months and 5 years. Factors that increase the risk of having recurrent febrile seizures are early onset of the first febrile seizure, frequent infection and fever, and familial history of febrile seizures among family members.

Investigators in Greece examined the recurrence of febrile seizures among 260 children with a first episode between 3 months and 6 years of age. The median follow-up was 4.3 years with evaluations every 4–6 months and at the time of each recurrence. The strongest risk factors for recurrence were early onset, familial history of febrile seizures, and low temperature prior to the initial seizure (Pavlidou, Tzitiridou, Kontopoulos, & Panteliadis, 2008).

Investigators in the United States examined the recurrence of febrile seizures among 428 children who were assessed every 3 months for at least 2 years after their first episode. Recurrent febrile seizures occurred in 126 (31.8%) of these children; 73 (17.1%) had only one recurrence, 38 (8.9%) had two recurrences, and 25 (5.8%) had three or more recurrences. Early age at onset, history of febrile seizures in a first-degree relative (parent or sibling), low fever preceding the first seizure, and brief interval between fever and seizure onset were strong independent predictors of recurrent febrile seizures. The investigators suggest that these four factors can be used to define groups of patients with high versus low probability of developing recurrent febrile seizures (Berg et al., 1997).

Febrile seizures were once considered to be an early warning sign of impending epilepsy. However, most children (over 90%) affected by febrile seizures recover completely over time without developing epilepsy. Furthermore, risk factors that predict subsequent febrile seizures (early onset, recurrent fever, and familial history) have not consistently been found to predict the development of epilepsy; and reciprocally, most risk factors associated with epilepsy have not been found to increase the risk of recurrent febrile seizures. Nevertheless, some studies suggest that certain types of recurrent febrile seizures do increase the risk of subsequently developing epilepsy, and the association remains under intense investigation (Berg, 1992).

A study conducted in Singapore examined neurological outcomes among 476 children initially hospitalized for febrile seizures during infancy. During more than 7 years of follow-up, 10 of these children (2.1%) had one or more unprovoked seizures and 5 children (1.1%) became epileptic. The incidence of epilepsy among children with a febrile seizure lasting 30 minutes or more was increased nearly ninefold compared to children with shorter seizures (12.1% vs. 1.4%); and the incidence of epilepsy was increased nearly sixfold among children with a familial history of epilepsy compared to those with no familial history (9.1% vs. 1.6%). Gender, ethnicity, age at onset, and number of recurrent febrile seizures did not influence the risk (Lee, 1989).

Investigators at Rotterdam in the Netherlands reexamined the risk factors for febrile seizures and associations with epilepsy in a pooled analysis of individual data from five follow-up studies that incorporated standardized definitions of febrile seizures, complex seizures, and risk factors. Among 2496 children with fever seizures, 32% had 1, 15% had 2, and 7% had 3 or more recurrent febrile seizures after a first episode. The hazard of recurrent febrile seizures was greatest between the ages of 12 and 24 months, and the risk of having additional febrile seizures more than doubled with each successive recurrence. Recurrence risk was also increased by a history of either *febrile or unprovoked seizures* in a first-degree relative (parent or sibling) and low temperature preceding the first febrile seizure. Notably, early onset of febrile seizure (less than 12 months), familial history of unprovoked seizures, and an initial partial fever seizure (affecting only one part of the body) were found to significantly increase the risk of subsequently developing complex seizures and epilepsy (Offringa et al., 1994).

In a landmark study, investigators in Denmark evaluated the association between febrile seizures and epilepsy in a long-term population-based cohort of 1.54 million persons born during 1978–2002, including 49,587 children with febrile seizures, 16,481 individuals with epilepsy, and 2149 individuals who developed epilepsy after febrile seizures. At 23 years of follow-up, the cumulative incidence of epilepsy among individuals who had childhood febrile seizures was 6.9%, more than five times higher than individuals with no history of febrile seizures (adjusted RR = 5.4). The risk remained high during the entire follow-up period but was particularly high shortly after the first febrile seizure (**FIGURE 51.1**). Familial history of epilepsy, history of cerebral palsy, and low APGAR score at birth were also found to independently elevate the risk of epilepsy development. The investigators suggest that febrile seizures may be the first sign of epilepsy, or share common risk factors with epilepsy, or may cause brain damage (edema of the hippocampus) predisposing to epilepsy in certain individuals (Vestergaard, Pedersen, Sidenius, Olsen, & Christensen, 2007).

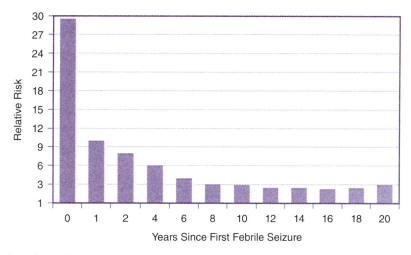

FIGURE 51.1 Epilepsy Risk and Febrile Seizures.

Data from Vestergaard, M., Pedersen, C. B., Sidenius, P., Olsen, J., & Christensen, J. (2007). The long-term risk of epilepsy after febrile seizures in susceptible subgroups. *American Journal of Epidemiology, 165*(8), 911–918.

▶ Isolated Seizures

Occasionally, an individual may experience a single solitary seizure or a cluster of seizures in a short span of time during or following an illness or injury without any further episodes. Such "isolated seizures" can be provoked by any number of factors such as head trauma, infection, stress, etc. Often no identifiable cause can be found. Such events clearly *do not* meet the criteria for the diagnosis of epilepsy: 2 or more unprovoked seizures separated by at least 24 hours in time.

▶ Circumstantial (Situation-Related) Seizures

Circumstantial seizures are stimulated by identifiable environmental or physiological causes such as stress, trauma, hormones, alcohol, drugs, sleep deprivation, infection, vascular disease, cancer, endocrine disorders, and a variety of other conditions. This "waste-basket" category includes *nonepileptic* patients with solitary seizures for which the cause can be concluded from patient-related circumstances and situations.

▶ Status Epilepticus

One seizure type that deserves special mention is *status epilepticus*, a catastrophic life-threatening continuous seizure lasting longer than 30 minutes. Status epilepticus can occur as an amplification of one of the aforementioned epileptic syndromes or it can occur spontaneously without warning due to a variety of other causes. Indeed, epilepsy is only *one* cause of status

epilepticus found in only about one-third of patients. Other predominant causes include infectious diseases (particularly in children), strokes, hemorrhage, brain tumors, metabolic diseases, drug overdose, alcohol abuse, and head trauma. Status epilepticus can be focal, generalized, or complex, involving both focal and generalized seizure activity. The condition is surprisingly common, particularly among infants and young children and older adults (**FIGURE 51.2**). Case fatality rates of status epilepticus range from 10% in children to nearly 50% in the elderly (DeLorenzo, Pelloch, Towne, & Boggs, 1995).

Status epilepticus has been found to have a strong genetic basis. Corey and colleagues examined the role of genetic factors in status epilepticus using the population-based *Virginia Twin Registry*. Their study included 70 individuals with at least 1 episode of status epilepticus and 318 individuals with verified seizures among 332 twin pairs. Status epilepticus occurred in 21 (13.2%) of 158 individuals with febrile seizures and 49 (22.0%) of 223 individuals with afebrile seizures. The age at first occurrence of status epilepticus ranged from 2 months to 59 years. The overall concordance rate of status epilepticus was 31% among monozygous twins and 0 among dizygous twins. Furthermore, among monozygous twin pairs with epilepsy, 67% were also concordant for status epilepticus. The investigators concluded that genetic factors contribute significantly to the genesis of status epilepticus (Corey, Pellock, Boggs, Miller, & DeLorenzo, 1998; Corey, Pellock, & DeLorenzo, 2004).

The twin studies of status epilepticus therefore reflect a definite genetic predisposition to this life-threatening condition. Nevertheless, causation is obviously multifactorial involving a combination

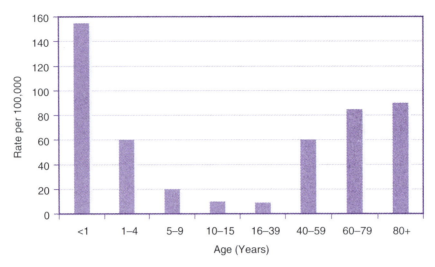

FIGURE 51.2 Age-Specific Incidence of Status Epilepticus.

Data from DeLorenzo, R. J., Pelloch, J. M., Towne, A. R., & Boggs, J. G. (1995). Epidemiology of status epilepticus. *Journal of Clinical Neurophysiology 12*, 316–325.

of genetic and environmental factors. As already discussed in this chapter, certain monogenic epileptic syndromes involving mutations in key genes have been identified (GABRA5, GABRB3, SCN1A, CHRNA7). However, these syndromes are relatively rare and as pointed out in a recent review, "*mutations in a single gene can produce different epilepsy phenotypes in different individuals as a result of modifying genetic or environmental factors*" (Schauwecker, 2009). Epigenetic effects might also contribute to the phenotypic heterogeneity of status epilepticus. Obviously, further studies are needed to elucidate major genes that contribute to the genesis of status epilepticus.

▶ Global Burden of Epilepsy

At the turn of the century, the World Health Organization reported that about 50 million people worldwide had epilepsy. Of these, 37 million people had primary epilepsy and 13 million had secondary epilepsy caused by other diseases or injury. At that time, 40 million people with epilepsy (80%) were residing in developing nations with little or no access to treatment, and it was estimated that 15–20 million people with this condition received no medication (Leonardi & Ustun, 2002; Scott, Lhatoo, & Sander, 2001; World Health Organization, 2001).

Current estimates from the World Health Organization suggest that epilepsy afflicts more than 50 million people worldwide, and most (80%) live in regions with poor economies and little access to health care. Globally, approximately 2.4 million new cases of epilepsy are diagnosed per year, and it is estimated that 30 million individuals who suffer from epilepsy are not receiving therapy for their condition (WHO, 2018).

Incidence of Epilepsy and Unprovoked Seizure

The worldwide distribution of epilepsy reflects marked variability. Socioeconomically deprived people are clearly at higher risk. The annual incidence rates are highest in resource-poor countries, particularly those in sub-Saharan Africa and Latin America, ranging from 100 to 200 per 100,000 (Scott et al., 2001; Singhal et al., 1998). Rates are much lower in industrialized countries such as the United States, the United Kingdom, Australia, and Western Europe ranging from 23 to 54 per 100,000 (Jallon, 2002). Relatively low annual incidence rates have also been reported for population samples from China (29–35 per 100,000) and India (38–60 per 100,000). However, studies of these populations are sparse, and additional prospective population-based studies are needed for confirmation (Li et al., 1985; Mac et al., 2007; Mani et al., 1998; Ray, Bhattacharya, Kundu, Saha, & Das, 2002; Sawhney, Singh, Kaur, Suri, & Chopra, 1999; Wang et al., 2003).

Kotsopoulos and colleagues reviewed reported estimates of the incidence of epilepsy and unprovoked seizures published during 1966–1999 and conducted a meta-analysis of these data. Forty studies of population samples from around the globe were included in their analysis. The median annual age-adjusted incidence rate was 47 per 100,000 for epilepsy and 56 per 100,000 for unprovoked seizures. Males had slightly higher rates of epilepsy than females (51 vs. 46 per 100,000) and developing countries had higher rates than developed countries (69 vs. 43 per 100,000). In developing countries, rates tended to be higher in children than in the elderly, perhaps due to shortened life expectancies and fewer survivors of stroke, tumors, and neurodegenerative conditions that heighten

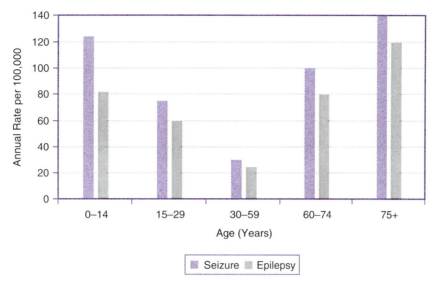

FIGURE 51.3 Age-Specific Incidence of Epilepsy and Unprovoked Seizure.

Data from Kotsopoulos, I. A. W., Van Merode, T., Kessels, F. G. H., De Krom, M. C. T. F. M., & Knottnerus, J. A. (2002). Systematic review and meta-analysis of incidence studies of epilepsy and unprovoked seizures. *Epilepsia, 43*(11), 1402–1409; Hauser, W. A., Annegers, J. F., & Kurland, L. T. (1993). Incidence of epilepsy and unprovoked seizures in Rochester, Minnesota: 1935–1984. *Epilepsia, 34*, 453–468.

susceptibility to seizure. As discussed later in this chapter, such populations are more prone to endemic infectious and parasitic conditions (neurocysticercosis, onchocerciasis) that increase the risk of childhood seizure. Childhood rates in some developed countries declined over the time span covered, perhaps due to improving prenatal and antenatal care; in contrast, rates in the elderly increased, likely due to better survival of stroke and other conditions that predispose to seizures (Kotsopoulos, Van Merode, Kessels, De Krom, & Knottnerus, 2002). The composite distribution of age-specific incidence is a U-shaped curve with high rates in children and the elderly (**FIGURE 51.3**).

▶ Global Prevalence of Epilepsy

Epilepsy is often a lifelong disorder that persists in an individual for many decades. Annual prevalence rates are therefore much higher than the incidence rates, varying widely worldwide from 1 to 20 per 1000 with a median rate of about 7 per 1000. High annual prevalence rates have been reported for impoverished nations in sub-Saharan Africa and Latin America (15–20 per 1000) whereas much lower values have been reported for industrialized nations. Rates in the United States, the United Kingdom, Australia, and European nations range from 1 to 10 per 1000 with a median of 5 per 1000. A recent review of reported prevalence rates for population samples from Asian nations found a range of 1.5 per 1000 in Japan to 10 per 1000 in Pakistan with a median of 6 per 1000 (Bharucha, 2003; Fong et al., 2003; Huang et al., 2002; Li et al., 1985; Mac et al., 2007; Mannan, 2004; Scott

et al., 2001; Singhal, 1998; Sridharan & Murthy, 1999; Wang et al., 2003).

Similar findings were reported from a meta-analysis comparing the prevalence of epilepsy in developed countries to the prevalence in urban and rural settings of developing countries. Estimates of the prevalence of *lifetime epilepsy* and *active epilepsy* were derived from 65 studies published during 1990–2006. Active epilepsy denotes the presence of seizure activity during the past 12 months whereas lifetime epilepsy refers to the presence of epileptic seizures at any time during the lifespan. The median prevalence of lifetime epilepsy was higher in rural settings of developing countries (15.4 per 1000) than in developed countries (5.8 per 1000), and the median prevalence of active epilepsy was also higher in rural settings of developing countries (12.7 per 1000) than in developed countries (4.9 per 1000). The median prevalence for all ages was 9.7 per 1000 (11.3 per 1000 in adults and 6.7 per 1000 in children). It was estimated that 51.8 million people suffer from epilepsy in the world population, 45 million (87%) in developing countries and 6.8 million (13%) in developed countries (Ngugi et al., 2010).

▶ Disability-Adjusted Life Years (DALY) Lost from Epilepsy

The DALY is the sum of *Years of Life Lost from Premature Death* (YLL) and *Years of Life Lost from Disability* (YDL): DALY = YLL + YDL. The DALY that are lost due to epilepsy reflect a public health burden of tremendous dimensions. In 2000, epilepsy contributed

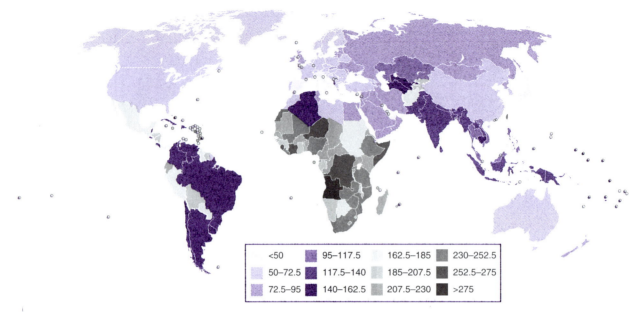

FIGURE 51.4 Disability-Adjusted Life Years Due to Epilepsy, 2004.

Data from World Health Organization. (2008). *The global burden of disease: 2004 update.* Geneva: WHO. Available at www.who.int/evidence/bod

0.5% of the total DALY from all diseases (de Boer, Mula, & Sancer, 2008). Rates are highest in impoverished nations where there is little access to treatment (**FIGURE 51.4**). On a positive note, according to recent data reported by Global Burden of Disease (GBD) investigators, the years of healthy lost due to disability from epilepsy declined by about 6% during 2005–2015 (Vos & 2015 GBD Collaborators, 2016). These results suggest that there has been progress in the early diagnosis of epilepsy and its effective therapy.

▶ Epilepsy Mortality

Individuals with epilepsy die from four major causes: *status epilepticus* (often due to lack of anticonvulsant medications), *suicide* associated with depression, trauma associated with seizures, and *sudden unexpected death in epilepsy*. Those at highest risk for epilepsy-related deaths usually have underlying neurological impairment or poorly controlled seizures whereas those with mild to moderate epilepsy are at much lower risk for epilepsy-related death.

Epilepsy Mortality in Developing Countries

The case fatality and mortality rates reported for epileptic patients appear to be highest in developing nations and rural areas where there is little access to treatment. For example, in a study of epileptic patients conducted in rural Ethiopia, most patients were treated with local herbs, holy water, and amulets, whereas less than 2% received antiepileptic drugs.

Injuries from burns or trauma suffered during seizures were found in 14% of patients. During the 2-year study period, eight of the nine reported deaths among patients were due to status epilepticus and 1 due to burns suffered when the patient fell into a domestic fire during a seizure (Tekle-Haimanot et al., 1990).

In a study conducted in a rural area of Cameroon in Central Africa, 37 (29%) of 128 patients with epilepsy died compared to 6 (5%) of 128 matched controls during 10 years of follow-up (RR = 6.2). The most frequent causes of death among epileptic patients were status epilepticus, sudden unexpected death in epilepsy, and drowning (Kamgno, Pion, & Boussinesq, 2003).

A recent study of patients living in a mountainous region of Laos revealed a *case fatality rate* of 91 deaths per 1000 person-years. No patients had access to standard therapy with antiepileptic medications (Tran et al., 2006).

An international team of investigators traced the mortality experience of 103 *untreated* epileptic patients from a rural area of Bolivia over a 10-year period. Ten deaths were recorded yielding an overall mortality rate of 10 deaths per 1000 person-years. The standardized mortality rate (SMR) was elevated among patients with *remote symptomatic epilepsy* (SMR = 3.0) but not among patients with idiopathic disease (Nicoletti et al., 2009).

Investigators in Shanghai examined the mortality experience of 2455 *prevalent* cases of epilepsy ascertained from eight rural counties of six provinces in China with a population of 3,185,000 people. Patients were older than 2 years with a history of at least 2

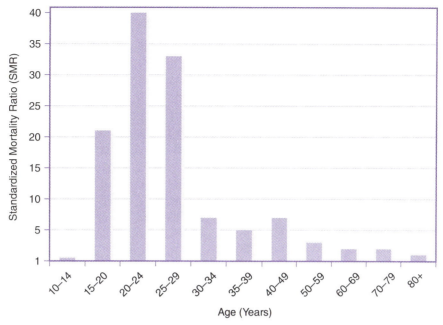

FIGURE 51.5 Epilepsy in Rural China: Age-Specific Standardized Mortality Ratios.

Data from Ding, D., Wang, W., Wu, J., Ma, G., Dai, Z., Yang, B., ... Sander, J. W. (2006). Premature mortality in people with epilepsy in rural China: A prospective study. *The Lancet Neurology 5*, 823–827.

convulsion seizures in the previous 12 months. Most were started on monotherapy with phenobarbital as part of a community-based intervention study (which is described in last section of this chapter on epileptic therapy). SMRs were computed by age using the 2004 Chinese population as the reference group. During the year of study, 35 deaths were recorded, 471 patients withdrew, and 91 patients were lost to follow-up. The SMR for all ages was 3.9, but estimates were much higher in the younger age groups (**FIGURE 51.5**). The principal causes of death among young patients were suicide or drowning, whereas older patients died primarily from myocardial infarction, stroke, cancer, or pneumonia (Ding et al., 2006).

Epilepsy Treatment Gap

The *epilepsy treatment gap*, defined as the proportion of people with active epilepsy who require treatment but do not receive it, has been proposed as a useful parameter to compare access to and quality of care for epilepsy patients across populations. Prior anecdotal and descriptive estimates suggest that the treatment gap is much higher in low-income than high-income countries.

Wang and colleagues carried out a door-to-door survey to determine the prevalence of epilepsy and the proportion of patients receiving treatment among 55,000 people living in rural areas of China. The lifetime prevalence was 7.0 per 1000, and 41% of all patients had not received any appropriate treatment. The prevalence of active epilepsy was 4.6 per 1000 and 63% of individuals with active epilepsy had not

received antiepileptic therapy in the week before the survey (Wang et al., 2003).

Meyer and colleagues at the World Health Organization recently examined the treatment gap for patients with active epilepsy in 54 populations from 28 countries based upon a comprehensive review of relevant published data. Their review encompassed studies spanning nearly 30 years, from 1978 to 2006 and included samples of patients from Africa, Asia, Europe, Australia, and North and South America. Results revealed a wide range of treatment gaps from 6% in Singapore to 100% in Bolivia. Treatment gaps of less than 10% were observed for patient populations in Taiwan, Norway, Singapore, the United Kingdom, Ireland, the United States, and selected populations in Argentina, Brazil, and France. In sharp contrast, treatment gaps greater than 95% were found in rural China, Ethiopia, the Gambia, the Lao People's Republic, Nigeria, Pakistan, Panama, Togo, Uganda, the United Republic of Tanzania, and Zambia. Wide variability was also noted within some countries. For example, treatment gaps in India ranged from 22% for patients in urban areas to 90% for patients living in rural villages. The results of this systematic review of the literature clearly reflect dramatic global disparities in the care and treatment of epilepsy patients. Treatment gaps for active epilepsy exceeded 75% in most low-income countries and 50% in most middle income countries, whereas high-income countries had treatment gaps of less than 10%. The investigators concluded their report with the following statement: "*Increased commitment by the global health community is needed to reduce the treatment gap and thereby reduce the potentially devastating social consequences and poor health outcomes resulting from untreated epilepsy*" (Meyer, Dua, Ma, Saxena, & Birbeck, 2010).

Epilepsy Mortality in Developed Countries

The case fatality and mortality rates due to epilepsy are markedly lower in developed nations than developing nations. For example, long-term studies in the United States, the United Kingdom, Australia, several European nations, some South American nations, and urban populations in China and India have found case fatality rates ranging from 1 to 10 deaths per 1000 person-years (Mac et al., 2007). As one might expect, survival is significantly better among patients who achieve early long-term remission from epileptic symptoms without reliance on medications. Recent studies are discussed below suggesting that more than half of patients who receive early treatment successfully achieve long-term remission without seizure activity.

Sillanpää and Shinnar examined the mortality experience of a Finnish cohort of 245 cases with childhood epilepsy (160 incident cases and 95 prevalent cases) followed for more than 40 years. Follow-up examinations were conducted every fifth year, and detailed information was collected including the age and cause of death. A total of 60 patients died during follow-up yielding an overall case fatality rate of 24%. The overall death rate was 6.9 deaths per 1000 person-years (5.3 deaths per 1000 person-years for incident cases only). Subjects with *remote symptomatic epilepsy* secondary to neurological impairment (cognitive impairment, developmental delay, cerebral palsy, or autism) or neurological insult (head trauma, stroke, or meningitis) were compared to those with idiopathic or cryptogenic epilepsy (of indeterminate origin). Mortality among subjects with *remote symptomatic epilepsy* was more than threefold higher than among subjects with idiopathic or cryptogenic epilepsy (11.1 vs. 3.2 deaths per 1000 person-years, RR = 3.5). Among the 60 deaths observed in the cohort, 33 (55%) were attributed to epilepsy per se and 26 (43%) were attributed to the underlying neurologic condition. Among the epilepsy-related deaths, 18 were due to *sudden unexplained death in epilepsy*, 9 were due to seizure or *status epilepticus*, and 6 were due to drowning. Notably, only 4 deaths occurred among 103 patients who achieved 5-year remission and were not receiving medication at last follow-up (1.5 deaths per 1000 person-years), compared to 5 deaths among 35 patients in 5-year remission and receiving medication at last follow-up (11.2 deaths per 1000 person-years), and 51 deaths among 107 subjects who did not achieve

5-year remission (15.9 deaths per 1000 person-years). Early deaths (during childhood) were primarily due to underlying neurologic conditions whereas later deaths (during adulthood) were mostly due to epilepsy-related events (Sillanpää & Shinnar, 2010).

A team of Swedish investigators conducted a comprehensive review of epilepsy mortality data reported in the literature for developed countries. In population-based cohorts of incident disease with 7–29 years of follow-up, standardized mortality ratios ranged from 1.6 to 3.0, and survivorship following the diagnosis of epilepsy was 91%, 85%, and 83% at 5, 10, and 15 years, respectively. Mortality in patients from Iceland, France, Sweden, and the United Kingdom did not differ significantly from the general population, whereas mortality among U.S. patients was increased. Notably, all studies reported increased standardized mortality ratios for patients with *remote symptomatic epilepsy* ranging from 2.2 to 6.5. The highest mortality ratios occurred among patients diagnosed with epilepsy or other neurological disorders at birth. Excess mortality was also high among elderly patients, primarily due to underlying disorders such as stroke, cancer, other neurodegenerative conditions, and pneumonia. The most common seizure-related cause of death among epileptic children and adolescents was sudden unexpected death (Forsgren et al., 2005).

▶ Suicide and Epilepsy

Suicide is a major cause of death among patients with epilepsy and its impact is often underestimated. Pompili and colleagues recently examined this phenomenon in a meta-analysis of 29 published studies. Their analysis included 50,814 patients, 187 of whom committed suicide. Overall, the annual suicide rate among patients with epilepsy was estimated at 32.5 per 1000, which was 8.5 times higher than in the general population (matched by age group, country, and year). However, rates varied widely and perhaps surprisingly, some cohorts of epileptic patients actually had lower suicide rates than their comparison populations. Suicide risk appears to be increased by intractable epilepsy, depression, and surgical intervention, particularly temporal lobectomy, whereas low rates are associated with early therapy and freedom from seizure activity, particularly without medication. The investigators state that "*despite intensive efforts, effective prediction and prevention strategies remain elusive*" and they encourage further studies to address "*the role played by mood disorders, treatment-resistant epilepsy, and surgical treatment in the precipitation of suicide*" (Pompili, Girardi, Ruberto, & Tatarelli, 2005).

▶ Epilepsy Risk Factors

From the preceding discussion, it is obvious that the term "*epilepsy*" encompasses a vast collection of syndromes and conditions, each having its own defining features and characteristics. Likewise, multiple risk factors have been implicated in the etiopathogenesis of the epilepsies. Indeed, the risk of developing epilepsy varies widely according to age, gender, genetic predisposition, physiology, medical history, behavior, and external environment.

By definition, *idiopathic epileptic syndromes* have a significant genetic basis whereas *circumstantial (situation-related) epilepsy* is associated with environmental exposures and/or physiological processes or disturbances. Risk factors for circumstantial epilepsy include age (epilepsy is most commonly diagnosed in children and elderly adults), male gender, head trauma, stroke, cardiovascular disease, encephalitis (infection of the brain), brain tumors and other cancers, certain metabolic conditions, alcohol and other drugs, and prolonged febrile seizures in childhood. Frankly, any exposure that causes brain damage or interrupts normal brain function should be regarded as a potential risk factor for the development of epileptic seizures.

The risk factors for early onset disease during childhood and late onset disease in the elderly are dramatically different. Young patients develop epilepsy as a consequence of genetic predisposition, trauma, infection, and febrile seizures, whereas elderly patients develop epilepsy secondary to cerebrovascular disease (stroke), metabolic conditions (type 2 diabetes), cancer, other neurodegenerative conditions (Alzheimer's disease), and alcohol abuse and/or withdrawal. It is also noteworthy that about 30% of first acute seizures among the elderly are *status epilepticus* requiring emergency care. It is emphasized that about 50% of epilepsy cases in children and 30%–50% of elderly patients are not classifiable with respect to known causes or risk factors (Forsgren, Bucht, Eriksson, & Bergmark, 1996; Hauser, Annegers, & Kurland, 1993; Hauser & Kurland, 1975; Sirven, 1998; Wirrell et al., 2011). Selected studies of the risk factors for epilepsy are discussed in the following paragraphs.

Fetal Alcohol Syndrome and Epilepsy

Investigators at Queens University in Ontario, Canada, examined the association between *fetal alcohol spectrum disorder* and the subsequent development of epilepsy. The investigation identified 425 exposed subjects, 86 with fetal alcohol syndrome, and 339 with alcohol-related neurodevelopmental disorder. Among all 425 subjects, 25 (5.9%) developed confirmed epilepsy, approximately 10 times the prevalence in the general population. Exposure during the first trimester was the predominant pattern of fetal alcohol exposure among the epileptic patients. The investigators suggest the need for future studies to clarify the pathogenic mechanisms that link prenatal alcohol exposure to a reduced seizure threshold (Bell et al., 2010).

Alcohol Abuse and Epilepsy

Samokhvalov and colleagues conducted a systematic review and meta-analysis of published epidemiologic data to characterize the association between alcohol consumption and the risk of developing epilepsy. Their analysis is based upon 18 published studies that quantified the association between alcohol consumption and epilepsy risk. Results reveal a significant dose response in the risk of epilepsy with increasing alcohol consumption (**FIGURE 51.6**). The data suggest that a threshold level of about four alcoholic drinks per day (48 g of pure alcohol) is sufficient to significantly elevate the risk (Samokhvalov, Irving, Mohapatra, & Rehm, 2010).

Various hypotheses have been advanced to explain the link between alcohol abuse and epilepsy risk. These include alcohol toxicity to neurons, hypoxia due to alcohol-related cerebrovascular disease, brain damage due to traumatic injury, and a "*kindling theory*." The kindling theory suggests that repeated episodes of withdrawal from alcohol including natural withdrawal during sleep over many years gradually reduces the epileptogenic threshold (Ballenger & Post, 1978).

Stroke and Epilepsy

Stroke is a major risk factor for the development of epileptic seizures. In an international prospective multicenter study, Bladin and colleagues followed 1897 consecutive patients with acute stroke to

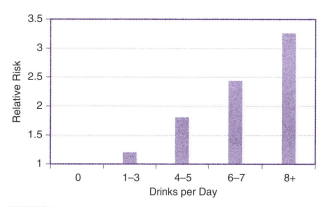

FIGURE 51.6 Epilepsy Risk and Alcohol Consumption.

Data from Samokhvalov, A. V., Irving, H., Mohapatra, S., & Rehm, J. (2010). Alcohol consumption, unprovoked seizures, and epilepsy: A systematic review and meta-analysis. *Epilepsia, 51*(7), 1177–1184.

determine the incidence of seizures overall and by type of stroke. They found that 8.6% of 1632 patients with ischemic stroke had seizures, compared to 10.6% of 265 patients with hemorrhagic stroke. Among patients who suffered an ischemic stroke, 4.8% had seizures within 2 weeks (3.4% within 24 hours); and among patients who suffered hemorrhagic strokes, 7.9% had seizures within 2 weeks (6.0% within 24 hours). Epilepsy was diagnosed in 47 (2.5%) of stroke patients (Bladin et al., 2000). Similar results have been observed in several other studies (Kilpatrick et al., 1990; Olsen, Hagenhaven, & Thage, 1987; Reith, Jorgensen, Nakayama, Raaschou, & Olsen, 1997; So, Annegers, Hauser, O'Brien, & Whisnant, 1996).

Longer-term studies suggest that the risk of developing epileptic seizures persists for several years following stroke (Awada, Omojola, & Obeid, 1999). In a British prospective study of 675 patients with a first stroke (545 of whom had cerebral infarction), the 5-year actuarial risk of seizure was 11.5% (Burn et al., 1997). In a U.S. study of stroke patients in Olmstead County, Minnesota, the cumulative risk of seizure development was 7.4% at 5 years and 8.9% at 10 years (So et al., 1996). Such population-based studies have found 20–40-fold increases in seizure risk relative to the general population. Status epilepticus can also occur following a stroke, involving 31% of stroke patients with seizures in 1 large study. Status epilepticus was the initial seizure type in more than half of these patients (Rumbach et al., 2000).

Type 1 Diabetes Mellitus and Epilepsy

Idiopathic generalized epilepsies, which account for about 30% of all patients with epilepsy, have no apparent cause other than genetic predisposition. Due to a long-term clinical impression that epilepsy and type 1 diabetes are possibly related, investigators in the United Kingdom reviewed the medical histories of 518 patients with confirmed idiopathic generalized epilepsy to quantify their prevalence of type 1 diabetes compared to the general population. Seven cases of type 1 diabetes were identified among the patient cohort which was 4.4 times the number expected. In six of the seven patients, the onset of type 1 diabetes preceded the development of epilepsy. These results suggest there may be an etiologic link between the two conditions, possibly due to precipitation of seizures by hypoglycemic episodes; however, additional studies are needed for confirmation (McCorry et al., 2006).

Type 2 Diabetes and Epilepsy

Patients with type 2 diabetes have been found in a number of studies to be at increased risk for the development of acute epileptic seizures. Investigators in Stockholm, Sweden, conducted a nested case–control study of 933 patients 15 years or older with newly diagnosed unprovoked seizures and 6039 controls matched to the cases by gender, year of diagnosis, and catchment area. Results revealed significant increases in the odds of seizure associated with prior hospitalization for diabetes (OR = 1.9), myocardial infarction (OR = 1.7), cerebral infarction (OR = 9.4), intracerebral hemorrhage (OR = 7.2), subarachnoid hemorrhage (OR = 7.2), and transient ischemic attack (OR = 3.2) (Adelöw, Andersson, Ahlbom, & Tomson, 2011).

In patients with type 2 diabetes, the onset of epileptic seizure is often associated with nonketotic hyperglycemia. Several types of epileptic seizures have been reported in patients with nonketotic hyperglycemia, and early recognition and swift correction of the condition by administration of insulin and rehydration are essential to prevent serious morbidity and mortality (Brick, Gutrecht, & Ringel, 1989; Scherer, 2005; Singh, Gupta, & Strobus, 1973).

Glucose Homeostasis and Epilepsy

Acute seizures including status epilepticus have been reported for diabetic patients at both ends of the spectrum of inadequate glucose control: those with *nonketogenic hyperglycemia* and those with *hypoglycemia*. Numerous reports have appeared in the literature describing epileptic seizures in diabetic children and adults associated with hypoglycemia (Lahat, Barr, & Bistritzer, 1995; Malouf & Brust, 1985) and with hyperglycemia (Askenasy, Streifler, & Carasso, 1977; Singh et al., 1973; Sirven, 1998).

Body Mass and Epilepsy

Investigators in the United Kingdom conducted a retrospective cohort study using the data from *The Health Improvement Network (THIN)* to examine incidence rates of seizures by different levels of body mass index (BMI). Individuals with BMI of 30 or more were classified as obese. The annual incidence of seizures among obese subjects (34.8 cases per 100,000) was similar to the rate among subjects with normal weight (35.8 cases per 100,000). However, underweight subjects with BMI less than 18.5 and gravidly obese subjects with BMI greater than 40 had elevated seizure rates (RR = 1.6 and 1.8, respectively). These findings suggest that individuals at the extremes of body mass are susceptible to seizure development (Gao, Juhaeri, & Dai, 2008).

Parasitic Infection and Epilepsy

Cysticercosis is a systemic infection caused by the pork tapeworm *Taenia solium*. Humans acquire the parasite by ingesting its eggs in food or water contaminated by feces of infected individuals. Neurocysticercosis is caused by infection of the central nervous system and/or brain by the larval stage of *Taenia solium*. This condition is a major cause of neurologic disease in developing countries of Latin America, South America, Africa, and Asia. Neurocysticercosis is the underlying cause of many seizures in these populations and is primarily responsible for the higher incidence of epilepsy in developing versus industrialized nations.

Human *toxocariasis* is another parasitic zoonotic infection found primarily in populations of developing nations. Infection is caused by *Toxocara canis*, a common roundworm found in dogs and cats. Humans ingest eggs of the parasite in contaminated food and fomites. The larvae of *Toxocara canis* can migrate into the central nervous system and cause neurologic symptoms including epilepsy.

Nicoletti and colleagues have conducted extensive studies of zoonotic infections and epilepsy throughout the world. In rural Bolivia, they compared serologies of 113 cases with confirmed epilepsy (59 with partial seizures and 54 with generalized seizures) to 233 controls matched by age, gender, and location. Cases and controls were assessed serologically for antibodies against both *T. canis* and *T. solium*. Results revealed significant increases in the odds of epilepsy among individuals seropositive for *T. solium* (OR = 1.85) and *T. canis* (OR = 2.85). Stronger associations were found for epileptic individuals with late onset partial seizures diagnosed after age 15 years (OR = 3.66 for *T. solium* and OR = 18.2 for *T. canis*). Findings suggest that both neurocysticercosis and toxocariasis contribute to the high rates of epilepsy in developing countries (Nicoletti et al., 2002).

Additional studies of epileptic patients from the same region of Bolivia using both neuroradiologic and serologic testing confirmed the presence of neurocysticercosis in 27% of cases. The investigators note that cysticercosis and other zoonotic conditions are preventable and treatable. The results therefore suggest that elimination of these parasitic infections could markedly reduce the morbidity and mortality due to epilepsy in endemic areas (Nicoletti et al., 2005).

Onchocerciasis, also known as *river blindness*, is a parasitic infection caused by *Onchocerca volvulus*, a small nematode (roundworm) that is transmitted to humans through the bite of a blackfly of the genus *Simulium*. The larval nematodes spread to many tissues of the body including the retina of the eye and in some cases the brain. The worms carry a symbiotic bacterium, *Wolbachia pipientis*, and when the worms die, Wolbachia symbionts are released triggering a host immune response that causes intense itching and necrosis of infected tissues. The vast majority of these infections occur in populations living along the riverbanks of sub-Saharan Africa where the blackfly lives, hence the term "*river blindness*." An estimated 18 million people suffer from onchocerciasis and approximately 270,000 are blind. Onchocerciasis can be effectively treated with two doses of an antiparasitic drug called ivermectin taken 6 months apart every 3 years (World Health Organization, 2010).

Due to the high prevalence of onchocerciasis in regions with high rates of epilepsy and the predilection of this parasite for neural tissues, a number of epidemiologic investigations have been conducted in search of a cause-and-effect relationship; albeit, the results of these studies have been inconsistent.

A team of investigators conducted a matched case–control study 187 cases and 374 controls in three northwestern towns of the Central African Republic. Each case was matched to two controls by gender, age, residence, treatment with ivermectin, date of last use, and the number of doses. Onchocerciasis infection was assessed by the presence of microfilaria in a skin biopsy. Active infections were detected in 39.6% of cases and 35.8% of controls. The mean dermal parasitic load was 26 microfilaria per mg of skin in cases and 24 microfilaria per mg of skin in controls, and the odds of epilepsy due to infection was only marginally elevated (OR = 1.21) (Druet-Cabanac et al., 1991).

Investigators in Cameroon compared 72 patients with epilepsy to 72 controls matched by age, gender, and location. Cases were ascertained from 14 villages in central Cameroon where onchocerciasis is endemic. On average, the microfilarial load per skin snip was twice as high among cases compared to controls (288 vs. 141), supporting the existence of a link between onchocerciasis infection and the development of epilepsy. The investigators speculate that null results observed in some populations may be due to ivermectin control measures implemented in the past two decades (Boussinesq, Pion, Demanqa-Nqanque, & Kamqno, 2002).

More recently, Druet-Cabanac and colleagues conducted a meta-analysis of available data from epidemiologic studies of onchocerciasis and epilepsy. Nine African studies were included in the analysis. The combined estimate of relative risk barely missed statistical significance (RR = 1.21, $p < 0.06$), and the investigators suggest that additional research is needed to confirm a causal relationship and clarify the neurological pathogenicity of onchocerciasis (Druet-Cabanac et al., 2004).

Estrogen and Estrogen Replacement Therapy

Catamenial epilepsy is when partial seizures cluster around certain phases of a woman's menstrual cycle. Three major types of catamenial epilepsy have been defined: perimenstrual, periovulatory, and periluteal. In each type, seizure activity is increased by about twofold during the corresponding time of the menstrual cycle. The perimenstrual type is associated with drastic decreases in serum levels of both estrogen and progesterone, the periovulatory type coincides with a spike in serum estrogen just before ovulation, and the periluteal type is associated with abnormally low levels of progesterone throughout the luteal phase of the menstrual cycle. All three types are characterized by heightened serum levels of estrogen relative to progesterone, and most treatment regimens for catamenial epilepsy involve the administration of progestins (Herzog, 2008).

Hormone replacement therapy has traditionally been used in menopausal women with epilepsy to alleviate their menopausal symptoms such as hot flashes and vaginal dryness. However, recent studies suggest that hormone therapy may actually increase seizure activity.

Investigators at Cornell University in New York City conducted a small randomized double-blind placebo-controlled clinical trial to evaluate the effects of estrogen and medroxyprogesterone in postmenopausal women with epilepsy. Investigators randomized 21 eligible epileptic patients, aged 42–62 years, to receive either estrogen plus progesterone or placebo. Five of seven women receiving high-dose hormone therapy and four of eight women receiving low-dose hormone therapy had worsening seizure frequency compared to one of six women receiving placebo. The investigators concluded there was a dose-related increase in seizure frequency in postmenopausal women who received hormone replacement therapy (Harden et al., 2006).

Epilepsy: Treatment and Prognosis

The cornerstone of epileptic treatment is administration of anticonvulsant and antipsychotic medications antecedent to seizures or during times of high stress. In the United States, there are more than 20 medications that are approved for the treatment of epilepsy. Recent studies suggest that with early diagnosis and accurate differentiation between generalized and partial seizures coupled with administration of targeted anticonvulsant medications as needed to inhibit seizures and minimize side effects, the majority of patients with idiopathic or cryptogenic disease are able to achieve sustained freedom from seizure activity. In patients with symptomatic epilepsy (with known etiology), effective treatment involves not only the management of seizure activity but also intervention to address the underlying pathology.

Investigators at the Mayo Clinic compared long-term outcomes in children with newly diagnosed epilepsy identified in Olmstead County, Minnesota, during 1980–2004. Among 359 cases, 215 (60%) had nonidiopathic focal epilepsy and of these, 206 were followed to determine recurrent seizure activity over time. Cases were classified as having symptomatic epilepsy if their disease had a known structural or metabolic etiology and cryptogenic if not. Ninety-five cases were classified as cryptogenic and 111 as symptomatic. Median follow-up exceeded 11 years in both groups. Long-term outcome was significantly better among cases with cryptogenic epilepsy than those with symptomatic epilepsy. At last follow-up, only 7% of patients with cryptogenic epilepsy were experiencing intractable seizures compared to 40% of patients with symptomatic epilepsy, and of those achieving freedom from seizure activity, 68% of the cryptogenic group were off antiepileptic medications compared to 46% of the symptomatic group. Furthermore, approximately one-third of children with cryptogenic epilepsy experienced no further seizures after the initiation of treatment. The investigators concluded that more than half of nonidiopathic epilepsy is cryptogenic (without an identifiable cause), and children with this epileptic subtype have an excellent long-term prognosis (Wirrell, Grossardt, So, & Nickels, 2010).

Early epilepsy diagnosis and intervention has also proven successful in rural communities. Investigators at the Beijing Neurosurgical Institute conducted a community-based intervention study to evaluate the efficacy of monotherapy with phenobarbital in patients diagnosed with convulsive epilepsy in primary healthcare clinics in eight rural counties of China. Local physicians who completed a specialized training course carried out the screening, treatment, and follow-up. The study enrolled 2455 patients. In 68% of patients who completed 12 months of treatment, seizure frequency was decreased by at least 50%, and a third of patients became seizure-free. Furthermore, 72% of patients who completed 24 months' treatment had at least 50% reduction in seizure frequency, and a quarter of patients remained seizure-free. The study confirms the value of intervention and monotherapy in treating rural patients with convulsive epilepsy (Wang et al., 2006).

Persisting seizure activity in patients with epilepsy places them at risk for sudden expected death. This catastrophic outcome may occur without warning in patients with frequent generalized tonic-clonic seizures and/or convulsive seizures. A recent synthesis of published clinical trials and observational studies found that nocturnal supervision to detect and treat seizure activity during sleep was effective in reducing the risk of sudden death in patients with epilepsy (Maguire, Jackson, Marson, & Nevitt, 2016).

Many developing countries have instituted novel programs of early detection and therapy to decrease the epilepsy treatment gap, and large community-based trials have shown that epilepsy can be controlled and cured with inexpensive and effective antiepileptic drugs administered by primary care physicians. Indeed, early detection and intervention to prevent death from epileptic seizure is a major public health priority (Jette & Trevathan, 2014; Kar, 2016).

References

Adelöw, C., Andersson, T., Ahlbom, A., & Tomson, T. (2011). Prior hospitalization for stroke, diabetes, myocardial infarction, and subsequent risk of unprovoked seizures. *Epilepsia, 52*(2), 301–307.

Askenasy, J. J., Streifler, M., & Carasso, R. (1977). Moderate nonketotic hyperglycemia—A cause of focal epilepsy: Report of two cases and review of literature. *European Neurology, 16*, 51–61.

Awada, A. M., Omojola, M. F., & Obeid, T. (1999). Late epileptic seizures after cerebral infarction. *Acta Neurologica Scandinavica, 99*, 265–268.

Bali, B., Kull, L. L., Strug, L. J., Clarke, T., Murphy, P. L., Akman, C. I., … Pal, D. K. (2007). Autosomal dominant inheritance of centrotemporal sharp waves in rolandic epilepsy families. *Epilepsia, 48*(12), 2266–2272.

Ballenger, J. C., & Post, R. M. (1978). Kindling as a model for alcohol withdrawal syndromes. *The British Journal of Psychiatry, 133*, 1–14.

Bell, S. H., Stade, B., Reynolds, J. N., Rasmussen, C., Anderew, G., Hwang, P. A., & Carlen, P. L. (2010). The remarkably high prevalence of epilepsy and seizure history in fetal alcohol spectrum disorders. *Alcoholism: Clinical and Experimental Research, 34*(6), 1084–1089.

Berg, A. T. (1992). Febrile seizures and epilepsy: The contributions of epidemiology. *Paediatric and Perinatal Epidemiology, 6*(2), 145–152.

Berg, A. T., Shinnar, S., Darefsky, A. S., Holford, T. R., Shapiro, E. D., Salomon, M. E., … Hauser, A. W. (1997). Predictors of recurrent febrile seizures: A prospective cohort study. *Archives of Pediatrics & Adolescent Medicine, 151*(4), 371–378.

Berkovic, S. F., & Scheffer, I. E. (1997). Epilepsies with single gene inheritance. *Brain and Development, 19*, 13–18.

Bharucha, N. E. (2003). Epidemiology of epilepsy in India. *Epilepsia, 44*, 9–11.

Bladin, C. F., Alexandrov, A. V., Bellavance, A., Bornsetin, N., Chambers, B., Coté, R., … Seizures After Stroke Study. (2000). Seizures after stroke: A prospective multicenter study. *Archives of Neurology, 57*, 1617–1622.

Boussinesq, M., Pion, S. D. S., Demanqa-Nqanque, & Kamqno, J. (2002). Relationship between onchocerciasis and epilepsy: A matched case-control study in the Mbam Valley, Republic of Cameroon. *Transactions of the Royal Society of Tropical Medicine and Hygiene, 96*(5), 537–541.

Brick, J., Gutrecht, J., & Ringel, R. (1989). Reflex epilepsy and non-ketotic hyperglycemia in the elderly: A specific neuroendocrine syndrome. *Neurology, 39*, 394–349.

Burn, J., Dennis, M., Bamford, J., Sandercock, P., Wade, D., & Warlow, C. (1997). Epileptic seizures after a first stroke: The Oxfordshire community stroke project. *BMJ, 315*, 1582–1587.

Chen, Y., Lu, J., Pan, H., Zhang, Y., Wu, H., Xu, K., … Wu, X. (2003). Association between genetic variation of CACNA1H and childhood absence epilepsy. *Annals of Neurology, 54*, 239–243.

Clarke, M., Gill, J., Noronha, M., & McKinlay, I. (1987). Early infantile epileptic encephalopathy with suppression burst: Ohtahara syndrome. *Developmental Medicine & Child Neurology, 29*, 520–528.

Commission on Classification and Terminology of the International League against Epilepsy. (1989). Proposal for revised classification of epilepsies and epileptic syndromes. *Epilepsia, 30*, 389–399.

Commission on Epilepsy and Prognosis, International League against Epilepsy. (1993). Guidelines for epidemiologic studies on epilepsy. *Epilepsia, 34*, 592–596.

Corey, L. A., Pellock, J. M., Boggs, J. G., Miller, L. L., & DeLorenzo, R. J. (1998). Evidence for a genetic predisposition for status epilepticus. *Neurology, 50*(2), 558–560.

Corey, L. A., Pellock, J. M., & DeLorenzo, R. J. (2004). Status epilepticus in a population-based Virginia twin sample. *Epilepsia, 45*(2), 159–165.

Cowan, L. D., & Hudson, L. S. (1991). The epidemiology and natural history of infantile spasms. *Journal of Child Neurology, 6*, 355–364.

de Boer, H. M., Mula, M., & Sander, J. W. (2008). The global burden and stigma of epilepsy. *Epilepsy & Behavior, 12*(4), 540–546.

DeLorenzo, R. J., Pelloch, M., Towne, A. R., & Boggs, J. G. (1995). Epidemiology of status epilepticus. *Journal of Clinical Neurophysiology: Official Publication of the American Electroencephalographic Society, 12*, 316–325.

Depieene, C., Trouillard, O., Saint-Martin, C., Gourfinkel-An, I., Bouteiller, D., Carpentier, W., … LeGuern, E. (2009). Spectrum of SCN1A gene mutations associated with Dravet syndrome: Analysis of 333 patients. *Journal of Medical Genetics, 46*, 183–191.

Ding, D., Wang, W., Wu, J., Ma, G., Dai, Z., Yang, B., … Sander, J. W. (2006). Premature mortality in people with epilepsy in rural China: A prospective study. *The Lancet Neurology, 5*, 823–827.

Druet-Cabanac, M., Boussinesq, M., Dongmo, L., Farnarier, G., Bouteille, B., & Preux, P. M. (2004). Review of epidemiological studies searching for a relationship between onchocerciasis and epilepsy. *Neuroepidemiology, 23*(3), 144–149.

Druet-Cabanac, M., Preux, P. M., Bouteille, B., Bernet-Bernady, P., Dunand, J., Hopkins, A., … Dumas, M. (1991). Onchocerciasis and epilepsy: A matched case-control study in the Central African Republic. *American Journal of Epidemiology, 149*, 565–570.

Elmslie, F. V., Rees, M., Williamson, M. P., Kerr, M., Kjeldsen, M. J., Pang, K. A., … Gardiner, R. M. (1997). Genetic mapping of a major susceptibility locus for juvenile myoclonic epilepsy on chromosome 15q. *Human Molecular Genetics, 6*(8), 1329–1334.

Feucht, M., Fuchs, K., Pichlbauer, E., Hornik, K., Scharfetter, J., Goessler, R., … Aschauer, H. (1999). Possible association between childhood absence epilepsy and the gene encoding GABRB3. *Biological Psychiatry, 46*(7), 997–1002.

Fong, G. C. Y., Mak, W., Cheng, T. S., Chan, K. H., Fong, J. K. Y., & Ho, S. L. (2003). A prevalence study of epilepsy in Hong Kong. *Hong Kong Medical Journal, 9*, 252–257.

Forsgren, L., Bucht, G., Eriksson, S., & Bergmark, L. (1996). Incidence and clinical characterization of unprovoked seizures in adults: A prospective population-based study. *Epilepsia, 37*, 224–229.

Forsgren, L., Hauser, W. A., Olafsson, E., Sander, J. W., Sillanpää, M., & Tomson, T. (2005). Mortality of epilepsy in developed countries: A review. *Epilepsia, 46*(Suppl. 11), 18–27.

Fotheringham, J., Donati, D., Akhyani, N., Fogdell-Hahn, A., Vortmeyer, A., Heiss, J. D., … Jacobson, S. (2007). Association of human herpesvirus-6B with mesial temporal lobe epilepsy. *PLoS Medicine, 4*(5), e180.

Gao, S., Juhaeri, J., & Dai, W. S. (2008). The incidence rate of seizures in relation to BMI in UK adults. *Obesity, 16*(9), 2126–2132.

Gastaut, H. (1982). A new type of epilepsy: Benign partial epilepsy of childhood with occipital spike-waves. *Clinical Electroencephalogrphy, 13*, 13–22.

Harden, C. L., Herzog, A. G., Nikolov, B. G., Koppel, B. S., Christos, P. J., Fowler, K., … Hauser, W. A. (2006). Hormone replacement therapy in women with epilepsy: A randomized, double-blind, placebo-controlled study. *Epilepsia, 47*(9), 1447–1451.

Hauser, W. A., Annegers, J. F., & Kurland, L. T. (1993). Incidence of epilepsy and unprovoked seizures in Rochester, Minnesota: 1935–1984. *Epilepsia, 34*, 453–468.

Hauser, W. A., & Kurland, L. T. (1975). The epidemiology of epilepsy in Rochester, Minnesota, 1935 through 1967. *Epilepsia, 16*, 1–66.

Herzog, A. G. (2008). Catamenial epilepsy: Definition, prevalence, pathophysiology and treatment. *Seizure, 17*(2), 151–159.

Huang, M., Hong, Z., Zeng, J., Rong, X., Sheng, Y., & Lu, C. (2002). The prevalence of epilepsy in rural Jinshan in Shanghai. *Zhonghua Liu Xing Bing Xue Za Zhi, 23*, 345–346.

Jallon, P. (2002). Epilepsy and epileptic disorders, an epidemiological marker? Contribution of descriptive epidemiology. *Epileptic Disorders, 4*, 1–13.

Janz, E. (2000). Epilepsy with grand mal on awakening and sleep-waking cycle. *Clinical Neurophysiology, 111*(Suppl. 2), S103–S110.

Jette, N., & Trevathan, E. (2014). Saving lives by treating epilepsy in developing countries. *Neurology, 82*(7), 552–553. doi:10.1212/WNL.0000000000000133.

Joensuu, T., Lehesjoki, A. E., & Kopra, O. (2008). Molecular background of EPM1-Unverricht-Lundborg disease. *Epilepsia, 49*, 557–563.

Kalviainen, R., Khyuppenen, J., Koskenkorva, P., Eriksson, K., Vanninen, R., & Mervaala, E. (2008). Clinical picture of EPM1-Unverricht-Lundborg disease. *Epilepsia, 49*, 549–556.

Kamgno, J., Pion, S. D. S., & Boussinesq, M. (2003). Demographic impact of epilepsy in Africa: Result of a 10-year cohort study in a rural area of Cameroon. *Epilepsia, 44*, 956–963.

Kar, S. K. (2016). Epilepsy treatment in developing countries: Constraints and possibilities. *International Journal of Neurorehabilitation, 3*, e123. doi:10.4172/2376-0281.1000e123.

Kilpatrick, C. J., Davis, S. M., Tress, B. M., Rossiter, S. C., Hopper, J. L., & Vandendriesen, M. L. (1990). Epileptic seizures in acute stroke. *Archives of Neurology, 47*(2), 157–160.

Kotsopoulos, I. A. W., Van Merode, T., Kessels, F. G. H., De Krom, M. C. T. F. M., & Knottnerus, J. A. (2002). Systematic review and meta-analysis of incidence studies of epilepsy and unprovoked seizures. *Epilepsia, 43*(11), 1402–1409.

Kuzniecky, R., & Rosenblatt, B. (1987). Benign occipital epilepsy: A family study. *Epilepsia, 28*(4), 346–350.

Lahat, E., Barr, J., & Bistritzer, T. (1995). Focal epileptic episodes associated with hypoglycemia in children with diabetes. *Clinical Neurology and Neurosurgery, 97*(4), 314–316.

Lee, W. L. (1989). Long-term outcome of children with febrile seizures. *Annals of the Academy of Medicine, Singapore, 18*(1), 32–34.

Leonardi, M., & Ustun, T. B. (2002). The global burden of epilepsy. *Epilepsia, 43*(Suppl. 6), 21–25.

Li, S. C., Schoenberg, B. S., Wang, C. C., Cheng, X. M., Zhou, S. S., & Bolis, C. L. (1985). Epidemiology of epilepsy in urban areas of the People's Republic of China. *Epilepsia, 26*, 391–394.

Mac, T. L., Tran, D. S., Quet, F., Odermatt, P., Preux, P. M., & Tan, C. T. (2007). Epidemiology, aetiology, and clinical management of epilepsy in Asia: A systematic review. *The Lancet Neurology, 6*, 533–543.

Maguire, M. J., Jackson, C. F., Marson, A. G., & Nevitt, S. J. (2016). Treatments to prevent Sudden Unexpected Death in Epilepsy (SUDEP). *Cochrane Database of Systematic Reviews, 7*, CD011792. doi:10.1002/14651858.cd011792.pub2.

Malouf, R., & Brust, J. C. M. (1985). Hypoglycemia: Causes, neurologic manifestations, and outcomes. *Annals of Neurology: Official Journal of the American Neurological Association and the Child Neurology Society, 17*, 421–430.

Mani, K. S., Rangan, G., Srinivas, H. V., Kalyanasundaram, S., Narendran, S., & Reddy, A. K. (1998). The Yelandur study: A community-based approach to epilepsy in rural South India: Epidemiological aspects. *Seizure, 7*, 281–288.

Mannan, M. A. (2004). Epilepsy in Bangladesh. *Neurol Asia, 9*, 18.

McCorry, D., Nicolson, A., Smith, D., Marson, A., Feltbower, R. G., & Chadwick, D. W. (2006). An association between type 1 diabetes and idiopathic generalized epilepsy. *Annals of Neurolgy, 59*(1), 204–206.

Meyer, A. C., Dua, T., Ma, J., Saxena, S., & Birbeck, G. (2010). Global disparities in the epilepsy treatment gap: A systematic review. *Bulletin of the World Health Organization, 88*, 260–266.

Neubauer, B. A., Fiedler, B., Himmelein, B., Kämpfer, F., Lässker, U., Schwabe, G., … Stephani, U. (1998). Centrotemporal spikes in families with rolandic epilepsy: Linkage to chromosome 15q14. *Neurology, 51*(6), 1608–1612.

Ngugi, A. K., Bottomley, C., Kleinschmidt, I., Sander, J. W., & Newton, C. R. (2010). Estimation of the burden of active and lifetime epilepsy: A meta-analytic approach. *Epilepsia, 51*(5), 883–890.

Nicoletti, A., Bartoloni, A., Reggio, A., Bartalesi, F., Roselli, M., Sofia, V., … Hall, A. J. (2002). Epilepsy, cysticercosis, and toxocariasis: A population-based case-control study in rural Bolivia. *Neurology, 58*, 1256–1261.

Nicoletti, A., Bartoloni, A., Sofia, V., Bartalesi, F., Rosdao Chavez, J., Osinaga, R., … Hall, A. J. (2005). Epilepsy and neurocysticercosis in rural Bolivia: A population-based survey. *Epilepsia, 46*(7), 1127–1132.

Nicoletti, A., Sofia, V., Vitale, G., Bonelli, S. I., Bejarano, V., Bartalesi, F., … Bartoloni, A. (2009). Natural history and mortality of chronic epilepsy in an untreated population of rural Bolivia: A follow-up after 10 years. *Epilepsia, 50*(10), 2199–2206.

Offringa, M., Bossuyt, P. M., Lubsen, J., Ellenberg, J. H., Nelson, K. B., Knudsen, F. U., … Larsen, S. (1994). Risk factors for seizure recurrence in children with febrile seizures: A pooled analysis of individual patient data from five studies. *The Journal of Pediatrics, 124*(4), 574–584.

Olsen, T. S., Hagenhaven, H., & Thage, O. (1987). Epilepsy after stroke. *Neurology, 37*, 1209–1212.

Panayiotopoulos, C. P. (2007). The birth and evolution of the concept of Panayiotopoulos syndrome. *Epilepsia, 48*, 1041–1034.

Panayiotopoulos, C. P., Michael, M., Sanders, S., Valeta, T., & Koutroumanidis, M. (2008). Benign childhood focal epilepsies: Assessment of established and newly recognized syndromes. *Brain, 131*(Pt 9), 2264–2286.

Pavlidou, E., Tzitiridou, M., Kontopoulos, E., & Panteliadis, C. P. (2008). Which factors determine febrile seizure recurrence? A prospective study. *Brain and Development, 30*(1), 7–13.

Phillips, H. A., Scheffer, L. E., Crossland, K. M., Bhatia, K. P., Fish, D. R., Marsden, C. D., … Mulley, J. C. (1998). Autosomal dominant nocturnal frontal-lobe epilepsy: Genetic heterogeneity and evidence for a second Locus at 15q24. *The American Journal of Human Genetics, 63*(4), 1108–1116.

Pompili, M., Girardi, P., Ruberto, A., & Tatarelli, R. (2005). Suicide in the epilepsies: A meta-analytic investigation of 29 cohorts. *Epilepsy & Behavior, 7*(2), 305–310.

Ray, B. K., Bhattacharya, S., Kundu, T. N., Saha, S. P., & Das, S. K. (2002). Epidemiology of epilepsy-Indian perspective. *Journal of the Indian Medical Association, 100*, 322–326.

Reith, J., Jorgensen, H. S., Nakayama, H., Raaschou, H. O., & Olsen, T. S. (1997). Seizures in acute stroke: Predictors and prognostic significance. The Copenhagen Stroke Study. *Stroke, 28*, 1585–1589.

Rumbach, L., Sablot, D., Berger, E., Tatu, L., Vuiller, F., & Moulin, T. (2000). Status epilepticus in stroke: Report on a hospital-based cohort. *Neurology, 54*, 350–354.

Samokhvalov, A. V., Irving, H., Mohapatra, S., & Rehm, J. (2010). Alcohol consumption, unprovoked seizures, and epilepsy: A systematic review and meta-analysis. *Epilepsia, 51*(7), 1177–1184.

Sander, T., Bockenkamp, B., Hildmann, T., Blasczyk, R., Kretz, R., Wienker, T. F., … Ziegler, A. (1997). Refined mapping of the epilepsy susceptibility locus EJM 1 on chromosome 6. *Neurology, 49*, 842–847.

Sander, T., Hildmann, T., Kretz, R., Fürst, R., Sailer, U., Bauer, G., … Janz, D. (1997). Allelic association of juvenile absence epilepsy with a GluR5 kainate receptor gene (GRIK1) polymorphism. *American Journal of Medical Genetics, 74*(4), 416–421.

Sander, J. W., & Shovron, S. D. (1996). Epidemiology of the epilepsies. *Journal of Neurology, Neurosurgery, and Psychiatry, 61*(5), 433–443.

Sawhney, I. M., Singh, A., Kaur, P., Suri, G., & Chopra, J. S. (1999). A case control study and one year follow-up of registered epilepsy cases in a resettlement colony of North India, a developing tropical country. *Journal of the Neurological Sciences, 165*, 31–35.

Schauwecker, P. E. (2009). The genetics of status epilepticus. *Epilepsia, 50*(Suppl. 12), 22–24.

Scherer, C. (2005). Seizures and non-ketotic hyperglycemia. *Presse Médicale (Paris, France: 1983), 34*(15), 1084–1086.

Schmitz, B., Gardiner, R. M., Janz, D., & Beck-Mannagetta, G. (1997). Linkage analysis between idiopathic generalized epilepsies and the GABA a receptor α5, β3 and γ3 subunit gene cluster on chromosome 15. *Acta Neurologica Scandinavica, 96*, 1–7.

Scott, R. A., Lhatoo, S. D., & Sander, J. W. (2001). The treatment of epilepsy in developing countries: Where do we go from here? *Bull World Health Organ, 79*, 344–351.

Sillanpää, M., & Shinnar, S. (2010). Long-term mortality in childhood-onset epilepsy. *New England Journal of Medicine, 363*, 2522–2529.

Singh, B. M., Gupta, D. R., & Strobus, R. J. (1973). Nonketotic hyperglycemia and Epilepsia, partialis continua. *Archives of Neurology, 29*, 1887–1900.

Singhal, B. S. (1998). Neurology in developing countries: A population perspective. *Archives of Neurology, 55*, 1019–1021.

Sirven, J. I. (1998). Epilepsy in older adults: Causes, consequences and treatment. *Journal of American Geriatrics Society, 46*, 1291–1301.

So, E. L., Annegers, J. F., Hauser, W. A., O'Brien, P. C., & Whisnant, J. P. (1996). Population-based study of seizure disorders after cerebral infarction. *Neurology, 42*, 350–355.

Sridharan, R., & Murthy, B. M. (1999). Prevalence and pattern of epilepsy in India. *Epilepsia, 40*, 631–636.

Steinlein, O. K., Mulley, J. C., Propping, P., Wallace, R. H., Phillips, H. A., Sutherland, G. R., … Berkovic, S. F. (1995). A missense mutation in the neuronal nicotinic acetylcholine receptor α4 subunit is associated with autosomal dominant nocturnal frontal lobe epilepsy. *Nature Genetics, 11*, 201–203.

Takahashi, Y., Mori, H., Mishina, M., Watanabe, M., Kondo, N., Shimomura, J., … Fujiwara, T. (2005). Autoantibodies and cell-mediated autoimmunity to NMDA-type GluRepsilon2 in patients with Rasmussen's encephalitis and chronic progressive Epilepsia, partialis continua. *Epilepsia, 46*(Suppl. 5), 152–158.

Taylor, I., Berkovic, S. F., Kivity, S., & Scheffer, I. E. (2008). Benign occipital epilepsies of childhood: Clinical features and genetics. *Brain, 131*(9), 2287–2294.

Tekle-Haimanot, R., Forsgren, L., Abebe, M., Gebre-Mariam, A., Heijbel, J., Holmgren, G., & Ekstedt, J. (1990). Clinical and electroencephalographic characteristics of epilepsy in rural Ethiopia: A community-based study. *Epilepsy Research, 7*(3), 230–239.

Tran, D. S., Odermatt, P., Le, T. O., Huc, P., Druet-Cabanac, M., Barennes, H., … Preux, P. M. (2006). Prevalence of epilepsy in a rural district of central Lao PDR. *Neuroepidemiology, 26*, 199–206.

Trevathan, E., Murphy, C. C., & Yeargin-Allsopp, M. (1997). Prevalence and descriptive epidemiology of Lennox-Gastaut syndrome among Atlanta children. *Epilepsia, 38*(2), 1283–1288.

Turk, V., & Bode, W. (1991). The cystatins: Protein inhibitors of cysteine proteinases. *FEBS Letters, 285*(2), 213–219.

Vestergaard, M., Pedersen, C. B., Sidenius, P., Olsen, J., & Christensen, J. (2007). The long-term risk of epilepsy after febrile seizures in susceptible subgroups. *American Journal of Epidemiology, 165*(8), 911–918.

Vos, T., & GBD 2015 Disease and Injury Incidence and Prevalence Collaborators. (2016). Global, regional, and national incidence, prevalence, and years lived with disability for 310 diseases and injuries, 1990–2015: A systematic analysis for the Global Burden of Disease Study 2015. *The Lancet, 388*(10053), 1545–1602.

Wang, W. Z., Wu, J. Z., Ma, G. Y., Dai, X. Y., Yang, B., Wang, T. P., … Sander, J. W. (2006). Efficacy assessment of phenobarbital in epilepsy: A large community-based intervention trial in rural China. *The Lancet Neurology, 5*, 6–52.

Wang, W. Z., Wu, J. Z., Wang, D. S., Dai, X. Y., Yang, B., Wang, T. P., … Sander, J. W. (2003). The prevalence and treatment gap in epilepsy in China: An ILAE/IBE/WHO study. *Neurology, 60*, 1544–1545.

Wirrell, E. C., Grossardt, B. R., So, E. L., & Nickels, K. C. (2010). A population-based study of long-term outcomes of cryptogenic focal epilepsy in childhood: Cryptogenic epilepsy is probably not symptomatic epilepsy. *Epilepsia, 52*(4), 738–745.

Wirrell, E. C., Grossardt, B. R., Wong-Kisiel, L. C., & Nickels, K. C. (2011). Incidence and classification of new-onset epilepsy and epilepsy syndromes in children in Olmsted County, Minnesota from 1980 to 2004: A population-based study. *Epilepsy Research, 95*(1–2), 110–118.

World Health Organization. (2001). *Epilepsy: Epidemiology, aetiology and prognosis*. WHO Factsheet, 165. Geneva, Switzerland: World Health Organization.

World Health Organization. (2010). *Water-related diseases: Onchocerciasis*. Geneva, Switzerland: World Health Organization, Geneva, Switzerland.

World Health Organization. (2018). International Epilepsy Day. Retrieved from http://www.who.int/mental_health/neurology/epilepsy/en/

CHAPTER 52

Epidemiology of Schizophrenia

▶ Introduction

Schizophrenia is a mental condition characterized by hallucinations, delusions, suicidal ideation, paranoia, and other disturbances of thought processes and cognition. The signs and symptoms of schizophrenia are highly variable and often categorized as positive, negative, and cognitive.

A century ago, the noted Swiss psychiatrist, Eugen Bleuler, coined the term "*schizophrenia*" from the Greek roots for schizo (split) and phrene (mind). However, the term was not meant to imply split personality but rather the fragmented thinking process of patients with the disorder. Bleuler was also the first to categorize schizophrenia according to its positive and negative symptoms (Bleuler, 1911, 1931).

Positive symptoms refer to abnormal and sometimes bizarre psychotic thoughts and behaviors including auditory and visual hallucinations and "*delusions of grandeur*" and "*delusions of persecution*." Afflicted persons often exhibit unusual, dysfunctional, and/or disorganized thought processes, and agitated repetitive body movements. Patients with severe "*end-stage*" disease develop catatonia, a mental state of immobilization and failure to respond.

Negative symptoms include a *flat affect* of expression and speech, lack of pleasure in ordinary life, inability to carry out planned activities, and failure to speak and communicate with others. Cognitive symptoms refer to memory deficits, failure to focus, and inability to use information in a logical fashion.

The onset of schizophrenia differs by gender, peaking during late adolescence and young adulthood in males, and 10–20 years later in females (**FIGURE 52.1**).

Following the peak times of onset, the rates gradually decline with age, although the condition may develop at any time during the lifespan. The onset is highly variable and may be either acute or preceded by a long prodromal phase. For example, negative symptoms may precede the development of the more overt positive signs by several years (Beiser, Erickson, Fleming, & Iacono, 1993; Hafner, Maurer, & Loffler, 1999).

▶ Global Burden of Schizophrenia

Global Burden of Disease (GBD) investigators recently examined 129 data sources representing 21 regions of the world to obtain global estimates of the prevalence of schizophrenia and the years of life lost from disability (YDL) during 2016. The global age-standardized point prevalence of schizophrenia was 0.28% which translates to 20.9 million people living with the disease. Prevalence estimates ranged from less than 0.22% in sub-Saharan Africa to 0.42% in China. Most prevalent cases (70%) were young adults, aged 25–54 years. Globally, the estimated number of prevalent cases of schizophrenia rose more than 50% during 1990–2016 (from 13.1 million in 1990 to 20.9 million in 2016), and during 2016, 13.4 million years of healthy life were lost due to disability associated with schizophrenia (1.7% of the total YDL from all diseases). Notably, lower- and middle-income nations had the greatest burden of schizophrenia accounting for more than 80% of the YDL. Results suggest that the global burden of schizophrenia is rising, particularly among young adults where the risk is greatest (Charlson et al., 2018).

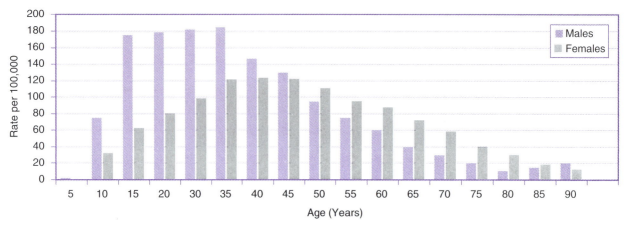

FIGURE 52.1 Age at Diagnosis of Schizophrenia.

Data from Center for Chronic Disease Prevention and Control, Health Canada, Hospital Morbidity File, Canadian Institute for Health Information, 1999/2000.

Global Incidence of Schizophrenia

In past years, there was a long-standing dogmatic opinion that the prevalence and the incidence of schizophrenia varied little from population to population (Eaton, 1985, 1991; Jablensky, 2000). However, recent studies based upon rigorously compiled data using standardized techniques of diagnosis and case reporting have revealed wide variability in both the incidence and prevalence among populations (McGrath, 2005, 2006).

McGrath and colleagues systematically reviewed and compared published incidence rates of schizophrenia for the period 1965–2001. Their review included 1458 rate estimates derived from 100 core population studies, 24 migrant studies, 23 cohort studies, and 14 studies of special populations from 33 different countries. Results revealed an asymmetric distribution of annual incidence rates with a median value of 15.2 per 100,000. Omitting the upper and lower 10% of all estimates, the rates still varied fivefold from 7.7 to 43.0 per 100,000. On average, rates were higher in males than females (RR [Relative Risk] = 1.40) and tended to be higher in urban areas than rural areas. Rates were also higher in migrants than native-born persons (RR = 4.6). These findings indicate the presence of considerable variation in the incidence rates of schizophrenia around the world due to the influence of cultural, urban, and geographic factors (McGrath et al., 2004).

Global Prevalence of Schizophrenia

McGrath and colleagues also systematically reviewed published estimates of the prevalence of schizophrenia.

They identified 188 studies that provided 1721 prevalence estimates, 132 from population-based core studies, 15 from migrant studies, and 41 from studies of special populations. The median point prevalence was 4.6 per 1000 with a range from 3.1 to 10.0 for the 10th and 90th percentiles. In contrast to the incidence which is higher in males, there was no difference in prevalence between males and females. However, migrants had 1.8-times higher prevalence values than native-born individuals, and populations of developed countries had higher values than those of less-developed countries (median estimates: 3.3 vs. 2.6 per 1000, respectively). Furthermore, the prevalence rates were approximately twofold higher for populations living at higher altitudes (McGrath, Saha, Chant, & Welham, 2008).

Prevalence of Schizophrenia in the United States

There is considerable controversy regarding the prevalence of schizophrenia in the United States. In 1993, the U.S. National Institute of Mental Health (NIMH) reported an annual prevalence of 1.1% among U.S. adults which is equivalent to 11 cases per 1000 adults or 2.8 million afflicted individuals for the U.S. population during the survey years. This early estimate was based upon a major epidemiological study of mental illness in five U.S. catchment areas (Los Angeles, St. Louis, New Haven, Baltimore, and rural counties in North Carolina). The study, which was conducted during the 1980s, included data from households, mental hospitals, prisons, nursing homes and other institutions (Regier et al., 1993).

More recently, an international team of investigators analyzed data from the *U.S. National Comorbidity Survey Replication* (NCS-R) and reported a much lower prevalence of schizophrenia and related nonaffective psychotic disorders (0.3% or 3 per 1000) (Kessler et al., 2005). The NCS-R estimate was based upon a nationally representative, face-to-face household survey of 9282 adults using a standardized questionnaire designed to accurately detect the presence of schizophrenia and related conditions (Gordan, 2018). However, the survey focused only on households and excluded data from psychiatric hospitals, nursing homes, prisons, and other facilities. The estimate from the NCS-R reflects a startling deficit of 2.0 million individuals afflicted with schizophrenia in the U.S. population compared to the older estimate and has therefore been widely disputed (Tasman, 2018; Torrey & Sinclair, 2018).

During 2001–2002, an analysis team in Boston derived a U.S. prevalence rate of 5.3 per 1000 utilizing claims data from health insurance groups including Medicaid, Medicare, and the Veterans Administration (Wu, Shi, Birnbaum, Hudson, & Kessler, 2006). But since the data did not include cases that were uninsured, this value may also underestimate the U.S. prevalence of schizophrenia. Clearly, there is an urgent need for comprehensive studies of the U.S. population to resolve the wide discrepancies in estimates of the prevalence of schizophrenia (Gordon, 2018; Tasman, 2018; Torrey & Sinclair, 2018).

▶ Excess Mortality from Schizophrenia

The systematic literature review by McGrath and colleagues identified 37 studies that estimated the standardized mortality rate (SMR) for patients with schizophrenia. A total of 561 SMR estimates were derived from these studies for analysis. The median SMR for all-cause mortality was 2.6 with a range of 1.2–5.8 for the 10th and 90th percentiles. Mortality from suicide was elevated nearly 13-fold (SMR = 12.9). The results also revealed a secular trend of age-SMRs during the period 1970–1990, increasing from 1.8 to 3.2 (McGrath et al., 2008). Nevertheless, a recent Global Burden of Disease study reported that since 1990, age-SMRs from schizophrenia have declined by about 60% (Murray & 2013 GBD Collaborators, 2015).

Other systematic literature reviews show that people with schizophrenia have elevated standardized mortality ratios for cardiovascular disease (SMR = 2.6), cancer (1.5), pulmonary diseases (SMR = 5.0), and gastrointestinal disease (SMR = 2.9). Patients with schizophrenia have high rates of risk factors for these comorbid conditions (e.g., smoking, alcohol abuse, diabetes, hypertension, obesity, and elevated lipids), all of which are potentially modifiable. The observed decline in age-standardized mortality due to schizophrenia since 1990 may reflect improved prevention and control of these factors in patients with the disease (Kilbourne et al., 2009; Murray & GBD 2013 Collaborators; Tran et al., 2009; Wildgust & Beary, 2010).

Disability-Adjusted Life Years (DALY) Lost: Schizophrenia

The DALY is the sum of *Years of Life Lost from Premature Death* (YLL) and *Years of Life Lost from Disability* (YDL): DALY = YLL + YDL. The *DALY* lost due to schizophrenia tend to be highest in Oceania, the Middle East, and Southeast Asia, while the nations of Australia, Japan, United States, and Western Europe have lower values (**FIGURE 52.2**). Marked differences are apparent in some populations despite their relative geographical proximity. For example, the DALY for schizophrenia in Indonesia is nearly twice that of Australia (the nations with the highest and lowest respective DALY).

Overall, the divergent pattern of lower DALY in more developed nations may reflect significant advances that have been made in the treatment of schizophrenia in recent decades; in fact, many patients treated judiciously with antipsychotic medications for acute schizophrenic episodes have been found to recover and lead relatively normal lives with little disability or increased mortality (Bleuler, 1972; Harding & Zahniser, 1994). Nevertheless, in a recent international study of 1633 cases of schizophrenia from 18 participating centers, patients from developing nations such as India, Nigeria, and Columbia were found to have a 40% higher recovery rate than patients from developed nations in Europe, the United States, and Japan (Leff, Sartorius, Jablensky, Korten, & Ernberg, 1992; Sartorius et al., 1986; Sartorius, Jablensky, & Shapiro, 1977). This surprising result is discussed in greater detail in the next section of this chapter.

▶ Course of Schizophrenia

The course of schizophrenia is highly variable from patient to patient. In a classic investigation, Manfred Bleuler (the son of Eugen Bleuler) followed 100 male and 108 female patients in *Burghölzli Psychiatric Hospital* in Zurich, Switzerland during 1942–1965. Patients ranged in age from 17 to 67 years at the time the study began and were followed up to 23 years. Bleuler differentiated patients according to onset (acute vs. chronic) and progression or regression of disease. Among 194 evaluable patients, 76 (39%) manifested a simple

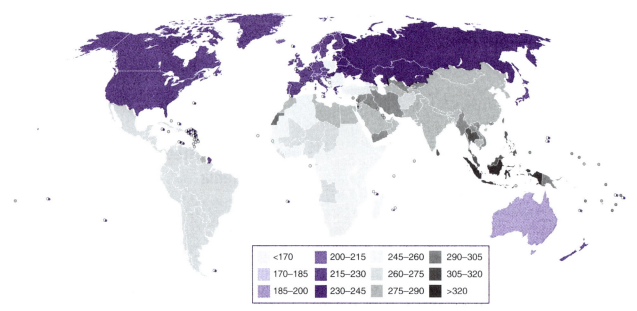

FIGURE 52.2 Disability-Adjusted Life Years: Schizophrenia, 2004.

Data from World Health Organization. (2008). *The global burden of disease: 2004 update.* Geneva: WHO. Available at www.who.int/evidence/bod

course of unrelenting disease progression and 118 (61%) manifested an undulating course characterized by periods of remission interspersed with episodic disease. At the end of follow-up, 45 patients (23%) had progressed to severe end-stage disease (catatonia), 105 (54%) were stable with mild to moderate disease, and 44 (23%) had recovered (Bleuler, 1972).

Many other studies have been conducted to examine the course of schizophrenia in patients ascertained from populations throughout the world. Most of these have found even higher rates of recovery than observed in the classic investigation by Bleuler, thus dispelling the myth that schizophrenia is an incurable mental illness. Selected studies are summarized in the following paragraphs.

In the *Iowa 500 Study* in the United States, 186 patients were followed for an average of 35 years and 46% either improved or recovered (Clancy, Tsuang, Norton, & Winokur, 1974). In the *Bonn Hospital Study* in Germany, 502 patients were followed for an average of 22.4 years. Findings revealed that 22% of patients had complete remission of symptoms and 43% had remission with mild cognitive disturbances (Huber, Gross, & Schüttler, 1978). In the *Lausanne Study* in Switzerland, findings were reported for 289 patients followed up to 64 years. Results indicated that 27% of patients recovered, 22% reached an end-stage of mild disease, 24% reached an end-stage of moderately severe disease, and 18% suffered severe end-stage disease (Ciompi & Müller, 1976). At the *Chestnut Lodge Psychiatric Hospital* in the United States, 446 patients received long-term residential psychotherapy for an average of 15 years. At the end

of study, 36% of patients had recovered and 64% were either chronically ill or marginally functional (McGlashan, 1984). In the *Japanese Long-Term Study*, 105 patients ascertained at Gunma University Hospital were followed up to 27 years. Of these, 31% recovered, 46% improved, and 23% regressed (Ogawa et al., 1987). The *Vermont Longitudinal Research Project* followed 269 patients for an average of 32 years. The study involved an innovative rehabilitation program with community and social support of all patients. Results revealed that 45% of patients recovered and 68% were assessed as having good social and psychological function at last contact (Harding, Brooks, Ashikaga, Strauss, & Breier, 1987). A comparative cohort of 269 patients from Maine received standard psychiatric care and were followed an average of 36 years. Results revealed that 49% of patients improved and demonstrated good social and psychological function at follow-up (DeSisto, Harding, McCormick, Ashikaga, & Brooks, 1995). The *Cologne Long-Term Study* in Germany followed 148 patients for an average of 25 years. Results revealed complete recovery among 7% of patients and better than expected outcomes for 58% of patients (Marneros, Deister, Rohde, Steinmeyer, & Jünemann, 1989).

The World Health Organization *International Study of Schizophrenia (ISOS)* was designed to examine disease outcomes in 18 culturally diverse cohorts of schizophrenia patients. The study included 14 cohorts of incident cases and 4 cohorts of prevalent cases, a total of 1633 patients with schizophrenia or related psychotic diseases. Patients were evaluated for disease status after 15 and 25 years of follow-up.

Results revealed a recovery rate of 56% among patients in the incident cohorts and 60% among patients in the prevalence cohorts. A notable finding was that the recovery rate was higher among patients in centers of developing nations than in developed nations (56% vs. 39%) (Leff et al., 1992; Sartorius et al., 1977, 1986). This surprising result was reconfirmed in a reanalysis of the ISOS data, suggesting the presence of factors in developing nations that favor recovery from schizophrenia (Hopper & Wanderling, 2000).

Findings of the *ISOS* have prompted other investigations of mortality and morbidity associated with schizophrenia in developing nations. Cohen and colleagues at Harvard University conducted a literature review and tabulation of data from 23 longitudinal studies of schizophrenia in 11 low- and middle-income countries. Clinical outcomes including suicide, patterns of disease course, disability, and social outcomes such as marital status and occupation, and access to treatment were reviewed. Results revealed wide variation in clinical outcomes, standard of care, patterns of disease course, disability, social dysfunction, and suicide rates with relatively high levels of "poor outcomes" reported in some developing countries (Brazil, China, and Nigeria) but not in others (India and Indonesia). The investigators suggest the need for continuing studies "*to better understand how neuropsychiatric processes and social worlds interact to shape the lives of persons with schizophrenia in low- and middle-income countries*" (Cohen, Patel, Thara, & Gureje, 2008). It is important to note that a variety of comorbid conditions such as depression, cardiovascular disease, diabetes mellitus, metabolic syndrome, and cancer are common in patients with schizophrenia and may contribute to the progression of disease. Variability in the risk factors and comorbidities associated with these conditions may help explain the disparities in the course and long-term outcomes in patients with schizophrenia (Holla & Thirthall, 2015).

▶ Suicide in Schizophrenia

Suicide is the leading cause of premature death among patients with schizophrenia. However, there is some controversy concerning the magnitude of suicide risk that apparently arose from early reports of *proportionate mortality* (the fraction of deceased patients who committed suicide), which is not the same as the *case fatality rate from suicide* or the *cumulative incidence of suicide* among all patients. Based on his studies in Switzerland, Bleuler reported that 12.8% of *deceased patients* died from suicide (Bleuler, 1972). Tsuang later

reported a similar estimate of 10.1% among decedents in the United States (Tsuang, 1978).

It is important to note that these early estimates reflect *proportionate mortality* due to suicide among only deceased patients rather than the case fatality or cumulative incidence of suicide among all patients. Estimates of proportionate mortality and case fatality due to suicide would yield similar results only when either all patients are observed until death or if suicides occur at a constant rate over time relative to other causes of death.

Investigators at the Mayo Clinic in Rochester, Minnesota, conducted a meta-analysis of cohort studies of patients with schizophrenia to accurately quantify their lifetime (cumulative) suicide risk. Studies included 32 studies of prevalent cases ($n = 25,578$ patients) and 29 studies of incident cases ($n = 22,958$ patients). The lifetime prevalence of suicide was estimated at 5.6% and the cumulative lifetime incidence of suicide was estimated at 4.9%. The approximate pattern of the cumulative suicide risk among schizophrenics is depicted in **FIGURE 52.3**. The cumulative risk of suicide rises linearly in the early years after diagnosis of schizophrenia, but then plateaus at approximately 5% after about 20 years. These results demonstrate that unless all subjects are followed until death, the proportionate mortality estimated from only decedents would markedly exceed the case fatality, since nearly all suicides are committed within a few years of diagnosis and the majority of schizophrenic patients exhibit long-term survival with 95% ultimately dying from other causes. As pointed out, this pattern "highlights the significant effect of suicide concentrated early in the course of illness" and "implies that suicide-prevention interventions are best directed at persons early in the course of their schizophrenic illness" (Palmer, Pankratz, & Bostwick, 2005).

Numerous investigations have been conducted to identify and treat those schizophrenic patients who have suicidal ideation and are at high risk of committing suicide. In the *Chestnut Lodge Study* of 322 patients diagnosed with schizophrenia or related disorders, 40% of patients reported suicidal ideation, 23% reported suicide attempts, and 6.5% died from suicide. The suicide rate among patients with paranoid schizophrenia was higher (12%) than among other patients. The investigators concluded that "*suicide may emerge from a nondelusional but acutely painful awareness of the illness process, negative expectations of the future, depleted self-esteem, and hopelessness*" (Fenton, McGlashan, Victor, & Blyler, 1997).

Investigators at Oxford conducted a meta-analysis of studies of suicide among patients with schizophrenia to elucidate the risk factors and

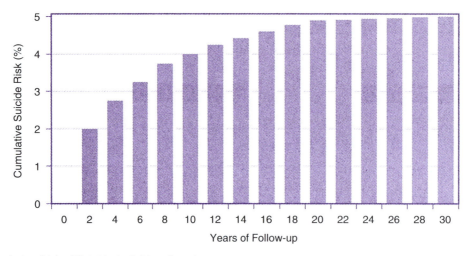

FIGURE 52.3 Cumulative Risk of Suicide in Schizophrenia.

Data from Palmer, B. A., Pankratz, V. S., & Bostwick, J. M. (2005). The lifetime risk of suicide in schizophrenia: A reexamination. *Archives of General Psychiatry 62*, 247–253.

formulate preventive measures. Systematic review of the literature identified 29 studies for analysis including 5 cohort studies and 24 case–control studies. Findings revealed an increased risk of suicide among patients with fear of mental disintegration (OR = 12.1), previous suicide attempts (OR = 4.09), recent loss (OR = 4.03), poor adherence to treatment (OR = 3.75), drug misuse (OR = 3.21), depression (OR = 3.03), and agitation or motor restlessness (OR = 2.61). Hallucinations and delusions were associated with reductions in risk (OR ~ 0.50). Based on these results, the investigators suggested that

prevention of suicide is thus likely to result from active treatment of affective symptoms and syndromes, improving adherence to treatment, use of medication that may have special anti-suicidal effects, and maintaining special vigilance in patients with risk factors, especially when faced with significant loss events (Hawton, Sutton, Haw, Sinclair, & Deeks, 2005).

In 1997, Mark Williams published his *"Cry of Pain"* model of psychological conditions under which suicide is more likely together with possible intervention strategies. According to this model, suicidal risk is elevated by untoward environmental stressors; intractable feelings of hopelessness, defeat, and entrapment; negative perceptions of oneself, others, and circumstances; a perceived absence of rescue factors; and access to methods of suicide (Williams, 1997). Various approaches involving cognitive-behavioral psychotherapy are currently being explored for the treatment of depression and suicidal ideation (Johnson, Gooding, & Tarrier, 2008; Rasmussen et al., 2010).

▶ Models of Pathogenesis: Schizophrenia

A long-standing hypothesis proposes that schizophrenia is caused by excess *dopamine* production and release by the mesolimbic neurons of the *substantia nigra* in the midbrain. This hypothesis links the hallucinatory and delusional symptoms of schizophrenia to hyperactivity of dopaminergic circuits in the forebrain. The dopamine hypothesis of schizophrenia is supported by pharmacologic evidence that phenothiazines and other drugs that reduce dopaminergic activity show therapeutic efficacy in patients with schizophrenia, whereas drugs such as amphetamines and cocaine that promote dopaminergic activity induce psychotic symptoms. Furthermore, the administration of levodopa to patients with Parkinson's disease induces paranoid ideation and auditory hallucinatory symptoms that are indistinguishable from those observed in some patients with schizophrenia. Indeed, the antidopaminergic impact of neuroleptic drugs is the cornerstone of the dopamine hypothesis of schizophrenia (Meltzer & Stahl, 1976).

A corollary of the dopamine hypothesis of schizophrenia suggests there are increased levels of *dopamine receptors* in neurons of the basal ganglia. There are two major types of dopamine receptors, D1 and D2, and several subtypes. Antipsychotic drugs directed against D2 have shown some therapeutic efficacy in the treatment of schizophrenia (Girault & Greengard, 2004).

A second hypothesis that has gained credibility in recent years postulates an imbalance of dopamine and a second neurotransmitter, glutamate, that works through activation of its cell membrane receptor, *N-methyl-D-aspartate (NMDA).* This hypothesis is based upon the effects of phencyclidine (PCP), a general anesthetic that was abandoned for clinical use because a significant fraction of patients who received it experienced disturbing thoughts and feelings on emergence from anesthesia. Specifically, PCP was found to induce the full spectrum of psychotic symptoms (disorganized thinking, hallucinations and delusions, flat affect, and social withdrawal) that characterize patients with schizophrenia.

Molecular studies have since revealed that PCP inhibits the activity of glutamate by blocking the NMDA receptor. Glutamate normally serves as the *"brake"* for dopaminergic activity in the brain, and blockade of the NMDA receptor results in hyperactivity of dopaminergic pathways. Thus, both the dopaminergic and the glutamate neurotransmitter systems appear to be involved in the pathogenesis of schizophrenia. Specifically, if NMDA receptors are either deficient or fail to function properly, the regulation of dopamine by glutamate is interrupted leading to schizophrenic symptoms (Goff & Coyle, 2001; Jentsch & Roth, 1999; Mechri et al., 2001).

▶ Risk Factors of Schizophrenia

Genetics of Schizophrenia

Genetic factors undoubtedly play an important role in the development of schizophrenia. Studies of schizophrenia in twins reveal that the risk approaches 50% in monozygous twins which is about threefold higher than in dizygous twins, and familial studies reflect 6- to 13-fold increases in the risk among first-degree relatives of cases (probands) compared to relatives of disease-free controls (**TABLE 52.1**). Nevertheless, spouses of patients have a twofold increase in risk, and adopted children of affected mothers have roughly the same risk as dizygotic twins, indicating the importance of shared environmental factors (Tsuang, 2000).

Investigators at the University of North Carolina conducted a meta-analysis of 12 twin studies in order to estimate the *heritability of additive genetic effects* that influence the liability to schizophrenia. Results revealed a heritability estimate of 81%, although there was also evidence of significant common or shared environmental influences. The investigators concluded that *"schizophrenia is a complex trait that results from genetic and environmental etiological influences"* (Sullivan, Kendler, & Neale, 2003).

Intensive research is now focused on finding genes that influence predisposition to the development of schizophrenia. To date, several genes have

TABLE 52.1 Genetic Risk of Schizophrenia

Genetic Risk Category	Risk (%)
General population	1
Spouse of patient	2
Parent of patient	6
Sibling of patient	9
Offspring of patient	13
Adopted child of patient	17
Dizygotic twin	17
Monozygotic twin	48

Data from Tsuang, M. (2000). Schizophrenia: Genes and environment. *Biological Psychiatry 47*(3), 210–220.

been discovered that show significant linkage with schizophrenia.

Catechol-O-methyltransferase is one of several enzymes that methylates and inactivates catecholamine neurotransmitters such as dopamine, epinephrine, and norepinephrine. In humans, catechol-O-methyltransferase is encoded by the *COMT* gene on the long arm of chromosome 22. Some studies have suggested that dysfunctional genetic variants of *COMT* predispose to the development of schizophrenia, particularly on exposure to cannabis during adolescence (Caspi et al., 2005).

The *Neuregulin 1 gene* (*NRG1*) on the short arm of chromosome 8 encodes a glycoprotein that modulates neuronal migration and formation of synapses during fetal development. Neuregulin is also involved in regulating myelination of neurons and signaling between glia and neurons. Dysfunctional genetic variants of *NRG1* have been found in association with the development of schizophrenia (Harrison & Law, 2005).

Other candidate schizophrenia liability genes include *dysbindin, disrupted-in-schizophrenia 1 (DISC1), regulator of G-protein signaling 4 (RGS4), and metabotropic glutamate receptor-3 (GRM3)*, all of which likely encode proteins that influence NMDA-receptor-mediated glutamate transmission and/or signaling by dopamine and gamma-aminobutyric acid (GABA). These genes and the proteins they encode could serve as specific molecular targets for therapy (Harrison & Weinberger, 2005; Straub & Weinberger, 2006).

Male Gender and Schizophrenia

In 1919, Emil Kraepelin, one of the founders of modern psychiatry, asserted that *"the male sex appears in general to suffer somewhat more frequently from dementia praecox than the female"* (Kraepelin, 1919). Nevertheless, the general view that there is no gender difference in the lifetime risk of developing schizophrenia persisted throughout most of the 20th century.

André Aleman and colleagues at the University of Amsterdam re-examined the issue of male gender as a risk factor based on a meta-analysis of gender-specific estimates of the incidence of schizophrenia derived from 49 studies published during 1980–2002. Results revealed a 42% increase in the incidence in males compared to females (RR = 1.42). Furthermore, the increased risk in males persisted for individuals diagnosed after the age of 65 years (RR = 1.32) (Aleman, Kahn, & Selten, 2003).

Apart from the 40% excess of schizophrenia in males compared to females, other distinct gender differences have been noted in the onset, symptoms, and outcomes of the disorder. Female patients are characterized by later onset of symptoms, depression and mood changes, a better ability to adjust to their environment, higher familial risk, and response to lower dosages of antipsychotic medications. In contrast, male patients are more likely to manifest a flat affect, lack of communication, and social isolation (Cannon & Clarke, 2005).

Season of Birth and Schizophrenia

Multiple studies of patients with schizophrenia conducted in different climates and in different populations consistently reveal a slightly higher frequency of patients that are born during the winter months (Carrion-Baralt et al., 2006; Davies, Welham, Chant, Torrey, & McGrath, 2003).

Torrey and colleagues at the NIMH Neuroscience Center in Washington DC reviewed 86 studies including 437,710 cases, 411,874 from in the Northern Hemisphere countries, and 25,836 from countries in the Southern Hemisphere. Despite methodological differences among studies, the results were remarkably consistent in showing a 5%–8% excess of cases born during the winter and spring months and a similar deficit of cases born during the summer and fall months. This effect was not influenced by gender, social class, race, pregnancy or birth complications, clinical subtypes, or neurological measures. Although unproven, it is hypothesized that heightened seasonal exposure of the developing fetal brain to environmental toxins, infectious agents, and/or nutritional/energy deficiencies during the second trimester, when early differentiation and maturation of neurons and neuronal circuits are occurring, may elevate the risk of subsequently developing schizophrenia (Torrey, Miller, Rawlings, & Yolken, 1997).

Obstetric Complications and Schizophrenia

Many studies have focused on obstetric complications during labor and delivery as risk factors for the subsequent development of schizophrenia. Rosanoff and colleagues first suggested there may be a link between cerebral birth trauma during delivery and the development of schizophrenia based upon a study of 142 twin pairs that were either concordant or discordant for the disorder (Rosanoff, Handy, Plesset, & Brush, 1934). More than 20 years later, Pasamanick and colleagues published their classic study of mental disorders diagnosed among individuals with a history of obstetric complications in Baltimore. Based upon the results, they suggested a *"continuum of reproductive causality"* whereby brain damage incurred during pregnancy and birth complications can lead to a gradient of subsequent injury and mental disorders including fetal and neonatal death, cerebral palsy, epilepsy, mental deficiency, and behavioral disorders (Pasamanick, Rogers, & Lilienfeld, 1956). In 1967, Stabenau and Pollin published an analysis of the birth histories of 100 pairs of monozygotic twins discordant for schizophrenia and reported that significantly more of the schizophrenic twins had been the lighter of the two at birth and had experienced birth complications, particularly asphyxia (Stabenau & Pollin, 1967).

Subsequent studies have also revealed associations between serious pregnancy or obstetric complications and the development of schizophrenia. In a meta-analysis of data from 16 published case–control studies and two cohort studies, a past history of obstetric complications increased the odds of developing schizophrenia by twofold. Subgroup analyses revealed significant risk increases for a number of obstetric complications including premature rupture of membranes, prematurity, resuscitation at time of delivery, low birth weight (<2500 g), preeclampsia, and forceps delivery (Geddes & Lawrie, 1995; Geddes et al., 1999).

In a later meta-analysis of eight prospective cohort studies, multiple obstetric complications were found to significantly increase the risk of developing schizophrenia. Of these, the strongest risk factor was gestational diabetes (RR = 7.76) followed by placenta abruption (RR = 4.02), very low birth weight (RR = 3.89), and emergency Cesarean section (RR = 3.24). Significant risk increases were also noted for uterine atony, rhesus incompatibility, asphyxia, bleeding in pregnancy, and preeclampsia. The investigators categorized obstetric risk into three groups: (1) complications of pregnancy (bleeding, preeclampsia, diabetes, and rhesus incompatibility), (2) abnormal fetal growth and development (low birth weight, congenital malformations, and small head circumference), and (3) complications of delivery (asphyxia, uterine atony, and emergency Cesarean section) (Cannon, Jones, & Murray, 2002).

Maternal Infection and Schizophrenia

Infection during fetal development has been linked to the subsequent occurrence of schizophrenia in a number of epidemiologic investigations. Various infectious agents with predilection for evolving neural tissues have been implicated. Selected studies are discussed below.

Influenza and Schizophrenia

Mednick and colleagues at the University of Southern California were the first to find a link between *prenatal* infection and schizophrenia. The investigation involved long-term follow-up of a birth cohort of individuals from Helsinki, Finland, whose birth dates coincided with the 1957 A2 influenza epidemic. Results revealed that potential fetal exposure to influenza during the second trimester of pregnancy (the period of rapid neuron formation) significantly elevated the risk of subsequently being diagnosed with schizophrenia (Mednick, 1970; Mednick, Machon, Huttunen, & Bonett, 1988).

Since this initial investigation, many others have examined maternal influenza as a risk factor for schizophrenia in offspring. Recently, investigators in Denmark conducted a nested case–control study of schizophrenia and obstetric complications in which they compared 1039 incident cases to 24,826 individually matched controls. Participants were ascertained from the *Danish National Longitudinal Registry System*. Though several obstetric risk factors were identified, maternal influenza was by far the strongest, increasing the risk more than eightfold (RR = 8.2). Risk estimates ranged from 1.5 to 2.9 for other obstetrical factors such as lack of prenatal care, prematurity, preeclampsia, hemorrhaging during delivery, manual extraction, and maternal sepsis. These results suggest that fetal neurodevelopment may be significantly compromised by maternal influenza as well as other obstetric complications, and such effects may persist and manifest later in life in the form of schizophrenia (Byrne, Agerbo, Bennedsen, Eaton, & Mortensen, 2007).

Rubella and Schizophrenia

The *Rubella Birth Defects Evaluation Project* was established at New York University Medical Center in 1964 to examine the clinical manifestations of congenital rubella and formulate appropriate management techniques. The project identified a birth cohort of 214 individuals whose mothers tested positive for rubella, and these individuals were followed over time to assess psychiatric outcomes. Psychiatric evaluations were conducted after 20 years to determine the incidence of nonaffective psychosis in comparison to an unexposed birth cohort of 766 individuals from Saratoga County and Albany, New York. Results revealed more than a fivefold increase in the incidence of nonaffective psychosis in rubella-exposed subjects compared to nonexposed subjects (16% vs. 3%, RR = 5.2). Since the rubella virus is known to cross the placenta, infect the fetal brain, disrupt organogenesis, and cause encephalitis, these findings suggest that rubella infection during fetal development causes schizophrenia-like neurodevelopmental disorders (Brown, Cohen, Greenwald, & Susser, 2000).

Toxoplasmosis gondii and Schizophrenia

There is consistent evidence that individuals with antibodies to the feline protozoan parasite, *Toxoplasmosis gondii*, have a higher prevalence of schizophrenia than those without. Since 1953, a total of 19 studies of *Toxoplasmosis gondii* antibodies in persons with schizophrenia and other severe psychiatric disorders versus controls have been published. Among these, 18 reported a higher percentage of antibodies in the affected persons, and in 11 studies the difference was statistically significant (Torrey & Yolken, 2003). In the two largest studies, Kozar and colleagues reported antibodies in 495 (52%) of psychiatric inpatients compared with 170 (25%) of 681 controls (Kozar, 1953), and Roch and Varela detected antibodies in 836 (86%) of 973 patients with schizophrenia versus 30% in the general population (Roch & Varela, 1966).

Two case–control studies have examined childhood exposure to cats as a risk factor for the development of schizophrenia. In one study, 84 (51%) of 165 cases versus 65 (38%) of 165 matched controls had owned a house cat in childhood (OR = 1.59). In the other study, 136 (52%) of 262 cases versus 219 (42%) of 522 matched controls owned a cat between birth and age 13 (OR = 1.53) (Torrey, Rawlings, & Yolken, 2000; Torrey & Yolken, 1995).

In humans, *Toxoplasma* is an important cause of abortions and stillbirths after primary infection in pregnant women. The organism is capable of crossing the placenta and infecting the fetus and is known to cause a variety of congenital abnormalities and neurological symptoms including hydrocephaly, microcephaly, intracranial calcifications, deafness, seizures, cerebral palsy, damage to the retina, and mental retardation (Torrey & Yolken, 2003).

Notably, a recent study in the laboratories of Glenn McConkey at the University of Leeds found that *Toxoplasmosis gondii* produces and secretes two key enzymes needed for the biosynthesis of dopamine, *phenylalanine hydroxylase* and *tyrosine hydroxylase*. Conceivably, active infection with this parasite may contribute to the pathogenesis of schizophrenia and other forms of psychosis through over-stimulation of dopaminergic circuitry in the brain (Gaskell, Smith, Pinney, Westhead, & McConkey, 2009). As a consequence of these investigations, clinical trials are now being conducted to assess effects of antimicrobial agents specific for *Toxoplasma* in patients with schizophrenia.

These reports and many others suggest that a variety of infectious agents may elevate the risk of developing schizophrenia in the offspring of mothers who became infected during pregnancy. Infectious agents that cross the placenta and infect the fetal brain at a critical time in development may affect the differentiation and maturation of neurons, synapses, receptors, and other components of the central nervous system. Multiple factors could elicit such neurological changes including the direct impact of live viruses or bacteria, the influx of immune cells and release of inflammatory cytokines, temperature changes associated with fever and febrile illness, and antibodies that cross react with neurological tissues (Boksa, 2008).

▶ Prenatal Dietary Deficiency and Schizophrenia

Several investigations have focused on the association of prenatal dietary deficiencies with the later development of schizophrenia during adulthood. Perhaps the most famous of these was a study of the Dutch birth cohort prenatally exposed to severe famine by the Nazi blockade of the Western Netherlands during World War II. In a follow-up study of the birth cohort exposed to the "*hunger winter of 1944–1945*" compared to nonexposed birth cohorts, the relative risk (RR) for development of schizophrenia was significantly elevated in young women with severe prenatal caloric deprivation during the first trimester of pregnancy (RR = 2.6). The risk was attenuated with exposure in the second and third trimesters and was not significantly elevated (RR = 1.4) in young men

(Susser & Lin, 1992). This initial link between severe prenatal food deprivation and the subsequent risk increase in schizophrenia was later replicated in two regions of China which experienced famines during 1959–1961 (St Clair et al., 2005). Animal studies, ecological studies, and cohort studies provide evidence that prenatal deficiencies in specific nutrients (vitamin D, folic acid and iron) may be linked to the subsequent development of schizophrenia (McGrath, Brown, & St Clair, 2011).

Choline is a nutrient that is essential for normal brain development of the fetus during pregnancy. Choline and its metabolites help regulate DNA methylation and gene expression, membrane stability, and cholinergic neurotransmission during embryogenesis, and its prenatal influence on brain development may carry forward throughout life (Bekdash, 2016).

A randomized clinical trial of 100 pregnant women was conducted at the University of Colorado to evaluate the effects of supplemental choline on measures of brain development in newborns. Electroencephalographic (EEG) patterns of newborns were measured revealing significant beneficial changes in biomarkers of schizophrenia in the group receiving supplemental choline. Results suggest the need for further investigations of potential epigenetic effects of choline on brain development during embryogenesis (Ross et al., 2013).

Cannabis and Schizophrenia

The association between cannabis (also known as marijuana or hashish) and schizophrenia was recognized long ago (Moreau, 1973; Warnock, 1903). Though the exact mechanisms of action remain to be clarified, the results of several recent prospective studies provide compelling evidence of a cause and effect relationship between cannabis exposure and the development of this disorder (Hall & Degenhardt, 2000).

In a large longitudinal study, 45,570 Swedish male conscripts (persons enlisted in the military by compulsion) were followed over a 15-year period to determine the association of self-reported use of cannabis and the development of schizophrenia. A total of 246 cases were identified in the *Swedish National Register of Psychiatric Care* during follow-up. Results reflect a pronounced dose–response of the exposure-specific incidence with cannabis use, increasing more than sixfold among heavy users compared to nonusers (**FIGURE 52.4**). These effects persisted with adjustment for potential social and psychological confounders indicating "*that cannabis is an independent risk factor for schizophrenia*" (Andréasson, Allebeck, Engström, & Rydberg, 1987).

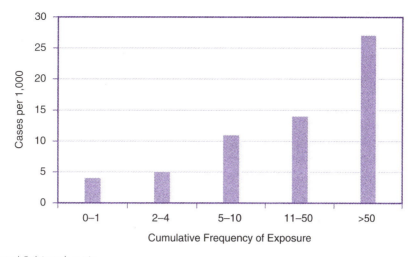

FIGURE 52.4 Cannabis and Schizophrenia.

Andréasson, S., Allebeck, P., Engström, A., & Rydberg, U. (1987). Cannabis and schizophrenia: A longitudinal study of Swedish conscripts. *Lancet 330*(8574), 1483–1486.

The association of cannabis and schizophrenia was also examined in the *Dunedin Multidisciplinary Health and Development Birth Cohort* of 1037 individuals born in Dunedin, New Zealand, during 1972–1973. Information on adolescent drug use was obtained by self-report at ages 15 and 18 years of age, and psychiatric status was assessed at 26 years of age. The analysis focused on a subset of 759 subjects with complete data on adult psychiatric outcomes, adolescent use of illicit substances (including cannabis), and childhood psychotic syndromes. The findings revealed that individuals who began regular cannabis use before age 15 years were nearly seven times more likely to be diagnosed with symptoms of schizophrenia (OR = 6.91). This effect persisted with adjustment for the presence of psychotic symptoms during childhood. Based on results, the investigators advised that "*cannabis use among psychologically vulnerable adolescents should be strongly discouraged by parents, teachers, and health practitioners*" (Arseneault et al., 2002).

In the *Netherlands Mental Health Survey and Incidence Study*, a population sample of 4045 individuals was followed during 1997–1999 to assess effects of cannabis exposure on the development of psychotic disorders. Baseline cannabis use was found to be a risk factor for the development of psychotic symptoms in a dose–response pattern. Compared to nonuse, any level of cannabis use increased the risk more than threefold (OR = 3.25) and daily use increased the risk nearly sevenfold (OR = 6.81) (van Os et al., 2002).

In a retrospective cohort study, investigators in Denmark identified 535 patients treated for cannabis-induced psychosis through the Danish Psychiatric Central Register and followed their course for at least 3 years to determine their risk of developing schizophrenia. Among these individuals, 44.5% developed schizophrenia-spectrum disorders. In a separate analysis, individuals in the cannabis-exposed cohort developed disease earlier than who had no history of exposure (24.6 years vs. 30.7 years in males and 28.9 years vs. 33.1 years in females). The investigators concluded that cannabis-induced psychosis is a strong prognostic factor for the development of schizophrenia-spectrum disorders (Arendt, Rosenberg, Foldager, Perto, & Munk-Jorgensen, 2005).

Henquet and colleagues examined the association of cannabis use and psychosis in a meta-analysis of published prospective studies. Seven studies were included in their analysis, all of which focused on either schizophrenia per se or psychotic outcomes related to schizophrenia. Prior history of cannabis use increased the risk of psychosis by about twofold (Pooled OR = 2.1). There was no evidence of heterogeneity among studies (Henquet, Murray, Linszen, & van Os, 2005).

An international team of investigators conducted a meta-analysis to clarify the timing of onset of psychotic disorders among individuals exposed to cannabis compared to those with no exposure. Data were extracted from 83 studies for analysis. The combined data revealed that the mean onset of psychosis occurred 2.7 years earlier in individuals who used cannabis (Large, Sharma, Compton Slade, & Nielssen, 2011).

In summary, observational studies are consistent in finding that individuals with higher frequency and longer duration of cannabis use are at increased risk of developing schizophrenia, and patients with cannabis-induced psychosis are at particularly high risk for the development of schizophrenia-spectrum disorders. The available epidemiologic evidence, therefore, suggests that regular cannabis use is a component cause *of schizophrenia in some individuals (D'Souza, Sewell, and Ranganathan, 2009). Nevertheless, recent clinical trials suggest that medicinal cannabinoids have positive effects in relieving pain and nausea in patients with cancer and other debilitating diseases, and more studies are needed to clarify the benefit to risk ratios of these compounds. (Modified from Gunnell, D., & Frankel, S. (1994). Prevention of suicide: Aspirations and evidence. BMJ, 308(6938), 1227–1233).*

Parental Age and Schizophrenia

Advanced *paternal age* was first proposed as a risk factor for schizophrenia in a report by Gregory in 1959. In the study, fathers of 1000 patients newly admitted to Canadian hospitals were, on average, 2–3 years older than fathers in the general population (Gregory, 1959). Results of most subsequent studies lend support to this association (Brown et al., 2002; Byrne, Agerbo, Ewald, Eaton, & Mortensen, 2003; Dalman & Allebeck, 2002; Granville-Grossman, 1966; Hare & Moran, 1979; Kinnell, 1983).

In Israel, Malaspina and colleagues studied the association of paternal age and schizophrenia in a population birth cohort of 87,907 individuals born in Jerusalem from 1964 to 1976. Cases were identified in the cohort by linking records to the *Israel Psychiatric Registry*. During the follow-up period which ended in 1998, a total of 658 cases were diagnosed with either schizophrenia or nonaffective psychosis. Compared with offspring of fathers younger than 25 years of age, the relative risk of schizophrenia increased monotonically with each successive 5-year paternal age group, reaching 2.02 and 2.96 in offspring of fathers aged 45–49 years and 50 years or older, respectively. In contrast, *maternal age* had no effect on the risk (Malaspina et al., 2001).

In Sweden, Sipos and colleagues conducted a population-based cohort study of 712,014 individuals born in Sweden between 1973 and 1980 to investigate the association of paternal age at conception and the risk of developing schizophrenia in the offspring. A total of 639 cases of schizophrenia and 1311 cases of nonaffective psychosis were identified in the cohort by linking records to the *Swedish Inpatient Discharge Register* during 1989–2001. After adjustment for obstetric complications, socioeconomic factors, family history, and other factors, the overall hazard ratio for each 10-year increase in paternal age was 1.46. The association was present only in patients without a family history of schizophrenia, suggesting that accumulation of de novo mutations in sperm may elevate the risk (Sipos et al., 2004).

Autoimmune Diseases and Schizophrenia

Various autoimmune disorders have been linked to schizophrenia, some that apparently increase the risk and others that either have no effect or may even decrease the risk. The evidence appears strongest for a positive association with celiac disease and a negative association with rheumatoid arthritis (Ganguli, Brar, & Rabin, 1994).

Celiac disease is a rare autoimmune disorder caused by immunoreactivity of cells lining the small intestine to gliadin, a prolamin (gluten protein) found in wheat and other grains such as barley and rye. Symptoms include malabsorption of gluten-containing products, inflammatory bowel disease, chronic diarrhea, and failure to thrive in infants. The condition occurs primarily in genetically susceptible individuals that inherit specific alleles of the *human leukocyte antigen (HLA)* locus on chromosome 6. Nearly half a century ago, celiac disease was proposed as a risk factor for schizophrenia based primarily on case reports and ecological data showing a correlation between national changes in wheat intake and hospital admissions of schizophrenic patients (Dohan, 1966, 1980).

An international team of investigators recently examined the association of celiac disease and schizophrenia in a case–control study of 7997 incident cases admitted to Danish psychiatric facilities during 1981–1998 and nearly 20,000 disease-free controls from the general population matched by year of birth and gender. Only celiac disease diagnosed before the onset of schizophrenia was considered in the study. The rate of celiac disease was found to be threefold higher among cases than controls (1.5 vs. 0.5 per 1000, adjusted RR = 3.2). These results suggest that patients with celiac disease who develop schizophrenia may respond to removal of gluten from the diet (Eaton et al., 2004). Though the mechanism of action is not fully understood, studies of celiac disease in humans show the presence of circulating gluten antibodies and T-cells activated by gluten breakdown products with neurotoxic and psychoactive effects (Hadjivassiliou et al., 2010).

In a subsequent investigation, William Eaton and colleagues in Denmark used the *Danish National Medical Register System* to examine the association of schizophrenia with any form of antecedent autoimmune disease. The dataset included 7704 cases of schizophrenia diagnosed during 1981–1998 and a matched sample of controls from the general population. Data were also ascertained for the parents of cases and controls. Only autoimmune diseases occurring before the diagnosis of schizophrenia were considered in the analysis. Findings revealed a 45% increase in the risk of schizophrenia among individuals with a medical or familial history of *any form of autoimmune disease*. Risk increases were noted for celiac disease, thyrotoxicosis (Grave's disease), hemolytic anemia (antibodies against red blood cells), and several other forms of autoimmunity. These results suggest that some autoimmune conditions have risk factors in common with schizophrenia (Eaton et al., 2006).

In contrast to the positive associations observed between schizophrenia and several autoimmune disorders, many studies have consistently shown that individuals with schizophrenia are *less* likely to develop *rheumatoid arthritis*. For example, Eaton and colleagues reviewed data from 14 epidemiologic investigations and concluded that "*there is sufficient evidence for the negative association between the two disorders to justify further research*" (Eaton, Hayward, & Ram, 1992). In a subsequent meta-analysis of 15 epidemiologic studies, the risk of developing rheumatoid arthritis in schizophrenic patients was well below that in patients with other psychiatric conditions (OR = 0.29) (Oken & Schulzer, 1999).

Rheumatoid arthritis is a chronic systemic inflammatory condition of the synovial joints and other tissues that eventually leads to the massive destruction of synovial membranes and cartilage. This disorder is associated with the sustained presence of *rheumatoid factor*, an autoantibody that binds to synovial membranes, collagen, and articular cartilage thus promoting persistent inflammation, complement activation, and other destructive and lytic processes. Conceivably, one or more infectious agents are capable of inducing the production of rheumatoid factor in susceptible individuals which in turn incites a recursive autoimmune reaction directed primarily against synovial membranes and articular cartilage (Robbins & Cotran, 1979).

Allelic combinations of the *HLA* loci on chromosome 6 have been examined in autoimmune and psychiatric conditions. These genetic loci are components of the *major histocompatibility complex (MHC)* of genes on chromosome 6 which encode antigens and other components of the immune system. Since there are six major HLA loci (A, B, C, DP, DQ, and DR) as well as a large number of other genes within the MHC, thousands of genotypic combinations are possible.

Notably, certain HLA alleles have been found in association with the development of several of the autoimmune conditions that apparently influence schizophrenia risk (e.g., celiac disease with *HLA-DQ2 and DQ8*; thyroiditis with *HLA DR3*; and rheumatoid arthritis with *HLA DR4*) (Thorsby & Benedicte,

2005). Furthermore, preliminary results of linkage studies suggest there are genes that influence susceptibility to schizophrenia located on the short arm of chromosome 6 (Mayilyan & Weinberger, 2008). It is therefore plausible that certain HLA genotypic configurations may either predispose to both autoimmunity and schizophrenia, or reciprocally, have divergent impact on the etiopathogenesis of these disorders. Identification of such genes, the antigens they encode, and the cellular functions influenced may elucidate molecular targets for effective molecular intervention.

▶ Primary Prevention of Schizophrenia

Modifiable risk factors for schizophrenia include obstetrical complications, infection and poor nutrition during the prenatal and antenatal periods, and cannabis use. Potential interventions must be effective, safe, inexpensive, and acceptable to the public. Of foremost importance is ready access to adequate prenatal nutrition for all women of reproductive age in order to support optimal fetal brain development and reduce the risk to offspring of developing schizophrenia and other neurological conditions. As first pointed out by John McGrath, "*Vaccinations and interventions related to improving prenatal nutrition and antenatal care appear to be the most plausible options for universal prevention*" (McGrath, 2000). Nevertheless, more research is required to clarify preventive effects of specific nutrients (e.g., iron, vitamin D, and folate), and demonstrate the plausibility of implementing broad programs of supplementation, fortification and/or food-based approaches to correct micronutrient deficiencies in large populations (Bailey, West, & Black, 2015; McGrath et al., 2011).

▶ Tertiary Prevention in Schizophrenia

Guidelines for the treatment of patients with schizophrenia have been comprehensively reviewed by several authorities in the field (Royal Australian and New Zealand College of Psychiatrists, 2005). There is general agreement that the judicious use of antipsychotic agents plays a significant role in the treatment of schizophrenia and other psychotic disturbances. However, as noted by Manfred Bleuler, among his patients who maintained long-standing remission or a stable recovery, not a single one had received chronic neuroleptic medication. Instead, the patients were given medication during acute phases and never for longer than a few weeks after recovery from their acute episode (Bleuler, 1972). More recently, in their assessment of the long-term follow-up literature on schizophrenic patients, Harding and Zahniser found that 25%–50% of patients in recovery were completely off medications and functioning well without further symptoms (Harding & Zahniser, 1994).

Coexistent substance abuse is common in patients with schizophrenia and is potentially responsible for a myriad of collateral health problems including deterioration of psychiatric symptoms. Substance abuse should therefore be candidly addressed with the aim of tapering and ultimately eliminating exposure. An integrated motivational approach to care is advocated with family and community support and intensive case management by a psychiatrist during acute episodes of psychosis and periods of vulnerability (Ziedonis et al., 2005).

References

Aleman, A., Kahn, R. S., & Selten, J. P. (2003). Sex differences in the risk of schizophrenia: Evidence from meta-analysis. *Archives of General Psychiatry, 60*(6), 565–571.

Andréasson, S., Allebeck, P., Engström, A., & Rydberg, U. (1987). Cannabis and schizophrenia: A longitudinal study of Swedish conscripts. *Lancet, ii,* 1483–1485.

Arendt, M., Rosenberg, R., Foldager, L., Perto, G., & Munk-Jorgensen, P. (2005). Cannabis-induced psychosis and subsequent schizophrenia-spectrum disorders: Follow-up study of 535 incident cases. *British Journal of Psychiatry, 187,* 510–515.

Arseneault, L., Cannon, M., Poulton, R., Murray, R., Caspi, A., & Moffitt, T. E. (2002). Cannabis use in adolescence and risk for adult psychosis: Longitudinal prospective study. *BMJ (Clinical Research Edition), 325*(7374), 1212–1213. doi:10.1159/000371618. Epub 2015 Jun 2

Bailey, R. L., West, K. P., Jr., & Black, R. E. (2015). The epidemiology of global micronutrient deficiencies. *Annals of Nutrition & Metabolism, 66*(Suppl. 2), 22–33.

Beiser, M., Erickson, D., Fleming, J. A., & Iacono, W. G. (1993). Establishing the onset of psychotic illness. *The American Journal of Psychiatry, 150*(9), 1349–1354.

Bekdash, R. A. (2016). Choline and the brain: An epigenetic perspective. *Advances in Neurobiology, 12,* 381–399.

Bleuler, E. (1911). Dementia Praecox oder Gruppe der Schizophrenien. Leipzig, Germany: Deuticke.

Bleuler, M. (1931). Schizophrenia: Review of work of Professor Eugen Bleuler. *Archives of Neurology and Psychiatry, 26,* 610–627.

Bleuler, M. (1972). *The schizophrenic disorders: Long-term patient and family studies.* London, UK: Yale University Press.

Boksa, P. (2008). Maternal infection during pregnancy and schizophrenia. *Journal of Psychiatry & Neuroscience, 33*(3), 183–185.

Brown, A. S., Cohen, P., Greenwald, S., & Susser, E. (2000). Nonaffective psychosis after prenatal exposure to rubella. *The American Journal of Psychiatry, 157*(3), 438–443.

Brown, A. S., Schaefer, C. A., Wyatt, R. J., Begg, M. D., Goetz, R., Bresnahan, M. A., ... Susser, E. S. (2002). Paternal age and risk of schizophrenia in adult offspring. *The American Journal of Psychiatry, 159*(9), 1528–1533.

Byrne, M., Agerbo, E., Bennedsen, B., Eaton, W. W., & Mortensen, P. B. (2007). Obstetric conditions and risk of first admission with schizophrenia: A Danish national register based study. *Schizophrenia Research, 97*(1–3), 51–59.

Byrne, M., Agerbo, E., Ewald, H., Eaton, W. W., & Mortensen, P. B. (2003). Parental age and risk of schizophrenia: A case-control study. *Archives of General Psychiatry, 60*(7), 673–678.

Cannon, M., & Clarke, M. C. (2005). Schizophrenia: Epidemiology and risk factors. *Psychiatry, 4*(10), 7–10.

Cannon, M., Jones, P. B., & Murray, R. M. (2002). Obstetric complications and schizophrenia: Historical and meta-analytic review. *The American Journal of Psychiatry, 159*(7), 1080–1092.

Carrion-Baralt, J. R., Smith, C. J., Rossy-Fullana, E., Lewis-Fernandez, R., Davis, K. L., & Silverman, J. M. (2006). Seasonality effects on schizophrenic births in multiplex families in a tropical island. *Psychiatry Research, 142*(1), 93–97.

Caspi, A., Moffitt, T. E., Cannon, M., McClay, J., Murray, R., Harrington, H., ... Craig, I. W. (2005). Moderation of the effect of adolescent-onset cannabis use on adult psychosis by a functional polymorphism in the catechol-Omethyltransferase gene: Longitudinal evidence of a gene x environment interaction. *Biological Psychiatry, 57*(10), 1117–1127.

Center for Chronic Disease Prevention and Control, Health Canada, Hospital Morbidity File, Canadian Institute for Health Information, 1999/2000.

Charlson, J. F., Ferrari, A. J., Santomauro, D. F., Diminic, S., Stockings, E., Scott, J. G., ... Whiteford, H. A. (2018). Global epidemiology and burden of schizophrenia: Findings from the Global Burden of Disease Study 2016. *Schizophrenia Bulletin,* sby058. doi:10.1093/schbul/sby058.

Ciompi, L., & Müller, C. (1976). *Lebensweg und alter der schizophrenen, eine katamnestische langzeitstudie bis ins senium.* Berlin, Germany: Springer.

Clancy, J., Tsuang, M. T., Norton, B., & Winokur, G. (1974). The Iowa 500: A comprehensive study of mania, depression and schizophrenia. *Journal of Iowa Medical Society, 64*(9), 394–396.

Cohen, A., Patel, V., Thara, R., & Gureje, O. (2008). Questioning an axiom: Better prognosis for schizophrenia in the developing world? *Schizophr Bull, 34*(2), 229–244.

Dalman, C., & Allebeck, P. (2002). Paternal age and schizophrenia: Further support for an association. *The American Journal of Psychiatry, 159*(9), 1591–1592.

Davies, G., Welham, J., Chant, D., Torrey, E. F., & McGrath, J. (2003). A systematic review and meta-analysis of Northern Hemisphere season of birth studies in schizophrenia. *Schizophrenia Bulletin, 29*(3), 587–593.

DeSisto, M. J., Harding, C. M., McCormick, R. V., Ashikaga, T., & Brooks, G. W. (1995). The Maine and Vermont three-decade studies of serious mental illness. Matched comparison of cross-sectional outcome. *The British Journal of Psychiatry, 167,* 331–338.

Dohan, F. (1966). Cereals and schizophrenia-data and hypothesis. *Acta Psychiatrica Scandinavica, 42,* 125–152.

Dohan, F. C. (1980). Hypothesis: Genes and neuroactive peptides from food as cause of schizophrenia. *Advances in Biochemical Psychopharmacology, 22,* 535–548.

D'Souza, D. C., Sewell, R. A., & Ranganathan, M. (2009). Cannabis and psychosis/schizophrenia: Human studies. *European Archives of Psychiatry and Clinical Neuroscience, 259*(7), 413–431.

Eaton, W. W. (1985). Epidemiology of schizophrenia. *Epidemiologic Reviews, 7*, 105–126.

Eaton, W. W. (1991). Update on the epidemiology of schizophrenia. *Epidemiologic Reviews, 13*, 320–328.

Eaton, W. W., Byrne, M., Ewald, H., Mors, O., Chen, C. Y., Agerbo, E., & Mortensen, P. B. (2006). Association of schizophrenia and autoimmune diseases: Linkage of Danish national registers. *American Journal of Psychiatry, 163*(3), 521–528.

Eaton, W. W., Hayward, C., & Ram, R. (1992). Schizophrenia and rheumatoid arthritis: A review. *Schizophrenia Research, 6*(3), 181–192.

Eaton, W. W., Mortensen, P. B., Agerbo, E., Byrne, M., Mors, O., & Ewald, H. (2004). Coeliac disease and schizophrenia: Population based case control study with linkage of Danish national registers. *BMJ (Clinical Research Edition), 328*(7437), 438–439.

Fenton, W. S., McGlashan, T. H., Victor, B. J., & Blyler, C. R. (1997). Symptoms, subtype, and suicidality in patients with schizophrenia spectrum disorders. *American Journal of Psychiatry, 154*, 199–204.

Ganguli, R., Brar, J. S., & Rabin, B. S. (1994). Immune abnormalities in schizophrenia: Evidence for the autoimmune hypothesis. *Harvard Review of Psychiatry, 2*(2), 70–83.

Gaskell, E. A., Smith, J. E., Pinney, J. W., Westhead, D. R., & McConkey, G. A. (2009). A unique dual activity amino acid hydroxylase in Toxoplasma gondii. *PLoS ONE, 4*(3), e4801.

Geddes, J. R., & Lawrie, S. M. (1995). Obstetric complications and schizophrenia: A meta-analysis. *British Journal of Psychiatry, 167*, 786–793.

Geddes, J. R., Verdoux, H., Takei, N., Lawrie, S. M., Bovet, P., Eagles, J. M., … Murray, R. M. (1999). Schizophrenia and complications of pregnancy and labor: An individual patient data meta-analysis. *Schizophrenia Bulletin, 25*(3), 413–423.

Girault, J.-A., & Greengard, P. (2004). The neurobiology of dopamine signaling. *Archives of Neurology, 61*, 641–644.

Goff, D. C., & Coyle, R. J. (2001). The emerging role of glutamate in the pathophysiology and treatment of schizophrenia. *American Journal of Psychiatry, 158*, 1367–1368.

Gordon, J. (2018). On the prevalence of schizophrenia and transforming care through research. *Psychiatric Times, 35*(3), 11.

Granville-Grossman, K. L. (1966). Parental age and schizophrenia. *British Journal of Psychiatry, 112*(490), 899–905.

Gregory, I. (1959). Factors influencing first admission rates to Canadian mental hospitals: III. An analysis by education, marital status, country of birth, religion, and rural-urban residence, 1950–1952. *Canadian Journal of Psychiatry, 4*, 133–151.

Gunnell, D., & Frankel, S. (1994). Prevention of suicide: Aspirations and evidence. *BMJ, 308*(6938), 1227–1233.

Hadjivassiliou, M., Sanders, D. S., Grünewald, R. A., Woodroofe, N., Boscolo, S., & Aeschlimann, D. (2010). Gluten sensitivity: From gut to brain. *Lancet Neurology, 9*, 318–330.

Hafner, H., Maurer, K., & Loffler, W. (1999). Onset and prodromal phase as determinants of the course. In W. F. Gattaz, & H. Hafner (Eds.), *Search for the causes of schizophrenia: Vol IV, Balance of the century* (pp. 35–58). Darmstadt, Germany: Steinkopf Springer.

Hall, W., & Degenhardt, L. (2000). Cannabis use and psychosis: A review of clinical and epidemiological evidence. *The Australian and New Zealand Journal of Psychiatry, 34*(1), 26–34.

Harding, C. M., Brooks, G. W., Ashikaga, T., Strauss, J. S., & Breier, A. (1987). The Vermont longitudinal study of persons with severe mental illness, I: Methodology, study sample, and overall status 32 years later. *American Journal of Psychiatry, 144*, 718–726.

Harding, C. M., & Zahniser, H. (1994). Empirical correction of seven myths about schizophrenia with implications for treatment. *Acta Psychiatrica Scandinavica Supplement, 384*, 140–146.

Hare, E. H., & Moran, P. A. (1979). Raised parental age in psychiatric patients: Evidence for the constitutional hypothesis. *British Journal of Psychiatry, 134*, 169–177.

Harrison, P. J., & Law, A. J. (2005). Neuregulin 1 and schizophrenia: Genetics, gene expression, and neurobiology. *Biological Psychiatry, 60*(2), 132–140.

Harrison, P. J., & Weinberger, D. R. (2005). Schizophrenia genes, gene expression, and neuropathology: On the matter of their convergence. *Molecular Psychiatry, 10*, 40–68.

Hawton, K., Sutton, L., Haw, C., Sinclair, J., & Deeks, J. J. (2005). Schizophrenia and suicide: Systematic review of risk factors. *The British Journal of Psychiatry, 187*, 9–20.

Henquet, C., Murray, R., Linszen, D., & van Os, J. (2005). The environment and schizophrenia: The role of cannabis use. *Schizophrenia Bulletin, 31*(3), 608–612.

Holla, B., & Thirthall, J. (2015). Course and outcome of schizophrenia in Asian countries: Review of research in the past three decades. *Asian Journal of Psychiatry, 14*, 3–12.

Hopper, K., & Wanderling, J. (2000). Revisiting the developed versus developing country distinction in course and outcome in schizophrenia: Results from ISOS, the WHO-collaborative follow-up project. *Schizophrenia Bulletin, 26*(4), 835–846.

Huber, G., Gross, G., & Schüttler, R. (1978). *Schizophrenie: Eine verlaufsund sozialpsychiatrische langzeitstudie.* Berlin, Germany: Springer.

Jablensky, A. (2000). Epidemiology of schizophrenia: The global burden of disease and disability. *European Archives of Psychiatry & Clinical Neuroscience, 250*, 274–285.

Jentsch, J. D., & Roth, R. H. (1999). The neuropsychopharmacology of phencyclidine: From NMDA receptor hypofunction to the dopamine hypothesis of schizophrenia. *Neuropsychopharmacology, 20*, 201–225.

Johnson, J., Gooding, P., & Tarrier, N. (2008). Suicide risk in schizophrenia: Explanatory models and clinical implications, the schematic appraisal model of suicide (SAMS). *Psychology and Psychotherapy: Theory, Research and Practice, 81*, 55–77.

Kessler, R. C., Birnbaum, H., Demler, O., Falloon, I. R. H., Gagnon, E., Guyer, M., … Wu, E. Q. (2005). The prevalence and correlates of non-affective psychosis in the National Comorbidity Survey Replication (NCS-R). *Biological Psychiatry, 58*(8), 558–676.

Kilbourne, A. M., Morden, N. E., Austin, K., Ilgen, M., McCarthy, J. F., Dalack, G., & Blow, F. C. (2009). Excess heart-disease-related mortality in a national study of patients with mental disorders: Identifying modifiable risk factors. *General Hospital Psychiatry, 31*, 555–563.

Kinnell, H. G. (1983). Parental age in schizophrenia. *British Journal of Psychiatry, 142*, 204.

Kozar, Z. (1953). Badania nad toksoplazmoza wsród umyslowo chorych. *Biuletyn Panstwowego Instytutu Medycyny Morskiej i Tropikalnej w Gdansku, 5*, 134–145.

Kraepelin, E. (1919). *Dementia Praecox and Paraphrenia.* R. M. Barclay (Trans.). New York, NY: Krieger.

Large, M., Sharma, S., Compton Slade, T., & Nielssen, O. (2011). Cannabis use and earlier onset of psychosis: A systematic meta-analysis. *Archives of General Psychiatry.* doi:10.1001/archgenpsychiatry.2011.5.

Leff, J., Sartorius, N., Jablensky, A., Korten, A., & Ernberg, G. (1992). The international pilot study of schizophrenia: Five-year follow-up findings. *Psychological Medicine, 22*(1), 131–145.

Malaspina, D., Harlap, S., Fennig, S., Heiman, D., Nahon, D., Feldman, D., & Susser, E. S. (2001). Advancing paternal age and the risk of schizophrenia. *Archives of General Psychiatry, 58*(4), 361–367.

Marneros, A., Deister, A., Rohde, A., Steinmeyer, E. M., & Jünemann, H. (1989). Long-term outcome of schizoaffective and schizophrenic disorders: A comparative study. *European Archives of Psychiatry and Clinical Neuroscience, 238*(3), 118–125.

Mayilyan, K. R., & Weinberger, D. R. (2008). Involvement of the HLA diversity in schizophrenia, supporting data and perspectives. *ASHI Quarterly,* Third Quarter, 74–77.

McGlashan, T. H. (1984). The chestnut lodge follow-up study II. Long-term outcome of schizophrenia and the affective disorders. *Archives of General Psychiatry, 41*(6), 586–601.

McGrath, J. (2000). Universal interventions for the primary prevention of schizophrenia. *Australian & New Zealand Journal of Psychiatry, 33*(Suppl. 1), A58–A64.

McGrath, J., Brown, A., & St Clair, D. (2011). Prevention and schizophrenia—The role of dietary factors. *Schizophrenia Bulletin, 37*(2), 272–283.

McGrath, J., Saha, S., Chant, D., & Welham, J. (2008). Schizophrenia: A concise overview of incidence, prevalence, and mortality. *Epidemiological Reviews, 30*(1), 67–76.

McGrath, J., Saha, S., Welham, J., El Saadi, O., MacCauley, C., & Chant, D. (2004). A systematic review of the incidence of schizophrenia: The distribution of rates and the influence of sex, urbanicity, migrant status and methodology. *BMC Medicine, 2*, 13. doi:10.1186/1741-7015-2-13.

McGrath, J. J. (2005). Myths and plain truths about schizophrenia epidemiology, the NAPE lecture 2004. *Acta Psychiatrica Scandinavica, 111*(1), 4–11.

McGrath, J. J. (2006). Variations in the incidence of schizophrenia: Data versus dogma. *Schizophrenia Bulletin, 32*, 195–197.

Mechri, A., Saoud, M., Khiari, G., d'Amato, T., Dalery, J., & Gaha, L. (2001). Glutaminergic hypothesis of schizophrenia: Clinical research studies with ketamine. *Encephale, 27*(1), 53–59.

Mednick, S. A. (1970). Breakdown in individuals at high risk for schizophrenia: Possible predispositional perinatal factors. *Mental Hygiene, 54*, 51–63.

Mednick, S. A., Machon, R. A., Huttunen, M. O., & Bonett, D. (1988). Adult schizophrenia following prenatal exposure to an influenza epidemic. *Archives of General Psychiatry, 45*(2), 189–192.

Meltzer, H. Y., & Stahl, S. M. (1976). The dopamine hypothesis of schizophrenia: A review. *Schizophrenia Bulletin, 2*, 19–76.

Moreau, J. (1973). *Hashish and mental illness.* New York, NY: Raven.

Murray, C. L., & GBD 2013 Mortality and Causes of Death Collaborators. (2015). Global, regional, and national age–sex specific all-cause and cause-specific mortality for 240 causes of death, 1990–2013: A systematic analysis for the Global Burden of Disease Study 2013. *The Lancet, 385*, 117–171.

Ogawa, K., Miya, M., Watarai, A., Nakazawa, M., Yuasa, S., & Utena, H. (1987). A long-term follow-up study of schizophrenia in Japan with special reference to the course of social adjustment. *The British Journal of Psychiatry, 151*, 758–765.

Oken, R. J., & Schulzer, M. (1999). Schizophrenia and rheumatoid arthritis: The negative association revisited. *Schizophrenia Bulletin, 25*, 625–638.

Palmer, B. A., Pankratz, V. S., & Bostwick, J. M. (2005). The lifetime risk of suicide in schizophrenia: A reexamination. *Archives of General Psychiatry, 62*, 247–253.

Pasamanick, B., Rogers, M. E., & Lilienfield, A. M. (1956). Pregnancy experience and the development of behavior disorder in children. *American Journal of Psychiatry, 112*, 613–618.

Rasmussen, S., Fraser, L., Gotz, M., MacHale, S., Mackie, R., Masterton, G., … O'Connor, R. C. (2010). Elaborating the cry of pain model of suicidality: Testing a psychological model in a sample of first-time and repeat self-harm patients. *British Journal of Clinical Psychology, 49*, 15–30.

Regier, D. A., Narrow, W. E., Rae, D. S., Manderscheid, R. W., Locke, B. Z., & Goodwin, F. K. (1993). The de facto US mental and addictive disorders service system. Epidemiologic catchment area prospective 1-year prevalence rates of disorders and services. *Archives of General Psychiatry, 50*, 85–94.

Robbins, S. L., & Cotran, R. S. (1979). *Pathologic basis of disease.* Philadelphia, PA: W.B. Saunders Company.

Roch, E., & Varela, G. (1966). Diversos aspectos de la investigación sobre toxoplasmosis en México. Resultados obtenidos en 29 883 reacciones de Sabin y Feldman efectuadas de 1953 a 1965. *Revista de Investigacion en Salud Publica (Méx), 26*, 31–49.

Rosanoff, A. J., Handy, L. M., Plesset, I. R., & Brush, S. (1934). The etiology of so-called schizophrenic psychoses: With special reference to their occurrence in twins. *American Journal of Psychiatry, 91*, 247–286.

Ross, R. G., Hunter, S. K., McCarthy, L., Beuler, J., Hutchison, A. K., Wagner, B. D., … Freedman, R. (2013). Perinatal choline effects on neonatal pathophysiology related to later schizophrenia risk. *American Journal of Psychiatry, 170*(3), 290–298.

Royal Australian and New Zealand College of Psychiatrists Clinical Practice Guidelines Team for the Treatment of Schizophrenia and Related Disorders. (2005). Royal Australian and New Zealand College of Psychiatrists clinical practice guidelines for the treatment of schizophrenia and related disorders. *Australian & New Zealand Journal of Psychiatry, 39*(1–2), 1–30.

Sartorius, N., Jablensky, A., Korten, A., Ernberg, G., Anker, M., Cooper, J. E., & Day, R. (1986). Early manifestations and first-contact incidence of schizophrenia in different cultures. A preliminary report on the initial evaluation phase of the WHO Collaborative Study on determinants of outcome of severe mental disorders. *Psychological Medicine, 16*(4), 909–928.

Sartorius, N., Jablensky, A., & Shapiro, R. (1977). Two-year follow-up of the patients included in the WHO International Pilot Study of Schizophrenia. *Psychological Medicine, 7*(3), 529–541.

Sipos, A., Rasmussen, F., Harrison, G., Tynelius, P., Lewis, G., Leon, D. A., & Gunnell, D. (2004). Paternal age and schizophrenia: A population based cohort study. *BMJ (Clinical research Edition), 329*(7474), 1070.

Stabenau, J. R., & Pollin, W. (1967). Early characteristics of monozygotic twins discordant for schizophrenia. *Archives of General Psychiatry, 17*, 723–734.

St Clair, D., Xu, M., Wang, P., Yu, Y., Fang, Y., Zhang, F., … He, L. (2005). Rates of adult schizophrenia following prenatal exposure to the Chinese famine of 1959–1961. *JAMA, 294*, 557–562.

Straub, R. E., & Weinberger, D. R. (2006). Schizophrenia genes: From famine to feast. *Biological Psychiatry, 60*, 81–83.

Sullivan, P. F., Kendler, K. S., & Neale, M. C. (2003). Schizophrenia as a complex trait: Evidence from a meta-analysis of twin studies. *Archives of General Psychiatry, 60*(12), 1187–1192.

Susser, E. S., & Lin, S. P. (1992). Schizophrenia after prenatal exposure to the Dutch Hunger Winter of 1944–1945. *Archives of General Psychiatry, 49*(12), 983–988.

Tasman, A. (2018). Lies, damn lies, and statistics. *Psychiatric Times, 35*(3), 3.

Thorsby, E. M., & Benedicte, A. L. (2005). HLA associated genetic predisposition to autoimmune diseases: Genes involved and possible mechanisms. *Transplant Immunology, 14*(3–4), 175–182.

Torrey, E. F., Miller, J., Rawlings, R., & Yolken, R. H. (1997). Seasonality of births in schizophrenia and bipolar disorder: A review of the literature. *Schizophrenia Research, 28*(1), 1–38.

Torrey, E. F., Rawlings, R., & Yolken, R. H. (2000). The antecedents of psychoses: A case-control study of selected risk factors. *Schizophrenia Research, 46*, 17–23.

Torrey, E. F., & Yolken, R. H. (1995). Could schizophrenia be a viral zoonosis transmitted from house cats? *Schizophrenia Bulletin, 21*(2), 167–171.

Torrey, E. F., & Yolken, R. H. (2003). Toxoplasma gondii and schizophrenia. *Emerging Infectious Diseases, 9*(11), 1375–1380.

Torrey, E. F., & Sinclair, E. (2018). Hocus Pocus: How the NIMH made 2 million people with schizophrenia disappear. *Psychiatric Times, 35*(3), 1, 10.

Tran, E., Rouillon, F., Loze, J. Y., Casadebaig, F., Philippe, A., Vitry, F., & Limosin, F. (2009). Cancer mortality in patients with schizophrenia: An 11-year prospective cohort study. *Cancer, 115*, 3555–3562.

Tsuang, M. (2000). Schizophrenia: Genes and environment. *Biological Psychiatry, 47*(3), 210–220.

Tsuang, M. T. (1978). Suicide in schizophrenics, manics, depressives, and surgical controls: A comparison with general population suicide mortality. *Archives of General Psychiatry, 35*, 153–155.

van Os, J., Bak, M., Hanssen, M., Bijl, R. V., de Graaf, R., & Verdoux, H. (2002). Cannabis use and psychosis: A longitudinal population-based study. *American Journal of Epidemiology, 156*(4), 319–327.

Warnock, J. (1903). Insanity from hasheesh. *Journal of Mental Science, 49*, 96–110.

Wildgust, H. J., & Beary, M. (2010). Are there modifiable risk factors which will reduce the excess mortality in schizophrenia? *Journal of Psychopharmacology, 24*(11) Supplement 4, 37–50.

Williams, J. M. G. (1997). *Cry of pain.* Harmondsworth, UK: Penguin Psychology.

Wu, E. Q., Shi, L., Birnbaum, H., Hudson, T., & Kessler, D. (2006). Annual prevalence of diagnosed schizophrenia in the USA: A claims data analysis approach. *Psychological Medicine, 36*(11), 5135–1540.

Ziedonis, D. M., Smelson, D., Rosenthal, R. N., Batki, S. L., Green, A. I., Henry, R. J., … Weiss, R. D. (2005). Improving the care of individuals with schizophrenia and substance use disorders: Consensus recommendations. *Journal of Psychiatric Practice, 11*(5), 315–339.

© Andrew Brookes/Getty Images

CHAPTER 53

Epidemiology of Suicide

▶ Introduction

Suicide accounts for 1.5% of all deaths and is now the 15th leading cause of death in the world population. Each year, approximately 800,000 individuals die by their own hand (Wang & GBD 2015 Collaborators, 2016; World Health Organization (WHO) 2002, 2008, 2009, 2016, 2018, 2018). In young people, suicide has become a public health crisis, ranking second among all causes of death in individuals between 10 and 24 years of age. During 2004, the worldwide death toll from suicide among adolescents and young adults was 164,000 (93,000 males and 71,000 females) accounting for more than 6% of all deaths in this age group (Patton et al., 2009). Recent data reflect an increasing global trend in the number of suicides among young people, for example, in 2016, more than 222,000 suicides (28% of all suicides in that year) were committed by adolescents and young adults aged 10–29 years. Current estimates suggest that nearly 80% of suicides are committed by individuals living in low- and middle-income nations (WHO, 2018).

Suicide is often committed out of perceived despair and hopelessness due to an underlying chronic mental disorder such as depression, bipolar disorder, schizophrenia, epilepsy, multiple sclerosis, alcoholism, and drug abuse. Indeed, the presence of a mental disorder is the predominant risk factor for suicide, and it is generally acknowledged that more than 95% of those who committed suicide had a psychiatric diagnosis at the time of death (Bertolote & Fleischmann, 2002a). Emerging evidence also suggests that post-traumatic stress disorder (PTSD) and traumatic brain injury

(TBI) increase suicide risk. Undesirable circumstances (financial crises, interpersonal conflicts, terminal disease, chronic pain, debilitation, and other untoward situations) also play a significant role. The most common methods of committing suicide are by firearms, poisons, knives, drowning, hanging, suffocation, and jumping from heights.

Suicide rates are based upon death certificates and likely reflect underreporting in certain populations. As pointed out by Bertolote and Fleischmann in their review of global suicide,

> The official figures on suicide made available to WHO by its Member States are based on death certificates signed by legally authorized personnel, usually doctors and, to a lesser extent, police officers. Generally speaking, these professionals do not misrepresent the information. However, suicide may be hidden and underreported for several reasons, e.g., as a result of prevailing social or religious attitudes. In some places, it is believed that suicide is underreported by a percentage between 20% and 100%. This underlines the importance of bringing about corrections and improvement on a worldwide basis (Modified from Bertolote & Fleischmann, 2002a).

▶ Global Burden of Suicide

Worldwide, 793,000 people died from suicide in 2016. In that year, the global age-standardized suicide rate was 10.5 per 100,000, a decline of 23% from the rate reported in 2005 (13.7 per 100,000). Nevertheless, the number of suicides in the world population has

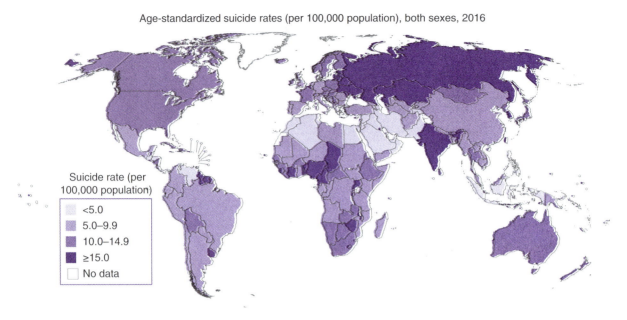

Age-standardized suicide rates (per 100,000 population), both sexes, 2016

Suicide rate (per 100,000 population)
- <5.0
- 5.0–9.9
- 10.0–14.9
- ≥15.0
- No data

FIGURE 53.1 Global Distribution of Suicide Rates, 2016.

Reproduced from World Health Organization. (2018). *Mental health: Suicide data*. Geneva, Switzerland: World Health Organization. Retrieved from http://www.who.int/mental_health/prevention/suicide /suicideprevent/en

remained relatively constant (~800,000 per year) for the past decade (WHO, 2008, 2009, 2016, 2018).

The global distribution of suicide for 2016 shows considerable variability among nations ranging from less than 1 to more than 30 suicides per 100,000 (**FIGURE 53.1**). Rates exceeding 15 per 100,000 were observed in Russia, India, and clusters of nations in Central Europe, Asia, and Western Africa. The highest suicide rates were observed in Lithuania (32.7 per 100,000), the Russian Federation (31 per 100,000), the small nation of Guyana in South America (29 per 100,000), the small nation of Lethoso in South Africa (28.9 per 100,000), and South Korea (28.3 per 100,000).

High suicide rates (~20 per 100,000 or higher) continue to burden the populations of many nations in Central Europe and Asia (Russian Federation, Lithuania, Belarus, Kazakhstan, Latvia, Slovenia, Ukraine, Hungary, and Belgium). Over the years, many of these nations have been ravaged by famine, war, and poverty, conditions that are inescapably associated with depression, hopelessness, and despair. Rates tended to be lower in populations with a higher standard of living, although there were notable exceptions. For example, rates were high in Japan (18.5 per 100,000), France (17.7 per 100,000), and Switzerland (17.2 per 100,000) and low in Islamic countries of the Middle East. The lowest suicide rates in the world (less than 2 per 100,000) were observed in the Caribbean Islands of the Bahamas (Jamaica, Grenada, and Barbados). The U.S. suicide rate in 2016 was intermediate (13.7 per 100,000) (WHO, 2009, 2016).

One notable exception to the rates that are routinely reported in WHO and Global Burden of Disease (GBD) reports is Greenland. Rates of suicide began to rise in Greenland during the 1970s and by 1990–1994, Greenland had the highest rate of suicide in the world (107 per 100,000). The number of suicides in Greenland shows a seasonal pattern with clustering in the summer months in boys and young men between the ages of 15 and 24 years. The most common methods used to commit suicide were by hanging (46%) or self-inflicted gunshot (37%). Potential reasons for the high suicide rate in Greenland include high rates of alcoholism, depression, poverty, and familial strife. The spiking number of suicides in the summer months may also be related to sleeplessness due to incessant daylight (Björkstén, Kripke, & Bjerregaard, 2009).

▶ Gender and Suicide

In the majority of nations, the suicide rate in males far exceeds the rate in females. In the impoverished country of Lithuania, which has the highest rate in the world (32 suicides per 100,000), the male rate is nearly seven times higher than the female rate (47.5 per 100,000 versus 6.5 per 100,000). Male to female ratios of suicide rates are in the range of 3–4 for most other countries (**TABLE 53.1**). One notable exception is China, where reported suicide rates in females have consistently been higher than males. During 2004, the female suicide rate in China (14.8 per 100,000) was the highest in the world and about 15% higher than

TABLE 53.1 Age-Adjusted Suicide Rates by Gender, 2015

Country	Males	Females	Ratio
Lithuania	47.5	6.7	7.1
Russian Federation	48.3	7.5	6.4
Kazakhstan	40.1	7.7	5.2
United States	21.1	6.4	3.3
Finland	20.8	6.8	3.1
France	17.9	6.5	2.8
Canada	17.9	5.4	3.3
Australia	17.4	6.0	2.9
United Kingdom	11.9	3.5	3.4
India	12.2	9.1	1.3
China	7.9	8.3	0.9

Data from World Health Organization. (2002). *Mortality and burden of disease estimates for WHO member states in 2002.* Geneva, Switzerland: World Health Organization.

the male rate (13.3 per 100,000) (WHO, 2008). In 2015, the rates for Chinese men and women decreased more than 40%, but the female rate remained about 5% higher than the male rate (8.3 versus 7.9 per 100,000) (WHO, 2016). Potential reasons for the gender differences in suicide rates in China are discussed in a later section of this chapter.

▶ Age Distribution of Suicide

Bertolote and Fleischmann compared the age-specific distributions of suicide rates for males and females based upon rates reported by 62 WHO member nations in 1998 (**FIGURE 53.2**). These average rates highlight the predominance of suicide in males compared to females throughout the lifespan. Rates increase dramatically during adolescence and early adulthood, and worldwide, suicide is the second leading cause of death among individuals aged 10–24 years. After age 50 years, suicide rates in men and women rise exponentially and are highest among the elderly (Bertolote & Fleischmann, 2002b; Patton et al., 2009).

Hawton and van Heeringen recently reviewed 144 studies of suicide in order to identify and evaluate significant risk factors in different populations

and formulate preventive strategies. While differences were noted by age, gender, and population, they found general agreement regarding the significance of several major suicide risk factors.

The major risk factors for suicide among the young include suicidal thoughts, psychiatric disorders (such as depression, impulsive aggressive behavior, bipolar disorders, and anxiety disorders), and drug and/or alcohol abuse. Other important contributory factors include previous suicide attempts and/or episodes of self-harm; family disruption and discord; familial history of suicide; violence and/or drug abuse; recent loss of a parent, sibling, or close friend; physical and sexual abuse; homelessness; and homosexual and/or bisexual orientation. There is also a large body of evidence indicating that *PTSD* is a significant independent risk factor for suicide, and that *TBI* may modify the risk. The risk is also increased if there is ready access to firearms.

Major risk factors for suicide among the elderly include a previous suicide attempt, presence of chronic depression or other psychiatric disorder, chronic debilitating disease, unemployment, lack of independence, social isolation (some studies have shown this is especially so in older males who are recently widowed), and access to means, such as the availability of firearms in the home (Hawton & van Heeringen, 2009).

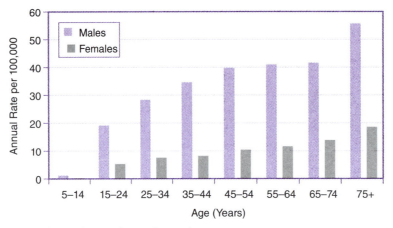

FIGURE 53.2   Age-Specific Rates of Suicide in Males and Females, 1998.

Data from Bertolote, J. M., & Fleischmann, A. (2002). Suicide and psychiatric diagnosis: A worldwide perspective. *World Psychiatry, 1*(3), 181–185.

▶ Time Trends in Suicide Rates

Bertolote and Fleischmann also examined the gender-specific time trends in global suicide rates between 1950 and 1995. In their analysis, suicide rates reported by WHO member nations were averaged by gender and year, and plotted. During this 45-year time span, the suicide rate increased by 49% in males and 33% in females. The investigators cautioned, however, that the 1950 data are based on only 11 countries whereas the later estimates are the average rates for 62 countries that reported on suicide (Bertolote & Fleischman, 2002b).

Investigators associated with the Karolinska Institute in Sweden investigated gender differences and time trends in global suicide rates among adolescents, ages 15–19 years, using data reported by the WHO. Data were available from 90 countries representing most regions of the world. Across all countries, suicide accounted for 9.1% of all reported deaths. The mean annual suicide rate in males was 2.5 times higher than females (10.5 per 100,000 versus 4.1 per 100,000) and the male rate was higher than the female rate in 85 of the 90 countries. Exceptions were noted in China, Cuba, Ecuador, El Salvador, and Sri Lanka, where females had a slightly higher rate than males. Time trends and patterns were also examined for 26 countries that reported suicide data during 1965–1999. Eighteen of these were European countries of Western Europe, Central Europe, and Scandinavia and eight were non-European countries (United States, Canada, Australia, New Zealand, Japan, Singapore, and Mauritius). The data revealed twofold higher suicide rates among young males of non-European nations and a disturbing rising trend in suicide among young males of both sets of countries (**FIGURE 53.3**). Female rates were also higher in the non-European countries but remained relatively stable over time. The investigators

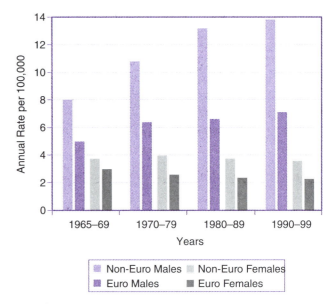

FIGURE 53.3   Time Trends in Global Suicide Rates, Ages 15–19 Years.

Data from Wasserman, D., Cheng, Q., & Jian, G.-X. (2005). Global suicide rates among young people aged 15–19. *World Psychiatry, 4*(2), 114–120; Roh, B. P., Jung, E. H., & Hong, H. J. (2018). A comparative study of suicide rates among 10–19-year-olds in 29 OECD countries. *Psychiatry Investigation, 15*(4), 376–383.

conclude that "*suicide among young people is a major health problem in many societies, and preventive measures are strongly recommended*" (Wasserman, Cheng, & Jian, 2005).

Investigators at Hallym University in the Republic of South Korea examined suicide rates among teenagers, ages 10–19 years, reported by 29 countries of the *Organization for Economic Cooperation and Development* (OECD) during 1995–2012. The estimates for European and non-European males and females during 2000–2010 are consistent with the pattern evident from earlier estimates for 1965–1999 (Figure 53.3). The mean annual suicide rate in males, ages 15–19 years, was 2.4 times higher than females, and mean rates for non-European males and females were

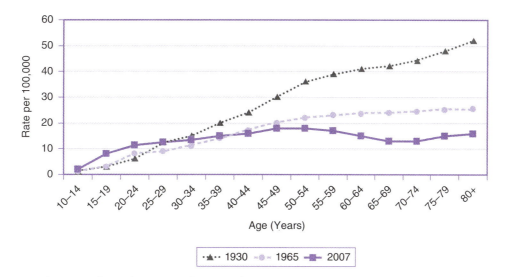

FIGURE 53.4 Age Distributions of Suicide Rates in the United States, 1930–2007.

Data from Stockard, J., & O'Brien, R. M. (2003). Cohort variations and changes in age-specific suicide rates over time: Explaining variation in youth suicide. *Social Forces, 81*(2), 605–642. Centers for Disease Control. (2007). Atlanta, Georgia, USA.

higher than European males and females. Suicide rates were markedly higher for ages 15–19 years than ages 10–14 years, 8-fold higher in males and 5-fold higher in females. New Zealand had the highest mean annual rate (8.7 per 100,000) and Sweden the lowest (3.9 per 100,000) (Roh et al., 2018).

FIGURE 53.4 depicts the age-specific rates of suicide in the United States for three periods spanning 1930–2007. As noted by several investigators, there has been a dramatic shift in the pattern of age-specific rates in recent decades (O'Brien & Stockard, 2006; Stockard & O'Brien, 2003; Wasserman et al., 2005). In 1930, the suicide rate increased monotonically with age and the highest levels occurred among the elderly. In contrast, the patterns of 1965–2007 reflect increases in the rates of suicide during adolescence and young adulthood and declines in the rates among the elderly. In 2007, the highest suicide rates in the United States occurred during middle age. The rise in suicide rates among middle-aged U.S. adults is likely due to a combination of factors including circumstantial depression because of retirement, unemployment, declining health, and/or the heavy use of prescription drugs.

▶ Risk Factors for Suicide

Suicide and Mental Disorders

In order to discuss the implications of psychiatric diagnosis for suicide prevention, Bertolote and Fleischmann reviewed the psychiatric literature on mental disorders and suicide published during 1959–2001. Their review included 31 reports with information on the presence/absence of mental disorders among 15,629 cases of suicide. Of these, 7424 cases (47.5%)

had been admitted at least once to a psychiatric hospital or ward whereas 8205 cases (52.5%) had not. All diagnoses of mental disorders were coded according to either the *International Classification of Diseases* (ICD) or the *Diagnostic and Statistical Manual of Mental Disorders* (DSM). The investigators noted that more than 90% of the cases included for study were from developed nations of North America, Europe, Australia, and New Zealand. As expected, 99.9% of previously hospitalized cases had an established psychiatric disorder; but surprisingly, the vast majority (96.8%) of the cases who had never been hospitalized were also found to have an antecedent mental disorder. The frequency of mental disorders among suicide cases with and without a history of being a psychiatric inpatient is compared in **FIGURES 53.5A** and **53.5B**.

The predominant psychiatric disorder in both sets of suicide cases was mood disorder. This condition includes depression, bipolarity, and mania. Schizophrenia, substance abuse (particularly alcohol abuse), and personality disorders were also present in 10% or more of cases in both groups. Organic conditions (e.g., epilepsy, Parkinson's disease, multiple sclerosis, strokes, and tumors) were prominent among previously hospitalized cases (15%) but not cases from the general population (1%). It is important to note that these conditions are not mutually exclusive and may combine to accentuate the risk of suicide. For example, schizophrenia in combination with a psychotic disorder was present in more than 30% of suicide victims that had been previously hospitalized for a psychiatric condition. Based upon these results, the investigators recommend a multifaceted approach to suicide prevention including appropriate therapy for mental disorders, control of the availability of toxic substances

(A)

(B)

FIGURE 53.5 (A) Mental Disorders and Suicide: Psychiatric Inpatients and (B) Mental Disorders and Suicide: General Population.

Data from Bertolote, J. M., & Fleischmann, A. (2002). Suicide and psychiatric diagnosis: A worldwide perspective. *World Psychiatry, 1*(3), 181–185.

and medicines, restricted access to firearms and other weapons, preventive public health measures (detoxification of domestic gas and car emissions, erection of barriers to deter jumping from high places), and responsible media reporting about suicide (Bertolote & Fleischmann, 2002b).

Similar results were reported by Arsenault-Lapierre and colleagues based upon their review of 3275 suicides from 27 studies in which psychological autopsy studies of cases were performed. In a psychological autopsy, interviews are conducted with key informants and official medical records are examined to extract information regarding demography, psychiatric disorders, comorbidity, and other relevant data. Among all suicide cases, 87.3% had been diagnosed with a mental disorder prior to suicide. However, in comparisons of males and females, major gender differences became apparent. Male suicide cases had higher odds of substance abuse (OR [Odds

Ratio] = 3.58), personality disorders (OR = 2.01), and childhood disorders (OR = 4.95), whereas female cases had higher odds of affective disorders (OR = 1.52) and depression (OR = 1.89). Results suggest that most suicides are committed by those with a history of psychiatric illness, but that suicidal males and females have differential psychiatric profiles (Arsenault-Lapierre, Kim, & Turecki, 2004).

Post-traumatic Stress Disorder and Suicide

The term "stress" was coined by the Dutch pathologist, Hans Selye, in 1936 to define the non-specific response of the body to demand for change. Selye noted in numerous experiments that laboratory animals subjected to noxious physical and emotional stimuli all exhibit the same pathological changes of stomach ulceration, shrinkage of lymphoid tissue, and enlargement of the adrenal glands. Selye demonstrated that persistent stress caused laboratory animals to develop diseases similar to those seen in humans such as heart attacks, stroke, kidney disease, and rheumatoid arthritis (Selye, 1936).

Twenty years earlier, Walter Cannon first described the "fight or flight" response and identified hormonal changes associated with response to acute emergencies (Cannon, 1914). Acute stress activates the sympathetic nervous system that incites elaboration of the adrenal hormones: epinephrine, norepinephrine, and cortisol.

PTSD develops after a terrifying ordeal that involved physical harm or the threat of physical harm. The person who develops PTSD may have been the one who was harmed, or the harm may have happened to a loved one, or the person may have witnessed a harmful event that happened to loved ones or strangers. PTSD was first brought to public attention in relation to war veterans (shell shock). Nevertheless, PTSD can result from a variety of traumatic incidents, such as mugging, rape, torture, being kidnapped or held captive, child abuse, car accidents, train wrecks, plane crashes, bombings, or natural disasters such as floods or earthquakes.

Patients with PTSD are "psychologically traumatized" due to chronic activation of the sympathetic nervous system by adrenal hormones. The psychological trauma of PTSD is described by psychiatrists Jonathan Sherin and Charles Nemeroff in the following statement:

> *Though transient, such reactions can be quite unpleasant and are typically characterized by phenomena that can be grouped for the most part into three primary domains: (1) reminders of the exposure (including flashbacks, intrusive thoughts, nightmares); (2) activation (including hyperarousal, insomnia, agitation, irritability, impulsivity and anger); and (3) deactivation (including numbing, avoidance, withdrawal, confusion, derealization, dissociation, and depression) (Sherin & Nemeroff, 2011).*

A large body of research has documented a significant elevation in the risk of suicide, suicide attempts, and suicidal ideation among PTSD patients. Selected examples include studies from different populations, cultures, and age groups.

Davidson, Hughes, Blazer, & George (1991) studied PTSD among 2985 subjects in the Piedmont region of North Carolina. The lifetime prevalence of PTSD in the community was 1.3%. In comparison to subjects without PTSD, those with disease had significantly higher rates of attempted suicide as well as increased rates of comorbid conditions including bronchial asthma, hypertension, and peptic ulcers.

In a nested case–control study of 9612 cases and 199,306 age-gender-matched controls ascertained from the Danish National Health Registry, the odds ratio (OR) for PTSD and suicide was 9.8 (Gradus et al., 2010). In a U.S. cohort study of young adults, individuals with PTSD were at increased risk of attempting suicide (RR = 2.7) whereas those with traumatic injuries were not (Wilcox, Storr, & Breslau, 2009). In a U.S. cohort of 1433 adults with major depression, PTSD increased the hazard ratio for a suicide attempt by 2.5-fold (Stevens et al., 2013). In the United Kingdom, 94 patients suffering from chronic PTSD were assessed for suicidal ideation and suicide attempts following the index traumatic event. Of these, 53 patients (56%) reported elements of suicidality and 9 patients attempted suicide. Six of the nine patients who had attempted suicide had made more than one attempt (Tarrier & Gregg, 2004).

In military veterans, depression, PTSD and suicidal ideation are relatively common and often occur together. During the Iraq and Afghanistan wars, the U.S. Army's suicide rate increased from 12.4 per 100,00 in 2003 to 29.8 per 100,000 in 2012. In a survey of 407 veterans of these wars, those with PTSD (*n* = 202) were fourfold more likely to report suicidal ideation than those without PTSD (Jakupcak et al., 2009).

Collaborators in the *Army Study to Assess Risk and Resilience in Service members* (Army STARRS) examined suicidal risk factors among 9650 soldiers who had attempted suicide during 2004–2009. Risk estimates for suicide attempts were highest for soldiers in their second month of service (103 per 100,000 person-months) and after return from deployment (40 per 100,000 person-months). On return from deployment, soldiers with PTSD were at increased risk of attempting suicide (OR = 2.4) compared to those without PTSD (Ursano et al., 2016).

The above sampling of investigations shows a clear causal association between PTSD and suicide. Certainly, PTSD is often one of the major components of the web of causation that leads to suicidal ideation, suicide attempts and ultimately the commission of suicide.

Traumatic Brain Injury and Suicide

Studies in Denmark and Sweden provide evidence of an association between TBI and the risk of suicide. Madsen and colleagues recently examined prior diagnosis of TBI as a risk factor for suicide in a retrospective cohort study that included all 7.4 million people in Denmark aged 10 years or older during 1980–2014. Cross-linking with the Danish Cause of Death Registry revealed 34,529 suicides. Of the suicides, 2536 (10.2%)

had a medical history of TBI, and the incidence of suicide among persons with TBI was twofold higher than individuals without TBI (Madsen et al., 2018).

Similar findings were reported by Swedish investigators in a nested case–control study of 218 cases with TBI and 2163 controls without TBI. Results showed more than a threefold increase in suicide risk among patients with TBI compared to controls without TBI (Fazel, Wolf, Pillas, Lichtenstein, & Långström, 2014).

These findings suggest that TBI may be related to persisting neurological sequelae after injury that may either independently or in combination with other factors elevate the risk of suicide (Goldstein & Diaz-Arrastia, 2018).

Opioids, Chronic Pain, and Suicide

During 2017, more than 72,000 individuals in the United States died from drug overdose, and of these 42,000 were attributed to opioid overdose. The term "opioid" refers to natural opiates such as heroin and morphine as well as synthetic forms of opiates such as fentanyl and oxycodone. While these compounds are highly effective for pain relief, the misuse of and addiction to opioids, particularly prescription opioids such as fentanyl, has resulted in an epidemic of accidental deaths due to opioid overdose in the United States. Furthermore, in addition to accidental deaths, suicide from opioid overdose is increasing among patients suffering from chronic pain (NIDA, 2018).

The *National Violent Death Reporting System* (NVDRS) is an active surveillance system initiated by the Centers for Disease Control to collect data regarding violent deaths, including suicide, in the United States. The NVDRS contains data on suicide cases including demographic characteristics, instrument of death, toxicology results, as well as personal health information based on interviews with informants who knew the decedent, such as precipitating circumstances (chronic pain, mental health, substance use, interpersonal problems, life stressors), and suicide planning and intent. Among 123,181 individuals who committed suicide during 2003–2014, 10,780 (8.8%) had evidence of chronic pain, and the percentage increased from 7.7% in 2003 to 10.2% in 2014. While the majority (54%) of individuals in chronic pain who committed suicide used firearms, 16.2% committed suicide by opioid overdose. These results indicate that chronic pain is an important contributor to suicide with either firearms or opioid overdose as primary instruments of death (Petrosky et al., 2018).

In a retrospective cohort study of suicide in the general population of Maryland, opioid levels were tested in blood samples of 5900 suicide cases ascertained through the state medical examiner's office during 2006–2017. The fraction of cases with detectable blood opioid levels increased more than 90% during this period, from 8.8% in 2006 to 17.7% in 2017. Results suggest that opioid addiction is not only increasing death rates by accidental overdose, but also as cofactor or the method of choice for suicide in some individuals (Nestadt, Mojtabai, & Borota, 2018).

The current veteran population in the United States is 20.7 million (18.9 million men and 1.8 million women). Approximately 6 million veterans receive their health care through the VA healthcare system thereby providing an enormous resource for studies of all diseases and conditions, including suicide.

More than 6000 U.S. veterans commit suicide annually, a rate of 22 per 100,000, which is more than double that of the non-veteran U.S. population. The prevention of suicide among U.S. veterans was given the highest clinical priority in the U.S. Department of Veterans Affairs Strategic Plan for 2018–2024. Monitoring and epidemiological evaluation of suicide cases among veterans is an essential component of this strategy, and important findings have emerged from these studies (U.S. Department of Veterans Affairs, 2018).

In a follow-up study of 123,946 U.S. veterans who were prescribed opioids for chronic pain during 2004–2005, 2601 individuals committed suicide during the follow-up period, 2004–2009. Among suicide cases, 1669 (64%) died by firearms, 532 (20%) by opioid overdose, and 252 (9.7%) from strangulation. The annual rate of suicide by any method was 44 per 100,000 for individuals who received a dosage of 0 mg per day (in morphine equivalents) versus 90 per 100,000 for individuals receiving at least 100 mg per day. The rate of suicide by intentional opioid overdose was also highest for the maximum opioid dosage prescribed. These findings indicate that greater opioid dose is a marker for increased suicide risk regardless of the method used (Ilgen et al., 2016).

Bohnert and colleagues examined associations of substance abuse disorders and suicide in a retrospective cohort of 4.86 million veterans (4.46 million men and 402,000 women) who received medical services through the U.S. Veterans Health Affairs system during 2005. Among members of the cohort, 8.4% of men and 3.4% of women had at least one diagnosis of a substance abuse disorder. The addictive substances studied included alcohol, cocaine, cannabis, opioids, amphetamines, and sedatives including hypnotic or anxiolytic agents. During 6 years of follow-up, 9087 cases of suicide were identified in the cohort by link-age to the U.S. National Death Index. For patients with a history of substance use disorder, suicide rates were higher in men than women (76 per 100,000 person-years in men and 63 per 100,000 person-years in women). Suicide rates ranged from 171 per 100,000 person-years for sedative abuse to 49 per 100,000 person-years for cocaine abuse. The age-adjusted hazard ratio for any form of substance abuse was higher in women (HR = 4.8) than men (HR = 2.3), and the estimates for each form of substance abuse in women were two to three times higher than for men. Hazard ratios for individual substances were attenuated with adjustment for psychiatric comorbid conditions, except for opioid abuse and alcohol abuse the individual effects of which were stable and statistically significant even after adjustment. The investigators concluded that substance abuse, regardless of type, may be an important marker for suicide risk and that opioid abuse and alcohol abuse are independent risk factors for suicide (Bohnert, Ilgen, Louzon, McCarthy, & Katz, 2018).

Alcohol and Suicide

Alcohol abuse has consistently been found to heighten the risk of suicide. Harris and Barraclough conducted an early empirical review and meta-analysis of 249 cohort studies focused on alcohol abuse and suicide that were published during 1966–1993. They found marked elevations in standardized mortality ratios (SMRs) for suicide associated with alcohol abuse (SMR = 9.2), opioid abuse (SMR = 14.0), and mixed drug abuse (SMR = 19.2). Females with alcohol abuse were found to be at fivefold greater risk for suicide than males (SMR = 18.5 for women versus SMR = 3.9 for men) (Harris & Barraclough, 1997).

In a subsequent review of the literature through 2002, Wilcox and colleagues identified 42 additional studies for inclusion in an updated meta-analysis. Based on pooled results from all studies, the estimated SMR for suicide due to alcohol abuse was elevated nearly 10-fold (SMR = 9.8) and was three times higher in women (SMR = 16.9) than men (SMR = 4.8). The estimated SMR for suicide due to opioid abuse was elevated more than 13-fold (SMR = 13.5) and was higher in men (SMR = 7.6) than women (SMR = 3.6). The estimated SMR for suicide due to mixed drug use was elevated overall (SMR = 16.9) and was higher in women (SMR = 10.0) than men (SMR = 3.3). Results were consistent with findings of the earlier meta-analysis showing that individuals who have disorders of alcohol abuse, opioid abuse, or intravenous drug

abuse have markedly elevated risks of committing suicide (Wilcox, Conner, & Caine, 2004).

Psychological autopsy refers to data collected from interviews with key informants and official medical records to extract information regarding demography, psychiatric disorders, comorbidity, and other relevant data pertaining to the decedent. Conner and colleagues conducted a recent meta-analysis of 35 case–control psychological autopsy studies to quantify and compare the suicide risk due to mood disorders with the risk due to alcohol abuse and other substance abuse disorders. ORs were highest for suicide cases with mood disorders (OR = 14.3) or major depression (OR = 9.1). Drug use disorders not involving alcohol increased the suicide risk more than sevenfold (OR = 7.1) and disorders involving alcohol increased the risk approximately fourfold (mean OR = 4.0 for alcohol abuse, alcohol dependence, or alcohol use disorder). These results underscore the importance of targeting mood disorders, major depression, and all forms of drug abuse in suicide prevention strategies (Conner, Bridge, Davidson, Carly Pilcher, & Brent, 2017).

Geographic Patterns of Suicide
Suicide in China

Investigators from Harvard University and the Beijing *Suicide Research and Prevention Center* examined suicide rates in China by gender, age, and region (urban or rural) based upon mortality data provided for 1995–1999 by the Ministry of Health of the People's Republic of China. Suicide was found to be the fifth leading cause of death in China, accounting for 3.6% of all deaths and claiming 287,000 victims per year. The mean annual suicide rate was 23 per 100,000. The suicide rate was 25% higher in females than males, mainly because of the large number of suicides in young women living in rural communities. Gender-specific suicide rates in rural communities were threefold higher than in urban communities, and in rural areas, ingestion of lethal pesticides that are readily accessible in the homes of most residents is the preferred method of committing suicide (Phillips, Li, & Zhang, 2002).

Investigators in Beijing conducted a case–control study of 152 individuals who attempted suicide and 152 matched controls to evaluate the role of mental illness and other potential risk factors. Three independent risk factors were identified for suicidal behavior: severe acute stress (OR = 67.5), presence of mental illness (OR = 13.9), and depression due to negative life events in the previous year (OR = 5.3). In contrast to findings in other populations, the relative frequency of mental illness among Chinese suicide cases was relatively low (38%). The investigators concluded that mental illness is an important risk factor of attempted suicide, but not an essential precondition (Li, Yang, & Zhang, 2001).

The Chinese government policy that restricts the number of children and favors male versus female progeny has also been suggested as a risk factor for suicide in Chinese women. David Reardon provides an interesting discussion of the high suicide rate among Chinese women and the potential role of strictly enforced birth quotas in China. Chinese women face the prospect of being pressured into having abortions, particularly in rural areas. Reardon states that *"the preference for boys in rural areas has led to infanticide and selective abortion of female fetuses which may cause impacted grief and sense of devaluation of women's self worth"* (Reardon, 2002). Notably, induced abortion has been found to significantly increase the risk of suicide (Morgan, Evan, Peter, & Currie, 1997) and suicidal ideation after abortion is likely related to unresolved grief and depression rather than preexisting psychiatric illness (Burke & Reardon, 2002; Law & Liu, 2008).

United States Suicide Belt

Suicide is the 11th leading cause of death in the United States, responsible for 34,598 deaths in 2007. As in other populations, rates are three to four times higher in males than females, and the *"web of causation"* usually involves some combination of the following conditions and risk factors: psychiatric illness (particularly depression), substance abuse (particularly alcohol abuse), debilitating/terminal illness (cancer, HIV disease), familial history of mental disorder, substance abuse, violence, physical and/or sexual abuse, and other undesirable circumstances (financial and/or interpersonal crises). Firearms are readily accessible in the United States and are the instrument of destruction in 55% of all suicides (Moscicki, 2001).

It has long been recognized that the western intermountain region of the United States (Montana, Idaho, Wyoming, Colorado, Utah, Nevada, Arizona, and New Mexico) has a higher suicide rate than the rest of the country in what has been labeled the *suicide belt* **FIGURE 53.6**). Factors contributing to the high rates in these populations include widespread poverty and depression, abuse of alcohol and other drugs, easy access to firearms and other weapons, and circumstances that can quickly fuel financial crises and interpersonal conflicts. For example, individuals who experience a major losing spree at the gambling tables and amass insurmountable debt have been known to commit suicide on site.

Individuals at the University of California examined the relative mortality from suicide among out-of-state visitors to three standardized metropolitan statistical areas with long-standing legalized gambling: Atlantic City in Atlantic County, New Jersey; Las Vegas in Clark County, Nevada; and Reno in Washoe County, Nevada. The relative mortality from suicide among *"out-of-state visitors"* to these three counties

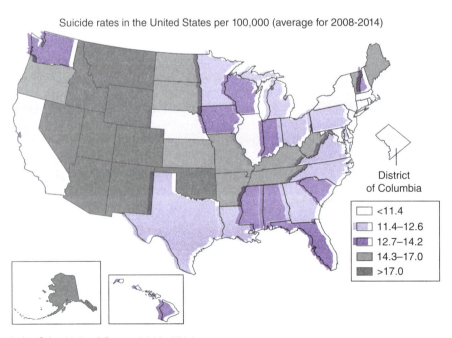

Suicide rates in the United States per 100,000 (average for 2008-2014)

District of Columbia

- ☐ <11.4
- ☐ 11.4–12.6
- ☐ 12.7–14.2
- ☐ 14.3–17.0
- ☐ >17.0

FIGURE 53.6 Suicide Belt of the United States, 2008–2014.

Reproduced from National Institute of Mental Health. (2018). *Transforming the understanding and treatment of mental illnesses.* Bethesda, MD: NIMH. www.nimh.nih.gov/health/statistics/suicide.shtml; Data from Centers for Disease Control and Prevention. (2017). *CDC WISQARS Leading causes of death reports, 1981–2016.* Atlanta, GA: CDC.

was compared to the average relative mortality from suicide among "*out-of-state visitors*" to all other counties in the United States. The relative mortality rates due to suicide for visitors to Las Vegas, Reno, and Atlantic City were 4.3%, 2.3%, and 1.9%, respectively, compared to 1.0% for other U.S. counties. The corresponding proportionate mortality ratios adjusted for age, gender, race, and geographic location were 160, 149, and 152 for the three gambling counties. These results suggest that gamblers are more suicide-prone than other interstate travelers of the same gender, age, race, and geographic region. The investigators suggest three explanations of results: gambling prompts some individuals to commit suicide; gambling settings attract suicidal people; or both processes are at work (Phillips, Welty, & Smith, 1997).

Ethnicity and Suicide

Bertolote and Fleischmann examined rates of suicide prior to the turn of the 20th century according to the predominant religious denomination of countries. Results revealed a remarkable difference between countries of Islamic faith and countries of other prevailing religions. In Muslim (Islamic) countries where suicide is strictly forbidden and/or illegal, the reported suicide rates for men and women are very near zero (**FIGURE 53.7**). These data suggest that religious preference is a major determinant of suicidal ideation (Bertolote & Fleischmann, 2002b).

However, in stark contrast to the very low estimates of suicide rates in Islamic countries shown in Figure 53.7, recent GBD investigations suggest that the number of suicides has risen significantly during the past 25 years in populations that are predominantly of Islamic faith. During 2015, approximately 30,000 suicides were reported in Muslim-majority countries, approximately double the number reported

in 1990. The study focused on the 600 million people living in 22 countries of the Eastern Mediterranean region: Afghanistan, Egypt, Bahrain, Djibouti, Iraq, Iran, Jordan, Saudi Arabia, Kuwait, Lebanon, Libya, Morocco, Oman, Pakistan, Palestine, Qatar, Yemen, Somalia, Sudan, Syria, Tunisia, and the United Arab Emirates. By comparison, the average increase in suicides for other nations increased only 19% over the same period. The increase in number of suicides in Muslim-majority populations has occurred concurrently with a sharp increase in mental health conditions such as depression, anxiety, bipolar disorder, and schizophrenia (Charara, Mokda, Murray, & 2015 GBD Collaborators, 2018).

It is also important to note that studies of subpopulations of Islamic faith find suicide rates that are similar to the rates among people of other religions. For example, in Wayne County, Michigan, which has the largest population of Arab Americans in the United States, annual suicide rates during 1990–2007 were 12.4 per 100,000 and 4.9 per 100,000 among Arab-American men and women, respectively. While these rates are approximately 50% lower than corresponding rates for men and women in Wayne County, Michigan, the annual rate of suicide among Arab-American men is similar to the rate for men of Hindu faith and only about 25% less than men of Christian faith (El-Sayed, Tracy, Scarborough, & Galea, 2011) (Figure 53.7).

Suicide Attempts and Completed Suicide

The strongest known predictor of suicide is a suicide attempt. The suicide risk among individuals who have attempted suicide is hundreds of times higher than the general population. Approximately 10%–15% of individuals who attempt suicide will eventually commit suicide. The risk is highest shortly after an attempt and

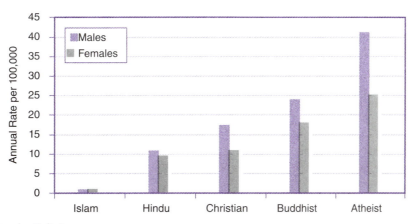

FIGURE 53.7 Suicide Rates by Religion.

Data from Bertolote, J. M., & Fleischmann, A. (2002). A global perspective in the epidemiology of suicide. *Suicidologi, 7*(2), 6–8; El-Sayed, A. M., Tracy, M., Scarborough, P., & Galea, S. (2011). Suicide among Arab-Americans. *PLoS ONE, 6*(2), e14704. https://doi.org/10.1371/journal.pone.0014704

gradually declines over time (Schmidtke, Bille-Brahe, De Leo, Kerkhof, & Wasserman, 2001).

Parasuicide refers to suicide attempts or gestures where there is no actual intention of completing the act. Parasuicide is difficult to distinguish from an actual attempt to commit suicide and should be considered a major risk factor for a future completed suicide.

Investigators in Helsinki, Finland, conducted a long-term study of morbidity and mortality among 100 patients who attempted suicide by self-poisoning. Patients were followed for up to 37 years to determine their cause-specific mortality and the relative frequency of completed suicide. Two of the patients were lost to follow-up. Among the 98 remaining subjects, 13 (13.2%) committed suicide (7 women and 6 men), 8 by drug overdose, 4 by hanging, and 1 by jumping. Eight of the thirteen suicides were committed 15 or more years after the first attempt, and suicides continued to accumulate in the cohort over nearly 40 years of follow-up. These results clearly show that a first suicide attempt is an indicator of high risk for completed suicide throughout the adult lifetime (Suominen et al., 2004).

Genetics of Suicide

Several lines of evidence suggest that suicidal behavior has a significant genetic component. For example, suicidal behavior has been shown to cluster in families, and twin studies have demonstrated that monozygous twins have greater concordance for suicidal behavior than dizygous twins. Recently, molecular studies have found associations of suicidal risk with polymorphisms of the gene encoding *tryptophan hydroxylase* (Roy, Rytander, & Sarchiapone, 1997). Notably, tryptophan hydroxylase is the rate-limiting enzyme in the biosynthetic pathway of *serotonin* (5-hydroxytryptamine or 5-HT). Serotonin functions as neurotransmitter in the brain and central nervous system and is well known for its *"mood elevating"* effects. Several molecular studies have also noted associations of suicidal behavior with polymorphisms of genes encoding serotonin transporters and serotonin receptors. Results of these early molecular studies therefore suggest that genetic variation in the serotonin regulating genes may be associated with depression, suicidal ideation, and completed suicide (Du, Faludi, Palkovits, Bakish, & Hrdina, 2001). However, it has been pointed out that the genetics of suicidal behavior is undoubtedly complex, and likely involves post-transcriptional, post-translational, and/or epigenetic phenomena as well as genetic mutations and polymorphisms (Arango, Huang, Underwood, & Mann, 2003).

Antidepressant Drugs and Suicide

Though little objective evidence exists on the impact of antidepressant drugs on suicide ideation, there is a long-standing concern that antidepressants might actually induce suicidality early in treatment. Debate on this question intensified in 1990 with a report of six adult patients who became suicidal after treatment with fluoxetine (Prozac), a *selective serotonin reuptake inhibitor (SSRI)* (Teicher, Glod, & Cole, 1990). This report prompted a meta-analysis of data from randomized clinical trials of fluoxetine to assess possible adverse effects, but the results *did not* reveal increased suicidality among patients who received the drug (Beasley et al., 1991).

Subsequently, three separate meta-analyses of data from a large number of placebo-controlled randomized clinical trials of antidepressant drugs *did not* find significant differences between those assigned to drug versus placebo in rates of attempted or completed suicide (Hammad, Mosholder, Boehm, Racoosin, & Laughren, 2003; Khan, Warner, & Brown, 2000; Storosum, van Zweiten, van den Brink, Gersons, & Broekmans, 2001). It is important to note that these findings are based upon trials of adults and may not be relevant to children and adolescent patients.

Published reports of the emergence of self-destructive behavior in children and adolescents treated with fluoxetine and other antidepressants motivated a renewed concern about potential drug-induced suicide ideation in pediatric patients (King et al., 1991; Olfson, Shaffer, Marcus, & Greenberg, 2003). In 2006, investigators from the U.S. Food and Drug Administration reported the results of their meta-analysis of 23 placebo-controlled randomized clinical trials of antidepressants used in the treatment of pediatric patients with major depressive or anxiety disorders. Evaluable data were available for 4582 patients enrolled in these studies. *While there were no completed suicides in any of the trials,* the findings suggested an increase in the risk of suicidality across all antidepressant drugs tested (RR = 1.95). The risk increase with *SSRIs* was slightly less than other classes of antidepressants but remained significant (RR = 1.66). The investigators concluded that *"the use of antidepressant drugs in pediatric patients is associated with a modestly increased risk of suicidality."* However, they also pointed out that other pertinent data seem inconsistent with these findings (Hammad, Laughren, & Racoosin, 2006).

For example, the rate of suicide in adolescent males aged 15–19 years declined by 31% in the United States during 1992–2002, concurrent with increased prescriptions for antidepressants in this age group (CDC, 2017; Stockard & O'Brien, 2003). Furthermore, suicide autopsy studies have failed to find evidence of antidepressant drug use in adolescent victims (Leon, Marzuk, Tardiff, & Teres, 2004). Nevertheless, as a precautionary measure, the FDA has modified antidepressant drug labeling to include a *"black box"* warning regarding risk of suicide ideation. The warning states that *"antidepressant medicines may increase suicidal thoughts or actions in some children, teenagers, and young adults when the medicine is first started"* (USFDA, 2007).

Recently, a team of investigators from The Ohio State University conducted an independent meta-analysis to assess the suicidal effects of antidepressants used for the treatment of pediatric depression and obsessive compulsive and anxiety disorders. Their analysis included data from 27 trials enrolling a total of 5310 patients. There were no completed suicides in these trials and medication produced significant symptom relief for all types of disorders. Nevertheless, consistent with the findings of the FDA meta-analysis, there was a small overall increase in the risk of treatment-emergent suicidal ideation and/or suicide attempt (Bridge et al., 2007).

Classification of Suicide

Various types of suicide have been defined in the literature. One of the most famous classifications of suicide types was published in 1897 by the famous French sociologist, Emile Durkeim. He categorized suicide into four types (egoistic, altruistic, anomic, and fatalistic) according to integration and regulation in social groups rather than by individual characteristics (Durkheim, 1897). Durkheim's social theory of suicidal behavior suffers from the "ecological fallacy" whereby the diseases contracted by individuals do not necessarily reflect the populations that they live in. Despite its limitations, Durkheim's work on suicide has influenced proponents of control theory and is often mentioned as a classic sociological study (Pope, 1976).

In modern epidemiology, diseases (including suicide) are most accurately described and classified by the special characteristics of afflicted individuals rather than the general characteristics of groups or populations. As discussed already, suicidal behavior usually involves a complex web of causative factors, and conceivably, combinations of these factors could be used to derive a workable classification scheme. However, there is no consensus among experts in the field of suicide research regarding standardized nomenclature for the classification of suicide. Most recently, David Lester has proposed an interesting classification scheme that parallels the classification of murder and manslaughter. According to his scheme, there are

five basic types of *"self-inflicted"* murder: first-degree suicide (the act was premeditated with intent to kill), second-degree suicide (the act was not premeditated with intent to kill), third-degree suicide (an act of self-harm that was not intended to kill but did), voluntary suicide (the act was provoked by severe psychiatric stress, such as intended rape), and involuntary suicide (the act was due to negligence or recklessness, such as alcohol or drug overdose). It is suggested that the majority of cases of suicide can be classified according to this scheme (Lester, 2009). Albeit, this classification would have to be extended to encompass some special forms of suicidal behavior, all of which directly involve *other individuals as either accessories or victims.*

Assisted Suicide and Euthanasia

Assisted suicide is when an individual solicits the help of another person to commit suicide. There is considerable debate regarding legal, religious, and moral issues surrounding assisted suicide versus one's personal *"right to die."* Medically assisted suicide (*euthanasia*) is currently a controversial ethical issue involving people who are terminally ill, in extreme pain, or have (perceived or construed) minimal quality of life due to injury or illness. While euthanasia is illegal in most jurisdictions, the practice is legal with certain restrictions in Belgium, Switzerland, the Netherlands, and the state of Oregon. Recently, the *Social, Health, and Family Affairs Committee* of the *Council of Europe,* representing 45 nations, issued a report which called upon European nations to consider decriminalizing euthanasia (Marty, 2003). Three statements from the report are of primary interest.

1. Nobody has the right to impose on the terminally ill and the dying the obligation to live out their life in unbearable suffering and anguish where they themselves have persistently expressed the wish to end it.
2. There is no implied obligation on any health worker to take part in an act of euthanasia, nor can such an act be interpreted as the expression of lesser consideration for human life.
3. Governments of Council of Europe member states are asked to collect and analyze empirical evidence about end-of-life decisions; to promote public discussion of such evidence; to promote comparative analysis of such evidence in the framework of the Council of Europe; and, in the light of such evidence and public discussion, to consider whether enabling legislation authorizing euthanasia should be envisaged.

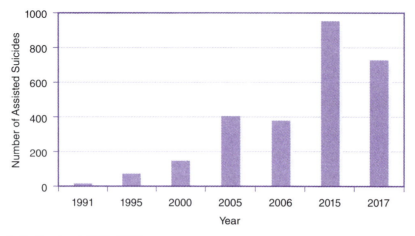

FIGURE 53.8 Euthanasia in Switzerland, 1991–2017.

Data from Bosshard, G. (2010, May). *Assisted suicide and euthanasia (EAS) in Europe with special regard to Switzerland.* Briefing Report to End of Life Assistance (Scotland) Bill Committee.

In Switzerland where euthanasia was legalized in 1941, the number of assisted suicides has risen dramatically in the past two decades (**FIGURE 53.8**). Furthermore, in recent years, increasing numbers of individuals from other countries have entered Switzerland to undergo euthanasia, a practice called *tourist suicide* (Bosshard, 2010).

Investigators at the University of Zurich analyzed all cases of assisted suicide in Switzerland facilitated by two "right to die" organizations during 2001–2004. Their objective was to quantify the predominant reasons for euthanasia and characterize its epidemiologic features. Among 421 assisted suicides, 65% were women, 61% were from outside Switzerland, and 75% were suffering from fatal diseases such as multiple sclerosis or amyotrophic lateral sclerosis. Among the 25% of cases who did not have a fatal illness, chronic pain, and debilitation, depression and "*weariness of life*" were common reasons given for undergoing euthanasia (Fischer et al., 2008).

Murder-Suicide

Murder-suicide is an act of murder followed by suicide of the perpetrator. *Familicide* is a type of murder-suicide in which a spouse and one or more children are murdered, or in which parents and/or other relatives are murdered followed by suicide of the perpetrator. Spree killings are another form of murder-suicide that ends in suicide by the perpetrators, such as in several school shootings that have occurred in the United States and elsewhere.

Peter Marzuk and colleagues reviewed the epidemiology, patterns, and major determinants of murder-suicide with the objective of identifying individuals who either commit this type of violence or are at greatest risk to become a victim. Data and relevant information were obtained from articles, books, and monographs published during 1966–1992. In the United States, the annual incidence of murder-suicide episodes was about 2 per million person-years accounting for 1000–1500 deaths per year. Incidence rates were relatively constant in those populations reporting data and no significant time trends were noted. The investigators found that "*the principal perpetrators are young males with intense sexual jealousy, depressed mothers, or despairing elderly men with ailing spouses. The principal victims are female sexual partners or consanguineous relatives, usually young children*" (Marzuk, Tardiff, & Hirsch, 1992).

Rare Forms of Suicide

Other rare types of suicide have been described. Fortunately, such episodes are extraordinarily rare and as a consequence, there is little epidemiologic data pertaining to any of them.

A *copycat suicide* is defined as emulation of another suicide based on accounts or depictions of the original suicide in the media or elsewhere.

A *cult suicide* is a term used to describe mass suicide by the members of groups that have been considered cults. In some cases, all or nearly all members have committed suicide at the same time and place as ordered by the cult leader.

Mass suicide is when a number of people kill themselves for the same ideological reason. Suicide missions, kamikaze, and suicide terrorist attacks are military or paramilitary forms of mass suicide. An *honor suicide* is when a person commits suicide to escape the shame of an immoral or cowardly action.

An *Internet suicide* is a suicide conducted in full view of the public via the Internet, or pursuant to a suicide pact made between individuals who meet on the Internet. The majority of Internet suicides have been reported in Japan.

Suicide by cop is when a suicidal individual deliberately threatens a law enforcement officer or other armed official with the goal of provoking a lethal response.

A *suicide pact* describes suicide in two or more individuals who agree to die together. Such pacts usually involve married or romantic partners, particularly elderly couples.

It is stressed that these forms of suicide are extraordinarily rare with a very low lifetime risk, perhaps less than 1 per million. Despite this, such episodes are often sensationalized by exhaustive media coverage which may in fact influence suicidal and violent behavior in others. One of the earliest known associations between the media and suicide arose from Goethe's novel *Die Leiden des Jungen Werthers* (*The Sorrows of Young Werther*) published in 1774, in which the hero shoots himself after an ill-fated love affair. Shortly after its publication, there were many reports of young men who committed suicide by the same method. Hence the term *"Werther effect"* has persisted in the literature to describe imitation (or copycat) suicides. Obviously, sensationalized reporting of such cases in the media is to be discouraged (Schmidtke & Schaller, 1998).

Prevention of Suicide

Prevention of suicide is a major public health challenge in all countries of the world. In 1993, six broad guidelines were proposed by the WHO to prevent suicidal behavior: timely diagnosis and effective treatment of those with depression and other mental disorders, restricting possession of firearms and other weapons, detoxification of domestic gas, detoxification of car emissions, control of availability of poisons and toxic substances, and *"toning down"* sensationalized reports of suicide in the press (WHO, 1993).

Shortly thereafter, Gunnell and Frankel reviewed the literature on the efficacy of various methods of suicide prevention. Though evidence of efficacy was found lacking for single interventions, the investigators advocated further testing of a multifaceted approach that includes restricting access to firearms and weapons of self-destruction, educating general practitioners on how to recognize and treat depression

and other psychiatric disorders, limiting over-the-counter and prescription drugs that are most often taken in fatal overdoses, implementing population-based registries of parasuicide and suicide, and modifying car exhaust design to prevent exposure to carbon monoxide. The investigators also noted that patients recently discharged from psychiatric hospitals and those with a history of parasuicide are at particularly high risk; hence, such patients should be carefully monitored and managed appropriately with antidepressant medications (Modified from Gunnell & Frankel, 1994).

> *Suicide is often the consequence of longstanding suffering that has made life unbearable. For example, those with severe disabling and incurable diseases may decide to end their struggle with the unrelenting pain and mental anguish brought about by their medical condition. Other individuals contemplating suicide may be in the throes of depression brought about by circumstantial events, perhaps a broken relationship, heavy financial burden, death of a loved one, or other major crises they perceive as irreparable and cause for self-destruction. It is important to reach out to suicidal individuals who are in crisis; do not leave them alone, encourage them to talk, remove access to firearms or other lethal means, and take action to get emergency medical care for psychiatric assessment and therapy.*

In 2012, the *U.S. Surgeon General* in collaboration with the *National Action Alliance for Suicide Prevention* released the "*Revised National Strategy for Suicide Prevention.*" The revised national strategy has three major priorities: (1) changing the narrative about suicide to promote hope, connectedness, social support, resilience, treatment, and recovery, (2) transforming healthcare delivery for individuals at risk for suicide to promote "zero suicides", and (3) developing comprehensive, integrated, community-based suicide prevention resources for states and communities (U.S. Surgeon General, 2012). It is stressed that the early recognition and effective treatment of mental disorders and substance abuse disorders are paramount for effective suicide prevention.

References

Arango, V., Huang, Y. Y., Underwood, M. D., & Mann, J. J. (2003). Genetics of the serotonergic system in suicidal behavior. *Journal of Psychiatric Research, 37*, 375–386.

Arsenault-Lapierre, G., Kim, C., & Turecki, G. (2004). Psychiatric diagnoses in 3275 suicides: A meta-analysis. *BMC Psychiatry, 4*, 37.

Beasley, C. M., Jr., Dornseif, B. E., Bosomworth, J. C., Sayler, M. E., Rampey, A. H., Jr., Heiligenstein, J. H., … Masica,

D. N. (1991). Fluoxetine and suicide: A meta-analysis of controlled trials of treatment for depression. *BMJ, 303*, 685–692.

Bertolote, J. M., & Fleischmann, A. (2002a). Suicide and psychiatric diagnosis: A worldwide perspective. *World Psychiatry, 1*(3), 181–185.

Bertolote, J. M., & Fleischmann, A. (2002b). A global perspective in the epidemiology of suicide. *Suicidologi, 7*(2), 6–8.

Björkstén, K. S., Kripke, D. F., & Bjerregaard, P. (2009). Accentuation of suicides but not homicides with rising latitudes of Greenland in the sunny months. *BMC Psychiatry, 9*, 20. doi:10.1186/1471-244X-9-20.

Bohnert, K. M., Ilgen, M. A., Louzon, S. L., McCarthy, J. F., & Katz, I. R. (2018). Substance use disorders and the risk of suicide mortality among men and women in the US Veterans Health Administration. *Addiction, 112*(7), 1193–1201.

Bosshard, G. (2010, May). *Assisted suicide and euthanasia (EAS) in Europe with special regard to Switzerland.* Briefing Report to End of Life Assistance (Scotland) Bill Committee.

Bridge, J. A., Iyengar, S., Salary, C. B., Barbe, R. P., Birmaher, B., Pincus, H. A., … Brent, D. A. (2007). Clinical response and risk for reported suicidal ideation and suicide attempts in pediatric antidepressant treatment: A meta-analysis of randomized controlled trials. *JAMA, 297*(15), 1683–1696.

Burke, T., & Reardon, D. C. (2002). *Forbidden grief: The unspoken pain of abortion.* Springfield, IL: Acorn Books.

Cannon, W. B. (1914). The emergency function of the adrenal medulla in pain and the major emotions. *American Journal of Physiology-Legacy Content, 33*, 356–372.

Centers for Disease Control and Prevention. (2017). QuickStats: Suicide rates for teens aged 15–19 years, by sex — United States, 1975–2015. *Morbidity and Mortality Weekly Report, 6*, 816. doi: 10.15585/mmwr.mm6630a6.

Charara, R., Mokda, A., Murray, C. L., & 2015 GBD Eastern Mediterranean Region Collaborators. (2018). The burden of mental disorders in the Eastern Mediterranean region, 1990–2015: Findings from the global burden of disease 2015 study. *International Journal of Public Health, 63*(Suppl. 1), 25–37.

Conner, K. R., Bridge, J. A., Davidson, D. J., Carly Pilcher, C., & Brent, D. A. M. D. (2017). Meta-analysis of mood and substance use disorders in proximal risk for suicide deaths. *Suicide and Life Threatening Behavior.* doi:10.1111/sltb.12422.

Davidson, J. R., Hughes, D., Blazer, D. G., & George, L. K. (1991). Posttraumatic stress disorder in the community: An epidemiological study. *Psychological Medicine, 21*, 713–721.

Du, L., Faludi, G., Palkovits, M., Bakish, D., & Hrdina, P. D. (2001). Serotonergic genes and suicidality. *Crisis, 22*(2), 54–60.

Durkheim, E. (1897). *Le Suicide.* Paris, France: Les Presses universitaires de France.

El-Sayed, A. M., Tracy, M., Scarborough, P., & Galea, S. (2011). Suicide among Arab-Americans. *PLoS ONE, 6*(2), e14704. doi:10.1371/journal.pone.0014704.

Fazel, S., Wolf, A., Pillas, D., Lichtenstein, P., & Långström, N. (2014). Suicide, fatal injuries, and other causes of premature mortality in patients with traumatic brain injury: A 41-year Swedish population study. *JAMA Psychiatry, 71*(3), 326–333.

Fischer, S., Huber, C. A., Imhof, L., Imhof, R. M., Furter, M., Ziegler, S. J., & Bosshard, G. (2008). Suicide assisted by two Swiss right-to-die organisations. *Journal of Medical Ethics, 34*, 810–814.

Goldstein, L., & Diaz-Arrastia, R. (2018). Traumatic brain injury and risk of suicide. *JAMA, 320*(6), 554. doi:10.1001/jama.2018.10825.

Gradus, J. L., Qin, P., Lincoln, A. K., Miller, M., Lawler, E., Sørensen, H. T., & Lash, T. L. (2010). Posttraumatic stress disorder and completed Suicide. *American Journal of Epidemiology, 171*(6), 721–727.

Gunnell, D., & Frankel, S. (1994). Prevention of suicide: Aspirations and evidence. *BMJ, 308*(6938), 1227–1233.

Hammad, T., Mosholder, A., Boehm, G., Racoosin, J. A., & Laughren, T. (2003). Incidence of suicide in randomized

controlled trials of patients with major depressive disorder [abstract]. *Pharmacoepidemiol Drug Safety, 12*, S156.

Hammad, T. A., Laughren, T., & Racoosin, J. (2006). Suicidality in pediatric patients treated with antidepressant drugs. *Archives of General Psychiatry, 63*, 332–339.

Harris, E. C., & Barraclough, B. (1997). Suicide as an outcome for mental disorders. A meta-analysis. *The British Journal of Psychiatry, 170*, 205–228.

Hawton, K., & van Heeringen, K. (2009). Suicide. *The Lancet, 373*(9672), 1372–1381.

Ilgen, M. A., Bohnert, A. S. B., Ganoczy, D., Bair, M. J., McCarthy, J. F., & Blow, F. C. (2016). Opioid dose and risk of suicide. *Pain, 157*(5), 1079–1084.

Jakupcak, M., Cook, J., Imel, Z., Fontana, A., Rosenheck, R., & McFall, M. (2009). Posttraumatic stress disorder as a risk factor for suicidal ideation in Iraq and Afghanistan war veterans. *Journal of Traumatic Stress: Official Publication of the International Society for Traumatic Stress Studies, 22*, 303–306.

Khan, A., Warner, H. A., & Brown, W. A. (2000). Symptom reduction and suicide risk in patients treated with placebo in antidepressant clinical trials. *Archives of General Psychiatry, 57*, 311–317.

King, R. A., Riddle, M. A., Chappell, P. B., Hardin, M. T., Anderson, G. M., & Lombroso, P. (1991). Emergence of self-destructive phenomena in children and adolescents during fluoxetine treatment. *Journal of the American Academy of Child & Adolescent Psychiatry, 30*, 179–186.

Law, S., & Liu, P. (2008). Suicide in China: Unique demographic patterns and relationship to depressive disorder. *Current Psychiatry Reports, 10*(1), 80–86.

Leon, A. C., Marzuk, P. M., Tardiff, K., & Teres, J. J. (2004). Paroxetine, other antidepressants, and youth suicide in New York City: 1993 through 1998. *Journal of Clinical Psychiatry, 65*, 915–918.

Lester, D. (2009). A proposal for a nomenclature for suicide. *Psychological Reports, 105*, 685–686.

Li, X. Y., Yang, R. S., & Zhang, C. (2001). A case-control study of the risk factors in attempted suicide. *Chinese Journal of Epidemiology, 22*, 281–283.

Madsen, T., Erlangsen, A., Orlovska, S., Mofaddy, R., Nordentoft, M., & Benros, M. E. (2018, August). Association between traumatic brain injury and risk of suicide. *JAMA, 320*(6), 580. doi:10.1001/jama.2018.10211.

Marty, D. (2003). *Euthanasia. Report: Social, health and family affairs committee*, Doc 9898, September 10, 2003. Strasbourg, France: Council of Europe.

Marzuk, P. M., Tardiff, K., & Hirsch, C. S. (1992). The epidemiology of murder-suicide. *JAMA, 267*, 3179–3183.

Morgan, C. M., Evan, M., Peter, J. R., & Currie, C. (1997). Mental health may deteriorate as a direct effect of induced abortion. *BMJ, 314*, 902.

Moscicki, E. K. (2001). Epidemiology of completed and attempted suicide: Toward a framework for prevention. *Clinical Neuroscience Research, 1*, 310–323.

Nestadt, P., Mojtabai, R., & Borota, D. (2018, May). *Opiates and suicide. P1-216.* Presented at American Psychiatric Association Annual Meeting, New York.

NIDA. (2018). *Overdose death rates.* Bethesda, MD: National Institute on Drug Abuse (NIDA).

O'Brien, R. M., & Stockard, J. (2006). A common explanation for the changing age distributions of suicide and homicide in the United States, 1930 to 2000. *Social Forces, 84*(3), 1539–1557.

Olfson, M., Shaffer, D., Marcus, S. C., & Greenberg, T. (2003). Relationship between antidepressant medication treatment and suicide in adolescents. *Archives of General Psychiatry, 60,* 978–982.

Patton, G. C., Coffey, C., Sawyer, S. M., Viner, R. M., Haller, D. M., Bose, K., … Mathers, C. D. (2009). Global patterns of mortality in young people: A systematic analysis of population health data. *The Lancet, 374*(9693), 12–18.

Petrosky, E., Harpaz, R., Fowler, K. A., Bohm, M. K., Helmick, C. G., Yuan, K., & Betz, C. J. (2018). Chronic pain among suicide decedents, 2003 to 2014: Findings from the National Violent Death Reporting System. *Annals of Internal Medicine, 169*(7), 448–455.

Phillips, D. P., Welty, W. R., & Smith, M. M. (1997). Elevated suicide levels associated with legalized gambling. *Suicide and Life Threatening Behavior, 27*(4), 373–378.

Phillips, M. R., Li, X., & Zhang, Y. (2002). Suicide rates in China, 1995–1999. *Lancet, 359,* 835–840.

Pope, W. (1976). *Durkheim's suicide: A classic analyzed.* Chicago, IL: University of Chicago Press.

Reardon, D. C. (2002). Suicide rates in China. *Lancet, 359,* 2274.

Roh, B. P., Jung, E. H., & Hong, H. J. (2018). A comparative study of suicide rates among 10–19-year-olds in 29 OECD countries. *Psychiatry Investigation, 15*(4), 376–383.

Roy, A., Rytander, G., & Sarchiapone, M. (1997). Genetics of suicide: Family studies and molecular genetics. *Annals of the New York Academy of Sciences, 836,* 135–157.

Schmidtke, A., Bille-Brahe, U., De Leo, D., Kerkhof, A., & Wasserman, D. (2001). *Suicidal behaviour in Europe: Results from the WHO/EURO multicentre study on suicidal behaviour.* Bern, Switzerland: Hogrefe & Huber.

Schmidtke, A., & Schaller, S. (1998). What do we do about media effects on imitation of suicidal behaviour. In D. De Leo, A. Schmidtke, & S. Schaller (Eds.), *Suicide prevention: A holistic approach* (pp. 121–137). Dordrecht, The Netherlands: Kluwer Academic Publishers.

Selye, H. (1936). A syndrome produced by diverse nocuous agents. *Nature, 138*(3479), 32.

Sherin, J. E., & Nemeroff, C. (2011). Posttraumatic stress disorder: The neurobiological impact of psychological trauma. *Dialogues in Clinical Neuroscience, 13*(3), 263–278.

Stevens, D., Wilcox, H. C., MacKinnon, D. F., Mondimore, F. M., Schweizer, B., Jancic, D., … Potash, J. B. (2013). Posttraumatic stress disorder increases risk for suicide attempt in adults with recurrent major depression. *Depress Anxiety, 30*(10), 940–946.

Stockard, J., & O'Brien, R. M. (2003). Cohort variations and changes in age-specific suicide rates over time: Explaining variation in youth suicide. *Social Forces, 81*(2), 605–642.

Storosum, J. G., van Zweiten, B. J., van den Brink, W., Gersons, B. P. R., & Broekmans, A. W. (2001). Suicide risk in placebo-controlled studies of major depression. *American Journal of Psychiatry, 158,* 1271–1275.

Suominen, K., Isometsa, E., Suoka, J., Haukka, J., Achte, K., & Lonnquiest, J. (2004). Completed suicide after a suicide attempt: A 37 year follow-up study. *American Journal of Psychiatry, 161,* 563–564.

Tarrier, N., & Gregg, L. (2004). Suicide risk in civilian PTSD patients: Predictors of suicidal ideation, planning and attempts. *Social Psychiatry and Psychiatric Epidemiology, 39*(8), 655–661.

Teicher, M. H., Glod, C., & Cole, J. O. (1990). Emergence of intense suicidal preoccupation during fluoxetine treatment. *The American Journal of Psychiatry, 147,* 207–210.

Ursano, R. J., Kessler, R. C., Stein, M. B., Naifeh, J. A., Aliaga, P. A., Fullerton, C. S., … Army STARRS Collaborators. (2016). Risk factors, methods, and timing of suicide attempts among US Army soldiers. *JAMA Psychiatry, 73*(7), 741–749.

U.S. Department of Veterans Affairs. (2018). *National strategy for preventing veteran suicide, 2018–2014.* Washington, DC: Office of Mental Health and Suicide Prevention.

US FDA. (2007). *Antidepressant use in children, adolescents, and adults. Revisions to medication guide, antidepressant medicines, depression and other serious mental illnesses, and suicidal thoughts or actions.* United States Food and Drug Administration, Silver Spring, Maryland

U.S. Surgeon General. (2012). *National strategy for suicide prevention: Goals and objectives for action, 2012, a report of the U.S. surgeon general and of the national action alliance for suicide prevention.* Washington, DC: U.S. Department of Health and Human Services.

Wang, H., & GBD 2015 Mortality and Causes of Death Collaborators. (2016). Global, regional, and national life expectancy, all-cause mortality, and cause-specific mortality for 249 causes of death, 1980–2015: A systematic analysis for the Global Burden of Disease Study 2015. *The Lancet, 388*(10053), 1459–1544.

Wasserman, D., Cheng, Q., & Jian, G. X. (2005). Global suicide rates among young people aged 15–19. *World Psychiatry, 4*(2), 114–120.

Wilcox, H. C., Conner, K. R., & Caine, E. D. (2004). Association of alcohol and drug use disorders and completed suicide: An empirical review of cohort studies. *Drug Alcohol Depend, 76,* S11–S19.

Wilcox, H. C., Storr, C. L., & Breslau, N. (2009). Posttraumatic stress disorder and suicide attempts in a community sample of urban American young adults. *Archives of General Psychiatry, 66*(3), 305–311.

World Health Organization. (1993). *Guidelines for the primary prevention of mental, neurological and psychosocial disorders: Suicide.* Geneva, Switzerland: Division of Mental Health, World Health Organization.

World Health Organization. (2002). *Mortality and burden of disease estimates for WHO member states in 2002.* Geneva, Switzerland: World Health Organization.

World Health Organization. (2008). *The global burden of disease: 2004 update.* Geneva, Switzerland: WHO. Retrieved from www.who.int/evidence/bod.

World Health Organization. (2009). *Mortality and burden of disease estimates for WHO member states in 2004.* Geneva, Switzerland: World Health Organization.

World Health Organization. (2016). *Suicide rates: Data by country.* Geneva, Switzerland: World Health Organization.

World Health Organization. (2018). *Mental health: Suicide data.* Geneva, Switzerland: World Health Organization. Retrieved from http://www.who.int/mental_health/prevention/suicide/suicideprevent/en

Epidemiology of Chronic Infectious Diseases

© Andrew Brookes/Getty Images

CHAPTER 54

Epidemiology of Tuberculosis

▶ Introduction

Tuberculosis is a common infectious disease caused by *Mycobacterium tuberculosis.* The infection typically attacks the lungs but can also spread to other organs including the meninges, lymph nodes, skeletal system, and genitourinary tract. Tuberculosis is a communicable disease that is disseminated by coughing and sneezing. Most infections in humans are asymptomatic and become latent, but about 10% of latent infections eventually progress to active disease. Without treatment, active tuberculosis has a case fatality rate exceeding 50% (Jasmer, Nahid, & Hopewell, 2002).

Classic symptoms of active tuberculosis are chronic cough with blood-tinged sputum, fever, night sweats, and profound weight loss. Historically, tuberculosis was called "consumption" since patients were virtually consumed from within by the disease. The definitive diagnosis of tuberculosis relies on chest X-rays, a tuberculin skin test (Mantoux test), blood serology, and microscopic examination of cultures of biological specimens (Konstantinos, 2010).

▶ Historical Record of Tuberculosis

Tuberculosis has ravaged the human population for thousands of years. The causative microbe, *M. tuberculosis,* has been detected in mummies (3000 BC), prehistoric human remains (7000 BC), and the remains of bison (15000 BC) (Hershkovitz et al., 2008; Rothschild et al., 2001; Zink et al., 2003). Hippocrates identified

phthisis (the Greek term for tuberculosis) as the most widespread disease of his time (460 BC). Afflicted patients had intractable fever and hemoptysis (pulmonary hemorrhage), which was almost always fatal (Herzog, 1998).

Discovery of *Mycobacterium tuberculosis*

The bacillus causing tuberculosis, *M. tuberculosis,* was identified and described in 1882 by the famed German microbiologist, Robert Koch. It has been estimated that during the 18th and 19th centuries, tuberculosis was responsible for the deaths of more than *1 billion people.* In the year that Koch made his discovery, 7 million people died from tuberculosis (Waddington, 2004). Koch also synthesized a vaccine from killed bacteria that he called *"tuberculin."* Although ineffective as a treatment, tuberculin testing became routine in detecting bovine tuberculosis leading to the elimination of the disease in livestock (Waddington, 2004). Robert Koch's discovery of the *tubercle bacillus* and his subsequent development of measures to prevent the spread of tuberculosis have had a profound impact on human history and undoubtedly spared many lives. The Nobel Prize in Physiology or Medicine was awarded to Dr. Koch in 1905 *"for his investigations and discoveries in relation to tuberculosis"* (Koch, 1905).

Tuberculosis in the 19th and 20th Centuries

Tuberculosis was one of the leading causes of death in the United States, Europe, and many other countries throughout the 19th century and the early

20th century. Those infected with tuberculosis were isolated from society and placed in sanatoriums to prevent dissemination of the disease. Therapies for the *"white plague"* were of little benefit until the development of an effective vaccine in France and the subsequent discovery of streptomycin in the United States.

The anti-tuberculosis *Bacille Calmette–Guérin vaccine* was conceived and developed between 1905 and 1921 at the Pasteur Institutes in France by Albert Calmette and Camille Guérin. Their vaccine was eventually proven to be of value in preventing tuberculosis in humans, but was not widely used until after World War II (Bonah, 2005; Comstock, 1994).

Selman Waksman was an American biochemist and microbiologist whose research promoted the discovery of streptomycin and several other antibiotics. In 1952, Waksman was awarded the Nobel Prize in Physiology or Medicine in recognition of *"his discovery of streptomycin, the first antibiotic active against tuberculosis"* (Waksman, 1952).

Due to the effective use of antibiotics for patients with latent and active disease during the last half of the 20th century, the death rates from tuberculosis plummeted in the United States and other developed countries. Nevertheless, with the emergence of multidrug-resistant strains of *M. tuberculosis* (MDR-TB) and coinfections with human immunodeficiency virus (HIV), there has been a resurgence of tuberculosis that has become a global public health emergency in many regions of the world (World Health Organization, 2007).

▶ Global Burden of Tuberculosis in the 21st Century

Based upon recent global surveys of member nations and territories, the World Health Organization (WHO) reports that approximately *one-quarter of the world population* is infected with *M. tuberculosis*. As shown in **FIGURE 54.1**, most of the nearly *2 billion* individuals who are seropositive for *M. tuberculosis* (~80%) are found in 30 developing countries of Asia and sub-Saharan Africa (Houben & Dodd, 2016; WHO, 2007, 2009, 2010, 2018).

The prevalence of seropositive individuals varies by location and also by age. In developed countries such as the United States, Canada, European, and Australasian nations, the rates remain low (less than 1%) throughout the lifespan. In contrast, rates in endemic areas, such as sub-Saharan Africa, India, China, and Russia rise dramatically with age approaching nearly 100% in some populations. **FIGURE 54.2** shows the prevalence of seropositive individuals by age based upon tuberculin testing among 1061 individuals in Cape Town, South Africa. All individuals surveyed were HIV-negative. Note that by age 35, the prevalence of seropositive individuals is nearly 90% (Wood et al., 2010).

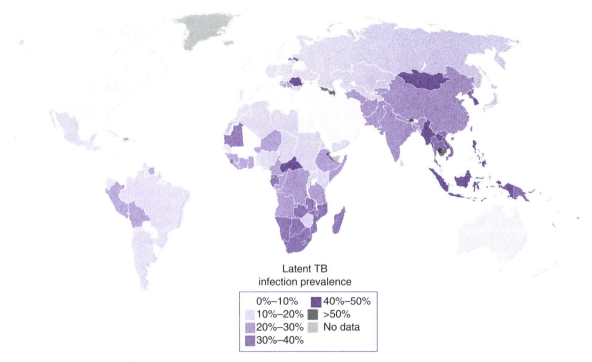

Latent TB infection prevalence

0%–10% 40%–50%
10%–20% >50%
20%–30% No data
30%–40%

FIGURE 54.1 Global Prevalence of *M. tuberculosis*.

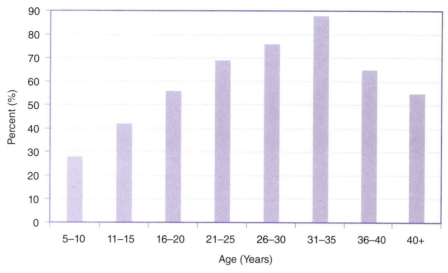

FIGURE 54.2 Age-Specific Prevalence of Tuberculin Seropositivity in South Africa.

Data from Wood, R., Liang, H., Wu, H., Middelkoop, K., Oni, T., Rangaka, M. X., … Lawn, S. D. (2010). Changing prevalence of TB infection with increasing age in high TB burden townships in South Africa. *The International Journal of Tuberculosis and Lung Disease, 13*(4), 406–412.

▶ Tuberculosis: Incidence, Prevalence, and Mortality, 2007

During 2007, the World Health Organization (WHO) conducted a comprehensive global survey to determine the incidence, prevalence, and mortality of tuberculosis among its 196 member nations and territories. The survey captured nearly all (99.7%) of the world population (WHO, 2007, 2009). The following statistics quoted from the 2009 WHO Report capture the essence of the global burden of tuberculosis and related conditions. These data refer to "active" cases of tuberculosis (TB).

Globally, there were an estimated 9.27 million incident cases of TB in 2007. This is an increase from 9.24 million cases in 2006, 8.3 million cases in 2000, and 6.6 million cases in 1990. Most of the estimated numbers of cases in 2007 were in Asia (55%) and Africa (31%), with small proportions of cases in the Eastern Mediterranean Region (6%), the European Region (5%), and the Region of the Americas (3%). The five countries that rank first to fifth in terms of total numbers of cases in 2007 are India (2.0 million), China (1.3 million), Indonesia (0.53 million), Nigeria (0.46 million), and South Africa (0.46 million). Of the 9.27 million incident TB cases in 2007, an estimated 1.37 million (15%) were HIV-positive; 79% of these HIV-positive cases were in the African Region and 11% were in the South-East Asia Region…

There were an estimated 13.7 million prevalent cases of TB in 2007 (206 per 100 000 population), a decrease from 13.9 million cases (210 per 100 000 population) in 2006…

An estimated 1.3 million deaths occurred among HIV negative incident cases of TB (20 per 100 000 population) in 2007. There were an additional 456,000 deaths among incident TB cases who were HIV-positive; these deaths are classified as HIV deaths in the International Statistical Classification of Diseases (ICD-10). The 456,000 deaths among HIV-positive incident TB cases equate to 33% of HIV-positive incident cases of TB and 23% of the estimated 2 million HIV deaths in 2007 (WHO, 2009).

The 9.3 million incident (new) cases of tuberculosis observed in 2007 converts to an annual global incidence rate of 139 per 100,000, slightly less than the incidence observed in 2004 (142 per 100,000). However, the annual incidence rates varied by tenfold among nations, from less than 25 per 100,000 in developed nations of North America, Europe, and Australasia to more than 300 per 100,000 in many of the impoverished nations of sub-Saharan Africa. Swaziland in Central Africa had the highest incidence (1200 per 100,000), and Canada one of the lowest (2 per 100,000).

Relatively high national incidence rates were observed in India (168 per 100,000) and China (98 per 100,000), yielding 2 million and 1.3 million new cases, respectively. Rates were also high in Indonesia (530,000 new cases), Nigeria (460,000 new cases), and South Africa (460,000 new cases). The highest incidence in South America was observed in Brazil (48 per 100,000). Portugal and Spain had the highest incidence rates among Western European nations (30 cases per 100,000). Rates were comparatively low in the United Kingdom (15 per 100,000) and the United States (4 per 100,000).

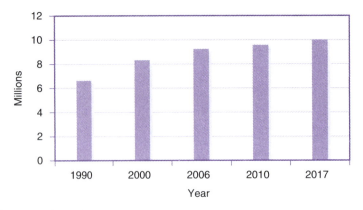

FIGURE 54.3 Global Cases of Active Tuberculosis, 1990–2017.

Data from World Health Organization. (2009). *Epidemiology. Global tuberculosis control: Epidemiology, strategy, financing* (pp. 6–33). Geneva, Switzerland: World Health Organization; World Health Organization. (2018). *Global tuberculosis report 2018.* Geneva, Switzerland: World Health Organization.

Annual mortality rates ranged from less than 10 per 100,000 in North America, Europe, and Australasia to greater than 70 per 100,000 in sub-Saharan Africa. Rates were intermediate in Southeast Asia (31 per 100,000), Eastern Mediterranean countries (18 per 100,000), and the islands of the West Pacific (13 per 100,000). The global pattern of mortality due to tuberculosis is similar to the pattern of *disability-adjusted life years* (DALY) shown in **FIGURE 54.3**

More than 80% of deaths from tuberculosis occurred in Southeast Asia and sub-Saharan Africa where coinfection with HIV is common. As discussed in the following section on HIV-tuberculosis coinfection, case fatality rates are markedly elevated in co-infected patients who do not have access to both highly active antiretroviral therapy (HAART) and combination antibiotic therapy for tuberculosis.

The WHO investigators estimated that about 110,000 deaths were caused by multidrug-resistant tuberculosis (MDR-TB) or extensively drug-resistant tuberculosis (XDR-TB). In high-burden regions of the world, these strains have been found in 10%–20% of patients with active tuberculosis, compared to less than 5% of patients in other areas. Resistant strains of *M. tuberculosis* require special regimens of antibiotics taken for long periods of time. Such antibiotics are expensive and not readily available in most societies, and as a consequence, the case fatality rates are inordinately high (50% or more) among individuals infected with MDR-TB or XDR-TB (WHO, 2009).

▶ Tuberculosis: Incidence, Prevalence, and Mortality, 2017 Update

Globally, 10.0 million people developed active tuberculosis in 2017 (5.8 million men, 3.2 million women,

and 1.0 million children). Since 1990, the annual number of incident cases increased more than 50%. The upward trend in the number of incident cases of tuberculosis during 1990–2017 is shown in Figure 54.3 (WHO, 2009, 2018).

Overall, 90% of cases diagnosed during 2017 were adults, 9% were people living with HIV and two-thirds were in eight countries: India (27%), China (9%), Indonesia (8%), the Philippines (6%), Pakistan (5%), Nigeria (4%), Bangladesh (4%), and South Africa (3%). These 8 countries plus 22 other countries constitute a list of 30 high-burden countries established by the WHO that account for 87% of all cases of tuberculosis worldwide. Only 6% of global cases were in the WHO European Region (3%) and WHO Region of the Americas (3%). Of the cases with coinfection involving tuberculosis and HIV, 72% were living in Africa.

In 2017, there were fewer than 10 new cases per 100,000 population in most high-income countries, 150–400 per 100,000 in most of the 30 high TB burden countries, and above 500 per 100,000 in a few countries including Mozambique, the Philippines, and South Africa.

Tuberculosis caused approximately 1.3 million deaths among HIV-negative people during 2017, and an additional 300,000 deaths among HIV-positive people. Among HIV-negative cases of tuberculosis, the number of deaths per year fell 28% during 2000–2017, from 1.8 million to 1.3 million. Among HIV-positive cases of tuberculosis, the number of deaths per year fell 44% during 2000–2017, from 534,000 to 300,000. The total number of deaths from tuberculosis per year fell approximately 30% during 2000–2017 from 2.3 million to 1.6 million.

The annual age-adjusted mortality rate for HIV-negative cases of tuberculosis in 2017 was 17 per 100,000. Inclusion of HIV-positive cases increased the rate to 21 per 100,000. Mortality rates ranged from 1 per 100,000 in high-income nations to over 40 per

100,000 in high-burden nations of Africa and Asia. The annual mortality rate fell 42% during 2000–2017.

Substantial progress has been made in reducing mortality from HIV-positive tuberculosis in many African nations where anti-retroviral HIV therapy has been combined with first-line drugs for tuberculosis. During 2000–2017, the annual mortality rate for HIV-negative tuberculosis in Africa fell from approximately 60 per 100,000 to less than 25 per 100,000, a reduction of nearly 60%. The overall case fatality rate of tuberculosis in 2017 was 17% compared to 23% in 2000, a reduction of 26%.

Drug-resistant tuberculosis continues to be a public health crisis. During 2017, 558,000 people developed tuberculosis resistant to rifampicin, the most effective first-line drug, and of these, 82% had multidrug-resistant tuberculosis (MDR-TB). Three countries accounted for almost half of all cases of MDR-TB: India (24%), China (13%), and the Russian Federation (10%). Globally, 3.5% of new tuberculosis cases and 18% of previously treated cases had multidrug resistance to rifampin and other first-line drugs. Conversion to multidrug resistance was observed in more than 50% of treated patients living in several countries of the former Soviet Union. Among cases with multidrug resistance, 8.5% had extensively drug-resistant tuberculosis (XDR-TB, defined as resistance to all first-line drugs).

The declining trend in the annual number of deaths from tuberculosis reflects the impact of early diagnosis and effective therapy in some nations that has averted approximately 54 million deaths during 2000–2017. Nevertheless, tuberculosis is currently the ninth leading cause of global death and the leading cause of death due to a single infectious agent. Large gaps remain in the diagnosis and treatment of tuberculosis in populations of many underdeveloped nations that have little access to health care. Furthermore, it is estimated that approximately 1.7 billion people (23% of the world population) have latent tuberculosis and are at high risk of developing active tuberculosis during their lifetimes. Thus, national comprehensive screening programs for detection of latent disease coupled with effective therapy are urgently needed in order to further reduce the global burden of tuberculosis (WHO, 2018).

▶ Disability-Adjusted Life Years: Tuberculosis

The pattern of *DALY* lost due to premature death and disability from tuberculosis reflects high rates in sub-Saharan Africa, Southeast Asia, the Russian Federation, and some countries in South America (Figure 54.3). Childhood deaths from tuberculosis contribute heavily to the DALY. Of the 2 million total deaths from tuberculosis in 2007, nearly one-fourth (470,000) occurred in children under the age of 15 years. Furthermore, without adequate treatment, tuberculosis is a progressive disease that causes significant disability. The pattern of DALY due to tuberculosis therefore reflects early childhood death and progressive disability among afflicted adults in the impoverished populations of Africa, Asia, and other regions with high incidence and prevalence rates (**FIGURE 54.4**) (WHO, 2008a).

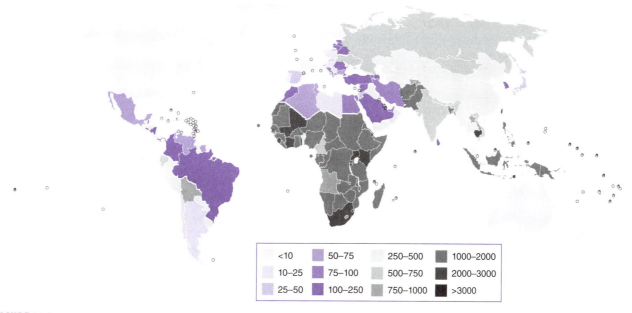

<10	50–75	250–500	1000–2000
10–25	75–100	500–750	2000–3000
25–50	100–250	750–1000	>3000

FIGURE 54.4 Disability-Adjusted Life Years: Tuberculosis, 2004.
Data from World Health Organization. (2008). *The global burden of disease: 2004 update.* Geneva: WHO. Available at www.who.int/evidence/bod

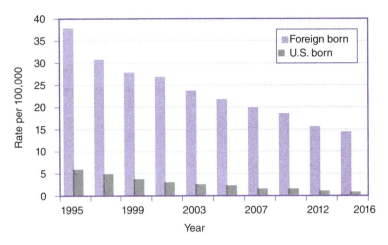

FIGURE 54.5 Rates of Tuberculosis in the United States, 1995–2016.

Data from Centers for Disease Control. (2017). *Reported tuberculosis in the United States, 2016.* Atlanta, GA: U.S. Department of Health and Human Services, CDC.

Tuberculosis in the United States

Every year, the United States Centers for Disease Control (CDC) reports results from the *National Tuberculosis Surveillance System* for the previous year (CDC, 2017). In 2016, a total of 9272 new cases of active tuberculosis were reported in the United States, a reduction of 60% from the 22,726 cases reported in 1995. The overall annual incidence rate in 2016 was 2.9 cases per 100,000, a reduction of 66% from the rate of 8.5 per 100,000 reported in 1995. The 2016 rate in foreign-born persons was 14.7 per 100,000, over 13 times higher than in U.S.-born persons (1.1 per 100,000). The rate of tuberculosis in foreign-born persons has decreased 61% from the rate of 38 per 100,000 reported in 1995 (**FIGURE 54.5**).

There are marked ethnic differences in the rates of active tuberculosis in the United States. The average rate among Hispanics and African Americans (4.7 per 100,000) was approximately eight times higher than among non-Hispanic Caucasians (0.6 per 100,000), and rates among Asians were nearly 30 times higher (18 per 100,000). Four countries account for more than 50% of the tuberculosis cases in foreign-born persons: Mexico (23%), the Philippines (12%), India (8%), and Vietnam (8%). In 2016, among persons with tuberculosis and a known HIV test result, 5.6% were co-infected with HIV (CDC, 2017).

Transmission of Tuberculosis

When people suffering from active pulmonary tuberculosis cough, sneeze, speak, or spit, they expel infectious aerosolized droplets 0.5–5 μm in diameter. A single sneeze can release up to 40,000 droplets, each of which may transmit the disease since the infectious dose of tuberculosis is very low and inhaling fewer than 10 bacteria may cause an infection.

People with prolonged, frequent, or intense contact with patients who have active tuberculosis are at particularly high risk of becoming infected. A person with active untreated tuberculosis can infect 10–15 other people per year. Others at risk include people in areas where tuberculosis is common, people who inject drugs using unsanitary needles, residents and employees of high-risk congregate settings, medically underserved and low-income populations, high-risk racial or ethnic minority populations, children exposed to adults in high-risk categories, patients immunocompromised by conditions such as HIV/AIDS, people who take immunosuppressant drugs, and healthcare workers serving these high-risk clients (Cole & Cook, 1998).

In endemic areas, community acquisition of latent tuberculosis infection is common. In a recent study of school children in South Africa where *M. tuberculosis* and HIV are endemic, the annual rate of new infection based upon tuberculin skin testing was 4.1% resulting in a prevalence of 52% among adolescents by 17 years of age (Middlekoop, Bekker, Myer, Dawson, & Wood, 2008).

M. tuberculosis can only be transmitted by patients with active disease. The probability of transmission from one person to another depends upon the number of infectious droplets expelled by a carrier, the effectiveness of ventilation, the duration of exposure, and the virulence of the *M. tuberculosis* strain. The chain of transmission can be broken by isolating patients with active disease and by starting effective therapy. After 2 weeks of treatment, patients with nonresistant active tuberculosis generally cease to be contagious. In newly infected individuals, there is a 21- to 28- day incubation period before the bacterium can be transmitted to others. Tuberculosis is also a "food-borne" infectious disease and can be transmitted by ingestion of contaminated meat and milk. *Mycobacterium bovis*, once a common cause of tuberculosis, was virtually eliminated from human populations of developing countries after the introduction of pasteurized milk (Robbins & Cotran, 1979; Thoen, Lobue, & de Kantor, 2006; Tweddle & Livingstone, 1994).

▶ Pathogenesis of Tuberculosis

Infection begins when mycobacteria reach the pulmonary alveoli where they invade and replicate within the endosomes of alveolar macrophages. Within macrophages, mycobacteria are shielded from oxidative and enzymatic damage by their highly resistant lipid cell walls. Macrophages, lymphocytes, and fibroblasts aggregate around infected cells to form a granuloma which is characteristic of *latent* tuberculosis infection. Tuberculosis is thus classified as a *granulomatous* inflammatory condition. In many patients with tuberculosis, the infection waxes and wanes. Over time, the cores of tuberculous granulomas become necrotic with the texture of soft white cheese, a pathologic feature known as *caseous necrosis*. Tissue destruction and necrosis are balanced by healing and fibrosis. With successful therapy, granulomatous lesions are totally replaced by scar tissue. However, upon eruption from granulomas, live mycobacteria can disseminate through the bloodstream to other tissues and organs causing the formation of secondary lesions in peripheral lymph nodes, kidneys, brain, and bone. Disseminated tuberculosis (miliary tuberculosis) is most common in infants and the elderly. Without early treatment, the case fatality rate of this condition approaches 100% (Kim et al., 2003; Robbins & Cotran, 1979).

▶ Risk Factors for Tuberculosis

Risk factors for tuberculosis are divisible into those that influence transmission of the mycobacterium, and those modulate the course of latent versus active infection. Individual studies of mycobacterial transmission and resistance to infection in humans are complicated by a variety of issues including the

ethics and morality of conducting such investigations and the absence of a validated measure of exposure. Epidemiologic studies are therefore limited to ecological studies of the prevalence of coinfection by *M. tuberculosis* and HIV, and individual studies of other noninfectious factors that heighten or lessen the risk of developing active disease among those who have latent tuberculosis.

HIV and Tuberculosis

Among the 9.27 million incident cases of tuberculosis in 2007, an estimated 1.37 million (14.8%) were HIV-positive. Of these, 79% were found in sub-Saharan Africa and 11% in Southeast Asia. The heaviest burden of this co-epidemic of tuberculosis and HIV infections is in sub-Saharan Africa. In South Africa and Swaziland, approximately 1% of the population develops tuberculosis annually and these two nations account for more than 40% of all cases of HIV-associated tuberculosis. In 2007, more than 465,000 deaths were attributed to HIV-tuberculosis coinfections. Most of these deaths (~70%) occurred in five countries: 131,000 in India, 112,000 in China, 43,000 in Russia, 16,000 in South Africa, and 15,000 in Bangladesh (WHO, 2009, 2010).

For patients with HIV infection, the risk of developing active tuberculosis is contingent upon prophylaxis and therapy. In Barcelona, Spain, Guelar and colleagues conducted a prospective study of 839 HIV-infected patients to examine effects of immune status (tuberculin positivity) and prophylaxis with isoniazid among patients with a positive tuberculin test. During 52 months of follow-up, active tuberculosis developed in 23 (3.1%) of 733 patients with a negative tuberculin test (2.4 cases per 100 patient-years). Among tuberculin positive patients, active tuberculosis developed in 7 of 26 patients who did not receive isoniazid prophylaxis (16.2 cases per 100 patient-years), 4 of 61 patients who completed 9 months of prophylaxis (8.9 cases per 100 patient-years), and none of 19 patients who continued prophylaxis until the end of study. These results suggest that sustained prophylaxis with isoniazid provides significant protection against the development of active tuberculosis in patients with HIV infection (Guelar et al., 1993).

In a study conducted at the University of Cape Town in South Africa, investigators compared the incidence rate of tuberculosis in 264 patients with HIV disease who were treated with HAART to the rate in 760 patients not receiving HAART. Results revealed that HAART reduced the incidence of tuberculosis by

81% in patients with HIV disease (2.4 vs. 9.7 cases per 100 patient-years); furthermore, the protective effect of HAART was greatest in symptomatic patients and those with advanced immune suppression (Badri, Wilson, & Wood, 2002).

The results of these and other trials indicate that with appropriate therapy and management, tuberculosis can be averted in HIV-infected patients. However, due to the high cost and intensive nature of patient management, most patients in developing countries simply do not have access to such therapy and therefore develop coinfections with HIV and tuberculosis. For example, the WHO survey of 2007 suggests that in regions with a high prevalence of HIV-positive individuals such as South Africa and Swaziland, the incidence of active tuberculosis is increased more than twentyfold in HIV-positive individuals compared to HIV-negative individuals (WHO, 2009). In co-infected patients, immunosuppression due to HIV often results in extra-pulmonary and disseminated tuberculosis; reciprocally, the presence of tuberculosis has been noted to increase the viral load of HIV. The case fatality rate among coinfected individuals is extraordinarily high.

Gandhi and colleagues recently examined the prevalence of MDR-TB and XDR-TB and the consequences of coinfection with HIV in a rural area of South Africa. During 2005 and 2006, sputum samples were collected from 1539 patients. Of these, 221 (14.3%) had MDR-TB and 53 (3.4%) had XDR-TB. More than half (55%) of patients with XDR-TB had never been previously treated for tuberculosis. Most notably, all XDR-TB cases tested positive for HIV. Among cases with XDR-TB, the median survival was only 16 days and nearly all (52 of 53) died within a few weeks. Results therefore suggest that XDR-TB is readily transmitted to HIV-infected patients in the South African population and coinfected patients have little chance of survival (Gandhi et al., 2006).

Childhood Tuberculosis

Accurate estimates of the burden of tuberculosis in children are unavailable for many populations. This is because cases with active pulmonary disease are detected by virtue of "positive smears" of sputum samples, and most children with active disease (up to 95%) simply do not produce enough sputum for testing. As a consequence, tuberculosis rates based upon "smear positive" cases probably only represent about 5%–10% of the actual cases (Lighter & Rigaud, 2009; Rekha & Swaminathan, 2007).

Infection rates in children can be monitored by periodic tuberculin skin tests; however, without such testing, primary infection in children is predominantly asymptomatic and goes unrecognized in the vast majority (~90%) of cases. Recent studies conducted in endemic areas have noted twofold higher seroconversion rates among young children with sustained exposure to female caregivers with HIV and tuberculosis coinfection compared to children without such exposure (Kenyon et al., 2002). However, the seroconversion rate is also high in children from endemic regions due to community acquisition of mycobacterial infection (see Figure 54.2).

Young children who become infected with *M. tuberculosis* are at high risk for the development of active disease. As shown in **FIGURE 54.6**, the risk is highest during the first year of life when the immune system is most immature and then declines dramatically in subsequent years as immunocompetence rises. Meningitis and military tuberculosis, conditions with high case fatality rates, are common in those infants with primary infection. Furthermore, infected

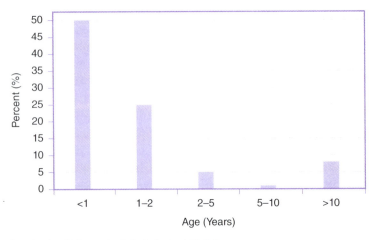

FIGURE 54.6 Risk of Developing Active Tuberculosis in Infected Children.

Data from Marais, B. J., Gie, R. P., Schaaf, H. S., Hesseling, A. C., Obihara C. C., Atarke, J. J., & Enarson, D. A. (2004). The natural history of childhood intra-thoracic tuberculosis: A critical review of literature from the pre-chemotherapy era. *International Journal of Tuberculosis and Lung Disease*, 9(4), 392–402.

children frequently manifest progression to these life-threatening conditions without significant prior symptoms (Marais et al., 2004).

Pregnancy and Tuberculosis

The greatest burden of tuberculosis in women occurs during the childbearing years. Eighty percent of all mortality due to tuberculosis in women occurs in this age group (WHO, 2009).

A number of studies have noted that HIV infection and tuberculosis during pregnancy are a particularly deadly combination and are independent risk factors for maternal mortality (Mofenson & Laughon, 2007; Tripathy & Tripathy, 2003). In communities where tuberculosis and HIV infection are endemic, pregnant women are at high risk of acquiring both infections. In Durban, South Africa, a dramatic increase in the case load of tuberculosis in pregnant women was observed from 1996 to 1998; notably, there was a tenfold increase in the rate of tuberculosis among the women who were HIV-positive and 72% of these cases were attributed to HIV infection. Furthermore, more than 10% of these young mothers died (Pillay et al., 2001).

In a study conducted in Zambia, tuberculosis accounted for 25% of all nonobstetric maternal deaths and AIDS was present in 92% of cases with tuberculosis (Ahmed et al., 1990).

In a study of maternal mortality in South Africa, there was a 3.2-fold increase in the relative risk of death in mothers with TB-HIV coinfection compared with HIV-uninfected mothers with tuberculosis infection, and 54% of maternal deaths caused by tuberculosis were attributable to coinfection with HIV. Furthermore, in tertiary care hospitals in South Africa, TB-HIV coinfection accounted for 14%–15% of all maternal mortality (Khan, Pillay, Moodley, & Connolly, 2001).

A team of investigators conducted a cross-sectional survey to identify HIV status and cases of active tuberculosis among pregnant women in six clinics in Sowet, South Africa. During 2008–2009, 3963 pregnant women were enrolled and screened for tuberculosis, of whom 1454 (36.7%) were HIV-seropositive. Active pulmonary tuberculosis was diagnosed in 10 HIV-seropositive women (6.9 per 1000) and 5 HIV-seronegative women (2.0 per 1000). Results suggest a threefold higher burden of active tuberculosis in pregnant women who are HIV-seropositive (Gounder et al., 2011).

The deadly combination of tuberculosis and HIV infection has also been noted among pregnant women in developed countries. In New York City, Margono and colleagues reviewed the medical records of 18 pregnant women diagnosed with tuberculosis between 1985 and 1992 at two metropolitan hospitals. Eleven of the women were tested for HIV and seven (64%) were positive. The investigators concluded that cases of active tuberculosis associated with HIV infection are increasing among pregnant women and recommended early tuberculin skin testing in HIV-positive women of reproductive age and the initiation of appropriate preventive strategies to reduce morbidity and mortality from tuberculosis (Margono et al., 1994).

Lynne Mofenson and Barbara Laughon of the United States National Institute of Child Health and Human Development point to five lines of evidence to support tuberculin testing among pregnant women who are HIV-positive to facilitate targeted prophylaxis in those found to have latent tuberculosis:

(1) TB-HIV coinfection is frequent in many resource-limited settings, (2) HIV infection is the strongest risk factor for progression of latent TB to active TB disease, (3) tests are available to identify TB infection, (4) there is an intervention available that is effective in preventing progression from infection to disease, (5) and the development of TB disease in HIV-infected pregnant and postpartum women is associated with significant maternal and infant mortality (Mofenson & Laughon, 2007).

Consensus guidelines have been issued regarding tuberculin testing and treatment of tuberculosis during pregnancy. The following statement is quoted from the Centers for Disease Control (CDC, 2010).

Untreated tuberculosis represents a greater hazard to a pregnant woman and her fetus than does its treatment. Treatment of pregnant women should be initiated whenever the probability of TB is moderate to high. Infants born to women with untreated TB may be of lower birth weight than those born to women without TB and, rarely, the infant may be born with TB. Although the drugs used in the initial treatment regimen cross the placenta, they do not appear to have harmful effects on the fetus. Tuberculin skin testing is considered both valid and safe throughout pregnancy. The special TB blood test is safe to use during pregnancy, but has not been evaluated for diagnosing M. tuberculosis infection in pregnant women. Other tests are needed to show if a person has TB disease (CDC, 2010).

Noninfectious Risk Factors

A number of noninfectious risk factors have been elucidated that heighten the risk of developing active tuberculosis among patients with latent disease. These include chronic smoking, pulmonary silicosis, chronic obstructive pulmonary diseases (emphysema, chronic bronchitis, asthma), immunosuppressive exposures other than HIV (chemotherapy for malignancy, immunosuppressive drugs), metabolic diseases (diabetes, autoimmune conditions), and other physiologic stressors (pregnancy, poor nutrition).

Silicosis and Active Tuberculosis

In 1948, J.H. Lee reported findings of a study of 100 miners who developed pulmonary silicosis. Of these 100 patients, 65 were proven to also have active tuberculosis by positive sputum, postmortem examination, or other bacteriological tests (Lee, 1948). Silica particles increase the risk of developing active tuberculosis by irritating the respiratory system and interfering with macrophage function (Robbins & Cotran, 1979).

Diabetes and Active Tuberculosis

Several studies have suggested that type 2 diabetes increases the risk of developing active tuberculosis. To clarify and quantify the association, Jeon and Murray conducted a meta-analysis of data from 13 observational studies containing 1,786,212 participants and 17,698 cases of active tuberculosis. In a random effects model, diabetes was found to increase the risk more than threefold (RR = 3.11). However, case–control studies were heterogeneous with odds ratios ranging from 1.16 to 7.83. Nevertheless, the results clearly show that diabetes increases the risk of developing active tuberculosis, and the investigators suggest that *active case finding and treatment of latent TB and efforts to diagnose, detect, and treat DM may have a beneficial impact on TB control*" (Jeon & Murray, 2008). Mechanistically, diabetes has been found to modulate chemotaxis, phagocytosis, activation, and antigen presentation by phagocytes in response to *M. tuberculosis*. (Dooley & Chaisson, 2009; Moutschen, Scheen, & Lefebvre, 1992).

Smoking and Tuberculosis

An international team of investigators recently studied the association between tobacco smoking and active tuberculosis in a sizable cohort of the general population of Taiwan. The study included 17,699 participants who completed a standardized health interview survey and were followed during 2001–2004. Smoking status and other variables were measured by in-person interviews at baseline and incident cases of active tuberculosis were identified from the *Taiwan National Health Insurance* database. During 3.3 years of follow-up, 57 new cases of active tuberculosis were detected. Overall, current smoking was associated with an increase in the risk (OR = 1.94). These results are similar to findings of several case–control studies and suggest that tobacco smoking increases the risk of developing active tuberculosis (Lin, Ezzati, Chang, & Murray, 2009).

Bates and colleagues conducted a meta-analysis of the epidemiologic studies that provided relative risk estimates quantifying the association between tuberculosis infections and tobacco smoking. They included data from 24 studies in their analysis. Findings revealed that smoking increases the risk of developing active tuberculosis by up to 60% (RR = 1.6). The combined evidence from these studies therefore indicates that smoking is a risk factor for the development of active tuberculosis among individuals with latent disease (Bates et al., 2007).

Dietary Risk Factors

Certain other risk factors and conditions have been implicated in the genesis of active tuberculosis. As one might expect, pulmonary diseases such as emphysema, chronic bronchitis, and asthma, and exposure to immunosuppressive drugs during chemotherapy or organ transplant procedures have all been found to heighten the risk. Some studies have found vitamin deficiencies to be associated with risk. For example, in a review and meta-analysis of seven studies vitamin D and active tuberculosis yielded an overall risk reduction of 32% for individuals with high versus low serum levels (Nnoaham & Clarke, 2008). In addition, conditions reflecting poor nutrition or malnutrition are two to three times more common among patients with active tuberculosis than among patients with latent disease (Schaible & Kaufmann, 2007).

Genetic Susceptibility to Tuberculosis

Studies of monozygous and dizygous twins have found some evidence that genetic factors may modulate susceptibility or resistance to the development of tuberculosis. One recent genetic study of 516 cases and 514 healthy controls in the Hong Kong Chinese population revealed that specific polymorphisms of the interleukin 12 gene may influence the risk (Tso, Lau, Tam, Wong, & Chiang, 2004). Nevertheless, these preliminary findings await independent confirmation in other laboratories.

Multidrug-Resistant Tuberculosis and Extensively Drug-Resistant Tuberculosis

By definition, *multidrug-resistant tuberculosis* (*MDR-TB*) does not respond to first-line drugs (isoniazid and rifampicin) and *extensively drug-resistant tuberculosis* (*XDR-TB*) is also resistant to three or more of the six classes of second-line drugs (and often does not respond to any drug). Drug-resistant tuberculosis is rapidly disseminating throughout the world. In a recent survey of 109 member nations conducted by WHO, cases of MDR-TB were found in all participating countries, and cases of XDR-TB were found in 55 (50%) of the countries sampled (Donald & van Helden, 2009).

A team of investigators recently examined characteristics of MDR-TB and XDR-TB in Shanghai, one of the largest cities in Asia (population ~23 million). In the study, MDR-TB cases were identified by testing for resistance to first-line drugs (isoniazid and rifampicin) in all culture-positive cases of tuberculosis, and XDR-TB cases were identified by testing for resistance to second-line drugs in the MDR-TB cases. During 2004–2007, 4379 culture-positive cases of tuberculosis were diagnosed. Of these, 247 (5.6%) were infected with MDR-TB, and 11 (6.3%) of 175 MDR-TB cases tested were found to carry XDR-TB. Among patients with MDR-TB, 57% responded to treatment with second-line drugs. It is notable that more than half of the patients infected by resistant strains of tuberculosis were newly diagnosed without any history of treatment for tuberculosis. Thus, community acquisition of resistant tuberculosis strains is a serious public health problem in Shanghai (Zhao et al., 2009).

Antibiotic Resistance in *Mycobacterium tuberculosis*

The development of antibiotic resistance by *M. tuberculosis* has been extensive studied and reviewed. Dartmouth microbiologist Jay Dalton provides a succinct but thorough treatise in which he states:

> Tuberculosis has become a threat again in the modern era of antimicrobial warfare, because its unique characteristics give it enormous potential for developing resistance to even the strongest antibiotics. Tuberculosis combines one of the slowest division rates among bacteria with a hardy cell wall defense system. Both of these factors stretch treatment into a multiple month process, creating a massive window for human error in the form of incorrect or missed dosages. Similarly, this slow pace of infection increases the possibility of evolution-based antimicrobial resistance by giving tuberculosis bacteria time to mutate. For these reasons, multi-drug resistant tuberculosis is one of the biggest health threats of this generation and the discovery of new treatment methods will be essential in the ongoing fight against this disease (Dalton, 2009).

Dalton points out that the cell wall of *M. tuberculosis* is a major determinant of its virulence due to a high content of mycolic acid and other lipids that form a protective shield against cationic proteins, lysozymes, and oxygen radicals of phagocytosis. This waxy hydrophobic cell wall resists sustained exposure to acids, detergents, oxidants, and antibiotics, thereby facilitating survival of the bacterium for long periods of time. Indeed, even a *short* treatment course for active tuberculosis involves a minimum of 6 months of combined antibiotic therapy: 2 months of isoniazid, rifampin, and pyrazinamide followed by 4 months of isoniazid, rifamate, and rimactane. The long period of treatment required for success is due to the slow reproductive rate and resistant cell wall of the bacterium and it is within this time period that mutations may accumulate and confer bacterial resistance (Dalton, 2009).

Prevention of Tuberculosis

Tuberculosis, malaria, and HIV/AIDS are the three major infectious diseases of poverty. Together they account for nearly 5 million deaths per year. Notwithstanding, all three of these conditions are preventable, and among those infected, death can be averted with early diagnosis and effect treatment.

The control and prevention of tuberculosis involves primary, secondary, and tertiary prevention. While no vaccine is available that provides reliable protection for adults, vaccination using the *Bacille Calmette–Guérin vaccine* (*BCG*) offers significant protection in children and is widely used throughout the world. Approximately 85% of infants in 172 countries were immunized in 1993 (WHO, 1995).

One country that *does not* widely administer BCG is the United States where tuberculosis remains relatively uncommon. Vaccination is only recommended for infants or children with negative skin test results who are continually exposed to untreated or ineffectively treated patients or will be continually exposed to multidrug-resistant tuberculosis (MDR-TB); and for healthcare workers considered on an individual basis in settings in which a high percentage of MDR-TB patients have been found, transmission of MDR-TB is likely, and TB control precautions have been implemented and were not successful (CDC, 2010).

Mantoux tuberculin skin tests are widely used for routine screening of children and high-risk individuals. Early detection and effective treatment of active cases are essential for prevention and control.

In 2008, the WHO implemented a *STOP TB Strategy* for its member nations, with the objective of dramatically reducing the global burden of tuberculosis. The WHO strategy has six principal components:

1. Pursue high-quality *DOTS* (*Directly Observed Treatment Short-course*) expansion and enhancement.
2. Address TB/HIV, MDR-TB, XDR-TB, and other special challenges.
3. Contribute to health system strengthening.
4. Engage all care providers.
5. Empower people with TB, and communities, through partnership.
6. Enable and promote research.

The program builds on the success of DOTS while also explicitly addressing the key challenges facing tuberculosis prevention and control. Its goal is to dramatically reduce the global burden of tuberculosis by ensuring that all patients with tuberculosis, including those co-infected with HIV and those with MDR-TB and XDR-TB, benefit from universal access to high-quality diagnosis and patient-centered treatment. The *STOP TB Strategy* also supports the development of new and effective tools to prevent, detect, and treat tuberculosis (WHO, 2008b).

Most recently, the WHO has extended the *STOP TB Strategy* to a more comprehensive *"End TB Strategy"* that incorporates three pillars for its member nations: (1) integrated patient-centered tuberculosis care and prevention, (2) political commitment, community engagement, social protection, and universal health coverage, and (3) intensified research and innovation with rapid translation of novel tools, interventions and strategies to reduce the global burden of tuberculosis (WHO, 2014).

References

Ahmed, Y., Mwaba, P., Chintu, C., Grange, J. M., Ustianowski, A., & Zumla, A. (1990). A study of maternal mortality at the University Teaching Hospital, Lusaka, Zambia: The emergence of tuberculosis as a major nonobstetric cause of maternal death. *The International Journal of Tuberculosis and Lung Disease, 3*, 675–680.

Badri, M., Wilson, D., & Wood, R. (2002). Effect of highly active antiretroviral therapy on incidence of tuberculosis in South Africa: A cohort study. *Lancet, 359*(9323), 2059–2064.

Bates, M. N., Khalakdina, A., Pai, M., Chang, L., Lessa, F., & Smith, K. R. (2007). Risk of tuberculosis from exposure to tobacco smoke: A systematic review and meta-analysis. *Archives of Internal Medicine, 167*(4), 335–342.

Bonah, C. (2005). The 'experimental stable' of the BCG vaccine: Safety, efficacy, proof, and standards, 1921–1933. *Studies in History and Philosophy of Biological and Biomedical Sciences, 36*(4), 696–721.

Centers for Disease Control. (2010). *Ethnographic guides: Promoting cultural sensitivity—A practical guide for tuberculosis programs.* Atlanta, GA: U.S. Department of Health and Human Services.

Centers for Disease Control. (2017). *Reported tuberculosis in the United States, 2016.* Atlanta, GA: U.S. Department of Health and Human Services, CDC.

Centers for Disease Control. (2018). *Reported tuberculosis in the United States, 2009.* Atlanta, GA: U.S. Department of Health and Human Services, CDC.

Cole, E., & Cook, C. (1998). Characterization of infectious aerosols in health care facilities: An aid to effective engineering controls and preventive strategies. *American Journal of Infection Control, 26*(4), 453–464.

Comstock, G. (1994). The International Tuberculosis Campaign: A pioneering venture in mass vaccination and research. *Clinical Infectious Diseases, 19*(3), 528–540.

Dalton, J. (2009). Antibiotic resistance of tuberculosis. *DUJS Online,* 22 Feb 2009.

Donald, P. R., & van Helden, P. D. (2009). The global burden of tuberculosis—Combating drug resistance in difficult times. *The New England Journal of Medicine, 360*(23), 2393–2395.

Dooley, K. E., & Chaisson, R. E. (2009). Tuberculosis and diabetes mellitus: Convergence of two epidemics. *The Lancet. Infectious Diseases, 9*(12), 737–746.

Gandhi, N. R., Moll, A., Sturm, A. W., Pawinski, R., Govender, T., Lalloo, U., … Friedland, G. (2006). Extensively drug-resistant tuberculosis as a cause of death in patients co-infected with tuberculosis and HIV in a rural area of South Africa. *The Lancet, 368*(9547), 1575–1580.

Gounder, C. R., Wada, N. I., Kensler, C., Violari, A., McIntyre, J., Chaisson, R. E., & Martinson, N. A. (2011). Active tuberculosis case-finding among pregnant women presenting to antenatal clinics in Soweto, South Africa. *Journal of Acquired Immune Deficiency Syndromes.* doi:10.1097/QAI.0b013e31821ac9c1.

Guelar, A., Gatell, J. M., Verdejo, J., Podzamczer, D., Lozano, L., Aznar, E., Miró, J. M., … González, J. (1993). A prospective study of the risk of tuberculosis among HIV-infected patients. *Acquired Immune Deficiency Syndrome, 7*(10), 1345–1349.

Hershkovitz, I., Donoghue, H. D., Minnikin, D. E., Besra, G. S., Lee, O. Y. C., Gernaey, A. M., … Spigelman, M. (2008). Detection and molecular characterization of 9000-year-old *Mycobacterium tuberculosis* from a neolithic settlement in the Eastern Mediterranean. *PLoS One, 3*(10), e3426.

Herzog, B. H. (1998). History of tuberculosis. *Respiration, 65,* 5–15.

Houben, R., & Dodd, P. J. (2016). The global burden of latent tuberculosis infection: A re-estimation using mathematical modelling. *PLoS Medicine, 13*(10), e1002152.

Jasmer, R. M., Nahid, P., & Hopewell, P. C. (2002). Clinical practice. Latent tuberculosis infection. *The New England Journal of Medicine, 347*(23), 1860–1866.

Jeon, C. Y., & Murray, M. B. (2008). Diabetes mellitus increases the risk of active tuberculosis: A systematic review of 13 observational studies. *PLoS Medicine, 5*(7), e152.

Kenyon, T. A., Creek, T., Laserson, K., Makhoa, M., Chimidza, N., Mwasekaga, M., … Binkin, N. (2002). Risk factors for transmission of *Mycobacterium tuberculosis* from HIV-infected tuberculosis patients, Botswana. *International Journal of Tuberculosis and Lung Disease, 6*(10), 843–850.

Khan, M., Pillay, T., Moodley, J. M., & Connolly, C. A. (2001). Maternal mortality associated with tuberculosis-HIV-1 co-infection in Durban, South Africa. *Acquired Immune Deficiency Syndrome, 15*, 1857–1863.

Kim, J., Park, Y., Kim, Y., Kang, S., Shin, J., Park, I., & Choi, B. (2003). Miliary tuberculosis and acute respiratory distress syndrome. *The International Journal of Tuberculosis and Lung Disease, 7*(4), 359–364.

Koch, R. (1905). The Nobel Prize in Physiology or Medicine, 1905. Retrieved from https://www.nobelprize.org/prizes/medicine/1905/summary/

Konstantinos, A. (2010). Testing for tuberculosis. *Australian Prescriber, 33*(1), 12–18.

Lee, J. H. (1948). Tuberculosis and silicosis. *Canadian Medical Association Journal, 58*(4), 349–353.

Lighter, J., & Rigaud, M. (2009). Diagnosing childhood tuberculosis: Traditional and innovative modalities. *Current Problems in Pediatric and Adolescent Health Care, 39*, 61–88.

Lin, H. H., Ezzati, M., Chang, H. Y., & Murray, M. (2009). Association between tobacco smoking and active tuberculosis in Taiwan: Prospective cohort study. *American Journal of Respiratory and Critical Care Medicine, 180*(5), 475–480.

Marais, B. J., Gie, R. P., Schaaf, H. S., Hesseling, A. C., Obihara, C. C., Atarke, J. J., & Enarson, D. A. (2004). The natural history of childhood intra-thoracic tuberculosis: A critical review of literature from the pre-chemotherapy era. *The International Journal of Tuberculosis and Lung Disease, 9*(4), 392–402.

Margono, F., Mroueh, J., Garely, A., White, D., Duerr, A., & Minkoff, H. L. (1994). Resurgence of active tuberculosis among pregnant women. *Obstetrics and Gynecology, 83*(6), 911–914.

Middlekoop, K., Bekker, L. G., Myer, L., Dawson, R., & Wood, R. (2008). Rates of tuberculosis transmission to children and adolescents in a community with a high prevalence of HIV Infection among adults. *Clinical Infectious Diseases, 47*(3), 349–355.

Mofenson, L. M., & Laughon, B. E. (2007). Human immuno-deficiency virus, *Mycobacterium tuberculosis*, and pregnancy: A deadly combination. *Clinical Infectious Diseases, 45*(2), 250–253.

Moutschen, M. P., Scheen, A. J., & Lefebvre, P. J. (1992). Impaired immune responses in diabetes mellitus: Analysis of the factors and mechanisms involved. Relevance to the increased susceptibility of diabetic patients to specific infections. *Diabetes & Metabolism, 18*, 187–201.

Nnoaham, K. E., & Clarke, A. (2008). Low serum vitamin D levels and tuberculosis: A systematic review and meta-analysis. *International Journal of Epidemiology, 37*(1), 113–119.

Pillay, T., Khan, M., Moodley, J., Adhikari, M., Padayatchi, N., Naicker, V., … Coovadia, H. M. (2001). The increasing burden of tuberculosis in pregnant women, newborns and infants under 6 months of age in Durban, KwaZulu-Natal. *South African Medical Journal, 91*(11), 983–987.

Rekha, B., & Swaminathan, S. (2007). Childhood tuberculosis—Global epidemiology and the impact of HIV. *Paediatric Respiratory Reviews, 8*(2), 99–106.

Robbins, S. L., & Cotran, R. S. (1979). *Pathologic basis of disease* (2nd ed.). Philadelphia, PA: WB Saunders Co.

Rothschild, B., Martin, L., Lev, G., Bercovier, H., Bar-Gal, G., Greenblatt, C., … Brittain, D. (2001). *Mycobacterium tuberculosis* complex DNA from an extinct bison dated 17,000 years before the present. *Clinical Infectious Diseases, 33*(3), 305–311.

Schaible, U. E., & Kaufmann, S. H. (2007). Malnutrition and infection: Complex mechanisms and global impacts. *PLoS Medicine, 4*(5), e115.

Thoen, C., Lobue, P., & de Kantor, I. (2006). The importance of *Mycobacterium bovis* as a zoonosis. *Veterinary Microbiology, 112*(2–4), 339–345.

Tripathy, S. N., & Tripathy, S. N. (2003). Tuberculosis and pregnancy. *International Journal of Gynaecology and Obstetrics, 80*, 247–253.

Tso, H. W., Lau, Y. L., Tam, C. M., Wong, H. S., & Chiang, K. S. (2004). Associations between *IL12B* polymorphisms and tuberculosis in the Hong Kong Chinese population. *The Journal of Infectious Diseases, 190*(5), 913–919.

Tweddle, N., & Livingstone, P. (1994). Bovine tuberculosis control and eradication programs in Australia and New Zealand. *Veterinary Microbiology, 40*(1–2), 23–39.

Waddington, K. (2004). To stamp out so terrible a malady: Bovine tuberculosis and tuberculin testing in Britain, 1890–1939. *Medical History, 48*(1), 29–48.

Waksman, S. A. (1952). The nobel prize in physiology or medicine 1952. Retrieved from https://www.nobelprize.org/prizes/medicine/1952/summary/

Wood, R., Liang, H., Wu, H., Middelkoop, K., Oni, T., Rangaka, M. X., … Lawn, S. D. (2010). Changing prevalence of TB infection with increasing age in high TB burden townships in South Africa. *The International Journal of Tuberculosis and Lung Disease, 13*(4), 406–412.

World Health Organization. (1995). *WHO statement on BCG revaccination for the prevention of tuberculosis*. Geneva, Switzerland: World Health Organization.

World Health Organization. (2007). *Tuberculosis*. Geneva, Switzerland: World Health Organization.

World Health Organization. (2008a). *The global burden of disease: 2004 update*. Geneva, Switzerland: World Health Organization.

World Health Organization. (2008b). *Implementing the STOP TB strategy*. Geneva, Switzerland: World Health Organization.

World Health Organization. (2009). *Epidemiology. Global tuberculosis control: Epidemiology, strategy, financing* (pp. 6–33). Geneva, Switzerland: World Health Organization.

World Health Organization. (2010). *WHO tuberculosis factsheet*. Geneva, Switzerland: World Health Organization.

World Health Organization. (2014). *The End TB Strategy, global strategy and targets for tuberculosis prevention, care and control after 2015*. Geneva, Switzerland: World Health Organization.

World Health Organization. (2018). *Global tuberculosis report 2018*. Geneva, Switzerland: World Health Organization.

Zhao, M., Li, X., Xu, P., Shen, X., Gui, X., Gui, X., … Gao, Q. (2009). Transmission of MDR and XDR tuberculosis in Shanghai, China. *PLoS One, 4*(2), e4370.

Zink, A., Sola, C., Reischl, U., Grabner, W., Rastogi, N., Wolf, H., & Nerlich, A. (2003). Characterization of *Mycobacterium tuberculosis* complex DNAs from Egyptian mummies by spoligotyping. *Journal of Clinical Microbiology, 41*(1), 359–367.

© Andrew Brookes/Getty Images

CHAPTER 55
Epidemiology of Malaria

▶ Introduction

Malaria is a zoonotic infectious disease transmitted to humans by *Anopheles* species of mosquitoes. The disease is caused by a plasmodium (microscopic worm) that is carried in mosquito saliva. Humans become infected when an infected mosquito inserts its long hollow needle-like proboscis through the skin and sucks up blood.

Four species of malaria infect and cause disease in humans. Severe life-threatening malaria is most commonly caused by *Plasmodium falciparum*. Other species, *Plasmodium vivax*, *Plasmodium ovale,* and *Plasmodium malariae* generally cause infections with milder symptoms that are rarely fatal. Parasitic *Plasmodium* species also infect birds, reptiles, monkeys, chimpanzees, and rodents.

Malaria is caused by the proliferation of malarial parasites within red blood cells (erythrocytes), typically producing fever and headache and in severe cases progressing to anemia, coma, and death.

Malaria is most common in tropical and subtropical regions of the world near the equator, including much of sub-Saharan Africa, Asia, and Central America. Significant rainfall and warm temperatures enable mosquitoes that serve as vectors of malarial transmission to breed continuously.

▶ History of Malaria

In 2700 BC, the symptoms of malaria were accurately described in ancient Chinese medical writings in the *Nei Ching,* the *Chinese Canon of Medicine.* During the 2nd century BC, the *Qinghao* plant *(Artemisia annua)* was described in the Chinese medical treatise, *52 Remedies.* Derivatives of this extract, known collectively as *artemisinins,* are very potent and effective antimalarial drugs that are still used today, especially in combination with other drugs (Wright, Linley, Brun, Wittlin, & Hsu, 2010).

Following their arrival in the New World, Spanish Jesuit missionaries learned from indigenous Indian tribes of a medicinal tree bark used for the treatment of fevers. The Countess of Chinchón, the wife of the Viceroy of Peru, was cured of fever by an extract of this bark and the tree was subsequently named *Cinchona* after the countess. The active compound in Cinchona bark is the antimalarial, quinine. Along with artemisinins, quinine is one of the most effective antimalarial drugs available today (Greenwood, 1992).

In 1880, Charles Louis Alphonse Laveran, a French army surgeon stationed in Constantine, Algeria, was the first to detect parasites in the blood of a patient suffering from malaria. Laveran was awarded the 1907 Nobel Prize (Laveran, 1907).

In 1897, Ronald Ross, a British officer in the Indian Medical Service, demonstrated that malaria parasites are transmitted to and from humans by mosquitoes. In further work, Ross showed that bird malaria is transmitted by mosquitoes and that the life cycle of the parasite involves a sporogonic cycle (the time interval during which the parasite developed in the mosquito). Ross also described in great detail the use of bed nets to protect against malarial transmission by mosquitoes. Ross was awarded the Nobel Prize in 1902 (Ross, 1902).

Camillo Golgi, an Italian neurophysiologist, established that malarial fever coincided with the rupture and release of merozoites into the blood stream. For their discoveries in the field of neurology, Golgi and his colleague, Santiago Ramón y Cajal, were awarded the Nobel Prize in 1906 (Golgi & Cajal, 1906).

Chloroquine was discovered by Hans Andersag in 1934 at Bayer laboratories in Germany. Chloroquine was established as an effective and safe antimalarial drug after World War II and is still being used today. Nevertheless, many malarial strains have now developed chloroquine resistance (Jensen & Melhorn, 2009).

Fred Soper, an American epidemiologist and public health administrator, was called the *"General Patton"* of mosquito eradication. During 1927–1962, Soper directed successful campaigns in several regions of the world to eliminate malaria and yellow fever by draining swamps and spraying insecticides to eradicate the mosquito population by reducing their breeding sites. One of his early successes was the total eradication of the *Anopheles gambiae* mosquito population and elimination of malaria from certain regions of Brazil. Soper spearheaded the *Global Malaria Eradication Program* that helped eliminate the disease from the developed world and from many parts of the developing world. He was a strong advocate of the *judicious* use of the insecticide, dichlorodiphenyltrichloroethane (DDT), to selectively eliminate species of *Anopheles* mosquitoes, the vectors of malaria transmission. Fred Soper, the *mosquito killer,* directed massive campaigns to eliminate malaria by the eradication of plasmodium-infected mosquitoes and his efforts undoubtedly spared the lives of millions of people (Gladwell, 2001).

The insecticidal property of DDT was discovered in 1939 by Paul Müller in Switzerland. This compound was widely and successfully used for malaria elimination and control in many countries at the end of World War II. For example, targeted spraying with DDT had virtually eliminated malaria from the U.S. population by 1951. Müller was awarded the Nobel Prize in 1948 (Müller, 1948).

In 1955, members of the World Health Organization (WHO) submitted an ambitious proposal at the World Health Assembly for the eradication of malaria worldwide. This global program involved house spraying with insecticides (DDT), antimalarial drug treatment, and surveillance. Though the initial efforts of this program were successful in some populations, it was eventually abandoned due to lack of funding and various other reasons. Strong opposition to the use of DDT was voiced in the book *Silent Spring* by Rachel Carson who emphasized its persistence in the environment and potential for causing long-term damage to the ecosystem (Gladwell, 2001).

Life Cycle of Plasmodia

Female mosquitoes of the Anopheles genus are primary hosts and the vectors of transmission. Humans and other vertebrates are considered secondary (intermediate) hosts. The life cycle of plasmodia is extraordinarily complex and involves both sexual and asexual replication (**FIGURE 55.1**).

Young pregnant Anopheles female mosquitoes ingest the malaria parasite by feeding on the blood of an infected human carrier. Infected mosquitoes carry *Plasmodium sporozoites* in their salivary glands. Sporozoites differentiate into male or female gametes that undergo *sexual recombination* in the gut of the mosquito. Sexual fusion of gametes produces an *ookinete* that penetrates the gut lining and produces an *oocyst* in the gut wall. When the oocyst ruptures, it releases new sporozoites that migrate through the mosquito's body to the salivary glands, where they can infect a new human host. The sporozoites are injected into the skin and blood with the mosquito's saliva when the mosquito ingests a human blood meal.

Upon entering the human bloodstream, sporozoites migrate to the liver where they infect liver cells (hepatocytes). Within the cytoplasm of hepatocytes, sporozoites undergo transformation into merozoites that multiply asexually for 1–4 weeks. Infected hepatocytes eventually rupture releasing thousands of merozoites into the blood stream where they infect erythrocytes (red blood cells). Within erythrocytes, merozoites continue to multiply *asexually,* periodically rupturing their host cells and invading other erythrocytes. Various forms of merozoites have been detected in red blood cells (ring forms, trophozoites, and schizonts). Clinically, waves of fever are associated with repeating cycles of erythrocytic infection, rupture, and release of merozoites in the same individual.

Pathogenesis of Malaria

The clinical symptoms of malaria are caused by the asexual erythrocytic (blood stage) parasites. When merozoites invade erythrocytes, they digest hemoglobin, the oxygen-carrying molecule of the body. A toxic breakdown product of hemoglobin (hemozoin pigment) and other toxic factors accumulate and are released into the bloodstream along with newly invasive merozoites when the infected cells lyse (rupture). The hemozoin and other toxic factors stimulate macrophages and other immune cells to produce cytokines and other soluble factors which incite fever, rigors, and potentially fatal immunoreactive pathophysiology.

Life Cycle of the Malaria Parasite

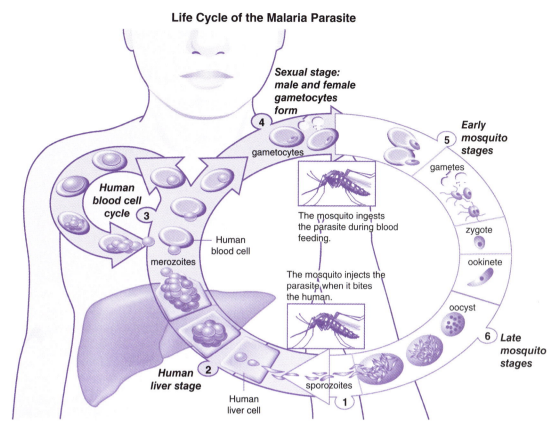

FIGURE 55.1 Life Cycle of Malaria.

Plasmodial parasites spend most of their human life cycle within hepatocytes and erythrocytes and are therefore protected from attack by the immune system. One exception is in the spleen where infected erythrocytes are immobilized, identified, and destroyed. However, *P. falciparum* has developed a mechanism to avoid passage through the spleen whereby infected erythrocytes, particularly those with mature trophozoites, adhere to the vascular endothelium of venular blood vessel walls and do not freely circulate in the blood. The sequestration of infected erythrocytes in the small blood vessels of the brain is the pathogenic mechanism of *cerebral malaria.*

Two malarial species, *P. vivax* and *P. ovale,* can remain dormant for long periods of time in hepatocytes. The dormant liver stage parasites are called *hypnozoites.* Reactivation and relapse are particularly characteristic of subspecies of *P. vivax,* which are endemic in India and the equatorial regions of Central and South America (Chin, 1973; Cogswell, 1992).

Plasmodium malariae is the most persistent of the malarial species and can coexist in the human system as a chronic infectious disease over a period of many years. Infections in untreated or inadequately treated individuals are often asymptomatic and can induce the formation of antigen–antibody complexes that deposit in the glomeruli of the kidneys. Chronic *P. malariae* infections are commonly detected in individuals living in the equatorial regions of South America and Africa and are a primary cause of the nephrotic syndrome and kidney failure (Chin, 1973).

Malarial infection, particularly due to *P. falciparum,* can quickly turn fatal. Life-threatening complications include cerebral malarial infection, hyperparasitemia when more than 5% of erythrocytes are infected by malarial parasites, severe anemia due to hemolysis (massive destruction of red blood cells), splenic rupture, acute respiratory distress syndrome, abnormalities in blood coagulation, low blood pressure due to cardiovascular collapse, acute kidney failure, metabolic acidosis (excessive acidity in the blood and tissues), and/or hypoglycemia (Chen, Schlichtherle, & Wahlgren, 2000).

▶ Global Burden of Malaria

Malaria: Incidence and Mortality, 2006

In 2006, the WHO conducted a survey of 109 of its member nations and territories to characterize the global incidence, prevalence, and mortality of malaria.

Only those countries classified as "malaria-endemic" participated in the survey. Estimates of the number of cases of malaria were obtained by adjusting the reported cases for coverage of the population and the parasite-positivity rate. Estimates of the number of deaths from malaria were obtained by multiplying the estimated number of *P. falciparum* malaria cases by a fixed case fatality rate for each country.

Results revealed that malaria causes 250 million cases of fever and nearly 1 million deaths annually. Most cases (98%) were diagnosed in sub-Saharan Africa (86%), Southeast Asia (9%), or the Eastern Mediterranean region (3%). It is notable that more than half of all cases occurred in just five African countries (Nigeria, Democratic Republic of Congo, Ethiopia, United Republic of Tanzania, and Kenya). Of the 250 million cases, 230 million (92%) were due to *P. falciparum,* and in Africa, 98% of cases were due to this strain of malaria.

The vast majority of malarial deaths (91%) occurred in sub-Saharan Africa and 85% occurred in children under the age of 5 years of age. Pregnant women, individuals with HIV/AIDS, and elderly individuals (over 65 years of age) were especially vulnerable accounting for 8%, 5%, and 2% of malarial deaths, respectively. Southeast Asia and the Eastern Mediterranean region each contributed about 4% of malarial deaths.

These data reflect little change since 1992 when the WHO conducted a similar survey of malaria in these same nations. Furthermore, these figures are likely underestimates of the global burden of malaria, since many cases occur in rural areas where there is no access to health care, and as a consequence, they are undocumented (WHO, 2008).

▶ Malaria: Incidence and Mortality, 2013–2016 Update

Using new methodologies, Murray and Global Burden of Disease (GBD) collaborators developed estimates of incidence and mortality for malaria during the period 1990–2013. Their estimates were based on nationally available numbers of cases and deaths and models of incidence as a function of mortality, age, sex, and region. Mortality estimates were derived from vital statistics as well as verbal autopsies. Global Burden of Disease investigators have reported estimates for subsequent years, 2014–2016, utilizing similar methods (Murray & GBD 2016 Causes of Death Collaborators, 2017; Murray, Ortblad, Guinovart, & Global Burden of Disease Collaborators, 2014; Wang & Naghavi, 2016).

FIGURE 55.2 shows the global trends in numbers of cases of and deaths from malaria during 1990–2015. The annual number of new cases of malaria peaked during 2003 at 232 million and then fell to less than 200 million in subsequent years. Notably, there has been an uptick in new cases during recent years. During 2016, 216 million new cases of malaria were detected worldwide (Murray & GBD 2016 Causes of Death Collaborators, 2017; Murray et al., 2014; Wang & Naghavi, 2016).

The annual number of deaths from malaria peaked in 2004 at about 1.2 million and declined to 0.73 million in 2015. The largest number of cases of

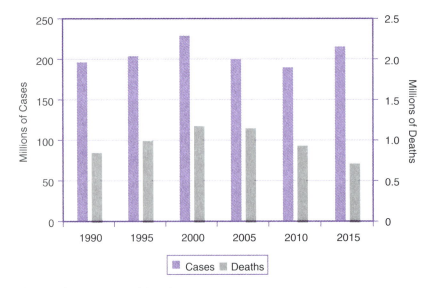

FIGURE 55.2 Global Trends in Malaria, Cases and Deaths, 1990–2015.

Data from Murray, C. J. L., Ortblad, K. F., Guinovart, C., & Global Burden of Disease Collaborators. (2014). Global, regional, and national incidence and mortality for HIV, tuberculosis, and malaria during 1990–2013: A systematic analysis for the Global Burden of Disease Study 2013. *The Lancet, 384*(9947), 1005–1070; Wang, H., Naghavi, M., & GBD 2015 Mortality and Causes of Death Collaborators. (2016). Global, regional, and national life expectancy, all-cause mortality, and cause-specific mortality for 249 causes of death, 1980–2015: A systematic analysis for the Global Burden of Disease Study 2015. *The Lancet, 388*(10053), 1459–1544; Murray, C. J. L., & GBD 2016 Causes of Death Collaborators. (2017). Global, regional, and national age-sex specific mortality for 264 causes of death, 1980–2016: A systematic analysis for the Global Burden of Disease Study 2016. *The Lancet, 390*(10100), 1151–1210; World Health Organization. (2017). *World malaria report.* Geneva, Switzerland: World Health Organization.

malaria (80%) developed in children and adolescents under 15 years of age. Children under 5 years of age have the greatest number of deaths from malaria (55%–65%). Age standardized incidence and mortality rates rose between 1990 and 2000 and have since declined. The global age standardized incidence rate of malaria is approximately 11.9 per 100,000, ranging from near zero in developed nations to rates exceeding 85 per 100,000 in Western sub-Saharan Africa. Three nations account for nearly 50% of malaria cases, India (~60 million cases), Nigeria (~30 million cases) and DR Congo (~6 million cases) (Murray et al., 2014; Wang & Naghavi, 2016; WHO, 2017).

▶ Global Incidence of *Plasmodium falciparum*: Controversial Findings

Using different methodology, Robert Snow, Guerra, Noor, Myint, and Hay (2005) estimated the number of incident cases of *P. falciparum* malaria during 2002 to be 515 million, more than double the number reported by the WHO in 2006. These investigators also suggest that a higher fraction of new cases (30%) occur outside Africa (**FIGURE 55.3**). Their estimates were based upon reported clinical attack rates of only the most virulent malarial strain, *P. falciparum*. Estimates were derived from 83 studies conducted in 22 countries of 5 WHO regions. Using these data, a classification scheme was developed according to the *median annual attack rates*

(*cases per 1000*) observed in different geographic areas: 39 areas were classified as hypoendemic (43 per 1000), 25 as mesoendemic (171 per 1000), and 8 were holo/hyperendemic (873 per 1000). The number of new cases for each WHO region was estimated by weighting attack rates by the corresponding populations of the geographic areas within that region (Snow et al., 2005).

Snow et al. (2005) chose not to estimate mortality from *P. falciparum* using their methodology "*because of the paucity of prospective epidemiological descriptions of cause-specific mortality outside Africa.*" Nevertheless, they point out that the risk of death after a clinical attack of *P. falciparum* may be tenfold higher in sub-Saharan Africa than nations outside of Africa, likely because of lack of access to prompt treatment.

More recently, Snow and colleagues estimated the global number of incident cases of *P. falciparum* in 2007. Among 87 countries endemic for malaria, estimates of transmission rates (attack rates) were modeled to estimate incidence rates for countries, regions, and worldwide. The combined global estimate for all areas of transmission risk was 451 million new cases of disease during 2007, nearly twofold higher than estimates utilizing more conventional surveillance methods. More than half of the cases of *P. falciparum* were found in just four countries: India, Nigeria, DR Congo, and Burma. The investigators suggest the need to scale-up investment in improved surveillance methods in order to construct an accurate and detailed global map of "*malarial transmission intensity*" to facilitate the implementation and

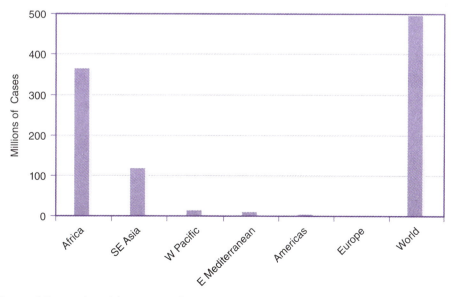

FIGURE 55.3 New Cases of *Plasmodium falciparum* Malaria, 2002.

Data from Snow, R. W., Guerra, C. A., Noor, A. M., Myint, H. Y., & Hay, S. I. (2005). The global distribution of clinical episodes of *Plasmodium falciparum* malaria. *Nature, 434*, 214–217.

evaluation of improved malaria control programs (Hay et al., 2010).

Snow and colleagues also conducted an extensive review of the literature and extracted data from more than 50,000 surveys at 37,000 locations to update their estimates of the global burden of malaria during the last century. Their results show that the prevalence of malaria due to *P. falciparum* in Africa has declined from approximately 40% during 1900–1929 to less than 24% during 2010–2015. They suggest the presence of two precipitous declines in malarial infections, the first, during 1945–1949, was attributed to widespread spraying of *dichlorodiphenyltrichloroethane* (DDT) to eliminate mosquitoes and early chloroquine treatment of infections. The more recent decline, during 2005–2010, was attributed to widespread distribution of long-lasting insecticide-treated bed nets and a major change in the treatment of infections from chloroquine to artemisinin-based combination therapy (Snow et al., 2017).

Case Fatality: *Plasmodium falciparum* Malaria

Malaria represents a medical emergency and may rapidly progress to severe complications and death without prompt and appropriate treatment. Severe malaria is almost exclusively caused by *P. falciparum*. Major complications of severe malaria include cerebral malaria, pulmonary edema, acute renal failure, severe anemia, and/or bleeding. Acidosis and hypoglycemia are the most common metabolic complications. Any of these complications can develop rapidly and progress to death within hours or days. In many patients, several of these complications exist together or evolve in rapid succession within a few hours.

Malaria can be particularly devastating in infants and young children. Among 1357 Gambian children hospitalized with malaria, 179 (13.2%) died within 6 months of admission. Case fatality rates were high in patients with cerebral malaria plus severe anemia (17%), cerebral anemia (16%), severe anemia (8%), or hypoglycemia (33%). Among those with cerebral malaria, 11% suffered major residual neurological deficits such as hemiplegia, cortical blindness, aphasia, and/or ataxia. Onset of severe anemia tended to occur before the age of 3 years whereas onset of cerebral malaria was more typical during ages 3–5 years (**FIGURE 55.4**) (Brewster, Kwiatkowski, & White, 1990).

Murphy and Breman conducted an extensive review and analysis of published case fatality rates for children of sub-Saharan Africa who were less than 5 years of age when diagnosed with malaria. Their review included 3275 cases of cerebral malaria and 3723 cases of malarial anemia diagnosed and treated in multiple centers in sub-Saharan Africa. Results revealed that cerebral malaria has an overall case fatality rate of 19% and malarial anemia has a case fatality rate of 13%. The case fatality rate was also high among children presenting with respiratory distress, hypoglycemia, or overlapping symptoms due to malaria (18%). Furthermore, low birth weight babies born to infected mothers had a case fatality rate of 38%. Based on these case fatality rates, the investigators suggest that the annual death toll from early childhood malaria in sub-Saharan Africa could be as high as 2.26 million (Murphy & Breman, 2001).

Both fetal and maternal mortality are elevated among pregnant women who develop malarial infections. In a review of published data on maternal mortality due to anemia, severe malarial anemia was

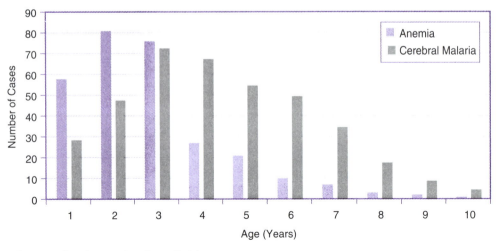

FIGURE 55.4 Age Distribution of Malaria in Gambian Children.

Data from Brewster, D. R., Kwiatkowski, D., & White, N. J. (1990). Neurological sequelae of cerebral malaria in children. *Lancet, 336*(8722), 1039–1043.

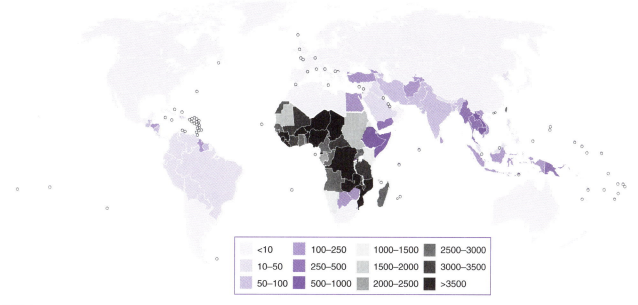

FIGURE 55.5 Disability-Adjusted Life Years: Malaria, 2007.

Data from World Health Organization. *The global burden of disease: 2004 update.* Geneva: WHO. Retrieved from www.who.int/evidence/bod

found to elevate maternal mortality more than three-fold (Brabin, Hakimi, & Pelletier, 2001).

Disability-Adjusted Life Years: Malaria

The *disability-adjusted life years* (*DALY*) lost from malaria reflect the high burden of deaths in early child-hood plus disability due to chronic infection, particularly neurological deficits due to cerebral malaria. As shown in **FIGURE 55.5**, the highest DALY are evident in sub-Saharan Africa, similar to other infectious diseases of poverty such as tuberculosis and HIV/AIDS.

▶ Genetic Resistance to Malaria

The devastation wreaked upon the human population by malaria has taken some unexpected twists and turns. Due to the predilection of plasmodium species for infants and children who often died of malaria before reaching reproductive age, *malarial resistance genes* have been fixed at high frequencies in populations residing in endemic areas.

Sickle Cell Anemia and Malaria

Sickle cell anemia is an autosomal recessive genetic disorder characterized by red blood cells that assume an abnormal, rigid, sickle shape. The condition was discovered in 1910 by Chicago physician James Herrick in the blood of a young boy with anemia from the West Indies (Herrick, 1910). A later report demonstrated that the sickling was associated with low erythrocyte oxygen content (Hahn & Gillespie, 1927).

Epidemiologic studies soon revealed that the trait was relatively common in populations with endemic malaria because it protects red blood cells from infection by *P. falciparum*. The sickle cell trait is caused by a single base pair change in the gene for hemoglobin on chromosome 11 (Ashley-Koch, Yang, & Olney, 1998; Pauling, Itano, Singer, & Wells, 1949). Individuals homozygous for the mutated gene have a morphologically altered form of hemoglobin (hemoglobin S) that forms "tactoid" crystals in red blood cells causing them to transform into a "sickle" shape. Hemoglobin S is not particularly efficient at carrying oxygen to tissues; hence individuals who are homozygous for the sickle cell gene usually become anemic. However, the sickled cells are not favorable hosts for the *P. falciparum* merozoites, and consequently, individuals with sickle cell anemia who live in regions endemic for malaria are protected from falciparum infection during childhood and survive to reproduce and pass the gene to subsequent generations. Recent studies have confirmed that the sickle cell gene is most common in populations of sub-Saharan Africa, the Middle East, and India, coincident with the historically high rates of malaria in these regions (Piel et al., 2010).

Glucose-6-Phosphate Dehydrogenase Deficiency and Malaria

Glucose-6-phosphate dehydrogenase (G6PD) is an X-linked enzyme that protects red blood cells from oxidative stress. Infants with deficiencies in G6PD can develop neonatal jaundice and hemolytic anemia following certain environmental stimuli.

Populations endemic for malaria have high rates of G6PD deficiencies that may afford protection against certain types of plasmodium infections. Louicharoen and colleagues investigated the effects of a common G6PD deficiency variant in Southeast Asia, the *G6PD-Mahidol* variant, in patients with *P. vivax* or *P. falciparum* malariae. They examined parasite density in blood samples from 400 individuals with *P. falciparum* infection and 227 individuals with *P. vivax* infection. They found that the density of vivax parasites was reduced by 30% in heterozygous females and by 61% in homozygous females for the Mahidol G6PD mutation. The G6PD-variant had no effect on parasite density among patients with falciparum infection. Their results suggest that *P. vivax* has been a driving force behind the strong selective advantage conferred by this mutation (Louicharoen et al., 2009).

▶ Control of Malaria

The complex life cycle of the malarial plasmodia presents several opportunities for intervention including mosquito eradication, prevention of mosquito strikes, plasmodium eradication, and treatment of malarial infections. Recently, the WHO launched a global program designed to reduce the burden of malaria worldwide (WHO, 2010). The program advocates combinations of four basic components.

Vector Control

Vector control remains the most generally effective measure to prevent malaria transmission and therefore the cornerstone of the four basic technical elements of the WHO Global Malaria Control Strategy. Elements of vector control include distribution of insecticide-treated bed nets, targeted spraying of insecticides and larvicides, and drainage of mosquito breeding sites to reduce populations of Anopheles mosquitoes. Malaria transmission can be reduced substantially by preventing mosquito bites by distribution of inexpensive mosquito nets and insect repellents, or by mosquito-control measures such as spraying insecticides inside houses and draining standing water where mosquitoes lay their eggs.

The malaria life cycle involves plasmodial infection of not only humans, but also mosquitoes. Obviously, curbing infection in the susceptible mosquito population could have a major impact in preventing spread into humans and other species. As pointed out by George Dimopoulos and colleagues of the Johns Hopkins Malaria Research Institute:

Prevention and control measures for malaria and other mosquito-borne diseases depend upon mosquito biology and the effectiveness, cost, safety, and acceptability of intervention in high-risk populations. Current measures are focused on reduction of contact between mosquitoes and humans by elimination of mosquito larvae by environmental management (draining swamps) and judicial spraying with larvicides. Because of the nocturnal feeding habits of mosquitoes, malaria transmission occurs primarily at night. Protection against mosquito bites, therefore, mandates the use of insecticide-treated bed nets, wearing clothes that cover most of the body, and use of insect repellent on exposed skin. Novel methods for prevention of malaria that are currently being tested involve genetic manipulation of mosquito immunity to inhibit infection by the malarial plasmodium (Modified from Cirimotich, Dong, Garver, Sim, & Dimopoulos et al., 2010).

Early Diagnosis and Treatment

Early diagnosis of malaria and its effective and timely treatment reduce morbidity and prevents death from malaria. Advanced diagnostic tools (microscopy and rapid diagnostic tests) and effective drug therapies (artemisinin-based combination treatments) administered by highly trained healthcare personnel facilitate effective case management with a high probability of cure.

Identification of High-Risk Groups

Some population groups are at considerably higher risk of contracting severe malaria than others. High-risk groups include pregnant women, patients with HIV/AIDS, nonimmune travelers, and in high transmission areas, children less than 5 years of age. Such individuals warrant special measures for prevention and treatment of malaria, and to mitigate their risk, consideration should be given to their specific circumstances and the tools and strategies available.

Coinfection with HIV has been found to increase the severity and case fatality of malaria in a number of studies. A team of international investigators recently assessed the impact of coinfection by HIV-1 and malaria in 41 countries of sub-Saharan Africa. Overall, the data suggest that the HIV-1 epidemic had increased the incidence of malaria by 1.3% and malarial deaths by 4.9%. However, in the countries of southern Africa that have high rates of HIV-1 infections in

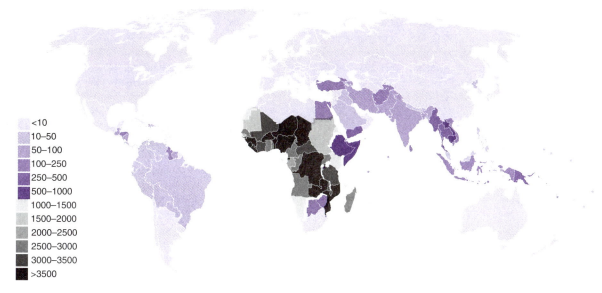

FIGURE 55.6 Global Malarial Resistance to Chloroquine, 2004.
Data from World Health Organization. (2004). *World malaria report*. Geneva, Switzerland: World Health Organization.

rural areas (Botswana, Zimbabwe, Swaziland, South Africa, and Namibia), the incidence of clinical malaria increased by 28% and the mortality from malaria increased by 114% (Korenromp et al., 2005).

Mounting evidence has also revealed pathologic interactions between HIV and malaria in coinfected patients. A transient (one-log) elevation in the HIV viral load had been observed during febrile malaria episodes; and reciprocally, the severity and symptoms of malaria are enhanced in HIV-infected patients (Abu-Raddad, Patnaik, & Kublin, 2006).

Surveillance, Monitoring, and Evaluation

Monitoring and evaluation are essential components of the WHO Global Malaria Program. Monitoring measures the implementation of the range of strategic activities, while evaluation measures the extent to which objectives are being reached.

Chloroquine Resistance of Malaria

A disturbing feature in the fight against malaria is the development of large-scale resistance by *P. falciparum* to several antimalarial drugs, most notably chloroquine (**FIGURE 55.6**). Nevertheless, a variety of antimalarial medications are available and most recently, the treatment of *P. falciparum* infections in endemic countries has been transformed by the use of combinations of drugs containing an *artemisinin* derivative. Severe malaria is treated with intravenous or intramuscular quinine, or increasingly, the artemisinin derivative *artesunate* which appears to be superior to quinine in both children and adults.

References

Abu-Raddad, L., Patnaik, P., & Kublin, J. (2006). Dual infection with HIV and malaria fuels the spread of both diseases in sub-Saharan Africa. *Science, 314*(5805), 1603–1606.

Ashley-Koch, A., Yang, Q., & Olney, R. S. (1998). Hemoglobin S allele and sickle cell disease. *American Journal of Epidemiology, 151*(9), 839–845.

Brabin, B. J., Hakimi, M., & Pelletier, D. (2001). An analysis of anemia and pregnancy-related maternal mortality. *Journal of Nutrition, 131*(2S–2), 604S–614S.

Brewster, D. R., Kwiatkowski, D., & White, N. J. (1990). Neurological sequelae of cerebral malaria in children. *Lancet, 336*(8722), 1039–1043.

Chen, Q., Schlichtherle, M., & Wahlgren, M. (2000). Molecular aspects of severe malaria. *Clinical Microbiology Reviews, 13*(3), 439–450.

Chin, W. (1973). Malaria. In J. M. Last (Ed.), *Maxey-Rosenau public health and preventive medicine* (12th ed., pp. 361–370). Norwalk, CT: Appleton-crofts.

Cirimotich, C. M., Dong, Y., Garver, L. S., Sim, S., & Dimopoulos, G. (2010). Mosquito immune defenses against Plasmodium infection. *Development & Comparative Immunology, 34*(4), 387–395.

Cogswell, F. B. (1992). The hypnozoite and relapse in primate malaria. *Clinical Microbiology Reviews, 5*(1), 26–35.

Gladwell, M. (2001, July). The mosquito killer. Annals of Public Health. *The New Yorker*. Retrieved from www.newyorker.com /magazine/2001/07/02/the-mosquito-killer/

Golgi, C., & Cajal, S. R. (1906). The nobel prize in physiology or medicine, 1906. Retrieved from www.nobelprize.org/prizes /medicine/1906/summary/

Greenwood, D. (1992). The quinine connection. *Journal of Antimicrobial Chemotherapy, 30*(4), 417–427.

Hahn, V. E., & Gillespie, E. B. (1927). Report of a case greatly improved by splenectomy. Experimental study of sickle cell formation. *Archives of Internal Medicine, 39*(2), 233–254.

Hay, S. I., Okiro, E. A., Gething, P. W., Patil, A. P., Tatem, A. J., Guerra, C. A., & Snow, R. W. (2010). Estimating the global clinical burden of *Plasmodium falciparum* malaria in 2007. *PLoS Medicine.* doi:10.1371/journal.pmed.1000290.

Herrick, J. B. (1910). Peculiar elongated and sickled shaped corpuscles in a case of severe anemia. *A.M.A Archives of Internal Medicine, 6,* 517.

Jensen, M., & Mehlhorn, H. (2009). Seventy-five years of Resochin in the fight against malaria. *Parasitology Research, 105*(3), 609–627.

Korenromp, E. L., Williams, B. G., de Vlas, S. J., Gouws, E., Gilks, C. F., Ghys, P. D., & Nahlen, B. L. (2005). Malaria attributable to the HIV-1 epidemic, Sub-Saharan Africa. *Emerging Infectious Diseases, 11*(9), 1410–1419.

Laveran, C. L. (1907). The Nobel Prize in Physiology or Medicine, 1907.

Louicharoen, C., Patin, E., Paul, R., Nuchprayoon, I., Witoonpanich, B., Peerapittayamongkol, C., … Sakuntabhai, A. (2009). Positively selected *G6PD*-Mahidol mutation reduces *Plasmodium vivax* density in Southeast Asians. *Science, 326*(5959), 1546–1549.

Müller, P. H. (1948). The nobel prize in physiology or medicine 1948. Retrieved from Nobelprize.org

Murphy, S. C., & Breman, J. G. (2001). Gaps in the childhood malaria burden in Africa: Cerebral malaria, neurological sequelae, anemia, respiratory distress, hypoglycemia, and complications of pregnancy. In J. G. Breman, A. Egan, & G. T. Keusch (Eds.), The intolerable burden of malaria: A new look at the numbers. Supplement to Volume 64(1) of the *American Journal of Tropical Medicine and Hygiene.*

Murray, C. J. L., & GBD 2016 Causes of Death Collaborators. (2017). Global, regional, and national age-sex specific mortality for 264 causes of death, 1980–2016: A systematic analysis for the Global Burden of Disease Study 2016. *The Lancet, 390*(10100), 1151–1210.

Murray, C. J. L., Ortblad, K. F., Guinovart, C., & Global Burden of Disease Collaborators. (2014). Global, regional, and national incidence and mortality for HIV, tuberculosis, and malaria during 1990–2013: A systematic analysis for the Global Burden of Disease Study 2013. *The Lancet, 384*(9947),1005–1070.

Pauling, L., Itano, H. A., Singer, S. J., & Wells, I. C. (1949). Sickle cell anemia, a molecular disease. *Science, 110,* 543–548.

Piel, F. B., Patil, A. P., Howes, R. E., Nyangiri, O. A., Gething, P. W., Williams, T. N., … Hay, S. I. (2010). Global distribution of the sickle cell gene and geographical confirmation of the malaria hypothesis. *Nature Communications, 1*(8), 104–108.

Ross, R. (1902). The Nobel Prize in Physiology or Medicine, 1902.

Snow, R. W., Guerra, C. A., Noor, A. M., Myint, H. Y., & Hay, S. I. (2005). The global distribution of clinical episodes of *Plasmodium falciparum* malaria. *Nature, 434,* 214–217.

Snow, R. W., Sartorius, B., Kyalo, D., Maina, J., Amratia, P., Mundia, C. W., … Noor, A. M. (2017). The prevalence of *Plasmodium falciparum* in sub Saharan Africa since 1900. *Nature, 550*(7677), 515–518.

Wang, H., Naghavi, M., & GBD 2015 Mortality and Causes of Death Collaborators. (2016). Global, regional, and national life expectancy, all-cause mortality, and cause-specific mortality for 249 causes of death, 1980–2015: A systematic analysis for the Global Burden of Disease Study 2015. *Lancet, 388*(10053), 1459–1544.

World Health Organization. (2004). *World malaria report.* Geneva, Switzerland: World Health Organization.

World Health Organization. (2008). *World malaria report.* Geneva, Switzerland: World Health Organization.

World Health Organization. (2010). *World malaria report.* Geneva, Switzerland: World Health Organization.

Wright, C. W., Linley, P. A., Brun, R., Wittlin, S., & Hsu, E. (2010). Ancient Chinese methods are remarkably effective for the preparation of artemisinin-rich extracts of qing hao with potent anti-malarial activity. *Molecules, 15*(2), 804–812.

© Andrew Brookes/Getty Images

CHAPTER 56

Epidemiology of HIV/AIDS

▶ Introduction

The *acquired immunodeficiency syndrome* (*AIDS*) is a disease of the immune system caused by infection with the *human immunodeficiency virus (HIV)*. The condition is therefore called HIV/AIDS. The infection progressively reduces the integrity of the immune system and renders afflicted individuals susceptible to opportunistic infections and certain types of cancer.

HIV can be transmitted from person to person in blood, semen, or vaginal fluid. Viral entry into the adult human system typically occurs when bodily fluids containing live virus come into contact with mucous membranes of the vagina, anus, or oral cavity. AIDS is therefore classified as a sexually transmitted disease (STD). HIV can also be transmitted by contaminated hypodermic needles, and from an infected mother to her baby during pregnancy, childbirth, or in breast milk.

HIV/AIDS is a modern-day pandemic, causing death and disability throughout the world. The most recent global survey conducted by the World Health Organization (WHO) in 2009 found that 33.3 million individuals worldwide are living with HIV/AIDS. In that year, 2.6 million new HIV infections were detected, and 1.8 million people died from HIV/AIDS. Most of the deaths from HIV/AIDS (76%) occur in sub-Saharan Africa. In this region, 22.5 million people are living with HIV/AIDS.

▶ History of HIV/AIDS

AIDS Outbreaks, United States

The initial report of the condition now known as HIV/AIDS described five homosexual young men in Los Angeles who had developed multiple opportunistic infections including a rare type of pneumonia caused by *Pneumocystis carinii* (MMWR, 1981a). This was quickly followed by reports of homosexual men living in New York, San Francisco, and Los Angeles who had developed various opportunistic infections plus a rare tumor characteristic of immunodeficiency, Kaposi sarcoma (MMWR, 1981b, 1982a). The combination of opportunistic infections and Kaposi sarcoma was subsequently reported in Haitians, drug addicts, hemophiliacs and other transfusion recipients, infants, female sex contacts of afflicted men, prisoners, and Africans (Masur et al., 1981, 1982; MMWR, 1982b, 1982c, 1982d, 1982e, 1983a, 1983b). Many other complications were typical of these patients including candidiasis, cytomegalovirus infection, mycobacterial infection, herpes infection, toxoplasmosis, fungal infection, varicella, and non-Hodgkin's lymphoma.

Discovery of HIV

Early theories of causation that were advanced to explain these outbreaks included exposure to multiple viruses and agents such as cytomegalovirus, Epstein–Barr virus (Sonnabend, Witkin, & Purtilo, 1983), sperm cell antibodies (Mavligit et al., 1984), and amyl nitrite (Goedert, Neuland, & Wallen, 1982). The prominence of homosexual men and intravenous drug addicts with opportunistic infections among the early cases of AIDS suggested an etiologic agent that was blood-borne, sexually transmitted, and caused severe immunosuppression.

The search for a novel virus responsible for AIDS was highly competitive and widely publicized. The causal RNA retrovirus, later named the *human immunodeficiency virus (HIV)* was first isolated in France in 1983 by Françoise Barré-Sinoussi and colleagues in the laboratory of Luc Montaignier (Barré-Sinoussi et al., 1983). The same virus was also isolated from several AIDS patients by Robert Gallo and colleagues at the National Institutes of Health and by Jay Levy and colleagues in San Francisco (Gallo et al., 1984; Levy et al., 1984). Shortly thereafter, Montaignier's group isolated a closely related virus in West African patients; hence the original virus was designated *HIV-1* and the West African virus *HIV-2*. Based upon their discovery of HIV-1 and HIV-2, the French group suggested that "these viruses existed long before the current AIDS epidemics. Their biological properties are conserved in spite of limited sequence homology; this may help the determination of the structure-function relationships of the different viral elements" (Guyader et al., 1987).

▶ Human Immunodeficiency Virus Life Cycle

The life cycle of HIV can be succinctly described in six steps.

1. Binding and Fusion: HIV begins its life cycle when it binds to a CD4 receptor and one of two co-receptors on the surface of a CD4+ T-lymphocyte. The virus then fuses with the host cell. After fusion, the virus releases RNA, its genetic material, into the host cell.
2. Reverse Transcription: An HIV enzyme called *reverse transcriptase* converts the single-stranded HIV RNA to double-stranded HIV DNA.
3. Integration: The newly formed HIV DNA enters the host cell's nucleus, where an HIV enzyme called integrase integrates the HIV DNA within the host cell's DNA. The integrated HIV DNA is called *provirus*. The provirus may remain inactive for several years, producing few or no new copies of HIV.

4. Transcription: When the host cell receives a signal to become active, the provirus uses a host enzyme called RNA polymerase to create copies of the HIV genomic material, as well as shorter strands of messenger RNA (mRNA). The mRNA is used as a blueprint to make long chains of HIV proteins.
5. Assembly: An HIV enzyme called *protease* cuts the long chains of HIV proteins into smaller individual proteins. As the smaller HIV proteins come together with copies of HIV's RNA genetic material, a new virus particle is assembled.
6. Budding: The newly assembled virus "buds" from the host cell. During budding, the new virus incorporates part of the cell's outer envelope. This envelope, which acts as a covering, is studded with protein/sugar combinations called HIV glycoproteins. These HIV glycoproteins are necessary for the virus to bind CD4 and co-receptors. The new copies of HIV can now move on to infect other cells (**FIGURE 56.1**).

The RNA genome of HIV contains nine genes that regulate its cell cycle. Three genes, *gag*, *pol*, and *env* encode structural proteins to make new virus particles. The six remaining genes (*tat*, *rev*, *nef*, *vif*, *vpr*, and *vpu*) are regulatory genes that control specific processes such as binding to CD4 cells, entry into the host cell, integration into the host cell DNA, activation and transcription of viral genes, regulation of viral replication, and the budding process (Hope & Trono, 2000).

▶ Global Burden of HIV/AIDS

The global surveillance of HIV/AIDS and other sexually transmitted infections is a combined effort of the WHO and the *Joint United Nations Program on HIV/AIDS* (UNAIDS). The *UNAIDS/WHO Working Group* on Global HIV/AIDS was formed in 1996 to strengthen national, regional, and global structures and networks for improved monitoring and surveillance of HIV/AIDS. The UNAIDS/WHO Working Group collaborates with investigators at six WHO Regional Offices (Africa, Europe, Asia, America, Middle East, and Western Pacific) in order to compile and improve the quality of data needed for informed decision-making and planning at national, regional, and global levels. Data on HIV are collected from each of the 194 member nations of WHO and used to produce an HIV

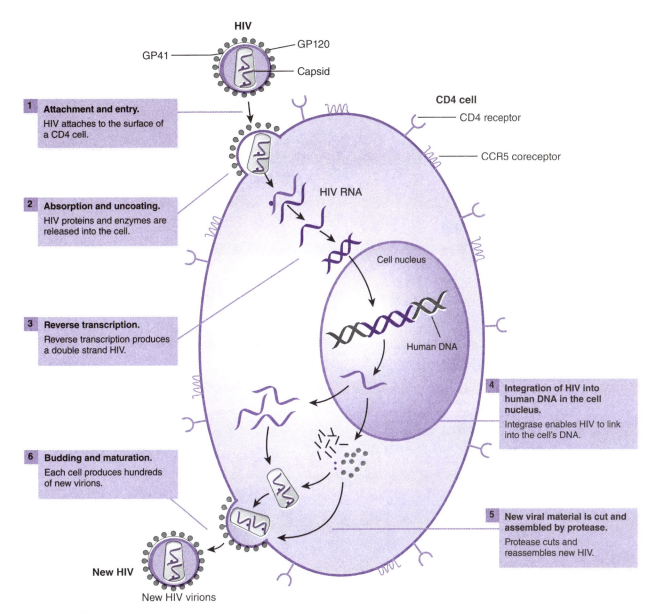

FIGURE 56.1 HIV Life Cycle.

epidemiological fact sheet for each nation. These data are updated and used to derive annual estimates of HIV incidence, prevalence, and mortality for the six WHO regions and worldwide (UNAIDS, 2017; WHO, 2017).

The global pattern of HIV/AIDS is shown in **FIGURE 56.2**. Though HIV/AIDS is widely distributed throughout the world, the prevalence ranges from less than 1% in more developed nations to greater than 15% in less developed nations, particularly those of sub-Saharan and Eastern Africa. It is important to realize that HIV/AIDS afflicts populations in two major ways. In the Americas and nations of Western Europe, HIV/AIDS strikes predominantly high-risk groups (e.g., males who have sex with males, bisexual males, female sex workers, and intravenous drug abusers). In sharp contrast,

HIV/AIDS in Africa strikes more women than men and is consistent with a heterosexually transmitted infection.

The cumulative number of deaths from HIV/AIDS and the number of prevalent cases are plotted for the period 1990–2016 in **FIGURE 56.3**. In 2017, there were approximately 36.9 million people living with HIV/AIDS in the world population, and of these, 1.8 million were children under the age of 15 years. Over half of infected children and adults live in sub-Saharan Africa. Children become infected via transmission of the virus by HIV-infected mothers during pregnancy, childbirth, or breastfeeding (UNAIDS, 2018).

During 2017, 1.8 million new cases of HIV/AIDS were reported including 160,000 cases among children. The number of new HIV infections has fallen

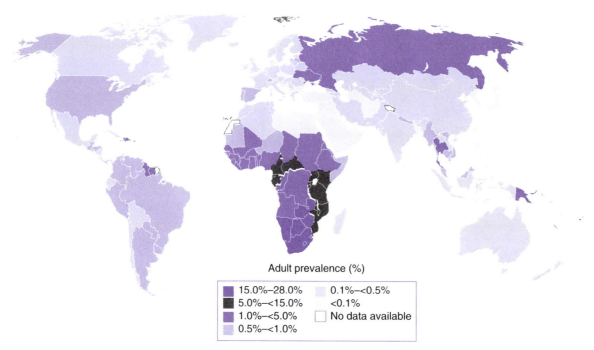

Adult prevalence (%)

- 15.0%–28.0%
- 5.0%–<15.0%
- 1.0%–<5.0%
- 0.5%–<1.0%
- 0.1%–<0.5%
- <0.1%
- No data available

FIGURE 56.2 Global Prevalence of HIV/AIDS.
WHO/UNAIDS, 2010.

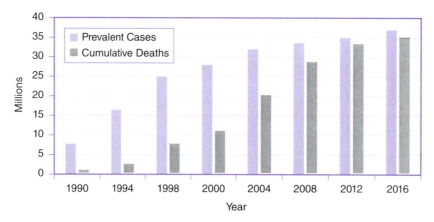

FIGURE 56.3 Global Epidemic of HIV/AIDS.
Prevalent Cases and Cumulative Deaths, HIV/AIDS, 1990–2016.

Data from UNAIDS. (2018). *Global HIV & AIDS statistics — 2018 fact sheet*. Geneva, Switzerland: UNAIDS.

by 47% from the peak of 3.4 million new infections reported in 1996.

Worldwide, approximately 940,000 deaths were attributed to HIV/AIDS in 2017, bringing the cumulative number of deaths since the start of the epidemic to 35.4 million. The annual number of deaths has fallen by more than 50% since reaching a peak of 1.9 million deaths in 2004 (UNAIDS, 2018).

The reductions in new HIV infections and HIV-related deaths are due primarily to decreased rates of viral transmission among high-risk individuals and greater access to anti-retroviral therapy among infected individuals. Prevention and therapy of HIV/AIDS is discussed in more detail later in this chapter (UNAIDS, 2018).

HIV/AIDS in Africa

According to the 2017 survey results on HIV/AIDS from the UNAIDS/WHO Working Group, approximately 19.6 million people living in sub-Saharan African have HIV/AIDS. This constitutes about 53% of all people living with HIV/AIDS worldwide. In that year, 800,000 new cases were detected and 380,000 died (approximately 44% of all new infections and 40% of all HIV-related deaths).

The adult prevalence (5%) in sub-Saharan Africa is fivefold higher than any other region in the world, and AIDS continues to be the leading cause of mortality in this region (**FIGURE 56.4**). Unlike other regions where HIV occurs predominantly in high-risk groups of males

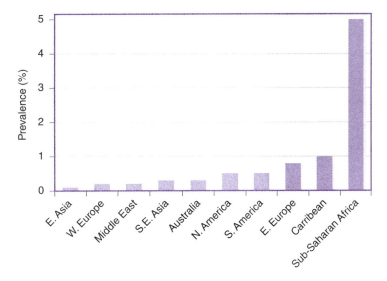

FIGURE 56.4 Global Prevalence of HIV/AIDS, 2009.

Data from WHO. (2010). *World Health Statistics 2010*. Geneva, Switzerland: World Health Organization Statistical Information System (WHOSIS).

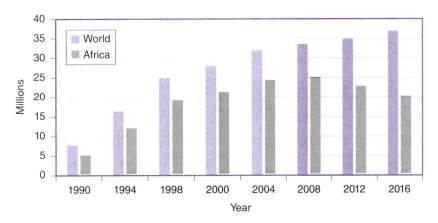

FIGURE 56.5 Prevalent Cases of HIV/AIDS, Africa, 1990–2016.

Data from UNAIDS. (2018). *Global HIV & AIDS statistics — 2018 fact sheet*. Geneva, Switzerland: UNAIDS.

who have sex with males, most people living with HIV in sub-Saharan Africa are women (61%). The gender difference is particularly striking in young adults (e.g., for ages 15–24 years), the ratio of HIV-infected women compared to men is approximately 3 to 1.

The relative proportion of HIV/AIDS cases in Africa among all cases worldwide has declined in recent years from over 75% in 2008 to 54% in 2016 (**FIGURE 56.5**). The recent decline in the relative cases of HIV/AIDS in the sub-Saharan and Eastern Africa is due to the introduction and widespread use of *highly active antiretroviral therapy* (HAART).

The *disability-adjusted life years* (*DALY*) attributable to HIV/AIDS is shown in **FIGURE 56.6**. The pattern reflects extraordinarily high values for most of the 47 countries in sub-Saharan Africa. Life expectancy has fallen dramatically in the countries with the highest incidence and prevalence of HIV/AIDS; for example, during the period 1980–2005, it is estimated that

life expectancy fell from 65 to 35 years in Botswana (Kallings, 2008).

Notably, the global pattern of DALY due to HIV/AIDS shows substantial overlap with the DALY due to other common infectious diseases such as tuberculosis, hepatitis B, hepatitis C, and malaria. Indeed, the clustering of such infectious agents in poverty-stricken regions of the world has led to dramatic increases in coinfections that contribute significantly to the global toll of death and disability.

▶ HIV/AIDS in the United States

The discovery of a new syndrome of severe immunodeficiency was first reported in 1981 by the United States Centers for Disease Control (CDC) based upon reports of *Pneumocystis carinii pneumonia* and *Kaposi sarcoma* in homosexual males living in New York and

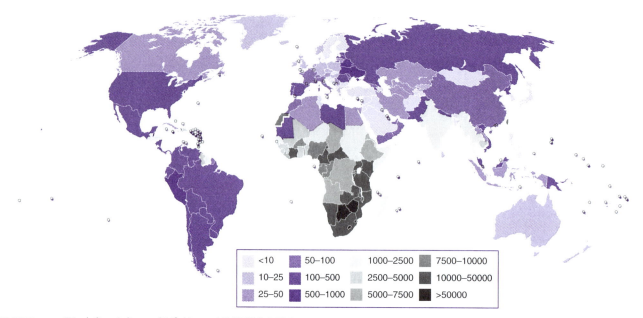

FIGURE 56.6 Disability-Adjusted Life Years, HIV/AIDS, 2004.

Data from World Health Organization. (2008). *The global burden of disease: 2004 update*. Geneva: WHO. Available at www.who.int/evidence/bod

San Francisco (MMWR, 1982f). By the end of the year, 270 similar cases had been reported resulting in 121 deaths. In 1983, the causative virus of HIV/AIDS was discovered and the mode of transmission elucidated. Over the next decade, HIV/AIDS cases were detected throughout the world.

In 1993, the definition of AIDS was modified to include those patients with a CD4-lymphocyte count below 200 cells per cubic millimeter or below 14% of the lymphocytic population. The epidemic peaked in the United States during 1993–1995, but with the introduction of HAART, the epidemic has since declined (**FIGURE 56.7**) (Fauci & Folkers, 2012).

Despite the impact of HAART in reducing the annual incidence and mortality of HIV/AIDS, the disease has persisted as a chronic infection in certain high-risk groups. **FIGURE 56.8** shows the number of prevalent cases and the cumulative number of deaths from HIV/AIDS in the United States during 1980–2016. During that period, 675,000 people died from HIV/AIDS in the U.S. population, and in 2016, over 1.3 million people were living with the disease. Notably, approximately 15% of HIV-positive individuals (162,500) are unaware of their status (CDC, 2018).

In 2016, 39,782 new cases of HIV/AIDS were diagnosed in the U.S. population and 6465 deaths were attributed to HIV-related conditions. During that year, the HIV infection rate was 12.3 per 100,000, and the mortality rate from HIV was 8.9 per 100,000. On average since 2011, the annual numbers of cases and deaths have declined by about 1% per year, and the annual incidence and mortality rates have declined by about 1.6% per year (CDC, 2018).

The mode of transmission of HIV has changed dramatically over the course of the epidemic in the United States. The largest proportionate increase occurred in cases attributable to heterosexual transmission, from 5% in 1983 to 23% in 2016 (**FIGURE 56.9**). Most heterosexual cases (76%) were women, suggesting a marked preeminence of male to female transmission. In contrast, the relative frequency of cases identified as men who have sex with men has decreased from over 90% to around 68%. The proportion of cases identified as acquiring HIV by intravenous drug abuse has stabilized at approximately 9% (CDC, 2007, 2018; Fenton, 2007; Osmond, 2003).

The race and ethnicity of new cases of HIV/AIDS has also changed dramatically over time (**FIGURE 56.10**). The relative frequency of Caucasian cases dropped from 60% in 1981 to 28% in 2005 whereas the frequency of African-American cases rose from 25% to 50% over the same time period. Hispanics also account for a high fraction of cases (~20%). Currently, men who have sex with men and African-American men and women bear a disproportionate burden of death and disability from HIV/AIDS (CDC, 2007; Fenton, 2007; Osmond, 2003).

▶ Origin of HIV

It is likely that HIV/AIDS existed in sub-Saharan Africa long before its recognition in the United States. In West Africa, viruses similar to HIV-1 and HIV-2 have been found in chimpanzees and monkeys. It is hypothesized that such viruses entered the human

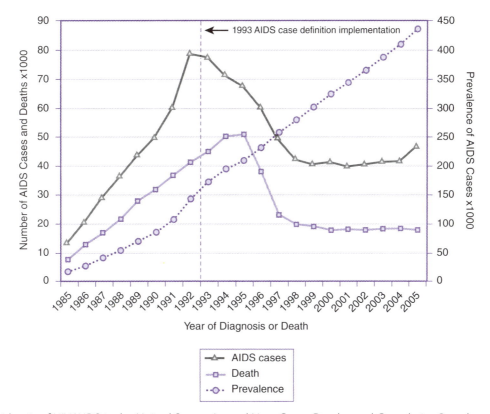

FIGURE 56.7 Epidemic of HIV/AIDS in the United States, Annual New Cases, Deaths, and Cumulative Prevalence, 1985–2005.

Prevalent cases include only physician-diagnosed HIV infections.

Reproduced from CDC. (2007). *Epidemiology of HIV infection (through 2005). Slide 2: Diagnoses of HIV infection among adults and adolescents, by sex, 2006–2009—40 states and 5 U.S. dependent areas.* Atlanta, GA: Centers for Disease Control and Prevention, U.S. Department of Health and Human Services. http://www.cdc.gov/hiv/topics/

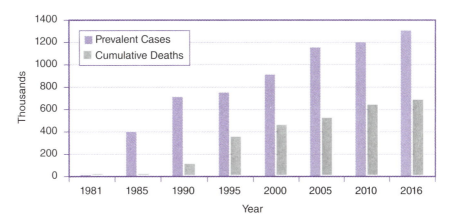

FIGURE 56.8 Epidemic of HIV/AIDS in the United States, 1981–2016. Prevalent Cases and Cumulative Deaths, 1980–2016.

Prevalence estimates include diagnosed and undiagnosed HIV infections.

Data from CDC. (2018). *HIV surveillance report: Diagnoses of HIV infection in the United States and dependent areas, 2016* (Vol. 28). Atlanta, GA: Centers for Disease Control and Prevention, U.S. Department of Health and Human Services.

population by direct exposure to contaminated blood and tissues during the slaughter of primates for meat (Hahn, Shaw, De Cock, & Sharp, 2000).

▶ Coinfections Involving HIV

The geographic pattern of HIV/AIDS overlaps with several other infectious conditions. The *disability-adjusted life years* (*DALY*) lost due to HIV/AIDS shown in Figure 56.5 is largely a consequence of death

and disability due to coinfection of HIV patients with human herpes virus 8, hepatitis B, hepatitis C, tuberculosis, and malaria.

HIV and Human Herpes Virus 8 (HHV-8)

Kaposi sarcoma has already been discussed in Chapter 35 of this text. This tumor occasionally develops in individuals who are severely immunocompromised such as those with HIV infection. Kaposi sarcoma became widely known as one of the defining conditions

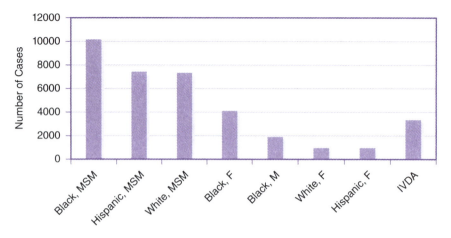

FIGURE 56.9 High-Risk Groups, United States HIV/AIDS, 2016.

Data from CDC. (2018). *HIV surveillance report: Diagnoses of HIV infection in the United States and dependent areas, 2016* (Vol. 28). Atlanta, GA: Centers for Disease Control and Prevention, U.S. Department of Health and Human Services.

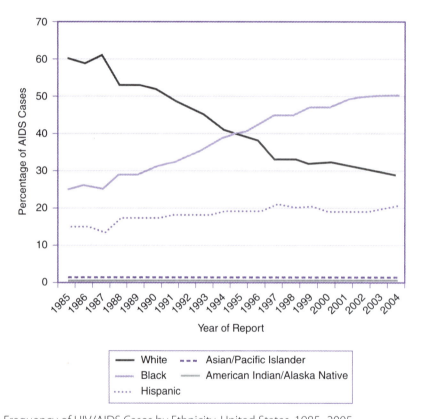

FIGURE 56.10 Relative Frequency of HIV/AIDS Cases by Ethnicity, United States, 1985–2005.

Reproduced from Centers for Disease Control and Prevention, National Center for HIV/AIDS, Viral Hepatitis, STD, and TB Prevention. (2009). *2007 disease profile*. Atlanta, GA: Centers for Disease Control and Prevention, 12

of AIDS during the 1980s. Although associated with HIV disease, Kaposi sarcoma is actually caused by another virus, *human herpes virus 8* (*HHV-8*).

In 1994, Yuan Chang, Patrick Moore, and Ethel Cesarman at Columbia University in New York isolated a novel herpes virus from the tumor cells of a Kaposi sarcoma. They later sequenced the virus and identified it as the eighth human herpes virus; hence it was given the name, HHV-8. This virus has since been found in all Kaposi sarcomas tested and is considered the cause of the disease (Cesarman et al., 1995; Chang et al., 1994; Moore & Chang, 1995; Moore et al., 1996).

Kaposi sarcoma arises from the endothelial cells that line lymphatic vessels. The tumor is characterized by the formation of vascular channels engorged with red blood cells giving it a dark red papular appearance. Kaposi sarcoma is typically found on the skin, but metastatic spread to other sites is common, especially the mouth, the gastrointestinal tract, and the respiratory tract. Kaposi sarcoma is associated with significant morbidity and mortality worldwide (Parkin, Bray, Ferlay, & Pisani, 2005).

Herpes viruses can be transmitted by intimate sexual contact and by transplantation of contaminated organs. *In sub-Saharan Africa where high rates of HHV-8 prevail, Kaposi sarcoma is the most common of all cancers.* As with other herpes viral infections, HHV-8 may persist in a dormant state for many years, only to be reactivated by conditions of severe immunosuppression such as HIV disease. Active HHV-8 infection specifically initiates and promotes malignant transformation of the lymphatic endothelium in the genesis of Kaposi sarcoma (Cesarman et al., 1995; Chang et al., 1994; Moore & Chang, 1995).

Before the epidemic of AIDS, Kaposi sarcoma was rare in Western countries, comprising only 0.3% of all cancers in men and 0.1% in women in the United States and Europe. Following onset of the HIV epidemic, rates of Kaposi sarcoma increased dramatically among men in developed nations. In the United States, the annual incidence rates peaked in 1989 at 9.6 per 100,000. Since that time, rates have declined to pre-AIDS levels, presumably in response to effective combined chemotherapy for HIV disease by HAART (Stebbing, Portsmouth, & Bassard, 2003).

In many parts of Africa, post-AIDS rates of Kaposi sarcoma have continued to increase in populations with high endemic rates and little access to effective therapy, such as Uganda, Malawi, Zimbabwe, and Swaziland. Indeed, *Kaposi sarcoma is now the most common cancer in men and the second most common cancer in women in many nations of sub-Saharan Africa* (Parkin et al., 2005).

HIV and Hepatitis B Virus

Coinfection with HIV and hepatitis B virus (HBV) is common due to shared modes of transmission. In areas of low HBV endemicity, such as North America, Australia, and Europe, HBV and HIV infection are usually acquired in adolescence or adulthood through sexual contact or intravenous drug injection. In areas of low HBV endemicity, the prevalence of chronic coinfection is around 5%–7% among HIV-infected individuals (Alter, 2006). In countries with intermediate and high HBV endemicity, the main routes of transmission of HBV are perinatal or in early childhood; in these countries, HBV and HIV coinfection rates are 10%–20% (Diop-Ndiaye & Touré-Kane, 2008; Lee, Ko, & Lee, 2008; Nyirenda, Beadsworth, & Stephany, 2008).

The rate of progression and complications from viral hepatitis are accelerated in patients with HIV coinfection (Puoti, Torti, & Ripamonti, 2003; Thio, Seaberg, & Skolasky, 2002). After acquiring HBV infection, HIV-infected individuals are six times more likely to develop chronic hepatitis B than HIV-negative individuals (Bodsworth, Cooper, & Donovan, 1991; Gatanaga et al., 2000; Hadler, Judson, &

O'Maeely, 1991). This risk of progressive HBV disease and liver cirrhosis and failure is higher with lower CD4 lymphocyte counts (Biggar, Goedert, & Hoofnagle, 1987; Laukamm-Josten, Muller, & Bienzle, 1988). There is also evidence that HIV-infected individuals with low CD4 counts are at a greater risk of developing hepatocellular carcinoma (Clifford, Rickenbach, & Polesel, 2008).

HIV and Hepatitis C Virus

Approximately one-third of HIV-infected patients in Europe and the United States are coinfected with hepatitis C virus (HCV). Such patients have been found to be at high risk for the development and progression of liver disease, particularly those receiving HAART. Treatment with HAART has been found to reduce morbidity and mortality from HIV; however, the adverse effects of HAART include liver toxicity, which may hasten the progression of liver cirrhosis in patients coinfected with HCV. Notably, the introduction of *pegylated interferon* in combination with ribavirin has improved the treatment options for patients with HIV and HCV coinfection (Rockstroh & Spengler, 2004).

HIV and Tuberculosis

Tuberculosis is the leading cause of death among individuals with HIV infection. In 2017, tuberculosis accounted for more than 300,000 (32%) of the 940,000 deaths due to HIV-related diseases. Furthermore, recent data reported by the WHO and UNAIDS suggest that rates of coinfection with HIV and the *Mycobacterium tuberculosis* are increasing in many populations. In 2017, approximately 1.2 million individuals were coinfected with HIV/AIDS and tuberculosis, most of whom (~80%) were living in sub-Saharan and Eastern Africa. The risk of developing tuberculosis is 20 times greater among individuals with HIV than those without HIV, and without therapy targeting both infectious agents, coinfected patients are at high risk for the development of multidrug-resistant tuberculosis (MDR-TB) (UNAIDS, 2018; WHO, 2010).

In patients with HIV/AIDS who are tuberculin-positive, the risk of developing active tuberculosis is high and prophylaxis with isoniazid is warranted (Guelar et al., 1993). Furthermore, HAART has been found to reduce the incidence of tuberculosis in patients with HIV/AIDS (Badri, Wilson, & Wood, 2002). Results suggest that appropriate therapy can reduce the onset of active tuberculosis in patients with HIV/AIDS. However, without therapy, immunosuppression due to HIV often results in disseminated forms of multidrug-resistant tuberculosis (MDR-TB) or extensively resistant tuberculosis (XDR-TB) and rapid demise of coinfected patients (Gandhi et al., 2006).

HIV and Malaria

Coinfection with HIV has been found to increase the severity and case fatality of malaria, particularly in sub-Saharan African where the most virulent malarial strain, *Plasmodium falciparum*, is endemic. In nations with high rates of HIV-1 infections, the incidence of clinical malaria has increased nearly 30% and malaria-related mortality has increased more than 100% (Korenromp et al., 2005). Synergistic increases have been noted in the HIV viral load and the severity of malarial symptoms in coinfected patients (Abu-Raddad, Patnaik, & Kublin, 2006).

▶ Prevention and Control of HIV/AIDS

The successful prevention and control of HIV/AIDS depends upon interrupting transmission of the virus. The main features of prevention are avoiding sexual contact with any HIV-infected individual, avoiding use of injectable drugs, avoiding contact with contaminated bodily fluids, and (for healthcare workers) practicing universal precautions. All blood products and blood donors should be carefully screened to avoid contamination. Accurate information about HIV/AIDS prevention and control should be disseminated to the general public, preferably before sexual activity begins.

The majority of HIV infections are acquired through unprotected sexual activity between partners, one of whom has HIV. The primary mode of HIV infection worldwide is through sexual contact between members of the opposite sex. The male latex condom, if used correctly without oil-based lubricants, is the single most effective available technology to reduce the sexual transmission of HIV and other sexually transmitted infections. Studies of couples where one partner is infected show that with consistent condom use, HIV infection rates for the uninfected partner are below 1% per year (Cayley, 2004).

Antiretroviral treatment of infected patients has been found to significantly reduce the sexual transmission of HIV by reducing the level of virus in bodily fluids. In a recent multicenter study conducted in Botswana, Brazil, India, Kenya, Malawi, South Africa, Thailand, Zimbabwe, and the United States,

1763 couples discordant for HIV-positivity were randomly assigned to either a treatment group where the HIV-positive partner received antiretroviral drugs immediately or a control group where no drug was given. Out of 28 HIV infections that developed among study participants who were HIV-negative at baseline, 27 developed among members of the untreated couples. The early preventive treatment therefore led to a 96% reduction in HIV transmission to HIV-negative partners, strong evidence of the value of early intervention with antiretroviral therapy in such couples (Warren, 2011).

During 2017, UNAIDS investigators estimated that approximately 59% of people infected with HIV (21.7 million) were accessing antiretroviral therapy, an increase of 8 million since 2010 and 2.3 million in the past year (UNAIDS, 2018). Due to the high rates of coinfections among HIV-infected individuals (e.g., hepatitis, tuberculosis, malaria, and cryptococcosis), there is an urgent need for vaccination programs and therapeutic regimens that target multiple infectious agents without further damage to the immune system (Chang et al., 2013).

Healthcare workers should follow universal precautions to reduce their risk of exposure to contaminated blood. These precautions include wearing gloves, masks, protective eyewear or shields, and gowns or aprons that prevent exposure of the skin or mucous membranes to blood-borne pathogens. Frequent and thorough washing of the skin immediately after being contaminated with blood or other bodily fluids reduces the chance of infection. Sharp objects like needles, scalpels, and glass are carefully disposed of to prevent needle-stick injuries with contaminated items (Kerr et al., 2007).

Injection of illicit drugs using contaminated needles and syringes is a major mode of HIV transmission among intravenous drug abusers. Harm reduction strategies such as needle-exchange programs have been used with some success in reducing rates of HIV infection associated with intravenous drug abuse (Wodak & Cooney, 2006).

To avoid mother-to-child transmission, HIV-infected mothers are encouraged to avoid breastfeeding their infant and instead use replacement feeding that is acceptable, feasible, affordable, sustainable, and safe. However, if replacement feeding is unavailable, exclusive breastfeeding is recommended during the first months of life and discontinued as soon as possible (WHO, 2006).

One way to change risky behavior is health education. Several studies have shown the positive impact of culturally adapted educational programs advocating cautious sexual behavior. In 2010, a United Nations AIDS Inter-Agency Task Team encouraged more research on the actual implementation of sex-education programs (such as teacher training, access to related services through schools and the community,

or parental attitudes to HIV and AIDS education), and more longitudinal studies on the deeper complexities of the relationship between education and HIV prevention and control (Lakhanpal & Ram, 2008; Rindermann & Meisenberg, 2009).

References

Abu-Raddad, L., Patnaik, P., & Kublin, J. (2006). Dual infection with HIV and malaria fuels the spread of both diseases in sub-Saharan Africa. *Science, 314*(5805), 1603–1606.

Alter, M. J. (2006). Epidemiology of viral hepatitis and HIV co-infection. *Journal of Hepatology, 44*(1 Suppl.), S6–S9.

Badri, M., Wilson, D., & Wood, R. (2002). Effect of highly active antiretroviral therapy on incidence of tuberculosis in South Africa: A cohort study. *Lancet, 359*(9323), 2059–2064.

Barré-Sinoussi, F., Chermann, J. C., Rey, F., Nugeyre, M. T., Chamaret, S., Gruest, J., … Montagnier, L. (1983). Isolation of a T-lymphotropic retrovirus from a patient at risk for acquired immune deficiency syndrome (AIDS). *Science, 220,* 868–871.

Biggar, R. J., Goedert, J. J., & Hoofnagle, J. (1987). Accelerated loss of antibody to hepatitis B surface antigen among immnodeficient homosexual men infected with HIV. *The New England Journal of Medicine, 316,* 360–361.

Bodsworth, N. J., Cooper, D. A., & Donovan, B. (1991). The influence of human immunodeficiency virus type 1 infection on the development of the hepatitis B carrier state. *The Journal of Infectious Diseases, 163,* 1138–1140.

Cayley, W. E., Jr. (2004). Effectiveness of condoms in reducing heterosexual transmission of HIV. *American Family Physician, 70*(7), 1268–1269.

CDC. (2007). *AIDS surveillance—General epidemiology (through 2005).* Atlanta, GA: Centers for Disease Control and Prevention, U.S. Department of Health and Human Services.

CDC. (2018). *HIV surveillance report: Diagnoses of HIV infection in the United States and dependent areas, 2016* (Vol. 28). Atlanta, GA: Centers for Disease Control and Prevention, U.S. Department of Health and Human Services.

Cesarman, E., Chang, Y., Moore, P. S., Said, J. W., & Knowles, D. M. (1995). Kaposi's sarcoma-associated herpesvirus-like DNA sequences in AIDS-related body-cavity-based lymphomas. *The New England Journal of Medicine, 332*(18), 1186–1191.

Chang, C. C., Crane, M., Zhou, J. L., Mina, M., Post, J. J., Cameron, B. A., … Lewin, S. R. (2013). HIV and co-infections. *Immunological Reviews, 254*(1), 114–142.

Chang, Y., Cesarman, E., Pessin, M. S., Lee, F., Culpepper, J., Knowles, D. M., & Moore, P. S. (1994). Identification of herpesvirus-like DNA sequences in AIDS-associated Kaposi's sarcoma. *Science, 266,* 1865–1869.

Clifford, G. M., Rickenbach, M., & Polesel, J. (2008). Influence of HIV-related immunodeficiency on the risk of hepatocellular carcinoma. *AIDS, 22,* 2135–2141.

Diop-Ndiaye, H., & Touré-Kane, C. (2008). Hepatitis B, C seroprevalence and delta virus in HIV-1 Senegalese patients at HAART initiation (retrospective study). *Journal of Medical Virology, 80,* 1332–1336.

Fauci, A. S., & Folkers, G. K. (2012). Toward and AIDS-free generation. *JAMA, 308*(5), 343–344.

Fenton, K. A. (2007). Changing epidemiology of HIV/AIDS in the United States: Implications for enhancing and promoting HIV testing strategies. *Clinical Infectious Diseases, 45*(Suppl. 4), S213–S220.

Gallo, R. C., Salahuddin, S. Z., Popovic, M., Shearer, G. M., Kaplan, M., Haynes, B. F., … Safai, B. (1984). Frequent detection and isolation of cytopathic retroviruses (HTLV-III) from patients with AIDS and at risk for AIDS. *Science, 224*(4648), 500–503.

Gandhi, N. R., Moll, A., Sturm, A. W., Pawinski, R., Govender, T., Lalloo, U., … Friedland, G. (2006). Extensively drug-resistant tuberculosis as a cause of death in patients co-infected with tuberculosis and HIV in a rural area of South Africa. *The Lancet, 368*(9547), 1575–1580.

Gatanaga, H., Yasuoka, A., Kikuchi, Y., Tachikawa, N., & Oka, S. (2000). Influence of prior HIV-1 infection on the development of chronic hepatitis B infection. *European Journal of Clinical Microbiology & Infectious Diseases, 19,* 237–239.

Goedert, J. J., Neuland, C. Y., & Wallen, W. C. (1982). Amyl nitrite may alter T lymphocytes in homosexual men. *Lancet, 1,* 412–416.

Guelar, A., Gatell, J. M., Verdejo, J., Podzamczer, D., Lozano, L., Aznar, E., … González, J. (1993). A prospective study of the risk of tuberculosis among HIV-infected patients. *AIDS, 7*(10), 1345–1349.

Guyader, M., Emerman, M., Sonigo, P., Clavel, F., Montagnier, L., & Alizon, M. (1987). Genome organization and transactivation of the human immunodeficiency virus type 2. *Nature, 326*(6114), 662–669.

Hadler, S. C., Judson, F. N., & O'Maeely, P. M. (1991). Outcome of hepatitis B virus infection in homosexual men and its relation to prior human immunodeficiency virus infection. *The Journal of Infectious Diseases, 163,* 454–459.

Hahn, B. H., Shaw, G. M., De Cock, K. M., & Sharp, P. M. (2000). AIDS as a zoonosis: Scientific and public health implications. *Science, 287,* 607–614.

Hope, T. J., & Trono, D. (2000). *Structure, expression and regulation of the HIV genome. HIV InSite.* San Francisco: University of California.

Kallings, L. O. (2008). The first postmodern pandemic: 25 years of HIV/AIDS. *Journal of Internal Medicine, 263*(3), 218–243.

Kerr, T., Kimber, J., Debeck, K., & Wood, E. (2007). The role of safer injection facilities in the response to HIV/AIDS among injection drug users. *Current HIV/AIDS Reports, 4*(4), 158–164.

Korenromp, E. L., Williams, B. G., de Vlas, S. J., Gouws, E., Gilks, C. F., & Ghys, P. D. (2005). Malaria attributable to the HIV-1 epidemic, Sub-Saharan Africa. *Emerging Infectious Diseases, 11*(9), 1410–1419.

Lakhanpal, M., & Ram, R. (2008). Educational attainment and HIV/AIDS prevalence: A cross-country study. *Economics of Education Review, 27,* 14–21.

Laukamm-Josten, U., Muller, O., & Bienzle, U. (1988). Decline of naturally acquired antibodies to hepatitis B surface antigen in HIV-1 infected homosexual men. *AIDS, 2,* 400–401.

Lee, H. C., Ko, N. Y., & Lee, N. Y. (2008). Seroprevalence of viral hepatitis and sexually transmitted disease among adults with recently diagnosed HIV infection in southern Taiwan, 2000-5: Upsurge in hepatitis C virus infections among injection drug users. *Journal of the Formosan Medical Association, 107*, 404–411.

Levy, J. A., Hoffman, A. D., Kramer, S. M., Landis, J. A., Shimabukuro, J. M., & Oshiro, L. S. (1984). Isolation of lymphocytopathic retroviruses from San Francisco patients with AIDS. *Science, 225*(4664), 840–842.

Masur, H., Michelis, M. A., Greene, J. B., Onorato, I., Stouwe, R. A., Holzman, R. S., … Cunningham-Rundles, S. (1981). An outbreak of community-acquired *Pneumocystis carinii* pneumonia: Initial manifestation of cellular immune dysfunction. *The New England Journal of Medicine, 305*(24), 1431–1438.

Masur, H., Michelis, M. A., Wormser, G. P., Lewin, S., Gold, J., Tapper, M. L., … Cunningham-Rundles, S. (1982). Opportunistic infection in previously healthy women. Initial manifestations of a community-acquired cellular immunodeficiency. *Annals of Internal Medicine, 97*(4), 533–539.

Mavligit, G. M., Talpaz, M., Hsia, F. T., Wong, W., Lichtiger, B., Mansell, P. W., & Mumford, D. M. (1984). Chronic immune stimulation by sperm alloantigens: Support for the hypothesis that spermatozoa induce immune dysregulation in homosexual males. *JAMA, 251*, 237–241.

MMWR. (1981a). Pneumocystis pneumonia—Los Angeles. *Morbidity and Mortality Weekly Report, 30*, 250–252.

MMWR. (1981b). Kaposi's sarcoma and Pneumocystis pneumonia among homosexual men—New York City and California. *Morbidity and Mortality Weekly Report, 30*, 305–308.

MMWR. (1982a). A cluster of Kaposi's sarcoma and *Pneumocystis carinii* pneumonia among homosexual male residents of Los Angeles and Orange Counties, California. *Morbidity and Mortality Weekly Report, 31*, 305–307.

MMWR. (1982b). Opportunistic infections and Kaposi's sarcoma among Haitians in the United States. *Morbidity and Mortality Weekly Report, 31*, 353–354.

MMWR. (1982c). Pneumocystis carinii pneumonia among persons with hemophilia A. *Morbidity and Mortality Weekly Report, 31*, 365–367.

MMWR. (1982d). Possible transfusion-associated acquired immune deficiency syndrome (AIDS)—California. *Morbidity and Mortality Weekly Report, 31*, 652–654.

MMWR. (1982e). Unexplained immunodeficiency and opportunistic infections in infants—New York, New Jersey, California. *Morbidity and Mortality Weekly Report, 31*, 665–667.

MMWR. (1982f). Update on acquired immune deficiency syndrome (AIDS)—United States. *Morbidity and Mortality Weekly Report, 31*(37), 507–508, 513–514.

MMWR. (1983a). Immunodeficiency among female sexual partners of males with acquired immune deficiency syndrome (AIDS)—New York. *Morbidity and Mortality Weekly Report, 31*, 697–698.

MMWR. (1983b). Acquired immune deficiency syndrome (AIDS) in prison inmates—New York, New Jersey. *Morbidity and Mortality Weekly Report, 31*, 700–701.

Moore, P. S., & Chang, Y. (1995). Detection of herpesvirus-like DNA sequences in Kaposi's sarcoma in patients with and without HIV infection. *The New England Journal of Medicine, 332*(18), 1181–1185.

Moore, P. S., Gao, S. J., Dominguez, G., Cesarman, E., Lungu, O., Knowles, D. M., … Chang, Y. (1996). Primary characterization of a herpesvirus agent associated with Kaposi's sarcoma. *The Journal of Virology, 70*(1), 549–558.

Nyirenda, M., Beadsworth, M. B., & Stephany, P. (2008). Prevalence of infection with hepatitis B and C virus and co infection with HIV in medical inpatients in Malawi. *Journal of Infection, 57*, 72–77.

Osmond, D. H. (2003). *Epidemiology of HIV/AIDS in the United States. HIV InSite*. San Francisco: University of California.

Parkin, D. M., Bray, F., Ferlay, J., & Pisani, P. (2005). Global cancer statistics, 2002. *CA A Cancer Journal for Clinicians, 55*, 74–108.

Puoti, M., Torti, C., & Ripamonti, D. (2003). Severe hepatotoxicity during combination antiretroviral therapy treatment: Incidence, liver histology, and outcome. *Journal of Acquired Immune Deficiency Syndromes, 32*, 259–267.

Rindermann, H., & Meisenberg, G. (2009). Relevance of education and intelligence at the national level for health: The case of HIV and AIDS. *Intelligence, 37*, 383–395.

Rockstroh, J. K., & Spengler, U. (2004). HIV and hepatitis C virus co-infection. *The Lancet Infectious Diseases, 4*(7), 437–444.

Sonnabend, J., Witkin, S. S., & Purtilo, D. T. (1983). Acquired immunodeficiency syndrome, opportunistic infections, and malignancies in male homosexuals. A hypothesis of etiologic factors in pathogenesis. *JAMA, 249*(17), 2370–2374.

Stebbing, J., Portsmouth, S., & Bassard, B. (2003). How does HAART lead to the resolution of Kaposi's sarcoma? *Journal of Antimicrobial Chemotherapy, 51*(5), 1095–1098.

Thio, C. L., Seaberg, E. C., & Skolasky, R. L. (2002). HIV-1, hepatitis B virus, and risk of liver-related mortality in the Multi-Center AIDS Cohort Study (MACS). *Lancet, 360*, 1921–1926.

UNAIDS. (2017). *Global AIDS monitoring 2018*. Geneva, Switzerland: UNAIDS Joint United Nations Program on HIV/AIDS.

UNAIDS. (2018). *Global HIV & AIDS statistics—2018 fact sheet*. Geneva, Switzerland: UNAIDS Joint United Nations Program on HIV/AIDS.

Warren, M. (2011). Earlier initiation of HIV treatment led to a 96 percent reduction in HIV transmission to the uninfected partner. AIDS Vaccine Advocacy Coalition (AVAC).

WHO. (2006). *HIV and infant feeding technical consultation, consensus statement*. Geneva, Switzerland: World Health Organization.

WHO. (2010). *Report on the global AIDS epidemic*. Geneva, Switzerland: World Health Organization.

WHO. (2017). *The UNAIDS/WHO working group on global HIV/AIDS and STI surveillance*. Geneva, Switzerland: World Health Organization.

Wodak, A., & Cooney, A. (2006). Do needle syringe programs reduce HIV infection among injecting drug users: A comprehensive review of the international evidence. *Substance Use & Misuse, 41*(6–7), 777–813.

Index

Page numbers followed by *f* and *t* indicate figures and tables, respectively.